THE TRAUMA MANUAL:
TRAUMA AND ACUTE CARE SURGERY

Third Edition

THE TRAUMA MANUAL: TRAUMA AND ACUTE CARE SURGERY

Third Edition

Andrew B. Peitzman, MD, FACS
Professor & Chief
Division of General Surgery
Department of Surgery
University of Pittsburgh School of Medicine
Vice Chair for Clinical Services
Department of Surgery
University of Pittsburgh Medical Center—
Presbyterian Hospital
Pittsburgh, Pennsylvania

Michael Rhodes, MD, FACS
Professor of Surgery
Thomas Jefferson University
Chairman
Department of Surgery
Christiana Care Health Services
Wilmington, Delaware

C. William Schwab, MD, FACS
Professor of Surgery
Department of Surgery
University of Pennsylvania School of Medicine
Chief, Division of Traumatology & Surgical
Critical Care
Hospital of the University of Pennsylvania
Philadelphia, Pennsylvania

Donald M. Yealy, MD, FACEP
Professor and Vice Chair
Department of Emergency Medicine
University of Pittsburgh
Chief of Emergency Services
University of Pittsburgh Medical Center—
Presbyterian University Hospital
Pittsburgh, Pennsylvania

Timothy C. Fabian, MD, FACS
Harwell Wilson Professor & Chairman
Department of Surgery
University of Tennessee Health Science
Center
Attending Surgeon
Presley Regional Trauma Center
Memphis, Tennessee

 Wolters Kluwer | Lippincott Williams & Wilkins
Health
Philadelphia · Baltimore · New York · London
Buenos Aires · Hong Kong · Sydney · Tokyo

Acquisitions Editor: Brian Brown
Managing Editor: Nicole T. Dernoski
Project Manager: Nicole Walz
Senior Manufacturing Manager: Benjamin Rivera
Marketing Manager: Lisa Parry
Design Coordinator: Terry Mallon
Cover Designer: Becky Baxendell
Production Services: GGS Book Services

Library of Congress Cataloging-in-Publication Data
The trauma manual: trauma and acute care surgery / [edited by] Andrew B. Peitzman
[et al.]. 3rd ed.
   p. ; cm.
   Includes bibliographical references and index.
   ISBN-13: 978-0-7817-6275-5 (pbk. : alk. paper)   1. Traumatology—Handbooks, manuals, etc.   2. Wounds and injuries—Handbooks, manuals, etc.   3. Surgical emergencies—Handbooks, manuals, etc.   I. Peitzman, Andrew B.
   [DNLM: 1. Wounds and Injuries—Outlines. 2. Emergency Medicine—Outlines.
3. Traumatology—Outlines. WO 18.2 T7768 2008]
   RD93.T6895 2008
   617.1—dc22

                                                                    2007007923

This book is dedicated to those who have given their lives, and those who daily risk their lives, in the care of the injured.

CONTENTS

Louis H. Alarcon, MD
Assistant Professor, Critical Care and
Surgery, Associate Medical Director,
Trauma Surgery, Director of Education,
Trauma Surgeon, University of Pittsburgh
School of Medicine, Pittsburgh,
Pennsylvania

Juan A. Asensio, MD
Professor of Surgery, Director of Trauma
Clinical Research, Training and
Community Affairs, Director, Trauma
Surgery and Surgical Critical Care
Fellowship, University of Miami

Kodi Azari, MD
Assistant Professor, Department of
Surgery, Division of Plastic and
Reproductive Surgery, University of
Pittsburgh, Pittsburgh, Pennsylvania

Randall L. Beatty, MD
Assistant Professor, Department of
Opthalmology, Chief, Orbital and
Oculoplastic Surgery, University of
Pittsburgh Medical Center, Pittsburgh,
Pennsylvania

Vishal Bansal, MD
Assistant Professor of Surgery, Division of
Trauma and Critical Care, University of
California, San Diego

Joel E. Barbato, MD
Vascular Surgery Fellow, Department of
Vascular Surgery, University of Pittsburgh,
Pittsburgh, Pennsylvania

Philip S. Barie, MD
Professor of Surgery and Public Health,
Chief, Division of Critical Care and
Trauma, Weill Cornell Medical College;
Director, Anne and Max A. Cohen
Surgical Intensive Care Unit, New York
Presbyterian Hospital, New York,
New York

Tiffany K. Bee, MD
Assistant Professor, University of
Tennessee Health Science Center;
Attending Surgeon, Department of
Surgery, University of Tennessee,
Memphis, Tennessee

Timothy R. Billiar, MD
George Vance Foster Professor and Chair,
Department of Surgery, University of
Pittsburgh, UPMC Presbyterian,
Pittsburgh, Pennsylvania

Tracy Bilski, MD, FACS
Fellow, Division of Traumatology
and Surgical Critical Care, Department
of Surgery, University of Pennsylvania
School of Medicine, Philadelphia,
Pennsylvania

Kenneth D. Boffard, MD
Professor and Head, Department of
Surgery, Johannesburg Hospital,
University of the Witwatersand,
Johannesburg, South Africa

Charles C. Branas, PhD
Assistant Professor of Epidemiology,
Biostatistics and Epidemiology, University
of Pennsylvania, Assistant Professor of
Epidemiology in Surgery, Department
of Surgery, Hospital of the University of
Pennsylvania, Philadelphia, Pennsylvania

Susan M. Briggs, MD, MPH, FACS
Associate Professor of Surgery,
Department of Surgery, Harvard Medical
School, Director, International Trauma
and Disaster Institute, Department of
Surgery, Massachusetts General Hospital,
Boston, Massachusetts

L.D. Britt, MD
Brickhouse Professor and Chairman,
Eastern Virginia Medical School, Norfolk,
Virginia

Percival O. Buenaventura, MD
Attending Thoracic Surgeon, Wellspan
Cardiothoracic Surgery, York, Pennsylvania

Jeffrey A. Claridge, MD
Department of Surgery, Metro Health,
Cleveland, Ohio

Michael Christian Coello, MD
Cardiothoracic Surgery Resident,
Department of Cardiothoracic Surgery,
Massachusetts General Hospital, Boston,
Massachusetts

Stephen M. Cohn, MD, FACS
Professor and Chairman, The Dr. Witten B.
Russ Professor, Department of Surgery,
University of Texas Health Science Center,
San Antonio, Texas

John S. Cole, MD
Assistant Professor, Department of
Emergency Medicine, University of
Pittsburgh Medical Center, Medical
Director, Stat Medivac, Pittsburgh,
Pennsylvania

David C. Cone, MD
Associate Professor of Emergency
Medicine and Public Health, Section of
Emergency Medicine, Yale University
School of Medicine, New Haven,
Connecticut

Martin A. Croce, MD
University of Tennessee Health Science
Center, Professor of Surgery, Department
of Surgery, Regional Medical Center at
Memphis, Chief, Trauma and Critical
Care, Department of Trauma, Memphis,
Tennessee

Kimberly A. Davis, MD, FACS
Associate Professor and Chief of the
Section of Trauma, Surgical Critical Care
and Surgical Emergencies, Vice Chair for
Clinical Affairs, Department of Surgery,
Yale University School of Medicine,
Yale-New Haven Hospital, New Haven,
Connecticut

Theodore R. Delbridge, MD, MPH
Professor and Chair, Department of
Emergency Medicine, Brody School of
Medicine at East Carolina University,
Chief of Emergency Services, Pitt
County Memorial Hospital, Greenville,
North Carolina

**Frederick J. Denstman, FACS,
FASCRS**
Assistant Section Chief, Colon and
Rectal Surgery, Department of Surgery,
Christiana Care, Wilmington,
Delaware

William F. Donaldson, MD
Associate Professor, Department of
Orthopaedic Surgery, Associate Professor,
Departments of Orthopedic Surgery and
Neurological Surgery, Chief, Division of
Spinal Surgery, Department of Orthopedic
Surgery, University of Pittsburgh,
University of Pittsburgh Medical Center,
Pittsburgh, Pennsylvania

Suomitra R. Eachempati, MD, FACS
Associate Professor of Surgery and Public
Health, Director of Quality Improvement,
Division of Critical Care and
Trauma, Weill Cornell Medical College,
NewYork Presbyterian Hospital, Weill
Cornell Medical Center, New York,
New York

Timothy C. Fabian, MD
Harwell Wilson Professor and Chairman,
Department of Surgery, University of
Tennessee Health Science Center;
Attending Surgeon, Presley Regional
Trauma Center, Memphis, Tennessee

Samir M. Fakhry, MD, FACS
Professor, Department of Surgery,
Virginia Commonwealth University–Inova
Campus, Chief, Trauma and Surgical
Care, Associate Chair for Research and
Education, Department of Surgery,
Inova Fairfax Hospital, Falls Church,
Virginia

Linda M. Farkas, MD, FACS, FASCRS
Assistant Professor of Surgery, University
of Pittsburgh, Shadyside Hospital–UPMC,
Pittsburgh, Pennsylvania

Michael P. Federle, MD
Professor of Radiology, Radiology
Department, University of Pittsburgh
Medical Center, Chief of Abdominal
Imaging, Department of Radiology,
UPMC, Pittsburgh, Pennsylvania

Anthony Fiorillo, MD
University of Pittsburgh Medical
Center, Pittsburgh, Pennsylvania

Henri Ronald Ford, MD
Professor of Surgery and Vice-Chairman, Department of Surgery, University of Southern California Keck School of Medicine, Vice-President and Surgeon-in-Chief, Department of Surgery, Children's Hospital of Los Angeles, Los Angeles, California

Racquel H. Forsythe, MD
Assistant Professor of Surgery and Critical Care Medicine, University of Pittsburgh Medical Center, Pittsburgh, Pennsylvania

Heidi Lee Frankel, MD
Professor, Division of Burn, Trauma, and Critical Care, UT Southwestern Medical Center, Dallas, Texas

Paul Thomas Freudigman, Jr., MD
Orthopedic Trauma Surgeon, Department of Orthopedics, Baylor University Medical Center, Dallas, Texas

Eric R. Frykberg, MD
Professor of Surgery, Department of Surgery, University of Florida College of Medicine, Chief, Division of General Surgery, Department of Surgery, Shands Medical Center, Jacksonville, Florida

Gerald J. Fulda, MD
Associate Professor of Surgery, Department of Surgery, Jefferson Medical College, Philadelphia, Pennsylvania, Director, Surgical Critical Care, Department of Surgery, Christiana Care Health Services, Newark, Delaware

Barbara A. Gaines, MD
Assistant Professor, Department of Surgery, University of Pittsburgh School of Medicine, Attending Surgeon, Division of Pediatric Surgery, Children's Hospital of Pittsburgh, Pittsburgh, Pennsylvania

Fred Giberson, MD
Clinical Associate Professor of Surgery, Department of Surgery, Jefferson Medical College of Thomas Jefferson University; Program Director, General Surgery Residency Program, Department of Surgery, Christiana Care Health Services, Newark, Delaware

Vincente Gracias, MD
Division of Trauma and Surgical Critical Care, Hospital of the University of Pennsylvania, Pittsburgh, Pennsylvania

Gary S. Gruen, MD
Professor, Orthopaedic Surgery, University of Pittsburgh Medical Center, Orthopaedic Trauma Surgery, Presbyterian University Hospital, Pittsburgh, Pennsylvania

C. William Hanson, III, MD, FCCM
Professor of Anesthesia, Surgery, University of Pittsburgh; Director of Trauma Program, Department of Surgery, University of Pittsburgh Medical Center, Presbyterian Hospital, Pittsburgh, Pennsylvania

Brian G. Harbrecht, MD
Professor of Surgery, Chief of Trauma, Department of Surgery, University of Louisville, Louisville, Kentucky

David Heimbach, MD
Professor, Department of Surgery, University of Washington, Seattle, Washington

William S. Hoff, MD, FACS
Clinical Associate Professor of Surgery, Division of Trauma and Surgical Critical Care, University of Pennsylvania, Philadelphia, Pennsylvania, Trauma Program Medical Director, Division of Traumatology, St. Luke's Hospital, Bethlehem, Pennsylvania

James Hill Holmes, IV, MD
Assistant Professor of Surgery, Medical Director, Burn Services, Department of Surgery, Wake Forest University, Baptist Medical Center, Winston-Salem, North Carolina

John A. Horton, III, MD
Assistant Professor, Department of Physical Medicine and Rehabilitation, University of Pittsburgh; Director, Spinal Cord Injury Program, University of Pittsburgh Medical Center Rehabilitation Hospital, Pittsburgh, Pennsylvania

David B. Hoyt, MD
Professor and Chairman, Department of Surgery, University of California-Irvine, Irvine, California

Steven J. Hughes, MD
Assistant Professor of Surgery, Chief, GI Surgery, Chairman, Surgical Services Oversight Committee, University of Pittsburgh, Pittsburgh, Pennsylvania

Rao R. Ivatury, MD, FACS
Professor of Surgery, Emergency Medicine, and Physiology, Virginia Commonwealth University, Chief, Trauma, Critical Care, and Emergency Surgery, Department of Surgery, VCU Health System, Richmond, Virginia

Brian T. Jankowitz, MD
PGY2 Resident, Department of Neurosurgery, University of Pittsburgh Medical Center, Presbyterian Hospital, Pittsburgh, Pennsylvania

Geetha Jeyabalan, MD
General Surgery Resident, Department of General Surgery, University of Pittsburgh Medical Center, Pittsburgh, Pennsylvania

Gregory J. Jurkovich, MD
Professor of Surgery, Department of Surgery, University of Washington, Chief of Trauma, Harborview Medical Center, Seattle, Washington

Donald R. Kauder, MD, FACS
Associate Director, Trauma Services, Riverside Regional Medical Center, Newport News, Virginia

Patrick K. Kim, MD
Assistant Professor of Surgery, Department of Surgery, University of Pennsylvania School of Medicine, Attending Surgeon, Department of Surgery, Hospital of the University of Pennsylvania, Philadelphia, Pennsylvania

Paul R. Klepchick, MD
Surgery Resident, Department of Surgery, University of Pittsburgh, University of Pittsburgh Medical Center, Pittsburgh, Pennsylvania

James W. Krugh, MD
Clinical Associate Professor, Department of Anesthesiology, University of Pittsburgh, Anesthesiologist, University of Pittsburgh Medical Center, Pittsburgh, Pennsylvania

Kenneth K. Lee, MD
Associate Professor of Surgery, University of Pittsburgh Medical Center, Pittsburgh, Pennsylvania

John C. Lee, MD
Department of General Surgery, Lancaster General Hospital, Lancaster, Pennsylvania

W. P. Andrew Lee, MD, FACS
Professor of Surgery, University of Pittsburgh, Chief, Division of Plastic Surgery, University of Pittsburgh, Pittsburgh, Pennsylvania

Peter D. LeRoux, MD
Associate Professor and Vice Chairman, Department of Neurosurgery, Hospital of the University of Pennsylvania, Department of Neurosurgery, Philadelphia, Pennsylvania

Ryan M. Levy, MD
Surgery Resident, Department of Surgery, University of Pittsburgh, University of Pittsburgh Medical Center, Pittsburgh, Pennsylvania

James D. Luketich, MD, FACS
Sampson Family Endowed Professor of Surgery, Chief, Division of Thoracic and Foregut Surgery, University of Pittsburgh, Director, Heart, Lung, and Esophageal Surgery Institute, University of Pittsburgh Medical Center, Pittsburgh, Pennsylvania

James M. Lynch, MD, FACS
Associate Professor of Clinical Surgery, Department of Pediatric Surgery, University of Pittsburgh School of Medicine; Attending Surgeon, Department of Pediatric Surgery, Children's Hospital of Pittsburgh, Pittsburgh, Pennsylvania

Ellen J. MacKenzie, PhD
Professor and Director, Center for Injury Research and Policy, Johns Hopkins Bloomberg School of Public Health, Baltimore, Maryland

Ajai Malhortra, MD
Assistant Professor of Surgery, Department of Surgery, Virginia Commonwealth University Health Systems, MCV Hospitals & Physicians; Medical College of Virginia, Richmond, Virginia

Eric L. Marderstein, MD
Department of Surgery, University of Pittsburgh Medical Center, Pittsburgh, Pennsylvania

R. Shayn Martin, MD
Department of General Surgery, Wake Forest University School of Medicine, Winston-Salem, North Carolina

Kimball I. Maull, MD
Senior Scientist, Injury Control
Research Center, University of Alabama,
Chairman, Surgical Education, Carraway
Methodist Medical Center, Birmingham,
Alabama

Robert Maxwell, MD
Assistant Professor, University
of Tennessee–Chatanooga Unit;
Trauma Staff, Department of Surgery,
Erlanger Medical Center, Chatanooga,
Tennessee

J. Wayne Meredith, MD
Richard T. Myers Professor and Chair,
Department of Surgery, Wake Forest
University School of Medicine, Chief of
Surgery, Wake Forest University Baptist
Medical Center, Winston-Salem, North
Carolina

Kevin P. Mollen, MD
Resident, Department of Surgery,
University of Pittsburgh, University of
Pittsburgh Medical Center, Pittsburgh,
Pennsylvania

Forrest O. Moore, MD
Attending Trauma Surgeon, Division
of Trauma and Surgical Critical Care,
St. Joseph's Hospital Medical Center,
Phoenix, Arizona

Arthur James Moser, MD
Co-Director, UPMC Pancreas Cancer
Center, Department of Surgery,
University of Pittsburgh, Assistant
Professor of Surgery, Department
of Surgery, University of Pittsburgh
Medical Center, Pittsburgh,
Pennsylvania

Juan B. Ochoa, MD
Medical Director, Division of Trauma
Surgery, Professor of Surgery, Associate
Professor of Critical Care, University of
Pittsburgh Medical Center, Pittsburgh,
Pennsylvania

Mark Ochs, DMD, MD
Chair and Program Director,
Department of Oral & Maxillofacial
Surgery, University of Pittsburgh;
Chief, Department of Hospital
Dentistry, University of Pittsburgh
Medical Center, Pittsburgh,
Pennsylvania

Michael D. Pasquale, MD
Associate Professor, Department
of Surgery, Penn State University, Hershey,
Pennsylvania, Chief, Trauma/Surgical
Critical Care, Department of Surgery,
Lehigh Valley Hospital, Allentown,
Pennsylvania

Andrew B. Peitzman, MD, FACS
Professor and Chief, Division of General
Surgery, University of Pittsburgh School
of Medicine; Executive Vice Chair for
Clinical Services, Department of Surgery,
University of Pittsburgh Medical Center,
Presbyterian Hospital, Pittsburgh,
Pennsylvania

Louis E. Penrod, MD
Assistant Professor, Department of
Physical Medicine and Rehabilitation,
University of Pittsburgh School of
Medicine, Pittsburgh, Pennsylvania

Jose Manuel Prince, MD
Chief Resident, Department of Surgery,
University of Pittsburgh, University of
Pittsburgh Medical Center, Pittsburgh,
Pennsylvania

John P. Pryor, MD, FACS
Assistant Professor of Surgery, Division of
Trauma & Surgical Critical Care, Hospital
of Pennsylvania; Trauma Program
Director, Division of Surgical Care,
Philadelphia, Pennsylvania

**Juan Carlos Puyana, MD, FACS,
FRCSC, FACCP**
Trauma Surgeon, Associate Professor of
Surgery and Critical Care, Director of
Applied Research IMITs Center, Innovative
Medical & Information Technology Center,
University of Pittsburgh Medical Center,
Pittsburgh, Pennsylvania

Patrick M. Reilly, MD, FACS
Associate Professor, Department of
Surgery, University of Pennsylvania School
of Medicine, Vice-Chief, Division of
Traumatology and Surgical Critical Care,
Hospital of the University of Pennsylvania,
Philadelphia, Pennsylvania

Michael Rhodes, MD, FACS
Professor of Surgery, Thomson Jefferson
University; Chairman, Department of
Surgery, Christiana Care Health Services,
Wilmington, Delaware

Michael Rodricks, MD
Anesthesiologist and Intensivist,
Department of Anesthesiology and Critical
Care Medicine, Florida Hospital, Orlando,
Florida

Aurelio Rodriguez, MD
Director, Trauma Program, Trauma
Department, Allegheny General Hospital,
Pittsburgh, Pennsylvania

Matthew R. Rosengart, MD, MPH
Trauma Attending and Assistant Professor
of Surgery, Department of Surgery,
University of Pittsburgh, Pittsburgh,
Pennsylvania

Michael F. Rotondo, MD, FACS
Professor and Chairman, Department of
Surgery, East Carolina University, Chief,
Trauma & Surgical Critical Care, Center
for Excellence for Trauma & Surgical
Critical Care, Pitt County Memorial
Hospital, Greenville, North Carolina

Gregory D. Rushings, MD
Resident, Department of Surgery Eastern
Virginia Medical School, Norfolk, Virginia

James M. Russavage, MD, DMD
Assistant Professor, Department of
Surgery, Division of Plastic and
Maxillofacial Surgery, University of
Pittsburgh, Pittsburgh, Pennsylvania

Scott G. Sagraves, MD, FACS
Associate Professor, Department of Surgery,
The Brody School of Medicine, Greenville,
North Carolina; Director for Trauma,
University Health Systems of Eastern
North Carolina–Pitt County Memorial
Hospital, Greenville, North Carolina

Rohit Kumar Sahai, MD
Resident, Department of Surgery, University
of Pittsburgh, University of Pittsburgh
Medical Center, Pittsburgh, Pennsylvania

Michael G. Scheidler, MD
Chief Resident, Department of General
Surgery, Allegheny General Hospital,
Pittsburgh, Pennsylvania

Carol R. Schermer, MD, MPH
Associate Professor of Surgery, Division of
Critical Care, Loyola University
Chicago–Stritch School of Medicine,
Maywood, Illinois

Vaishali Dixit Schuchert, MD
Assistant Professor, Department of
Surgery and Critical Care, University of Pittsburgh, Pittsburgh,
Pennsylvania

C. William Schwab, MD, FACS
Professor of Surgery, Department of
Surgery, University of Pennsylvania
School of Medicine; Chief, Division
of Traumatology & Surgical Critical
Care, University of Pennsylvania
Medical Center, Philadelphia,
Pennsylvania

C. William Schwab, II, MD
Clinical Associate Surgery
Administration, University of
Pennsylvania Medical Center,
Philadelphia, Pennsylvania

Michael B. Shapiro, MD, FACS
Assistant Professor, Department of
Surgery, Division of Traumatology and
Surgical Critical Care, Hospital of the
University of Pennsylvania, Philadelphia,
Pennsylvania

Alan A. Simeone, MD
Fellow, Department of Surgical Critical
Care, Yale University School of Medicine,
New Haven, Connecticut

Carrie A. Sims, MD, FACS
Assistant Professor, Department of
Surgery, University of Pennsylvania
School of Medicine, Attending Staff,
Division of Traumatology and Surgical
Critical Care, Hospital of the University
of Pennsylvania, Philadelphia,
Pennsylvania

Francis X. Solano, Jr., MD
Clinical Professor, University of Pittsburgh
School of Medicine, Philadelphia,
Pennsylvania

Michael Stang, MD
Department of Surgery, University of
Pittsburgh, Pittsburgh, Pennsylvania

S. Tonya Stefko, MD
Assistant Professor, Department of
Ophthalmology & Otolaryngology,
University of Pittsburgh, University of
Pittsburg Medical Center, Pittsburgh,
Pennsylvania

Glen Tinkoff, MD, FACS
Medical Director, Trauma Program, Department of Surgery, Associate Director, Surgical Critical Care, Christiana Care Health Services, Newark, Delaware; Clinical Associate Professor of Surgery, Thomas Jefferson University, Philadelphia Pennsylvania

Samuel A. Tisherman, MD
Associate Professor, Departments of Surgery and Critical Care Medicine, University of Pittsburgh, Pittsburgh, Pennsylvania

Eric A. Toschlog, MD, FACS
Associate Professor, Department of Surgical Critical Care, The Brody School of Medicine; Director of Surgical Critical Care, University Health Systems of Eastern North Carolina–Pitt County Memorial Hospital, Greenville, North Carolina

Edith Tzeng, MD
Assistant Professor, Department of Surgery, University of Pittsburgh, Pittsburgh, Pennsylvania

Glenn Updike, MD
Assistant Professor, Department of Obstetrics, Gynecology, and Reproductive Services, University of Pittsburgh, Pittsburgh, Pennsylvania

Raghuveer Vallabhaneni, MD
General Surgery Resident, Department of Surgery, University of Pittsburgh, General Surgery Resident, Department of Surgery, University of Pittsburgh Medical Center, Pittsburgh, Pennsylvania

George Velmahos, MD, PhD, MSEd
Professor of Surgery, Harvard Medical School; Chief, Division of Trauma, Emergency Surgery and Surgical Critical Care Massachusetts General Hospital, Boston, Massachusetts

Henry E. Wang, MD, MPH
Assistant Professor, Department of Emergency Medicine, University of Pittsburgh, Pittsburgh, Pennsylvania

Andrew R. Watson
Assistant Professor of Surgery, Associate Residency Program Director, Division of Surgical Oncology, University of Pittsburgh Medical Center, Pittsburgh, Pennsylvania

Gregory A. Watson, MD
Resident, Department of Surgery, University of Pittsburgh, Pittsburgh, Pennsylvania

William C. Welch, MD, FACS, FICS
Professor, Department of Neurological Surgery, University of Pittsburgh School of Medicine, Chief, Neurological Surgery, University of Pittsburgh Medical Center, Pittsburgh, Pennsylvania

Anthony J. Wilson, MBChB
Clinical Professor, University of Washington School of Medicine, Seattle, Washington

Donald M. Yealy, MD, FACEP
Professor and Vice Chair, Department of Emergency Medicine, Chief of Emergency Services, University of Pittsburgh Medical Center, Pittsburgh, Pennsylvania

Ross D. Zafonte, DO
Professor and Chair, Physical Medicine and Rehabilitation, University of Pittsburgh, Vice President, Clinical Rehabilitation Services, UPMC Health System, Pittsburgh, Pennsylvania

Boris Zelle, MD
Resident, Orthopedic Surgery, University of Pittsburgh, Pittsburgh, Pennsylvania

Brian S. Zuckerbraun, MD
Assistant Professor of Surgery, Department of Surgery, University of Pittsburgh School of Medicine, Attending Surgeon, Department of Surgery, University of Pittsburgh Medical Center, VA Medical Center, Pittsburgh, Pennsylvania

*I*n reflecting on the other editions and publications from the vast experience in trauma care represented in the editors and authors of *The Trauma Manual*, and having used the manual with medical students, nurses, house staff, and attendings over the years, I find it difficult not to approach another edition of this book without being tempted to think it could not come up to, and certainly not exceed, the quality of the previous work. One *expects* this manual to be current, incisive, definitive in its advice, well-referenced, and authoritative. Above all, one expects it would never be a "cookbook."

Any reservations one could have about this edition falling short of previous ones are put to rest simply by perusing the listing of the editors and contributors to this third edition. Again, as with the previous two editions, this band of experts are truly that—clinical experts with national and international reputations who, on a daily basis, teach, do rounds, push the clinical envelope through academic research and, above all in authoring a "manual" of which the prime motive is to teach, they care for trauma patients and are part of a trauma *system*. No better credentials could be offered than those of this group.

Reflecting this experience and involvement in a trauma system is the approach taken to the broad spectrum of trauma care—from prevention, mechanism of injury, severity "scoring," to rehabilitation and evaluation of outcomes. And there is depth as well as breadth. The approach is current, well-researched, and *practical*. All of these qualities, including the clarity of the writing and organisation, will appeal to all students of medicine at every level—from first-year medicine to aging attending consultants. It will, as in past editions, also endear itself to other health professionals and caregivers of many stripes.

A welcome addition to the format of the manual is the inclusion of surgical emergencies presenting independently quite often as diagnostic dilemmas, or occasionally as a complication of trauma. The inclusion in the manual of GI haemorrhage, hernias, bowel obstruction, pancreatitis, biliary tract, disease and other surgical challenges has broadened the scope of the manual as well as its appeal.

In short, the measure of this third edition, as was the case with the previous efforts by these editors and authors, in reality will rest with those who use and need it most as an authoritative reference work. Judging from the response to previous editions among students at various levels and at several institutions with which I am familiar, this latest effort will be received with equal, or perhaps greater, enthusiasm. *The Trauma Manual: Trauma and Acute Care Surgery* will continue to occupy a place on the desk of the academic, on the quick-reference shelf in any modern emergency department, or in the pocket of any student or house staff on morning rounds or on the wards in the dead of night.

Ronald D. Stewart, OC, ONS, BA, BSc, MD, DSc
Professor of Emergency Medicine
Professor of Anaesthesia
Director of Medical Humanities
Faculty of Medicine, Dalhousie University
Halifax, Nova Scotia, Canada

$\mathcal{S}$ince the publication of the first edition of *The Trauma Manual*, there have been major changes in trauma care and trauma systems from a global standpoint. The last 10 years have seen emergency general surgery in many countries incorporated into trauma surgery. This is primarily due to the availability of trauma surgeons on a 24-hour basis. It also reflects that general surgery has become overly specialized, and many of the surgical specialists do not want to take emergency call or trauma call. In many countries, trauma surgeons are increasingly being called on to do emergency management of orthopedic injuries and even neurosurgical injuries.

From a trauma systems standpoint, there have also been major changes. Many European countries now have state-wide systems, as does Australia. China and India are also moving toward establishing trauma systems, but rural areas are still problematic. Sub-Saharan Africa continues to have major problems in trauma system development, except for South Africa. Unfortunately, trauma continues to be a major public health problem, due to increased road traffic accidents, war, and interpersonal violence. The Global Burden of Disease Study shows that by 2020, the death rate will have increased from trauma, as well as Disability Adjusted Life Years (DALYs).

The Trauma Manual, in its original form, has been very successful. This new edition addresses some of the issues listed above and continues to be a pragmatic, no-nonsense quick reference book for those people providing trauma care in sophisticated and austere environments. The book continues to emphasize the principles of injury mechanisms, pre-hospital care, resuscitative care, operative priorities, and critical care. It will be a useful reference for this evolving specialty of acute care surgery and trauma.

Donald D. Trunkey, MD, FACS
Professor Emeritus, Department of Surgery
Oregon Health & Science University
Portland, Oregon

$\mathcal{T}$he third edition of *The Trauma Manual: Trauma and Acute Care Surgery* is substantially different in scope and content than the first two editions of *The Trauma Manual*. As the new title reflects, the manual now includes what we have done in practice for decades: trauma, critical care, and emergency general surgery. The Emergency Department and the Trauma/Acute Care Surgery services at many hospitals are essentially the "safety nets" for the inpatients and the critically ill outpatients. *The Trauma Manual* now incorporates the diverse disease processes and care that we deliver everyday. We have built upon the success of the first two editions of *The Trauma Manual* by expanding the authorship of the chapters to more international and national experts. The chapters on trauma care have been updated and revised. The chapter on Intensive Care is completely rewritten. Chapters on all aspects of emergency general surgery have been added and include Evaluation of the Acute Abdomen, Preoperative Clearance, Bowel Obstruction, Anorectal Pain, GI Bleeding, Hernias, Infection, Cholecystitis, Cholangitis, and Pancreatitis, Esophageal Emergencies, Stomach, Duodenum, Small Intestine, Appendix and Colon, and Obstetric and Gynecologic Emergencies. As with the first editions, these chapters are written by experts in these fields. The recommendations made are backed by the extensive clinical experience of the authors.

The goal of *The Trauma Manual* remains to serve as a ready pocket reference for all who provide care for the patient with acute surgical diseases. The format of *The Trauma Manual* is that of a user-friendly pocket manual rather than a comprehensive textbook. With that said, this book contains a great deal of information covering all phases of *Trauma and Acute Care Surgery*.

The Trauma Manual is organized in a chronological fashion, following the usual events and phases of care after injury or acute surgical illness. Rather than listing every option in a clinical situation, a consensus recommendation is generally presented. Flow charts, sequential lists, and algorithms are used throughout as approaches to clinical problems. We have attempted to keep the content of *The Trauma Manual* practical and direct. The editors hope that this edition of *The Trauma Manual* again provides a clear, pragmatic approach to those providing care for the critically ill or injured patient.

Andrew B. Peitzman, MD, FACS
Timothy C. Fabian, MD, FACS
Michael Rhodes, MD, FACS
C. William Schwab, MD, FACS
Donald M. Yealy, MD, FACEP

INTRODUCTION TO TRAUMA CARE
R. SHAYN MARTIN AND
J. WAYNE MEREDITH

I. INTRODUCTION. Trauma is mechanical damage to the body caused by an external force. The trauma patient has been defined as "an injured person who requires timely diagnosis and treatment of actual or potential injuries by a multidisciplinary team of health care professionals, supported by the appropriate resources, to diminish or eliminate the risk of death or permanent disability." This chapter describes the current impact of injury on society, the structure of modern trauma systems, and finally the way injuries are measured and quantified.

II. EPIDEMIOLOGY

    A. Overall, trauma is the third leading cause of death in the United States and is the leading source of mortality for patients between 1 and 44 years of age. In 2003, 164,002 people died secondary to injury, representing 56 deaths per 100,000 population. Of these, 109,277 were unintentional in nature while 49,639 were caused by violence. A fatal injury occurs approximately every 5 minutes.

    B. Mortality after trauma can be characterized by a well-studied distribution that identifies three time periods during which the majority of deaths occur. Approximately 50% of deaths occur immediately and are usually secondary to severe neurologic injuries or exsanguination from major blood vessel injuries (Fig. 1-1). These deaths can be avoided only through injury prevention. The second peak of approximately 30% of all deaths occurs during the initial hours postinjury and preventing these deaths is the goal of modern trauma care, such as is taught through the Advanced Trauma Life Support (ATLS) course. Finally, 20% of deaths occur late (within 1–2 weeks) and are secondary to sepsis and multiple organ failure. It is believed that improved early management of injury and associated shock may prevent these late complications.

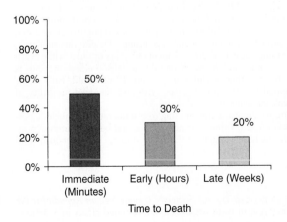

Figure 1-1. Distribution of death after injury. (Adapted from Trunkey DD. Trauma. Accidental and intentional injuries account for more years of life lost in the U.S. than cancer and heart disease. Among the prescribed remedies are improved preventive efforts, more expedient surgery and further research. *Sci Am* 1983; 249:28.)

C. In 2003, more than 29 million medically attended, nonfatal injuries occurred in the United States. Data from 2002 reveal an estimated 37.8 million injury-related emergency department and 99.2 million office-based visits. There were approximately 1.8 million hospital discharges for injured patients. Injury represents the greatest cause of years of potential life lost (YPLL) before age 65 totaling over 3.4 million years or 29.3% of all YPLL. The total cost for injuries occurring in 2003 including medical expenses, lost wages, property damage, cost to employers, fire losses, and all other costs was estimated to be $607.7 billion.

D. **Specific injury patterns and mechanism**
   1. **Age.** While people 44 years old and younger account for the majority of fatal and non-fatal injuries, the impact of trauma on the elderly is far more severe. The death rate for injuries among patients 0 to 44 years old is approximately 45 per 100,000 population, whereas this rate is 113 per 100,000 for people over 65 years old and 169 per 100,000 for people over 75 years old.
   2. **Gender.** Sixty-nine percent of all injury-related deaths occur in males, twice the number of female deaths. The distribution of nonfatal injuries is more equivalent with males representing 55%.
   3. **Mechanism**
      a. **Motor vehicle crashes (MVCs)** are the leading cause of injury-related death, accounting for 44,800 deaths in 2003 or 15.4 deaths per 100,000 population. Over 3.5 million people sustained nonfatal injuries secondary to MVC in 2003. Despite this, the death rate per vehicle miles traveled (VMT) has declined steadily throughout the century from 18 deaths per 100 million VMT in 1925 to approximately 5 per 100 million VMT in 1960 to as low as 1.56 per 100 million VMT in 2003. In the 2005 National Trauma Data Bank (NTDB), MVCs accounted for 43.1% of cases and 46% of the mortalities. MVC-related deaths occurred in 4.9% of NTDB cases.
      b. **Firearm-related injury** resulted in 28,827 deaths in 2003 and was the second leading cause of injury-related mortality for all ages in that year. Fifty-nine percent were the result of suicide, while 41% were homicide related. Nonfatal gunshot wounds were identified in 65,834 patients in 2003. Predominately, fatal shootings involve young males, with the number of deaths in the 15-to-34-year-old age range being over seven times that of females. Handguns were involved in 80% of all homicides with a firearm in 2003. Six percent of the injuries in the NTDB were associated with firearms; 16% of cases resulted in death. Firearm-related injuries peaked at 19 years of age.
      c. **Falls** are the leading cause of nonfatal injury resulting in approximately 8.1 million injuries and 17,229 deaths throughout all age groups. Falls are most common among the young and the elderly with both groups demonstrating injury rates of greater than 4,000 injuries per 100,000 population in 2003, twice that of people in the intermediate age groups. Despite this similarity, falls are the leading cause of death in patients 65 years or older while death in children is uncommon. The death rate due to falls in elderly patients is more than 170 times that of children less than 10 years old. Falls in the NTDB accounted for 26% of all cases, with an associated mortality of 3.5%. The peak incidence occurred at age 82.
      d. Other common mechanisms contributing to trauma mortality include poisoning, suffocation, drowning, cutting/piercing, and burns. Common non-fatal injuries include struck by/against injury, overexertion, and bites/stings.

III. **TRAUMA SYSTEMS**
   A. **Overview**
      1. As defined by the American Trauma Society's *Trauma System Agenda for the Future*, "A trauma system is an organized, coordinated effort in a defined

geographic area that delivers the full range of care to all injured patients and is integrated with the local public health system."

2. **Historical perspective.** The systematic care of trauma changed significantly with the publication of the National Academy of Science/National Research Council's *Accidental Death and Disability: The Neglected Disease of Modern Society* in 1966. This document revealed the deficiencies in injury management and initiated the development of systems to improve trauma care. The Emergency Medical Services Systems Act was passed in 1973 to support the development of regionalized Emergency Medical Services (EMS) systems. In 1976, the American College of Surgeons (ACS) Committee on Trauma (COT) published *Optimal Hospital Resources for the Care of the Seriously Injured* which established criteria that identified hospitals as trauma centers. This document has been revised as knowledge about trauma systems has evolved. More recently, the Model Trauma Care System Plan created by the Health Resources Services Administration (HRSA) was published to further define and guide trauma system development.

3. **Function.** Trauma systems have been designed to be *inclusive* in nature and therefore use all available resources to provide appropriate care to all injured patients and not only to the most severely injured.

4. **Designation and verification.** Facilities within a trauma system require identification of injury management capabilities so that resource assessments can be achieved. A process for designating trauma centers is needed to provide consistent and inclusive care within the trauma system. A government group designates a hospital as a trauma center after evaluating the facility's resources and the ability to provide a specific level of care. The ACS COT performs the process of verification which reviews a facility and ensures that the trauma care provided is in accordance with the *Resources for Optimal Care of the Injured Patient* document. The criteria for designation and verification may be similar but only designation is the active process of becoming approved to provide a specific level of care.

5. **Systems consultation.** The ACS COT as well as some private organizations provide consulting services that are valuable in evaluation of the status of trauma care either during the development or maintenance of a trauma system.

B. **Fundamental components**

1. **Injury prevention** has become an essential focus for all trauma systems in order to proactively reduce the impact of injury. Many systems have developed formal injury prevention programs and dedicated centers to better address this need.

2. **Pre-hospital care** includes community access and communication systems as well as EMS systems and triage protocols. Universal access to emergency care (i.e., 911) is essential to allow efficient activation of the system. A robust communication system provides for coordination of pre-hospital resources as well as proper transfer of information to receiving facilities. Standardized curricula for training EMS personnel provide a more consistent knowledge base and skills set. Developed trauma systems have ensured more efficient emergency response through improved geographical placement of EMS providers versus only facility-based responders.

3. **Acute care facilities** provide a range of injury management from initial stabilization and transfer to all-inclusive definitive care. Based on available resources, facilities are characterized by injury management capabilities and many are designated as trauma centers using a scale of 1 to 4, with Level 1 centers providing the most comprehensive level of care. Successful trauma systems benefit from the contributions of all available facilities to become more inclusive and to provide consistent care to all people within the system.

4. **Post-hospital care** is an important part of reducing disability and improving an injured patient's long-term outcome. Efficient transfer from the acute

care setting to rehabilitation is a necessary attribute of a well-developed trauma system.

C. Trauma system infrastructure elements
1. **Leadership.** A lead agency should be established to coordinate trauma system development and provide necessary administration.
2. **Professional resources.** Successful trauma systems rely on competent and energetic health care providers to ensure optimal injury care. Recruiting methods to identify and employ the highest quality health care professionals is a necessity.
3. **Education/Advocacy.** Trauma systems must improve public awareness about trauma as a disease state and the ability of injury prevention to reduce the societal impact of trauma.
4. **Information management.** Trauma data registries at the local and national levels provide an invaluable resource for performance improvement, research, and trauma system management. Ideally, trauma data should be consistently captured and incorporated into regional and national databases to provide the most accurate depiction of the status of injury care.
5. **Finances.** Adequate financial support is essential for both trauma system development and the continued provision of trauma care. Increased public and political awareness of the magnitude of the problem is required to improve governmental funding.
6. **Research.** To continue improving the care of the injured, research endeavors must be encouraged and efforts to increase financial support for trauma research is crucial.
7. **Technology.** The potential of novel and developing technologies must be adopted and applied to the field of trauma care. For example, technological advancements have decreased EMS response times and improved crash investigations.
8. **Disaster preparedness and response.** Trauma systems are charged with the task of being prepared to respond to potential disasters by developing a systematic and organized approach that can be implemented if the need arises.

D. State and regional trauma systems
1. Each hospital and prehospital agency within a state is encompassed by a state COT that coordinates the fundamental components of the trauma system and implements the infrastructural programs.
2. State COTs are grouped geographically into 14 regions that are overseen by a regional committee.
3. All state and regional trauma systems are represented by the ACS COT that develops necessary policies to improve trauma care at the national level.

IV. INJURY SCORING
A. Principles
1. **Purpose.** Injury scoring systems have been developed to accurately and consistently quantify the magnitude of injury from an anatomic, physiologic, or a combined standpoint. Scoring systems are used in triage decision making, quality improvement and benchmarking initiatives, prevention program analyses, and research endeavors.
2. **Database use.** Scoring systems are commonly included in trauma databases to provide a quantifiable means of patient comparison. Based on the purpose of the database, certain scoring systems may be more appropriate and relevant than others. For example, administrative databases would more appropriately contain *International Classification of Diseases (ICD-9)* based scoring systems (e.g., *ICD*-based Injury Severity Score [ICISS]) while trauma registry databases may contain Abbreviated Injury Score (AIS) based scoring systems. Identification of the specific needs of the database often reveals the type of scoring system that would be most applicable.
3. **Correct use of scoring.** While there are many available scoring systems, the use of some of these systems may be limited. Systems used for triage decision

making must be easy to calculate from rapidly available information. Scoring is commonly used in the research setting and in this case should be able to identify patients with comparable injuries. Evaluation of responses to therapy may benefit from applying a physiologic scoring system. The combined scores are valuable when assessing outcome after injury.

   4. **Limitations.** Since every injured patient is unique, there is no single scoring system that can provide a perfect description. Care must be taken when interpreting the results of injury severity scoring to recognize that there will always be aspects of the patient's condition that were not captured.

B. **Scoring systems**
   1. **Anatomic scores**
      a. **Abbreviated Injury Score (AIS).** First proposed in 1969 and updated last in 1990, the AIS assigns a severity level to the worst injury in each of six separate body regions: head/neck, face, thorax, abdomen/pelvic contents, bony pelvis/extremities, and external structures. Level of severity ranges from 1 (minimally injured) to 6 (fatal). The AIS does not account for multiple injuries in the same patient.
      b. **Injury Severity Score (ISS).** ISS was first introduced in 1974 to more accurately characterize severity when multiple injuries were present. ISS is calculated by squaring the AIS scores from the three most severely injured body regions and adding the results. If any AIS is 6, the ISS is automatically 75 and considered to be a fatal injury. ISS is commonly used for injury quantification, although it is limited in that its accuracy requires that all injuries be identified before calculation and it is unable to account for multiple injuries within the same body region.
         i. The 2005 NTDB categorized injuries based on ISS as minor (ISS 1–9), moderate (ISS 10–15), severe (ISS 16–24), and very severe (ISS >24). Minor injuries constituted about two thirds (68%) of the injuries with the remainder being nearly equal among the other groups. The average hospital length of stay increased by approximately 3 days for each severity grouping while intensive care unit (ICU) days also increased (moderate = 1.7 days, severe = 3.9 days, very severe = 7.7 days).
      c. **New Injury Severity Score (NISS).** In an attempt to improve on the shortcomings of ISS, NISS was developed in 1997. NISS is calculated similarly to ISS, but the three most severe injuries, regardless of body region, are used in the equation. As a result, NISS is more straightforward to calculate and has been shown to be more predictive of survival than ISS.
      d. **American Association for the Surgery of Trauma (AAST) Organ Injury Scale (OIS).** In 1987 the AAST organized the OIS committee to create an injury scoring system that accurately quantifies the severity of individual organ injuries for clinical investigation and outcomes research purposes. Scales were created from critical review of available literature as well as expert trauma surgeon consensus. Injuries to organs are graded from 1 to 5 to reflect severity and anticipated impact on outcome. Injury scales for abdominal organs—spleen, liver, kidney, pancreas, duodenum, small bowel, colon, and rectum—have been provided (Appendix A).
      e. **Survival Risk Ratios (SRR)/*ICD*-based Injury Severity Score (ICISS).** Recently, *ICD*-9 diagnostic codes have been employed to quantify injury severity. Using large trauma databases, SRRs are calculated by determining the mortality observed for each injury-related *ICD*-9 code. All SRRs for a given patient are then combined to yield ICISS. Because reimbursement depends on *ICD*-9 codes, the information needed to calculate ICISS is readily available in any hospital data repository. Despite its simplicity, ICISS has been found to be a better predictor of mortality than either ISS or the Trauma and Injury Severity Score (TRISS).
      f. **Anatomic Profile (AP).** The AP incorporates injuries from three body regions: head/spine, anterior neck and chest, and all other injuries. Scores

TABLE 1-1	Glasgow Coma Scale	
Eye opening	Spontaneous	4
	To voice	3
	To pain	2
	None	1
Verbal response	Oriented	5
	Confused	4
	Inappropriate	3
	Incomprehensible	2
	None	1
Motor response	Obeys commands	6
	Localizes pain	5
	Withdraws to pain	4
	Flexion	3
	Extension	2
	None	1
Total Glasgow Coma Score		3–15

for these regions are modified and used in an equation derived from logistic regression. The AP has recently been shown to demonstrate good injury model predictiveness compared to other scoring systems.

   g. **Penetrating Abdominal Trauma Index (PATI).** PATI is a scoring system designed to quantify the effects of penetrating abdominal injury. Each organ has a pre-determined risk factor score (1 to 5) and injured organs are assigned a severity score (1 to 5) based on published criteria. The severity score is multiplied by the risk factor score and the sum of all of these results is the PATI.

2. **Physiologic scores**
   a. **Glasgow Coma Score (GCS).** The GCS is the most widely used scoring system for the characterization of neurologic injury. A patient's status in terms of eye opening, verbal response, and motor activity is determined and summed to calculate the GCS (Table 1-1). A patient's GCS can be rapidly calculated in the field or in the emergency department and is commonly used for patient care decision-making and triage.
      i. A GCS of 8 or less is usually indicative of severe brain injury and suggestive of required intervention (e.g., intubation).
      ii. The motor component of the GCS has been found to correlate well with the entire GCS and be the most predictive of outcome.
   b. **Trauma Score (TS).** The TS was developed in 1981 to incorporate physiologic parameters in severity scoring. Quantification of respiratory effort, systolic blood pressure, capillary refill, and GCS are included in the determination of the TS. Use of the TS has been limited by the subjective nature of respiratory effort and capillary refill assessments.
   c. **Revised Trauma Score (RTS).** The RTS addressed the deficiencies of the TS by removing the ambiguous respiratory and perfusion components. As Table 1-2 demonstrates, coded values are assigned to quantify the GCS, systolic blood pressure, and respiratory rate parameters. The result is a score of 0 to 12 with 12 demonstrating normal physiology. Therefore, the RTS is simple to calculate and is used in making triage decisions and predicting hospital outcomes.
   d. **Systemic Inflammatory Response Syndrome Score (SIRS Score).** The SIRS score incorporates patient temperature, heart rate, respiratory rate, and white blood cell count to physiologically characterize injured patients

TABLE 1-2	Revised Trauma Score		
A **Glasgow** **Coma Score**	**B** **Systolic blood** **pressure (mmHg)**	**C** **Respiratory rate** **(breaths/min)**	**Coded value** **(CV)**
13–15	>89	10–29	4
9–12	76–89	>29	3
6–8	50–75	6–9	2
4–5	1–49	1–5	1
3	0	0	0

mmHg, millimeters of mercury.

(Table 1-3). The SIRS score can be calculated easily and has been demonstrated to be predictive of outcome on admission and further into a patient's hospital course.

3. **Combined scores**
   a. **Trauma and Injury Severity Score (TRISS).** Introduced in 1983, TRISS combines anatomic and physiologic parameters to arrive at a calculated probability of survival. TRISS incorporates the ISS, RTS, patient age, and injury mechanism into an equation that uses established coefficients determined using large trauma databases. TRISS is valuable in outcomes analyses and research but has no value in the patient care setting.
   b. **A Severity Characterization of Trauma (ASCOT).** ASCOT uses a methodology similar to TRISS but has been adapted to better characterize situations where the predictive ability of TRISS is deficient (e.g., penetrating torso injury). ASCOT uses the RTS, patient age, and an anatomic description similar to the AP. ASCOT also employs a logistic regression model to determine survival probabilities. The results of ASCOT assessments have been minimally more predictive than TRISS methodology.
   c. **Harborview Assessment for Risk of Mortality (HARM).** First published in 2000, HARM combines 80 variables such as *ICD-9* codes, age, injury mechanism, comorbidities, and injury associations to predict survival probabilities.

C. **Validation of scoring systems**
   1. After the development of a scoring system, a process of validation is required to confirm its accuracy and predictive nature. This can often be accomplished by challenging the scoring system against a large, well-constructed trauma database such as a state trauma registry, governmental database, or the NTDB.

TABLE 1-3	Systemic Inflammatory Response Syndrome Score	
Variable	**Positive result**	**Points**
Temperature	>38°C (100.4°F) or <36°C (96.8°F)	1
Heart rate	>90 beats/min	1
Respiratory rate	>20 breaths/min, $PaCO_2$ <32 mmHg	1
White blood cell count	>12,000/mm^3, <4,000/mm^3, or ≥10% bands	1
Total SIRS Score	SIRS defined as ≥2	0–4

$PaCO_2$, alveolar carbon dioxide.
mm^3, cubic millimeters.

AXIOMS

■ The impact of trauma on individuals and society as a whole is significant.
■ Organized trauma systems provide the greatest means of combating the substantial effects of injury.
■ Injury severity scoring is an important component of trauma care and careful selection of the most appropriate scoring system will provide the most accurate information.

Bibliography

American College of Surgeons Committee on Trauma. *Resources for Optimal Care of the Injured Patient: 1999.* Chicago, Ill: American College of Surgeons; 1998.

American Trauma Society. *Trauma System Agenda for the Future.* Upper Marlboro, Md: American Trauma Society; 2002.

Baker SP, O'Neill B, Haddon W, et al. The injury severity score: A method for describing patients with multiple injuries and evaluating emergency care. *J Trauma* 1974;14:187.

Champion HR, Copes WS, Sacco WJ, et al. A new characterization of injury severity. *J Trauma* 1990;30:539.

Champion HR, Sacco WJ, Carnazzo AJ, et al. Trauma score. *Crit Care Med* 1981;9:672.

Champion HR, Sacco WJ, Copes WS, et al. A revision of the trauma score. *J Trauma* 1989;29:623.

Champion HR, Sacco WJ, Hunt TK, et al. Trauma severity scoring to predict mortality. *World J Surg* 1983;7:4.

Federal Bureau of Investigation. *Uniform Crime Reports for the United States: 2003.* Washington, DC: U.S. Department of Justice; 2004.

Hoyt DB, Coimbra R, Potenza BM. Trauma systems, triage, and transport. In: Moore EE, Feliciano DV, Mattox KL, eds. *Trauma.* 5th ed. New York, NY: McGraw-Hill Co Inc; 2004:57–84.

MacKenzie EJ, Fowler CJ. Epidemiology in trauma. In: Moore EE, Feliciano DV, Mattox KL, eds. *Trauma.* 5th ed. New York, NY: McGraw-Hill Co Inc; 2004:21–38.

Malone DL, Kuhls D, Napolitano LM, et al. Back to basics: Validation of the Systemic Inflammatory Response Syndrome Score in predicting outcome in trauma. *J Trauma* 2001;51:458.

Meredith JW, Evens G, Kilgo PD, et al. A comparison of the abilities of nine scoring algorithms in predicting mortality. *J Trauma* 2002;53:621.

Moore EE, Cogbill TH, Jurkovich GJ, et al. Organ injury scaling: Spleen and liver (1994 revision). *J Trauma* 1995;38:323–324.

Moore EE, Cogbill TH, Jurkovich GJ, et al. Organ injury scaling: III—Chest wall, abdominal vascular, ureter, bladder, and urethra. *J Trauma* 1992;33:337–339.

Moore EE, Cogbill TH, Malangoni MA, et al. Organ injury scaling: II—Pancreas, small bowel, colon, rectum. *J Trauma* 1990;30:1427–1429.

Moore EE, Jurkovich GJ, Knudson MM, et al. Organ injury scaling: VI—Extrahepatic biliary, esophagus, stomach, vulva, vagina, uterus (nonpregnant), uterus (pregnant), fallopian tube, and ovary. *J Trauma* 1995;39:1069–1070.

Moore EE, Malangoni MA, Cogbill TH, et al. Organ injury scaling: IV—Thoracic vascular, lung, cardiac, and diaphragm. *J Trauma* 1994;36:299–300.

Moore EE, Malangoni MA, Cogbill TH, et al. Organ injury scaling: VII—Cervical vascular, peripheral vascular, adrenal, penis, testis, and scrotum. *J Trauma* 1996;41:532–534.

Moore EE, Shackford SR, Patcher HL, et al. Organ injury scaling: Spleen, liver, and kidney. *J Trauma* 1989;29:1664–1666.

National Center for Health Statistics. Fast stats A to Z. U.S. Department of Health and Human Services Web site. Available at: http://www.cdc.gov/nchs/fastats/Default.htm. Accessed October 6, 2006.

National Center for Injury Prevention and Control. WISQARS. CDC Web site. Available at: http://www.cdc.gov/ncipc/wisqars/default.htm. Accessed March 30, 2006.

National Safety Council. *Injury Facts, 2004 Edition.* Itasca, Ill: National Safety Council; 2004.

Osler T, Baker SP, Long W. A modification of the injury severity score that both improves accuracy and simplifies scoring. *J Trauma* 1997;43:922.

Osler T, Rutledge R, Deis J, et al. ICISS: An international classification of diseases-based injury severity score. *J Trauma* 1996;41:380.

Rutledge R, Osler T, Emery S, et al. The end of ISS and the TRISS: ICISS outperforms both ISS and TRISS as predictors of trauma patient survival, hospital charges and hospital length of stay. *J Trauma* 1998;44:41.

Sauaia A, Moore FA, Moore EE, et al. Epidemiology of trauma deaths: A reassessment. *J Trauma* 1995;38:185.

Trunkey DD. Trauma. Accidental and intentional injuries account for more years of life lost in the U.S. than cancer and heart disease. Among the prescribed remedies are improved preventive efforts, speedier surgery and further research. *Sci Am* 1983;249:28.

West TA, Rivera FP, Cummings P, et al. Harborview assessment for risk of mortality: An improved measure of injury severity on the basis of *ICD-9-CM. J Trauma* 2000;49:530.

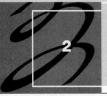

PATTERNS OF BLUNT INJURY

GREGORY D. RUSHINGS AND L. D. BRITT

 MECHANISM OF INJURY

Trauma is a physical injury with associated dissipation of energy to and within the person involved. Trauma can occur as a result of a blunt, penetrating, or thermal mechanism. The actual mechanism of injury often dictates the specific management approach. In addition to the mechanism, patterns of injury are important. Specific injuries can be anticipated based on some patterns of injury. Also, possible associated injuries must be considered for every diagnosed injury (Tables 2-1 and 2-2).

TABLE 2-1 Blunt Trauma: Documented and Possible Associated Injuries

Documented injury	Possible associated injuries
Neck injury (±cervical fracture)	Carotid artery injury
Sternal or first/second rib fracture	Thoracic aortic injury, myocardial contusion, atrial rupture
Scapula fracture	Pulmonary contusion, thoracic aortic injury
Chest wall injury (rib fractures 6–12)	Left side—splenic injury, right side—hepatic injury
Lumbar fracture (L_2–L_5)	Pancreatic contusion/transection, intestinal rupture
Abdominal wall abrasion/contusion ("seatbelt" sign)	Intestinal rupture, mesenteric rent
Severe pelvic fracture	Bladder rupture, urethral transection, rectal/vaginal injury
Shoulder dislocation (anterior)	Axillary nerve injury
Knee dislocation (posterior), supracondylar femur fracture	Popliteal artery injury (intimal tear/thrombosis)
Bilateral calcaneal fractures	Lower extremity and vertebral fractures, renal/thoracic aortic injuries

TABLE 2-2 Penetrating Trauma: Documented and Possible Associated Injuries

Documented injury	Possible associated injuries
Cervical (platysma penetration) injuries	Jugular vein/carotid artery injury, tracheal/esophageal injury
Transmediastinal injury	Cardiac/tracheobronchial and pulmonary/vascular/diaphragmatic/gastrointestinal injury
Thoracoabdominal injury	Pulmonary/diaphragmatic/cardiac/gastrointestinal injury
Transabdominal injury	Gastrointestinal/hepatic/vascular injury
Transpelvic injury	Bladder/intestinal/uterine/vascular injury
Flank injury	Genitourinary/intestinal injury

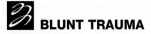

BLUNT TRAUMA

I. TYPES
   A. Motor vehicle crashes
   B. Motorcycle crashes
   C. Pedestrian–automobile impacts
   D. Falls
   E. Assaults

II. MOTOR VEHICLE CRASHES (MVCs)
   A. Injuries are produced by the rapid decrease in velocity over a short distance (deceleration). Severity of injury depends on energy transferred during deceleration as a result of a crash.
   1. MVCs account for over half of the deaths from unintentional causes.
   2. MVCs cause at least half of closed head and spinal cord injuries.
   3. The risk of a major injury increases 300% to 500% if the victim is ejected (including a 1 in 13 risk of spinal column injury).
   4. MVCs involve three types of collisions:
      a. Primary collision—motor vehicle impacts another object
      b. Secondary collision—victim strikes internal components of the car
      c. Deceleration-induced deformation—results in differential movement of fixed and nonfixed anatomic parts (e.g., shearing injury to the brain or transection of the thoracic aorta)
   B. Determinants of injury
   1. Magnitude of force (force = mass × acceleration)
   2. Location of victim (front seat versus back seat; driver versus passenger)
   3. Restraint devices (Table 2-3)
      a. Injury risk is greatest in the unrestrained victims.
      b. Lap belts alone decrease mortality by 50% (there is, however, an increased rate of abdominal injury).
      c. The lap belt is designed to fit across the pelvis (the anterior superior iliac spines). If inappropriately worn over the abdomen, compression fractures of the lumbar spine (Chance fractures) can occur. Lap belt injuries are associated with small bowel and colon injuries. Such injuries also include mesenteric tears and thrombosis of the abdominal aorta.
      d. Three-point constraints plus airbags provide the optimal protection, especially in front-end collisions.
      e. Secondary collisions of occupant with the vehicle are reduced with the utilization of three-point restraints. Ejection is prevented and mortality is substantially decreased.
      f. With three-point constraints, extremity injuries are not prevented. Also, there is no effect on major injury patterns with side impact collisions.
      g. Shoulder belt should not be worn without the lap component; the driver and passengers can slip under this restraint.
      h. Shoulder belt injuries are associated with multiple vascular injuries, including intimal damage or thrombosis of innominate, subclavian, carotid, or vertebral arteries.

TABLE 2-3	Restraint Devices

A. Lap belt
B. Shoulder belt
C. Shoulder and lap belts
D. Airbags (frontal and side impact)

    i. Airbags allow a less traumatic deceleration when compared to three-point restraints. The proportion and severity of lower extremity injuries are increased relative to torso and head injuries. However, airbags can cause injuries to occupants who are facing backward or leaning against the steering wheel or into another passenger's compartment.

4. Unrestrained (driver and front seat occupants)

  a. The majority of injuries in frontal crashes are a result of impact with the steering wheel, windshield, dashboard, or floorboards. These injuries include the following:

    i. cranial injuries (16%)
    ii. facial fractures (37%)
    iii. cervical spine injuries (10–15%)
    iv. major thoracic injuries (46%)
    v. abdominal injuries (5–10%)
    vi. femur fractures (65%)
    vii. distal lower extremity fractures (33%)
    viii. forearm fractures (46%)

  b. Lateral crashes ("T-bone")

    i. A lateral crash can result in direct impact between the vehicle and the occupant because of the limited space between the driver and the colliding vehicle.
    ii. Because there is very little substantive material to blunt such an impact, lateral impact collisions are associated with twice the mortality of frontal impacts.
    iii. Thoracic and abdominal injuries are most prevalent.
    iv. The occupant is projected into the next compartment.

  c. Rear-end impact collisions

    i. Rear-end impact collisions do not usually cause severe injuries, with only 8% of crashes resulting in serious injury.
    ii. An extension flexion injury ("whiplash") is common.

  d. Rollover collisions

    i. Because of the random nature of these collisions, force vectors vary.
    ii. Kinetic energy of the car is usually dissipated over a long distance.
    iii. Roof collapse can produce severe head injury.
    iv. Axial load forces can result in compression fractures of the spine.
    v. Ejection of the occupant can occur.

5. Unrestrained (backseat passenger)

  a. The rear seat passengers have the same risk of injury as those in the front seat except the direct injuries sustained from the steering wheel and dashboard impact.
  b. Rear seat passengers are less likely to be restrained.
  c. Unrestrained rear seat passengers can be a projectile, potentially causing injury to both themselves and occupants in the front seat.

III. MOTORCYCLE CRASHES

  A. Unlike motor vehicle crashes, the driver or passenger usually absorbs all the impact and the associated kinetic energy.
  B. The majority (75%) of motorcycle deaths are a result of cranial injuries.
  C. Spine, pelvis, and extremity injuries are also common.
  D. Less obvious fractures can occur.
  E. There is a high risk of limb loss with open or severe injuries to the tibia and fibula.

IV. PEDESTRIAN–AUTOMOBILE IMPACTS

  A. Although pedestrian–automobile impacts account for only 2% of traffic injuries, they account for 13% of traffic-related deaths. Children, the elderly, and the intoxicated, are more at risk for this mechanism of injury. The pattern of injury is depicted in Fig. 2-1. Torso trauma (chest, abdomen, and pelvis) represents 6% of the injuries; however, musculoskeletal and intraabdominal are more common (35% and 27%, respectively).

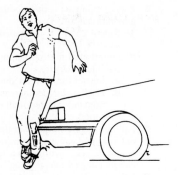

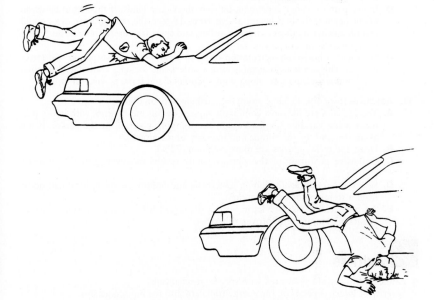

Figure 2-1. Pedestrian–automobile impact. (©Baylor College of Medicine 1986. Modified from Feliciano DV, Moore EE, Mattox KL, eds. *Trauma.* 3rd ed. Norwalk, Conn: Appleton and Lange, Englewood Cliffs, NJ; 1996:97, with permission.)

B. This type of impact often results in **Waddle's triad** of injury: (1) tibiofibular or femur fracture, (2) truncal injury, and (3) craniofacial injury. Therefore, a patient with two components of Waddle's triad of injury should be assumed to have the third component as well.

C. In general, small children tend to be "run over" and adults "run under" or thrown over the car with impact onto the street.

D. A lateral compression pelvic fracture can occur as a result of contact between the hip and the fender of the motor vehicle.

V. FALLS

A. Injuries sustained in falls depend on distance of fall, surface struck, and the position on impact.

B. Energy at impact is the product of the victim's weight times distance of fall times gravitational forces.

  1. Kinetic energy is dissipated, on impact, throughout the skeleton and soft tissues.

  2. Duration of impact (i.e., how quickly the victim stops) is critical in determining injury severity.

    a. Impact force over a shorter time increases the magnitude of injury.

    b. Harder surfaces increase severity of injury because of immediate deceleration and transfer of all energy to the body (e.g., concrete vs. grass, sand, or snow).

C. Fall injuries are frequent in the elderly. Comorbidities are major determinants of outcome and can also contribute to causing the fall.

D. Femoral neck fractures and head and cervical spine injuries can result from the elderly falling while walking.

E. Falls occurring from a height can involve a tumbling mechanism or a "free fall." Free falls imply a fall from a height directly to the ground.

F. Falls of 25 to 30 feet (three stories) have a mortality of 50%. Survival is rare in free falls from above five stories.

G. Injury patterns differ depending on how the victim lands. If the victim lands on his or her feet, from a height above 10 to 15 feet, the pattern of injuries could include calcaneal, lower extremity, pelvis, and spine fractures. Thoracic aorta and renal injuries can also occur.

H. Falls with a horizontal orientation result in greater energy dissipation and fewer injuries. This is a less predictable injury pattern and includes craniofacial trauma, hand and wrist fractures, along with abdominal and thoracic visceral injuries.

VI. Assaults (fisticuffs, kicking, stomping, striking with an object)

A. Young males are the most commonly injured by this mechanism, with injury patterns being variable (depending on the weapon, position of the person being assaulted, and the magnitude and intensity of the attack).

B. Head and facial injuries are more common (72%).

C. Defensive posturing of the victim usually results in lower extremity injuries (<10%).

D. Severe torso injuries (including pancreatic and hollow viscus injuries) can occur from a stomping or kicking injury.

E. An intoxicated assault victim with a depressed level of consciousness has an intracranial injury until proven otherwise.

AXIOMS

- Patterns of injury are associated with specific mechanisms.
- Severity of injury depends on the energy transferred to the injured person.
- Lateral impact collisions cause twice the mortality as compared to frontal crashes.
- Falls of 25 to 30 feet (three stories) have a mortality of 50%.

Bibliography

Benoit R, Watts DD, Dwyer K, et al. Windows 99: A source of suburban pediatric trauma. *J Trauma* 2000;49(3):477–482.

Dischinger PC, Cushing BM, Kerns TJ. Injury patterns associated with direction of impact: Drivers admitted to trauma centers. *J Trauma* 1993;35:454

Feliciano DV, Mullins RJ, Rozycki GS. Trauma and shock. In: Morris PJ, Wood WC, eds. *Oxford Textbook of Surgery.* 2nd ed. New York, NY: Oxford University Press USA; 2000:25–27.

Feliciano DV, Wall MJ Jr. Patterns of injury. In: Moore EE, Mattox KL, Feliciano DV, eds. *Trauma.* Norwalk, Conn: Appleton & Lange; 1988:81–96.

Lowenstein SR, Yaron M, Carrero R, et al. Vertical trauma: Injuries to patients who fall and land on their feet. *Ann Emerg Med* 1989;18:161–165.

Macpherson AK, Rothman L, McKeag AM, Howard A. Mechanism of injury affects 6-month functional outcome in children hospitalized because of severe injuries. *J Trauma* 2003; 55(3):454–458.

McGwin G Jr, Metzger J, Porterfield JR, et al. Association between side air bags and risk of injury in motor vehicle collisions with near-side impact. *J Trauma* 2003;55(3):430–436.

Peng RY, Bongard F. Pedestrian versus motor vehicle accidents: An analysis of 5,000 patients. *J Am Coll Surg* 1999;189:343.

3

PATTERNS OF PENETRATING INJURY
GREGORY J. JURKOVICH AND ANTHONY J. WILSON

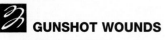

GUNSHOT WOUNDS

I. **INTRODUCTION.** To understand the mechanisms of gunshot injuries, it is important to understand the nature of firearms and their projectiles. **Ballistics** is defined as the scientific study of projectile motion and is divided into three categories: internal, external, and terminal ballistics. Internal ballistics has to do with the projectile within the firearm. External ballistics describes the projectile in the air. Terminal ballistics relates to actions of the projectile in its target. Wound ballistics is a subset of terminal ballistics and is the most important aspect of ballistics for physicians to understand. However, to completely understand the wounding process some knowledge of all aspects of ballistics is necessary.

II. **TYPES OF FIREARMS**
   A. Handguns, rifles, airguns, and shotguns are the major firearms encountered in civilian injuries in the United States. The wounding potential of each is different; it is important to be aware of these differences. Fully automatic weapons are illegal in the United States and injuries from these weapons are infrequent in civilian practice. Fully automatic weapons differ only from rifles and handguns in their ability to autoload and their resultant rapidity of fire. The injuries caused by the individual projectiles are essentially the same as those of handgun and rifle injuries. Handguns and rifles have many characteristics in common and will be discussed together. Airguns and shotguns, on the other hand, differ significantly in their wounding characteristics from other weapons and will be discussed separately.
   B. **Handguns and rifles.** Handguns and rifles fire bullets. Before firing, the lead bullet is held firmly in the end of a brass cartridge case. This cartridge case contains a flammable propellant (the charge) and has a primer at its base. When the firing pin of the gun strikes the primer, the primer is detonated, igniting the charge within the cartridge case. The burning gases expand and propel the bullet from the cartridge case and along the barrel of the gun. Spiral grooves within the barrel of the gun (rifling) grip the bullet causing it to spin around its long axis. This spinning creates a gyroscopic effect, which prevents yaw, or the deviation of the longitudinal axis of the bullet from its line of flight. This gives the bullet directional stability in the air, enabling it to travel more accurately than a nonspinning projectile, analogous to the stable flight of a football when a long pass is thrown with a "perfect" spiral, as compared with the wobble when thrown imperfectly. The longer the barrel, the more time the bullet has to accelerate and the faster it will be going when it leaves the gun. Because rifles have longer barrels than handguns, rifle bullets leave the gun with much higher velocities than handgun bullets (Tables 3-1, 3-2).
      1. Since the kinetic energy of the bullet is equal to half its mass multiplied by the square of its velocity, high-velocity bullets have much higher kinetic energy than low-velocity bullets.
      $$KE = 1/2\ mv^2$$
      (KE = kinetic energy in joules; m = mass in grams; v = velocity in feet/second.) This higher kinetic energy gives rifle bullets greater wounding potential than the handgun bullets.

TABLE 3-1	Ballistic Data for Four Handguns

Caliber (in)	Weapon type	Bullet weight (grains)	Muzzle velocity (ft/s)	Kinetic energy (ft-lb)
0.25	25 automatic	50	810	73
0.354	9-mm Luger	115	1,155	341
0.357	357 magnum	158	1,410	696
0.44	44 magnum	240	1,470	1,150

In, inches; ft/s, feet per second; ft-lb, foot-pounds; mm, millimeters.

TABLE 3-2	Ballistic Data for Four Rifles

Caliber (in)	Weapon type	Bullet weight (grains)	Muzzle velocity (ft/s)	Kinetic energy (ft-lb)
0.22	Remington 22	40	1,180	124
0.223	M-16	55	3,200	1,248
0.270	270 Winchester	150	2,900	2,810
0.308	30-0	150	2,910	2,820

In, inches; ft/s, feet per second; ft-lb, foot-pounds.

2. Wounding potential is only part of the equation. The type of projectile, type of tissue injured, and the distance (range) between the weapon and the victim all have major effect on these injuries. In direct contact injuries, not only does the energy of the bullet enter the victim but also most of the combustion gases, causing considerable tissue expansion and much more severe injuries than noncontact injuries.

3. The same handgun or rifle can often fire several different types of projectiles. The construction of these projectiles has a major effect on wounding. It is important to be aware not only of the behavior of projectiles before and after impact, but also of the manner in which various tissues respond to gunshot injuries. More elastic tissues, such as lung or fat, dissipate energy well. Less elastic tissues, such as brain, liver, or spleen (solid organs), do not dissipate energy well, with more tissue damage resulting from similar kinetic energy of the missile.

4. Although rifle bullets have greater energy available for wounding than handgun bullets, the wounding mechanisms of the two are similar in many respects. When the bullet strikes human tissue, it ceases spinning. Having lost its directional stability, it is now able to "tumble" (rotate around its short axis). A nondeformed bullet will usually be tapered at its tip and hence have more mass concentrated at its base. Momentum will cause the bullet to tumble through 180 degrees and continue through the tissue with its heavier base leading. If the bullet is deformed by impact with the tissue, this tendency to tumble will be modified and may even be eliminated completely. If there is sufficient width of tissue for the bullet to complete its 180-degree tumble, it will carve an elliptical-shaped tunnel of tissue damage, known as the *permanent cavity*. A shockwave is generated by this damage, compressing the adjacent tissue. This is known as the *temporary cavity* and is also elliptical in

shape. Damage in the temporary cavity varies from one tissue to another and generally increases with increasing tissue specific gravity.

5. Bullets are usually classified by caliber, which is a measurement of the diameter of the bullet, most commonly in decimals of an inch (e.g., 0.357) or in millimeters (e.g., 9 mm). The measurement of caliber does not address the weight of the bullet, construction of the bullet, or the size of the charge, all of which are important factors in determining the wounding potential (Tables 3-1, 3-2). Most bullets are made of lead. In some low-velocity weapons, the bullet is made entirely of lead. In medium- and high-velocity weapons, bullets usually have a metal jacket surrounding the lead to protect it from deformity, while the bullet is in the gun barrel. A copper jacket is most common, but occasionally other metals are used. If the bullet is entirely encased, it is said to have a *full metal jacket*; if the bullet is partially encased, it is said to be *semi-jacketed*. Semi-jacketed bullets typically have exposed lead at the tip, are also referred to as *soft-point bullets*, and are designed to deform on impact. Some bullets have an open cavity in their tips and are referred to as *hollow-point bullets*. Hollow-point bullets are also designed to deform on impact and typically transform into a mushroom shape. When bullets deform on impact, they decelerate faster, delivering more of their energy to a smaller volume of tissue. This is intended to increase tissue damage, making deforming bullets more effective at wounding than nondeforming bullets. A deformed bullet, particularly one with a mushroomed tip, tends not to tumble. High-velocity rifle bullets, particularly the soft- and hollow-point varieties, tend to fragment on impact with tissue. This fragmentation leads to an expanding conical pattern of permanent injury, as the fragments separate from one another.

6. Bullet injuries are most severe in friable solid organs (e.g., the liver and brain), where damage may be caused by temporary cavitation remote from the actual bullet track. Dense tissues (e.g., bone) and loose tissues (e.g., subcutaneous fat) are more resistant to bullet injury. Bones modify the behavior of bullets markedly, altering their course, slowing them down, and increasing their deformity and fragmentation.

7. In general, bullets and bullet fragments follow a straight trajectory, even after entering tissue. Bullets that strike rigid changes in tissue density, such as bone cortices and dense fascia, will often be deflected from their initial course. After this deflection the fragments will continue in a relatively straight trajectory unless they encounter another solid interface. Bullets that pass through intermediate targets (e.g., a door or wall) may already be deformed before they strike the victim and will always have reduced energy.

C. **Airguns.** Airguns do not use a flammable charge to propel their projectiles down the barrel but rely simply on air pressure from pumps, springs, or gas canisters. These weapons usually fire pellets in the form of round BBs or waisted lead slugs. In general these weapons have low muzzle velocity and therefore low wounding potential. The construction of airguns may resemble either rifles or handguns and once again, longer barreled weapons will impart more kinetic energy to their projectiles.

1. Low-velocity weapons, including both airguns and small-caliber handguns, have much lower wounding potential than high-velocity weapons. Whereas close-range injuries with low-velocity projectiles can be fatal, medium- and long-range injuries are often superficial. The subcutaneous tissue offers the path of least resistance for low-velocity projectiles, which may travel long distances through the subcutaneous tissue but fail to penetrate the fascia. This phenomenon is most common at medium to long range and when the entry wound is at a shallow angle to the skin surface.

D. **Shotguns**

1. Shotgun injuries differ substantially from rifle and handgun wounds. Unlike the single bullet of a rifle or handgun cartridge, shotgun shells usually contain multiple metal pellets, also known as shot. Typically, the shotgun shell is made

of plastic with a brass cap at the base, containing the primer. The charge is separated from the pellets by a wadding material that may be either paper or plastic. In contact or very close range injuries the wadding will be projected into the victim, along with the pellets and expanding gases. Shotguns do not have rifled barrels, and their pellets do not spin.

2. The size of shotgun cartridges is not measured in caliber but in *gauge*. The higher the gauge, the smaller is the diameter. Shotgun shells are usually much larger than rifle or handgun cartridges, containing a much bigger charge and a greater total mass of projectiles. Shotgun pellets separate after leaving the barrel of the gun and their velocity rapidly decreases. As the pellets spread with increasing range, their area of distribution increases and the energy in each pellet decreases. Thus, range differences affect the wounding potential of shotgun pellets far more than they affect the wounding potential of bullets. At close range (less than 15 feet) shotgun injuries are usually far more severe than bullet injuries because the total energy available is much greater.

3. The combined mass of multiple pellets spread over a small area can produce massive destruction of soft tissue and bone. At long range, the wider spread and lower velocity of the pellets produce multiple, widely separated, superficial injuries that are often painful but rarely life threatening. At intermediate range, shotgun injuries are less predictable, with severity being mainly a function of anatomic location and pellet density. Pellets come in many sizes, but each individual cartridge usually contains only one size. Larger pellets are known as *buckshot*, and smaller pellets are called *birdshot*. Most injuries encountered in clinical practice involve birdshot.

4. As with bullet injuries, the severity of shotgun injuries varies with tissue type and local anatomy. Vascular injuries are of particular concern because the smaller size of the pellets makes embolization more likely than with bullets. Such emboli can result in tissue infarction.

5. In the past, all shotgun pellets were made of lead. However, recent wildlife regulations require shotgun pellets to be made of steel, when they are used on waterfowl. Steel pellets are ferromagnetic and can move if the patient is exposed to a strong magnetic field, thus causing additional damage. Therefore, magnetic resonance (MR) imaging may be contraindicated in such patients. Fortunately, steel and lead pellets can usually be distinguished from one another at radiography. Lead pellets tend to be deformed and fragmented by impact with soft tissues and bone, whereas steel shot usually remains round. Simple analysis of a radiograph is all that is needed to determine if a patient with a shotgun injury can be safely placed in the MR imaging magnet.

III. GUNSHOT INJURY ASSESSMENT

A. Prompt and accurate assessment of the injuries is essential, both clinically and radiographically. While entrance and exit wounds have differing characteristics, distinguishing one from the other is unreliable. It is therefore best to refer to both simply as surface wounds, and characterize their appearance and location carefully. Both the surgical approach and appropriate planning of additional imaging are aided by the prompt acquisition of appropriate radiographs. These radiographs can often provide an accurate determination of the paths of the projectiles. Metallic markers should be put beside each surface wound, prior to obtaining the radiographs. Two perpendicular projections of the injured area are essential. If the projectiles are a long distance from the entry site, they may not be included in the field of view of the initial radiographs. If a low-velocity projectile is not found on the initial radiographs and there is no exit wound, additional radiographs over a wider field of view should be obtained.

B. With good imaging data, the organs at risk can be determined and the best possible action plan formulated. In hemodynamically unstable patients, there is often time only for conventional radiography before the patient must be taken to the operating room, but these essential initial films can provide important information as to bullet quality, fragmentation, pathway, or other unsuspected foreign bodies. However, in stable patients computed tomography (CT) offers a far more accurate road map of the injury. Careful evaluation of radiographs and CT images is generally more reliable than clinical examination for determining the direction of projectile travel and the tissue or tissues injured. Rapid acquisition of adequate images is essential in all patients. A rapid and accurate assessment of the path of the projectile and its direction of travel often aids the planning of surgical approach, particularly if the fragment has crossed body cavities, such as transmediastinal, transdiaphragmatic, or transpelvic. Any time the bullet or pellets are close to major vessels, conventional or CT angiography should be considered. Significant vascular injuries may be present, even when peripheral pulses are normal. To emphasize, **hemodynamic instability from presumed hemorrhagic shock precludes detailed imaging**.

C. In general, bullets that are not causing mechanical problems can safely be left in the tissues. There is one exception, however. Bullets left within synovial joints result in slow leeching of lead by the synovial fluid. This in turn leads to chronic inflammatory changes within the synovium and to a gradual increase in serum lead levels. After many years, the victim will develop not only a chronic, debilitating lead arthropathy but also systemic lead poisoning. Therefore, bullets and pellets within synovial joints should always be removed.

D. Imaging details. Evaluation of bone injuries and the distribution of bone and bullet fragments on radiographs can be helpful in determining the direction of travel, which is important not only for clinical assessment but also for forensic evaluation of the incident. Bone and bullet fragments are usually distributed along the bullet track within the soft tissues, beyond the defect in the bone. Careful examination of the images should reveal beveling of the bone toward the direction of travel.

1. The degree of bullet fragmentation is also readily visible on radiographs. Bullets with full metal jackets often remain in one piece and usually do not deform much. These projectiles typically do not leave a trail of lead fragments along their path. On the other hand, hollow-point, nonjacketed, and soft-point bullets tend to deform on impact or break apart, leaving a trail of metal fragments through the soft tissues. Hollow-point handgun bullets usually deform by simply mushrooming with minimal fragmentation, whereas high-velocity soft-point rifle bullets usually undergo marked fragmentation. This fragmentation of high-velocity bullets creates a "lead snowstorm" appearance on radiographs. The area over which the lead snowstorm fragments are deposited in the soft tissues widens as the distance from the entry site increases. Thus, a conical distribution of lead fragments is seen on radiographs, with the apex of the cone pointing toward the entry site.

2. While the makeup of shotgun pellets (lead vs. steel) can usually be determined based on their radiographic image as stated previously, the same is not true for jacketed bullets. The type of metal used for the jacket cannot be determined from radiographs. Because bullet jackets are occasionally made of steel, it may not be safe to place a bullet wound victim into an MR imager when the nature of the bullet construction is unknown.

IV. STAB WOUNDS

A. Stab wounds result from "hand-driven" weapons, such as knives, but also include more unusual weapons or offending agents such as ice picks, glass shards, sharp edges of metal, or even wooden posts. A description of the stab wound includes the length, width, and the depth of penetration of the offending agent, although this last dimension is seldom known at the time of initial evaluation. It is helpful to have direct examination of the weapon, as the victim's or witnesses' perceptions may not be accurate given the heightened emotional states at the time of injury. Wound size and history of type of weapon do not necessarily correlate to depth of wound or wound trajectory.

B. **Slash wounds** are usually long lacerations of relatively shallow depth. These wounds tend to gape, allowing easy visual inspection of their depth. **Impalement wounds** are those in which the offending agent is plunged into the victim along the long axis of the blade, resulting in a small puncture wound of the skin and unknown depth. In common use, "stab" implies the use of a knife, whereas "impalement" connotes a larger object driven into the torso. If the wounding agent is still in the victim on arrival at the treatment facility, it is best removed in the operating room. An impaling object can be providing tamponade of major vessels and therefore should be removed under direct vision. Of stab wounds, 4% mortality rate is primarily from direct injury to the great vessels or the heart.

C. **Impalement** usually occurs secondary to a fall onto a piercing object or sustained from machinery or pneumatic tools (nail guns), but also includes low-velocity missiles such as arrows. The wound can be complicated by blunt deceleration from the fall, by secondary injuries resulting from extraction by untrained personnel, or by unintentional shifts of the impaling object during transport.

D. Arrows are fired for hunting and recreational pursuit. **Crossbows** generate bolt velocity of 61.0–84.4 meters per second (m/s) (200–275 feet per second [ft/s]). Bolts are usually unable to pass through weight-bearing bone, but easily penetrate ribs, sternum, posterior vertebral elements, and calvarium. **Archery and hunting bows** can generate arrow velocities up to 74 m/s (240 ft/s). Arrow penetration is a function of arrow momentum (weight and velocity) and type of tip (target vs. hunting). These wounds should be treated as an impalement.

 AXIOMS

- Trajectory defines anatomic injury.
- Do not describe bullet wounds as exit or entrance wounds; describe location and appearance of wounds only.
- Objects that are impaled in the victim should be removed in the operating room.

Bibliography

Adams DB. Wound ballistics: A review. *Mil Med* 1982;147:831–835.

Centers for Disease Control and Prevention. Deaths resulting from firearm- and motor-vehicle-related injuries—United States, 1968–1991. *JAMA* 1994;271:495–496.

Centers for Disease Control and Prevention. Firearm-related deaths—Louisiana and Texas, 1970–1990. *JAMA* 1992;267:3008–3009.

Centers for Disease Control and Prevention. Wonder Web site. Available at: http://wonder.cdc.gov. Accessed October 3, 2006.

Choi CH, Pritchard J, Richard J. Path of bullet and injuries determined by radiography. *Am J Forensic Med Pathol* 1990;11:244–245.

Collins KA, Lantz PE. Interpretation of fatal, multiple, and exiting gunshot wounds by trauma specialists. *J Forensic Sci* 1994;39:94–99.

Dimaio VJM. *Gunshot Wounds: Practical Aspects of Firearms, Ballistics, and Forensic Techniques.* Boca Raton, Fla: CRC Press; 1985:163–226, 257–265.

Fackler ML. How to describe bullet holes. *Ann Emerg Med* 1994;23:386–387.

Glezer JA, Minard G, Croce MA, et al. Shotgun wounds to the abdomen. *Am Surg* 1993;59:129–132.

Hollerman JJ, Fackler ML, Coldwell DM, Ben-Menachem Y. Gunshot wounds. I. Bullets, ballistics, and mechanisms of injury. *AJR* 1990;155:685–690.

Hollerman JJ, Fackler ML, Coldwell DM, et al. Gunshot wounds. II. Radiology. *AJR* 1990;155:691–702.

Padra JC, Barone JE, Reed DM, Wheeler G. Expanding handgun bullets. *J Trauma* 1997;43:516–520.

Phillips CD. Emergent radiologic evaluation of the gunshot wound victim. *Radiol Clin North Am* 1992;30:307–324.

Rouse DA. Patterns of stab wounds: A six-year study. *Med Sch Law* 1994;34:67–71.

Stern EJ. *Trauma Radiology Companion*. Philadelphia: Lippincott-Raven; 1997.

Swan KG, Swan RC. Principles of ballistics applicable to the treatment of gunshot wounds. *Surg Clin North Am* 1991;71:221–239.

Yoshioka H, Seibel RW, Pillai K, Luchette FA. Shotgun wounds and pellet emboli: Case reports and review of the literature. *J Trauma* 1995;39:596–601.

THE PHYSIOLOGIC RESPONSE TO INJURY

BRIAN S. ZUCKERBRAUN AND BRIAN G. HARBRECHT

4

I. INTRODUCTION. Trauma results in significant physiologic changes in nearly all organ systems. The sympathetic nervous system and the neurohormonal response systems, acting locally and systemically, mediate the physiologic compensation that normally occurs with traumatic injury. Fear, pain, hemorrhage, hypovolemia, hypoxemia, hypercarbia, acidosis, and tissue injury can contribute to the stress response in proportion to the extent of injury. An appropriate response maintains homeostasis and allows for healing, whereas deficiencies or excesses of these responses cause morbidity. Critical illness and death can result when the stress response is excessive and sustained after severe trauma.

  A. Stress response syndrome. Psychological and physical perceptions of pain, injury, and shock can contribute to the stress response. Afferent impulses from the injury site are transmitted to the central nervous system where they are processed. Efferent signals mediate the physiologic response designed to correct the inciting event.

II. AFFERENT STIMULI (SYMPATHOADRENAL AXIS AND HYPOTHALAMIC-PITUITARY-ADRENAL AXIS). Neural afferent signals via periphery sensory nerves converge on the brain and activate the reflex arcs, which initiate the sympathetic nervous system output and hypothalamic stimulation. Epinephrine and norepinephrine are released from the sympathetic nervous system, resulting in an immediate increase in blood pressure, heart rate, myocardial contractility, and minute ventilation. Hypothalamic release of corticotropin-releasing hormone results in the production of corticotropin from the anterior pituitary gland, which stimulates the adrenal cortex to synthesize the release of cortisol. The effects of these physiologic increases in cortisol, designed to restore lost circulatory volume and provide energy substrates to sustain vital organ function, include gluconeogenesis, lipolysis, insulin resistance, sodium retention, and protein catabolism. The sympathoadrenal axis and hypothalamic-pituitary-adrenal axis are designed to initiate corrective responses to maintain essential organ perfusion and function.

  A. Sensory neural input (pain). The perception of pain and pain itself are important activators of the sympathetic nervous system and the hypothalamic-pituitary axis. Afferent signals from the injured tissue project to the thalamus via the sympathetic tracts and result in activation of the hypothalamic-pituitary-adrenal axis and subsequent release of cortisol. In addition, catecholamine release from the adrenal medulla is increased by direct neural stimulation.

  B. Baroreceptors (hypovolemia). Hemorrhage and intravascular hypovolemia stimulate baroreceptors in the aorta and carotid bodies and volume receptors in the atria, which signal to the central nervous system. Atrial baroreceptors are activated, first with low-volume hemorrhage, whereas arterial baroreceptors respond to more severe hemorrhage. Baroreceptors normally exert tonic inhibition of the autonomic nervous system. With hypovolemia, there is a reduction in baroreceptor impulses, which results in increased neural activity and centrally mediated vasoconstriction.

  C. Chemoreceptors (hypoxemia, acidosis, hypercarbia, hypothermia). Chemoreceptors, located in the carotid bodies and aorta, are activated by hypoxemia, acidosis, and hypercarbia. These receptors activate the centrally mediated stress response systems. In addition, hypothermia is sensed by the preoptic area of the hypothalamus and triggers the hypothalamic-pituitary-adrenal axis.

D. Wound mediators (cytokines/chemokines). Wounded and ischemic tissues and vascular endothelium produce a number of both locally and systemically acting mediators. The extent of these responses, which is dependent on the size and the degree of injury at the tissue level, serves to initiate mechanisms important in coagulation, metabolism, and inflammation. These mediators are a less rapid response to injury than are the aforementioned neural inputs, and they frequently play a role in cell-to-cell communication (i.e., cytokines such as interleukin-6).

III. EFFERENT RESPONSE. The purpose of the efferent response is to reestablish homeostasis by restitution of the effective circulating plasma volume, to provide fuel, and to maintain vital organ function.

A. Autonomic nervous system. Increased sympathetic output directly stimulates arteries and veins to produce vasoconstriction leading to decreased venous capacitance and increased arterial resistance. These responses are rapidly initiated to correct hypovolemia and to maintain end-organ perfusion. In addition, sympathetic stimulation results in catecholamine release from the adrenal medulla, which produces a more sustained effect.

1. Catecholamines. Tyrosine from the diet or by the endogenous conversion of phenylalanine serves as the substrate for catecholamine synthesis. Tyrosine is hydroxylated to form dihydroxyphenylalanine (Dopa), which undergoes decarboxylation to form dopamine. Norepinephrine is then formed by the hydroxylation of dopamine. Epinephrine is subsequently produced by the methylation of norepinephrine in the adrenal medulla.

a. Norepinephrine is released from neurons and diffuses into the circulation from the synapses.

b. Epinephrine is released from the adrenal medulla.

c. $\alpha 1$-mediated peripheral vasoconstriction is increased.

d. $\beta 1$-mediated heart rate and contractility is increased.

e. Glucose availability is increased by stimulating hepatic glycogenolysis, gluconeogenesis, and ketogenesis.

f. Skeletal muscle glycogenolysis is increased and skeletal muscle glucose uptake is decreased.

g. Glucagon secretion is increased.

h. Insulin release is suppressed.

i. Fatty acids are immobilized.

2. Cholinergic anti-inflammatory pathway. Recent studies have demonstrated the efferent activity in the vagus nerve leads to acetylcholine release in organs of the reticuloendothelial system, including the liver, heart, spleen, and gastrointestinal tract. Acetylcholine interacts with nicotinic receptors on tissue macrophages, which inhibits release of TNF, IL-1, and other cytokines.

B. Hormonal response. Traumatic injury initiates multiple endocrine responses. The net effect of these endocrine responses to injury is an increased secretion of catabolic hormones. This promotes the catabolism of carbohydrate, fat, and protein. In evolutionary terms, this may have served as a survival mechanism that allowed injured animals to sustain until their injuries were healed. In current surgical practice, it is questionable whether some of these endocrine stress responses are necessary.

1. Corticotropin is released from the pituitary gland after stimulation by hypothalamic corticotropin-releasing hormone.

a. Corticotropin stimulates the adrenal release of cortisol, which stimulates hepatic gluconeogenesis and increases skeletal muscle amino acid release.

2. Vasopressin (antidiuretic hormone). The posterior pituitary gland releases vasopressin in response to increases in plasma osmolality that occur with hemorrhage (major stimulus) and decreases in the effective circulating plasma volume.

a. Increases peripheral vasoconstriction

b. Increases water reabsorption

    c. Increases hepatic gluconeogenesis and glycogenolysis

    d. Decreases hepatic ketogenesis

3. Growth hormone. Growth hormone is released from the anterior pituitary gland in response to hypothalamic release of growth hormone releasing hormone.

    a. Increases amino acid uptake and hepatic protein synthesis

    b. Mediates the biological activity of growth hormone by somatomedins

    c. Decreases hepatic glucose transport

4. Thyroxine (T_4). Release of T_4 from the thyroid in response to thyroid-stimulating hormone from the anterior pituitary gland increases after injury. The conversion of T_4 to T_3 (a more potent form) decreases following trauma.

    a. Increases oxygen consumption and sympathetic output

    b. Increases glycolysis and gluconeogenesis

    c. Increases metabolic rate and heat production

5. Renin, angiotensin, aldosterone. The major regulator of aldosterone production is the renin-angiotensin system. Decreases in renal arterial blood flow and renal tubular sodium concentration, and increased β-adrenergic stimulation serve to stimulate renin secretion from the juxtaglomerular cells of the renal afferent arteriole. Renin results in the enzymatic conversion of angiotensinogen in the liver to the inactive angiotensin I. Angiotensin-converting enzyme produced by the lung converts angiotensin I to angiotensin II. Besides acting as a potent vasoconstrictor, angiotensin II also stimulates the release of aldosterone.

    a. Angiotensin II

        i. Increases peripheral vasoconstriction

        ii. Increases splanchnic vasoconstriction

        iii. Decreases renal excretion of salt and water

    b. Aldosterone

        i. Produced in the adrenal zona glomerulosa

        ii. Increases distal tubular sodium and chloride resorption

        iii. Increases potassium secretion

6. Glucagon is released from pancreatic α-cells in response to α-adrenergic stimulation, hypoglycemia, and elevated circulating levels of amino acids.

    a. Increases hepatic glycogenolysis and gluconeogenesis

    b. Increases lipolysis

7. Insulin is released from pancreatic β cells in response to β-adrenergic stimulation, glucagon, elevated plasma glucose, and amino acid levels.

    a. Increases glycolysis and glycogenesis.

    b. Increases protein synthesis.

    c. Decreases gluconeogenesis.

    d. The initial hyperglycemia seen following injury is secondary to an increase in the glucagon:insulin ratio and peripheral insulin resistance.

C. Systemic mediators. A variety of mediators are released after injuries that have both local and systemic effects. In addition, many of these mediators are released as a result of reperfusion and can lead to amplification of the inflammatory response. Many of these mediators are also released in infection, sepsis, and inflammation.

    1. Complement. Ischemia and endothelial injuries result in the activation of this cascade of plasma proteins, which initiates the inflammatory response and results in the destruction and lysis of invading organisms. Complement activation, which results in leukocyte adherence, activation, and degranulation, can contribute to tissue destruction and damage as seen in acute respiratory distress syndrome.

    2. Oxygen radicals. Highly reactive and short-lived oxygen species are produced by leukocytes and parenchymal cells in many tissues in response to ischemia and hypoxia. The activation of endogenous xanthine oxidase and other cellular oxidases by injury produces hydrogen peroxide (H_2O_2), superoxide (O_2^-) and hydroxyl radical (OH^-). Endogenous antioxidant defenses (superoxide dismutase, catalase, glutathione, the bilirubin-biliverdin redox cycle) serve to protect against cellular injury.

3. **Cytokines.** Both local tissues and migratory inflammatory cells release a variety of polypeptide mediators that have paracrine effects and serve to amplify the inflammatory response and signal wound repair. The cytokines act on surface receptors on many different target cells and their effects are produced ultimately by influencing protein synthesis within these cells. Many of these substances reach the systemic circulation and initiate a systemic inflammatory response. These factors include the interleukins (IL-1, IL-2, IL-6), tumor necrosis factor, and the interferons.

4. **Eicosanoids** are a group of lipid mediators (prostaglandins, leukotrienes, and thromboxanes) derived from plasma membrane phospholipids by phospholipase A_2 (PLA_2). PLA_2 produces arachidonic acid, which is further metabolized to the specific isoforms (prostaglandin [PGE]$_2$, PGE_1, prostacyclin [PGI]$_2$, thromboxane A_2 [TXA_2], Leukotriene C_4 [LTC_4]). Different compounds have vasoactive properties and induce vasodilation (PGI_2) or vasoconstriction (TXA_2). They can also influence leukocyte function (LTC_4). Some prostaglandins are thought to modulate the immune response but their role in injury and hemorrhage is not fully known.

5. **Nitric oxide (NO).** Normally, constitutively produced NO from endothelial cells is a homeostatic regulator of blood pressure that provides second-to-second vasodilation. Inflammation produces increased NO from a variety of cells and may contribute to the profound hypotension typical of patients with decompensated hemorrhagic shock.

6. **Other mediators.** A variety of growth factors and other mediators are expressed after traumatic injury, which serve to regulate wound healing. These include platelet-derived growth factor, epidermal growth factor, transforming growth factors, bradykinins, endothelin, and platelet-activating factor.

IV. **METABOLIC RESPONSE.** The metabolic response to traumatic injury and hemorrhagic shock is directly related to the aforementioned neuroendocrine response. Oxygen consumption and carbon dioxide production increase secondary to increased catecholamine production from increased sympathetic activity and from increased expression of inflammatory mediators produced at the tissue level. The metabolic responses seen after trauma have traditionally been defined according to the definitions outlined by Cuthbertson.

A. **Cuthbertson's two phases**

1. **Ebb phase,** which occurs initially after traumatic injury, is characterized by physiologic responses designed to restore tissue perfusion and circulating volume.

2. **Flow phase** begins once the patient is successfully resuscitated.
   a. The flow phase can be further subdivided into catabolic and anabolic phases.
      i. The catabolic phase, which is characterized by the hyperdynamic response to trauma, includes hypermetabolism, hyperglycemia, and sodium and water retention. This response can last from days to weeks.
      ii. The anabolic phase, beginning after wounds have closed, is characterized by the return of normal homeostasis.

B. The metabolic response to trauma can also be divided into the following four phases.

1. **Shock phase.** Characterized by hypoperfusion secondary to hemorrhage and tissue injury.

2. The **resuscitation phase** is seen with active volume resuscitation and operation to control hemorrhage. It is characterized by elaboration of many of the inflammatory mediators.

3. The **hypermetabolic phase (postinjury)**, similar to the catabolic phase described by Cuthbertson, is characterized by an increased sympathetic and adrenal response. The increased secretion of catecholamines, cortisol, and

insulin causes increased protein catabolism, negative nitrogen balance, and lipolysis. Acutely, this response serves to protect the individual. However, with prolonged and sustained hypermetabolism, the patient can develop Systemic Inflammatory Response Syndrome (SIRS). Persistence of SIRS can lead to Multiple Organ Dysfunction Syndrome (MODS).

4. **MODS** can be caused by the sustained overexpression of injury-induced inflammatory mediators or the development of infectious complications. MODS is the most important cause of late death in the trauma intensive care unit. Mortality increases by approximately 20% to 25% per organ that fails.

V. **SUMMARY OF ORGAN SYSTEM RESPONSE TO STRESS.** The physiologic responses seen following trauma are designed to preserve organ blood flow and, if necessary, shunt cardiac output to the heart and brain.

A. **Cardiovascular system**
   1. Increases cardiac output by increasing heart rate and contractility (CO = HR × SV).
   2. Maintains perfusion to the heart and brain by shunting blood from the skeletal and splanchnic vascular beds.
   3. Increases peripheral vasoconstriction secondary to increased angiotensin II and vasopressin activity.
   4. Preserves effective circulating plasma volume by increasing transcapillary movement of fluid from the interstitium to the intravascular space.

B. **Renal system**
   1. Maintains glomerular filtration rate secondary to increased efferent arteriolar vasoconstriction.
   2. Increases aldosterone and vasopressin expression resulting in increased sodium and water absorption.
   3. Shunts blood flow from renal cortex to medulla.

C. **Adrenal system**
   1. Regulates stress response through increased catecholamine, cortisol, and aldosterone production.

D. **Pulmonary system**
   1. Increases minute ventilation from hyperventilation and increased tidal volume.
   2. Produces angiotensin-converting enzyme.

E. **Central nervous system**
   1. First interprets physiologic responses to trauma, and then initiates the physiologic responses.
   2. Coordinates afferent stimuli into a multisystem response.
   3. Increases sympathetic nervous system activity.
   4. Governs neuroendocrine response.

F. **Splanchnic system**
   1. Decreases blood flow secondary to shunting of blood to preserve blood flow to the heart and brain.
   2. Provides glucose from hepatic glycogen and gluconeogenesis as well as from the conversion of amino acids and free fatty acids.
   3. Produces mediators secondary to the low blood flow state that can contribute to the inflammatory response.

VI. **PHYSIOLOGIC RESPONSES**
A. **Altered mental status.** Belligerence, anxiety, immobilization, withdrawal, and antagonism are commonly seen after major trauma. It is important to be aware that this can signify severe hypovolemia, hypoxemia, or both.

B. **Altered vital signs.** Fever may be seen after fluid resuscitation, which can be caused by the sustained inflammatory response. It is critical to be vigilant for infectious causes.

C. **Blood pressure** may not become significantly decreased until the patient has lost 30% to 40% of circulating blood volume. Therefore, blood pressure correlates poorly with either blood volume or flow.

D. **Tachycardia** can persist even after fluid resuscitation and pain is adequately controlled.

E. **Increased minute ventilation** secondary to both tachypnea and increased tidal volume is common.

F. **Generalized edema** is common secondary to increased total body salt and water within the interstitium. This is a result of increased sympathetic vasoconstriction, altered capillary permeability, and hypoproteinemia. Also, local inflammation at the wound site leads to edema formation secondary to the release of locally acting chemokines.

G. **Increased cardiac output.** Heart rate and contractility increase with injury. However, with hypovolemia, preload may be decreased to a degree that significantly lowers cardiac output.

H. **Hypermetabolism.** Energy demands, oxygen consumption, and carbon dioxide production are all elevated following trauma.

I. **Altered protein, glucose, and fat metabolism.** Energy requirements are increased following injury, with the magnitude of the additional energy need dependent on the severity of injury, magnitude of tissue destruction, and lean body mass of the patient.

   1. **Protein loss** is approximately 300 to 500 grams per day (g/day) of lean body mass, with visceral proteins spared at the expense of skeletal muscle proteins.

   2. **Proteins** are broken down to constituent amino acids that are catabolized to ammonia (forms urea) and precursors of the tricarboxylic cycle (TCA).

   3. **Carbohydrates** provide 4 kilocalories per gram (kcal/g) when oxidized. Muscle glycogen (storage form of glucose) is used only by skeletal muscle (i.e., not released systemically), whereas hepatic glycogen provides glucose for glucose-dependent tissues (brain, leukocytes).

      a. **Gluconeogenesis** can occur from amino acids, glycerol, lactate, or pyruvate via TCA or Krebs' cycle.

   4. **Lipids**, which are used by tissues that are not glucose dependent, are the largest source of energy (9.4 kcal/g) in the body. Lipids are catabolized to form ketone bodies in the liver along with CO_2 and energy from glycerol and fatty acids.

J. **Leukocytosis.** Elevation in the white blood cell count can be seen after injury.

VII. **SUMMARY.** The physiologic effect of stress response is to maintain perfusion and function of the heart and brain. Acutely, this results in a survival advantage. However, with prolonged activation of the inflammatory response, deleterious effects can be seen including SIRS, MODS, and even death.

SHOCK
BRIAN G. HARBRECHT AND
TIMOTHY R. BILLIAR

5

$\mathcal{S}$hock has been recognized as an important pathophysiologic event in surgery and trauma since the late 1800s. Pioneering studies by Wiggers and Blalock formed the foundation for current scientific studies in the field of shock research. Although the definition of shock may have changed greatly since these early investigations, the clinical syndrome and its profound impact on the care of injured patients remains essentially the same.

I. **DEFINITION AND CLASSIFICATION.** Although the clinical syndromes responsible for shock can originate from a variety of causes, the different forms of shock have a number of common features.

   A. **Definition.** Shock occurs when tissue perfusion is inadequate to maintain normal cellular function and structure. It cannot be emphasized strongly enough that **shock does not equal hypotension** and, conversely, a "normal" blood pressure **does not exclude** the presence of hypoperfusion. Although direct cellular injury may become evident, its contribution to the sequelae of shock is unclear. Cellular dysfunction can become evident in a variety of ways.

   B. **Classification**

      1. **Hypovolemic shock** is caused by decreased circulating volume from loss of red cell mass, plasma, and extracellular fluid, or a combination of these. This form of shock is the most common cause of shock in injured patients, and usually results from acute blood loss.

      2. **Cardiogenic shock** represents decreased tissue perfusion due to ineffective pump function. Cardiogenic shock can result from direct cardiac injury (myocardial contusion) or intrinsic cardiac disease (myocardial infarction, dysrhythmia).

      3. **Vasogenic shock** is caused by decreased vascular resistance so that the normal blood volume fails to maintain adequate circulatory perfusion.

         a. **Neurogenic shock** is a form of vasogenic shock in which a high spinal cord injury (or spinal anesthesia) results in loss of sympathetic vascular tone, producing peripheral vasodilation. Bradycardia may also be present.

         b. **Septic shock** is a form of vasogenic shock in which proinflammatory mediator release results in peripheral vasodilation, decreased peripheral arterial resistance, and increased peripheral venous capacitance. Tachycardia often accompanies it.

      4. **Obstructive shock.** Mechanical obstruction to cardiac function from either direct cardiac compression or obstruction of venous return (**cardiac tamponade, tension pneumothorax**) results in decreased peripheral perfusion.

      5. **Traumatic shock** includes elements of the above mentioned causes of shock that may not be sufficient to induce hypoperfusion in isolation, but markedly impair peripheral perfusion when combined. Generally includes the sequelae of hypovolemia from blood loss and activation of proinflammatory mediators elaborated as a result of long bone or soft tissue injury.

II. PATHOPHYSIOLOGY

A. Cardiovascular response. The body's normal response to hypovolemia is to adjust peripheral arterial resistance, cardiac output, and heart rate to maintain perfusion to essential organs such as the heart and brain.

1. **Peripheral arterial resistance** increases in response to decreased circulatory volume or impaired pump function and decreases as a contributor to shock in septic states and with loss of sympathetic tone (neurogenic shock).

2. **Cardiac output** will be intrinsically diminished because of pump failure in cardiogenic shock. May also be diminished by low circulatory volume (hypovolemia) or mechanical impediments (cardiac tamponade). Often increased in response to diminished peripheral arterial resistance in septic shock.

3. **Heart rate** is increased in response to decreased circulatory volume, decreased peripheral arterial resistance, and mechanical impediments to cardiac function. Often unchanged in neurogenic shock because of loss of sympathetic cardiac input. The normal reflexive change to hypovolemia can be absent or impaired in elderly patients with significant intrinsic cardiac disease or those taking selected medications (β-blockers). If shock is sustained, tachycardia can evolve into bradycardia as a preterminal event.

B. Neuroendocrine response. The neuroendocrine response to shock, which is similar to that of injury, is covered in detail in Chapter 4.

C. Inflammatory mediators. Proinflammatory mediators, which can be produced in response to bacterial products, lead to decreased arterial resistance and impaired tissue perfusion (septic shock). In addition, other forms of shock can result in the production of a variety of systemic and local mediators such as cytokines, eicosanoids, and radical species (see Chapter 4).

D. Cellular response to shock is a result of decreased oxygen delivery from hypoperfusion and direct changes in cell function caused by neural (adrenergic), humoral (corticotropin, vasopressin, glucagon), and proinflammatory (cytokine) mediators. Oxygen radicals, either intrinsically (i.e., xanthine oxidase) or extrinsically (i.e., neutrophil) derived, are produced in shock and can alter cell function. Alterations in the local microcirculatory environment, metabolic derangements, and hypoxia at the cellular level lead to cell membrane depolarization, increased intracellular water and cell swelling, dysfunction of the Na-K-adenosine triphosphatase (ATPase) pump, increased anaerobic metabolism, uncoupling of oxidative phosphorylation, and increased intracellular calcium changes in intracellular signaling pathways that regulate cell metabolism. Changes in cellular gene expression in response to shock and alterations in cellular protein production occur. The development of apoptosis in animal models of shock has been described but its significance is unknown.

III. DIAGNOSIS AND TREATMENT.

While the end-organ manifestations of shock may be the same regardless of the specific cause of shock, the treatment depends on the specific cause of the impaired perfusion.

A. Hypovolemic shock, which represents the most common cause of shock in injured patients, is caused by acute blood loss. Severity of the shock insult depends on the depth and duration of shock. Mild shock of longstanding duration can be as lethal as acute, profound shock.

1. **Diagnosis.** Signs of inadequate end-organ perfusion depend on the degree of volume loss. Hypotension can be a relatively late manifestation of decreased circulating volume if compensatory mechanisms are adequate. Tachycardia, diminished urine output, decreased pulse pressure, restlessness and anxiety, and cold, clammy extremities can be manifestations of reduced circulatory volume. Lethargy and stupor caused by hypovolemia represent profound volume loss and can signal impending cardiovascular collapse. Hypotension is a sign that the compensatory mechanisms have been exceeded. Patients in shock may not be hypotensive, but patients who are hypotensive should always be considered to be in shock.

2. Treatment. Treatment of hypovolemia focuses on simultaneous cessation of ongoing hemorrhage and restoration of circulating blood volume. Treatment for hypovolemia is usually instituted before a cause is identified.

  a. ABCs. The airway should be secure and bilateral breath sounds present. Fluid resuscitation should be instituted with balanced crystalloid solution through two large-bore intravenous catheters. Patients who respond briefly or not at all to the above measures have a high likelihood of requiring operative intervention to control hemorrhage and early transfusion of blood should be considered.

  b. Source. The source of blood loss in victims of penetrating injury depends on the nature, location, and path of the projectile. For blunt trauma victims, the potential sources of blood loss may be more difficult to localize. For both, the search for sites of hemorrhage is identical. Four main sites of large volume blood loss exist.

  i. Chest. May be suspected in settings of penetrating chest wound or chest wall injury. May be identified by absent or reduced breath sounds, the presence of hemothorax on chest x-ray, or return of blood through a chest tube. Physical exam may be insensitive to exclude significant hemorrhage in the chest.

  ii. Abdomen. Physical examination is a relatively insensitive method for detecting significant hemoperitoneum. Hemoperitoneum may be identified in the resuscitation area by focused abdominal sonography for trauma (FAST) or diagnostic peritoneal lavage (DPL) or in the operating room by laparotomy.

  iii. Retroperitoneum or pelvis. Usually associated with pelvic fractures.

  iv. External. Visible on inspection, such as major vascular injuries from extremity wounds, large surface area wounds, or uncontrolled wounds in areas of increased vascularity (face, scalp).

  v. Other sources of blood loss include long bone fractures and extensive soft tissue injury. Patients on anticoagulants can bleed extensively from relatively minor injuries. If no bleeding site is identified, consider alternative causes of shock (cardiac tamponade, neurogenic, cardiogenic). Also consider repeating the assessment of the chest, abdomen, and pelvis to ensure that no possible sources have been overlooked.

B. Cardiogenic shock. In trauma patients, cardiogenic shock can be caused by either significant cardiac injury (myocardial contusion) or intrinsic cardiac disease (myocardial infarction, cardiac arrhythmia).

  1. Diagnosis. Suspicion of cardiogenic shock may be increased when hypovolemic shock has been excluded or risk factors are identified (elderly patient, known preexisting cardiac disease, dysrhythmias present on electrocardiogram [ECG] or monitor, presence of sternal fracture). The diagnosis of cardiac pump failure as a source of ongoing shock in injured patients requires exclusion of other causes and demonstration of diminished cardiac function (decreased cardiac output, echocardiographic evidence of cardiac dysfunction).

  2. Treatment of cardiogenic shock in trauma patients involves restoration of cardiac function in conjunction with the treatment of acute traumatic injuries.

  a. ABCs. The airway should be secure and bilateral equal breath sounds present. Fluid resuscitation should be instituted judiciously in patients with known cardiac dysfunction.

  b. Invasive hemodynamic monitoring. An arterial line and pulmonary artery catheter may help guide therapy and assess the success of treatment.

  c. Inotropic agents. Selective use can be guided by the results of invasive hemodynamic monitoring.

  d. Circulatory support. Consider intraaortic balloon pump for refractory cardiac dysfunction.

C. Neurogenic shock. In trauma patients, is usually caused by injuries to the cervical or upper thoracic spinal column. Rarely, spinal cord injuries without bony abnormality (epidural hematoma of the cord) can result in neurogenic shock.

1. **Diagnosis.** The classic description of neurogenic shock includes hypotension and bradycardia, with warm, perfused extremities and presence of a sensory or motor deficit consistent with cord injury. Tachycardia can be present. Hypovolemia, in addition to the neurogenic component, can contribute to hypotension. The diagnosis is often made once hypovolemia has been excluded and a vertebral fracture in the appropriate area identified.

2. **Treatment**

   a. **ABCs.** The airway should be secure and equal bilateral breath sounds present. Fluid resuscitation should be instituted and restoration of intravascular volume may be sufficient to restore blood pressure and perfusion.

   b. If the diagnosis of neurogenic shock is certain and hypotension persists, vasopressor support can be helpful. Phenylephrine or norepinephrine can be instituted as a continuous infusion. If vasopressor support is needed, its duration is typically brief (24–72 hours [h]). If vasopressor support is indicated, invasive hemodynamic monitoring (e.g., an arterial line, central venous pressure monitor, or pulmonary artery catheter) should be considered based on patient age, associated injuries, and preexisting medical condition.

D. **Septic shock.** In trauma patients, is an unlikely cause of shock in the emergency department or early in the hospital stay. Septic shock can develop later from infectious complications after injury.

1. **Diagnosis.** A hyperdynamic hemodynamic profile is often present, with hypotension, tachycardia, and increased cardiac output. Fever, leukocytosis, and tachypnea are often present. Delirium or obtundation can also be present. Evidence of localized infection (pneumonia, urinary tract infection, intra-abdominal abscess, empyema, soft tissue infection) should be sought. Bacteremia can be present and secondary infection of monitoring devices (continuous venous or arterial lines, intracranial pressure monitors) or prosthetic devices may need to be excluded.

2. **Treatment**

   a. **ABCs.** The airway should be secure and proper ventilatory mechanics established. Intravascular volume should be restored initially. If hypotension persists, pharmacologic support may be necessary. Invasive hemodynamic monitoring should be considered to guide therapy. A pulmonary artery catheter can assist in deciding if inotropic or vasopressor support should be instituted.

   b. Treatment of the primary infection is essential. Systemic antibiotics should be instituted, purulent fluid collections should be drained (percutaneously or operatively), infected monitoring or prosthetic devices should be removed, and necrotic nonviable tissue should be debrided. Antibiotic therapy should be appropriate to cover the likely responsible organisms, based on the infectious cause, common organisms in the particular unit or institution, and the patient's previous history of infectious episodes. Antibiotics should be tailored to appropriate culture data when available and long-term empiric antibiotic usage should be discouraged to avoid the development of resistant organisms.

   c. The use of most antiendotoxin strategies, cytokines, and anticytokine antagonists should be considered experimental. Their use has not proved to be effective in clinical trials. The use of activated protein C reduces mortality after sepsis but is an anticoagulant whose use in trauma patients that may have injuries that predispose to hemorrhage should be carefully evaluated.

   d. Tight regulation of plasma glucose with exogenous insulin improves mortality in critically ill adults. The mechanism for this effect in unknown. Whether a similar benefit exists in injured patients has not yet been rigorously studied, but the preliminary evidence is encouraging.

   e. Corticosteroids in large doses in septic patients may worsen infectious complications and outcome. Low-dose corticosteroid replacement in septic patients who may have hypoadrenalism is suggested to be beneficial. The precise utility of corticosteroid treatment in sepsis requires further study.

E. Obstructive shock. Mechanical obstruction to perfusion is usually caused by the development of tension pneumothorax or cardiac tamponade. The diagnosis of these entities is covered in detail in Chapters 22 and 23. Correction of the primary cause should restore perfusion or additional causes should be sought.

F. Traumatic shock is usually caused by a combination of hypovolemic, cardiogenic, neurogenic, septic, and obstructive shock. Treatment of the contributing components can require rapid, coordinated medical decision making. After securing the airway, prompt control of hemorrhage is generally the major objective.

IV. SUMMARY. The term *shock* represents a state of abnormal tissue and cellular perfusion. Reliance on predetermined blood pressure criteria can lead to substantially underestimation of shock states. In trauma patients, acute blood loss represents the most common form of shock but other causes should be kept in mind. Usually, treatment of shock is instituted before or in conjunction with steps to identify the underlying cause. Patients who are actively bleeding need prompt operative intervention and the need for operative treatment should be established early to avoid the potential end-organ dysfunction and death associated with continue tissue hypoperfusion.

Bibliography

Gutierrez G, Brown SD. Response of the microcirculation. In: Schlag G, Redl H, eds. *Pathophysiology of Shock, Sepsis, and Organ Failure.* Berlin: Springer-Verlag; 1993:215–229.

Harbrecht BG, Alarcon LH, Peitzman AB. Management of shock. In: Moore EE, Feliciano DV, Mattox KL, eds. *Trauma.* 5th ed. New York, NY: McGraw-Hill Co Inc; 2004:201–225.

Hotchkiss RS, Karl IE. The pathophysiology and treatment of sepsis. *N Engl J Med* 2003;348:138–150.

Peitzman AB, Billiar TR, Harbrecht BG, et al. Hemorrhagic shock. *Curr Probl Surg* 1995;32:925–1012.

6

PREHOSPITAL TRAUMA, TRIAGE, AND CARE
DAVID C. CONE

I. TRAUMA TRIAGE. Trauma triage involves the sorting of patients based on the **severity of their injuries** and the **availability of resources.** Generally, there are two different types of trauma triage used in the out-of-hospital setting.

A. Field triage involves determining if a trauma patient requires the services of a trauma center, based on an estimation of the severity of injury, or can safely be cared for at a non-trauma center. Trauma triage criteria are used in single-patient events, or events with small numbers of patients that do not exceed the capabilities of the trauma system.

1. Field triage guidelines. Knowledge of injury, mechanism, and existing co-morbid factors is key for optimal trauma triage. Unfortunately, no single factor will guarantee triage success. The following must be incorporated into the triage decision-making process: (Table 6-1)

a. Patient assessment. The initial patient survey identifies and treats immediately life-threatening injuries.

i. Abnormal physiologic signs strongly suggest the need for rapid treatment and transport to a trauma center.

ii. Anatomic locations and types of injuries can predict the need for emergent surgical or specialty care.

b. Mechanism of injury. Although not as strong a predictor for the need to operate immediately or receive intensive care as the anatomic and physiologic criteria, analysis of injury mechanism at the scene can improve triage accuracy by considering the forces involved and the kinetic energy transferred during the event. When encountering a patient-meeting mechanism of injury criteria that are neither anatomic nor physiologic, pre-hospital personnel should review the case with the direct medical oversight (DMO) physician by phone or radio to choose a destination.

c. Premorbid conditions. No formal system exists for assessing or ranking premorbid conditions, yet these are included in decision making. As with mechanism of injury criteria, discussion with the DMO physician may be helpful.

2. Field triage scoring. Several trauma scoring techniques determine the severity of injury of trauma victims both in the hospital and in the field. Examples include the Trauma Score, CRAMS Scale, Prehospital Index, and Trauma Triage Rule. Accurate trauma scoring is dependent on diagnostic skills and capabilities, and thus can be limited by field conditions, patient intoxication, and compensatory physiologic mechanisms masking major injuries. Trauma scoring systems typically look at combinations of the following:

a. Cardiovascular system
b. Respiratory system
c. Central nervous system
d. Type and location of injury
e. Abdominal examination

B. Mass casualty triage involves prioritizing patients when needs exceed available resources. In situations when the number of patients and their injuries exceed the

TABLE 6-1	Field Triage Guidelines

Patient assessment
–**Physiologic:** If yes, take to trauma center
  –Respiratory rate <10 or >29 breaths/min
  –Systolic blood pressure <90 mmHg
  –Glasgow Coma Scale score <14
  –Revised Trauma Score <11 (or Pediatric Trauma Score <8)
–**Anatomic:** If yes, take to trauma center
  –Penetrating injuries to head, neck, torso, or extremities proximal to the
   elbow, or:
  –Flail chest
  –Two or more proximal long bone fractures
  –Combination trauma with burn
  –Pelvic fractures
  –Limb paralysis
  –Amputation proximal to wrist or ankle

Mechanism of injury and high-energy impact
  –Ejection from automobile: If yes, contact medical oversight, consider transport to trauma center
  –Death of victim in the same passenger compartment
  –Extrication time >20 min
  –Fall >20 ft
  –Rollover accident
  –High-speed vehicle crash (>40 mph, deformity >20 in,
  or intrusion >12 in)
  –Pedestrian thrown or run over
  –Motorcycle crash >20 mph or separation of rider from bike

Pre- or comorbid conditions: If yes, contact medical oversight, consider transport to trauma center
  –Age <5 or >55 y
  –Cardiac or respiratory disease
  –Insulin-dependent diabetes mellitus, cirrhosis, or morbid obesity
  –Immunosuppressed
  –Pregnant
  –History of bleeding disorder or taking anticoagulants

resources of the field providers, transport capability, or local treatment facilities, triage is required to identify potentially salvageable patients with life-threatening conditions that require immediate treatment and transport.

1. Mass casualty triage is typically initiated by the first EMS personnel to arrive on scene, once scene safety is ensured and basic information regarding the incident is relayed to dispatchers so additional resources can be mobilized. The responsibility for patient triage is often delegated to more experienced personnel when they arrive. Field triage works best when victims are limited to a small geographic area. Large disaster sites (such as earthquakes and floods) or disasters with geographically distinct areas or "sides" (such as either side of a train crash, when mobility between and access to the two sides is limited by the wreckage) can require multiple triage sites.

2. **Principles.** While it is generally taught that the most critically injured patients are transported first, empiric data are lacking to support this principle. Triage is a continuous process, with frequent reassessment of patient status and resources. Patients are typically retriaged on arrival at the hospital.

3. **Simple Triage and Rapid Treatment (START)** is the most commonly used mass casualty triage system in the United States. Patients who are ambulatory are first removed from the area. Remaining patients are classified as "expectant" if obviously dead or if not breathing after one attempt to reposition the airway. Remaining patients are categorized as "immediate" or "delayed," based on the evaluation of respiratory rate, perfusion, and mental status. An abnormality in any one parameter places the victim in the "immediate" category.

4. **Triage tags** are often used to identify needs in both large and small multivictim incidents.
   a. **Problems** that can occur with triage tags include:
      i. Separation of the tag from the victim
      ii. Contamination by blood or body fluids
      iii. Limited space for documentation
      iv. Inability to "upgrade" a patient's triage categorization, since many tags use color-coded strips that are torn off (leaving the patient's categorization attached) and cannot be reattached if a patient's status worsens
   b. **Color codes** are traditionally used to identify patient categorization by injury severity and need for transport:
      i. **Red = "immediate"** or most critically injured. Includes patients with major injuries to the head, thorax, and abdomen for which immediate surgical or specialty care is required.
      ii. **Yellow = "delayed"** or less critically injured. Includes patients who are less seriously injured, who still likely require in-hospital treatment, but whose clinical condition permits a delay of this treatment without endangering life.
      iii. **Green = "ambulatory"** with no life- or limb-threatening injury identified. Ideally, all of the ambulatory patients who are initially moved away from the disaster scene will be reassessed by medical personnel to identify injuries.
      iv. **Black = "expectant"** or dead. Patients who would be triaged to "red" under certain circumstances might be triaged to "black" when resources are more limited to optimize resource use.

C. **Limitations to triage.** Perfect triage is difficult to achieve for a variety of reasons. In field triage and mass casualty events, over- and under-triage may occur.
   1. **Over-triage** (false positives) occurs when a patient who does not require a trauma center or high level of immediate care is transported to a trauma center. When resources are not constrained, this is not a problem aside from some degree of resource waste if activation of teams unnecessarily occurs. In a mass casualty situation, overtriage may limit the ability of a trauma center to provide optimal care for those who need it.
   2. **Under-triage** (false negatives) occurs when a patient who may benefit from trauma center/higher level of care is transported to a non-trauma/less capable center. This can impact ultimate outcomes, either in the single-patient or multiple-patient setting. In a mass casualty incident, undertriage may be unavoidable as trauma centers become saturated.
   3. Due to the balance between sensitivity (which considers false negatives) and specificity (which considers false positives) of any diagnostic test, increases in over-triage are needed to reduce under-triage. While it is commonly stated that 50% over-triage is acceptable to achieve 10% undertriage, there are no outcome data nor formal consensus for these figures.

II. **TRAUMATIC ARREST.** The term "traumatic arrest" refers to the end result of a variety of pathologic processes in response to injury and is not a single clinical entity.
   A. **Etiology.** EMS personnel should be trained to recognize the three **most common treatable causes of traumatic cardiopulmonary collapse in the prehospital setting: airway obstruction, hypoventilation or hypoxemia, and tension pneumothorax.**

1. **Airway. Loss of a patient airway is a common reason for immediate cardiorespiratory collapse after trauma**. The following causes must be sought and treated:
   a. **Occlusion by tongue or epiglottis**
      i. **Loss of tone** (head injury, hypoxia, drugs, stroke)
      ii. **Facial fracture**
      iii. **Direct inter-oral trauma**
   b. **Occlusion by foreign body** (blood, avulsed teeth or soft tissue, emesis)
   c. **Direct traumatic disruption** (laryngeal fracture, tracheal collapse)
2. **Breathing.** Even with a patent airway, inadequate gas exchange can rapidly lead to death. This can result from:
   a. Loss of respiratory effort, caused by:
      i. Severe head injury
      ii. High spinal cord disruption (phrenic nerve roots exit C_{2-5} to innervate the diaphragm)
      iii. Central nervous system (CNS) depression from toxins or drugs (including alcohol)
   b. Mechanical dysfunction
      i. Tension pneumothorax
      ii. Large or bilateral open pneumothorax ("sucking chest wound")
      iii. Flail chest
      iv. Thoracic compression
      v. Diaphragm rupture
      vi. Large hemothorax
   c. Systemic toxins (including drugs, alcohol, and inhalation of toxic products of combustion such as carbon monoxide and cyanides)
3. **Circulatory.** Impaired delivery of oxygenated blood to vital organs will cause rapid clinical deterioration. This can occur from:
   a. **Severe hemorrhage**
      i. External
      ii. Intra-thoracic (including disruption of great vessels)
      iii. Intra-abdominal
      iv. Pelvis or retroperitoneal
      v. Multiple long bones
      vi. **Not** intracranial (except possibly in children <1 year of age)
   b. **Obstruction of blood flow** (preventing venous return to the heart)
      i. Tension pneumothorax
      ii. Pericardial tamponade
   c. **Myocardial dysfunction**
      i. Contusion
      ii. Rupture
      iii. Infarction and ischemia
      iv. Dysrhythmia
         a) Electrical shock
         b) Commotio cordis (due to a high-energy blow to chest)
         c) Hypoxemia or global ischemia (e.g., hemorrhagic shock)
B. **Determination of viability**
   1. **Likelihood of survival.** The research on this topic often include a mixture of clinical conditions, making interpretation difficult. Nonetheless, all studies show a dismal prognosis. A few general guidelines can be gleaned from the available data.
      a. **Victims of penetrating trauma** have a greater likelihood of survival from cardiac arrest than victims of blunt trauma.
         i. Survival from arrest is more likely after stab wounds than after gunshot wounds.
         ii. Arrest before EMS arrival decreases the likelihood of survival, particularly if transport times are long.
         iii. Presence of recognized *and* quickly treated pericardial tamponade is a positive prognostic factor, but this is usually not done in the field.

    b. Victims of blunt trauma who suffer cardiopulmonary arrest have an extremely low likelihood of survival, approaching zero (unless witnessed and treated in the emergency department).

        i. Those found by pre-hospital personnel to be in arrest with no signs of life (absence of spontaneous movement or respirations, and absence of reflexes including pupillary) and no electrical activity on the electrocardiogram have a negligible chance of survival. Pre-hospital resuscitation is **not** indicated for these patients.

        ii. The presence of some life sign (eye movement, pupil reaction, corneal reflex, organized cardiac rhythm) in pulseless, nonbreathing patients confers a likelihood of survival no greater than 1% to 2%. Because aggressive interventions (e.g., intubation, ventilation, release of tension pneumothorax, and volume resuscitation) result in occasional long-term survival, resuscitation is attempted. Persistence of pulselessness (especially asystole) on hospital arrival is uniformly fatal and further resuscitation is not warranted.

        iii. Deterioration into cardiac arrest after EMS arrival but before hospital arrival also has dismal prognosis, but full resuscitative efforts should generally be undertaken. Most data suggest no benefit for emergency department thoracotomy for prehospital blunt traumatic arrest.

C. Criteria for attempting resuscitation. Resuscitation should be attempted on patients in arrest caused by major blunt or penetrating trauma, **unless** one or more of the following criteria are met:

    1. Injury obviously incompatible with life (e.g., decapitation, incineration)

    2. Absent signs of life (no respiratory effort, no pupillary response or eye movement, no response to deep pain) and ECG rhythm of asystole

    3. Documented, untreated pulselessness and apnea for >10 minutes (e.g., prolonged entrapment, hazardous scene) in a normothermic patient

    4. Rigor mortis or dependent lividity

    5. Transport time to an ED or trauma center of more than 15 minutes after the onset of cardiopulmonary arrest

D. Special conditions

    1. Electrical shock or lightning. Because arrest is usually caused by a cardiac dysrhythmia and may be reversible, aggressive resuscitation should be attempted. In cases of multiple casualties from an electrical incident, those in arrest should be given first priority.

    2. Drowning or hanging. Arrest is usually caused by asphyxia in these situations. Although appropriate trauma care, such as spinal immobilization, should be instituted, the decision to resuscitate can be based on criteria for "medical" arrests. Hypothermia should be considered in drowning victims.

    3. Hypothermia. The presence of hypothermia (core temperature <35°C) can result from or lead to a traumatic event. Hypothermia can make it difficult to detect signs of life. Patients who are severely hypothermic should generally undergo active core rewarming before cessation of resuscitative efforts unless injuries are clearly incompatible with life. Refer to Chapter 41 for more detail on this illness and treatment.

    4. Arrest secondary to medical cause. Caution should be taken to recognize patients who may have suffered cardiac arrest because of a medical condition, such as the driver of an automobile who develops ventricular fibrillation with a resultant crash. Unless evidence suggests a fatal injury, patients whose mechanism of injury does not correlate with the clinical condition should typically undergo resuscitative efforts similar to any other non-traumatic arrest patient.

E. Management of traumatic arrest

    1. At the scene. Time on scene (excluding extrication) should typically be <10 minutes.

        a. Ensure scene safety before entry, particularly in cases involving assaults, fire, hazardous materials, confined spaces, and vehicular traffic. Law enforcement or fire service assistance may be needed to secure the scene prior to EMS operations. Field personnel should not put themselves at risk for a patient with a negligible chance of survival.

b. **Recognize cardiac arrest.**
    i. Determine whether to initiate resuscitation (see Section C).
    ii. Assess for the presence of special conditions such as hypothermia or a primary medical cause that might influence decision or course of resuscitation.

c. **Maintain manual spinal immobilization.**

d. **Open airway using jaw thrust without head tilt.** Inspect oral cavity, and suction or manually remove debris (blood, teeth, etc.).

e. **Ventilate patient** with basic techniques (e.g., bag-valve-mask) at a rate of 12 to 16 breaths/minute. Use supplemental high-flow oxygen as soon as available.

f. **Perform chest compressions at rate of 100/minute.**

g. **Control severe external hemorrhage.**

h. **Determine ECG rhythm** (note that above steps may be carried out while assessing rhythm to decide whether to proceed with resuscitation):
    i. Defibrillate up to three times for ventricular fibrillation.
    ii. Note the presence of an organized rhythm (pulseless electrical activity) as this confers a greater likelihood of a reversible condition.

i. Attempt endotracheal intubation (refer to Chapter 11).
    i. If able to intubate, confirm proper tube position and carefully secure tube.
    ii. If unable to perform intubation, determine effectiveness of ventilation using basic techniques:
        a) If able to ventilate adequately (chest rise and fall), continue ventilation with basic maneuvers.
        b) If unable to ventilate adequately with a mask device, and *if* the rescuer is properly trained and qualified, either insert an alternative airway device (e.g., Combitube or laryngeal mask airway [LMA]) or perform jet ventilation or surgical cricothyroidotomy; otherwise (as is often the case in most EMS situations), initiate rapid transport and continue to attempt ventilation with basic maneuvers.

j. Assess patient for tension pneumothorax.
    i. Signs: unilateral (or bilateral) decreased breath sounds, poor or worsening lung compliance (especially with positive pressure ventilation), tracheal deviation, subcutaneous emphysema.
    ii. If pneumothorax is suspected, perform needle decompression.

k. Immobilize the patient's spine on long backboard with straps, rigid cervical collar, and head immobilization device.

l. Transfer the patient rapidly to the vehicle, and initiate transport.

2. **En route to the hospital**
    a. Ensure ongoing optimal ventilation (using means above, ensuring tube position if present).
    b. Reassess for tension pneumothorax.
    c. Contact direct medical oversight and/or receiving facility, based on local protocol.
    d. Initiate intravenous (IV) access, or intraosseous (IO) access if intravenous access cannot be obtained and the rescuer is qualified.
        i. Two large-bore IV lines ($\geq$16 gauge) are optimal.
        ii. The role of fluid resuscitation is controversial. A pragmatic approach is to guide EMS providers to control any external hemorrhage first, and provide isotonic crystalloid fluid to help approach normal circulating volume but not to seek "normal" vital signs until hemorrhage is controlled. In many cases, the latter cannot occur until after hospital arrival.

3. **Advanced interventions** for **physicians and other advanced providers** may be indicated in some situations, especially when transport time is >15 to 20 minutes, or there is prolonged entrapment:

a. **Surgical airway**
   i. **Cricothyroidotomy**
   ii. **Translaryngeal jet ventilation**
b. **Venous access**
   i. **Central vein access**
   ii. **Cutdown of saphenous vein at groin or ankle**
c. **Tube thoracostomy** Needle decompression can produce inadequate or only temporary decompression of pneumothorax and is inadequate for drainage of hemothorax.
4. **Termination of efforts.** Termination of resuscitation efforts should be considered for traumatic arrest patients with 15 minutes of unsuccessful resuscitation efforts and cardiopulmonary resuscitation (CPR).

III. NONARREST PREHOSPITAL TRAUMA MANAGEMENT
A. **Airway management**
1. **Introduction.** While it has traditionally been taught that airway management is the most important skill to be mastered by EMS personnel, and endotracheal intubation the most desirable method for those near or in extremis, there are conflicting data on outcomes and intubation attempts by paramedics. Regardless, conditions and circumstances encountered by EMS personnel contribute to the challenge of establishing an airway. These include adverse environmental conditions (rain, snow, darkness); limited patient access (entrapment); limited numbers of personnel (often only two providers, only one of whom is trained in advanced airway management techniques); concern for cervical spine injury (precluding or complicating certain airway maneuvers); and patients with full stomachs, head injury, or acute intoxication (each of which can increase complication rates).
2. **Patient assessment.** The airway is assessed by simultaneous evaluation of several simple clinical features. These include level of consciousness, physical findings, and vital signs.
   a. **Level of consciousness.** The patient's general condition of wakefulness is the best predictor of the ability to protect the airway from aspiration or occlusion. Specific simple features are commonly sought using the AVPU scale: Is the patient **awake**, eyes open, and conversing? Is the patient reacting to **verbal** stimuli? Is the patient arousable only to **painful** or noxious stimuli? Is the patient **unresponsive**? Abnormalities of mental status can be caused by hypoventilation, hypoxemia, hypoperfusion, drug or alcohol intoxication, or head injury. If the patient's ability to maintain adequate oxygenation, ventilation, or airway patency is impaired, airway interventions are required.
   b. **Physical findings.** Search for findings indicative of poor oxygen delivery to tissues: pale, cool, moist skin; delayed capillary refill (>2 seconds); noisy or labored respirations (too fast or too slow). Other physical findings more specific to a pure respiratory abnormality include asymmetric or shallow chest excursion, crepitus, thoracic ecchymosis, nasal flaring, accessory muscle use, abdominal breathing, or subcostal retraction.
   c. **Vital signs.** Abnormal vital signs (including pulse oximetry) must be addressed and appropriate therapy instituted. Normal vital signs do not guarantee adequate ventilation or airway protection.
3. **Resuscitation.** Airway resuscitation encompasses positioning and clearing the airway, delivering supplemental oxygen, using adjuncts or assist devices, and implementing tracheal intubation techniques.
   a. **Positioning the airway.** Manual techniques for opening the airway include the head tilt/chin lift, jaw thrust, and jaw lift. Each acts to manually displace oropharyngeal soft tissues and the tongue away from the posterior portion of the throat, allowing upper airway patency. In the trauma patient, presence of a cervical spine injury must almost always be suspected; therefore, the head tilt/chin lift is **contraindicated** in most trauma patients,

aside from those with isolated extremity injuries. The **jaw thrust** is accomplished by placing two hands at the angles of the mandible and lifting the jaw forward. The **jaw lift** is performed by placing a thumb inside the mouth on the mandibular incisors and fingers under the tip of the chin. The jaw and its attached soft tissues are then lifted forward. Semiconscious or combative patients may bite rescuers, precluding use of the jaw lift. Otherwise, when performed with cervical spine immobilization, jaw thrust and lift offer low risk and good yield for patients requiring assistance in maintaining airway patency. These maneuvers are also adjuncts for more advanced interventions, including assisted ventilation and tracheal intubation.

b. **Supplemental oxygen.** To maximize alveolar oxygen concentration, supplemental oxygen should be administered to all trauma patients. This can be accomplished by numerous devices. The high-flow devices, including the partial and nonrebreather masks, are best for delivering oxygen to the conscious, alert trauma patient. The fraction of inspired oxygen (FiO_2) delivery by nasal cannula is variable and limited by blood or secretions in the nares. For this reason, nasal cannula oxygen supplementation should not be used in place of high-flow mask devices.

c. **Airway adjuncts** are devices or maneuvers that aid in maintaining airway patency.

   i. **Suctioning.** The clearing of secretions, mucus, blood, debris, or vomitus is essential to establishing airway patency. Dentures, loose teeth, bone fragments, and other foreign material must be removed. Suctioning is performed with a plastic, rigid, large-opening device (e.g., a Yankauer or tonsil tip catheter) to allow rapid removal of materials without clogging of the device. Handheld pump-action devices or large-caliber suction tubing without a tip can also be used to clear the airway of debris. Care must be taken to avoid inducing or exacerbating oropharyngeal bleeding when using any suction device. Small-bore devices are not recommended for use in trauma patients.

   ii. **Nasopharyngeal airway** is a device to maintain airway patency in the semiconscious or unconscious patient. Nasal airways must be used in conjunction with manual positioning of the airway (jaw thrust or lift). The size of the patient's little finger can help guide choice of a nasal airway, and the most patent nostril should be used for insertion. The device is an uncuffed, pliable rubber tube with a beveled tip and a funnel-shaped top (hence the common nickname "nasal trumpet"). The device is inserted into the nose, and extends from the nostril to the nasopharynx, coming to rest behind the base of the tongue. **Advantages** of the nasopharyngeal airway are ease of insertion; aid in maintaining airway patency behind the tongue; ability for repeated suctioning without intense oropharyngeal stimulation; and usefulness in patients with a gag reflex or clenched teeth where oropharyngeal airways cannot be used. **Disadvantages** include inability to isolate the trachea, and obstruction by blood or secretions.

   iii. **Oropharyngeal airway** is a rigid, plastic, semicircular-shaped device with side ports that facilitate suctioning. **It is used only in unconscious patients who lack a gag reflex.** Oropharyngeal airways must be used in conjunction with manual positioning of the airway. The device is placed into the mouth following the curvature of the tongue (while holding the tongue with a gauze pad or using a wooden depressor) with the tip resting behind the base of the tongue. Alternatively, the airway can be inserted with the open curve of the "C" facing cephalad or lateral, with the tip then rotated to match the natural tongue curve after placement. With either placement method, pushing the tongue posteriorly will occlude the airway. The size of the oropharyngeal airway is chosen based on the distance from the lip angle to the ear lobe. In addition to maintaining or restoring airway patency, the **advantages** of an oropharyngeal airway include ease of suctioning and assistance of ventilation. **Disadvantages** are stimulation of the gag reflex in the semiconscious patient, inability to place the device in patients with clenched teeth, and inability to isolate or protect the trachea.

iv. Esophagotracheal Combitube (ETC) (Fig. 6-1)

    a) The ETC is placed through the mouth without direct hypopharyngeal or glottic visualization. Normally, the tip resides in the upper esophagus and hypopharynx. After inflating the balloon to obstruct the flow of gases to the esophagus, the esophageal port is ventilated. Gas exits from holes above the esophageal cuff or balloon and is directed the short distance toward the glottis, resulting in near normal tidal volumes delivered to the lungs, with attendant breath sounds and expired CO_2.

    b) Approximately 10% to 15% of insertion attempts result in the glottis being entered rather than the upper esophagus; resultant ventilation of the esophageal port yields lack of chest excursion or breath sounds. **This must be recognized**; in this situation, the second port should be ventilated. Similar to a standard endotracheal tube, this should provide direct oxygen to the trachea and produce symmetric breath sounds, CO_2 on exhalation, and a quiet epigastrium. Little neck manipulation is needed with the blind insertion. The major disadvantages include lack of tracheal isolation in most cases, and the need to identify the cases in which the glottis is entered (to allow ventilation through the correct port).

v. Laryngeal mask airway (LMA) (Fig. 6-2) The LMA is a pliable, silicone teardrop-shaped diaphragm with an inflatable, cuffed rim and a proximal ventilation tube. The diaphragm is placed through the oropharynx and rests above the glottis, with its tip in the esophagus. The diaphragm acts to isolate the posteriorly located esophageal structures from the anterior laryngeal opening. The proximal port is ventilated using a bag-valve device. **Advantages** of the LMA include rapidity and ease of placement, high success rates with training, and

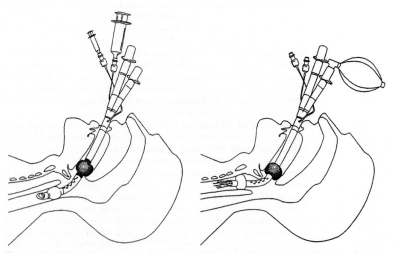

Figure 6-1. Esophagotracheal Combitube (ETC). (Modified from the Sheridan Catheter Corporation, Argyle, NY, with permission.)

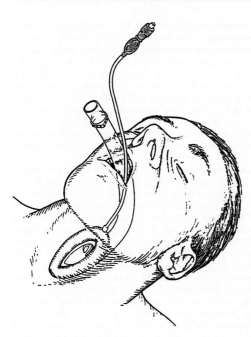

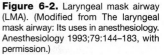

Figure 6-2. Laryngeal mask airway (LMA). (Modified from The laryngeal mask airway: Its uses in anesthesiology. Anesthesiology 1993;79:144–183, with permission.)

maintenance of inline cervical positioning during insertion. Its ability to prevent aspiration is controversial, particularly in patients with high airway pressures (e.g., asthma). **Disadvantages** include initial training requirements, little data on its use outside the operative suite or hospital, the requirement of an unconscious patient, and the necessity of "sizing" the device.

vi. **Sellick's maneuver.** Gentle manual pressure is placed on the cricoid cartilage, with the intent of occluding the esophagus that lies directly behind it. When correctly performed, cricoid pressure helps limit the risk of aspiration by impeding gastric insufflation and the movement of vomited material into the hypopharynx and glottis. It also can aid intubation by moving anterior laryngeal structures into view during laryngoscopy (e.g., backward, upward, rightward pressure, or BURP). Care must be exercised as aggressive pressure can transmit forces to the underlying cervical spine. Otherwise, this maneuver offers little risk and great potential benefit. One common mistake is to put pressure on the thyroid cartilage rather than the cricoid cartilage, which does not alter the risk of aspiration and can tilt the glottis out of view during laryngoscopy. Cricoid pressure is maintained until proper endotracheal tube position is confirmed.

d. **Advanced airway skills in the field**

i. All advanced airway techniques, from direct oral intubation to surgical airways, require a significant investment in training, equipment, and continuing education (to maintain competency). Each skill can be performed by physicians, paramedics, and nurses after proper training and with specific guidelines. However, it is not at all clear under what circumstances these techniques *should* be used, particularly in the nonarrest patient. Chapter 11 discusses general trauma airway issues; here, we highlight those specific to the prehospital setting.

ii. Endotracheal intubation. (Chapter 11 also discusses this topic.) **Orotracheal intubation** is the method of choice for most apneic patients, with **nasotracheal intubation** an alternative method in certain spontaneously breathing patients with clenched teeth or inability to open their mouths. In the field, the success rate of nasal intubation is lower than with oral intubation. Recent data strongly suggest that field intubation assisted by sedative and paralytic drugs ("rapid-sequence intubation") is associated with worse outcomes in patients with serious head trauma than is noninvasive management with bag-valve-mask techniques. No cause–effect relationship has been established, and optimal ventilation strategies for these patients remain unknown.

iii. Digital intubation may be useful when limited access to the patient or inability to directly visualize the airway structures exist. In the field, limited suction capabilities make this an attractive option for advanced providers. Digital intubation requires an unconscious patient and a "bite-block" (or other protective device) to prevent injury to the provider's fingers. The long finger of the nondominant hand is "walked" to the base of the tongue until a cartilaginous membrane (epiglottis) is encountered. While pushing the tongue downward with the long finger and elevating the epiglottis with the index finger, the endotracheal tube is guided blindly between the fingers into the glottic opening. Digital intubation has the advantage of being possible in cases where injury or foreign material limits direct visualization of the glottis. However, the technique requires dexterity, has risk of harming the provider, and causes uncertain motion of the cervical spine. There have been no organized studies of the efficacy or effectiveness of this technique.

iv. Transillumination (lighted stylet) intubation. Newly developed intubation devices take advantage of fiberoptic technology to aid in tracheal intubation. A bright light introduced into the larynx will transmit through the anterior neck soft tissues to allow the operator to visualize correct stylet positioning and subsequent endotracheal intubation.

v. Percutaneous translaryngeal catheter (jet) insufflation may be useful in either failed oral or nasal intubation or in those patients with incomplete upper airway obstruction unrelieved with standard maneuvers. The relevant techniques are discussed in Chapter 11.

vi. Cricothyroidotomy. Paramedics, flight nurses, and other providers can perform cricothyroidotomy for patients after failed intubation or with anatomic distortion that precludes other methods of gaining airway control. Several case studies regarding field use have been published. The techniques are discussed in Chapter 11.

e. Assist devices. Prehospital personnel provide ventilatory assistance using multiple methods.

i. Bag-valve devices. The bag-valve is an oblong, self-inflating rubber bag with two one-way valves. The bag has a standard (15 mm) connection that can attach to a face mask or endotracheal tube for ventilation. When used with room air, delivered FiO_2 is 21%. High-flow oxygen at 12 to 15 liters per minute (L/min) provided by a supplemental oxygen inlet with a reservoir bag can deliver up to 90% to 95% oxygen. The bag-valve-mask device can be used to assist spontaneous respirations or to ventilate apneic patients.

ii. Demand valve devices. The demand valve (manually triggered oxygen-powered breathing device) delivers 100% oxygen at high flow rates (40–60 L/min). A push-button valve allows oxygen to flow to the patient. **Advantages** include ease of use and high concentration of delivered oxygen. **Disadvantages** include lung barotrauma, inability to assess lung compliance, gastric distention, and inability to use in pediatric patients. Because of these disadvantages, demand valve use is discouraged.

iii. **Automatic ventilators** are time-cycled, constant-flow, gas-powered devices. These are small and portable, and usually have two controls—one for ventilatory rate and one for tidal volume. A standard (15 mm) adapter allows use with an endotracheal tube. While designed primarily for use in prolonged interfacility transports, some EMS systems use them in the prehospital setting.

4. **Field confirmation of tracheal tube placement.** Confirmation of proper endotracheal intubation is accomplished by multiple methods—**no single method is infallible**.

a. **Physical assessment** includes **visualization** of the vocal cords and trachea during intubation and **auscultation** of bilateral breath sounds in the anterior and axillary lung fields with lack of ventilatory sounds over the stomach (epigastrium). These are the first and easiest confirmatory methods for many patients, but are not definitive. Additional objective confirmation is needed.

b. **End-tidal carbon dioxide detectors (ETCO$_2$)**—electronic and colorimetric devices—are placed between the endotracheal tube and the ventilation device. These detect end-expiratory CO_2, with levels of 2% or greater indicating endotracheal placement. Semiquantitative CO_2 detectors may not be accurate in low pulmonary perfusion states such as cardiac arrest, massive pulmonary emboli, severe shock, or cardiac tamponade. Outside these situations, however, expired CO_2 is very useful to confirm correct tube location. All EMS systems should utilize ETCO$_2$ detection, and any endotracheal tube placed in the field should be assessed using an ETCO$_2$ device.

c. **Bulb and suction devices,** often referred to as esophageal detection devices, can be placed over the end of the endotracheal tube, creating negative expiratory pressure. These devices can be useful when ETCO$_2$ is unavailable or when it is negative, yet the provider believes the tube is properly placed in a patient with a low- or no-flow state that may limit or prevent delivery of CO_2 to the lungs. In general, these devices should not be the first-line confirmation device.

d. **Pulse oximetry** (oxygen saturation monitoring) is an adjunct to assess respiratory adequacy; however, arterial desaturation can be a late finding in respiratory failure. This, coupled with technical difficulties with sensing in the field, particularly with a hypotensive patient, limits the utility of pulse oximetry in rapid confirmation of tracheal tube placement, although it is valuable in identifying adequate arterial oxygenation.

B. **Other procedures and therapies**

1. **Intravenous access and fluid therapy**

a. **Intravenous (IV) access** allows the administration of crystalloids, blood products, and medications. Venous catheterization of trauma patients by paramedics is done routinely, even though outcome data supporting this practice are lacking. Currently, pragmatism suggests that IV access should be attempted while not delaying transport or other interventions (especially airway management and hemorrhage control). To limit the on-scene interval, attempts at IV placement should be made during extrication, while awaiting transport resources, or during transport to the hospital. Two large-bore ($\geq$16 gauge) peripheral IV lines are preferred for major trauma patients.

b. **Failures.** A number of trauma patients will arrive at the hospital without IV access because of short transport times, uncooperative patients, or other more pressing priorities (e.g., airway management, spine protection, or hemorrhage control).

c. **Fluid therapy in the field.** Significant controversy exists regarding the composition, amount, and ultimate clinical goals of fluid therapy in trauma patients. Specific heart rate or blood pressure targets to guide the amount of fluid are poorly understood. The issue does not appear to center on a "fluids: yes or no" question; rather, controlled or limited fluid resuscitation (sometimes referred to as "permissive hypotension") appears beneficial, although the endpoint and fluid makeup are still uncertain.

2. **Military antishock trousers (MAST)**

  a. **Background.** MAST, also referred to as the pneumatic antishock garment (PASG), have been in use by civilian EMS providers for many years. Their use grew out of the experiences during the Vietnam War and documented clinical effects on blood pressure in the hypotensive trauma patient. However, little positive outcome data (especially with respect to mortality or morbidity) are available to support MAST use, and they have generally fallen out of favor.

  b. **Effects.** Several mechanisms of action are proposed for the elevated blood pressure seen with MAST inflation. The major effect is to increase peripheral vascular resistance, accomplished by decreasing the perfusion of the capillary beds of the lower extremities by the external pressure provided via the inflated MAST. This may increase blood flow to more vital organs. MAST may help stabilize pelvic and femur fractures and limit blood loss.

  c. **Indications.** The following are current recommendations from the National Association of EMS Physicians (NAEMSP) regarding the use of MAST in trauma, using the American Heart Association's Emergency Cardiac Care "class" system:

  i. Class IIa. Acceptable, uncertain efficacy, weight of evidence favors usefulness and efficacy.

  a) Hypotension due to suspected pelvic fracture.

  b) Severe traumatic hypotension (palpable pulse, blood pressure not obtainable)

  ii. Class IIb. Acceptable, uncertain efficacy, may be helpful, probably not harmful.

  a) Penetrating abdominal injury.

  b) Pelvic fracture without hypotension.

  c) Spinal shock.

  iii. Class III. Inappropriate option, not indicated, may be harmful.

  a) Diaphragmatic rupture.

  b) Penetrating thoracic injury.

  c) To splint fractures of the lower extremity.

  d) Extremity trauma.

  e) Abdominal evisceration.

  d. **Application and removal**

  i. Remove any objects on the patient's lower body that might cause the MAST or the patient to be punctured. The MAST are slid under the patient and the three sections secured circumferentially. (Often, the MAST are laid on the long spine board before placing the patient on it.) The leg sections are inflated first, using a foot pump. Inflation continues until the Velcro crackles or the MAST pressure gauge reads 100 mmHg. The abdominal section is then inflated in a similar manner. The patient's respiratory efforts should be observed closely because inflation of the abdominal section can limit pulmonary reserve. Large-bore suction should be available in case the patient vomits.

  ii. Deflating the MAST prematurely or rapidly can lead to hypotension that may not respond to reinflation of the MAST. **As much as possible, the patient must be adequately volume resuscitated and/or have bleeding controlled before the device is removed.** The abdominal section should be deflated first, in a slow and deliberate manner. A small quantity of air is released and the patient's blood pressure is checked. If a fall of >5 to 10 mmHg occurs in the systolic blood pressure, deflation is halted. If no decrease in blood pressure ensues, deflation can proceed. Once the abdominal section is deflated, the leg sections are deflated, one at a time, in a similar fashion. **Under no circumstances** should the MAST be cut off a patient. This is both risky and renders the MAST unusable.

- e. **Complications.** The most common complication of MAST use is **interference with the physical examination** or gaining groin vascular access. Other complications include:
    - **i.** Shock after inappropriate removal
    - **ii.** Compartment syndrome
    - **iii.** Lactic acidosis
    - **iv.** Myoglobinuria
    - **v.** Ventilatory compromise
    - **vi.** Hyperkalemia
    - **vii.** Increased cerebral edema

3. **Needle thoracostomy**
    - a. **Indications.** Needle thoracostomy should be performed when a tension pneumothorax exists or is suspected. **Any trauma patient with severe respiratory distress should be evaluated immediately for tension pneumothorax.** In the field, the diagnosis is critical and must be treated before arrival at the hospital. Tension pneumothorax should be suspected in the trauma patient who is short of breath or hypotensive and with **any** of the following features:
        - **i.** Decreased breath sounds
        - **ii.** Tracheal deviation (away from the involved side)
        - **iii.** Distended neck veins (this may not be seen in the patient who is hypovolemic)
        - **iv.** Hyperresonance to percussion of the chest (on the involved side)—difficult to assess in the field environment.
        - **v.** If the patient is intubated, increasing difficulty in bag-valve ventilation can be the earliest or sole indication of a developing tension pneumothorax.
        - **vi.** Respiratory distress
    - b. **Procedure.** Treatment should proceed rapidly once the diagnosis is suspected; if incorrect, the only harm is creating the need for a formal tube thoracostomy in the receiving facility, whereas failing to recognize and treat can lead to death. Decompress the affected side of the chest by inserting a large-bore IV catheter (12 or 14 gauge) perpendicular to the skin at the second or third intercostal space in the midclavicular line, or the third or fourth interspace in the anterior axillary line. Advance the catheter until a rush of air occurs from the open distal end, or until the hub reaches the skin. Common errors include placing the needle either too close to the sternum or cephalad to the second intercostal space (making heart or great vessel puncture possible), or placing the needle under instead of over a rib (making puncture of the neurovascular bundle, which runs in a groove under each rib, possible). After placement, withdraw the needle, but leave the catheter in place to prevent reaccumulation of pleural gas. If the patient's condition worsens, suspect occlusion of the first catheter and place a second needle (Fig. 6-3).
    - c. **Bilateral decompression.** Occasionally, especially in the patient on positive pressure ventilation or with severe obstructive lung disease, bilateral tension pneumothorax can develop. The asymmetry described above with respect to tracheal and chest findings may not be present. If uncertain, both hemithoraces should be decompressed.
    - d. **Therapy after needle thoracostomy.** At the receiving facility, a chest tube is usually placed for definitive treatment once needle decompression is performed (whether or not clinical success occurred with the latter). Once the chest tube is in place, the catheter(s) can be withdrawn.

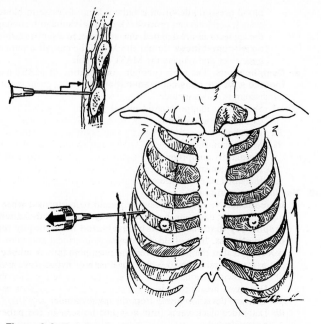

Figure 6-3. Technique for needle thoracostomy. (Modified from Champion HR, Robbs JV, Trunkey DD. Trauma surgery. In: Rob and Smith's Operative Surgery. London: Butterworth, 1989:57, with permission.)

4. Splinting
  a. Indications. The purposes of splinting are to prevent further injury, decrease blood loss, and limit the amount of pain the patient will have with movement of that extremity during extrication and transport. An injured extremity should be splinted in anatomic position *if possible*, with the splint extending to the joints above and below the fracture site for stabilization. If the patient refuses, or if resistance to straightening exists, splint in a position of comfort. Dressings should be applied to any open wounds before splinting.
  b. Splint types. A large variety of splint designs will appear on patients brought to the emergency department. They can be as simple as a rolled-up newspaper, or as complex as a vacuum or traction splint:
    i. Cardboard splints, with or without foam padding, are intended for single use.
    ii. Board splints, which are common and durable, are made of straight pieces of wood, metal, or plastic cut to various lengths.
    iii. Air splints, which encircle the injured extremity, are inflated with air to impart stiffness. They are usually clear to allow visualization of the underlying structures. Overinflation can cause neurovascular compromise.
    iv. Vacuum splints incompletely encircle the injured limb. Instead of air being blown into them, air is withdrawn and a vacuum is produced, which stiffens the splint.
    v. Traction splints are used for femur fractures. Thomas half-ring splints and Hare traction splints are those most commonly used. Specific training is required for proper placement.

vi. Ladder splints are made from heavy gauge wire in a ladder shape. They are useful for splinting extremities that cannot be straightened because they are bendable and can be shaped to match the extremity. The SAM Splint, with a flexible aluminum alloy core covered with closed-cell foam, is similarly flexible.

c. Complications. Although splinting is safe and effective in most patients, complications can develop, including:

  i. Neurovascular compromise. Whichever splint is used, distal neurovascular status must be checked before and after application of the splint. Also, if any patient movement has occurred, the patient reports more pain, or the extremity is noted to be cyanotic or edematous distal to the splint, reexamine the extremity and splint. It is also advisable to periodically check the neurovascular status, even if none of the above occur. When impaired neurovascular status is seen distal to an injury, the splint should be loosened or adjusted, and the neurovascular status rechecked.

  ii. Pain. When the patient reports pain, search for neurovascular compromise or malpositioning. Gentle repositioning should resolve this condition.

5. Axial spine immobilization

  a. Prehospital indications. Historically, despite the lack of supporting literature, the entire axial spine is immobilized by prehospital personnel whenever the mechanism of injury, injury pattern, or physical examination indicate the **possibility** of any spinal injury. Most major trauma patients have experienced kinematic forces that warrant the precautionary application of spinal immobilization devices until definitive clinical and/or radiographic examinations can be performed in the ED. Patients with obvious physical findings (e.g., bony crepitation, palpable step-offs) or those with neurologic findings (e.g., paresthesia, weakness, paralysis) consistent with spine or cord injury should always receive complete immobilization before transport.

  b. Clinical assessment of the spine often cannot be performed by field personnel because of time, space, distracting injury, altered consciousness, and other concerns (e.g., airway, bleeding control, vascular access) that can preclude adequate in-field evaluation to rule out spinal injury. While the rule in prehospital care is to maintain a high index of suspicion for such injuries with liberal application of spinal immobilization, it is well established that field personnel, with proper training and medical oversight, can safely assess which patients do and do not require spine immobilization. The protocols that EMS systems use for this purpose generally exclude major trauma patients from consideration for this assessment, requiring full spine immobilizing.

  c. The need for spinal immobilization occurs at the injury scene and continues through extrication, transportation, and stabilization in the ED. Immobilization is accomplished with the least possible neck movement, and ends only when physical and/or radiographic findings definitively rule out injury.

  d. Types of immobilization devices. No single method or combinations of methods of immobilization consistently place the spine in neutral position or prevent all motion in the axial spine.

  i. Cervical collars (c-collars) are numerous in design and efficacy. These rigid one- or two-piece devices encircle the cervical spine and soft tissues of the neck, providing (when properly fitted) a snug fit between the tip the chin and the suprasternal notch of the anterior chest, and between the occiput and the suprascapular region of the back. These collars limit movement of the head in the coronal and transverse planes, minimizing lateral and rotary motion. They do not, however, provide adequate immobilization in the sagittal plane (flexion-extension motion). For this reason, **a rigid cervical collar**

alone is inadequate for effective spinal immobilization and is always used in conjunction with a cervical immobilization device (CID) and a spine board (short or long). Soft neck collars (foam supports covered with loose-weave material) are ineffective at limiting motion of the head in all planes, and are not intended for use in spinal immobilization.

ii. **CIDs** are made of plastic, cardboard, or foam. They act to pad the lateral aspects of the head (limiting both lateral and rotary motion), and possess restraining straps that are positioned over the patient's forehead and chin, encircling the back of a short or long spine board. The CID affixes the patient's head and c-collar to a rigid spine board, limiting the head movements of flexion and extension. A CID can be fashioned from blanket rolls, blocks, or sandbags placed alongside the head, with fixation to the spine board via wide (2- to 3-inch) silk tape placed over the forehead and chin.

iii. **Spine boards** are termed "short" or "long," depending on the most distal portion of the patient immobilized. Short boards limit flexion and extension from the head to the hips, minimizing movement in all portions of the spine (cervical, thoracic, lumbar). Short boards are primarily used if patient access is limited (e.g., entrapment in a vehicle, or confined space extrication) and stability in the axial spine is needed before and during the extrication process. Once extrication is performed and complete access to the patient is achieved, the short board and patient are typically secured to a long spine board. Long spine boards limit flexion and extension from the head to the feet. Straps provide fixation points at the thorax, hips, and lower extremities (above the knees). Data suggest that including the lower extremities in the immobilization process aids in stabilizing the lumbosacral spine and limits lateral motion of the torso if lateral tilting of the board is needed to manage emesis. Padding between the lower extremities and under the knees enhances both stabilization and patient comfort.

a) **Secondary pain after immobilization.** With any of these devices, immobilization itself can produce symptoms of discomfort (e.g., occipital headache; neck, back, head, mandible pain). This should not preclude the liberal application of spinal immobilization devices in most patients with significant trauma. Padding behind the occiput and in the areas of lordosis and kyphosis make intuitive sense, and may be especially important in the pediatric and elderly population, given their anatomy.

AXIOMS

■ Recognizing trauma severity, assisting breathing in the simplest effective manner, controlling any bleeding, and rapidly transporting to an appropriate hospital are keys to good care.

■ Outcomes from out-of-hospital traumatic cardiac arrest are generally dismal, and each EMS system should have a protocol and procedure in place to optimally handle these difficult cases, recognizing the futility of attempting resuscitation in most such patients.

■ Effective trauma triage relies on the proficiency and accuracy of the assessment skills of field personnel.

■ The vast majority of trauma patients can be managed with basic life support skills, such as bag-valve-mask ventilation, splinting and spine immobilization, and hemorrhage control. There are no convincing data to support advanced life support interventions in trauma patients.

■ Objective confirmation of proper endotracheal tube placement, using end-tidal carbon dioxide detection supplemented by other means as needed, is mandatory for all patients intubated in the field.

■ The differences between field triage (for individual trauma patients) and mass casualty triage (for multipatient events) must be understood by both field and hospital personnel, and EMS systems must account for these two different types of triage when establishing or refining policies and procedures.

Bibliography

Bond RJ, Kortbeek JB, Preshaw RM. Field trauma triage: Combining mechanism of injury with the prehospital index for an improved trauma triage tool. *J Trauma* 1997;43(2):283–287.

Davis DP, Hoyt DB, Ochs M, et al. The effect of paramedic rapid sequence intubation on outcome in patients with severe traumatic brain injury. *J Trauma* 2003;54(3):444–453.

Domeier RM. Indications for prehospital spinal immobilization. National Association of EMS Physicians Standards and Clinical Practice Committee. *Prehosp Emerg Care* 1999;3(3):251–253.

Hopson LR, Hirsh E, Delgado J, et al. Guidelines for withholding or termination of resuscitation in prehospital traumatic cardiopulmonary arrest: A joint position paper from the National Association of EMS Physicians Standards and Clinical Practice Committee and the American College of Surgeons Committee on Trauma. *Prehosp Emerg Care* 2003;7(1):141–146.

O'Connor RE, Domeier RM. An evaluation of the pneumatic anti-shock garment (PASG) in various clinical settings. *Prehosp Emerg Care* 1997;1(1):36–44.

O'Connor RE, Swor RA. Verification of endotracheal tube placement following intubation. National Association of EMS Physicians Standards and Clinical Practice Committee. *Prehosp Emerg Care* 1999;3(3):248–250.

Rosemurgy AS, Norris PA, Olson SM, et al. Prehospital traumatic cardiac arrest: The cost of futility. *J Trauma* 1993;35(3):468–474.

Wang HE, O'Connor RE, Domeier RM. Prehospital rapid-sequence intubation. *Prehosp Emerg Care* 2001;5(1):40–48.

AIR MEDICAL AND INTERHOSPITAL TRANSPORT

JOHN S. COLE

AIR MEDICAL TRANSPORT

Based on the experience of the Korean and Vietnam Wars, air medical transport has grown to become an integral part of trauma care in the United States. Currently, over 650 private, hospital-based, public service, and military air medical helicopters transport more than 300,000 patients annually. Two thirds of the transports are interhospital, with the remaining one third transported directly from the scene. An air medical helicopter responding to an emergency takes off every 90 seconds in this country.

I. EQUIPMENT

    A. Most air medical transport today is accomplished with twin-engine helicopters specifically configured for medical missions. Some flight programs fly instrument flight rules (IFR) missions, allowing transport of trauma patients in weather conditions that previously prevented rotorcraft transport. Most aircraft with reconfiguration can transport two patients, in addition to two flight crew members and the pilot. The practical transport range for helicopter transfer is generally 150 miles. For longer distance transports or in poor weather conditions, fixed-wing aircraft are often utilized.

    B. The flight environment is noisy, making simple procedures such as auscultation of blood pressure and breath sounds difficult or impossible. Therefore, nonaudible-dependent monitoring is used. Most flight crews rely on noninvasive blood pressure monitoring, end-tidal CO_2, and pulse oximetry to monitor patients in flight. Rotorcraft rarely fly at altitudes above 2,000 feet above ground level (AGL). At these altitudes, pressure changes have only a minor impact on the volume of air-filled spaces such as a pneumothorax.

    C. The flight crew communicate with each other and the patient through headsets or helmets connected to internal communication systems. The crew must be able to communicate with the receiving hospital. Advance notification of patient assessment and changes in patient condition en route allow the receiving trauma center to be better prepared.

II. TRIAGE

    A. The transport of trauma patients directly from the scene should be supported by online medical control or preapproved protocols based on the factors of time, distance, geography, patient stability, and local resources. Although some literature is conflicting, a recent multicenter study demonstrated that air medical transport was associated with a significant reduction in blunt trauma mortality rates compared with ground transport. Undue delay of transport from the scene to the closest hospital while waiting for a helicopter should be avoided. Rendezvous at the hospital's helipad would be a more appropriate use of time.

    B. Interhospital transport of trauma patients usually involves moving a patient to a facility with a higher level of care.

    C. The National Association of EMS Physicians (NAEMSP) and the American College of Emergency Physicians (ACEP) have recommended triage guidelines for on-scene helicopter transport (Table 7-1).

TABLE 7-1	On-Scene Helicopter Triage

Trauma center candidate based on triage criteria
Trauma score <12
Unstable vital signs (e.g., hypotension or tachypnea)
Significant trauma in patients <12 or >55 y
Multisystem injury
Ground providers' perception based on mechanism of injury
Penetrating trauma to abdomen, pelvis, chest, head, or neck

    D. Weather, geography, logistics, or other factors determine flight suitability. **The final decision to accept the mission should lie solely with the pilot. Crew safety is paramount.**

III. FLIGHT CREW

    A. More than 70% of the medical flight crews consist of a nurse–paramedic team. Approximately 20% of programs use two nurses, and only 3% of programs use a flight physician. Respiratory therapists are also combined with nurses in a small percentage of programs.

IV. INTERVENTIONS

    A. Transport crews should be experienced in the care of critically ill patients. Crew members should be highly trained in airway management utilizing rapid sequence intubation, as well as resuscitation, vascular access, and control of hemorrhage. These interventions should be initiated prior to liftoff.

    B. Intravenous analgesia, sedation, and chemical paralysis, as well as administration of vasoactive substances and blood products, can be done in flight. These interventions must be performed under strict online medical direction or predetermined approved protocols.

V. HELIPAD ACCESS TEAM

    A. A helipad team trained in helicopter safety is usually designated to assist the flight crew in unloading and transporting the patient from the helicopter to the emergency department. Helipads should be in close proximity to the resuscitation area, limiting the need for therapeutic interventions on the helipad.

    B. When helipads are remote from the resuscitation area (e.g., rooftop with elevator and corridor transport), occasional therapeutic interventions may be required on the helipad. Only a limited number of resuscitative procedures should be performed on the helipad. Focus should be on identifying the need for immediate lifesaving procedures, establishing an airway, decompressing a tension pneumothorax, applying direct pressure to an open bleeding wound, or administering resuscitative drugs and countershocks for dysrhythmias. Other interventions (IV catheter placement for volume resuscitation or thoracotomy) are best performed in the emergency department.

VI. SAFETY

    A. The leading causes of accidents are weather, collision with an object or terrain, and loss of control of the aircraft. Pressure on pilots to fly and failure to observe minimum weather standards are contributing components to accidents. The pilot's decision to complete a mission should be based on aviation factors alone and not influenced by patient criteria.

    B. In general, a 500-foot ceiling and 1-mile visibility are required for daytime visual flight rules (VFR) flight. This may be geography-specific, depending on the presence of mountains and pockets of fog. Day-local is defined as <25 nautical miles from departure point to destination point, with generally the same terrain elevation.

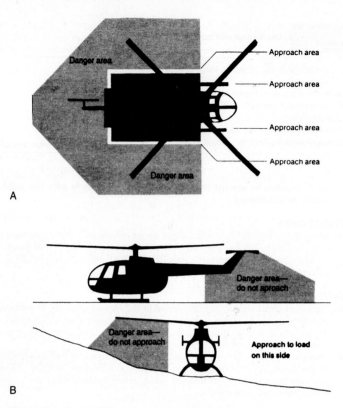

Figure 7-1. Air view **(A)** and ground view **(B)** of safe approaches.

TABLE 7-2	Safety Around the Helicopter

The same safety standards should be practiced whether the helicopter's engines are running or shut down.

- Do not approach the helicopter unless signaled to do so by a flight team member.
- Remain clear of the helicopter at all times unless accompanied by a flight team member.
- When approaching the helicopter, always approach from the front of the aircraft and move away in the same direction.
- When approaching the helicopter on a slope, **never** approach from the uphill side. Always approach from the downhill side because the main rotor to the ground clearance is much greater. Always be aware of the blade clearance.
- **Never** walk around the tail rotor area.
- No unauthorized personnel are allowed within 100 ft of the aircraft.
- No intravenous devices or other objects should be carried above the head, and long objects should be carried parallel to the ground.

C. Comprehensive safety orientation programs for local ground EMS personnel that include instruction covering helicopter communication, set-up of landing zones, patient preparation, and conduct around the aircraft are an essential part of any EMS air medical program (Fig. 7-1).

D. Table 7-2 outlines safety conduct around the helicopter.

INTERHOSPITAL TRANSPORT

I. INTRODUCTION. Emergent interhospital transport usually occurs after initial stabilization of the trauma patient and determination by the referring facility that the patient's needs for definite care are beyond the scope of local capabilities. This practice is in response to evidence supporting the view that trauma outcome is enhanced if critically injured patients are cared for in facilities dedicated to the needs of the acutely injured. A trauma center should have referral centers that facilitate transfers, outreach teams to provide referring facilities with continuing education, and public education programs about trauma systems and injury prevention.

A. Transfer of the trauma patient occurs with the expectation that care will continue en route to the receiving facility and that changes in patient status will be identified and treated. These goals frequently require specialized personnel and equipment. Coordination between referring and receiving institutions and medical direction during transport are fundamental to guarantee continuity of care.

II. BEFORE TRANSPORT. Interhospital transport can be performed by a transport team from the referring facility, the receiving facility, or by a third party. It is the responsibility of the **referring physician** to decide the best mode of transportation (air vs. ground) and to ensure that the transporting personnel have the necessary expertise and equipment to deal with the patient's condition and possible complications. For example, some non-hospital-based personnel may not be trained in the use of certain hospital equipment (intravenous pumps, ventilators, or other devices); this should be recognized and addressed before transport.

A. The transporting crew can be any combination of paramedics, nurses, or physicians, depending on the patient condition and local policies. If the referring physician is to provide medical direction during transport, transfer orders should be discussed before departure.

B. Complete documentation of all patient care records must be sent. This includes results of all therapeutic and diagnostic interventions, copies of all imaging studies performed, and patient consent for transfer. Teleradiology allows a trauma center to review a patient's studies before arrival. This also allows the center to help referring facilities manage patients who do not require transfer to a trauma center.

C. It is essential that the transport team establish direct communication with both referring and accepting physicians. Communication with the referring physician must detail the following information:

1. **Identification** of the patient and medical history
2. **Mechanism of injury** and circumstances about the incident
3. **Prehospital management** before arrival to the emergency department
4. **Interventions** performed during initial stabilization and patient's response
5. **Pertinent physical examination findings**
6. **Ongoing therapy**
7. **Potential complications** that may occur during transport

D. The transport team should then perform its own directed evaluation, equivalent to a primary survey, without delaying transport. This evaluation should include, but not be limited to, the following:

1. **Airway**
   a. **Recheck the airway** or assess adequate position of the endotracheal tube with appropriate methods that can include direct visualization, end-tidal CO_2, auscultation, esophageal detector device, or chest x-ray.

2. **Respiratory**
   a. **Document respiratory status** before initiation of transport.
   b. **Check for appropriate functioning of ventilatory equipment.**
   c. **Check or place nasogastric tube** to prevent aspiration in obtunded or intubated patients.
   d. **Check position of any tube** or device (e.g., thoracostomy). Chest tubes ideally should have pleuravacs attached and placed on suction for transport.
3. **Cardiovascular**
   a. **Document heart rate, pulse, pulse oximetry, and blood pressure** before initiation of transport.
   b. **Control external bleeding** and reevaluate bandages applied for bleeding control.
   c. **Secure two large-bore IV catheters.**
   d. **Secure adequate supply of blood products** for transfer.
   e. **Connect invasive lines** (e.g., arterial lines, central venous pressure [CVP] lines, and pulmonary artery catheters) to the transport monitor to allow continued hemodynamic monitoring during the transport.
   f. **Connect patient to electrocardiograph monitor.**
4. **Central nervous system**
   a. **Document neurologic examination and Glasgow Coma Scale (GCS)** score before initiation of transport or administration of paralytic or sedative agents.
   b. **Secure head, cervical, thoracic, and lumbar spine** with immobilization devices, as needed.

III. **DURING TRANSPORT.** The transport team must know before transport which physician is to be responsible for online medical direction. Responsibility for medical direction will vary, based on local practices and the policies of the transport service. The receiving physician, however, must always be made aware of changes in the patient's condition en route.
   A. Once the patient has been stabilized, the transport should be completed without delay. It is expected that care during transport be at the same level as received at the referring institution, within the obvious limitations of the out-of-hospital environment. Unstable patients should be accompanied by a provider capable of appropriate medical interventions; this may require a physician.
   B. The transporting unit must have the capability to continue cardiorespiratory support and blood volume replacement. Constant hemodynamic monitoring is essential. Communication via radio, cellular telephone, or satellite phone should occur to obtain medical direction and to provide updates to the receiving facility.
   C. When standing orders or protocols (the essential component of off-line medical direction) are given to the transport team, the referring physician must be sure that the orders match the team's capabilities and that the appropriate medications and equipment are present.

IV. **AFTER TRANSPORT.** On arrival at the receiving facility, the transport team must give a complete report to the receiving trauma team. This should include a brief summary of the initial history and treatments, followed by an update of any changes en route and any interventions. In addition, all documentation from the referring institution must be delivered to the receiving team leader. If the patient was transferred for diagnostic procedures and is to be transferred back to the original institution, the same transfer regulations apply now to the receiving hospital. If diagnostic procedures reveal new evidence of present or potential instability, the patient cannot be transferred back without appropriate stabilization.

V. **LEGAL CONSIDERATIONS.** The transfer of patients from one institution to another is regulated by federal statute. The legislation that created the patient stabilization and transfer requirements for hospitals and physicians is the **Consolidated Omnibus Budget Reconciliation Act (COBRA) of 1985,** also known as the "antidumping law." This is the current legal standard. One of the main objectives of this resolution is to guarantee equal access to emergency treatment to all citizens regardless of their ability to pay.

A. COBRA attributes responsibility for the patient's transfer to the referring hospital and physician.
   1. Violations can result in termination of Medicare privileges for the physician and hospital.
   2. A hospital can be fined between $25,000 and $50,000 per violation.
   3. A physician can be fined $50,000 per violation.
   4. A patient can sue the hospital for personal injury in civil court.

B. The Emergency Medical Treatment and Labor Act (EMTALA) established by COBRA legislation governs how patients can be transferred from one hospital to another. Hospitals cannot transfer patients unless the transfer is "appropriate," the patient consents to transfer after being informed of the risks of transfer, and the referring physician certifies that the medical benefits expected from the transfer outweigh the risks. Appropriate transfers must meet the following criteria:
   1. The transferring hospital must provide care and stabilization within its ability.
   2. Copies of medical records and imaging studies must accompany the patient.
   3. The receiving facility must have available space and qualified personnel and agree to accept the transfer.
   4. The interhospital transport must be made by qualified personnel with the necessary equipment.

AXIOMS

■ The outcome of air medical transport for trauma patients is dependent on appropriate triage and the skill of the flight crew.
■ Safety of crew and patient is paramount.
■ Never approach a helicopter without the assistance of the flight crew.
■ Transfers should be made for medical necessity and not financial reasons.
■ The medical benefits anticipated from the provision of specialized trauma care at the receiving facility should outweigh the risks of transfer.

Bibliography

Accreditation Standards of the Commission on Accreditation of Air Medical Services. 6th ed. Sandy Springs, SC: Commission on Accreditation of Air Medical Services.

American College of Emergency Physicians. *Appropriate utilization of air medical transport in the out-of-hospital setting.* Dallas, Tex: American College of Emergency Physicians; 1999.

Baxt WG, Moody P. The impact of rotorcraft aeromedical emergency care service on trauma mortality. *JAMA* 1983;22:249.

Emergency Medical Treatment and Active Labor Act of 1986: Consolidated Omnibus Budget Reconciliation Act of 1986, §9121, 42USC, §1395dd.

Hunt RC, Bryan DM, Brinkley VS, et al. Inability to assess breath sounds during air medical transport by helicopter. *JAMA* 1991;265:1982–1984.

Moylan J, Fitzpatrick KT, Beyer AJ, et al. Factors improving survival in multisystem trauma patients. *Ann Surg* 1988;6:207.

Omnibus Budget Reconciliation Act of 1989, §6018, 42USC, §1395cc (West Supp. 1990).

Thomas SH, Harrison TH, Buras WR, et al. Helicopter transport and blunt trauma mortality: A multicenter trial. *Ann Emerg Med* 2003;1:41.

Thomson DP, Thomas SH. Guidelines for air medical dispatch. *Prehosp Emerg Care* 2003;2:265–271.

8   TRAUMA TEAM ACTIVATION
THEODORE R. DELBRIDGE

I. **INTRODUCTION.** Health care facilities designated as trauma centers maintain the resources to provide initial definitive care, regardless of injury severity.
   A. As designated by the American College of Surgeons (ACS), **Level I trauma centers** possess the capabilities and physical resources necessary to provide comprehensive trauma care, including rehabilitation, education, prevention, and research components. **Level II centers** possess similar clinical resources, but have less ongoing commitments to research and education. **Level III centers** generally have limited staff and resources for clinical care. They provide care for many patients, and identify those with more serious injuries who are better treated at a Level I or II center.
   B. The most crucial triage decision for Emergency Medical Services (EMS) systems involves ensuring that injured patients are transported to appropriate-level trauma centers. The trauma centers must then decide for which patients the trauma team should be activated.
   C. The **trauma team** is at the hub of the trauma center activities. Ensuring the ongoing availability of a qualified trauma team represents a costly investment by the trauma center, indicating its commitment to providing quality trauma care for the community.

II. **ACTIVATION CRITERIA**
   A. Although the trauma team can be made available to all injured patients at the trauma center, it is a limited resource. It is important that the trauma team be activated for patients whose injuries, as reported by EMS personnel, are likely to demand an immediate operation, critical care, or multidisciplinary management.
   B. To some degree, "tiering," or grading of responses, occurs in all facilities that care for trauma patients. Not all injuries demand the attention of the entire trauma team (e.g., simple extremity fractures resulting from low-force mechanisms of injury). Varying levels of trauma team response may be developed to match patients' anticipated needs with available resources and expertise. These should be institution specific.
   C. Many Level I and II trauma centers currently employ triage criteria to guide the initial evaluation of trauma victims, including deployment of personnel and equipment. Development of such criteria follows recognition that primarily three categories of patients arrive at the trauma center.
      1. **Patients whose injuries are obviously severe and demand an immediate multidisciplinary approach.** The trauma team should be activated before arrival at the center. These patients have clear potential of life-threatening injury as evidenced by abnormal physiology (vital signs and sensorium) or penetrating truncal injury. Additionally, patients with less evidence of severe injuries, but who are arriving in numbers such that local resources would be overwhelmed, are often placed in this most serious category.
      2. **Patients whose injuries, or potential for injury, may not seem immediately life-threatening, but deterioration is possible.** These patients may not require the immediate activation of the entire trauma team, and most may be appropriately evaluated immediately by qualified emergency department

staff together with other trauma team members. Nevertheless, they are treated where multidisciplinary resources are immediately available should they be needed. Such patients may have experienced significant mechanisms of injury, but have no apparent serious anatomic or physiologic abnormalities.

3. **Patients who could be managed at most acute care facilities.** These patients require evaluations by qualified emergency department staffs, including consultation with other providers and similar resources needed to evaluate and treat most other acutely ill, non-trauma patients.

D. **Variations in activation criteria and responses**

1. Trauma team activation criteria, in general, include components similar to those of the ACS Triage Decision Scheme. Physiologic and anatomic factors, as strong predictors of the need for early operation or critical care, should be the primary determinants. Mechanism of injury information by itself is less predictive of the need for operation or critical care, but should be a consideration in activation criteria.

2. Trauma team activation criteria reflect each institution's patient volume and resources. In general, activation criteria identify the resources and personnel assembled initially to care for a seriously injured patient. Some centers choose a singular response type ("all or none"), which eases implementation but can expose the system to inefficient use of resources. Many trauma centers use a graded system of activation (e.g., full trauma team and modified trauma team) which helps ensure prompt response without waste.

3. An example of trauma team activation criteria is shown in Table 8-1. **Full team activation** occurs for patients whose injuries, as reported by EMS personnel, are or have potential to be severe. In such cases, the entire trauma team, including the attending trauma surgeon, responds to the emergency department. Partial or modified team activations do not require anesthesiology, respiratory therapy, and certain surgical housestaff to respond. Furthermore, the attending trauma surgeon is notified immediately via the paging system,

TABLE 8-1	Sample Trauma Team Activation Criteria

Level I trauma team activation
Full trauma team response: Attending emergency medicine physician, attending trauma surgeon, trauma fellow or senior surgical resident, two junior residents, radiology technician, respiratory technician, three emergency department nurses (attending or resident anesthesiologist immediately available).

Physiologic criteria:
-Intubated or question of airway security
-Respiratory distress
-Current decreased level of consciousness
-Any period of systolic blood pressure <100 mmHg

Anatomic criteria:
-Penetrating wound other than distal to the knee or elbow
-Amputation or degloving injury proximal to knee or elbow
-Spinal cord injury
-Flail chest
-Pelvic fracture
-Two or more long bone fractures

Other:
-Request by attending physician for Level I activation

(continued)

TABLE 8-1 *(Continued)*

Level II trauma team activation
Partial trauma team response: Attending emergency medicine physician, trauma fellow or senior surgical resident, one junior resident, two emergency department nurses, radiology technician; notification of attending trauma surgeon; others called as needed.

Physiologic criteria:
-History of loss of consciousness, now neurologically normal

Mechanism of injury criteria:
-Fall >15 ft
-Major deformity of vehicle
-Intrusion into passenger compartment of vehicle
-Death of another vehicle occupant
-Rollover vehicle crash
-Pedestrian struck at >20 mph
-Ejection from vehicle
-Extrication time >20 min

Other:
-Helicopter scene flight
-EMS personnel request for trauma team

but may not be required to respond initially for partial team activation. At any time, a partial response can be upgraded to a full response, if necessary. Similarly, a full response can be downgraded as the patient's condition permits.

4. Level I trauma centers using tiered trauma team activations have reported that 52% to 57% of trauma patients meet the criteria for lesser responses. Furthermore, such guidelines have achieved 85% to 95% sensitivity in terms of requiring full trauma team response for those patients who require early operations or admission to a critical care unit. Patients initially met by a partial team who subsequently require a full team response have outcomes comparable to those met initially by the entire trauma team. Thus, trauma centers have reported that the immediate availability of multidisciplinary expertise and resources is crucial, but that their deployment during the initial evaluation of all trauma patients is not always necessary. Performance improvement of level of team activation and patient outcome is essential.

5. For Level II trauma centers, which are often community hospitals with the trauma surgeon on call outside the facility, the issue of trauma team triage criteria is also important. Resources, including qualified surgeons, may not be as plentiful as at tertiary medical facilities. Their conservation for those situations when they are truly needed, while minimizing undertriage, is an important concern. When EMS personnel report that a trauma patient suffers respiratory compromise, altered mentation (e.g., Glasgow Coma Scale score <13), or hypotension, qualified emergency medicine and trauma surgery staff should be prepared to care for the victim on arrival. For other patients, evaluation by a qualified emergency physician and support staff, in consultation with an attending trauma surgeon, may be appropriate. When such guidelines have been used, no differences were found between observed and predicted mortality.

III. SUMMARY. The trauma team brings the comprehensive multidisciplinary capabilities of the trauma center to the emergency evaluation and management of injured patients. Its activation is crucial if the trauma center is to effect favorable outcomes for critically injured patients. However, judicious utilization of this resource is appropriate. As no standard criteria exist for trauma team activation, it is important for all centers to evaluate their trauma system components and quality and availability of resources, and prospectively create trauma team activation guidelines that are adequately dispersed and evaluated on an ongoing basis. Such efforts enhance the efficiency of care for trauma patients.

 AXIOMS

- Trauma team activation criteria must be developed locally, and consider the response capabilities and input of EMS, emergency medicine, trauma surgery, anesthesiology, and other related specialists.
- Grading of trauma team responses can help tailor resources, but guidelines should be planned, monitored, and adjusted, as needed.

Bibliography
Eastes LS, Norton R, Brand D, et al. Outcomes of patients using a tiered trauma response protocol. *J Trauma* 2001;50(5):908–913.
Helling TS, Nelson PW, Shook JW, et al. The presence of in-house trauma surgeons does not improve management or outcome of critically injured patients. *J Trauma* 2003;55(1):20–25.
Khetarpal S, Steinbrunn BS, McGonigal MD, et al. Trauma faculty and trauma team activation: Impact on trauma system function and patient outcome. *J Trauma* 1999;47(3):576–581.
Kohn MA, Hammel JM, Bretz SW, Stangby A. Trauma team activation criteria as predictors of patient disposition for the emergency department. *Acad Emerg Med* 2004;11(1):1–9.
Plaisier BR, Meldon SW, Super DM, et al. Effectiveness of a 2-specialty, 2-tiered triage and trauma team activation protocol. *Ann Emerg Med* 1998;32(4):436–441.
Simon B, Gabor R, Letourneau P. Secondary triage of the injured pediatric patient within the trauma center: Support for a selective resource-sparing two-stage system. *Ped Emerg Care* 2004;20(1):5–11.
Terregino CA, Reid JC, Marburger RK, et al. Secondary emergency department triage (supertriage) and trauma team activation: Effects on resource utilization and patient care. *J Trauma* 1997;43(1):61–64.
Thompson CT, Bickell WH, Siemens RA. Community hospital Level II trauma center outcome. *J Trauma* 1992;32(3):336–343.

ORGANIZATION PRIOR TO TRAUMA PATIENT ARRIVAL

WILLIAM S. HOFF

9

I. THE TRAUMA RESPONSE

A. Institutional capability. The resources available to manage trauma patients is institution-specific. The American College of Surgeons Committee on Trauma has designated trauma centers as follows:

1. Level I. Provides a 24-hour, in-house trauma team with the ability to fully resuscitate injured patients and provide definitive surgical care for the most complex injuries. The trauma team is usually led by an attending trauma surgeon, emergency physician, or senior-level surgical resident. Level I centers are typically located in population-dense areas. In addition to the clinical capabilities, Level I trauma centers also distinguish themselves through training, research, and prevention and outreach programs.

2. Level II. Clinical capabilities are similar to Level I centers. However, more specialized resources (e.g., cardiac surgery, microvascular surgery) are not required. Trauma team requirements are less stringent; an in-house trauma surgeon is not required, but must be available to meet the patient on arrival. Level II centers are frequently located in suburban areas.

3. Level III. These centers typically serve rural areas not easily accessible to Level I or II trauma centers. Surgical coverage must be available in a timely fashion and certain subspecialties (e.g., neurosurgery) are not required. Formal transfer agreements to higher level centers are paramount to optimize patient outcome.

4. Level IV. Designed to provide initial evaluation and assessment of injured patients, these centers are typically located in small hospitals or clinics serving the most remote areas. Surgical coverage is not mandatory and most patients will require transfer to higher levels of care.

5. Nondesignated. The majority of hospitals in the United States carry no specific trauma center designation. All hospitals should be aware of the resources available for management of trauma patients with clearly delineated plans for transfer of patients that exceed the "resource threshold."

B. Levels of response. All hospitals should have some established response to injured patients. In nondesignated hospitals, where a full trauma team is not available, an organized procedure (e.g., personnel, tasks, etc.) will facilitate resuscitation and optimize patient outcome. Many trauma centers use tiered levels of response based on established triage criteria. The composition of the trauma team varies based on the level of trauma response:

1. Full response (Trauma code, "code red"). Full trauma team response designed for patients with physiologic instability or who present with life-threatening injuries (e.g., abdominal gunshot wound).

2. Modified response (Level II trauma response, "trauma alert"). Modified response typically intended for stable patients with the potential for serious injury based on mechanism or anatomic findings. Exact composition of the trauma team will vary with the trauma center. Emergency physicians often provide the leadership role.

3. Trauma consultation. In most trauma centers, this response is reserved for low-energy or single system injuries in stable patients. Patients generally have their evaluation completed by the emergency physician prior to consultation with a trauma surgeon.

II. TRAUMA RESUSCITATION AREA
A. Physical plant
1. A dedicated trauma resuscitation area (TRA) is required for any Level I or II trauma center and should be considered in any hospital emergency department that receives a significant volume of injured patients or where injured patients may arrive without prior notification.
2. The TRA should be secure, with limited access to nonmedical personnel.
3. Convenient access to the operating room, radiology suite, intensive care unit, and staff call rooms are important considerations in TRA design.
4. The TRA must be sufficiently large to accommodate all members of the trauma team (i.e., 5–10 people). Ample space must be provided to allow free movement of prehospital providers into and out of the area, complete resuscitation, basic radiographic evaluation, orthopedic stabilization, and required emergency surgical procedures:
   - Airway intubation
   - Cricothyroidotomy
   - Insertion of central venous catheters
   - Tube thoracostomy
   - Placement of urinary catheters and nasogastric/orgogastric tubes
   - Resuscitative thoracotomy
   - Focused abdominal sonography for trauma (FAST)
   - Diagnostic peritoneal lavage (DPL)
   - Splinting of fractures
   - Wound irrigation and suturing
5. Other TRA considerations include:
   a. Lighting should be sufficient and must allow free access to the patient and easy movement of personnel and equipment through the workspace.
   b. Hypothermia must be actively prevented during trauma resuscitation. Specific measures to prevent hypothermia include individual TRA thermostats and overhead heat lamps.
   c. A mechanism to supply the TRA with uncrossmatched packed red blood cells (O-negative) should be implemented, especially for hospitals in which the blood bank is located a significant distance from the emergency department. Ideally, the laboratory or blood bank, as part of the trauma response, can deliver O-neg blood in a cooler to the TRA. This blood should be returned as soon as the need for early transfusion has been excluded.
   d. Each institution must have guidelines for resuscitation of multiple trauma patients within the confines of the defined TRA or emergency department.

B. Barrier precautions
1. Any **bodily fluid** should be considered a potential source of transmissible disease and, thus, barrier precautions should be mandated for all members of the trauma team. Specifically, non-sterile gloves, an impervious gown, surgical mask, protective eyewear, and shoe covers are necessary for all team members likely to come in contact with a patient.
2. **Barrier precaution items** should be available in a designated area adjacent to the TRA in full view of those who may enter the area. The trauma team leader or recorder should monitor and enforce compliance with barrier precautions.
3. Inevitably, **patients will arrive without notification.** In these cases, guidelines should be developed for relieving personnel who, by necessity, have entered the TRA without barrier precautions. Protected team members should provide rapid relief for those who have not had the opportunity to don protective equipment. The ultimate goal should be to minimize the total number of unprotected individuals during a given resuscitation.

C. Equipment. The minimal amount of equipment and supplies necessary to effectively resuscitate should be stored in the TRA. While frequent restocking may be necessary, eliminating superfluous inventory optimizes resuscitation space and facilitates standardization of care.

1. Equipment trays should contain only those instruments and materials absolutely necessary to perform a given procedure. Trays should be easily accessible, openly displayed, and clearly labeled for easy identification. One logical approach is to stock supplies in a head-to-toe configuration, with airway equipment and cervical collars stored near the head of the stretcher, thoracostomy trays near the midportion of the stretcher, and splinting materials at the foot of the stretcher.

2. Equipment necessary to manage immediately life-threatening conditions should be stocked close to the stretcher, in proximity to the trauma member most likely to use it (Table 9-1; Fig. 9-1).

3. Additional equipment and materials listed below can be stored along the walls of the resuscitation workspace. Large, portable equipment must be easily visible and accessible. Smaller items can be stored on shelves and counters or in designated trays or bins. Cabinets are not recommended, as closed doors impede rapid identification and ease of access.
   - Mechanical ventilator
   - Fluid warmer stocked with crystalloid solutions
   - Rapid infusion–warming device
   - Central venous catheter, pulmonary artery catheter kits
   - Instrument trays (e.g., basic surgical trays, plastic surgery trays)
   - Portable monitors
   - Suture cart
   - Traction devices
   - Preformed extremity splints
   - X-ray view boxes/monitors
   - Computers

4. A modest inventory of equipment and supplies to replace items used from other areas (e.g., angiocatheters, intravenous tubing) should be readily available.

5. Equipment and supplies should be stocked in a portable carrier that can be transported with the patient outside the TRA (e.g., radiology suite). Suggested contents include:
   - Nasal and oral airways
   - Cricothyroidotomy set
   - Suction equipment and tubing

TABLE 9-1	Immediately Accessible Equipment and Supplies
Head of Stretcher	Equipment for airway management, including multiple endotracheal tubes, oxygen, suction devices, oral/nasal airways, Ambu bags, and laryngoscopes
Tray #1	Equipment for intravenous access, intravenous tubing, phlebotomy, arterial blood gases
Trays #2 and #3	Thoracostomy trays, chest tubes (36 F, 40 F), appropriate suture material
Tray #4*	Diagnostic peritoneal lavage equipment
Foot of Stretcher	Chest drainage system (e.g., Pleurovac)
Left Side	Manual blood pressure cuff, electrocardiogram wires, pulse oximetry monitor

*Ultrasound machine.

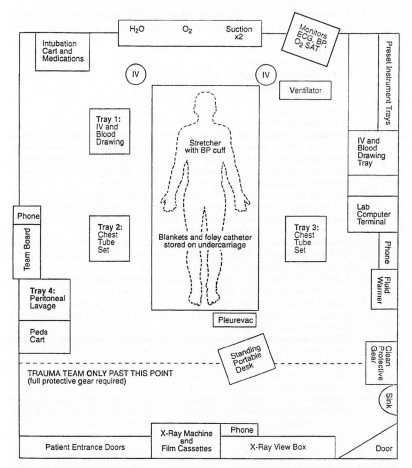

Figure 9-1. Layout of the trauma resuscitation area. (From Committee on Trauma, American College of Surgeons. *Resources for the optimal care of the injured patient*. Chicago, Ill: American College of Surgeons, 1999, with permission.)

- Pulse oximetry probe
- Manual blood pressure cuff
- Angiocatheters (14, 16, and 18 gauge)
- Intravenous tubing and adapters
- Syringes (3, 5, and 10 milliliters [mL])
- Phlebotomy supplies
- ABG syringes
- Irrigating syringe (60 mL)
- Dressings, gauze, tape
- Medications (Section II.E)
- Additional forms for documentation
- Telephone and pager lists

6. Equipment and medications specific for pediatric resuscitation should be stored on a separate cart. The cart should be equipped with a Broselow tape for rapid calculation of medication dosages and selection of appropriately sized equipment.

7. A resuscitation stretcher should be oriented in the center of the resuscitation workspace. Several items ideally should be stored under the stretcher:
   - Patient gowns
   - Blankets
   - Small oxygen tank
   - Nasogastric/orogastric tubes
   - Irrigation tray
   - Automatic blood pressure cuff
   - ECG leads
   - Pulse oximetry leads

D. Medications. In addition to standard medications stocked on the code cart, a small inventory of medications should be stocked in the TRA for immediate use:
   1. Drugs including those for airway management (e.g., succinylcholine, sodium thiopental, etomidate, vecuronium, midazolam). Ideally, these agents should be stored in labeled syringes for instant administration.
   2. Sedatives, analgesics, and antimicrobials including lorazepam, morphine sulfate, fentanyl, naloxone, tetanus toxoid, cefazolin, and an aminoglygoside.
   3. Medications including diphenylhydantoin, 50% dextrose, methylprednisolone, mannitol, thiamine, magnesium, and calcium.

E. Communication. Reliable communication among members of the trauma team and to areas outside the TRA is essential. Communication in the TRA can be facilitated by the following:
   1. A podium provides space to document resuscitation events and serves as an area from which the flow of activity in the TRA may be observed.
   2. Marker board can be useful to record history, physical findings, and test results, and to display pertinent pager numbers of on-call consultants and ancillary personnel.
   3. **Efficient communication throughout the hospital is essential.** Dedicated extensions to the operating room (OR), computed tomography (CT) suite, blood bank, and the ICU should be available and use of these extensions should be limited to the trauma team. In high-volume trauma centers a laboratory computer terminal and digital radiology station should be considered.
   4. Communication between the trauma team and the OR staff is facilitated by a patient classification system. Such a system allows the OR and blood bank staff to organize resources and allocate personnel. The trauma patient classification system described in Table 9-2 provides a template. Early in the

TABLE 9-2	Trauma Patient Classification System
Class A	Unstable patient: requires immediate surgical intervention; no further injury evaluation (e.g., x-ray or laboratory studies) required. Immediate access to the operating room is necessary. Initiate massive transfusion protocol for blood and blood products (e.g., fresh frozen plasma, platelets).
Class B	Unstable patient: high probability of surgical intervention within 15–30 min. Some injury evaluation in progress. Massive transfusion likely.
Class C	Stable patient: probability of surgical intervention within 2 h. Complete injury evaluation (e.g., CT scan) in progress. Crossmatched blood or type and screen sufficient.
Class D	Stable patient: minimal probability of surgical intervention (minor injuries).

resuscitation, a single individual should be responsible for communicating the OR classification to responsible OR staff.

III. TRAUMA TEAM
A. Definition.
The trauma team is an organized group of professionals who perform initial assessment and resuscitation of critically injured patients. Team composition, level of response, and responsibilities of each member are institution-specific. Personnel are outlined as follows:

1. **Trauma surgeon**—a general surgeon with demonstrated training and interest in trauma care. In designated trauma centers, the trauma surgeon typically functions as the trauma team leader.
2. **Emergency medicine physician**—in many hospitals, the emergency medicine physician functions as the trauma team leader depending on the perceived severity of injuries. Ideally, these physicians have Advanced Trauma Life Support (ATLS) certification.
3. **Anesthesiologist**—a physician with special skills in airway management, sedation, and analgesia. In many trauma centers, this role may be fulfilled by a certified registered nurse anesthetist (CRNA).
4. **Trauma nurses**—emergency department nurses with specialized training and demonstrated interest in trauma care.
5. **Resident physicians**—residents in emergency medicine or surgery and trauma fellows may assume active roles in the trauma team. In Level I and II trauma centers, senior surgical residents and trauma fellows may function as trauma team leaders.
6. **Respiratory therapist**—therapist available to assist in the evaluation and management of the patient's respiratory status.
7. **Radiology technicians**—technicians available to obtain x-rays as indicated by the initial assessment and secondary survey.
8. **Surgical subspecialists**—although not typically involved in the initial assessment, surgical consultants (e.g., orthopedic surgeons, neurosurgeons) are vital members of the trauma team.
9. **Other personnel**—the trauma team may also include OR nurses, laboratory technicians, ECG technicians, chaplains, social workers, transport personnel, and case managers.

B.
During periods of high volume or high acuity (e.g., multiple victims), some internal mechanism should be available to mobilize additional personnel. In addition, appropriate on-call personnel must be available.

C. Roles and responsibilities.
With adequate prenotification, the trauma team can be organized and positioned prior to arrival of the patient. A generic positioning scheme is illustrated in Fig. 9-2. Specific responsibilities of respective trauma team members are outlined in Table 9-3.

D. Multiple patient scenario
1. All hospitals must be prepared for the arrival of multiple trauma patients, a situation that can overwhelm the resources of the best-prepared trauma center. The definition of "multiple patients" is institution specific, based largely on the depth of personnel and the availability of resources.
2. The trauma team leader is responsible for assigning available personnel to ensure safe and effective resuscitation of each patient.
3. A triage plan for positioning patients and allocating resources should be formulated based on the prehospital report and early clinical findings; for example:
   a. Position patients based on perceived needs (e.g., patients with severe head injury should be positioned near the mechanical ventilator).
   b. Assign a primary resuscitator for each patient under the direct supervision of a trauma team leader. Effective communication between these individuals is of utmost importance.
   c. Recruit additional personnel. Properly trained nursing staff, prehospital providers, and technicians are potential sources of immediate in-house assistance.

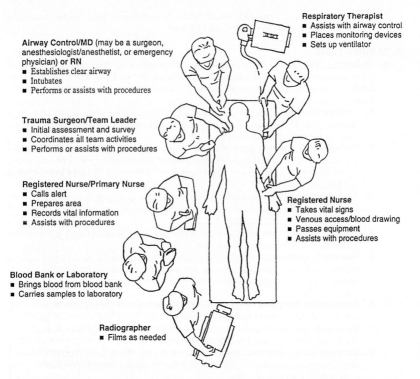

Respiratory Therapist
- Assists with airway control
- Places monitoring devices
- Sets up ventilator

Airway Control/MD (may be a surgeon, anesthesiologist/anesthetist, or emergency physician) or RN
- Establishes clear airway
- Intubates
- Performs or assists with procedures

Trauma Surgeon/Team Leader
- Initial assessment and survey
- Coordinates all team activities
- Performs or assists with procedures

Registered Nurse/Primary Nurse
- Calls alert
- Prepares area
- Records vital information
- Assists with procedures

Registered Nurse
- Takes vital signs
- Venous access/blood drawing
- Passes equipment
- Assists with procedures

Blood Bank or Laboratory
- Brings blood from blood bank
- Carries samples to laboratory

Radiographer
- Films as needed

Figure 9-2. Positions and roles of the trauma team members. (From *Resources for the optimal care of the injured patient.* Chicago, Ill: American College of Surgeons, 1999, with permission.)

On-call personnel (e.g., orthopedic surgeons) may also be mobilized to assist in the resuscitative phase.

   d. Reallocate personnel and resources based on results of each patient's primary survey.

   e. Move stable patients out of the TRA to other areas of the emergency department based on clinical assessment.

IV. TRANSFER OF PATIENT TO THE TRAUMA TEAM

   A. A formal report at the time of patient arrival signifies the transition of care from prehospital providers to the trauma team. Assuming adequate pre-notification, the trauma team can assemble prior to arrival of the patient to receive the pre-hospital report.

   B. With few exceptions (e.g., airway compromise), patients should be maintained on the transport stretcher until the pre-hospital report is completed. Once the patient has been moved to the resuscitation stretcher, the trauma team may not devote full attention to the report.

   C. The pre-hospital report should be a concise (30–45 seconds) summary given by a single pre-hospital provider and directed to the entire trauma team.

   D. Following the report and transfer of the patient, a designated member of the trauma team should attempt to get a more detailed history from the prehospital providers.

TABLE 9-3	Trauma Team Roles and Responsibilities

Trauma Team Leader	Primarily responsible for directing individual trauma team members, coordinating events of the resuscitation, and formulating the plans for definitive management. In larger centers, especially those with training programs, the trauma team leader may be an attending trauma surgeon, emergency physician, trauma fellow, or senior or chief surgical resident (i.e., command physician).
Primary Resuscitator	A surgeon or emergency medicine physician responsible for the initial assessment and performance of surgical procedures, as necessary. In smaller hospitals, this individual also assumes the role of team leader.
Airway Manager	Anesthesiologist, certified registered nurse anesthetist (CRNA), emergency physician, or surgeon primarily responsible for assessment and management of the airway. Required procedures can include endotracheal intubation, insertion of nasogastric or orogastric tubes, and assistance with cervical spine immobilization. Also expected to manage paralytics, sedatives, and analgesics relative to intubation and assist with medical management during code situations.
Assistant	The assistant is responsible for exposing the patient, placing electrocardiographic leads and pulse oximeter, and assisting with patient transfers. In addition, may be asked to assist with any necessary procedures. Depending on the institution, the assistant may be a physician (e.g., surgical resident) or, in nonteaching hospitals, a trauma nurse or emergency medicine technician.
Trauma Nurse	Prepares the trauma resuscitation area (TRA) for arrival of the patient. Serves as the patient's primary nurse during the resuscitative phase of care. Responsible for monitoring vital signs and performing select procedures (e.g., intravenous access, phlebotomy, urinary catheters). Assists with patient transfers, accompanies patient outside of TRA and reports to the receiving unit.
Recorder	Should be a nurse with extensive experience in trauma resuscitation. Responsible for documenting events of the resuscitation on an appropriate flowsheet. Facilitates communication and mobilization of additional resources (e.g., blood bank, operating room, consultants). May also assist in coordinating events of the resuscitation.
Respiratory Technician	Responsible for assessment of the airway and breathing and placement of appropriate monitoring devices (e.g., pulse oximeter). Assists airway manager with intubation and ventilator setup.
Radiology Technologist	Performs necessary radiographic studies. Assists with positioning the patient for the required studies. Processes films and returns completed radiographs to the TRA.
Laboratory Technician	Draws blood samples and transports samples to the laboratory for processing. Delivers blood to the TRA before arrival of the patient. Transports additional blood and blood products to the patient as necessary.
Chaplain/Social Worker/Case Manager	Assists with patient identification. Communicates between trauma team and patient's family.

✍ AXIOMS

■ Prior notification of patient arrival facilitates an organized response.
■ Barrier precautions should be utilized by all trauma team members who may come in direct contact with the patient.
■ Equipment and personnel placement in the TRA should be standardized.
■ During trauma resuscitation, verbal communication among trauma team members should be minimized.
■ The presence of an identified trauma team leader promotes efficiency and facilitates formulation of a definitive plan.
■ The trauma team leader should attempt to maintain a panoramic view of the resuscitation.

Bibliography

American College of Surgeons Committee on Trauma. *Resources for Optimal Care of the Injured Patient.* Chicago, Ill: American College of Surgeons; 1998.
Centers for Disease Control and Prevention. Recommendations for prevention of HIV transmission in health-care settings. *MMWR* 1987;36(suppl 2S):15–185.
DiGiacomo JC, Hoff WS. Universal barrier precautions in the emergency department. *Hosp Phys* 1997;33:11.
Driscoll PA, Vincent CA. Organizing an efficient trauma team. *Injury* 1992;23:107.
Fernandez L, McKenney MG, McKenney KL, et al. Ultrasound in blunt abdominal trauma. *J Trauma* 1998;45:841.
Gunnels D, Gunnels M. The critical response nurse role: An innovative solution for providing skilled trauma nurses. *J Trauma Nursing* 2001;7:3.
Hoff WS, Reilly PM, Rotondo MF, et al. The importance of the command-physician in trauma resuscitation. *J Trauma* 1997;43:772.
Maull KI, Rhodes M. Trauma center design. In: Feliciano DV, Moore EE, eds. *Trauma.* Norwalk, Conn: Appleton & Lange; 1996.
Moore EE. Resuscitation and evaluation of the injured patients. In: Zuidema GD, Rutherford RB, Ballinger WF, eds. *The Management of Trauma.* Philadelphia: WB Saunders; 1985.
Morgan T, Berger P, Land S, et al. Trauma center design and the OR. *AORN J* 1986;44:416.
O'Brien J, Fothergill-Bourbonnais F. The experience of trauma resuscitation in the emergency department: Themes from seven patients. *J Emerg Nursing* 2004;30:216.
Trauma Alert Policy, Ohio State University Hospitals, May 22, 1984. In: Chayet NL, Reardon TM, eds. *Trauma Centers and Emergency Departments.* Clifton, NJ: Law and Business Inc/Harcourt Brace Jovanovich; 1985.

ADULT TRAUMA RESUSCITATION
MICHAEL RHODES
10

I. INTRODUCTION

A. Resuscitation is an intense period of medical care in which initial and continuous patient assessment guides concurrent diagnostic and therapeutic procedures. As a dynamic period, resuscitation requires the trauma team to rapidly develop a differential diagnosis based on mechanism of injury, effectiveness of treatment, and results of available diagnostic studies. When possible, the attending surgeon and emergency physician should direct this crucial activity. The supervising physician must ensure that the optimal resuscitation space, personnel, and equipment are present.

B. Resuscitation of the trauma patient requires an organized, systematic approach utilizing a well-rehearsed protocol. Advanced Trauma Life Support (ATLS) is a single-physician resuscitation course of the American College of Surgeons that prescribes an initial approach to an unstable patient with life-threatening injury (Table 10-1). The principles of ATLS resuscitation are also applicable to the trauma center environment and should be supplemented by a **team approach** to the trauma patient. The approach of a trauma team should be multispecialty and protocol driven based on patient **"stability"** and mechanism of injury (blunt vs. penetrating) (Fig. 10-1). This chapter presents a team-oriented approach for trauma resuscitation.

II. PATIENT STABILITY

A. The term **"unstable"** has classically referred to physiologic parameters such as vital signs (pulse, blood pressure, and respiratory rate). Patients with abnormalities of these vital signs in essence are sending out a clear distress signal. However, in the context of trauma resuscitation, the definition of unstable can be expanded to include patients who are considered **metastable** (the capacity to change at any time). These patients exhibit subjective, objective, or anatomical findings that may predict need for specialized trauma care in the trauma center. These expanded criteria for *instability* and *metastability* are liberal and refer to the potential need for surgery or the intensive care unit (Table 10-2). Patients who meet these expanded criteria usually have injuries that are life or limb threatening. A subcategory of unstable patients, those who present *in extremis* (sometimes referred to as "agonal"), requires a tailored approach. All interventions in the patient in extremis must be therapeutic, rather than simply diagnostic. For example, evaluation of thoracic cavities in the multiply injured patient in extremis is best done with bilateral chest tube placement rather than chest radiograph. Chest tube placement is more expedient and will diagnose the presence of hemothorax or pneumothorax, but more importantly be definitive treatment for a tension pneumothorax.

B. Blood pressure response to initial fluid challenge is also a measure of stability. Hypotensive patients who sustain a normotensive response to the first 1 to 2 liters of fluid are responders and considered stable. **Transient responders** and **nonresponders** are **unstable** and should be treated accordingly. Their failure to correct abnormal physiology in response to treatment generally implies ongoing blood loss. Other causes for persistent hypotension despite fluid resuscitation include tension pneumothorax, cardiac tamponade, or neurogenic shock.

TABLE 10-1   Phases of Initial Assessment

Primary Survey (15 seconds)
- Airway with C-spine control
  - → Voice, air exchange, patency, cervical immobilization
- Breathing
  - → Breath sounds, chest wall, neck veins
- Circulation
  - → Mentation, skin color, pulse, blood pressure, neck veins, external bleeding
- Disability (neurologic)
  - → Pupils, extremity movement (site and type), voice
- Expose the patient

Resuscitation
- Generic—ECG leads, pulse oximetry, IV, draw labs
- Concurrent with life-threatening injuries identified on primary survey
- Include gastric and urethral catheters, or perform with secondary survey

Secondary Survey
- Head-to-toe examination (including spine)
- AMPLE history (A = allergies, M = medications currently taken, P = past illness, L = last meal, E = events related to injury)
- Imaging
- Second survey may be delayed until after OR in unstable patient or patient in extremis

Definitive Care
- Surgery (may be in resuscitation phase)
- Splinting
- Medications (3 A's): analgesics, antibiotics, antitetanus
- Consultants
- Transfer

Tertiary Survey
- Repeat primary and secondary surveys within 24 hours for occult or missed injuries.
- Create injury "problem" list with specific identification of physician handling each.

(Modified from American College of Surgeons Committee on Trauma. *Advanced Trauma Life Support Manual*. Chicago, Ill: American College of Surgeons; 2001.)

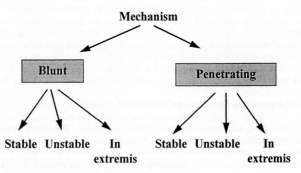

Figure 10-1. Initial emergency department triage.

TABLE 10-2	Criteria for Adult Unstable (and Metastable) Trauma Patient* (Blunt or Penetrating Trauma)

Altered Physiology
- Glasgow Coma Scale (GCS) score ≤14
- Pulse <60 or >120 beats/min
- Blood pressure <90 mmHg after 2-L fluid challenge
- Blood pressure >190 mmHg systolic
- Respiratory rate <12 or >24 breaths/min
- Poor gas exchange (e.g., SaO_2 <90%)
- Temperature <92°F (33°C)

Altered Physical Findings
- Paralysis
- Hoarseness/inability to talk
- Labored respirations
- Severe pain
- External hemorrhage site(s)
- Combative

Altered Anatomic Findings
- Severe deformit(ies): spine, neck, chest, extremities
- Penetrating wound from head to popliteal fossa

*Increased index of suspicion:
- Age >55 y
- Coronary artery disease
- Obstructive lung disease
- Liver disease
- Insulin-dependent diabetes mellitus
- Anticoagulation or history of coagulopathy
- History of mental illness
- Pregnancy

C. **Significant injury may also be suspected** from interpretation of key phrases verbalized by patients.
- "I'm choking"—airway dysfunction
- "I can't swallow"—airway dysfunction
- "I can't breathe"—ventilatory dysfunction
- "Let me sit up"—ventilatory dysfunction, hypoxia, cardiac tamponade
- "Please help me"—blood loss, hypoxemia
- "I'm going to die"—blood loss, hypoxemia
- "I'm thirsty"—blood loss
- "My belly hurts"—peritoneal irritation
- "I need to have a bowel movement"—hemoperitoneum
- "I can't move my legs"—spinal cord injury
- "Please do something for my pain"—significant injury

III. **MANAGEMENT OF THE STABLE ADULT WITH BLUNT TRAUMA**
   A. Assess for airway, breathing, circulation, and neurologic disability.
   B. Immobilize cervical spine.
   C. Administer O_2 nasally or by mask.
   D. Insert at least one peripheral intravenous (IV, 18 gauge or larger).
   E. Perform "stable patient" laboratory studies.
   F. Splint deformed extremities.
   G. Assess for occult injury.
      1. Head, neck, chest, abdomen, pelvis, spine, and extremities
      2. Selective rectal and pelvic examinations

H. Consider insertion of a nasogastric tube (unnecessary in most stable patients).

I. Insert urinary catheter (consider retrograde urethrogram prior to catheter insertion if patient is unable to void or pelvic fracture).

J. Limit IV fluid (e.g., 1 L in first 30 min). Fluid resuscitate the patient based on physiologic response to treatment.

K. Perform **select** radiologic studies as indicated by mechanism of injury and physical examination.

    1. Chest x-ray (usually routine)

    2. Cervical spine (C-spine)—no x-ray if no symptoms or signs and not intoxicated (Chapter 18)

    3. Pelvis—no x-ray if no symptoms or signs in an alert patient

    4. CT scan of head with any alteration in consciousness, headache, or history of anticoagulation

    5. CT scan of abdomen—if tenderness, macroscopic hematuria, or microscopic hematuria with signs and symptoms (Chapter 30)

    6. Ultrasound of abdomen (selective)—if abdominal tenderness

    7. CT chest (with CTA) if history of acceleration/deceleration injury (e.g., MVC >25 mph, fall >10 ft)

    8. CT angiogram of the neck (or carotid ultrasound) if seat-belt sign to neck

    9. Spine and extremity films (selective)—if tenderness

IV. MANAGEMENT OF THE UNSTABLE ADULT WITH BLUNT TRAUMA

  A. Assess airway (with C-spine immobilization).

    1. Patency, voice, stridor, foreign body, tongue, lacerations, O_2 saturation

    2. Treatment **options** (Chapter 11 gives specific indications)

      a. Administration of 100% O_2 (by mask)

      b. Suction

      c. Chin lift

      d. Oral airway (if obtunded)

      e. Nasopharyngeal airway

      f. Laryngeal mask airway (LMA)—very selective

      g. Endotracheal intubation

      h. Surgical airway

  B. Assess breathing.

    1. Facial expression (distress, anguish, flat), depth and quality of respiration (shallow or labored), skin pallor or cyanosis, use of accessory muscles (neck and abdomen)

    2. Trachea (midline, crepitus), neck veins (flat or distended), breath sounds (diminished or absent), chest symmetry (look for anterior or lateral flail, or splinting), respiratory rate, central cyanosis, O_2 saturation (pulse oximetry)

    3. Treatment **options** (Chapter 11 gives specific indications)

      a. Endotracheal tube

      b. Needle decompression of chest, unilateral or bilateral

      c. Chest tube(s), unilateral or bilateral

      d. Ventilator (manual or mechanical)

      e. Analgesia (systemic titrated opioids, inhalational opioids, intercostal block, epidural)

      f. Thoracotomy

  C. Assess circulation.

    1. Skin color, mentation, palpable pulse

    2. Quality of pulse, blood pressure, capillary refill, peripheral cyanosis, skin temperature, external hemorrhage, agitation, ECG monitoring, O_2 saturation

    3. Treatment **options** (Chapters 5 and 12 give specific indications)

      a. Two large-bore peripheral IVs, draw "unstable patient" labs.

      b. Central line if peripheral access unavailable—subclavian or femoral.

      c. If no IV access, consider adult IO (intraosseous) or cutdown at ankle or groin.

      d. One to 2 L of warmed Ringer's lactate IV as fast as possible (monitor response).

      e. With profound or persistent hypotension, early blood transfusion.

  f. Consider rapid focused abdominal ultrasound for trauma (FAST).
  g. If signs of persistent hypovolemia (e.g., thirst, base deficit, tachycardia, or hypotension), check for occult blood loss in one of six areas:
    i. External: (look under dressings), back, buttocks, occiput, axillae
    ii. Thoracic cavity: trachea, neck veins, stethoscope, early chest x-ray, chest tube
    iii. Abdominal cavity: palpation, ultrasound, diagnostic peritoneal lavage (DPL), exploratory laparotomy
    iv. Pelvis: physical examination, perineal laceration, unstable pelvic ring, pelvic binder, pelvic x-ray, arteriogram, or external fixation
    v. Extremities: fractures, particularly if bilateral or femoral
    vi. Spine: extensive fractures with hemorrhage (lumbar)
  4. If the search for bleeding is unrevealing, other **causes** of **hypotension** include the following:
  a. Tension pneumothorax
  b. Cardiac rupture and tamponade
  c. Neurogenic (e.g., spinal cord injury)
  d. Severe blunt cardiac injury with acute heart failure (very uncommon)

D. Neurologic disability
  1. Perform and document focused neurologic examination (Chapters 17 and 18) **before** patient is **intubated** and paralyzed: Glasgow Coma Scale (GCS) score, pupils, movement, and gross sensation of **all** extremities.
  2. Palpate head and spine (log roll).
  3. Treatment **options** (Chapters 17 and 18 give specific indications)
  a. Administration of O_2
  b. Intubation
  c. Mannitol
  d. Consider methylprednisolone (for blunt spinal cord injury with neurologic deficit)
  e. Emergency imaging of brain and/or spine
  f. Intracranial pressure monitoring
  g. Ventriculostomy
  h. Craniotomy

E. Extremities
  1. Palpate extremities and joints.
  2. Palpate pulses (Doppler if not palpable).
  3. Perform focused motor and sensory examination.
  4. Treatment **options** (Chapter 31 gives specific indications)
  a. Cover open wounds with sterile dressing.
  b. Apply direct pressure to control hemorrhage.
  c. Consider hemostatic composite pack for large bleeding wounds.
  d. Realign gross deformities and dislocated joints.
  e. Splint.
  f. Apply traction (femur fractures).

F. Place **nasogastric or orogastric tube** and **urinary catheter** at earliest opportunity **if not contraindicated** or **interfering** with assessment or stabilization of airway, breathing, circulation, or neurologic dysfunction.

G. Imaging in the **unstable blunt trauma patient**
  1. Suggested as time and clinical situation permit (in resuscitation area)
  a. Chest x-ray: Cassette under patient is preferred rather than under backboard; camera at maximal distance (lower resuscitation litter); inspiratory-hold.
  b. Cervical spine: If time permits, perform lateral (to rule out gross deformity only), delay full C-spine until stable.
  c. Pelvis: Anteroposterior (AP) to rule out site of occult hemorrhage.
  2. Selective (based on assessment and patient stability)
  a. Extremities
  b. Thoracic and lumbar spine

3. In general, **imaging** should be **delayed until airway, breathing, and circulatory dysfunctions** have been **stabilized**. Exceptions occur when chest x-ray or pelvic x-ray are needed to identify "occult" blood loss as previously stated.

   a. **CT scan (if stabilized hemodynamically). Sending the trauma patient if unstable for CT scan is dangerous**. Studies in the *metastable* trauma patient should be done only in CT scan units with full monitoring capability, easy full patient body viewing, and a nurse–physician team capable of performing any and all lifesaving procedures should a crisis arise (e.g., cricothyroidotomy, chest decompression, decision to operate). There is always risk in attempting to perform CT studies on the metastable trauma patient. Underestimating the patient's abnormal physiology will result in a patient decompensating in CT; never a good situation. Newer rapid helical or spiral scanners can image the head, chest, and abdomen rapidly allowing studies to be performed in select transient responders to fluid challenge when supported by clinical judgment and logistics.

      i. Head: if GCS <15
      ii. Chest: if suspected contusion or mediastinal anatomy uncertainty
      iii. Abdomen and pelvis: if signs or symptoms or unable to examine
      iv. Spine: if suspected by plain films or physical examination

V. MANAGEMENT OF THE STABLE ADULT WITH PENETRATING TRAUMA

A. Assess patient for airway, breathing, circulatory, and neurologic dysfunction.

B. Document **number** and **sites** of penetrating wounds.

C. Determine trajectory—this is vital in determining anatomic structures at risk from missiles, realizing that bullets often take an unpredictable course.

D. Treatment **options**
1. Administer O_2.
2. Secure at least one peripheral IV.
3. Selectively place nasogastric tube and urinary catheter (e.g., penetrating torso wound).
4. Perform "stable patient" **laboratory** studies.

E. Assess the patient for significant injury, depending on injury sites: physical examination and x-ray. Both plain film and CT are complementary to accurately determine precise trajectory. Diagnostic **options** include:

1. **Head:** CT scan without contrast.
2. **Neck:** CT scan with IV and oral contrast, AP and lateral x-rays, contrast swallow study, endoscopy, arteriogram, neck exploration. **(Caution: check airway repeatedly during diagnostic evaluations with low threshold for intubation.)**
3. **Chest:** chest x-ray; if transmediastinal, CT with IV and oral contrast, or angiography, bronchoscopy, esophageal contrast, cardiac window, echocardiography.
4. **Abdomen, back, or flank:** local wound exploration, DPL, ultrasound, CT scan with IV and oral contrast (including rectal), laparoscopy, laparotomy.
5. **Extremities:** pulses, motor and sensory examination, ankle brachial index, Duplex ultrasound, arteriogram, operative exploration.

VI. MANAGEMENT OF THE UNSTABLE ADULT WITH PENETRATING TRAUMA

A. Assess patient for airway, adequate gas exchange, circulatory or neurologic dysfunction.

B. Assess number and sites of penetrating wounds.

C. Determine trajectory—this is vital in determining anatomic structures at risk from missiles.

D. Treatment options
1. **Airway** (Chapter 11)
   a. Administration of 100% O_2
   b. Suction

   c. Chin lift
   d. Oral airway (if obtunded)
   e. Nasopharyngeal airway
   f. Endotracheal intubation
   g. Surgical airway (i.e., for shotgun wounds to face)
2. Breathing
   a. Needle decompression of chest, unilateral or bilateral
   b. Chest tube(s), unilateral or bilateral
   c. Ventilator (manual or mechanical)
   d. Thoracotomy or sternotomy
3. Circulatory
   a. Insert two large-bore IVs, draw **unstable** patient **laboratory studies,** consider large-bore central line, 1 to 2 L of warmed Ringer's lactate IV, blood transfusion with profound or persistent hypotension.
   b. IV access **above** and **below** diaphragm in penetrating **torso** trauma.
   c. Avoid IV placement such that the bullet wound is between the IV site and the heart.
   d. **If signs of hypovolemia occur (e.g., thirst, base deficit, tachycardia, or hypotension), search for sites of blood loss.**
      i. **Thoracic cavity:** tracheal deviation, neck veins, bilateral equal breath sounds, ultrasound, chest x-ray, chest tubes (bilateral if precise trajectory not known).
      ii. **Abdominal cavity:** exploratory laparotomy, ultrasound, or DPL (stab wounds).
      iii. If hypotension continues, look for cardiac tamponade, tension pneumothorax.
      iv. Occult spinal cord injury.
   4. Place nasogastric or orogastric tube and urinary catheter at earliest convenience.
E. Hemodynamically **unstable patient** with a **penetrating** wound to the **chest** may require chest tube(s) and thoracotomy in emergency department (ED) or operating room (OR).
   1. Chest tube may be diagnostic or therapeutic.
   2. If patient is hemodynamically unstable after chest tubes, perform thoracotomy in ED or OR.
   3. If stable after chest tubes and mediastinal or transmediastinal trajectory (Chapters 24 and 25), then perform the following:
      a. Ultrasound or pericardial window (repeat)
      b. Echocardiogram (transthoracic or transesophageal)
      c. Aortogram
      d. Bronchoscopy
      e. Esophageal contrast study
      f. CT scan with contrast in selected patients
F. The hemodynamically **unstable** patient with a **penetrating** wound to the **neck, abdomen,** or **extremity** requires prompt control of hemorrhage in the **OR.**

VII. MANAGEMENT OF THE PATIENT IN EXTREMIS
A. The patient in extremis presents with anatomic or physiologic findings that will result in **death within minutes** if not immediately corrected. These patients usually have signs of life such as reactive pupils, spontaneous respiratory efforts, spontaneous movement, or a palpable pulse, but otherwise present with profound shock or respiratory failure. This requires a **treat, then diagnose** approach (meaning **OR** now!).
B. If not intubated, **intubate.**
   1. If unable to intubate, **obtain a surgical airway.**
C. Penetrating injury, patient in extremis (Fig. 10-2)
   1. Neck
      a. Direct digital pressure if expanding hematoma or active bleeding

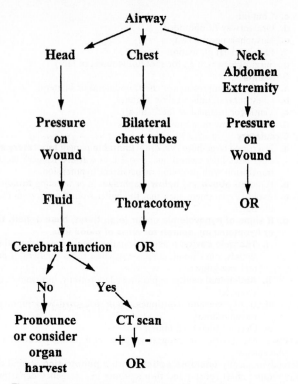

Figure 10-2. Penetrating trauma patient in extremis.

   b. IV fluid and blood
   c. OR
2. Chest
   a. Bilateral chest tubes
   b. IV fluid and blood
   c. Left thoracotomy or bilateral thoracotomy
   d. OR
3. Abdomen
   a. IV fluid and blood (avoid systolic blood pressure >80 mmHg until in the OR).
   b. Move to OR immediately.
      i. Left thoracotomy for aortic control within the chest if abdomen is expanding and blood pressure remains low despite volume resuscitation. Some prefer control of the aorta through a high midline abdominal incision.
4. Groin and extremities
   a. Applied pressure if expanding hematoma or active bleeding
   b. IV fluid and blood
   c. OR
5. Multiple penetrating wounds
   a. Applied pressure to sites of active bleeding
   b. Bilateral chest tubes
   c. IV fluid and blood

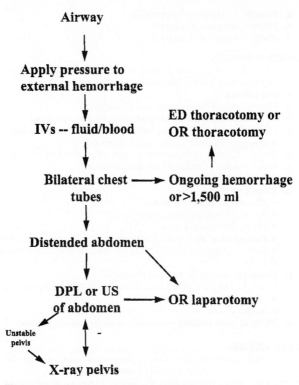

Figure 10-3. Blunt trauma patient in extremis.

    d. OR
    e. Left thoracotomy (Section C.3 above)
D. Blunt injury, patient in extremis (Fig. 10-3)
    1. Applied pressure to external hemorrhage (consider hemostatic composite pack for large wounds)
    2. IV fluid and blood
    3. Bilateral chest tubes
        a. If ongoing hemorrhage or >1,500 mL initial insertion of chest tubes, perform OR or resuscitative thoractomy.
    4. Ultrasound (US) or DPL of abdomen
        a. If grossly positive, move to OR.
        b. If negative DPL aspirate or US minimal or if no fluid, **x-ray pelvis**.
    5. X-ray of pelvis. One needs to identify the exsanguinating patient with pelvic fracture. (A small proportion of patients with major associated vascular injury must be taken to the OR.)
        a. If positive, place pelvic binder and move to angiography (consider aortography after pelvis).
        b. External fixation not usually appropriate for patient in extremis.
    6. Priorities with multiple injuries
        a. First → active thoracic hemorrhage or cardiac tamponade
        b. Second → abdominal hemorrhage
        c. Third → pelvic hemorrhage

      d. Fourth → extremity hemorrhage

      e. Fifth → intracranial injury

      f. Sixth → spinal cord injury

VIII. LABORATORY STUDIES

A. Recent data have suggested a more selective and cost-effective approach to laboratory studies in both blunt and penetrating trauma.

1. **Stable patient**
   a. Hemoglobin (Hb) and hematocrit (Hct)
   b. Blood ethanol (ETOH), depending on hospital protocol
   c. Urine dipstick for blood, human chorionic gonadotrophin (HCG) in women of childbearing age (urine or blood)
   d. Blood screening without cross-match unless condition changes
   e. Other studies as indicated by disease history

2. **Unstable patient**
   a. **Required**
      - Blood type and cross-match
      - Arterial blood gas and serum lactate
      - Hemoglobin/hematocrit
      - Prothrombin time, partial thromboplastin time, platelet count
      - Urine dipstick for blood, HCG for women of childbearing age
      - ECG
   b. **Selective** (based on hospital protocol)
      - Na, K, CO_2, Cl, blood urea nitrogen (BUN), creatinine, Ca^{2++}, Mg^{2++}
      - Serum amylase or lipase
      - Serum ETOH
   c. **Point of care testing**—available in many trauma centers

IX. MULTIPLE VICTIMS

A. When several trauma victims arrive in the resuscitation area simultaneously, priority should be given to the unstable trauma victims.

B. Trauma team leader (most senior physician) should assign physicians and nurses to specific areas, and designees should not cover several areas simultaneously.

C. The trauma team leader should rotate from patient to patient to oversee management, prioritize care, and supervise actions of individual trauma teams.

D. The team leader should decide the need for backup assistance or calling a disaster plan when demand outstrips immediate resources. The team leader should err on the side of calling for additional assistance.

AXIOMS

- The **unstable trauma patient** can be defined by potential requirement for surgery or the ICU as well as cardiopulmonary dysfunction.
- The trauma patient who remains unstable after initial resuscitation usually requires operative intervention.
- The trauma patient in extremis may require treatment before diagnosis.

Bibliography

American College of Surgeons Committee on Trauma. *Advanced Trauma Life Support Manual.* Chicago, Ill: American College of Surgeons; 2001.

Moore FA, Moore EE. Initial management of life threatening trauma. *ACS Surgery: Principles and Practice* [serial online]. February 2005; Section 7, Trauma and Thermal Injury. Available at: http://acssurgery.com.

AIRWAY MANAGEMENT
HENRY E. WANG AND DONALD M. YEALY

11

I. **GENERAL CONSIDERATIONS.** Ensuring adequate oxygenation, ventilation, and protection from aspiration are the cornerstones of airway management and the first priorities when treating the injured patient. Trauma patients have unique physiologic and anatomic challenges that significantly magnify the complexity of airway management. This chapter provides an overview of the basic principles of adult trauma airway management.

  A. Airway management consists of both basic (e.g., bag-valve-mask ventilation) and advanced (e.g., endotracheal intubation) airway interventions. **Basic airway interventions are more important than advanced interventions.**

  B. **Airway management must follow a clear, deliberate, systematic plan, including the anticipation for and use of alternative/rescue interventions.**

  C. **Assume all trauma patients have a cervical spine injury, head injury, and hypovolemia.** All airway management interventions must be performed with cervical immobilization.

  D. **Most trauma patients require the use of pharmacologic agents to facilitate endotracheal intubation (ETI).** Only properly trained and experienced personnel should use neuromuscular blocking agents (paralytics) to facilitate endotracheal intubation.

  E. **Airway procedures should be performed by the most experienced person available.** No other procedures should occur during intubation or other airway management efforts.

  F. **Airway management of the trauma patient is a team effort.** Communication between the airway manager and the trauma team leader is essential. The ultimate decision to perform endotracheal intubation or other advanced airway procedures should rest with the trauma team leader.

II. **ANATOMY.** The key structures that are visualized during endotracheal intubation include the epiglottis, vallecula, vocal cords, and aryepiglottic folds (Fig. 11-1). A cross-sectional view of airway structures during orotracheal intubation is depicted in Fig. 11-2. Anatomical landmarks for cricothyroidotomy are depicted in Fig. 11-3.

III. **BASIC AIRWAY INTERVENTIONS.** All patients should receive basic airway interventions. Basic airway interventions are more important than advanced interventions. All interventions must be performed with inline cervical immobilization. Two or three operators may be needed to maintain basic airway control.

  A. **In alert and spontaneously breathing patients,** apply a **non-rebreather mask** with 100% oxygen (10–15 L/min).

  B. **In semi-conscious or obtunded patients:**

    1. If possible, insert an **oropharyngeal** or **nasopharyngeal airway.** (Use extreme caution when inserting a nasopharyngeal airway in a patient with a suspected midface or basilar skull fracture.)

    2. Use the **jaw-thrust** maneuver to open the airway. Do not use head-tilt/chin-lift on trauma patients because of the risk of cervical spine injury.

    3. If the patient is spontaneously breathing, use a non-rebreather mask with 100% oxygen.

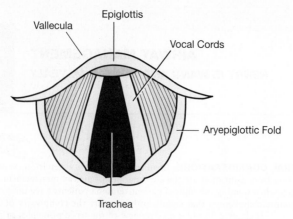

Figure 11-1. Pertinent laryngeal anatomy.

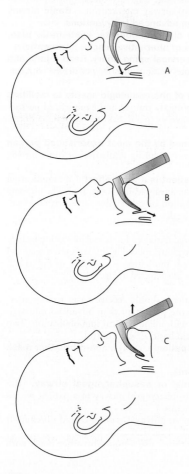

Figure 11-2. Laryngoscopy technique for orotracheal intubation of the trauma patient. Note that the cervical spine must be maintained inline—flexion and extension of the head are contraindicated.

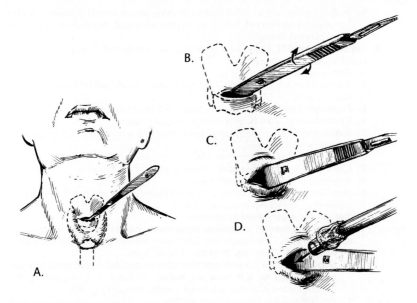

Figure 11-3. Cricothyroidotomy technique.
(From Trunkey DD, Guernsey JM. Cervicothoracic trauma. In: Blaisdell FM, Trunkey DD, eds. *Surgical Procedures in Trauma Management*. New York, NY: Thieme Inc; 1986:303, with permission.)

4. If the patient is not breathing spontaneously, if respiratory effort is inadequate, or if oxygen saturation cannot be maintained >90%, use **bag-valve-mask (BVM) ventilation.**
   a. BVM of the trauma patient requires at least two operators: one to perform a jaw thrust and seal the mask, and one to squeeze the bag.
   b. Consider applying cricoid pressure (or Sellick's maneuver) to lessen the risk of gastric distention during BVM ventilation (Chapter 6).
5. Use large-bore suction to keep the airway clear of blood and secretions.

IV. ADVANCED AIRWAY INTERVENTIONS—ENDOTRACHEAL INTUBATION (ORO-TRACHEAL).
After basic airway interventions have been instituted, advanced airway management may be considered. Endotracheal intubation (ETI) is the most common method of advanced airway management. ETI is believed to protect the airway from aspiration and to facilitate controlled ventilation. Orotracheal intubation is the most common and preferred method of ETI in trauma patients. Alternate/rescue and surgical airway techniques are described in Sections VII and VIII.

A. General considerations
1. ETI of the trauma patient is difficult and should be attempted by the most qualified operator available. There is high potential for ETI failure in trauma patients, and alternative strategies should be anticipated. Alternate/rescue airway management plans must always be formulated at the earliest stages of the patient encounter.
2. ETI must be performed with manual inline cervical immobilization. Flexion and extension of the head should never be used to facilitate ETI in trauma patients. Likewise, the sniffing position is contraindicated in trauma patients.
3. ETI requires the coordination of multiple tasks. At least three rescuers are usually needed to accomplish ETI on a trauma patient.
4. Most trauma patients will require pharmacologic agents (deep sedation or rapid-sequence intubation) to facilitate ETI (Section VI).

5. In the event of serious facial injury distorting oral or airway structures, it may be necessary to proceed directly to another advanced intervention (for example, a surgical airway).

B. Indications for ETI. These are general indications only and do not encompass all possible clinical scenarios.

1. Apnea or near apnea

2. Airway obstruction or respiratory compromise unrelieved with basic interventions

3. Depressed consciousness from head trauma or any other cause

4. Combativeness from head trauma or any other cause

5. Respiratory distress (severe tachypnea, increased work of breathing, cyanosis, hypoxemia, etc.)

6. Facial or neck injury with potential airway compromise

7. Chest wall injury or dysfunction with respiratory compromise

8. Persistent or refractory hypotension

9. Need for diagnostic or therapeutic procedures in patients at risk for deterioration (e.g., computed tomography, etc.)

C. Technique for orotracheal intubation

1. Prepare and test all intubation equipment *prior* to patient arrival.

a. For a typical 70-kilogram (kg) adult, use a **curved (Macintosh no. 3 or 4) or straight (Miller no. 3) blade**. Test the light.

b. **Use a no. 7.0 to 7.5 endotracheal tube on average-sized adult females and no. 7.5 to 8.0 tube on males**. Children may require smaller uncuffed tubes (Chapter 46). Insert a stylet, then test the cuff.

c. Prepare and test the large-bore suction.

d. Prepare the pharmacologic agents (Section VI).

e. Prepare an alternate/rescue airway plan (Sections VII and VIII).

2. Oral intubation requires at least three rescuers (Fig. 11-4).

a. Rescuer 1: The most experienced provider; performs laryngoscopy and placement of endotracheal tube.

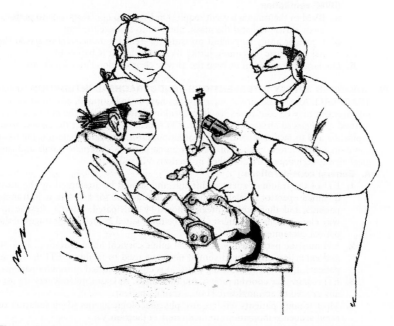

Figure 11-4. Positions of three rescuers for endotracheal intubation of the trauma patient.

    b. Rescuer 2: Performs manual cervical immobilization and applies cricoid pressure.

    c. Rescuer 3: Provides pre-oxygenation, assists rescuer 1 (handing equipment to intubator, etc.), and performs post-intubation ventilation.

3. Position the patient supine on the stretcher. **Rescuer 2 maintains manual cervical immobilization**. We recommend standing to the patient's side and facing the intubator—this gives the intubator more room while making it easier to use both hands to support the neck and jaw.

4. **Rescuer 3 should pre-oxygenate the patient** using a non-rebreather mask or BVM ventilation (Section III). Use 100% O_2 (10–15 L/min); if possible, optimize oxygenation and ventilation (spontaneous breathing or assisted) for 3 to 4 minutes; this technique maximizes pulmonary oxygen reserves. If possible, pre-oxygenate to $SaO_2 = 100\%$.

5. **Ensure a functioning intravenous catheter for drug administration.**

6. When directed, **rescuer 2 unfastens the cervical collar while maintaining cervical stabilization and applying cricoid pressure** (Sellick's maneuver; this technique minimizes gastric regurgitation and aspiration during intubation).

7. **Give sedative and/or paralytic drugs** (Section V).

8. **Perform the laryngoscopy** (insert the laryngoscope blade and expose the vocal cords) (Fig. 11.2).

    a. With a **curved (Macintosh) blade**, insert the blade in the right side of the patient's mouth and sweep the tongue to the left. Insert the tip of the blade in the vallecula (the space between the tongue and the epiglottis)—pressure placed on the hyo-epiglottic ligament will lift the epiglottis and expose the vocal cords. With a **straight (Miller) blade**, similarly insert the blade in the right side of the patient's mouth, but directly lift the epiglottis with the tip of the blade.

    b. Maintain in-line stabilization of the cervical spine. **Head-tilt/extension, neck flexion, and "sniffing position" are contraindicated in trauma patients**. Increased cricoid pressure (Sellick's maneuver) may be used to improve laryngoscopic view.

    c. **Limit the duration of each laryngoscopy attempt to 30 seconds. Stop earlier if SaO_2 drops <90%.**

    d. No other procedures should be performed while the laryngoscopy is being attempted.

9. **Insert the endotracheal tube.**

    a. Place the tip of the tube just past the vocal cords. In a typical 70-kg patient, the tube should be placed to a **depth of 21 to 22 centimeters (cm) for adult women and 22 to 23 cm for adult men** (denoted by depth markers on the tube) at the patient's teeth.

    b. Hold the tube manually—**do not release the tube until placement is confirmed and the assistant is prepared to secure the tube. Similarly, do not release cricoid pressure until proper tube position is confirmed**.

    c. Inflate the cuff with 10 mL of air, remove the stylet, and attach the bag-valve device.

    d. If tube placement fails, stop and reventilate with BVM. Re-attempt ETI. If unsuccessful after three total ETI attempts, go directly to alternate/rescue airway techniques. Proceed to an alternate/rescue airway sooner if clear barriers are encountered during initial ETI attempts.

10. **Confirm correct tube placement**. This step is essential—unrecognized tube misplacement (esophageal or hypopharyngeal) can be rapidly fatal. No singular method of monitoring or tube confirmation is infallible. Use a combination of focused examination and adjunct devices to confirm tube placement.

    a. Directed physical examination. Auscultate the epigastrium—it should be quiet. Auscultate the apices and bases of both lungs; breath sounds should be present and equal, and the chest should rise normally. Each of these findings can be misleading or difficult to appreciate, particularly under resuscitation conditions.

    b. End-tidal carbon dioxide detection. If the tube is correctly placed, carbon dioxide will be present in the endotracheal tube. This is likely the most accurate method for confirming tube placement. Note that these devices may be inaccurate in cardiac arrest or severe shock.

      i. The presence of expired CO_2 suggests correct tracheal placement. The absence of expired CO_2 means either incorrect placement (i.e., esophageal) or poor perfusion.

      ii. Colorimetric devices are widely used. These devices turn from purple to yellow in the presence of carbon dioxide. They are inaccurate when wet or exposed to air for extended periods.

      iii. Digital capnometers or **waveform capnographers** are the current standard. They are preferable because they are not susceptible to moisture and provide continuous information.

    c. Esophageal detector device (bulb detector or Toomey syringe)—may be used when CO_2 measuring devices are not available or as an adjunct for additional tube placement information.

      i. If using a bulb detector, squeeze the bulb and attach it to the endotracheal tube. Rapid and complete reinflation of the bulb (within 3–5 seconds) suggests correct tracheal placement.

      ii. If using a Toomey syringe, attach it to the endotracheal tube and aspirate quickly. Unimpeded aspiration suggests correct tracheal placement.

    d. If any uncertainty exists, laryngoscopy (direct revisualization) may be performed to visually confirm the tube passing through the vocal cords. **(Caution: this technique may be inaccurate, especially when airway structures are distorted from injury.)**

    e. Methods that should not be relied on for confirming tube placement: tube fogging (gastric contents can fog the tube), chest x-ray (identifies vertical position only, not intratracheal placement), and oxygen saturation (desaturation may not occur for several minutes after tube misplacement).

11. **Secure the tube** using adhesive tape, umbilical tape, or a commercial tube holder.

12. **Release cricoid pressure** and **replace the cervical immobilization collar**.

13. Place a nasogastric tube (oral if facial trauma is present) unless contraindicated.

D. Features suggesting difficult ETI. While the difficulty of an ETI is often relative to the experience of the operator, the following features are generally associated with ETI difficulty. The presence of multiple factors should lower the threshold for proceeding to alternate/rescue airway interventions. Note that this is not a comprehensive list of potential factors. In general, all trauma patients should be considered potentially difficult intubations.

    1. Anatomic features associated with ETI difficulty

      a. Obesity

      b. Short neck

      c. Small mouth

      d. Overbite or underbite

      e. Limited neck mobility

      f. Airway trauma or injury

    2. Clinical scenarios associated with ETI difficulty

      a. Head trauma or other major injury

      b. Hypotension

      c. Intoxicated or combative patient

E. Managing failed ETI efforts. ETI of the trauma patient is difficult. A common mistake is failing to recognize futile intubation attempts and failing to move immediately to alternate/rescue airway interventions.

    1. *Assume all attempts at intubation will fail.* Establish a clear alternate/rescue airway plan prior to the first ETI attempt.

    2. Reassess, oxygenate, and ventilate prior to each successive attempt.

    3. Change the ETI equipment, technique, or operator with each intubation effort—avoid repeating the same unsuccessful approach.

4. **Perform no more than three total laryngoscopy attempts** (regardless of the number of operators). If unsuccessful after three attempts, go directly to an alternate/rescue airway plan.

V. PHARMACOLOGIC ASSISTANCE DURING INTUBATION
A. General considerations

1. While deeply comatose or cardiac arrest patients can be intubated without drugs, **most trauma patients are awake, combative, or unrelaxed and must receive sedative and neuromuscular blocking agents to facilitate safe and rapid ETI**. A secondary purpose of pharmacologic assistance is to minimize hemodynamic response (e.g., blood pressure and intracranial pressure) to ETI, which can be stressful on a patient who is already in physiologic compromise from injury. The decision to use pharmacologic agents should be made on a case-by-case basis.

2. When choosing a drug regimen for the trauma patient, it is best to **assume that both hypovolemia and traumatic brain injury exist**. Although these conditions are often not present, this approach allows for a greater margin of safety because either condition can be difficult to exclude in the first minutes after patient arrival. Short-acting agents should be used to facilitate rapid recovery if ETI efforts fail.

3. The use of neuromuscular blocking agents (NMB) (rapid-sequence intubation, or RSI) is a helpful advanced technique but contains potential risks. A pharmacologically paralyzed patient has no airway tone or respiratory effort; if ETI cannot be readily accomplished, this condition can rapidly lead to death. **NMB agents should be used only by the most advanced and properly trained personnel**.

B. Preferred regimen—etomidate + succinylcholine.
The combination of short-acting sedative/inductive and neuromuscular blocking agents is preferred for injured patients. This will optimize intubation conditions while allowing for rapid recovery if ETI failure occurs. **Based on this consideration, while there are many potential drug regimens, we recommend the drug combination etomidate + succinylcholine**. Give both agents consecutively and in rapid sequence (IV over 3–5 seconds for each drug).

1. **Etomidate** (0.2–0.3 mg/kg IV; 15–20 mg in a 70-kg adult) facilitates deep sedation and has minimal side effects at these doses. Onset of action is 30 to 60 seconds, and duration is <10 minutes. Hypotension can occur with etomidate, particularly if severe hypovolemia is present, but is usually less frequent and profound than other agents. Etomidate is believed to be cerebroprotective.

   a. **Ketamine** (1–2 mg/kg IV; 70–140 mg in a 70-kg adult), a dissociative agent, is an alternative agent. Onset of action is 30 to 60 seconds, and duration of action is 5 minutes. Because it can raise intracranial pressure in head-injured patients, some authors discourage the use of ketamine in the presence of a head injury. Emergence reactions can occur with ketamine, but this side effect is of limited concern in the context of trauma resuscitation.

   b. **Fentanyl** (2–5 micrograms per kilogram [μg/kg] IV; 150–350 μg in a 70-kg adult), an opioid, is not an induction agent but may be used as an alternate for this role. Onset of action is 1 to 2 minutes, duration of action is 30 to 40 minutes. Fentanyl does not cause as much histamine release as other opioids and therefore is less likely to cause hypotension. Fentanyl can cause chest wall rigidity, but this effect is rare and has uncertain clinical significance in the setting of trauma resuscitation. Note that fentanyl provides no amnestic effect.

   c. **Barbiturates** can also be used for induction of isolated head injured patients; for example, thiopental (3–5 mg/kg IV; 210–350 mg in a 70-kg adult) or methohexital (1–3 mg/kg IV; 70–210 mg in a 70-kg adult). These agents have rapid onset (<1 minute) and short duration (thiopental, 5–10 minutes; methohexital, 4–6 minutes). We urge caution with this class of agents due to their hypotensive effects and do not use them in our trauma resuscitation area.

2. Succinylcholine (1–2 mg/kg IV; 70–140 mg in a 70-kg adult) is the preferred neuromuscular blocking agent for trauma airway management because of its rapid onset (1 minute) and short duration (5–7 minutes). Succinylcholine is a depolarizing paralytic; it causes transient muscle fasciculations prior to onset of paralysis. An important side effect of succinylcholine is hyperkalemia, which may cause cardiac arrest. While usually subclinical, this effect may be significant in renal failure patients, patients with burns >24 to 48 hours old, and patients with >1 week of paresis or motor dysfunction (e.g., CVA, spinal cord injury, etc.). Other relative contraindications to succinylcholine include globe (eye) injury and impending cerebral herniation.

  a. A variety of nondepolarizing neuromuscular blocking agents may be used where there are contraindications to succinylcholine. Note that these agents all have slower onset and longer duration of action. Two good choices are **vecuronium** (0.08–0.10 mg/kg IV; 5–7 mg in a 70-kg adult; onset 2–3 minutes, duration 30–35 minutes) and **rocuronium** (0.6–1.2 mg/kg IV; 45–85 mg in a 70-kg adult; onset 1.0–1.5 minutes, duration >30 minutes).

C. Pretreatment with other drug agents is often listed in RSI protocols but has unproven value.

  1. Intravenous lidocaine may blunt physiologic and intracranial response to ETI, but the benefit of this technique in trauma patients has not been demonstrated.

  2. Pretreatment with a nondepolarizing neuromuscular blocking agent may prevent succinylcholine fasciculations but offers little practical benefit.

  3. Atropine can help offset paralytic agent–associated bradycardia in pediatric patients (Chapter 46).

D. Postintubation paralysis and sedation

  1. Maintenance of paralysis may be required after intubation and may be accomplished by any conventional nondepolarizing agent. An initial dose of **vecuronium** (0.08–0.10 mg/kg IV; 5–7 mg in a 70-kg adult) will provide 30 to 35 minutes of paralysis. Repeating lower doses (0.01–0.02 mg/kg IV; 0.7–1.4 mg in a 70-kg adult) will provide an additional 12 to 15 minutes of paralysis. **(Caution: The effects of neuromuscular blocking agents are often cumulative, and repetitive dosages may cause prolonged paralysis.)**

  2. Provide concurrent sedation with a benzodiazepine such as **lorazepam** (0.025–0.05 mg/kg IV; 2–4 mg in a 70-kg adult) or **diazepam** (5–10 mg IV). **Propofol** (5–50 μg/kg/min constant infusion, adjusted as needed) may also be used.

E. Discouraged techniques

  1. Except for patients that are comatose, obtunded, or in cardiac arrest, we discourage intubation of trauma patients without drugs. Not only is this cruel, but it is technically difficult, is less likely to result in successful intubation, and may be hemodynamically stressful on a patient who is already in tenuous condition. We discourage the sole use of topical anesthetics (e.g., lidocaine, tetracaine, cetacaine) for the same reasons.

  2. We discourage "light sedation" only to facilitate ETI; for example, benzodiazepines (midazolam, lorazepam, or diazepam) or opioids (morphine, meperidine, hydromorphone). At conventional sedative doses, these agents have slow and unpredictable onset and often do not provide adequate intubating conditions. At higher deep sedation dosages, these agents can cause significant hypotension.

  3. It is important to recognize the patient who represents an anticipated difficult airway and high likelihood of failure of intubation with RSI. Examples are spontaneously breathing patients with major facial injuries and/or patients with significant bleeding into the airway. **RSI in this setting, making a spontaneously breathing patient an apneic patient, converts a difficult situation to a catastrophe.** In these situations, neuromuscular blocking agents are contraindicated (e.g., anticipated very difficult intubation, or the absence of personnel experienced with RSI), and we recommend the cautious use of deep sedation (anesthesia induction level) using etomidate (0.15–0.3 mg/kg IV; 10–20 mg in a 70-kg adult). Intubation must be by the team member with the most experience with difficult airways. The patient must be prepped and instrument trays open for immediate surgical airway if the attempt at awake (with sedation) fails. We discourage the routine use of this technique in trauma patients. However, patients who present with such tenuous airways must be recognized and managed appropriately.

VI. ALTERNATIVES TO OROTRACHEAL INTUBATION (ALTERNATE/RESCUE AIRWAYS).
As previously described, orotracheal intubation is the preferred method for ETI of trauma patients. In the event of failed ETI efforts, alternate or rescue airway techniques may be needed. Surgical airways are also considered forms of alternate/rescue airways and are described in Section VIII.

A. Combitube and **laryngeal mask airway (King Airway and LMA)** are alternatives to ETI. These devices are relatively easy to insert and are believed to ventilate almost as well as an endotracheal tube. (These alternatives are discussed in detail in Chapter 8.) Both devices may provide an adequate "bridge" airway until the execution of alternate ETI techniques or placement of a surgical airway.

B. Nasotracheal (nasal) intubation is usually performed in a "blind" fashion in patients who are spontaneously breathing. Although possible in many trauma patients, nasotracheal intubation is technically more difficult than orotracheal intubation, can cause significant airway trauma, and offers little advantage over oral intubation. Nasotracheal intubation is contraindicated in apneic patients or those with midface, nasal, or basilar skull fractures. A nasotracheal tube may cause significant sinusitis after 48 hours. Nasotracheal intubation requires the use of smaller diameter endotracheal tubes which may complicate ventilator management. Conversion of a nasotracheal to an orotracheal tube should be considered after the patient is stabilized; this may require specialized assistance from an anesthesiologist.

C. Other ETI techniques. There are a variety of alternate approaches to ETI; for example, tactile (**digital**) ETI, and **lighted-stylet** (transillumination) ETI. These approaches require specialized equipment or skill and may not be practical in the injured patient. Intubation over a flexible bronchoscope (**fiberoptic intubation**) requires special equipment and skill and is best left to specially trained operators (anesthesiologists who are facile with this technique). This technique is rarely appropriate in the trauma resuscitation area.

VII. SURGICAL AIRWAYS.
Surgical airways are required when basic interventions and ETI efforts are not likely to succeed or have failed. The equipment for these techniques is specialized and should be readily available in the resuscitation suite. Landmarks for these techniques are depicted in Fig. 11-3.

A. Percutaneous translaryngeal catheter insufflation ("needle cric" or "jet ventilation")

1. Technique
   a. Identify the cricothyroid membrane between the shield-shaped thyroid cartilage and the interiorly located, ring-shaped cricoid cartilage.
   b. Insert a large-bore over-the-needle catheter (12–14 gauge, preferably one with side holes specially designed for this procedure) with an attached syringe. Direct the needle caudad, penetrating the skin and cricothyroid membrane until air is aspirated.
   c. Thread the catheter into the airway and reaspirate to confirm intratracheal placement (evidenced by free gas withdrawal or "bubbles" if fluid is in the syringe).
   d. Attach a special jet insufflating device to the catheter. This device delivers high-flow oxygen at approximately 40 to 50 pounds per square inch (psi) (1 psi = 70 cm H_2O). This device can be a simple manually triggered one-way

valve or a more elaborate ventilator with multiple control settings. The hardware needed for jet insufflation is complex and must be identified and ready for use before the anticipated procedure, not improvised.

2. The trachea is used as a passive port for exhalation. Thus, the only absolute contraindication to jet ventilation is complete airway obstruction. Using the special jet ventilation device, tidal volumes of 700 to 1,000 mL can be achieved.

3. Contrary to popular misconceptions, correct jet ventilation can be used for unlimited periods of time, if used with the proper high-pressure source (40–50 psi) at an inspiration:expiration rate of 1:3 seconds.

4. Complications of jet ventilation include barotrauma, local hemorrhage, hypotension from overventilation and decreased venous return, inadvertent placement with resulting subcutaneous or mediastinal emphysema, hypoxia, hypercarbia, and dysrhythmias from prolonged attempts.

5. A transtracheal catheter can be easily converted to a conventional cricothyroidotomy. We recommend leaving the catheter in place and using it as a guide for identifying the cricoid membrane. A Seldinger-type guidewire can also be passed through the catheter to provide similar guidance.

B. **Cricothyroidotomy ("open cric")** is preferred to jet insufflation because of the simpler equipment, and the ability to provide optimal protection from aspiration and to place a large-bore airway for suctioning. Most clinicians are more familiar with this technique.

1. Technique (Fig. 11-3)

a. Palpate the thyroid cartilage—identify the depressed cricothyroid membrane immediately caudad.

b. Make a 3-cm midline, longitudinal incision over the membrane. In a thin neck with clear landmarks, it is acceptable to perform a transverse skin incision.

c. Spread the skin with fingers or retractors and identify key landmarks by palpation (thyroid cartilage, cricothyroid membrane). This procedure is performed by palpation, not visualization.

d. Make a transverse incision (1.5–2.0 cm) through the cricoid membrane. The procedure is essentially performed using tactile input; if the membrane cannot be seen, incise where the soft membrane is palpated. **Do not fracture the cricoid cartilage during the procedure**. Gain access through transverse spreading, not vertical.

e. Insert a no. 5 or 6 Shiley tracheostomy tube or a no. 5.5 or 6 endotracheal tube and inflate the cuff.

f. Attach a bag-valve device and confirm tube placement.

2. Complications include hemorrhage (avoid by limiting the size of incision and controlling bleeding with local pressure), misplacement, hypoxia secondary to prolonged procedure time, esophageal perforation, laryngeal fracture, and subcutaneous emphysema. Stenosis is often a problem if left in place for extended periods because of the narrow and contained diameter of the cricoid area; a cricothryoidotomy should be converted to a tracheostomy after the patient is stabilized.

3. Relative contraindications to cricothyroidotomy include laryngeal trauma or pediatric patients (age <10 to 12 years). Only needle techniques (jet ventilation) should be used on pediatric patients because the cricoid membrane is delicate and can be easily transected.

4. Percutaneous dilator-based cricothyroidotomy kits are available. These kits use a Seldinger guidewire technique with a series of dilators. These kits may be easier to insert by less experienced operators. However, familiarity with any technique is essential prior to the need to urgently attempt it.

C. **Tracheostomy** is generally reserved for nonemergent situations. A possible exception is the presence of laryngeal fracture or where the cricoid membrane integrity is compromised.

AXIOMS

- Basic airway interventions (e.g., bag-valve-mask ventilation) are more important than advanced interventions (e.g., endotracheal intubation).
- Airway management must follow a clear, deliberate, systematic plan, including the anticipation for and use of alternative/rescue interventions.
- Assume all trauma patients have a cervical spine injury, head injury, and hypovolemia. All airway management interventions must be performed with cervical immobilization.
- Most trauma patients require the use of pharmacologic agents to facilitate endotracheal intubation. Only properly trained and experienced personnel should use neuromuscular blocking agents (paralytics) to facilitate endotracheal intubation.
- Airway procedures should be performed by the most experienced person available. No other procedures should occur during intubation or other airway management efforts.
- Airway management of the trauma patient is a team effort. Communication between the airway manager and the trauma team leader is essential. The ultimate decision to perform endotracheal intubation or other advanced airway procedures should rest with the trauma team leader.

Bibliography

Benemouf JL, Scheller MS. The importance of transtracheal jet ventilation in the management of the difficult airway. *Anesthesiology* 1989;71:769–778.

Bivins HG, Ford S, Bezmalinovic Z, et al. The effect of axial traction during orotracheal intubation of the trauma victim with an unstable cervical spine. *Ann Emerg Med* 1988;17:25–30.

Roberts JR, Hedges JR, Chanmugam AS. *Clinical Procedures in Emergency Medicine.* 4th ed. Philadelphia: WB Saunders; 2004.

Woodard LL, Wolfson AB, Iorg EC, et al. Hemodynamic effects of etomidate for rapid sequence intubation (RSI) in emergency department trauma patients. *Acad Emerg Med* 1995;2:405.

Yealy DM, Paris PM. Recent advances in airway management. *Emerg Med Clin North Am* 1989;7:83–93.

Yealy DM, Plewa MC, Stewart RD. An evaluation of cannulae and oxygen sources for pediatric jet ventilation. *Am J Emerg Med* 1991;9:20–23.

VASCULAR ACCESS
MICHAEL D. PASQUALE
AND MICHAEL RHODES

12

I. VENOUS ACCESS
A. Flow through a catheter is determined by Poiseuille's law:

$$Q = \frac{r^4 \times (\Delta P)}{8 \times \text{viscosity} \times L}$$

where Q = flow in mL/min, r = radius, P = pressure gradient, and L = length. The best flow is obtained when dilute, warm (decreased viscosity) fluid is run through a short, wide catheter under pressure. The diameter of the catheter is the most important factor (Table 12-1).

B. Access to the vascular system should be obtained en route to the hospital or coincident with the primary survey in a horizontal resuscitation scheme. An intravenous (IV) line should not be placed with a vascular injury located between the IV access and the heart. For example, if a hypotensive patient has a gunshot wound to the upper right chest, IV access in the right arm can exacerbate bleeding from a subclavian vein injury.

C. Venous access is obtained in all trauma patients for initial blood sampling, fluid resuscitation, and administration of drugs.

D. Venous access is usually best obtained peripherally before consideration is given to placement of a central line.

1. Percutaneous

    a. Preferentially, two large-bore (14 or 16 gauge) IV catheters should be placed in large arm veins (e.g., the antecubital fossa). Blood should be drawn before initiation of fluid resuscitation via the catheter, provided the catheter has not been placed proximal to an infusing IV line. Sterile technique should always be used. Most peripheral lines placed for resuscitation in the prehospital setting or in the emergency department should be removed within 24 to 48 hours. These catheter sites need to be monitored for complications, particularly cellulitis and phlebitis.

2. Cutdown

    a. Surgical cutdowns are required infrequently in trauma patients, but can be invaluable in instances of difficult IV access, particularly in children.

    b. The **correct technique for venous cutdown** is essential for prompt, successful cannulation. Each cutdown site should be selected based on accessibility, vein size, and the urgency for venous access.

    c. Venous cutdowns for trauma have a higher infection rate and these lines should be removed when alternative access is secured.

    d. General technical principles

        i. The cutdown site should be immobilized, prepared, and draped.

        ii. Appropriate light and instruments should be available.

        iii. Mosquito hemostats and a no. 11 blade are recommended. In the small veins (<2 mm), venous wall elevators and dilators can be useful.

        iv. After anesthetizing the skin with a local anesthetic, a transverse skin incision is made, after which the fat and subcutaneous tissue is spread

TABLE 12-1	**Flow Rates Through Commonly Used Catheters or Infusion Systems**
Level I or rapid-infusion system	1,500 mL/min (high-flow tubing under pressure)
High-flow tubing*	250 mL/min
Standard tubing*	165 mL/min
7 F percutaneous sheath*	165 mL/min (high-flow tubing)
12-inch, central venous*	65 mL/min (14 gauge)
12-inch, central venous*	35 mL/min (16 gauge)
12-inch, central venous*	20 mL/min (18 gauge)
1.5-inch angiocatheter*	75 mL/min (16 gauge)
1.5-inch angiocatheter*	60 mL/min (18 gauge)

*Standard tubing with gravity flow at 1 m height.

in a longitudinal direction (i.e., along the course of the vein). A second hemostat or forceps is frequently necessary to secure the vein while it is being mobilized for a distance of approximately 1 to 2 cm.
- **v.** Two silk sutures are then placed under the vein as slings, tying the distal, looping the proximal, and holding each on tension.
- **vi.** With distal retraction, a partial venotomy is made in the anterior wall of the vein, with the 11-blade scalpel in a transverse fashion.
- **vii.** The catheter is then placed through the venotomy and secured with the proximal suture.
- **viii.** Special techniques for very small veins:
    - **a)** Consider using magnifying glasses or loupes.
    - **b)** Place a proximal tourniquet.
    - **c)** Use a longitudinal rather than a transverse venotomy.
    - **d)** Small pediatric feeding tubes (size 3 French [F] or 5 F catheter) have a rounded tip that can bluntly dilate the vein and negotiate proximal venous placement.
- **ix.** The skin incision should be carefully closed and dressed as a surgical wound.

- **e. Cutdown sites.** The saphenous vein is the preferred site for venous cutdown, with the arm veins as the secondary site.
    - **i. Saphenous vein at the ankle**
        - **a) Location:** 1 cm anterior and 1 cm proximal to the medial malleolus (Fig. 12-1)
        - **b) Advantages**
            - **1)** Performed at a location unencumbered by the rest of the resuscitation team
            - **2)** Low morbidity site
            - **3)** Safest site for the novice
        - **c) Disadvantages**
            - **1)** Small veins
            - **2)** Distal from the central circulation
            - **3)** Frequently inaccessible because of lower leg fractures, casts, splints, or military antishock trousers (MAST)
    - **ii. Proximal saphenous vein**
        - **a) Location:** 5 cm inferior to the inguinal ligament and 5 cm medial to the femoral pulse (or 5 cm medial to the midpoint of the inguinal ligament in a pulseless patient) (Fig. 12-2). This is a transverse **medial proximal thigh** incision and **not a groin** incision. The greater saphenous vein is somewhat variable in location because of the amount of fat in this area of the leg.

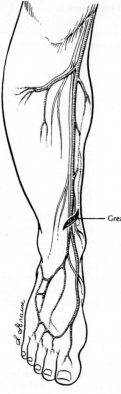

Greater saphenous vein

Figure 12-1. Saphenous vein cutdown at the ankle. (From Moore EE, Eisman B, van Way CW III. *Critical decisions in trauma.* St Louis, Mo: Mosby; 1984, with permission.)

b) Technique. After completing a 1- to 2-inch incision in the skin and subcutaneous fat, gentle cephalad and caudal retraction will help expose the vein. If performing this procedure alone, a small, self-retaining retractor is helpful.

In an adult, the vein can be identified rapidly by gentle palpation along the medial thigh fascia. The vein can frequently be mobilized longitudinally by spreading the hemostat under the vein while the index finger of the other hand is palpating the vein. The vein can then be immobilized over the hemostat, which can be left in place until the catheterization is complete.

Large catheters (8 F to 10 F) can be placed for rapid flow into the iliac vein. Less commonly, a no. 10 or 12 pediatric nasogastric tube (with its rounded tip) can be introduced into the inferior vena cava via the saphenous vein because the rounded tip can facilitate transversing the saphenofemoral junction. However, flow rate can be reduced by the length of the tube.

c) Advantages
   1) Large catheters can be placed quickly into the central circulation.
   2) Access can be obtained without interfering with resuscitative activities at the head and torso.
   3) Readily accessed in patients without a pulse.
   4) Can be obtained intraoperatively.
   5) Useful in experienced hands for infants and small children when no other access is obtainable.

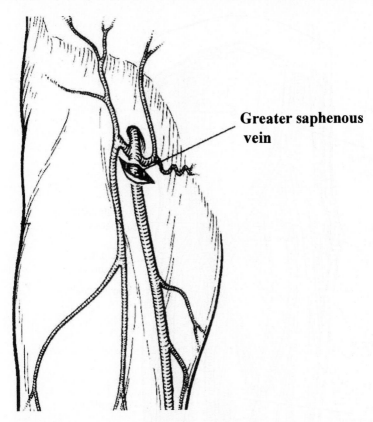

Greater saphenous vein

Figure 12-2. The greater saphenous vein is accessed at a location 1 inch inferior to the inguinal ligament and 1 inch lateral to the pubic tubercle.

    d) Disadvantages
        1) Requires experience and familiarity with the anatomy.
        2) Can be difficult in infants and children because of proximity to the femoral artery and vein.
        3) An incision in proximity to the groin is required.
iii. Antecubital region
    a) Venous cutdown in the arm is best obtained at a site slightly proximal to the antecubital fossa. Although veins can be identified in the antecubital fossa, this area is frequently inaccessible because of (*a*) previous attempts to obtain venous access and (*b*) because inadvertent injury to the brachial artery and median nerve can occur. The preferred sites are the basilic vein (located 1 inch proximal and 1 inch medial to the medial epicondyle of the elbow) and the cephalic vein (located 1 inch superior and 1 inch medial to the lateral epicondyle of the humerus) (Fig. 12-3). The technique of venotomy and placement is similar to that described for other sites.
    b) Advantage
        1) Easy access, particularly when the patient is draped

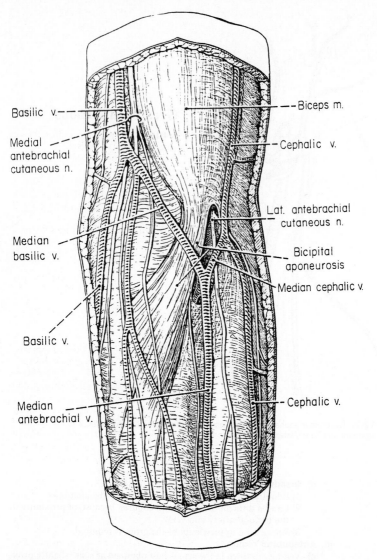

Figure 12-3. Upper arm cutdown.
(From Woodburne RT. *Essentials of human anatomy*. London: Oxford University Press;
1969:95, with permission.)

        c) Disadvantages
            1) More variable in location and somewhat more difficult than saphe-
               nous vein at the ankle
            2) In proximity to other members of the team
    E. Central access. Although central venous access was initially reserved for postre-
    suscitation stabilization, experience in many trauma centers has led to immediate
    central access for resuscitation of unstable trauma patients. With the advances of

the Seldinger technique (guidewire through needle, followed by catheter over guidewire), central resuscitation catheters (8 F to 12 F) placed over a dilator sheath have become common practice. These catheters provide very high flow rates because of their large diameters (2.5–4.0 mm), which are especially useful for rapid-infusion devices.

1. **Site**
   a. **Subclavian vein**
      i. **Advantages**
         a) Easily accessible and provides immediate filling of the heart from the superior vena cava.
         b) Allows measurement of the central venous pressure and access for subsequent placement of a pulmonary artery catheter.
         c) The site is easily accessible from the head of the bed for the anesthesia team (supraclavicular approach).
      ii. **Disadvantages**
         a) Initial resuscitation does not allow optimal positioning of the patient, such as the Trendelenburg position, placement of a roll between the shoulders, and rotation of the neck.
         b) Proximity of the pleural space, great vessels, and cervical nerve structures increases the risk of complications: pneumothorax, arterial puncture, hemothorax; and injury to the thoracic duct, phrenic artery, or brachial plexus.
         c) Radiologic confirmation of proper placement can be delayed.
         d) In proximity to other members of team.
      iii. **Technique** (Fig. 12-4)
         a) Ideally, the patient is placed in the Trendelenburg position with a roll between the shoulders, although this may not be possible in acute trauma resuscitation.
         b) If a cervical collar is in place, the anterior portion must be removed and the neck immobilized, to allow finger access to palpate the jugular notch. The subclavian area is prepared, and skin and subcutaneous local anesthesia is administered, using the needle to localize the subclavian vein.
         c) The access needle is then advanced beneath the clavicle, entering from lateral to medial under the middle third of the clavicle and aiming toward the index finger of the other hand, which is placed in the jugular notch of the sternum. The needle is advanced slowly, while hugging the undersurface of the clavicle and withdrawing on the syringe plunger until free blood flow is obtained.
         d) The guidewire should not be advanced unless blood flows freely in the syringe. It is usually helpful to advance the needle approximately 1 mm after obtaining rapid flow in the syringe before advancing the guidewire. The guidewire should be advanced slowly in short intervals, with the index finger and thumb close to the hub of the needle. If the guidewire meets resistance, the needle and guidewire should be removed together to avoid shearing the guidewire on the access needle.
         e) If the guidewire advances without resistance, the needle is removed, a small skin incision is made with the knife (11 blade), and the dilator and catheter sheath are advanced firmly but gently over the guidewire. **Some portion of the guidewire should be visible and secured at all times.**
         f) It is not necessary to advance the dilator its entire length because once it is in the vein, the catheter sheath can be advanced over the guidewire, which will help prevent perforation of the superior vena cava during placement.
         g) The ability to freely withdraw blood from the catheter sheath with gentle pressure should be ascertained before initiating IV flow.

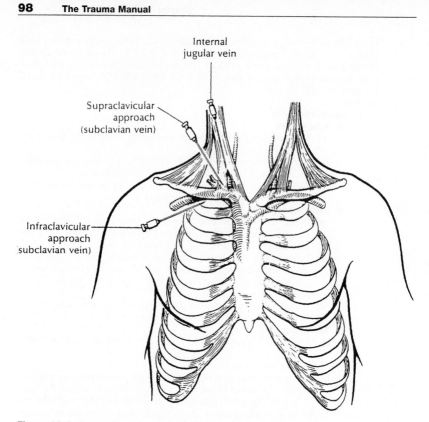

Figure 12-4. Approach to the subclavian and internal jugular veins.
(From Moore EE, Eisman B, van Way CW III. *Critical decisions in trauma.* St Louis, Mo: Mosby; 1984:513, with permission.)

Alternatively, free flow can be ensured by connecting the catheter to the IV delivery system and lowering the fluid bag toward the floor. If free backflow of blood is seen, IV fluids can be initiated. On occasion, the sheath will have to be withdrawn slightly to demonstrate blood flow.

h) A chest x-ray should be performed to confirm placement and rule out complications.

iv. **Complications**

a) **Arterial puncture.** When this occurs, the catheter should be withdrawn and digital pressure applied with the thumb below the clavicle and the index finger above the clavicle for a minimum of 5 minutes. Chest x-ray should be obtained to rule out a pleural effusion which would suggest bleeding.

b) **Pneumothorax** occurs in up to 5% of patients, even in experienced hands. Withdrawing air in the syringe can occur as a warning sign, but is present in only 20% of the cases in which pneumothorax occurs.

c) **Catheter malplacement into the internal jugular vein.** As long as free flow occurs, this catheter can still be used for resuscitation but should be repositioned at the first opportunity, which can usually be done without the need for an additional puncture.

Hypertonic solutions should not be infused until proper placement of the catheter tip in the superior vena cava is confirmed.

- **d) Exit from the superior vena cava** can result in life-threatening hemorrhage and is usually recognized by signs and symptoms of hemothorax, usually occurring in the opposite side of the chest.
- **e) Dysrhythmia,** particularly if the guidewire is advanced into the heart. In these cases, the guidewire should be slightly withdrawn. If the dysrhythmia does not resolve, the wire should be further withdrawn. **Caution** should be taken in patients with a known **left bundle branch block** because guidewire placement can precipitate a right bundle branch block leading to complete heart block requiring pacing.

  v. Subclavian site selection
  - **a)** No difference appears to exist in the success or complication rate between right and left subclavian catheter placement. This is more of an issue of judgment, comfort, and experience for the physician placing the catheter. It has been suggested that if a chest injury requiring a chest tube has already been identified, the catheter should be selectively placed on that side to avoid the possibility of an iatrogenic contralateral pneumothorax or injury. This intuitive approach has never been substantiated in the literature. More commonly, selection of the subclavian site is a practical determination based on resuscitative activities in progress on either side of the patient. For example, if a chest tube is being placed on the right side, it is much easier to simultaneously place a subclavian catheter on the left side.

- **b) Internal jugular vein.** In blunt trauma, the acute use of an internal jugular catheter is limited by the cervical collar, inability to properly position the neck, or inaccessibility to the head of the patient because of the airway team. However, in **penetrating trauma remote from the neck**, this approach has been found useful.

  i. Technique
  - **a) The Seldinger technique,** with the precautions noted previously for the subclavian vein, is the same. Most clinicians use the anterior approach through the supraclavicular triangle between the heads of the sternocleidomastoid muscle toward the ipsilateral nipple at an angle 45 degrees from the horizontal.

  ii. Advantage
  - **a)** Better access from the head when the patient is draped or having other resuscitative activity at the chest level

  iii. Disadvantages
  - **a)** Inability to position the neck and the presence of a cervical collar
  - **b)** Difficult to immobilize and maintain sterile dressing
  - **c)** Proximity of other members of team

  iv. Complications
  - **a)** Same as those for subclavian vein catheter (carotid artery injury rather than subclavian artery)

- **c. Femoral vein**

  i. Technique
  - **a)** The Seldinger technique, with placement of large-bore catheters through the femoral vein, is used frequently in trauma resuscitation. The femoral vein is located approximately 1 cm medial to the femoral artery just at or below the inguinal ligament.
  - **b)** It is generally easier for left-handed operators to access the patient's left femoral vein and vice versa.

  ii. Advantages
  - **a) Easy access,** particularly when other resuscitative efforts are occurring at the head or torso

b) Lower acute morbidity than the subclavian or internal jugular approach

iii. Disadvantages

  a) Difficult to locate the vein in a pulseless patient

  b) Does not guarantee high central flow in patients with intraabdominal or pelvic vascular injury

  c) Clot can develop at the puncture (frequently non-occlusive)

F. Intraosseous access

  1. In children who are aged 6 years or younger, intraosseous access should be established if reliable venous access cannot be established percutaneously after two attempts. It should be used for the initial resuscitation and should be removed when the child has been stabilized and alternative access has been obtained.

  2. In general, any IV drug or fluid required during the resuscitation of children can be safely administered by the intraosseous route. Fluids generally need to be administered under pressure. Specifically designed needles (modified bone marrow aspiration needles) have been developed for this purpose.

  3. Sites

  a. The flat anteromedial surface of the proximal tibia, approximately 1 to 3 cm below the tibial tuberosity, is the preferred site for infants and children, because the marrow cavity in this location is very large and the potential for injury to adjacent tissues is minimal (Fig. 12-5).

  b. The anterior surface of the distal tibia, approximately 2 cm above the medial malleolus, is the second preferred site.

  c. The anterior surface of the distal femur has also been used.

  4. Technique

  a. Identify the insertion site and prepare and drape in a sterile fashion.

  b. Infiltrate skin and subcutaneous with local anesthesia.

  c. Check the needle to ensure that the bevels of the outer needle and internal stylet are properly aligned.

  d. Stabilize the extremity without placing your hand behind the insertion site.

  e. Place the needle through the skin over the identified site, advancing the needle through the bony cortex, directing the needle perpendicular (90 degrees

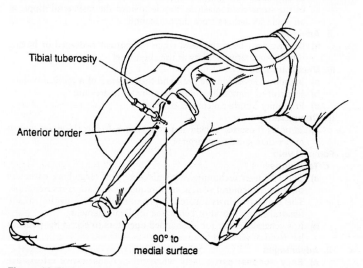

Tibial tuberosity

Anterior border

90° to medial surface

Figure 12-5. Intraosseous cannulation.

to the long axis of the bone). Use a gentle but firm twisting or drilling motion.

f. Stop advancing the needle when a sudden decrease in resistance to forward motion of the needle is felt. It is usually possible to aspirate bone marrow at this point. Aspiration of marrow should be followed by irrigation to prevent marrow obstructing the needle.

g. Unscrew the cap, remove the stylet, and stabilize the needle. A small inverted medicine cup (with the bottom removed) provides protection for the needle when placed over the site and taped in place.

h. Inject 10 mL of normal saline solution through the needle and check for signs of increased resistance to injection, increased circumference of the soft tissues of the calf, or increased firmness of the tissue.

i. If the test injection is successful, begin infusion.

j. If the test injection is unsuccessful, remove the needle and attempt the procedure on the other leg.

5. Complications are rare but include local cellulitis and abscess, osteomyelitis, fracture of the bone, pressure necrosis of the skin, compartment syndrome, epiphyseal plate injury, and hematoma.

II. ARTERIAL ACCESS. After the patient has been stabilized or during stabilization, insertion of an arterial catheter allows continuous blood pressure monitoring and frequent blood sampling. In general, the arterial line should be removed when the patient no longer requires continuous pressure monitoring and when frequent blood sampling is unnecessary.

A. Sites

1. The **radial artery** is the preferred site for arterial catheter placement, because the complication rate is lower than other sites. It has been suggested that the Allen test (simultaneous compression of the radial and ulnar arteries, followed by release of the ulnar artery, looking for a flush of perfusion in the hand) be performed before radial artery line puncture. This is not commonly done in most centers because the incidence of distal ischemia is rare, especially in young patients. However, this test should be considered in the elderly, especially under more elective conditions.

2. The **femoral artery** is a common line in trauma patients, but requires a somewhat longer catheter. The incidence of infection and distal ischemia is no greater than a radial artery catheter when used in initial resuscitation. However, after stabilization, these lines should be removed because the complication rate increases with time and the location can limit the mobility of the patient.

3. The **dorsalis pedis artery** is a more difficult site for percutaneous placement and is difficult to immobilize. This site is more useful in an elective environment, especially in younger patients with limited arterial access.

4. The **axillary artery.** Axillary arterial lines have been reported to be very successful in experienced hands in the elective intensive care unit (ICU) environment with low complication rates. They have not been used routinely as part of early resuscitation.

5. The **brachial artery should not be used** because it is an end artery with a relatively narrow lumen and a higher incidence of ischemic complications.

B. Technique

1. Immobilize the extremity and identify the pulse. Doppler or vascular access ultrasound can be helpful in this regard.

2. Prepare and drape the area in a sterile fashion.

3. Anesthetize the skin with a local anesthetic, even in the unconscious patient, to help reduce vasospasm.

4. A variety of arterial catheters have been developed and are typically 18 or 20 gauge for the radial artery and 16 or 18 gauge for the femoral artery for an adult. The incidence of thrombosis is related to the diameter of the catheter relative to the size of the artery.

5. Using the catheter-over-the-needle technique, advance the needle at a 30- to 45-degree angle through the skin at the site of maximal pulsation.
6. Two acceptable techniques have been described for the catheter-over-the-needle approach.
   a. The catheter and needle can be passed through both walls of the artery to transfix it, after which the needle is withdrawn, followed by slow withdrawal of the catheter until a pulsatile flow of blood is obtained. The catheter is then advanced slowly through the lumen of the artery. The catheter should not be advanced unless a pulsatile flow extends beyond the hub of the needle.
   b. A second technique is to puncture only the anterior wall of the artery, after which the catheter is slowly advanced until blood appears in the needle. The needle is then lowered to a nearly 10-degree angle from the horizontal, and the catheter is slowly advanced over the tip of the needle into the lumen of the artery.
   c. Both of these techniques can be facilitated by using a guidewire. The modified Seldinger technique uses a guidewire passed through a needle, followed by catheter placement over a guidewire. Commercial catheters with a self-contained guidewire are also available.
7. The catheter is connected to a **continuous** infusion of heparinized saline solution (the heparin can be withheld in patients with coagulopathy or head injury).
8. The catheter should be sewn into place and a sterile dressing applied.
9. Cutdown for arterial access is sometimes necessary. This is applicable only for the radial and dorsalis pedis areas. In general, a longitudinal skin incision is more useful than the transverse skin incision. The infection rate for an arterial cutdown site is high, and this site should be used only when no alternative exists. Small, curved forceps and vessel dilators (contained in cardiac catheterization kits) facilitate a successful arterial cutdown.

C. The incidence of complications from arterial access are low but can be serious. They include hematoma, cellulitis or abscess, systemic sepsis, ischemia, embolization, malposition, and nerve injury. The incidence of arterial thrombosis is proportional to the size of the catheter and duration of cannulation.

III. INITIAL FLUID RESUSCITATION

A. Details of fluid resuscitation are contained in Chapters 5, 10, 39, and 42.
B. Injury can result in a decrease in red blood cell mass and intravascular volume, with a reduction in cellular oxygen and nutrient delivery. This can worsen because of the increased metabolic demands of trauma. The goal of initial fluid resuscitation is to **restore effective circulating blood volume** and **avoid pulmonary and cerebral complications** of fluid overload.
C. **Key points** in initial fluid resuscitation include:
   1. Establish access in at least two venous sites. Examine all prehospital lines for catheter size, location, and function. Catheters in the back of the hand wrapped in gauze are commonly dislodged or infiltrated.
   2. Calculate the prehospital fluids as part of the initial resuscitation.
   3. Infuse warm fluid (40°C). Crystalloids (Ringer's lactate or normal saline solution) are the initial fluid of choice for most trauma patients.
   4. In hemodynamically normal patients without obvious injury, limit the initial fluid resuscitation (first hour) to 1 L in adults.
   5. In normotensive adults with tachycardia or obvious sources of blood loss, infuse 2 L of crystalloid as rapidly as possible. (Use some caution in this patient category in cases of an associated head injury.)
   6. In hypotensive adults who **respond** to initial fluid resuscitation, continue maintenance crystalloids (100–150 mL/h) after the initial 2 L.
   7. In hypotensive adults who are **transient** or **nonresponders** to initial fluid resuscitation, infuse **blood** as early as possible to avoid profound hemodilution from excessive crystalloid.

8. Blood component therapy (fresh frozen plasma and platelets) as part of initial fluid resuscitation should be given when clinical or laboratory evidence is seen of coagulopathy or in accord with the institutional massive transfusion protocol. Cryoprecipitate is usually reserved for documented hypofibrinogenemia. **Prophylactic** component therapy as part of initial fluid resuscitation has **not** been shown to be of **value**.

9. **Hypotensive pediatric** patients should have crystalloid infusion using boluses of 20 mL/kg, which can be repeated once. **Transient or nonresponders** should be given blood at **10 mL/kg**.

10. **Rapid-infusion devices** provide excellent tools for fluid resuscitation. Warmed fluids, including blood, can be infused at rates of up to 1.5 to 2.0 L/min. Care must be taken to monitor blood pressure, pulse, airway pressures, and arterial oxygen saturation to **avoid inadvertent fluid overload**.

11. Hypertonic saline solution has been shown to improve outcome in selected patients with head or thermal injury. Institutional protocols should be developed for safe and effective use.

AXIOMS

- Most trauma patients can be resuscitated with peripheral venous access only.
- Short, wide IV catheters and tubing are preferred.
- The technology for central venous access has lowered the threshold for placement of rapid-infusion catheters for resuscitation.
- Placement of large-bore catheters through central access during acute resuscitation should be done by experienced personnel, limiting the advancement of the dilator to avoid mediastinal or intrapleural hemorrhage, which can be fatal.
- Arterial lines can be placed as part of the early resuscitation to afford monitoring and frequent blood sampling. However, this can be delayed until the patient is in the OR or the ICU, using other noninvasive monitoring and sampling techniques in the resuscitation area.
- A venous line should not be placed at a site such that a penetrating wound is between the line and the heart. If the trajectory of a thoracic wound is not certain, place lines above and below the diaphragm.
- Establishing an IV cutdown on a small vein can be difficult. Light, loupes, and appropriate instrumentation and catheters are essential for success.
- Initial fluid resuscitation should be tailored to avoid the pulmonary and cerebral complications of fluid overload.

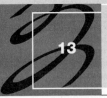

IMAGING OF TRAUMA PATIENTS
KEVIN MOLLEN AND MICHAEL P. FEDERLE

I. **INTRODUCTION.** The condition of the patient and the specific type of injury that is suspected determine the imaging modality that is most appropriate (e.g., plain-film radiography vs. computed tomography [CT] scan). In addition, the availability and location of imaging equipment as well as the clinical capabilities to support, monitor, and treat the patient during imaging are crucial in deciding how to proceed with imaging. Regardless of the type of imaging selected, the trauma patient requires constant monitoring and trauma team presence. **The trauma team should plan the sequence of the resuscitation to minimize time loss and avoid radiographs that are likely to be technically impossible or have minimal diagnostic yield.**

A. **Plain radiography** remains an essential component of the immediate evaluation of the injured patient, especially those with injuries to the chest or obvious fractures. The seriously injured patient should undergo lateral cervical spine, AP chest, and AP pelvis radiographs as a part of the primary survey. This set of films is commonly referred to as the **trauma series.** These films should be accomplished without moving the patient from the trauma resuscitation room. The need for further films or studies will be based on the mechanism of injury and findings during the primary and secondary assessments. Some authors advocate skipping the lateral C-spine series in patients without neurological deficit and routine use of CT of the neck.

Initial chest x-ray studies are usually performed in the supine position. After the initial stabilization of the patient, an upright film may be obtained to better assess for aortic injury, pneumothorax, or pleural effusion. In order to determine trajectory of missiles in the case of penetrating wounds, radiopaque markers should be placed over each skin penetration site and radiographs obtained.

B. **Computed tomography** has greatly advanced the diagnosis and management of the injured patient. The CT scan, which has become the standard modality used in the early diagnosis of head injury and pelvic fracture, provides a more comprehensive evaluation of chest injuries and maxillofacial fractures and allows for specific diagnosis of injury to the organs of the abdomen and retroperitoneum. The accuracy and speed of CT imaging has increased with development of spiral and multislice units. The increasing availability of multislice helical CT in or near the emergency department has expanded the role of CT in the trauma setting, allowing for a fast and comprehensive evaluation of the head, spine, thorax, abdomen, and pelvis, often in a single study. Newer **multidetector-row computed tomography (MDCT)** scanners allow for a thorough evaluation of the seriously injured patient in a single scan lasting only a few minutes.

C. **Magnetic resonance imaging (MRI)** has several advantages over CT scan, particularly in the evaluation of soft tissues. MRI offers the ability to obtain images in sagittal, coronal, and oblique planes without any contrast administration, and can be used to define shear injuries to the brain, injuries to the spinal column and cord, or vascular abnormalities that are not apparent on other films. However, MRI is time-consuming, allows minimal access to the patient during the procedure, and has limited application in the initial evaluation of the trauma patient. Although the duration of studies has decreased with the introduction of newer scanners, MRI has a limited role in the acute trauma setting.

D. **Ultrasonography** is being used more frequently in the management of trauma patients. The **focused abdominal sonography for trauma (FAST)** is routinely used in most trauma centers and has largely replaced the diagnostic peritoneal lavage (DPL) in unstable patients. A rapid diagnosis of hemoperitoneum can be made noninvasively in the trauma patient with a sensitivity of approximately 85%. Ultrasound (US) can also be used to assess the hemithoraces and, in experienced hands, peripheral vascular injury.

E. **Angiography** has been largely replaced by newer CT modalities in the diagnosis of vascular traumatic injury. It does, however, still play an important role in the definitive diagnosis of vascular injury, particularly when scans are equivocal or negative in the face of a high index of suspicion. In addition, its therapeutic role in such injuries has expanded. Angiography with embolization is the procedure of choice for difficult-to-access injuries (e.g., those to the vertebral artery, pelvic vessels, retroperitoneum) and selected vessels of the chest, abdomen, and large muscle masses.

II. SKULL AND BRAIN TRAUMA

A. **Plain-film radiography** (i.e., skull x-ray studies) has limited indications in patients with blunt head injury. Plain films are sometimes indicated for penetrating injuries of the skull to determine the course, location, or number of gunshots or foreign-body fragments, as well as possible depressed skull fragments.

B. Patients with a significant head injury, history of loss of consciousness (LOC), or postconcussive sequelae require immediate evaluation by CT scan. CT scan of the brain should be the initial screening tool for patients with symptoms indicating moderate to high risk of closed head injury. Technically, the CT scan images should be displayed with three windows: brain (shows edema, gray-white interface, ventricles, and cisterns), bone (outlines fractures, bony fragments), and blood (mass lesions, hemorrhage). Contrast enhancement is not used in the initial study.

1. **Common CT findings of brain injury**

   a. **Basilar skull fractures** can occur in 20% of craniofacial injuries, and CT is essential for complete evaluation. However, a negative CT scan does not exclude basilar skull fracture, especially with positive physical findings. Basilar skull fractures have significant associated morbidity, including cerebrospinal fluid (CSF) leak, damage to the internal carotid artery, and facial nerve injury. Multislice CT with multi-planar reconstruction of thin sections greatly improves the ease and accuracy of diagnosing basilar skull fractures.

   b. **Epidural hematomas** result from the rupture of arteries and large venous sinuses resulting in an accumulation of blood that strips the dura off the inner table of the skull. The temporal region of the skull is most commonly injured, resulting in a tear of the middle meningeal artery. The characteristic appearance of an epidural hematoma is a biconvex (lentiform) fluid collection that does not cross the skull suture lines but can cross the midline if venous sinuses are ruptured.

   c. **Subdural hematomas** result from the dissection of blood from ruptured veins that bridge through the subdural space. These hematomas are generally located between the dura and the arachnoid membrane. The typical subdural hematoma is a crescent-shaped fluid collection that conforms to the calvarium and underlying cerebral cortex. Recognition of atypical subdural hematomas is sometimes aided by coronal CT scan or repeat CT scan with enhancement.

   d. **Subarachnoid hemorrhage** is seen commonly in the basilar cisterns of patients following head trauma. Non-contrast-enhanced CT detects about 90% of subarachnoid bleeding within the first 24 hours, regardless of cause, as the higher density of blood replaces the water density of CSF in the cistern and sulci.

   e. **Shear injury or diffuse axonal injury (DAI).** Most brain parenchymal injuries are caused by shear-strain lesions; multiple and bilateral injuries are common. Linear and rotational acceleration–deceleration mechanisms cause shearing along interfaces of tissue of different densities, such as CSF and brain as well as gray-white junctions with the brain and meninges. Unenhanced CT scan may show multiple small focal hemorrhagic lesions with minimal mass effect, but it is an insensitive test. In a patient who is severely depressed neurologically with a relatively normal CT study, the possibility of diffuse brain injury (or cerebrovascular injury) should be considered. MRI is more accurate in diagnosing diffuse axonal brain injury.

f. **Cerebral contusions and intraparenchymal hematomas** are relatively common findings seen on brain CT after injury. Such injuries can coalesce or enlarge. Routine follow-up CT is recommended in these patients within 24 to 48 hours.

III. **FACIAL TRAUMA.** Facial injuries are seldom life threatening, but often are associated with more acute problems, such as airway obstruction, head or cervical spine injury, or globe injury. Occasionally, hemorrhage into the nose, nasopharynx, or mouth requires immediate attention.

A. **Plain radiographs** can be helpful for triage and initial management of facial injuries but are less comprehensive and confirmatory than other imaging modalities. Because of this, **CT is preferred to evaluate facial fractures**.

B. **CT scans of the face** can be obtained at the time of CT scan of the brain, but only as patient condition permits. Axial and coronal CT sections are obtained routinely in the stable patient. Computer-aided, three-dimensional (3D) reconstructions from thin axial sections provide optimal delineation of midfacial fractures and the spatial relationship of the fragments. These reconstructions have become much more available and valuable with access to multislice CT technology.

IV. **SPINE INJURIES.** Every patient with an appropriate mechanism of injury (MOI) must be considered to have a spine injury until such is proved otherwise, either radiographically or clinically.

A. **Cervical spine. An alert, communicative adult trauma victim without distracting injury who denies symptoms, such as neck pain, without drugs or alcohol on board, and has no signs, such as neck tenderness, may be "cleared" on the basis of clinical examination.** Patients with head injury often have accompanying cervical spine (C-spine) injuries, and radiographic evaluation of the C-spine is essential. The unconscious, intoxicated, noncommunicative, or multi-injured patient needs radiographic clearance. The cervical collar must not be removed until the C-spine has been evaluated and cleared.

1. **Techniques for obtaining adequate plain-film radiographs for C-spine clearance**

a. The plain-film lateral view of the C-spine is not adequate unless C1 through T1 are visualized. If the shoulders obscure the lower cervical and upper thoracic spine, caudal traction of the arms must be applied during filming, unless contraindicated on clinical grounds. Useful techniques to further define the C-spine include the "swimmer's view" or left and right oblique views. Failure to adequately visualize the cervicothoracic junction or the craniocervical junction will necessitate CT scan.

b. **Technically adequate lateral, anteroposterior (AP), and open-mouth odontoid C-spine films are the minimal views necessary to evaluate the C-spine radiographically.** A small percentage of patients with C-spine injury have only ligamentous injury and grossly normal static plain radiographs. Other studies, such as flexion-extension views, left and right oblique views, CT scan, or MRI, may be required to delineate these injuries or investigate areas that are not well visualized on plain films.

i. Active flexion-extension views are done voluntarily by the alert and cooperative patient only to the limit of pain tolerance. In the unconscious patient, fluoroscopic examination of passive flexion and extension of the C-spine can be performed. This examination requires a physician familiar with fluoroscopic technique and recognition of the ligamentous instability of the spine. Recent practice tends to use flexion-extension views less often and rely on CT with reformatting and MRI when needed.

  c. The purpose of the radiographic evaluation often is to identify possible C-spine bony injury that has not caused a neurologic deficit. In the hemodynamically unstable patient, protect and immobilize the spine, treat the condition causing instability, and clear the spine when the patient's condition permits. **Do not spend time attempting to clear the C-spine in a hemodynamically unstable patient**.

  d. The availability of a CT scan within or near the emergency department facilitates emergent evaluation of C-spine trauma. In particular, **MDCT offers the opportunity to obtain definitive and easily interpretable imaging of the C-spine quickly**. These scanners also offer greater flexibility in three-dimensional image reconstructing. Reliable coronal and sagittal reformations are easily obtained from the initial scan without the need for reimaging. CT scan is the imaging modality of choice for suspected fractures and fracture-dislocations of the spine in which plain films are not diagnostic. These scans are usually performed on an axial plane with thin (1 mm) cuts.

  e. MRI is the imaging procedure of choice for evaluation of injuries to the spinal column and cord but is a poor imaging technique for bone. In patients with myelopathy, MRI can establish the location, extent, and nature of the cord injury, as well as demonstrate the location and nature of nerve root injury in patients with radiculopathy. An MRI should be obtained to evaluate the spinal cord or suspected ligamentous injury, such as disruption of the posterior ligament complex due to anterior subluxation (whiplash).

B. Thoracic and lumbar spine. Plain films of the thoracic and lumbar spine should be obtained whenever signs or symptoms suggest a spine injury or when mechanism of injury indicates a high probability of spine injury. In the patient with distracting injuries (e.g., chest or pelvic fractures) or a concomitant C-spine injury, a complete thoracic and lumbar (T&L) spine series is necessary. Certain mechanisms of injury warrant radiographic evaluation of the T&L spine: automobile–pedestrian collisions, rollovers, ejections from a vehicle, collisions involving unrestrained automobile passengers, motorcycle crashes, or falls from a height.

  1. Radiographs must include two views of the area of concern: usually AP and lateral. Oblique views can be helpful, but CT scan directed to the suspected area of injury is preferred. At times, portable studies are not possible because of the patient's large size. In this circumstance, the patient should have these films done in the radiology department, with proper monitoring and trauma team presence. MDCT also offers the ability to reliably review areas of concern by reformatting images obtained from scans of the chest, abdomen, and pelvis. We routinely generate 3-D reconstruction of the CT thoracolumbar spine images as part of our chest/abdomen/pelvis CT.

V. CHEST TRAUMA

A. The chest x-ray is the fundamental and primary examination in chest trauma. A frontal AP chest radiograph should be obtained in all major trauma cases. Ideally, an erect chest film is obtained because the anatomic alterations caused by the supine position can simulate disease (e.g., a widened mediastinum or interstitial lung disease) and mask pleural effusions or pneumothorax. However, the upright position is often not possible. To decrease magnification artifacts, the distance from the x-ray tube (camera) to the film should be maximized to approximately 60 to 72 inches (5–6 ft) in either the supine or reverse Trendelenberg position.

1. **Acute aortic injury** should be suspected in any patient who suffers a significant deceleration injury. Among those patients who survive, the most common type and site of aortic injury is an incomplete tear through the intima and media of the descending thoracic aorta, just distal to the left subclavian artery. Mediastinal hemorrhage is present in most patients with aortic injury. However, 7% to 10% of patients with thoracic aortic injury have a normal admission chest x-ray study. In addition, only 10% to 20% of patients with plain chest film findings of mediastinal widening prove to have an aortic laceration.

   a. A patient who has radiographic evidence of mediastinal bleeding may be clinically stable enough to allow definitive imaging evaluation of the aorta. There are common radiographic findings on plain chest film that are associated with blunt thoracic aortic injury, including a widened mediastinum (>8 cm), obliteration of the aortic knob, aortopulmonary window opacification, left apical pleural cap, deviation of the trachea to the right, depression of the left mainstem bronchus, widened paraspinous stripe, and a left pleural effusion. Any of these findings alert the physician to the possibility of aortic injury. Due to limitations of plain-film radiography in the trauma setting, **any adult patient with significant blunt mechanism of injury should undergo CT evaluation of the thorax**.

2. **CT scan is now the imaging modality of choice for the definitive diagnosis of aortic injury.** Scanners using spiral and multislice technology are more accurate than earlier generation CT in the evaluation of the thoracic aorta and have been shown to accurately detect aortic injury. A complete scan of the chest plus the abdomen and pelvis can now be obtained without any increase in contrast exposure or time. CT findings of suspected aortic injury should be considered as representing:

   • Normal (no mediastinal blood, normal aortic contour)
   • Positive (mediastinal hemorrhage plus abnormal aortic contour)
   • Equivocal (mediastinal hemorrhage without an apparent aortic or arterial abnormality)

   Depending on other factors, including local experience and expertise and the degree of clinical concern, patients with unequivocally negative or positive studies can often be managed without aortography. Any uncertainty regarding aortic or major vascular injury requires catheter angiography, assuming adequate hemodynamic stability. CT may not be adequate in detecting injuries to the branches of the aortic arch. Therefore, a high level of clinical suspicion of an injury to the great vessels should lead to angiographic evaluation. Angiography remains an important diagnostic and therapeutic option for major vascular injury in trauma.

3. The diagnosis of **diaphragmatic rupture** is difficult to make on plain film. Apparent elevation and distortion of the hemidiaphragm (usually the left) can be evident along with ancillary findings such as pleural effusion or rib fractures. Disruption of the diaphragm, the presence of abdominal contents outside the contour of the diaphragm (i.e., abdominal organs lying in a dependent position near the ribs), nasogastric tube in the chest, and the "pinched" appearance of a herniated bowel are reliable signs. CT scan using sagittal and coronal reformations can be useful in appreciating the altered contour of the diaphragm, but even with CT scan, this diagnosis can be difficult. The optimal imaging procedure for diagnosis of equivocal diaphragmatic rupture is MRI in the sagittal and coronal planes. However, MRI should be employed in the trauma setting only after the patient has been stabilized. In the acute setting, with an unstable or marginal trauma patient, newer helical CT is the diagnostic procedure of choice.

4. **Most lung parenchymal and pleural space abnormalities** are adequately evaluated by plain radiograph examinations. CT scan can reveal unsuspected

pneumothorax or hemothorax, commonly seen on the upper cuts of an abdominal CT scan.

VI. ABDOMINAL TRAUMA

A. Penetrating trauma from gunshot wounds (GSWs) to the abdomen constitutes a special problem in preoperative evaluation. Chest and abdominal plain films are necessary to determine trajectory and localization of opaque foreign bodies and to identify injury in the stable patient. Large radiographs are used with radiographic markers placed over each skin penetration site. Two films are usually necessary, one under the chest and the second overlapping the chest slightly but covering the abdomen and pelvis.

1. Some authors advocate a "one-shot intravenous pyelogram (IVP)," which can assist in evaluating the GSW if the kidney or ureter has been injured. Specifically, it can prove both the presence and the function of the contralateral kidney. The yield however, is very low in the patient without hematuria. A more accurate study for the evaluation of renal injury is the **excretory phase** CT, which involves repeating the pertinent cuts after contrast has reached the collecting system. This accurate evaluation of the renal collecting system adds only a few minutes to the standard abdominal CT, and may also be valuable in evaluating blunt renal injury. The **technique** for an IVP is:

    a. Large-bore intravenous (IV) catheters are used to inject contrast material.

    b. 100 mL of 60% contrast is infused rapidly.

    c. A 2-minute postinjection film is obtained to show a bilateral nephrogram.

    d. Contrast material should be visualized in the renal collecting system and ureters on a 10-minute film.

    e. This study is contraindicated in patients with a severe intravenous allergy.

2. **Findings include:**

    a. Delayed function and visualization can be seen in renal contusion and minor parenchymal fractures.

    b. Nonvisualization of a portion of the kidney usually indicates injury to that specific area and may require additional studies (i.e., CT scan or angiography).

    c. Nonvisualization on one side is typical of major vascular injury such as renal artery injury, thrombosis, or renal pedicle avulsion. Unilateral nonvisualization prompts immediate arteriography or surgery to establish diagnosis.

    Many centers prefer plain-film evaluation and surgical exploration with on-table IVP. This is more expedient if the abdomen requires exploration and avoids unnecessary use of dye or delays in definite surgical evaluation and repair.

3. **Stable** patients with stab wounds to the back or flank can often be evaluated by **triple-contrast-enhanced CT scan.** Gunshot wounds that are thought to be tangential or extraperitoneal also can be evaluated with this study. Contrast material is administered orally, intravenously, and rectally prior to imaging.

B. Blunt trauma. In selecting the various diagnostic methods to evaluate blunt abdominal trauma, many factors are considered: clinical status of the patient, accuracy of the results, experience and expertise of those performing and interpreting the examination, cost, safety, and availability of the procedure.

1. **Plain radiography is not helpful for identification of significant abdominal injuries following blunt abdominal trauma.**

2. **CT scan has replaced diagnostic peritoneal lavage (DPL)** as the method for screening blunt abdominal trauma in **stable** patients. (**Focused abdominal sonography for trauma [FAST]** has replaced DPL as the screening tool for abdominal injury in **unstable** patients.) The major time factor in CT evaluation lies in the transport and positioning of the patient. Actual scanning and reconstruction of the images are done quickly. CT is accurate in identifying and quantifying hemoperitoneum, as well as identifying the site and extent of solid-organ injury; CT diagnosis of bowel injury is more challenging. A patient

who remains hemodynamically unstable following resuscitation is not a candidate for CT scan or other potentially time-consuming diagnostic imaging studies. In these patients, ultrasonography or DPL is recommended.

- **a.** CT provides valuable information regarding the depth and extent of abdominal visceral injuries, the extent of hemorrhage, and other criteria that correlate well with the American Association for the Surgery of Trauma (AAST) grade of injury and prognosis. A properly performed and interpreted CT scan reliably demonstrates active bleeding (extravasation), which usually indicates a need for surgery or transcatheter angiographic embolization.
- **b.** The technique for abdominal CT scan is
  - **i.** Intravenous contrast with or without oral contrast media. No IV contrast material should be given until the head scan is completed. The IV contrast (100–150 mL of 60% contrast) must be administered at a rate of 2.5 to 3.0 mL/second.
  - **ii.** The oral contrast material is a dilute solution (2%) of aqueous iodinated contrast medium (e.g., Gastrografin or Gastroview). Alert patients can drink the solution, whereas patients with an altered sensorium have the solution administered through a nasogastric or orogastric tube after evacuation of stomach contents. Although the safety of oral contrast has been demonstrated, there is still much debate about its utility in the trauma setting.
  - **iii.** If used, initial administration of "oral" contrast medium should be given as early as possible prior to the scan in order to facilitate bowel opacification and to minimize delays within the CT scan suite. Any delays in obtaining the scan in order to allow gastrointestinal passage of contrast material are not recommended.
- **c.** Routine scans are done with slices taken at 5-mm intervals from the nipple line (upper heart) to the upper thigh (lesser trochanter). Helical CT scanners allow faster acquisition of higher resolution scans. MDCT scanners may acquire contiguous 1.0- to 2.5-mm-thick sections. These are usually viewed as 5-mm-thick sections, while the thinner sections are utilized to construct high-resolution, sagittal, coronal, and 3-D images.

3. Ultrasonography (FAST) is useful in the diagnosis of hemoperitoneum. US is an alternative to DPL in the unstable patient, particularly if personnel with expertise in performance and interpretation are readily available. US is less accurate than CT in the diagnosis of injuries to solid abdominal viscera and does not depict bowel injuries nor the source of hemorrhage. **FAST** examination is used concomitantly with early resuscitation to rapidly determine hemoperitoneum, hemopericardium, or hemothorax. Due to the high false negative rate of this study, all stable patients with appropriate mechanism of injury should undergo abdominal CT.

4. The diagnosis of hollow viscous injury is probably the most challenging aspect of the radiographic evaluation of the trauma patient. CT has been proven to be highly accurate when there is a positive finding or in the setting of a completely negative scan. **If the CT is equivocal or there is a high clinical suspicion of bowel injury, close clinical monitoring with serial exams is mandatory.**

VII. PELVIC TRAUMA

A. The plain AP pelvic film is the key to the early diagnosis of pelvic fracture. If the alert and communicative patient is asymptomatic without distracting injuries, this x-ray study is not essential. This radiographic examination requires a frontal pelvic view that includes the iliac crests, both hip joints, and the proximal portion of both femurs. This can be supplemented by angled projections of the pelvis of the caudal ("inlet") and cephalad ("outlet") because these provide a more accurate delineation of the extent and relationship of pelvic fractures and joint disruptions.

B. **Traditionally, CT scan has had a minimal role** in the immediate evaluation of the acutely injured pelvis. However, helical CT is now an easy and fast way to accurately identify active hemorrhage associated with pelvic fractures. Therefore, it plays a valuable role in the identification of bleeding that will require intervention via angiography. CT scan is also the most accurate method for assessing the need for operation. Computer-generated 3-D images from the axial CT sections of the pelvis assist in preoperative display and reconstruction of complex pelvic fractures. No second scan is necessary; therefore using 3-D reconstructions will not delay any operative intervention. Pelvic CT scan is essential in determining:
1. Pelvic ring disruptions
2. The spatial orientation and relationship of complex or displaced pelvic ring fragments
3. The presence of joint instability
4. Intra-articular fragments
5. Fractures of the articular surface of the acetabulum or femoral head

C. Immediate pelvic angiography should be considered for patients with hemodynamic instability from pelvic fracture. Pelvic angiography assists in the identification of pelvic arterial bleeding sites secondary to fracture that are amenable to percutaneous transcatheter embolization. Between 6% and 18% of patients with unstable pelvic ring disruption have pelvic arterial injuries that warrant embolization. When pelvic arterial bleeding is found at angiography, embolization successfully occludes the bleeding artery in 80% to 90% of cases. Completion arteriography is required to ensure control of hemorrhage after therapeutic embolization. If the patient has a torn venous plexus or cancellous bone fragments are bleeding, angiographic embolization will not be of benefit, and immediate operative intervention may be required.

D. **Retrograde urethrography (RUG)** is essential in the evaluation of urethral injuries. Rupture of the bladder or urethral laceration occurs in approximately 20% of patients with significant pelvic ring disruptions. Therefore, RUG is the initial diagnostic procedure in patients with pelvic ring disruption and a clinical picture concerning for genitourinary injury. It is indicated for any male patient who has blood at the urethral meatus or a scrotal or perineal hematoma. When any of these findings are present, a RUG must be performed prior to insertion of a Foley catheter.
1. **Technique for RUG**
   a. An irrigating syringe filled with 10 mL of sterile 30% contrast material is inserted into the urethral meatus.
   b. The penis is stretched slightly to the side.
   c. The urethra is filled with the 10-mL bolus of contrast material.
   d. A film is shot just at the completion of the injection at a 30-degree oblique angle to demonstrate the prostatic and membranous urethra.
2. **Alternate technique**
   a. Pass an 8 F Foley catheter into the urethral meatus (approximately 3–4 cm).
   b. Position the balloon of the Foley catheter in the distal urethra with sufficient fluid to maintain a tight fit (usually 2–4 mL).
   c. Inject the sterile undiluted contrast material (10 mL) in a retrograde fashion, allowing for easy and complete filling of the urethra.
3. **Findings**
   a. **The most common site of urethral disruption** is the prostatomembranous urethral junction.
   b. **Extravasation of contrast** will be seen at the apex of the prostatic urethra, from the membranous urethra at the triangular ligament.
   c. **Partial visualization** indicates incomplete disruption.
   d. Complete disruption is indicated by an absence of contrast material in the bladder or prostatic urethra.

E. **If the urethrogram is negative, a cystogram is performed.**
1. **Technique for a cystogram**

    a. Pass a 16 F Foley catheter into the bladder.

    b. Gravity fill the bladder with 300 to 400 mL of sterile undiluted contrast material (i.e., Cystografin).

    c. Frontal and oblique radiographs of the bladder are obtained when the bladder is full.

    d. An AP post-void film is obtained to determine if an extraperitoneal bladder rupture is present.

  2. Findings

    a. Severe pelvic and lower abdominal pain, caused by extravasation of the contrast material, is a clinical indication of bladder rupture.

    b. In the unconscious patient, free flow of the diluted contrast fluid can indicate bladder rupture and intraperitoneal extravasation.

    c. These films detect bladder rupture with 98% accuracy.

VIII. IMAGING IN THE INTENSIVE CARE UNIT (ICU). The imaging techniques discussed in this chapter are applicable to the trauma patient in the ICU. Any trauma patients who are better cared for (monitoring, pharmacologic therapy, etc.) in the ICU may have many of their imaging studies performed in the ICU or as their condition permits.

A. Chest x-rays

  1. A daily chest x-ray may be indicated in any patient who has one or more of the following (can vary with hospital protocol):

    a. Acute respiratory failure

    b. Endotracheal intubation

    c. Positive end-expiratory pressure (PEEP) >5 cm H_2O

    d. FiO_2 >0.5

    e. Chest tube in place

    f. Under treatment for active disease (e.g., pneumonia, atelectasis, etc.)

  2. Selective daily chest x-rays in the ICU for the following patients:

    a. Weaning mode without change in cardiopulmonary status

  3. Chest x-ray is indicated after the following:

    a. Any acute cardiac or pulmonary deterioration

    b. Any invasive chest procedure (e.g., placement of a chest tube, central venous catheter, feeding tube, or endoscopy)

  4. Chest x-rays are not necessary when

    a. A central line was changed over a guidewire without difficulty

B. Computed tomography

  1. CT scan of the head may be indicated when an unexplained change occurs in neurologic status or as a follow-up for a previous CT scan of head injury. CT scan for encephalopathy or multiple-system organ failure has a low yield.

  2. CT scan of the chest can be helpful in delineating the pathology involved in acute pulmonary failure (e.g., consolidated lung, loculated collections, empyema).

  3. CT scan of the abdomen without history or physical examination suggesting intraperitoneal pathology is of little benefit. CT scan of the abdomen can be helpful if

    a. The patient has had previous surgery

    b. It is performed to confirm a presumptive clinical diagnosis

    c. It is necessary to direct a percutaneous study or procedure (i.e., abscess drainage)

    d. Missed intraperitoneal injury is suspected

    e. There is a suspicion of pancreatitis

C. Ultrasound

  1. Bedside US in the ICU is helpful to localize fluid collections and to diagnose acalculous cholecystitis.

  2. Duplex ultrasound can be useful in detecting venous thrombosis or arterial injury.

3. US is indicated if **pericardial tamponade is suspected**.

D. Fluoroscopy

    1. Fluoroscopy is being used in the ICU to guide the placement of invasive devices such as pulmonary artery catheters, central lines, inferior vena cava (IVC) filters, or enteral feeding tubes.

 AXIOMS

■ The more severely compromised the patient, the less time available for initial radiographic evaluation.

■ Specific images should be obtained to answer the most vital and highest priority questions.

■ Do not spend time attempting to clear the C-spine in an unstable patient.

■ Axial skeletal and pelvic films may not be indicated in an alert patient without signs or symptoms of these injuries.

■ Regional variations exist with regard to the availability of CT technology in emergency departments. However, MDCT has revolutionized the radiographic evaluation of the trauma patient, and there is a trend toward the institution of this technology in the ED.

Bibliography

Boone DC, Federle MP, Billiar TR, et al. Evolution of management of major hepatic trauma: Identification of patterns of injury. *J Trauma* 1995;39:344–350.

Butela ST, Federle MP, Chang PJ, et al. Performance of CT in detection of bowel injury. *AJR* 2001;176:129–135.

Dyer DS, Moore EE, Ilke DN, et al. Thoracic aortic injury: How predictive is mechanism and is chest computed tomography a reliable screening tool? *J Trauma* 2000;48:673–683.

Fabian TC, Davis KA, Gavant ML, et al. Prospective study of blunt aortic injury: Helical CT is diagnostic and antihypertensive therapy reduces rupture. *Ann Surg* 1998;227:666–677.

Federle MP, Courcoulas AP, Powell M, et al. Blunt splenic injury in adults: Clinical and CT criteria for management, with emphasis on active extravasation. *Radiology* 1998; 206:137–142.

Frankel H, Rozycki G, Ochsner M, et al. Indications for obtaining surveillance thoracic and lumbar spine radiographs in injured patients. *J Trauma* 1994;37(4):626–633.

Grogan EL, Morris JA, Dittus RS, et al. Cervical spine evaluation in urban trauma centers: Lowering institutional costs and complications through helical CT scan. *J Am Coll Surg* 2005;200:160–165.

Harris JP, Nelson RC. Abdominal imaging with multidetector computed tomography: State of the art. *J Comput Assist Tomogr* 2004;28:S17–S19.

Holmes JF, Mirvis SE, Panacek EA, et al. Variability in computed tomography and magnetic resonance imaging in patients with cervical spine injury. *J Trauma* 2002;53:524–530.

Mirvis SE, Shanmuganathan K, Miller BH, et al. Traumatic aortic injury: Diagnosis with contrast-enhanced thoracic CT—five-year experience at a major trauma center. *Radiology* 1996;200:413–422.

Novelline RA, Rhea JT, Rao PM, et al. Helical CT in emergency radiology. *Radiology* 1999;213:321–339.

Phillipp MO, Kubin TM, Hormann M, et al. Three-dimensional volume rendering of multidetector-row CT data: Applicable for emergency radiology. *Eur J Rad* 2003;48:33–38.

Ptak T, Rhea JT, Novelline RA. Radiation dose is reduced in a single-pass whole-body multi-detector row CT trauma protocol compared with a conventional segmented method: Initial experience. *Radiology* 2003;229:902–905.

Shackford SR, Wald SL, Ross SE, et al. The clinical utility of computed tomographic scanning and neurologic examination in the management of patients with minor head injuries. *J Trauma* 1992;33(3):385.

Shanmuganathan K, Mirvis SE, Sherbourne CD, et al. Hemoperitoneum as the sole indicator of abdominal visceral injuries: A potential limitation of screening abdominal US for trauma. *Radiology* 1999;212:423–430.

Shuman WP. CT of blunt abdominal trauma in adults. *Radiology* 1997;205:297–306.

Wechsler RJ, Spettell CM, Kurtz AB, et al. Effects of training and experience in interpretation of emergency body CT. *Radiology* 1996;29:1299–1310.

Yao DC, Jeffrey RB, Mirvis SE, et al. Using contrast-enhanced helical CT to visualize arterial extravasation after blunt abdominal trauma: Incidence and organ distribution. *AJR* 2002;178:17–20.

INTERVENTIONAL RADIOLOGY IN TRAUMA

PATRICK K. KIM AND C. WILLIAM SCHWAB

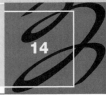

14

I. INTRODUCTION. The role of interventional radiology is rapidly evolving. As a diagnostic and therapeutic modality, interventional radiology (IR) is an important adjunct in every body region and for a wide variety of injuries.

II. GENERAL CONSIDERATIONS

  A. The IR suite should be staffed and equipped as an intensive care unit (ICU) setting. Where the trauma team or ICU team continue are aspects of critical management. Full monitoring with easy viewing, audible alarms, and user-friendly phone communication must be ensured at the patient's side and in the viewing room. Other personnel and resources should include critical care nursing, respiratory therapy, fluid warmers, external warming devices, and environmental control.

  B. IR access in the injured patient is typically via femoral approach. Imaging progresses from general to selective. Aortogram should be performed initially to identify the patient's anatomy, preexisting conditions, and unsuspected injuries. This is followed by a more selective "run" demonstrating the organ or region of interest. Finally, selective catheterization is performed for diagnosis and embolization as needed.

  C. If embolization is indicated, it is done as selectively as possible to minimize the amount of tissue under perfision and infarction. Embolization with absorbable gelatin (Gelfoam) slurry is temporary, allowing recanalization of the vessel after a period of time. Embolization with metal coils results in permanent occlusion. Embolization is highly effective (95% success rate) for hemorrhage control and has a low complication rate (approximately 5%). Postembolization rebleeding occurs rarely, and repeat embolization is usually effective.

  D. Risks of arteriography include groin hematoma/pseudoaneurysm, retroperitoneal hematoma, intravenous contrast allergy, and intravenous contrast nephropathy. The incidence of each complication is less than 5%. Anaphylaxis is rare, but airway and pharmacologic adjuncts should be immediately available in each room of the IR suite. Although studies have suggested that a history of seafood allergy does not accurately predict adverse reaction to intravenous contrast, most radiologists avoid routine use of intravenous contrast with this history. Cerebral arteriography carries a <1% risk of stroke. Regarding contrast nephropathy, oral N-acetylcysteine (NAC) and intravenous isotonic sodium bicarbonate may decrease the incidence of this complication, but in the trauma population, the benefit of either agent is not clear.

  E. Although arteriography is considered the gold standard of vascular imaging, it has limitations (Table 14-1). False negatives studies are due to vasospasm, spontaneous thrombosis, or technical factors that hinder selective catheterization. False positives arteriographic studies are often errors in interpretation due to overlying vessels or venous stasis.

iii. SPECIFIC CONSIDERATIONS

  A. Aorta and great vessels

   1. Accurate identification of thoracic aortic and great vessel injury is imperative to plan the potential operative approach and the details of circulatory support. Thoracic aortography and great vessel arteriography are still considered the gold

115

TABLE 14-1	Signs of Vascular or Parenchymal Injury

Arterial cutoff
Mural irregularities or flap
Laceration
Thrombosis
Dissection
Free-flow contrast extravasation
Stagnant intraparenchymal accumulation of contrast
Parenchymal blush
Stagnant arterial or venous flow
Diffuse vasoconstriction
Pseudoaneurysm
Arteriovenous fistula
Vessel displacement
Intraparenchymal avascular zones
Disruption of visceral contour
Displaced organ

(Adapted from Dondelinger RF, Trotteur G, Ghaye B, Szapiro D. Traumatic injuries: Radiological hemostatic intervention at admission. *Eur Radiol* 2002;12:979–993.)

standards for imaging vascular structures in the chest. Aortography generally includes frontal and left anterior oblique projections. The most common site of injury from blunt trauma is the proximal descending aorta at the ductus arteriosus.

2. In the traditional algorithm, the patient with an abnormal mediastinal silhouette on chest radiograph proceeded directly to thoracic aortography. Rapid, multi-slice chest computed tomography (CT) with properly timed contrast injection has become the screening study of choice for the thorax. Arteriography is reserved for patients whose CT demonstrates mediastinal hematoma, abnormality of the aorta or great vessels such as dissection or pseudoaneurysm, or is indeterminate for injury.

3. Patients with instability due to known or suspected thoracic aortic injury require immediate operative intervention. Experience in endovascular treatment of thoracic aorta is accumulating. At centers with experience in endovascular thoracic aortic techniques, stable trauma patients with known or suspected thoracic aortic injury must undergo a chest CT using a dedicated endovascular protocol. The three-dimensional reconstruction of the aorta is used to determine whether stent grafting is technically feasible, and if so, how to construct the stent graft. Although early reports have been promising, other results suggest that the technologic advancements of the stents for placement in the thoracic aortas of the younger trauma patients may be imperfect at this time. Proximal stent collapse has been seen in patients at several centers.

4. IR is useful in the diagnosis and treatment of subclavian artery injury, which is challenging to expose surgically. In the stable patient, endovascular stenting of subclavian and axillary artery injury compares favorably in terms of operative times and short-term outcomes. Also, IR intraluminal balloon occlusion has been described to obtain proximal control of subclavian artery injury, followed by operative exposure and injury repair.

B. **Carotid and vertebral arteries.** Arteriography is the gold standard in diagnosis of cerebrovascular injury. Traditionally, penetrating injury to zone I or zone III of the neck mandated cervical four-vessel arteriography (bilateral carotid and vertebral arteries). For zone I injuries, in the presence of normal physical exam and chest radiograph, routine arteriography has been questioned. Arteriography has utility in zone III by aiding operative planning and identifying injuries amenable to embolization.

TABLE 14-2	High Risk for Blunt Cerebrovascular Injury

- Severe cervical hyperextension/rotation/hyperflexion, especially with displaced or complex midface or mandible fracture
- Closed head injury with diffuse axonal injury
- Near-hanging with cerebral anoxia
- "Seat belt sign" of anterior neck
- Basilar skull fracture involving the carotid canal
- Cervical vertebral body fracture or distraction (except isolated spinous process fracture)

(Adapted from Biffl WL, Moore EE, Offner PJ, Burch JM. Blunt carotid and vertebral arterial injuries. *World J Surg* 2001;25:1036–1043.)

In blunt mechanism of injury, several patterns of injury have been suggested as being high risk for blunt cerebrovascular injury (BCVI) and probably warrant aggressive screening (Table 14-2). Arteriography remains a gold standard, but most centers have adopted CT angiography or magnetic resonance angiography (MRA) as the initial screening procedure.

C. Maxillofacial injury

1. Profuse hemorrhage from maxillofacial injury usually responds to direct compression, reduction of fractures, suture ligation, and nasal packing. Persistent maxillofacial hemorrhage may necessitate arteriography and embolization. Surgical ligation of the external carotid artery may not control hemorrhage because of extensive contralateral collateral flow. After arteriogram of the common carotid artery, selective arteriogram of the external carotid artery is performed, with selective embolization of bleeding branches of the external carotid artery. Of the branches of the external carotid artery, the most common source of hemorrhage is the maxillary artery.

2. Complications include stroke, facial nerve palsy, trismus, and tissue necrosis (including tongue).

3. Carotid artery–cavernous sinus fistula should be considered in patients with facial trauma and proptosis, abnormal visual acuity, and pulsating globe. Arteriography has the capability to diagnose and treat this condition by means of detachable balloon occlusion.

D. Peripheral vascular injury

1. In blunt or penetrating lower extremity injuries, arteriography is generally indicated when a pulse deficit is present on physical exam or when ankle-brachial index (or ankle-ankle index) is less than 0.9. Arteriography is generally **not** indicated for penetrating injury with "hard sign" of vascular injury (absent pulse, expanding hematoma, bruit/thrill, obvious distal ischemia). In these situations, immediate operative exploration is indicated.

2. Proximity or trajectory per se do not mandate arteriography if the pulse exam is normal and the ankle-brachial or ankle-ankle index are greater than 0.9.

3. The extremity with penetrating wounds at multiple levels or multiple projectiles (such as shotgun wounds or multiple bone fragment) and where multilevel injury is possible arteriography is usually indicated and helpful and may be warranted even with hard sign of vascular injury. Arteriography aids operative planning by identifying the level and extent of arterial injury.

4. In blunt injuries, arteriography is a useful adjunct in the evaluation of the mangled extremity. Absence of at least one-vessel flow into the foot or hand precludes limb salvage. Traditionally, posterior knee dislocation mandated routine arteriography, but recent literature questions routine arteriography in absence of ischemia, hard signs of vascular injury, or signs of peripheral embolization.

5. Each case should be individualized and if consults are used, orthopedic surgeons or vascular surgeons discussed.

E. Liver

1. Hepatic arteriography and embolization is a crucial component of the management of hepatic injuries. Arteriography assesses the anatomy of the individual's hepatic arterial system. The portal venous phase allows diagnosis of portal vein injury. Laparotomy followed by hepatic arteriography/embolization (or in the reverse sequence, depending on patient hemodynamics) should be considered complementary techniques to identify and control hepatic hemorrhage. Most hepatic vascular injuries can be controlled in the operating room with surgical techniques such as direct ligation and packing. In particular, perihepatic and intrahepatic packing is effective for venous injuries. However, after surgical control, arteriography with embolization is often the only effective method short of anatomic resection to control unrecognized and intraparenchymal hepatic arterial hemorrhage. Immediate postoperative hepatic arteriography/embolization should be considered in all patients who require perihepatic packing and damage control laparotomy for hepatic injuries.

2. In select patients, embolization can be primary therapy. Among hemodynamically stable patients with CT evidence of liver injury (and no evidence of hollow viscus injury), pseudoaneurysm, large hemoperitoneum, and extravasation of intravenous contrast are associated with a high failure rate of nonoperative management. These patients should undergo hepatic arteriography and embolization.

3. Routine arteriography for patients with grade IV or V hepatic injuries without contrast extravasation, pseudoaneurysm, or significant hemoperitoneum is controversial.

4. Patients chosen for initial nonoperative management of high-grade hepatic injury should be monitored in an ICU setting. Those who subsequently develop signs or symptoms of ongoing hemorrhage should undergo immediate hepatic arteriography and embolization, preferably selective.

5. Although the liver has a dual blood supply, embolization of the common hepatic artery should be considered a last resort when more selective embolization is not possible. Embolization of the main right hepatic artery should also be avoided if possible, as this necessitates subsequent cholecystectomy.

6. Late sequelae of hepatic injury includes hepatic necrosis, abscess, biloma, hematoma, and hemobilia. Postinjury collections can be treated by IR percutaneous drainage.

F. Spleen

1. **Splenectomy remains the safest therapy for hemodynamically unstable patients with splenic injury.** Among hemodynamically stable patients with splenic injury, the current indications for splenic arteriography and embolization vary widely by institution. Suggested criteria for performing arteriography are one or more of the following CT findings: splenic injury with hemoperitoneum, high-grade injury, intravenous contrast extravasation, or pseudoaneurysm. In most centers, splenic arteriography and embolization for splenic salvage is highly selective and reserved for young patients; in other centers, it is used more liberally. The optimal role of arteriography/embolization for splenic injury is still evolving. The two major types of splenic embolization are main artery embolization and selective embolization.

2. The overall failure rate (rebleeding) after embolization is 14%. Failure of splenic embolization warrants splenectomy, although repeat embolization has been described. Complications of splenic embolization also include abscess (4%) and infarction (21%).

3. Vaccinations for encapsulated organisms are routinely administered after main artery embolization. The role of vaccination after selective embolization is unclear.

G. Pelvis

1. Arteriography plays a critical role in identification and control of pelvic arterial hemorrhage and is a crucial component of the management of pelvic injuries. Depending on the injury pattern, embolization is effective as either primary therapeutic intervention or as an adjunct to external pelvic fixation or

laparotomy. The internal iliac (hypogastric) arteries and its branches are amenable to embolization.

2. The initial management of pelvic fracture with diastasis should be an attempt to "close" the pelvic ring, which can be achieved by placing a pelvic binder (using a bedsheet or Trauma Pelvic Orthotic Device [T-POD]) or by external fixation. These measures theoretically reduce hemorrhage by promoting tamponade of venous hemorrhage. Mechanism of injury, hemodynamic stability, physical exam findings, focused abdominal sonography for trauma (FAST), and radiography of chest and pelvis determine the subsequent evaluation and treatment. Pelvic arteriography and embolization should be considered in the following patients:

   a. Hemodynamically *unstable* blunt injury with pelvic fracture on x-ray and negative FAST or diagnostic peritoneal lavage (DPL).

   b. Hemodynamically *stable* blunt injury with CT demonstrating a large pelvic hematoma or pelvic contrast extravasation, pseudoaneurysm, or arteriovenous fistula.

   c. Immediately following trauma laparotomy for intra-abdominal hemorrhage and ongoing pelvic hemorrhage.

3. Pelvic embolization is largely safe and effective. Risks of pelvic embolization include rectal ischemia and gluteal necrosis. Sexual dysfunction occurs rarely in males and may be related to the pelvic fracture.

4. Repeat pelvic arteriography should be considered if hypotension or acidosis persist after initial arteriogram is negative and other sources of hemorrhage have been excluded.

5. Although selective embolization is preferable to proximal internal iliac artery embolization, selective embolization may be quite time-consuming. Unstable patients with multiple sites of pelvic arterial hemorrhage may best be served by unilateral (or bilateral) internal iliac artery embolization, which can be performed rapidly. However, bilateral internal iliac artery embolization increases the risk of rectal and gluteal ischemia and necrosis.

H. **Kidney.** Stable patients with evidence of renal injury on intravenous contrast CT may benefit from selective embolization. Infarction of large areas of the kidney is well-tolerated, presuming a functional contralateral kidney. Urinoma is a known complication of renal embolization and is treated by IR percutaneous drainage.

I. **Inferior vena cava filter.** Injured patients who are at extremely high risk for deep venous thrombosis and pulmonary embolism can be predicted (Table 14-3) (Chapter 50). In this group, inferior vena cava (IVC) filters reduce the risk of pulmonary embolism; placement of prophylactic IVC filter should be considered.

TABLE 14-3	Indications for Prophylactic IVC Filter

Patient who cannot receive anticoagulation because of increased bleeding risk* *and* has injuries resulting in immobility, such as:
Severe closed head injury (Glasgow Coma Scale score <8)
Paraplegia or quadriplegia
Complex pelvic fractures with long bone fractures
Multiple long bone fractures

*Intracranial hemorrhage, ocular injury with hemorrhage, solid organ injury, pelvic or retroperitoneal hematoma, cirrhosis, active ulcer disease, end-stage renal disease, preexisting or postinjury coagulopathy. (Adapted from Rogers FB, Cipolle MD, Velmahos G, et al. Practice management guidelines for the prevention of venous thromboembolism in trauma patients: The EAST Practice Management Guidelines Work Group. *J Trauma* 2002;53:142–164.)

However, it is unclear how long caval interruption is beneficial. Both permanent and retrievable IVC filters are available. Retrievable filters require manipulation at varying intervals to remain retrievable.

J. Other procedures. Other interventional procedures include percutaneous drainage of postoperative or postinjury collections (intra-abdominal/pelvic abscesses, hematomas, bilomas, urinomas, and thoracic empyemas), exchange of surgical drains and catheters, and insertion of peripherally-inserted central catheters (PICCs). These procedures are usually performed under guidance of fluoroscopy, CT, or ultrasound.

Bibliography

Asensio JA, Roldan G, Petrone P, et al. Operative management and outcomes in 103 AAST-OIS grades IV and V complex hepatic injuries: Trauma surgeons still need to operate, but angioembolization helps. *J Trauma* 2003;54:647–654.

Biffl WL, Moore EE, Offner PJ, Burch JM. Blunt carotid and vertebral arterial injuries. *World J Surg* 2001;25:1036–1043.

Bynoe RP, Kerwin AJ, Parker HH III, et al. Maxillofacial injuries and life-threatening hemorrhage: Treatment with transcatheter arterial embolization. *J Trauma* 2003;55:74–79.

Carrillo EH, Spain DA, Wohltmann CD, et al. Interventional techniques are useful adjuncts in nonoperative management of hepatic injuries. *J Trauma* 1999;46:619–624.

Dondelinger RF, Trotteur G, Ghaye B, Szapiro D. Traumatic injuries: Radiological hemostatic intervention at admission. *Eur Radiol* 2002;12:979–993.

Dunham MB, Zygun D, Petrasek P, et al. Endovascular stent grafts for acute blunt aortic injury. *J Trauma* 2004;56:1173–1178.

Haan JM, Bochicchio GV, Kramer N, Scalea TM. Nonoperative management of blunt splenic injury: A 5-year experience. *J Trauma* 2005;58:492–498.

Johnson JW, Gracias VH, Gupta R, et al. Hepatic angiography in patients undergoing damage control laparotomy. *J Trauma* 2002;52:1102–1106.

Mohr AM, Lavery RF, Barone A, et al. Angiographic embolization for liver injuries: Low mortality, high morbidity. *J Trauma* 2003;55:1077–1082.

Pryor JP, Braslow B, Reilly PM, et al. The evolving role of interventional radiology in trauma care. *J Trauma* 2005;59:102–104.

Rogers FB, Cipolle MD, Velmahos G, et al. Practice management guidelines for the prevention of venous thromboembolism in trauma patients: The EAST Practice Management Guidelines Work Group. *J Trauma* 2002;53:142–164.

Sclafani SJ, Shaftan GW, Scalea TM, et al. Nonoperative salvage of computed tomography-diagnosed splenic injuries: Utilization of angiography for triage and embolization for hemostasis. *J Trauma* 1995;39:818–827.

Velmahos GC, Toutouzas KG, Vassiliu P, et al. A prospective study on the safety and efficacy of angiographic embolization for pelvic and visceral injuries. *J Trauma* 2002;52:303–308.

Xenos ES, Freeman M, Stevens S, et al. Covered stents for injuries of subclavian and axillary arteries. *J Vasc Surg* 2003;38:451–454.

15

DOCUMENTATION, CODING, COMPLIANCE, AND EMTALA
DONALD M. YEALY
AND SAMIR M. FAKHRY

I. **INTRODUCTION.** Documentation and coding have clinical, legal, reimbursement, and performance improvement implications. Compliance in this setting refers to the proper match between documentation and coding. While specific rules and interpretations may change over time, we highlight the current basics of these important efforts.
   A. Scribing the events of trauma care requires attention to detail to allow performance assessment and to avoid coding/billing errors. All physician documentation **must** be legible.
   B. Failure to properly document or bill for services (**noncompliance**) has legal and financial risks for physicians and hospitals, irrespective of intent. Physicians comply best when the documentation of "who did what and when" is clear.
   C. **Coding** is assigning a numeric descriptor for the work done (CPT code) and matching it with one or more diagnosis numeric (ICD-9) codes. CPT codes include evaluation and management codes (E&M codes) and procedural codes. The **E&M** codes describe "cognitive" services such as admission evaluation, ongoing in-hospital care, critical care, and other nonprocedural services provided in the inpatient or outpatient setting. **Procedural codes** describe operations, bedside procedures, and other noncognitive activities such as outpatient excisions of lesions in the office. Without accurate coding supported by adequate and legible documentation, a physician cannot bill for services effectively.

II. **DOCUMENTATION.** Documentation should be carried out from prehospital through resuscitation, operating room, intensive care unit, ward, and outpatient care. The requirements for documentation in these areas differ, and tools should be tailored to each phase of trauma care.
   A. In many institutions, the **trauma resuscitation record** is a separate document from the trauma history and physical examination. The trauma resuscitation record is usually a nurse-driven tool, whereas the **trauma history and physical examination** is physician-driven. Frequently, these documents resemble each other and contain much of the same data, but they have distinct purposes. As the electronic medical record emerges, this duplication may not be necessary because the ideal trauma record would include the history, physical examination, and resuscitation. However, for the purposes of discussion in this chapter, they will be considered separately.
   B. **Trauma resuscitation record.** The trauma resuscitation record is generally two to three pages in length and is a permanent record (Appendix C). Frequently completed in duplicate by a clerk or nurse recorder, it is designed to minimize writing by use of check boxes and directed queries. Although most are institution-specific, the following elements are usually included:
      1. **Demographic information** should include the patient's name, age, sex, time and mode of arrival, allergies, medications, and significant medical history.
      2. **Initial assessment**
         a. Initial vital signs and "ABC" notations
         b. The Revised Trauma Score (RTS) and/or the Glasgow Coma Scale (GCS) score

    c. Mechanism of injury

    d. The trauma team members present (and time arrived) as well as consultants

    e. A serial record of vital signs, GCS, cardiac rhythm, pulse oximetry, pupil examination, and procedure times

    f. Injury description (anatomic diagram of the body, anterior and posterior, is helpful)

    g. Initial procedures and studies

    h. An accurate account of fluid infused and blood products transfused

    i. Disposition of the patient and notation of family contacts

C. Trauma history and physical examination (Appendix C)

    1. The trauma history and physical examination can be written in a standard hospital history and physical examination format. However, most trauma centers have developed a preprinted format similar to the resuscitation record to minimize writing and improve data collection.

    2. The classic components of a history often cannot be obtained during resuscitation, especially the social history, review of systems, and medical history. Rather than ignoring these (which has coding and billing effects), these items must be documented as "unobtainable" with a reason why this is the case (e.g., "Patient was intubated," "Patient was nonverbal," "Patient was critically ill"). To avoid ambiguity, do not use the term "noncontributory."

    3. In many hospitals, a formatted, preprinted checklist or flowchart form is used for the admitting history and physical examination. Although a dictated note is not mandatory, dictation using the flowchart as a reference improves legibility and can enhance reimbursement. The history of the present illness should include the major elements of the resuscitation, including the following information:

        a. Mechanism of injury

        b. Time of the accident

        c. Presence or absence of intrusion, entrapment, restraint, or airbag deployment

        d. Prehospital assessment and evaluation

        e. Inclusion of allergies, medications, past medical history, social history, family history, and review of systems will allow a higher level of coding and reimbursement. These can be recorded in nursing or physician notes, but if the former is used alone, a clear notation of physician review (or "link") is needed to support coding and billing.

    4. A format employing the Advanced Trauma Life Support (ATLS) initial assessment outline is used in many trauma centers:

        a. Primary survey

        b. Resuscitation

        c. Secondary survey

        d. Definitive care

        e. Interpretation of the radiographs, scans, and pertinent laboratory studies

        f. When and who removed immobilization devices (e.g., cervical spine) or placed devices (e.g., long leg splint)

    5. Teaching physician requirements. To generate a bill for services in a teaching setting, the attending physician who supervises house staff must personally provide the service or be present during that service. For the history and examination, the attending physician must either obtain or be present for this, **or** review the resident history and examination and affirm the key aspects independently, noting the latter in the teaching physician attestation note. This allows the teaching physician to link to the resident documentation, supporting optimal billing. **The phrase "Seen and agree with above" is inadequate.** Teaching physicians can link to resident histories and physical exams (if done together or confirmed). On the other hand, the teaching physician can link only to nurse, student, or other extender histories **but not to physical exams.**

        a. The trauma history and physical examination record should have a separate area for the attending physician to sign with the accompanying (or similar) statement: "I have evaluated this patient, including a review of the history, physical examination, and laboratory and x-ray studies, and have performed or supervised the procedures outlined in this resuscitation record." However, an additional terse note by the attending that includes brief detail on the four components of care is preferred: history and medications, physical examination, studies, and plan.

b. If billing is planned for any procedures, the attending or supervising physician must either clearly note that he or she performed the procedure or was present "elbow to elbow" (or using another clear statement of bedside presence) with any trainee during the procedure. **Simply stating "I supervised the chest tube insertion" is inadequate.** For those procedures that take 5 minutes or less, the attending physician must be present **and** document his or her presence for the entire procedure. For those requiring more time, the attending physician must note the "key portion(s)" of each and his or her bedside presence plus note immediate availability for remaining portions of the procedure. For example, skin opening and closure is often not a key portion, whereas intra-abdominal exploration or repair is a key portion. A supervising physician cannot attest to two key portions occurring simultaneously in different patients (i.e., one cannot "be present or supervising" in two places simultaneously). There are no clear guidelines on what portions of procedures are "key"—the supervising physician must be clear and reasonable when defining this part of care.

c. Critical care time is that spent by a **teaching physician** in the care of one patient with life- or limb-threatening or impending life- or limb-threatening illness or injury (Section III). It includes bedside care, consultations, laboratory and radiograph interpretations, and discussion with family or other health care providers. **Only the attending physician can provide and document billable critical care**, and the time can be summarized. Any note should be specific (e.g., "I spent xx minutes of critical care time providing care, excluding procedures"). Similar to procedures, critical care time cannot be billed for two patients at the same time interval, although it can occur sequentially.

d. All notations must be clearly generated by the attending physician—either handwritten and signed, dictated and signed (some insurers allow electronic signatures), or personally checked off (if a template used) and signed, with clear dates and times included.

e. **Procedural analgesia and sedation** documentation must be distinct from any procedure note (and cannot be performed by the same attending doing the procedure if separate billing is desired). It must include a pre- and post-procedure exam, a brief description of the regimen and effects (augmented by nursing notes/checklist), and note recovery time/status and total time spent by the attending physician (the latter analogous to critical care documentation).

6. The following guidelines should be used to document injuries. Diagnoses should be as specific as possible, because the severity scores assigned are affected by the documentation provided by the physicians.

a. Central nervous system (CNS) diagnoses
  i. Document the size of brain lesion, in centimeters.
  ii. Specify type of brain lesion—epidural, subdural, parenchymal.
  iii. Indicate duration of loss of consciousness.
  iv. Include neurologic deficits.
  v. Document cerebrospinal fluid (CSF) leak, hemotympanum, perforated tympanum, Battle's sign, and raccoon's eyes.
  vi. Specify cord syndromes as incomplete (anterior, posterior, central, or lateral) or complete, and note their level, if possible.
  vii. Note vertebral body compression fractures.

b. External injuries
  i. Document size and location of contusions and abrasions.
  ii. Document length and depth of lacerations.

     iii. Specify involvement of ducts and vessels.

     iv. Document volume of blood loss.

     v. Specify avulsions and tissue loss >25 cm^2.

     vi. Specify suspected bullet wounds by size, location, and presence of soot or powder burns. **Do not use the terms *exit wound or entrance wound.***

  c. Injuries to internal organs

     i. Classify length and depth of laceration or perforation of internal organs. Use a grading system if applicable (Appendix B).

     ii. Specify size and location of hematomas.

     iii. Document involvement of vascular system.

     iv. Specify blood volume loss (recognizing variability).

     v. Document any urinary extravasation or fecal contamination associated with injuries to urinary and gastrointestinal (GI) tracts.

  d. Blood vessel injuries

     i. Specify complete versus incomplete transection of the vessel.

     ii. Document any segmental loss.

     iii. Name the specific vessel, if possible.

  e. Orthopedic injuries

     i. Specify fractures as open or closed.

     ii. Document comminution or displacement, angulation.

     iii. When making the diagnosis of crush injury, document degree of destruction of bone, muscle, nerve, and vascular system of the extremity.

  f. Facial injuries

     i. Describe all lacerations, swelling, tenderness, deformity, and fracture, and try to use the designation of Le Fort I, II, and III fractures if applicable.

     ii. When intra-oral lacerations occur with facial fractures, indicate communication with the fracture.

D. Operating room dictation. The operating room dictation should include efforts at ongoing resuscitation and, if dictated by a resident, should have a notation as to the presence of the attending surgeon during the key portions of the case. A written brief operative note should be placed in the patient's chart to help guide the intensive care unit (ICU) team and other consultants who may be asked to see the patient until the dictated operative report is returned.

  1. Similar to other documentation, an attending/teaching physician note should be authored independent of any trainee note to attest to the procedure and presence (whole event or key portions) and availability during non-key portions. Again, this latter note need not be lengthy.

  2. The surgeon may request a higher than usual fee for an operative procedure under certain circumstances by appending the –22 modifier to the CPT code. These circumstances include increased risk, difficult procedure, over 600-mL blood loss, contamination control, prolonged operation, and obesity. The operative note dictation should clearly indicate the circumstances for the increased fee request.

E. Intensive care unit

  1. ICU notes should follow a prescribed template outlining the complexities of care. All entries should document the date and time. If written by a resident, a notation should be made that the patient was seen with an attending physician when that occurred.

  2. The **ICU note** should be structured to include

    a. Hospital day

    b. Diagnoses

    c. Surgical procedures

    d. Consultants

    e. Current problems

    f. System review

     i. CNS

     ii. Pulmonary

  iii. Hemodynamic
  iv. GI
  v. Musculoskeletal
  vi. Infectious disease
  vii. Skin and wounds
  g. Laboratory studies and other studies (not covered in the system review)
  h. Medications
  i. Plans
 3. The structured ICU note can be written or typed into a computer template and attached to the chart.
 4. A notation from the resident that the attending physician was present at rounds is useful, when appropriate. However, a supplemental note by the attending physician is necessary for reimbursement of critical care codes and should include the following five components:
  a. Diagnosis or problem
  b. History, including medications, major events, and other information relating to the patient's hospital course
  c. Physical examination, with specific mention of the head, chest, abdomen, and extremities and inclusion of laboratory and other diagnostic studies
  d. Plan, which reflects the complexity of the decision making
  e. Time spent providing critical care with a notation excluding time spent on procedures that are not bundled (included) with the critical care code
 F. Ward. Record date and time of all entries. The ward note also should contain the five components just listed and, when written by the house staff, should acknowledge the presence of the attending physician. The attending must, however, include a note detailing his or her specific care or actions.

III. CODING
A. Overview
 1. Basically, two coding systems are used. **CPT (current procedural terminology),** published by the American Medical Association (AMA), is widely accepted as the physician component of billing. There are three components of the CPT codes:
  a. Procedures
  b. E&M (evaluation and management)
  c. Modifiers. ICD-9-CM (*International Classification of Diseases, Ninth Revision*), developed by the World Health Organization, provides the diagnosis codes necessary to support both physician and hospital billing (ICD-9 procedure codes are also used for hospital billing). Lack of understanding by physicians that a **CPT code** (for procedure or evaluation and management by a physician) **must be accompanied by an ICD-9 diagnosis code(s)** is a major obstacle in reimbursement for trauma and critical care.
 2. Most CPT procedure codes are straightforward. Use of **modifiers** to indicate special situations is challenging because payers vary considerably in their recognition and acceptance of modifiers. Examples of these special situations include two surgeons, multiple or bilateral procedures, discontinued procedures, surgical team, distinct procedure, repeat procedure, shared procedure, preoperative evaluation only, surgery only, and so forth. However, it is the **E&M coding for trauma and critical care** that presents the **greatest challenge** for providers because of the ever-changing and complex rules for documentation. **The documentation components, rather than the severity of injury or illness, determine the code.** With this in mind, what follows are typical patient examples and potential use of E&M codes for trauma and critical care, assuming appropriate documentation (these rules are too lengthy to include).
 3. Global surgical fee or package. There is a long-standing surgical tradition that the surgeon should provide appropriate pre-and post-operative care to

patients as an integral part of the procedure. This tradition has become standard operating practice for payers. Payers pay surgeons one lump sum, the global surgical fee, for both the operation performed and the postoperative care delivered (beginning on the day of the operation). Postoperative visits in the hospital and in the office are included in this fee, as is any service that would normally be provided in the postoperative period (such as removing sutures). Typically this includes activities in the 90 days following the procedure. Centers for Medicare and Medicaid Services (CMS) guidelines define a postoperative visit as a follow-up visit during the postoperative period of the surgery that is related to routine recovery from the surgery. Complications following surgery are also included in the global surgical package. Per CMS guidelines, complications following surgery are defined as all additional medical and surgical services required of the surgeon during the postoperative period of the surgery that do not require additional procedures in the operating room. In general, this refers to complications directly related to the surgical procedure.

    a. There are many instances when a patient develops a problem in the postoperative period that is either out of the scope of the normal postoperative course or unrelated to the surgical procedure. A wound infection would be an example of a complication that is directly related to the surgical procedure and falls under the global surgical package. A postoperative myocardial infarction after a colectomy is not a routine complication and is unrelated to the surgical procedure itself and therefore a separately billable entity. To distinguish a service as not being part of the global surgical package, a physician must use a modifier so that the payer recognizes the service as distinct from the surgical procedure.

B. CPT coding for evaluation and management of the trauma patient

    1. Critical care codes are used for evaluation and management of a critically injured patient requiring constant attendance (includes peripheral IV, venous and arterial blood draw, NG and urinary catheters, arterial blood gases, interpretation of hemodynamic or cardiopulmonary monitoring and chest x-ray, and ventilatory management).

    2. (99291: 30–74 min, **99292:** 75–104 minutes). These codes are used when a critically injured patient requires continued bedside management during initial resuscitation or subsequent critical care. This includes continuous physician attention during transport to CT scan suite, angiography, operating room, or ICU. Three major requirements for using the critical care E&M codes are:

        a. Clinical condition criterion: "There is a high probability of sudden, clinically significant, or life threatening deterioration in the patient's condition which requires the highest level of physician preparedness to intervene urgently."

        b. Treatment criterion: Critical care services require direct personal management by the physician. They are life and organ supporting interventions that require frequent, personal assessment and manipulation by the physician. Withdrawal of or failure to initiate these interventions on an urgent basis would likely result in sudden, clinically significant or life threatening deterioration in the patient's condition.

        c. Documentation of time: For example, "Critical care time: 45 minutes excluding procedures."

        d. Procedures such as chest tube, central line, diagnostic peritoneal lavage (DPL), and arterial line are not included in this code and should be billed separately. A modifier (–25) should be added to the E&M code if a procedure is done on the same day to clarify that the global surgical package does not apply.

        e. These codes are also applicable to subsequent daily critical care management, utilizing the same time parameters.

   f. Critical care codes (99291 and 99292) may be used to describe care provided in the postoperative period if the care is for conditions not included in the global surgical package as long as the documentation clearly describes the condition for which critical care is required, the appropriate level of critical care delivered, and lists the diagnoses supporting this level of care. Note that the diagnoses must be different from those used for the operative coding and that an appropriate modifier must be used to indicate that the assumptions under which the global surgical package is applied have changed. In other words, the patient has developed a condition (described by the new diagnoses) that is not generally encountered in the routine postoperative care of patients undergoing the operation in question.

3. If initial resuscitation does not rise to the level of critical injury and the care rendered is not critical (by the surgeon's judgment and documentation), then the codes for **initial hospital care (99221–23)** should be used, depending on the complexity of decision making and time spent with the patient.

4. **(99233): Subsequent hospital care, often used in the ICU or step-down unit for patients with complex conditions requiring a high level of care.** This code can be used if the ICU care is for reasons other than specific postoperative care. For example, this code can be used for a patient with a closed head injury, multiple rib fractures, and a femoral fracture who had an exploratory laparotomy and splenectomy because the ICU care is primarily for reasons other than postoperative splenectomy.

   a. Postoperative care for an isolated splenectomy would be included in the operative code.

   b. Procedures such as chest tube, central line, DPL, and arterial line are not included in this code and should be billed separately (modifier required).

   c. **Time** spent **off the unit** in review of patient's data **cannot be reported**, so it is useful to review laboratory studies and images, write or dictate notes, **coordinate patient's care** (e.g., discussion with consultants), and conduct family conferences **in or near** the **unit** where the patient is located.

5. **(99232): Subsequent hospital care characteristically performed in the intermediate or step-down unit** when evaluated for reasons other than postoperative care (i.e., a postsplenectomy patient with a head injury, pulmonary contusion, and pelvic injury who has been extubated and is in a step-down unit for cardiac or neurologic monitoring).

   a. These codes do not apply to care of isolated postoperative injuries because they are included in the operative code.

6. **(99231): Subsequent hospital care, usually rendered on the floor or ward.** This is for follow-up evaluation on the medical surgical floor of the nonoperative or operative trauma patient for reasons other than the postoperative care. Total time is typically 15 minutes.

7. **(99223): Initial hospital care for stable trauma patient with significant injury.** Includes history and physical examination and **complex** decision making. An example is a 24-year-old man with a fracture-dislocation of the cervical spine, neurologically intact, or a 54-year-old woman with stable vital signs, awake, with multiple contusions and abrasions with a seat-belt sign without peritoneal signs who undergoes an abdominal CT scan. The documentation must reflect the level of care rendered as it is the documentation, not the patient's condition, that determines the level of the code applicable.

8. **(99222): Initial hospital care for a stable trauma patient with a potentially significant injury.** Includes a history and physical examination and moderate decision making. An example is a 65-year-old man with a cerebral concussion and multiple contusions and abrasions.

9. **(99221): Initial hospital care for a stable trauma patient who has no apparent significant or potentially significant injury but will require hospitalization.** This includes history and physical examination and straightforward decision making. For example, this code may be used for a 22-year-old

man, intoxicated, with multiple contusions and abrasions, triaged to the trauma center primarily on the mechanism of injury.

C. Trauma ICD diagnostic coding

1. **Introduction.** Billing for professional services begins with diagnoses for which care was rendered. Most claim forms accommodate four diagnoses. Since 1988, the Health Care Financing Administration (now called Centers for Medicare and Medicaid Services, CMS) mandates the use of the International Classification of Diseases (ICD) for diagnosis reporting; most other payers have followed suit. Proper ICD coding can decrease the number of claims sent to manual review, thereby optimizing timely reimbursement. Several principles should be applied whenever possible to ICD coding.

2. **Principles and examples**

   a. ICD coding is contained in two volumes, Volume I (the tabular list) and Volume II (the alphabetical list); use both.

   b. "Unspecified" and "other" codes should be avoided.

      i. Example: You wish to code for blunt hepatic injury. Volume II reveals "Injury, internal, liver 864.00" and "Laceration 864.09." Volume I, however, lists the entire classification scheme for closed hepatic injury with detailed descriptions for each code (e.g., "864.03 Injury to liver, laceration involving parenchyma but without major disruption of parenchyma; i.e., <10 cm long and <3 cm deep"). Using Volume I lets you choose the best description and avoid "other" (864.09) or "unspecified" (864.00).

   c. Diagnoses should reflect information known to you at the time the billed service was rendered. Each CPT code is linked to only those ICD codes related to that CPT code.

      i. Example: You are consulted regarding a patient who has been assaulted and also stabbed in the abdomen. He was unresponsive in the field but is awake, although incoherent during your evaluation. He has right lower quadrant tenderness. Diagnoses accompanying your emergency department consultation claim are (1) "879.2 Open wound, anterior abdominal wall, uncomplicated"; (2) "789.63 Abdominal tenderness, right lower quadrant"; and (3) "850.1 Concussion with brief loss of consciousness." You perform a DPL. For this procedure, your diagnoses are 1 and 2. DPL is positive, and at laparotomy you repair two distal ileal holes and one ascending colon hole. For the operation, you list (1) "863.39 Open injury, small intestine, other or multiple for CPT 44603 (repair multiple small bowel)" and (2) "863.51 Open injury, ascending colon for 44604 (repair colon)." Remember to use the −51 modifier to specify which procedure will be paid at 50% (Medicare no longer requires this but other payers may).

   d. ICD diagnoses must contain fourth or fifth digits where required. Failure to use required digits often leads to manual review.

      i. Examples: 789.63 Abdominal tenderness, right lower quadrant compared with 789 Abdominal pain and tenderness. 863.51 Open injury, ascending colon compared with 863.50 Open wound, colon.

   e. Thorough ICD coding supports CPT coding for critical care services and for complex evaluation and management services. Not all ICU patients require critical care services daily, and auditors are likely to visit physicians with perceived excess critical care or complex visit charges.

   f. Initial diagnostic code selection can have an impact on reimbursement for services provided later in the patient's course. For example, critical care services performed by the operating surgeon are normally not reimbursed during a postoperative global period. However, if the diagnostic codes for the operation are for injury, fracture, burns, open wounds, or other trauma, that surgeon also can charge and collect for critical care services.

   g. Use of E or V codes as primary diagnoses often leads to manual review or to automatic denial. E or V codes can be appropriately used in addition to other ICD codes, although they should not replace non-E or non-V codes. V codes can be appropriate as primary diagnoses for "no charge" visits.

IV. **EMTALA.** Beginning in the mid-1980s, federal legislation evolved to protect patients seeking emergency care. Initially referred to as "antidumping" laws, these actions have evolved into the Emergency Medical Treatment and Active Labor Act (EMTALA). All hospitals and providers that offer emergency services through a dedicated emergency department are bound by EMTALA. In 2005, clarifications and alterations to the act were disseminated.

A. EMTALA states that any person seeking care for an *emergency condition* (including trauma care) **must** receive a screening examination and stabilization, irrespective of the ability to pay. Simply arriving at an emergency department for care of a clearly nonemergency condition **does not** trigger an EMTALA obligation.

B. The providers and hospitals must provide and document care, or document refusal by a patient with capacity and the knowledge that care will be provided without financial concerns. All life- and limb-threatening injuries must be sought and stabilizing care given.

C. Hospitals must have policies that ensure physician availability (including functional on-call lists of providers across specialties) to provide this initial emergency care. EMTALA does not proscribe specific call regulations, but requires policy that addresses needs and local resource concerns.

D. Scheduled outpatient ED visits (done to ease care delivery), direct admissions to the hospital (who may traverse the ED), and inpatients no longer trigger for an EMTALA obligation (though previous interpretations included these populations).

E. The screening examination and stabilizing actions are not defined in the statute. Based on interpretations and case law, these should be similar to those provided to any patient presenting with the same symptoms or findings. This means the same or similar tests by the same or similar providers (e.g., a nurse screening examination would not suffice unless this was the only examination done routinely for all patients with that complaint). Definitive care is not mandated. The only exception to the stabilization requirement is when attempts to do so would jeopardize the patient's health or outcome.

F. Transfer to a more appropriate facility can occur after this screening and stabilization have occurred if the receiving facility offers services not available at the original site. Trauma centers often receive patients for this reason from nontrauma centers or lower level centers. The transfer must be accompanied by notification and acceptance between providers, documented agreement by the patient (if capable), and all pertinent medical records. Local policy and practice must ensure these steps and documentation.

G. EMTALA covers *any* hospital property—including clinics and other care sites, attached or offsite—held out to provide emergent care. A recent interpretative clarification states that *sites that do not provide emergent care are excluded* (e.g., dialysis centers, radiology facilities, etc.).

H. The obligation begins with patient arrival to the facility. That includes patients who reach the hospital security entrance, waiting room, driveway, and sidewalks (if for the purpose of seeking care). Also, patients in an ambulance requesting transport to a hospital are covered if the ambulance is owned or directed by the desired destination hospital's personnel, but not if under other conditions such as a municipal service (another change from previous interpretations).

I. The possible penalties for failure to comply with EMTALA include imprisonment, fines (with multiple violations possible in a given case), and potential exclusion from Medicare for up to 5 years. The fines can be tripled in selected circumstances where egregious behavior exists. These penalties are separate and unrelated to civil actions (i.e., malpractice).

J. Providers who send or receive patients have an obligation to report violations when they have direct knowledge of a violation (no obligation exists for informal or secondhand awareness).

K. The best ED and trauma bay approach is to evaluate and treat all patients the same, and ask insurance information only after the initial care and plan is complete.

AXIOMS

- Notes should be factual. Avoid the temptation to express nonmedical judgment or disappointment (e.g., "sequential compression boots found at foot of bed because of poor instruction" or "patient not taken for scan because of inadequate number of staff on floor").
- All documents, and any changes, should be dated and timed, and single strikethrough used to correct text (rather than attempts to remove) when handwritten charts are employed.
- Realize that payers recognize what you do **and** document, not just what you do. To minimize audits and denials, complete notes—especially for operative services, procedures, and critical care—as soon as possible (within hours rather than days to weeks).
- Teaching physicians must personally provide care to bill professional fees in a training setting. They must view care or review housestaff notes and independently confirm findings, **or** do a complete examination alone.
- Teaching physician notes need not be lengthy and should link to any resident and nursing documentation. Do not write "Seen and agree with above" alone if billing is planned.
- To avoid EMTALA problems, care for all patients first, leaving payment or insurance questions until after the resuscitation and emergent care is complete.

Bibliography

American College of Surgeons Committee on Trauma. *Resources for Optimal Care of the Injured Patient.* Chicago, Ill: American College of Surgeons; 1998.

American Medical Association. *International Classification of Diseases, Ninth Revision, Clinical Modification.* Chicago, Ill: American Medical Association; 1999.

American Medical Association. *Physicians' Current Procedural Terminology 2000.* Chicago, Ill: American Medical Association; 1999.

American Medical Association and US Health Care Financing Administration. *Documentation Guidelines for Evaluation and Management Services.* Washington, DC: American Medical Association and US Health Care Financing Administration; May 1997.

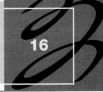

OPERATING ROOM PRACTICE
MICHAEL RHODES

16

I. CONDUCTING A TRAUMA OPERATION

A. The ideal location for a trauma operating room (OR) is adjacent to the resuscitation area. However, this depends on hospital-specific geography and resources. In general, it is more practical to have the trauma OR within the main OR suite for more flexibility of equipment and personnel. **It is better to take the patient and the resuscitation team to an OR than try to bring the OR to the patient.** A protocol for elevator standby and priority transport must be in place.

B. A trauma OR should have a minimum space of 400 to 450 square feet with an optimum space of 600 square feet. The following equipment should be available:
   1. A large, high-quality OR light with two peripheral satellite lights for patients requiring multiple, simultaneous procedures
   2. Dedicated imaging equipment (built-in, if possible) to move in and out of the operative field
   3. An OR table that is capable of radiography and fluoroscopy
   4. A minimum of four suction connections
   5. A minimum of eight electrical outlets
   6. Warm intravenous fluids
   7. A rapid-infusion device
   8. A blood salvage device
   9. A multipurpose anesthesia machine capable of high minute ventilation (up to 30 L/min), 20 cm H_2O of positive end-expiratory pressure (PEEP), and pressure-support inverse-ratio ventilation
   10. Multichannel pressure monitoring with a remote slave monitor
   11. Multiple x-ray view boxes (minimum eight) or PACS screens
   12. Patient heating devices
   13. Electrocautery with argon beam capability
   14. Rapid access to prepared hemostatic agents
   15. General trauma tray that includes aortic compressor, rib spreader, sternal retractor, and a variety of vascular clamps
   16. Head light, face shields and/or goggles, boots, and impervious gowns for the operating team

C. **The critically injured patient must be accompanied by the resuscitation team to the OR.** Adequate assistance should be available to move the patient from the resuscitation litter to the OR table; this movement should be directed by the trauma team. In general, the patient should be removed from the backboard, military anti-shock trousers (MAST), or pelvic binder prior to the start of the operation.

D. For urgent exploratory laparotomy, the patient should have both arms available for adequate access during the operative procedure. Access to the central veins should be in place for most critically injured patients. A **cervical collar** can be removed after the patient is anesthetized and **replaced with two 5-pound sandbags** on each side of the head with large **tape** across the forehead. This allows exposure of the lower neck and clavicular area for central access or subsequent thoracic incisions.

E. Pulse oximetry, capnometry, pressure monitoring, and electrocardiographic (ECG) monitoring should be applied. The ECG pads should be strategically placed to

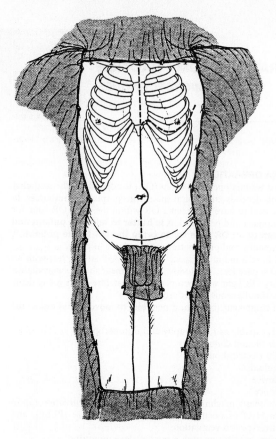

Figure 16-1. OR patient preparation. (From Champion HR, Robbs JV, Trunkey DD. Trauma surgery (parts 1 and 2). In: Dudley H, Carter D, Russell RCG, eds. *Rob and Smith's Operative Surgery.* Boston, Mass: Butterworth; 1989:540, with permission.)

avoid interference with subsequent operative intervention. Warming devices should be placed over those areas not in the surgical field. The patient should be **prepped from midthighs to midneck and laterally to the table** (Fig. 16-1). In agonal patients, even a 15-second painting or spray with antiseptic is superior to no prep. Draping should be wide and secured in place with staples or sutures.

F. In a **hypotensive** patient with an obtainable blood pressure, the **abdomen** should **not** be **opened until** blood is available in the room. Thus, it is essential to have adequate intravenous access in place, blood immediately available in the room, and the **anesthesia team prepared** to deal with possible sudden cardiovascular collapse.

G. A number of techniques are utilized in the OR for trauma care depending on the body region and stability of the patient. In general, the following are useful guidelines:

1. Adequate help, light, and suction should be ensured.

2. The incision should be large enough for rapid and thorough exploration. **The operation should not be compromised by inadequate exposure.**

3. Blood salvage capability should be ready before opening a body cavity suspected of massive hemorrhage.

4. Hemorrhage in most areas can be controlled by precise packing before attempting definitive repair.

5. In an unstable patient, frequent monitoring of hematocrit, arterial blood gases, ionized calcium, and potassium is necessary. A tableside point-of-service analyzer can be useful.

6. OR procedures presented in topic-specific chapters in this manual should be followed.

II. OPERATING ROOM TEAM

A. A physician team includes the trauma surgeon, the resident or assistant surgeons, and the anesthesiologist and residents. Continuous communication between the physician members of the team is essential. In a **persistently unstable** patient, a **second trauma surgeon** may be valuable to participate in resuscitative and technical aspects of the patient's care.

B. An OR scrub nurse, a circulating nurse, a nurse anesthetist, an emergency department nurse, and a critical care nurse are essential participants in a major OR resuscitation. OR technicians, perfusionists, laboratory technicians, and respiratory therapists should have assigned vital responsibilities as part of the OR resuscitation.

III. OPERATING ROOM COMMUNICATION

A. The OR should be notified of all Level I trauma patients arriving to the hospital. This occurs whether or not the need for immediate operative intervention is known. The **OR personnel** should be notified and on **standby** when the trauma team is activated. The OR personnel should communicate with the trauma team to determine the need for operative intervention.

B. A system should be in place for the operating team to be able to provide periodic updates to family members.

C. Direct communication between the OR and the blood bank/laboratory should be available.

IV. PRIORITIES FOR MULTIPLE PROCEDURES

A. The decisions as to prioritization of operative procedures can be challenging. Following are some general guidelines:

1. After airway and ventilatory control, major hemorrhage—either external or body cavity—takes priority.

2. External hemorrhage from the face, scalp, and extremities can be controlled by pressure, packing, or temporary suture closure until major body cavity hemorrhage is controlled.

3. In general, uncontrolled thoracic hemorrhage takes priority over uncontrolled abdominal hemorrhage.

4. Damage-control techniques with hemorrhage control, stapling of intestine, and packing should be seriously considered in the massively injured patient who is coagulopathic, acidotic, and hypothermic (Chapter 28).

5. Craniotomy without a preceding imaging study in the OR is rarely required, especially in the absence of lateralizing signs.

6. Body cavity hemorrhage (chest, abdomen, pelvis) takes priority over head injury.

7. A patient with a wide mediastinum and active intraabdominal hemorrhage should undergo exploratory laparotomy and simultaneous evaluation of the mediastinum with transesophageal echocardiography.

 AXIOMS

■ The resuscitation initiated in the emergency department should be continued in the OR. **Actively bleeding patients should be resuscitated in the OR**; control of the hemorrhage and resuscitation should occur simultaneously.

■ Severely injured trauma patients may require a specially designed OR with a team of physicians and nurses trained to respond in a flexible fashion to a variety of operative and logistic challenges.

- Trauma OR personnel should anticipate multiple visits by selected trauma patients, especially those managed with damage-control techniques.
- Advanced imaging resources, such as angiography and stenting, should be configured into trauma ORs when feasible.

Bibliography

Lafreniere R, et al. Preparation of the operating room ACS surgery, principles and practice. Section 1. Basic surgical and perioperative considerations. October 2003. Available at: http://www.acssurgery.com.

VINCENTE H. GRACIAS AND
PETER D. LEROUX

17

TRAUMATIC BRAIN INJURY

Central nervous system (CNS) injury is the most common cause of death from injury. Two million people per year in the United States suffer traumatic brain injuries (TBIs), many as the result of motor vehicle crashes and falls. Approximately 50,000 deaths per year and 500,000 hospital admission are attributable to head injury. Most of these victims are between the ages of 16 and 30 years. The increasing use of seat belts and airbags has resulted in an estimated 20% to 25% reduction in these traffic fatalities. However, the incidence of penetrating injury to the brain and spinal cord is increasing. As awareness of the correct methods for brain injury management grows, guidelines for TBI have developed and been shown to improve outcome.

I. ANATOMY AND PHYSIOLOGY
   A. The skull is particularly thin in the temporal region and thick in the occiput. The floor of the cranial cavity is divided into three regions: anterior (frontal lobes), middle (temporal lobes), and posterior (lower brainstem and cerebellum).
   B. The **meninges** cover the brain in three layers: dura mater (fibrous membrane that adheres to the internal surface of the skull), arachnoid membrane, and pia mater (attached to the surface of the brain). Cerebrospinal fluid (CSF) circulates between the arachnoid and pia mater in the subarachnoid space.
   C. The brain is composed of the cerebrum, cerebellum, and the brainstem. The brainstem consists of the midbrain, pons, and medulla. The reticular activating system (responsible for state of alertness) is within the midbrain and upper pons. The cardiorespiratory centers reside in the medulla. Small lesions in the brainstem can cause profound neurologic deficit.
   D. The Monro-Kellie doctrine states that the total volume of intracranial contents must remain constant because of the rigid bony cranium. With an expanding mass lesion, the intracranial pressure (ICP) is generally within normal limits. As cerebral edema worsens and brain swelling increases, CSF and blood volume within the skull decrease to compensate until the point of decompensation on the pressure-volume curve is reached; ICP then dramatically increases.
   E. Cerebral perfusion pressure (CPP) = Mean arterial pressure – ICP. Maintenance of cerebral perfusion is essential in the management of patients with severe closed head injury. Normal **cerebral blood flow (CBF)** is approximately 50 mL/100 g brain/minute. CBF <20 mL/100 g brain/minute represents cerebral ischemia, and cell death occurs at approximately 5 mL/100 g brain/minute. In addition to cerebral ischemia in response to injury, the injured brain loses its ability to autoregulate blood flow, increasing susceptibility of the injured brain to further ischemia. The generally acceptable range during active therapy in traumatic brain injury is CPP >60 to 70 mmHg.

II. TBIs are categorized as mild (80%), moderate (10%), or severe (10%), depending on the level of neurologic dysfunction at the time of initial evaluation. **Determination of the Glasgow Coma Scale (GCS) score as early as possible and then serially**

is essential. **Loss of consciousness (LOC)** is an important indicator of TBI. Classification of TBI is based on the GCS.

A. Mild head injury
   1. GCS score of 13 to 15
   2. Brief period of LOC
   3. Prognosis is excellent
   4. Mortality rate <1%
B. Moderate head injury
   1. GCS score of 9 to 12
   2. Typically, confused and may have focal neurologic deficits; able to follow simple commands
   3. Prognosis is good
   4. Mortality rate <5%
C. Severe head injury
   1. GCS of ≤8—generally, the accepted definition of coma
   2. Unable to follow commands
   3. Until recently, mortality >40%
   4. Most survivors have significant disabilities
   5. Airway control is essential
   6. Elevated ICP is a common cause of death and neurologic disability

III. INITIAL EVALUATION AND TREATMENT OF HEAD INJURY
A. General
   1. Patients suspected of having suffered a head injury, particularly if confused or unresponsive, require emergency evaluation and treatment at a center with capabilities for immediate neurosurgical intervention. **General objectives are rapid diagnosis and evacuation of intracranial mass lesions, expedient treatment of extracranial injuries, and avoidance of secondary brain injury due to hypoxia and hypotension.** Other secondary insults such as hyperglycemia, hypothermia, and anemia may also exacerbate outcome during the hospital course.
   2. Severe brain injury is associated with cerebral ischemia. Therefore, a principal therapeutic goal is to enhance cerebral perfusion and oxygenation and avoid further ischemic injury to the brain.
B. Initial management of the unresponsive patient with head injury
   1. **Intubation** with controlled ventilation (avoid routine hyperventilation). If possible, a focused neurologic examination, including assessment of GCS, pupillary response, and all four extremity movement, is critical before intubation and pharmacologic paralysis.
   2. **Venous access**
      a. Restore intravascular volume, blood pressure, and perfusion.
      b. Avoid hypotonic or dextrose-containing solutions.
   3. **Immobilize the patient with rigid backboard and cervical spine (C-spine) collar.** Assume that all patients with TBI have a spine injury until proved otherwise.
   4. **Pharmacologic paralysis** and sedation, if agitated or combative
      a. Short-acting agents are recommended.
         i. Vecuronium bromide, cisatracurium, or succinylcholine
         ii. Opioid sedation: fentanyl or morphine
         iii. Avoid benzodiazepines
   5. **Monitor blood pressure and O_2** saturation continuously.
   6. Check arterial blood gases (ABG), blood glucose, electrolytes, prothrombin time (PT), partial thromboplastin time (PTT), hematocrit, and platelet count. With active therapy, serum sodium levels and osmolality should be tracked.
   7. **Initiate medical management of the head injury.** Proceed with rapid acquisition of a computed tomographic (CT) scan of the head and complete cervical spine (if time permits). Based on time, distance, and local capabilities, transfer may be necessary Rapid referral to a center capable of immediate

neurosurgical intervention may be required. Do not delay transport to definitive care to obtain a CT scan of the head. Early diagnosis and evacuation of cranial mass lesions are critical.

   8. Repeated neurologic examination and assessment of GCS. Documentation of the GCS in patients who are intubated, or "tubed," should be noted by a *T* (i.e., 11[T]) patients who are intubated and pharmacologically paralyzed are noted by a *TP* (i.e., 3[TP]). This is needed for meaningful interpretation of the GCS values.

   9. Hyperventilation causes cerebral vasoconstriction and can worsen cerebral ischemia. **Routine hyperventilation should no longer be used.** Hyperventilation is indicated only in the setting of abrupt neurologic deterioration with suspected herniation.

C. Secondary management

   1. The avoidance of secondary brain injury is essential. Secondary brain injury is produced by hypoxia and hypotension. A single episode of hypotension (systolic blood pressure <90 mmHg) in the adult will worsen prognosis and can increase mortality up to 50%.

   2. The GCS obtained in the emergency department may be a more reliable assessment of the severity of brain injury than the GCS obtained in the field.

   3. The GCS cannot be assessed by simple observation and requires stimulation of the patient. In cases of asymmetry in either eye opening or motor scores, the best score is used.

   4. If time permits, a lateral cervical spine x-ray study usually can be obtained during secondary survey of the patient, which may detect gross injury or malalignment of the cervical spine (Fig.17-1). If available rapid C-spine CT should be used to detect fractures as well.

D. Indications for ICP monitoring. As a general approach, liberal use of ICP monitoring in patients with severe TBI (GCS ≤8) is recommended. An ICP monitor should be used with a brain oxygen monitor. ICP monitoring is not routinely indicated for patients with moderate or mild closed head injury. An ICP monitor should also be considered in a patient with moderate head injury who is going to the OR for other injuries. **ICP monitoring is indicated for:**

   1. Severe closed head injury (GCS ≤8) and abnormal CT of head

      a. Definition of abnormal CT:

         i. Hematoma

         ii. Contusion

         iii. Edema

         iv. Compressed basal cisterns

   2. Severe closed head injury (GCS ≤8) and normal CT of head, particularly if two or more of the following exist:

      a. Age >40 years

      b. Unilateral or bilateral flexor or extensor posturing

      c. Systolic blood pressure <90 mmHg (rapid correction of hypotension is essential)

E. Intensive care management of patients with severe TBI (GCS ≤8). The goal is to prevent secondary brain injury by limiting focal cerebral ischemia, preventing cerebral hypoxia and maintaining adequate cerebral perfusion. This can be accomplished only by the continuous monitoring of several physiologic parameters and the judicious use of therapies to lower elevated ICP.

   1. Recommendations for physiologic monitoring of the patient with severe TBI

      a. Arterial blood pressure. Noninvasive monitoring can be used, but an arterial catheter is preferred.

      b. Heart rate, electrocardiogram (ECG), temperature, and pulse oximetry.

      c. Central venous pressure or pulmonary artery catheter monitoring if the patient's volume status is in question.

      d. ICP monitoring.

      e. Brain tissue O_2 (and if available, cerebral microdialysis).

      f. Fluid balance (intake and output).

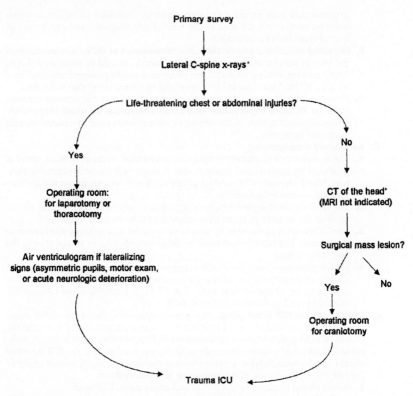

Figure 17-1. Emergency department triage of severe brain injury.
* can be deleted if CT of the cervical spine can be accomplished rapidly with CT of the brain

    g. Arterial blood gases every 4 to 6 hours initially; electrolytes, glucose, and serum osmolality (if receiving mannitol) every 6 hours; hematocrit, PT, PTT, platelets every 12 hours.

    h. Jugular venous O_2 saturation or O_2 content by local protocol if hyperemia or intractable ICP elevation suspected.

2. Goals of therapy

    a. Mean arterial blood pressure >80 mmHg. No role for hypertension control in TBI unless CT scan brain and/or ICP monitoring performed first.

    b. O_2 saturation (arterial) 100%.

    c. ICP <20 mmHg.

    d. CPP >60 to 70 mmHg (this can be individualized according to the patient's brain oxygen).

(Note: CPP = mean arterial pressure [MAP] − ICP.)

    e. $PaCO_2 = 35 \pm 2$ mmHg.

    f. Hematocrit = $32 \pm 2\%$.

    g. Central venous pressure = 8 to 14 cm H_2O.

    h. Avoid dextrose-containing intravenous solutions for first 24 hours; avoid free water for extent of active therapy unless diabetes insipidus present. Tight glucose control; avoid hyperglycemia.

    i. Maintain jugular venous O_2 saturation >50% or O_2 content of 4 to 6 vol%.

    j. Maintain direct brain O_2 greater than 20 mmHg.

k. Ensure normal PT, PTT, and platelet count.

l. Maintain a normal temperature.

3. **Management of elevated ICP**

   a. Improved outcomes can be expected if ICP is kept below 20 mmHg. Analgesia, sedation, fever control, and head position should be adjusted as needed immediately when first treating intracranial hypertension.

   b. Fiberoptic parenchymal catheters inserted through a bolt are accurate. They monitor ICP and allow the use of direct brain oxygen monitoring. They are easier to insert than ventricular catheters and are associated with a lower risk than ventriculostomies. However, they are more expensive and do not allow for CSF drainage (Fig. 17-2).

   c. A ventriculostomy catheter coupled with a strain gauge can be used to monitor ICP, particularly when there is hydrocephalus. This system is relatively inexpensive, accurate, and allows CSF drainage when needed to control ICP.

   d. Continuous CSF drainage is not recommended; the ventricular walls can collapse around the catheter tip and occlude its ports.

HEAD OF BED ELEVATED

Systemic neuromuscular paralysis

(Vecuronium bromide or pancuronlum)

and

Narcotic sedation

↓

Intermittent ventricular CSF drainage

↓

Bolus manniol 25–50 g IV/4 h

(Do not use if serum osms >315 mOsm, or sodium >150 mEq/L

↓

Lasix 20–40 mg IV/4 h

↓

Hyperventilation (PaCO$_2$ 28–30 mmHg)

↓

Barbiturates

(Pentobarbital 400–1,000 mg IV over 1 h, then 40–100 mg/h)

Titrate to maintain normal cardiac output

Figure 17-2. Steps for the management of elevated intracranial pressure (ICP).

    e. A repeat CT scan of the head should be obtained within 24 hours after the initial scan to detect delayed posttraumatic hematomas. A CT scan should be obtained with any abrupt increase in ICP or worsening of the neurologic examination. GCS declines by two or more or the patient develops hypoxia.

    f. Barbiturates are a second line therapy for ICP control when other treatments such as sedation, mannitol, CSF drainage, or optimized hyperventilation are not effective or their use is associated with deleterious side effects. When using barbiturates, patients should receive a pulmonary artery catheter and undergo continuous EEG monitoring. The depression of myocardial contractility can be minimized by maintenance of a high-normal intravascular volume. All patients receiving barbiturate therapy (for elevated ICP) should have frequent measurements of cardiac output and preload. EEG monitoring to observe burst suppression should be used.

    g. Avoid hypovolemia and hyperosmolality if mannitol is used. Bolus therapy (0.5–1.0 gm/kg) should be used with observed effect in 20 to 60 minutes. Repeat dosing if no effect within 20 minutes. Osmolality should be maintained at <310 to 320 milliosmol (mOsm). Mannitol has no effect above 320 mOsm.

    h. Optimized hyperventilation may be used to treat some patients with high ICP particularly when there is hyperemia (elevated brain oxygen or narrow arteriovenous oxygen content difference [$AVDO_2$] on jugular bulb). However, hyperventilation should be be used *only* when a measure of its effects (e.g., brain oxygen or cerebral blood flow) is in place; hyperventilation should be stopped if it adversely affects these parameters.

    i. A decompressive hemicraniectomy should be considered, particularly when elevated ICP is associated with cerebral hypoxia.

4. Anticonvulsant prophylaxis. Prolonged use of anticonvulsant therapy is not indicated for patients with TBI. Current recommendations are for the use of phenytoin during the first 7 days following injury in patients at high risk for early posttraumatic seizures. These risk factors include cortical contusion, subdural hematoma, penetrating head wound, epidural hematoma, depressed skull fracture, intracerebral hematoma, and seizure within 24 hours of injury. Seizure activity not related to acute injury event requires prolonged anticonvulsant therapy. Phemytoin should always be administered by giving a test dose and subsequently, monitoring for myocardiac depression.

5. Begin nutritional supplementation within 48 hours of the injury. TBI may increase caloric requirements by 25%. Aim for approximately 25 to 30 kcal/kg/day with either enteral (preferred) or parenteral supplementation. Most of these patients will tolerate postpyloric gut feeding.

6. Prognosis

    a. The outcome following severe TBI is strongly correlated with initial GCS score, pupil reactivity and size, age, ICP (pressures >20 mmHg or inability to reduce elevated ICP), surgical intracranial mass lesions (extent of midline shift), hypotension (systolic blood pressure <90 mmHg), and jugular venous O_2 saturation <50%.

    b. The establishment and availability of dedicated head injury rehabilitation facilities have greatly improved long-term outcome for these patients. Every effort should be made to transfer these patients to such a rehabilitation facility for aggressive inpatient therapy once they are medically and neurologically stable.

IV. MILD TO MODERATE HEAD INJURIES

    A. The distinction between mild and moderate head injuries is based on the initial Glasgow Coma Scale score and appearance of the initial CT scan of the brain. Patients who have an initial GCS score of 13 to 15 are considered to have a mild brain injury. Those patients with a GCS score of 9 to 12 are classified as having a moderate brain injury. Some recommend that any patient who has a posttraumatic abnormality such as contusion or subdural or epidural hematoma on initial

CT scan should be classified categorically as either a moderate or severe head injury patient regardless of initial GCS score. As many as 10% to 35% of those patients with GCS scores of 13 to 15 will have posttraumatic abnormalities on CT scan, and 2% to 9% ultimately will require a craniotomy for these lesions. Except for these empiric classification systems, the distinction between mild and moderate head injury is one of degree of severity of parenchymal injury. Thus, these two categories will be considered together in this section.

B. Most patients with **mild head injury** can be observed safely in the emergency department and discharged, although a few are at risk for delayed posttraumatic intracerebral hematomas or brain swelling. Identification of these patients requires careful neurologic assessment and liberal use of the CT scan.

  1. Clinical characteristics associated with an increased risk for subsequent brain swelling or hemorrhage are loss of consciousness associated with posttraumatic or retrograde amnesia. These patients should have a CT scan of the head.

  2. Patients with an abnormal CT scan or those who have a focal neurologic deficit on evaluation in the emergency department should be admitted for observation.

  3. PTS with a coagulopathic state or taking anticoagulants.

C. Decision on return to play after **sports-related head injuries** is determined by loss of consciousness or amnesia (Tables 17-1 and 17-2). The following guidelines are recommended (asymptomatic refers to no symptoms after provocative testing (e.g., a neurologic exam after 10 pushups or 10 situps) and based on their grade:

TABLE 17-1   Grading of Sports-Related Head Injury

Author	Grade I	Grade II	Grade III
AAN 1997	No LOC Symptoms <15 min	No LOC Symptoms >15 min	LOC
Cantu 1998	No LOC PTA <1 h	LOC <5 min PTA 1–24 h	LOC >5 min PTA >24 h
Colorado Medical Society 1991	No LOC Confusion No amnesia	No LOC Confusion and amnesia	LOC
Torg 1985	No LOC PTA only	LOC <few min PTA or retrograde amnesia	LOC Confusion and amnesia

TABLE 17-2   Return to Competition

Concussion Grade	First Concussion	Second Concussion	Third Concussion
Grade I	Return if asymptomatic >30 min	Return after 2 weeks and asymptomatic for 1 week	End season
Grade II	Return after 2 weeks and asymptomatic for 1 week	Return after 4 weeks and asymptomatic for 1 week	End season
Grade III	Return in 1 month and asymptomatic for 1 week	End season	End season? End career?

1. No loss of consciousness and no amnesia following a minor head injury: The patient can return 5 to 15 minutes after becoming completely lucid and asymptomatic.

2. Posttraumatic amnesia but no loss of consciousness or retrograde amnesia: No return to play that day.

3. Posttraumatic and retrograde amnesia with loss of consciousness: No return to play for 1 week after becoming completely lucid and asymptomatic and only after a detailed neurologic examination and CT scan.

4. Posttraumatic and retrograde amnesia and prolonged loss of consciousness: No return to play for 1 month and only after detailed neurologic evaluation and CT scan.

D. The likelihood of sustaining one or more head injuries after an initial minor head injury is increased, and subsequent head injuries have an additive, deleterious effect on complex processing abilities and reaction times.

V. PENETRATING BRAIN INJURIES

A. Penetrating injuries can be subcategorized into gunshot wounds and lower velocity injuries; the prognosis between the two is very different.

1. **Gunshot wounds to the brain** carry a high mortality rate. As the bullet traverses the brain tissue, it causes a cylinder of tissue destruction extending perpendicular from the bullet tract to a distance of as much as 10 times the diameter of the bullet.

2. General management of gunshot wounds to the brain follows the same principles of cerebral resuscitation as other brain injuries. The incidence of elevated ICP is high.

3. Superficial debridement of the entrance and exit wounds is generally recommended, although it is usually not necessary to retrieve all deep-seated bullet and bone fragments.

4. Broad-spectrum intravenous antibiotics and prophylactic anticonvulsant therapy are recommended.

5. Prognosis depends largely on the trajectory of the bullet through the brain. If the bullet traverses deep brain structures (e.g., the basal ganglia or brainstem), traverses the posterior fossa, or has a transcranial trajectory, the mortality rate is high. If the bullet avoids these structures, the outcome can be more optimistic.

6. Patients with an initial GCS score of 3 to 4 will have a high mortality rate (>80%). Conversely, 80% of patients who are able to follow commands on admission to the hospital (GCS >8) will have mild or no disability.

B. Lower velocity missile wounds. The most important factor determining outcome from lower velocity missile wounds (e.g., stab or arrow wounds) to the head is the location of brain injury. If the missile damages the motor cortex, for example, contralateral motor weakness should be confined to the area of cortex that was damaged.

1. The missile may be tamponading a major intracranial arterial injury, so it is best to remove protruding knives or other objects only in the operating room and only when the surgeon is prepared to deal with the consequences of major arterial bleeding.

2. A 7- to 14-day course of broad-spectrum antibiotics and prophylactic anticonvulsants (7 days) is indicated.

C. Following a penetrating head injury—including high- or low-velocity missile or nonmissile injury (e.g., stab wound)—it is important to perform an angiogram to exclude a traumatic aneurysm.

VI. SKULL FRACTURES

A. Linear skull fractures are most common and typically occur over the lateral convexities of the skull. The squamous portion of the temporal bone in this region is thin and closely associated with the middle meningeal artery. Fractures in this area can tear the artery, which is the most common cause for epidural hematoma.

For most skull fractures, it is not the fracture but rather the underlying blood clot or brain contusion that raises concern. Because these associated lesions are best detected with CT and are not recognized with plain skull x-rays, **a CT of the head is the diagnostic study of choice for patients suspected of having a skull fracture.**

B. Depressed skull fractures. The surgical elevation and repair of these fractures will not lead to a change in associated neurologic deficit or a decrease the risk for subsequent seizures. These fractures may be open (associated with an overlying scalp laceration) or closed. Indications for surgical repair of depressed skull fractures are evidence of CSF leak, cosmetic deformity, or contaminated bone or scalp fragments pushed into the brain. In addition, when a dural tear is suspected—usually indicated by the bone being depressed beyond the inner table—then repair should be considered. Other treatment includes:

  1. Broad-spectrum antibiotics for 7 to 14 days if the wounds are contaminated or the fracture involves a facial sinus
  2. Prophylactic anticonvulsant therapy for 7 days

C. Basilar skull fractures, which occur most commonly through the floor of the anterior cranial fossa, can disrupt the ethmoid bones and lead to CSF leak through the nose (rhinorrhea). Fractures also can occur through the petrous bones posteriorly, leading to CSF drainage through the ear (otorrhea). Cranial nerve injuries are commonly associated with posterior basilar skull fractures, and findings should be sought on clinical examination.

  1. The primary concern with basilar skull fractures is associated CSF leak and risk of meningitis.
  2. Prophylactic antibiotic treatment is not recommended. Several investigations have found that morbidity is increased with prophylactic antibiotics because of selection of more virulent organisms.
  3. Attempts to stop the leak should begin with elevation of the head of the bed to 60 degrees. If the leak does not stop within 6 to 8 hours, a lumbar CSF drainage catheter should be placed (provided there are no contraindications on CT such as edema or a mass lesion), and 50 to 100 mL of CSF should be drained every 8 hours. If this fails to stop the leak within 72 hours, the patient should be taken to surgery for repair of the dural laceration. When a patient deteriorates while undergoing lumbar CSF drainage it may be associated with overdrainage or meningitis. The lumbar drain should be closed if this happens.

VII. POSTCONCUSSION SYNDROME

  A. Postconcussion syndrome can result from relatively minor head injuries.
  B. Most commonly involves headaches, tinnitus, vertigo, gait unsteadiness, emotional lability, sleep disturbances, intermittent blurring of vision, and irritability.
  C. Symptoms can continue for weeks, months, or several years, but are rarely permanent.
  D. Of patients who suffer postconcussion syndrome, 90% have spontaneous resolution of their symptoms within 2 weeks of injury. Beta-blocking agents, tricyclic antidepressants, or nonsteroidal anti-inflammatory agents may be beneficial, as well as psychotherapy and physical therapy.
  E. For those with persistent symptoms referral to a brain rehabilitation specialist is necessary.

 AXIOMS

■ Loss of consciousness is an important indicator of brain injury.
■ Determine the GCS score as early as possible.
■ A principal therapeutic goal is to enhance cerebral perfusion and avoid further ischemic injury.
■ Early diagnosis and evacuation of mass lesions are critical.
■ CT scan is the diagnostic test of choice for patients with all brain injuries.

Bibliography

American College of Surgeons Committee on Trauma. *Advanced Trauma Life Support.* Chicago, Ill: American College of Surgeons; 1998.

Bouma GJ, Muizelaar JP, Choi SC, et al. Cerebral circulation and metabolism after severe traumatic brain injury: The elusive role of ischemia. *J Neurosurg* 1991:685–693.

Chesnut RM, Marshall LF, Klauber MR, et al. The role of secondary brain injury in determining outcome from severe head injury. *J Trauma* 1993;34:216–222.

Chesnut RM, Marshall SB, Piek J, et al. Early and late systemic hypotension as a frequent and fundamental source of cerebral ischemia following severe brain injury in the traumatic coma data bank. *Acta Neurochir Suppl (Wien)* 1993;59:121–125.

Clifton GL, Kreutzer JS, Choi SC, et al. Relationship between Glasgow outcome scale and neuropsychological measures after brain injury. *Neurosurgery* 1994;33:34–39.

Fletcher JM, Ewing-Cobbs L, Miner ME, et al. Behavioral changes after closed head injury in children. *J Consult Clin Psychol* 1990;58:93–98.

Gracias VH, Gullomondegui OD, Steifel MF, et al. Cerebral cortical oxygenation: A pilot study. *J Trauma* 2004;56(3):469–474.

Joint Section on Neurotrauma and Critical Care. *Guidelines for the Management of Severe Head Injury.* New York, NY: Brain Trauma Foundation; 1996.

Levin HS, Grossman RG, Rose JE, et al. Long-term neuropsychological outcome of closed head injury. *J Neurosurg* 1979;50:412–422.

Levin HS, Williams DH, Eisenberg HM, et al. Serial MRI and neurobehavioral findings after mild to moderate closed head injury. *J Neurol Neurosurg Psychiatry* 1992;55:255–262.

Marion DW, ed. *Traumatic Brain Injury.* New York, NY: Thieme Medical Publishers; 1999.

Marion DW, Carlier PM. Problems with initial Glasgow Coma score assessment caused by the prehospital treatment of head-injured patients: Results of a national survey. *J Trauma* 1994;36:89–95.

Marion DW, Darby J, Yonas H. Acute regional cerebral blood flow changes caused by severe head injuries. *J Neurosurg* 1991;74:407–414.

Muizelaar JP, Marmarou A, Ward JD, et al. Adverse effects of prolonged hyperventilation in patients with severe head injury: A randomized clinical trial. *J Neurosurg* 1991;75:731–739.

Smith MJ, Stiefel MF, Gracias VH, et al. Packed red blood cell transfusion increases local cerebral oxygenation. *Crit Care Med* 2005;33(5):1104–1108.

Vollmer DG, Torner JC, Jane JA, et al. Age and outcome following traumatic coma: Why do older patients fare worse? *J Neurosurg* 1991;75:S37–S49.

INJURIES TO THE SPINAL CORD AND SPINAL COLUMN

BRIAN T. JANKOWITZ, WILLIAM C. WELCH, AND WILLIAM F. DONALDSON, III

18

I. **INTRODUCTION.** Each year, approximately 10,000 new spinal cord injuries result in paralysis, with an estimated societal cost of $10 billion. The average age of the injured is 32 years with a 4:1 male-to-female ratio. Motor vehicle accidents account for 50% of the spinal cord injuries, sports 14%, falls 21%, and violence 15%. Of patients with spinal cord injuries, 44% also suffer from other significant trauma, with 14% having head and facial trauma. Half of all spinal cord injuries involve the cervical spine, most occurring between C4 and C7, with a 3-month mortality of 20%. Half of spinal cord injuries involve complete quadriplegia.

II. **ANATOMY AND BIOMECHANICAL DEFINITIONS**
   A. The spinal cord is a continuation of the brainstem (medulla). This area is the cervicomedullary junction, which is located at the foramen magnum of the skull. The spinal cord continues through the vertebral canal of the cervical, thoracic, and upper lumbar vertebra, generally ending at the L1 to L2 space. The spinal cord contains the upper motor neurons (UMNs) that synapse with lower motor neurons (LMNs) to form the nerve roots and cauda equina. The nerve roots in the cervical and lumbar regions fuse as the cervical and lumbar plexuses before separating again as specific nerves. Generally speaking, UMN lesions carry a worse prognosis than LMN lesions, as nerve roots have better capacity for repair than does the spinal cord.
   B. The spinal column is composed of 7 cervical, 12 thoracic, 5 lumbar, and 5 fused sacral vertebrae. With the exception of the sacral vertebra, the vertebral bodies articulate with each other across the intervertebral disc and facet joints, forming a functional spinal unit. The facet joints, associated ligamentous structures, and other bone articulations (e.g., the rib cage) determine the motion across two vertebral bodies. The motions are considered in the sagittal plane (flexion and extension), coronal plane (lateral flexion), and in the transverse plane (rotation). In the cervical spine, about 50% of flexion and extension occurs between the occiput and C1, whereas 50% of rotation occurs between C1 and C2. The remainder of cervical movement takes place in the subaxial (below C2) region. The thoracic spine has little motion because of the facet joint orientation and added stabilization of the rib cage. The facet joints of the lumbar spine have a more sagittal orientation and allow moderate motion in the sagittal plane while resisting rotation. The transition from the stiff thoracic spine to a mobile lumbar area accounts for the high number of injuries at the thoracolumbar junction.
   C. Injuries to the spinal column occur as a result of excessive forces applied to the spine. These forces can cause axial loading, hyperflexion, hyperextension, distraction, rotation, or a combination of forces. Injury to the spinal column can cause spinal instability, which can be defined on radiographic or clinical grounds. In the acute setting, radiographic features are most commonly used to determine spinal stability. This is reviewed later in the chapter.
   D. The conceptualization of the spine as a series of support columns increases our biomechanical understanding of stability. **Three columns of the spine** have been described for the lower thoracic and lumbar spine. The **anterior column** (anterior longitudinal ligament and the anterior two thirds of the vertebral body and disc),

145

the **middle column** (posterior third of the vertebral body and disc, the posterior longitudinal ligament), and the **posterior column** (the facet joints, capsule, ligamentum flavum, and posterior ligaments) describe the main columns of overall biomechanical support (Fig. 18-1). The three-column theory may not be completely applicable to the cervical spine, but it is still generally used. Injuries or deficits of two of three columns denotes biomechanical instability.

  E. Spinal cord injuries can be separate and distinct from spinal column injuries. The diagnosis of a spinal cord injury (SCI) is made on clinical grounds and supplemented with diagnostic tests such as magnetic resonance imaging (MRI), myelography, or electrodiagnostic studies. The level of SCI frequently correlates with the level of spinal column injury. However, **SCI can occur without spinal column injury**.

  F. **Spinal column injuries** are bone or ligamentous disruptions that result in bone fractures or ligamentous instability. The loss of these stabilizing and supporting elements can result in compression and injury of neural elements. The diagnosis of spinal column injury is based on clinical and radiographic criteria, such as pain and ecchymosis at the level of fracture and plain film evidence of fracture. Spinal column injuries can occur without spinal cord injury.

III. PREHOSPITAL CARE

  A. Treatment in the field of patients with spinal column and spinal cord injuries follows the basic prehospital protocols (Chapter 6). Treatment is directed to establishment of an adequate airway, ventilation of the lungs, and maintenance of circulatory support to prevent secondary neurologic injuries.

  B. Intubation is best accomplished by using manual inline immobilization, avoiding flexion of the neck. Fiberoptic intubation may also reduce spine manipulation. The patient's neurologic status as well as pulmonary function should be assessed and recorded, especially patients with high quadriplegia.

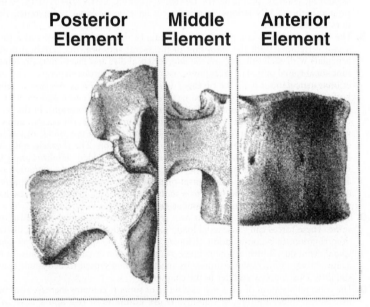

Posterior Element   **Middle Element**   **Anterior Element**

Figure 18-1. Drawing showing the three columns of support in the spine.

C. Hypovolemic and neurogenic shock can occur in the setting of SCI. The cause of hypotension must be determined and treated immediately. Hypotension should be regarded as a sign of abdominal bleeding, aortic or cardiac injury, external blood loss, or occult injury before considering neurogenic shock. Regardless of the cause, shock should be aggressively treated to prevent further ischemic injury to the spinal cord. Treatment consists of fluid administration and vasopressors to maintain the mean systemic blood pressure at approximately 90 mmHg. The patient is reevaluated continuously in the emergency department. Resuscitative measures are continued and modified as needed.

D. An estimated 3% to 25% of spinal cord injuries occur iatrogenically after the initial trauma, either in transport or during early resuscitation. After medical stabilization on the scene, the cervical spine should be immobilized in a rigid collar in any patient who is unconscious or suspected of having a cervical injury. A scoop stretcher or similar backboard with supportive blocks and straps should be used rather than logrolling to prevent uncontrolled motion. The patient should remain on a backboard until evaluated in the emergency department. Transport to a definitive treatment center should be the goal, as delays can incur worse outcomes, longer hospitalization, and higher costs.

IV. NEUROLOGIC EVALUATION

A. A standard neurologic examination is performed on each patient. This includes evaluation of mental status, cranial nerves, motor testing, sensory testing, and reflex assessment. Further specialized testing can be deferred.

B. The Glasgow Coma Scale (GCS) score is determined and recorded. The mental status is established as to person, place, and dates, surrounding the events. Cranial nerve evaluation is done with special attention directed to pupillary size and symmetry. Acute changes in the pupillary diameter can indicate a brain herniation syndrome and may require emergent surgery, hyperventilation, or diuresis.

C. Motor evaluation is performed for the GCS and SCI evaluation. The patient is asked to move all extremities individually and strength is assessed according to the American Spinal Injury Association/International Medical Society of Paraplegia (ASIA/IMSOP) protocol. Normal strength is graded 5/5, with mild weakness graded as 4/5. The ability to fully overcome gravity through a full range of motion is graded 3/5. Movement throughout a range of motion but unable to overcome gravity is graded 2/5. Flicker motion of muscles is 1/5 and no movement is 0/5. Patients with C5 levels of spinal cord function will be able to flex only their arms and should not be confused with pathological flexor posturing.

D. Sensory testing is performed with regard to light touch and pain perception (Fig. 18-2). Useful examination tools include a cotton swab broken in half or safety pins. Pay close attention to the level of sensation and asymmetry.

E. Reflex testing is performed at the biceps (C5), triceps (C7), brachioradialis , knee (L4), and ankle areas (S1). Special reflex testing including jaw jerk, deltoid (C5), pectoral, superficial abdominal (T9–T12), bulbo- or cliterocavernositis (S3–S4), anal wink (S5), and Babinski. The extremity reflexes are graded on a scale of 0 to 4, where 0 = absent reflex activity, 1 = decreased reflex activity, 2 = normal reflex activity, 3 = increased reflex activity, and 4 = grossly exaggerated reflex activity with sustained clonus. An exaggerated jaw jerk indicates injury at or above the pons. Deltoid and pectoral reflexes are usually associated with significant hyperreflexia. Bulbo- or cliterocavernosis reflexes may be retained in complete injury, but lost during spinal shock. Their reappearance may indicate that a period of spinal shock has ended. Babinski responses are recorded as present or absent. The presence of UMN findings (hyperreflexia, loss of superficial abdominal reflexes, Babinski responses) indicates spinal cord or conus medullaris injury. Decreased reflexes imply LMN (cauda equina and nerve root) injury. Weakness, sensory loss, and bladder, bowel, and sexual dysfunction can be seen with either UMN or LMN injuries. Of note, acute UMN injuries often present with reflex stunning or areflexia, which may last for 24 to 48 hours.

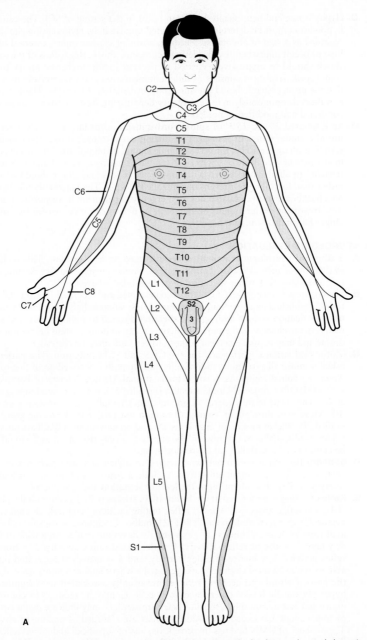

Figure 18-2. Anterior **(A)** and posterior **(B)** cervical, thoracic, lumbar, and sacral dermatomes. (From McDonald JV, Welch WC. Patient history and neurologic examination. In: Welch WC, Jacobs GB, Jackson RP, eds. *Operative Spinal Surgery*. Stamford, Conn: Appleton & Lange; 1999;3:15, with permission.) (*continued*)

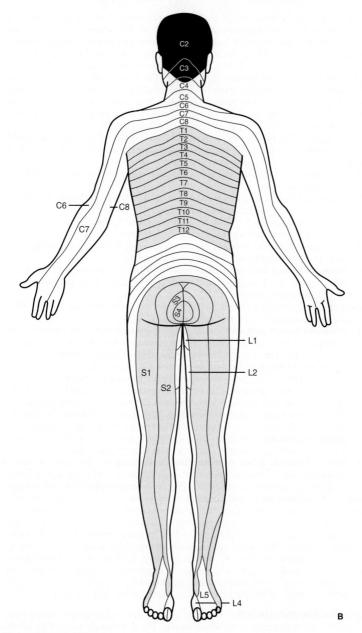

Figure 18-2. (continued)

F. The most sensitive predictor of prognosis is the severity of neurologic injury as characterized by level and completeness of deficit. The neurologic sensory levels are determined and recorded based on the lowest segment with normal sensory and motor function bilaterally. Complete injury is seen in the patient without sensory or motor function below the level of neurologic injury, including loss of perianal sensation and sphincteric function. The patient with incomplete injury has partial preservation of sensory or motor function below the level of neurologic injury, with preservation of perianal sensation and motor function. This is often referred to as sacral sparing, and does not include an intact bulbo/clitoro cavernosus reflex which can be present in complete injuries.

G. In the acute setting, the use of specific terms denoting neurologic level is preferable to more general terms (e.g., paraparesis, quadriplegia). The ASIA impairment scale, consisting of a five-point grading scale, is as follows:

1. Complete loss of sensory and motor function (including the sacral area) below the neurologic level.
2. Incomplete injury, whereby sensory function is preserved below the level of neurologic injury including the sacral area.
3. Incomplete injury with motor function preserved below the neurologic level and most preserved groups exhibiting strength of ≤ 3.
4. Incomplete injury with motor function preserved below the neurologic level and most preserved groups exhibiting ≥ 3 strength.
5. **Normal sensory and motor examination.** Even patients with ASIA 1 scores can improve neurologically, although few of these patients will achieve functional motor recovery.

H. Another useful descriptor of spinal cord injuries involves pathologic criteria. These syndromes correlate to anatomic areas of injury.

1. **Posterior cord injury** with loss of position sense (posterior columns) is rarely traumatic. This injury is usually related to vitamin deficiencies and infections (e.g., syphilis). The patients develop a loss of position and vibratory sense.
2. **Central cord injury** is common in patients who experience excessive motion in the sagittal plane (e.g., hyperflexion and hyperextension), particularly those with preexisting cervical stenosis. These injuries represent a centripetal force applied to the spinal cord with resultant central necrosis secondary to vascular compromise. The hallmark features are hand weakness more than leg weakness, bladder dysfunction, and variable degrees of sensory loss below the level of the lesion.
3. **Anterior cord injury** suggests anterior spinal artery occlusion and results in loss of all motor and sensory function other than proprioception.
4. **Brown-Sequard (cord hemisection) syndrome** is identified by loss of ipsilateral motor function, ipsilateral position sense, and contralateral loss of pain and temperature sensation two to three segments below the level of injury.

I. **Conus medullaris and cauda equina syndromes** occur at the thoracolumbar levels and result in varying degrees of weakness, sensory loss, bladder, bowel, and sexual dysfunction. Conus injuries affect UMNs, which may precipitate hyperreflexia. Conus injuries may also cause reflex stunning with the loss of the bulbocavernosus reflex. The cauda equina syndrome typically results from a compressive lesion below the level of the spinal cord with resultant bowel/bladder dysfunction, saddle paresthesias, and lower extremity weakness. This represents one of the few operative emergencies and should be alleviated as soon as safely possible to attain maximal recovery and prevent further deterioration.

V. RADIOGRAPHIC EVALUATION. The diagnosis of spinal cord or spinal column injury is of paramount importance in the acute setting. The diagnosis is reached by obtaining a history of the events, performing a neurologic evaluation of the patient, and obtaining the appropriate radiographic evaluation. The initial studies should cover the area of suspected injury. Patients with persistent complaints of pain along the spine should be assumed to have a spinal column injury until proven otherwise. Patients with a normal x-ray study and severe neck pain should remain in a rigid cervical collar. MRI should be obtained in this setting. Follow-up flexion/extension films can be completed about 3 days after injury to rule out instability that was masked by muscle spasm. Keep in mind that 10% to 15% of patients with one spine fracture will have another fracture elsewhere in the spine. The "skeletal level" is used to denote the area of greatest vertebral injury and can be different from the neurologic level(s).

A. Cervical spine

1. The cervical spine can be clinically cleared without radiography in patients who present with a GCS of 15, with no evidence of drug or alcohol use, normal neurologic exam, without midline cervical pain, and without distracting or significant injuries. The Canadian C-spine rules provide a well-validated algorithm to avoid unnecessary imaging with a sensitivity of 100%. For the majority of trauma patients who do not meet these guidelines, evaluation starts with plain films. The sensitivity and specificity of plain radiography to detect a fracture remain below 90%. This compares to a reported sensitivity and specificity of 96.0% and 96.5%, respectively, for CT. With a 14.5% probability of paralysis for missed injuries, CT has emerged as the diagnostic modality of choice. However, the negative predictive value of CT combined with plain films exceeds 99%, prompting our institution to always obtain at least a lateral C-spine. Fractures may be missed with CT if they extend horizontally in the axial plane, parallel to the tomographic imaging slice. While cost remains a point of contention, in moderate- to high-risk patients in urban trauma centers, CT can be cost-effective. Of note, the most commonly missed cervical fractures are at the C1 to C2 and C7 to T1 levels, usually the result of inadequate imaging.

2. The basic lateral radiographic studies must include the skull base and T1 vertebral body for adequate interpretation. A "swimmer's view" may be required to fully assess C7 to T1. Oblique views may also help assess C7 to T1, although a CT is usually obtained after two attempted failures to obtain adequate plain films. The films are reviewed with careful attention to three lines:
   a. Posterior vertebral body line
   b. Anterior vertebral body line
   c. Spinolaminar line (Fig. 18-3)
   These lines should be uninterrupted and smooth. The appearance of a straight spine (loss of the normal cervical lordosis) indicates extensor muscular spasm and can suggest spinal injury. A rigid cervical collar can also cause loss of lordosis. The vertebral canal is defined as the distance from the spinolaminar line to the posterior vertebral body line. This space available for the cord should be >13 mm at every level. A narrower canal may represent injury or congenital cervical stenosis.

3. Soft tissues are then examined. The trachea contains air and provides a line of contrast against the vertebral bodies. Prevertebral swelling indicates a hematoma consistent with spinal column injury. The hematoma can also compromise the patient's airway, leading to respiratory collapse. An easy rule to remember is that the soft-tissue space should be no greater than 6 mm in front of the C2 vertebral body and no greater than 22 mm anterior to C6. Another important distance is the atlantodens interval. This is the space between the anterior aspect of the odontoid (dens) and the ring of C1. This space should not exceed 3.5 mm in the adult and 5 mm in the child. Distances greater than those indicate disruption of the transverse ligament, with resultant instability.

4. Vertebral height is examined next, including vertebral body morphology. The vertebral bodies should be similar in appearance, without evidence of compression or fracture. The distance between the posterior spinous processes, or interspinous distance, should be similar at each level.

5. Other radiographs obtained of the cervical spine include the open mouth view of C1 to C2. This study shows the base of the odontoid and helps determine whether a type I, II, or III odontoid fracture (discussed below) is present. The lateral masses of C1 are examined with regard to their relationship to C2.

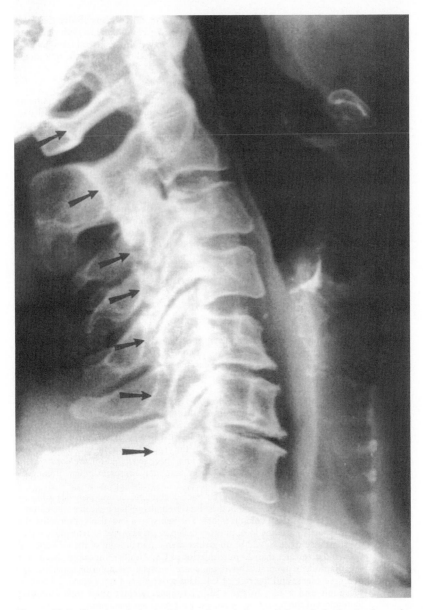

Figure 18-3. Normal cervical spine lateral radiograph demonstrating spinolaminar line (*arrows*).

Little or no overhang of the lateral masses should be seen. A combined, bilateral overhang ≥6.9 mm indicates a fracture of the ring of C1, with probable disruption of the transverse ligament. The odontoid bone should be symmetrically located between the lateral masses of C2.

6. The anteroposterior (AP) view of the spine is examined for the distance between spinous processes, alignment, and rotation. Facet anatomy is more closely observed with oblique views of the cervical spine. Areas suspected of having fracture can be further assessed with fine-cut CT. MRI is indicated in patients with neurologic deficits or significant fractures that will require reduction. The MRI yields information as to ligamentous integrity, subtle compression fractures, traumatic disc rupture, and SCI. Signal change on long TR images help differentiate acute injury from those that are chronic. Patients with neurologic deficits should be evaluated in consultation with the spine surgery service.

7. If a conscious patient has no neck pain to palpation and can voluntarily flex, extend, and rotate without pain, and initial x-rays are normal, the collar may be removed. Should a patient have neck pain and yet have normal preliminary x-rays, further studies should be undertaken. At a minimum, flexion and extension films should be performed to rule out ligamentous instability. These must visualize C7 to T1. A normal three-view films and flex-extension series has a negative predictive values greater than 99%. Further radiographs, including magnetic resonance imaging (MRI) and even bone scan, can be appropriate to rule out possible bone or ligamentous injury. The rigid collar should remain in place until the neck is cleared clinically and radiographically.

B. Thoracolumbar spine

1. The thoracolumbar spine is commonly injured at the T12 to L1 levels. This occurs because of the large lever arm created by the inflexible thoracic spine as it joins the lumbar spine. This area of the spine is well examined with lateral and AP views. Three lines are observed along the anterior and posterior aspects of the vertebral bodies, and along the posterior aspect of the spinous processes. The distance between these processes should also remain equal.

2. On the AP view, the distance between pedicles is determined as is the distance between the posterior spinous processes. The transverse processes and ribs are evaluated for fractures and the soft tissues are examined for swelling.

3. More specialized imaging studies are obtained as necessary. CT is useful for a closer examination of bone anatomy. These studies can be ordered with 1- to 3-mm cuts, and sagittal and coronal reconstruction to better define bony anatomy. MRI provides excellent visualization of the spinal cord and nerve roots and helps define spinal cord and ligamentous injury.

4. AP and lateral films are indicated in those patients with symptoms referable to the thoracic area or those who have a mechanism that is consistent with such an injury. This would include patients involved in motorcycle accidents, falls from height, ejection from vehicle, or pedestrian–automobile collisions. Flexion and extension films are not as helpful in this area as compared with the cervical spine. Thoracic spine CT is indicated for those patients with fractures noted on x-ray film or when the anatomy is not well seen on plain films. MRI is indicated for all patients with neurologic findings.

C. Lumbar spine

1. The lumbar spine is subjected to injurious forces in falls, motor vehicle crashes, and by other means. Because the spinal cord ends at the L1 to L2 level, true SCI from lumbar fractures is infrequent. Injuries to the conus medullaris and cauda equina can occur if the spinal canal is compromised. Commonly, no neurologic injury is noted with lumbar spine fractures.

2. The lumbar spine is evaluated similar to the thoracolumbar spine. AP and lateral spine films are the initial studies.

3. CT can be useful to determine the amount of canal compromise in cases of burst fracture. MRI and myelography are also helpful in cases of traumatic nerve root injury, canal compression, and conus medullaris and cauda equina syndromes.

VI. MEDICAL MANAGEMENT OF SCI.
Once the patient has arrived in the trauma resuscitation area, more sophisticated medical management can begin. The goal is to prevent secondary cord injury, which can be exacerbated by hypotension, shock, hypoxia, hypercoaguability, and hyperthermia. Management protocols include

definitive treatment of other injuries; maintenance of adequate blood pressure; detailed radiographic studies; high-dose steroids, if appropriate; determination of the need for surgical intervention; and postoperative rehabilitation.

A. Methylprednisolone. A number of studies have suggested that neurologic improvement can occur following the administration of high-dose steroids after blunt injury to the spinal cord. Penetrating trauma to the spine, such as gunshot wounds, are not appropriate candidates, considering the increased risk of infection. The second National Acute Spinal Cord Injury Study (NASCIS 2) showed that methylprednisolone given in a dose of 30 mg/kg intravenously (IV) over 45 minutes within 8 hours after injury in those with incomplete or suspected incomplete SCI improved neurologic outcome. The initial dose is followed by 5.4 mg/kg/h IV given over the next 23 hours by continuous drip. The NASCIS 3 study reported that if patients begin treatment between 3 and 8 hours postinjury, the steroid infusion must be extended to 48 hours to attain the same benefit as 24 hours of steroids given within 3 hours of injury. Significant, functional benefit remains inconclusive and there is no defined standard of care. Currently, the *Guidelines for the Management of Acute Cervical Spine and Spinal Cord Injuries* (AANS) state that administration of steroids "is recommended as an option in treatment of patients with acute spinal cord injuries that should be undertaken only with the knowledge that the evidence suggesting harmful side effects is more consistent than any suggestion of clinical benefit." In practice, the protocol is often initiated at referring hospitals prior to transfer. We routinely complete the regimen in these circumstances.

B. Hemodynamic instability is common in acute SCI. Approximately 70% of patients with high cervical SCI will have severe bradycardia (<45 beats per minute [bpm]) and hypotension with an associated 16% incidence of cardiac arrest. Animal models have shown hypotension can exacerbate spinal cord ischemia and worsen neurologic outcome. Extensive class III data supports blood pressure augmentation to maintain mean arterial pressure (MAP) at 85 to 90 mmHg for 5 to 7 days postinjury. This therapy can be sustained with minimal morbidity and has shown improved outcomes compared to historical controls. **Hypotension and hypoxia should be avoided at all costs.**

C. Other medical issues to be considered in patients with SCI include prevention and treatment of pulmonary complications. Aggressive pulmonary toilet, specialized rotating beds, and antibiotics are often appropriate. Early tracheostomy can reduce length of stay and facilitate care. After evaluating 178 patients with ASIA A SCI, 70% required a tracheostomy; 100% for injuries at or above C3 and none at or below C8. Urinary tract infections are common in paralyzed patients because of repeated catheterization. Decubitus ulcers can occur rapidly in insensate patients. Aggressive nursing care is the mainstay of treatment. Stress gastric and duodenal ulcers are common and prophylaxis is recommended. Joint contractures and heterotopic ossification are common in paralyzed patients. These complications can be reduced by physical therapy. SCI patients are more sensitive to acetylcholine and the use of succinylcholine can precipitate a hyperkalemic crisis. Autonomic dysreflexia occurs in up to 90% of patients with lesions above T6. Distension of hollow viscera or cutaneous stimulation can produce rapid fluctuations in blood pressure, vasoconstriction, bladder spasm, flushing, sweating, encephalopathy, seizures, congestive heart failure, and arrhythmias. Treatment involves removal of the stimulus and aggressive blood pressure control.

D. The risk of deep venous thrombosis (DVT) and pulmonary embolus (PE) are 39% to 100% and 4% to 10%, respectively. Unfractionated or low-molecular-weight heparin and serial compression devices should be instituted as soon as medically feasible. These interventions provide a 50% reduction in incidence of thromboembolism.

E. Patients with suspected vertebral artery injury should have a CT, MR, or catheter-based angiogram. The lower sensitivity of a computed tomography angiography (CTA) is balanced by the ease with which it is obtained, particularly for unstable patients or those receiving CT imaging of other regions.

Indications for angiogram include a complete cervical spine injury, fracture of the foramen transversarium, facet dislocation, subluxation, or suspicious neurologic exam. Symptomatic injuries presenting with a stroke may be anticoagulated for 3 to 6 months. Asymptomatic patients should be observed and followed closely as delayed ischemia is common. Antiplatelet agents remain a viable option that will require further study, particularly for asymptomatic patients.

F. Obtunded patients represent a particular dilemma. Prolonged cervical immobilization has been associated with decubitis ulcers, elevated ICP, pain, and pulmonary complications. Patients who have suffered neurologic injury rendering them comatose or who have other conditions that prevent them from fully cooperating with the examining physician should have complete spine radiographic evaluation. Approximately 1% of patients who are obtunded will have ligamentous instability that is missed when x-ray studies are normal. Classically, passive flexion-extension under fluoroscopy with negative plain films was utilized to rule out instability. However, visualization is inadequate in up to 30% of patients. Combined with the rare but serious potential for permanent morbidity, MRI has emerged as the study of choice to clear the cervical spine in this population. Protocols designed with limited, specialized imaging sequences can reduce time in the scanner and ultimately cost when applied routinely. Sensitivity may be increased by imaging within 48 hours to maximize visualization of edematous tissue. Without access to MRI, a collar can be left in place for 30 days, allowing time for occult ligamentous injury to heal.

VII. SURGICAL MANAGEMENT OF CERVICAL SPINAL COLUMN INJURIES. The timing of a surgical intervention remains debated. Data are accumulating in support of early (<3 days) surgery. Safety, decreased morbidity, shorter length of stay, and lower rates of pneumonia have been documented. There is no consistent evidence to show improved neurologic outcome.

A. Occiput C1 to C2 injuries

1. Occipital C1 injuries are an uncommon but often missed injury. Otherwise known as atlantooccipital dislocation, these typically cause a disruption between the occipital condyles and C1. Patients who survive typically exhibit lower cranial neuropathies, mono/para/quadraplegia, and respiratory dysfunction, although 20% may have normal exams. Craniocervical subarachnoid blood or cervical prevertebral edema can provide an early clue to the diagnosis. Treatment involves craniocervical fusion with internal fixation.

2. C1 to C2 injuries, which are common, are frequently missed because of the relatively complex anatomy of the C1–C2 junction and the difficulty in obtaining a full set of films in the multiply injured patient. The bony odontoid fractures can be divided into types I, II, and III (Fig. 18-4).

a. Type I fractures are oblique fractures through the upper portion of the odontoid process that can be managed with a rigid cervical collar. These are rare and often confused with os odontoidium, an isolated bony ossicle with smooth margins and no osseous connection to the body of C2. Os odontoidium likely represents an acquired nonunion of C2 secondary to prior trauma. This stable fracture can be managed with observation.

b. Type II fractures are those that occur at the base of the dens. These fractures are considered to be unstable in the acute setting, although most can be managed with external stabilization (rigid cervical collar or halo-vest device). Surgical intervention should strongly be considered in patients over 50 years old, after failure to achieve anatomic alignment with external fixation, with >5 mm dens displacement, or with significant comminution. Fractures with posterior displacement provide increased morbidity as they may impinge on the spinal cord. Surgical options include an odontoid screw, posterior fixation incorporating a Gallie-or Brooks-type construct, and transarticular screws. Airway management is critical in these patients

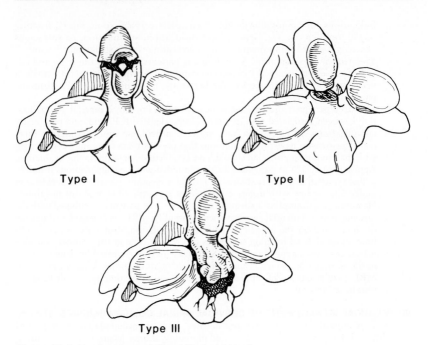

Type I

Type II

Type III

Figure 18-4. Drawing of types I, II, and III odontoid fractures.

as upper airway swelling and subsequent respiratory compromise can occur (Fig. 18-5).

   c. Type III fractures extend from the odontoid into the vertebral body of C2. They generally have a better healing rate than type II fractures with external fixation, and rarely need surgery.

3. Jefferson fractures occur when an axial load is placed on the head. The C1 bone, which is circular in nature, is forced apart. Fractures occur anteriorly or posteriorly. Stability depends on the integrity of the transverse ligament as described below. A fracture with evidence of ligamentous disruption can be treated with a halo orthosis for 3 months or a C1–C2 fusion. Stable fractures can be treated with a rigid cervical collar for 2 to 3 months.

4. It is important to consider that the main ligament stabilizing the dens within the ring of C1 is the transverse ligament. This ligament keeps the dens in close approximation to the ring of C1. The space between the posterior aspect of the ring of C1 and the anterior border of the dens is called the atlantodens interval. This space should not exceed 3.5 mm in the adult (Fig. 18-6).

   a. The ligament can be torn whenever the ring of C1 is fractured. The amount of medial-lateral displacement of the ring of C1 can be measured on AP radiographs or CT reconstructions. Normally, the C1 lateral masses do not overlap the C2 vertebral body. Should the combined amount of lateral mass overlap of C1 on C2 exceed 6.9 mm, consider the transverse ligament to be torn and the C1–C2 area unstable (Fig. 18-7). MRI can also identify ligamentous injury or avulsion.

5. Hangman's fracture refers to spondylolisthesis of the C2 pedicle. This type of fracture is also unstable and requires external fixation with a collar or halo vest, or rarely, internal fixation. Anterior C2–C3 fusion or posterior C1–C3 fusion should be

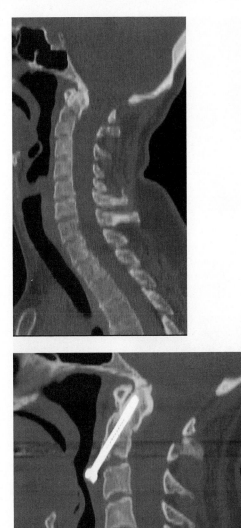

Figure 18-5. Radiograph type II odontoid fracture.

considered in cases of severe angulation, C2–C3 disc disruption, fracture/dislocation, or failure to achieve anatomic alignment with external fixation.

B. C3 to C7 injuries

1. Most of the C3 to C7 injuries can be diagnosed from a lateral film using the three lines to determine alignment and stability. On flexion and extension views, no >3.5 mm of listhesis should be seen between two vertebrae and no >11 degrees of angulation between vertebral bodies, as measured at the adjoining endplates. The spinous process distances should be symmetric. CT will define the bone anatomy and MRI will better show the ligamentous injury, cord anatomy, and disc pathology. In most injuries, both studies should be obtained. In all injuries requiring traction, delay in treatment reduces the chance of nonoperative reduction.

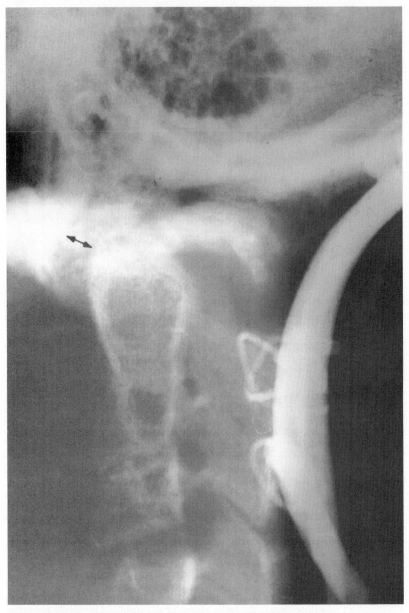

Figure 18-6. Lateral radiograph demonstrating excessive atlantodens interval.

  2. A common type of injury involves unilateral and bilateral facet injuries. These injuries include both fractures of the facet joints and injury to the capsules with resultant "perched" facets. Both types of injuries are noted on plain films and CT. The presence of 25% subluxation of one vertebra on another can represent a unilateral facet fracture or dislocation. The CT scan appearance of this frac-

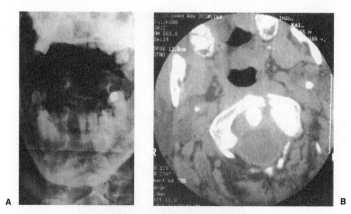

Figure 18-7. C1 fracture with overhanging of the C1 lateral masses as seen on anteroposterior plain film **(A)** and axial computed tomography scan **(B)**.

ture has the appearance of "opposing hamburger buns" (Fig. 18-8). Subluxation of 50% generally means that a bilateral facet injury has occurred. Patients with these injuries should have MRI to diagnose any disc herniation that could interfere with reduction of the two vertebral bodies, potentially causing a neurologic catastrophe if the disc compromises the cord during reduction. Those patients may need anterior discectomy before reduction.
   3. Generally, unilateral and bilateral facet dislocations are reduced in tong or halo traction under close supervision by the spine surgeon. Awake reduction in a stable, alert patient with no distracting injury is both feasible and preferred. The reduction can also be performed intraoperatively with electrodiagnostic monitoring. A prereduction plain film or CT should be obtained to provide baseline anatomy. MRI should be obtained prior to reduction to rule out a ruptured cervical disc. Unilateral facet fractures can be stable, with pure bony injuries handled by halo-vest immobilization. An irreducible injury, ligamentous injury, >20% subluxation, or spinal cord compression necessitates anterior or posterior surgical fixation and possible decompression.
   4. Bilateral facet injuries are unstable because the spinal canal is generally severely compromised. Closed reduction with traction may be unsuccessful. Intraoperative reduction and surgical stabilization is the treatment method of choice if awake reduction fails. Once again, MRI is essential prior to reduction to prevent cord injury from a traumatically herniated disc.
   C. Burst fractures generally occur as a result of flexion or axial loading. The columns may appear well aligned at first glance on the lateral radiograph. Generally noted is an expansion of the prevertebral space and loss of vertebral height. The CT scan will show the vertebral comminution which can cause canal compromise and subsequent neurologic deficit. Fracture compression of 40% or more and subluxation of 20% or more indicate definitive instability. These will require surgical stabilization but should have gentle traction or collar immobilization during studies and before surgery.
   D. Teardrop fractures must be differentiated from the less ominous extension injury with a small fragment off the anterior cortex of the vertebral body. The true teardrop injury is highly unstable; CT will show the sagittal split in the vertebral body. MRI will often demonstrate an early spinal cord contusion. Most of these patients are neurologically impaired and will need surgery to stabilize the neck and decompress the spinal cord.

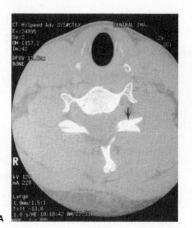

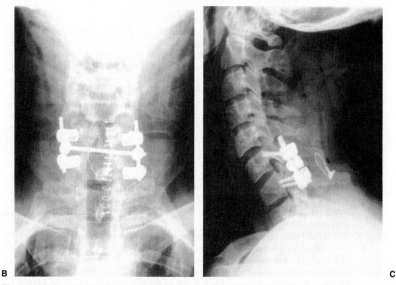

Figure 18-8. Preoperative axial computed tomography scan demonstrating a unilateral jumped and locked facet fracture and dislocation **(A)**. The left jumped facet has the appearance of two opposing hamburger buns (*arrow*). Anteroposterior **(B)** and lateral **(C)** radiographs demonstrating the instrumented fusion using lateral mass screws and rods with interspinous wiring and bone grafting.

E. Spinal cord injuries without radiographic abnormality (SCIWORA). A number of patients will appear to be neurologically impaired without fractures or ligamentous injuries noted on initial radiographic studies. Generally, patients in this group are at the ends of the age spectrum. Young patients are susceptible to this type of injury because of the elasticity of their ligaments. In the older patient, underlying degenerative or congenital cervical stenosis is usually found. Mild hyperflexion or hyperextension injuries will cause spinal cord compression without bony fracture. Early spinal cord changes are often noted on the MRI.

A central cord-type injury is often the result in these types of injuries. Although some of these patients will slowly recover, a number will need surgical decompression of the spinal cord to promote recovery. Conservative therapy involves a rigid cervical collar and activity restriction for 2 to 3 months followed by flexion-extension films.

F. Ankylosing spondylitis is an inflammatory arthropathy that affects the spine and sacroiliac joints. Care of these patients is extremely difficult and should be guided by a spine specialist to avoid iatrogenic injury. The ligaments and intervertebral discs become calcified and fuse to form a "bamboo spine" that often results in a flexion contracture. The rigid and weakened bone, which is prone to bleed, fractures easily. Fractures often occur in the low cervical region, and can be difficult to identify on plain radiographs. Frequently, the underlying deformity is not known, positioning is difficult and dangerous for imaging studies, and these patients can deteriorate neurologically because of malposition of the neck and their propensity to develop epidural hematomas. Excessive extension must be avoided. Prepositioning x-rays are essential to determine the baseline anatomy.

VIII. SURGICAL MANAGEMENT OF THORACOLUMBAR SPINAL COLUMN INJURIES

A. Compression fractures typically involve the anterior column only. CT will differentiate a one-column injury from a more unstable two-column injury. The lateral film will show the loss of vertebral height (Fig. 18-9). Greater than 40% loss of height can signal an unstable fracture requiring surgical treatment. This amount of wedging associated with posterior tenderness generally signals a ligamentous injury to the posterior column. Multiple compression fractures can be unstable and should be watched closely. Higher fractures (T1–T9) require much more

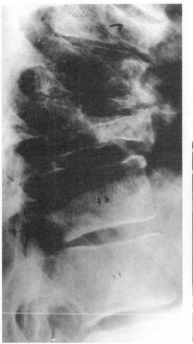
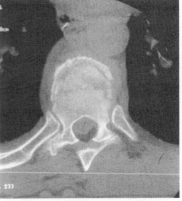

A   B

Figure 18-9. T9 compression fracture as seen on lateral radiograph **(A)** and axial computed tomography scan **(B)**.

energy to fracture because of rib cage stability and are associated with more serious injury. Multiple rib fractures and sternal fractures are associated with instability. Most T10–L5 compression fractures with <40% loss of height and no posterior tenderness can be managed in a brace. Kyphoplasty and vertebroplasty, which involve injection of viscous cement into the fracture bed, are emerging as therapeutic options. Their role is still being defined in the acute setting.

1. Imaging (CT, MRI) is indicated for any compression fracture associated with neurologic injury, >30% loss of height of vertebral body, and any patient with posterior tenderness or widening of the pedicles on an AP view. These patients should be evaluated by a spine surgeon.

B. Burst fractures involve the anterior two columns and are generally considered unstable. X-ray findings are positive when the lateral view shows loss of vertebral height, widening of the spinous processes, or interruption of the posterior vertebral body line. The AP view shows widening of the pedicles, widening between the spinous processes, and loss of vertebral height. Many of these patients have neurologic injury. All of these fractures should have detailed imaging studies and the patients should receive spine service consultation. Although surgical fusion remains the standard of care, neurologically intact patients without evidence of damage to the posterior osteoligamentous complex may be managed in an extension brace for 3 months. Patients receive close radiographic follow-up with concern for progressive kyphosis. Patients with a progressive deficit require emergent operative intervention. Surgery may be deferred in those with a stable deficit for the theoretical benefit of allowing progression and resolution of cord edema and inflammation, which may reduce the risk of iatrogenic injury.

C. Flexion or distraction (seat belt or Chance) fractures. This axially oriented fracture is caused by a flexion injury around an anterior fulcrum (lap belt without shoulder harness). The fracture can split the pedicles in half, tear open the disc space, or spare bone elements and be ligamentous in nature. The excessive flexion motion places the spine in kyphosis. This injury is associated with a 30% to 45% incidence of abdominal injury and 13% risk of paralysis. Some of the pure bony injuries can be managed nonoperatively by placing the patients in an extension brace to bring the fractured bony elements into apposition, but ligamentous injuries require surgery. These injuries require detailed imaging studies.

D. Fracture-dislocations are highly unstable and require imaging studies on all patients. Most occur at the thoracolumbar junction. The more cephalad the injury, the more likely paraplegia will result (90% above T10 and 60% below T10). The AP and lateral views will show translation of the spine as well as fractures in the facets, dislocations, or comminution fraction. These injuries require detailed radiographic studies, followed by surgical stabilization.

E. Sacral fractures are difficult to see on x-ray film and will require CT for delineation. Fractures lateral to the sacral foramen have a 6% incidence of neurologic injury (L5 root) and fractures through the foramen have a 28% incidence. Fractures medial to the foramen through the canal have an associated neurologic injury in 57%, most involving bowel and bladder function. Displaced fractures can require surgery.

IX. GUNSHOT WOUNDS TO THE SPINE

A. Penetrating injuries to the spine should be treated as elsewhere in the body. The standard surgical principles of debridement and closure can be applied. The caveat is that patients with cerebrospinal fluid (CSF) leaks are at risk of meningitis and paravertebral abscess formation, unless CSF egress is controlled. Steroid therapy is contraindicated in this population due to the risk of infection.

B. In general, large penetrating wounds require exploration and debridement. Wound cultures are taken and all potentially contaminating material (e.g., clothing fragments or shotgun wadding) is removed. Passage through the esophagus, pharynx, or colon before traversing the spine has the potential to cause spinal sepsis. Radical debridement of the spine is no longer advocated in this situation. Minimal debridement of bullet tract and 1 to 2 weeks of broad-spectrum antibiotics is sufficient to decrease the chance of spinal infection to about 10% of cases when the bullet traverses the colon, esophagus, or pharynx.

C. Removing bullet fragments may necessarily be delayed if an abnormal lead level develops. Removal of a bullet from the spinal canal is recommended with a worsening neurologic picture or evidence of neurologic compression on radiographic studies. These procedures can be facilitated if performed in a delayed fashion to allow easier dural repair. CSF diversion (e.g., lumbar, cervical, or ventricular drainage) may be required for persistent leakage. Neurologic deterioration mandates a more urgent approach to debridement.

D. Few civilian spinal injuries caused by the bullet striking the spinal column are unstable enough to require surgical stabilization. The three-column theory can be used to dictate treatment. If two of three columns are involved, a rigid orthosis is necessary. Flexion or extension films may be necessary to determine stability.

AXIOMS

■ The most important factors when treating injuries to the spine are attention to the mechanism of injury, understanding the level of neurologic function at the time of injury compared to later presentation, maintaining a continual awareness of other injuries to the spine, confounding injuries, and patient variables.

■ The most commonly missed fractures occur at the C1 to C2 and C7 levels.

■ The general assumption is that all patients have an unstable spine until proven otherwise.

■ Patients with continued complaints of spine-related pain must be thoroughly evaluated and this evaluation must be repeated if the symptoms persist.

■ Patients with ankylosing spondylitis have a significant risk of missed or iatrogenic injury and should be managed closely by a spine specialist.

■ Should any doubt about the injury persist, evaluation by a spine surgeon is necessary.

Bibliography

American College of Surgeons Committee on Trauma. *Advanced Trauma Life Support Instructor Manual*. Chicago, Ill: American College of Surgeons; 1997.

Bracken MB, Holford TR. Effects of timing of methylprednisolone or naloxone administration on recovery of segmental and long-tract neurologic function in NASCIS 2. *J Neurosurg* 1993;79:500–507.

Bracken MB, Shepard MJ, Collins WF, et al. A randomized, controlled trial of methylprednisolone or naloxone in the treatment of acute spinal-cord injury. Results of the Second National Acute Spinal Cord Injury Study. *N Engl J Med* 1990;332:1405–1411.

Bracken MB, Shepard MJ, Holford TR, et al. Administration of methylprednisolone for 24 or 48 hours or tirilazad mesylate for 48 hours in the treatment of acute spinal cord injury. Results of the Third National Acute Spinal Cord Injury Randomized Controlled Trial. *JAMA* 1997;277:1597–1604.

Burney RE, Waggoner R, Maynard FM. Stabilization of spinal injury for early transfer. *J Trauma* 1989;29:1497–1499.

Carlson GD, Gorden C. Invited review. Spinal cord injury research: Current status and clinical implications. *SpineLine* 2000;1:7–18.

Grogan EL, Morris JA, Dittus RS, et al. Cervical spine evaluation in urban trauma centers: Lowering institutional costs and complications through helical CT scan. *J Am Coll Surg* 2005;200:160–165.

Harrop JS, Sharan AD, Scheid EH Jr, et al. Tracheostomy placement in patients with complete cervical spinal cord injuries: American Spinal Injury Association Grade A. *J Neurosurg Spine* 2004;100(1):20–23. Available from: http://www.asia-spinalinjury .org/publications/index.html.

International Standards for Neurological and Functional Classification of Spinal Cord Injury. 4th ed. Chicago, Ill: American Spinal Injury Association, International Medical Society of Paraplegia (ASIA/IMSOP); 1992.

Neurosurgery 2002;50(suppl).

O'Keeffe T, Goldman RK, Mayberry JC, Rehm CG, Hart RA. Tracheostomy after anterior cervical spine fixation. *J Trauma* 2004;57(4):855–860.

Przybylski G, Welch WC, Jacobs GB. Spinal instability and biomechanics. In: Welch WC, Jacobs GB, Jackson RP, eds. *Operative Spinal Surgery*. Stamford, Conn: Appleton & Lange; 1999;7:104–112.

Stiell IG, Wells GA, Vandemheen KL, Clement CM, Lesiuk H. The Canadian C-spine rule for radiography in alert and stable trauma patients. *JAMA* 2001;286(15):1841–1848.

I. GENERAL

A. Careful examination and evaluation of the wound should be made prior to any treatment. Lacerations or contusions should be considered evidence of underlying bone injury and alert the clinician to inspect the radiographs of the bones in that area. Fractures of the underlying bone should be detected and, in many cases, treated before definitive soft tissue management. Treatment of the fracture after soft-tissue management often disrupts the soft-tissue closure and further damages the soft tissue. If the fractures are exposed through soft-tissue injuries, perform the fracture repair through the lacerations rather than use the standard incisions for facial fracture treatment.

B. Injuries to associated nerves, ducts, glands, and sinuses require assessment. Thorough investigation of the structural functions in the vicinity of the laceration is important.

C. Tissue that is contaminated and damaged by crush and contusion present a hazard for infection if primary repair is undertaken. The probability of contamination increases rapidly and is directly proportional to the length of time that has elapsed since injury. The history and circumstances of the injury provide evidence signaling the possibility of deeply embedded foreign material.

D. Delayed primary wound closure

  1. Indications

    a. Patient seen late after injury

    b. Extensive tissue edema

    c. Subcutaneous hematoma

    d. Crush injury

    e. Wound edges are badly contused

    f. Tissue is devitalized

  2. Treatment

    a. Limited debridement to remove devitalized tissue

    b. Wet dressings

    c. Antibiotic therapy

  3. Treatment is continued until resolution of edema and acute inflammation and a clean appearance of the wound; delayed primary closure is likely to be successful.

E. Primary closure under unsatisfactory conditions can contribute to increased tension, soft-tissue loss, infection, and soft-tissue necrosis. Healing by secondary intention should be avoided if possible.

II. PHOTOGRAPHY should be done for:

A. Accurate record keeping

B. Insurance and legal purposes

C. Supplementing the written evaluations

D. Assessing the effectiveness of therapy

III. ANESTHESIA. An attitude of reassurance and sympathy, together with adequate premedication, permits extensive operation under local anesthesia.

A. Nerve blocks can be used to establish regional anesthesia in a wide field, with reduced dosage of medication and less discomfort. Less complicated wounds (e.g., small cuts, bruises, lacerations) and some uncomplicated fractures of the facial bones (e.g., the nose) can be treated under local anesthesia, either in the operating room or in an outpatient treatment area.

B. More extensive injuries may require general anesthesia.

IV. **DEBRIDEMENT AND CARE.** Thorough cleansing of soft-tissue wounds is imperative before any definitive treatment is attempted. All blood and debris should be carefully washed from the tissues with copious amounts of water and mild detergents. Remove any foreign materials such as glass, hair, clothing, tooth structures, pieces of artificial dentures, paint, grease, gravel, and dirt.

A. Except for the removal of obviously devitalized portions of tissue, extensive debridement of soft tissue has little place in management of facial injuries. All tissues that can participate in a satisfactory repair should be retained.

  1. Err on the side of retaining tissues that may not survive rather than to debriding or destroying any tissues that might be important in a final result. The excellent blood supply of the face usually makes extensive debridement unnecessary.

V. **CLEANING OF THE WOUND.** All wounds should be carefully inspected for foreign material. Its removal is imperative to prevent separation, infection, delayed healing, and subsequent pigmentation of the skin. The presence of foreign material and hematoma reduces the bacterial inoculum necessary for infection to develop.

A. The tissue edges can be cleansed with dilute antiseptics, detergent soaps, and water.

B. In rare cases, solvents (e.g., ether, benzene, or alcohol) can be used and are necessary to remove materials not soluable in water or removable by scrubbing or debridement. Scrubbing with a brush under anesthesia may be required to remove foreign material and prevent the development of infection and "traumatic tattoo." The material can be removed initially with scrubbing, the point of a no. 11 blade, or a small dermatologic curette.

VI. **WOUND TYPE**

A. Abrasions

  1. Clean with mild, nonirritating soap or dilute Hibiclens (Zeneca; Wilmington, Delaware), Betadine (Purdue Frederick; Norwalk, Connecticut), or Technicare (Care Tech Laboratories; St. Louis, Missouri).

  2. Carefully scrub dirt, grease, carbon, and other material out of the wound.

  3. Apply a light lubricating dressing.

  4. Apply moist compresses (wet to wet) or an antibacterial ointment to prevent drying and dessication of the exposed wound surfaces.

B. Contused wounds

  1. Generally subside without active treatment.

  2. Most hematomas are diffuse and absorb gradually.

  3. Eyelid, cheek, or forehead hematoma may require drainage.

  4. Nasal septal hematoma needs to be evacuated through a small incision in the septal mucosa or with a large-bore needle.

C. Simple lacerations

  1. Repair should be undertaken after underlying structures have been assessed and foreign bodies removed.

  2. Time lapse between injury and repair is important relative to risk of infection and choice of repair technique.

  3. With the exception of animal bites and traumatic tattoo, most soft-tissue wounds of the face, properly cleansed and dressed, can await primary repair up to 24 hours without serious risk of infection.

  4. Tissue that is devitalized must be excised, regardless of its location or how important it was.

    a. Although debridement should be conservative, it must be adequate. Ragged, severely contused wound edges should be conservatively excised to provide perpendicular skin edges that will heal primarily with minimal scarring.

5. Closely parallel lacerations can be converted to a single wound by excising the intervening skin bridge, facilitating repair and reducing scar formation.
6. Displaced tissue should be returned to its original position.
7. Occasionally, immediately changing the direction of a wound by Z-plasty or making tissue allowance for scar contracture at the time of primary wound repair is appropriate.
8. If the contused marginal tissues are of anatomic importance, it is best to avoid debridement and consider secondary reconstructive surgery.
D. Deep lacerations. The muscles of facial expression (Fig. 19-1) are so closely associated with the skin that careful closure of the wound in layers gives adequate approximation of the muscle.
  1. If possible, facial muscle layers should be identified and closed separately with fine absorbable sutures.
  2. Closure of the muscle and fascia in layers, including the subcutaneous tissue, restores adequate function and prevents adherence of cheek skin to the muscle.

VII. ANATOMIC CONSIDERATIONS IN REPAIRING SOFT TISSUE
  A. Facial nerve. It is often impractical and unnecessary to identify and suture the terminal branches of the facial nerve. The plexus of nerve fibers makes regeneration of activity a common occurrence, despite the absence of direct facial nerve suturing. Reasonably accurate approximation of the tissues usually allows some element of nerve regeneration by neurotization of muscle.

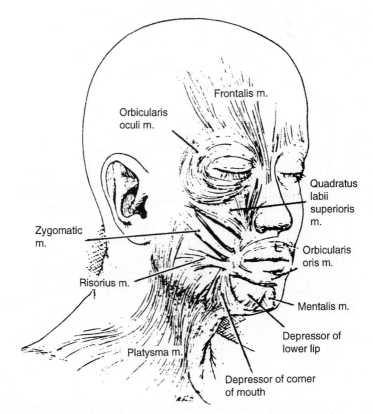

Figure 19-1. Muscles of facial expression.

1. Nerve repair need not be performed anterior to a line drawn at the lateral canthus of the eyelids.

2. Suture of named branches of the facial nerve should be performed and the branches should be sought (Fig.19-2). Primary repair at the time of the initial treatment is recommended.

B. Trigeminal nerve. The sensory branches of the trigeminal nerve (Fig. 19-3) in the region of the skin are small, and approximation is impractical and unnecessary. Partial or complete recovery of sensation usually occurs within a few months to a year, with slight hypesthesia often present. Contusion of trigeminal nerve branches also occurs as a result of fractures.

C. Parotid duct lacerations. Lacerations of the parotid duct should be repaired at the time of wound closure to prevent fistula to the skin or to the mucous membrane of the mouth.

1. To identify the course of the parotid duct, a line is drawn from the tragus of the ear to the midportion of the upper lip. The duct traverses the middle third of the line.

2. The parotid duct travels adjacent to the buccal branch of the facial nerve. Buccal branch paralysis with an overlying laceration should suggest the possibility of a parotid duct injury.

3. The parotid duct empties into the mouth opposite the maxillary second molar.

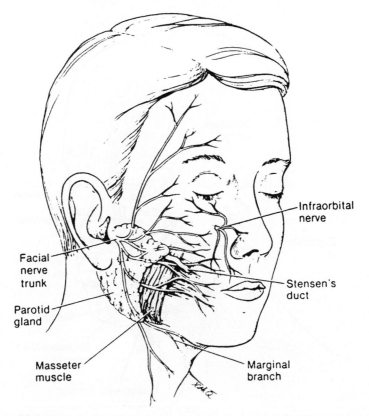

Figure 19-2. Deep anatomy of the cheek showing facial nerve, parotid gland, Stensen's duct, and masseter muscle.

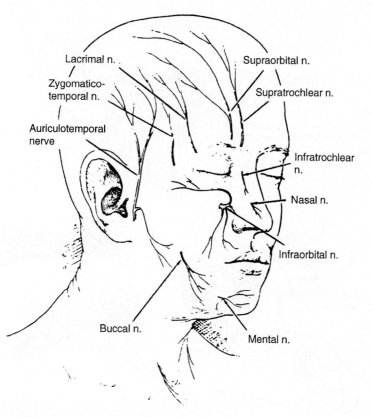

Figure 19-3. Trigeminal sensory nerve distribution to the face.

      a. A Silastic tube or silver probe can be inserted into the opening of the duct and the course of the duct followed. The duct can be irrigated with saline using a no. 22 angiocath sleeve. The appearance of saline in the wound indicates that the duct is injured. The proximal end of the duct can be identified in the wound expressing secretion of saliva.

      b. A silastic catheter is placed in the duct and the wound repaired with fine sutures. The tube is left in for a 2-week period, as tolerated (Fig. 19-4).

VIII. REGIONAL CONSIDERATIONS IN REPAIRING SOFT TISSUE
A. Forehead and brow
    1. Preserve the eyebrow.
    2. Do not shave the eyebrow.
    3. Repair the muscle layer.
B. Ears.
Assess adjacent wounds and the middle and inner ear. The presence of hearing loss, hemorrhagic otorrhea, cerebrospinal fluid (CSF) leak, or facial nerve injury suggests middle- or inner-ear injury.
    1. Ecchymosis over the mastoid area is known as **Battle's sign**, a finding associated with basilar skull fracture.
    2. The ear may be involved in abrasions, contusions, lacerations, and hematomas.
      a. Abrasions heal with the continued application of light dressing and ointment. A well-designed dressing, suitably padded (with mineral oil–soaked

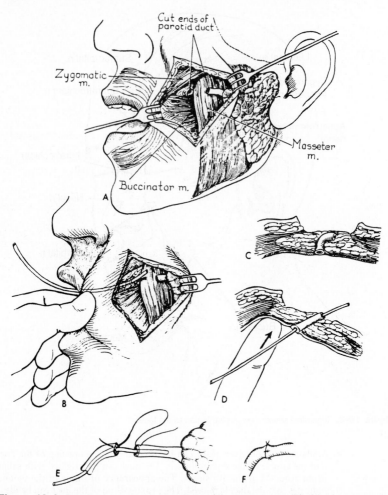

Figure 19-4. Repair of a severed parotid duct **(A)**, severed duct **(B)**, Silastic tube in duct **(C)**, angulation of Stensen's duct in cheek **(D)**, stretching of mucosa facilitating stent placement **(E)**, suturing of duct under magnification **(F)**, stent remaining in 10 to 14 days.

cotton), minimizes edema and hemorrhage. Care must be taken not to exert inordinate pressure that prevents circulation to the auricle.

  b. Lacerations of the auricle are usually associated with lacerations of the cartilage. The ear can be totally or incompletely avulsed, but is often viable when even a small pedicle remains. Appropriate debridement and cleansing of the wound minimizes the likelihood of subsequent chondritis or deformity.

  i. The ear should be carefully sutured into place and adequately supported with dressings.

  ii. The ear canal can be stented with Xeroform (Sherwood-Davis & Geck; St. Louis, Missouri) gauze.

  iii. The cartilage should be trimmed accurately to the skin margin.

  iv. The auricle has numerous landmarks that allow accurate placement of skin sutures, providing excellent realignment and minimal deformity.

3. Repair
   a. Conservative debridement.
   b. Return tissues to point of origin.
   c. Repair cartilage with 5-0 **clear** monofilament nonabsorbable suture.
   d. Repair skin with 6-0 monofilament nonabsorbable suture.
C. Nose. Lacerations of the nose can involve the skin, the lining in the vestibule of the nose, or the mucous membrane of the nasal cavity, most commonly at the junction of the bone and the cartilages.
   1. Wounds must be **approximated with anatomic accuracy**, aligning the nostril borders precisely.
   2. Septal hematomas can be diagnosed easily with a nasal speculum examination. Immediately evacuate the hematoma through a small mucosal incision or by needle aspiration. An untreated septal hematoma will typically resorb and destroy septal cartilage, especially when becoming infected; **a saddle nose deformity results**.
   3. When treating injuries that penetrate all soft-tissue layers of the nose, it is easiest to repair the mucous membrane lining first, with 4-0 plain catgut or other resorbable suture.
   4. Torn septal, upper lateral, alar, and collumellar cartilages can usually be reapproximated under direct vision through the wound and held in good position simply by accurate repair of the underlying mucoperichondrium and the overlying skin. Interrupted sutures with 6-0 monofilament polypropylene are ideal for such skin closure.
      a. The nose is sometimes packed with a petroleum-impregnated gauze to maintain position of cartilaginous or bony fragments.
D. Lips
   1. Lacerations of the lips can involve only the superficial skin and subcutaneous tissues or extend into the orbicularis oris muscle. Full thickness lacerations can also be encountered.
   2. Bleeding can be profuse if the labial artery is severed. Local pressure or ligation of the vessel controls the bleeding.

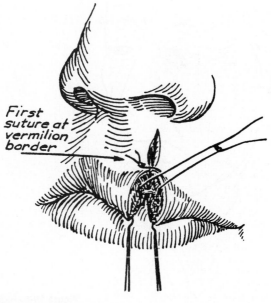

Figure 19-5. Repair of vertical laceration of lip.

3. The vermilion-cutaneous margin and the vermilion-mucosal margin provide accurate landmarks that must be accurately approximated.
    a. Lip musculature should be closed first, using 4-0 or 5-0 absorbable sutures.
    b. Blood and debris should be completely cleaned from the vermilion border and an accurate approximation made.
    c. The mucous membrane should be closed with 4-0 or 5-0 absorbable suture.
    d. Skin closure is with 6-0 nonabsorbable suture (Fig. 19-5).

IX. NONSUTURE TECHNIQUE OF WOUND CLOSURE. Some superficial wounds, especially in children, respond well to approximation with commercially available sterile adhesive strips or skin adhesive (cyanoacrylate). Benzoin or mastisol can be placed along the wound edges to assist tape adherence. The tape is reinforced and provides strong resistance to traction in the lateral direction.
    A. Adhesive strapping can provide uniform approximation of tissue margins and eliminates trauma from sutures.
    B. The disadvantage is the potential for uneven alignment of the wound edges. Adhesive strips may be left in place for 2 to 3 weeks if indicated, and the wound, thus reinforced, prevents lateral pull on the incision.

X. SUTURING. The most satisfactory scars after repair of facial lacerations are seen in cases in which the laceration parallels the relaxed skin tension lines (Fig. 19-6). The

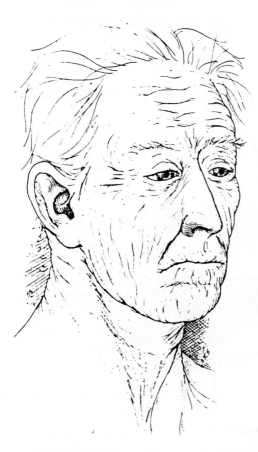

Figure 19-6. Relaxed skin tension lines.

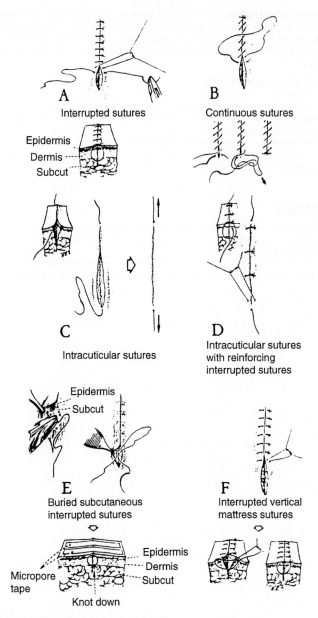

Figure 19-7. Basic suture techniques.

basic techniques are best described by illustration (Fig. 19-7). Choice of suture materials and surgical needles is wide.

A. If proper closure of the subcutaneous and dermal tissues has been achieved, minimal tension in the skin closure should result. Skin sutures, therefore, should be removed as soon as possible to prevent suture hole scarring.

XI. REMOVAL OF SUTURES. Facial wounds have the advantage of a rich vascular supply, which contributes to early healing. Where the skin is thin, as in the eyelids, sutures can be removed in 3 days. Elsewhere on the face, sutures can be left in 4 to 6 days. Sutures in ears can remain 10 to 14 days when associated with injury to underlying cartilage.

XII. ANIMAL AND HUMAN BITES
- **A.** The surgical creation of a clean wound is an essential prerequisite prior to primary wound closure. Irrigate the wound with large amounts of saline.
- **B.** Alternatively, surgical debridement and excision of the wound can convert the wound to a clean injury.
- **C.** Broad-spectrum antibiotic coverage is mandatory.
- **D.** Because the risk of infection from human bites is significant, some surgeons perform only secondary closures in such injuries.

AXIOMS

- Careful assessment of a facial wound is required before treatment.
- Extensive debridement of soft tissues is rarely required for facial injuries; preserve as much tissues as possible.
- Scars from facial wounds are determined less by suture materials and needles than by the character of the wound, appropriate debridement, and skill of the surgeon.

BONY ORAL-MAXILLOFACIAL INJURIES
MARK W. OCHS

I. EVALUATION OF THE PATIENT WITH SUSPECTED FACIAL TRAUMA
A. Initial evaluation
1. Relieve airway obstruction.
2. Control hemorrhage.
3. Search for more immediately life-threatening injuries (thoracic, abdominal, intracranial, extremity).
4. Assume cervical spine (C-spine) injury and stabilize until it is cleared.
5. Perform a neurologic assessment.

B. Secondary evaluation
1. Complete head, eye, ear, nose, throat (HEENT) examination.
   a. Scalp and skull evaluation (palpate)
   b. Cranial nerve evaluation (especially optic, CN II)
   c. Otologic evaluation (external ear, otoscopic examination)
   d. Ophthalmologic evaluation (pupil symmetry, reactivity, visual acuity, and ocular movement)

II. DENTOALVEOLAR TRAUMA
A. Anatomy
1. Adult dentition is composed of 32 teeth, including bilateral maxillary and mandibular central and lateral incisors, canines, first and second bicuspids, and three molars. Typically, the third molars (wisdom teeth) are either absent or impacted. The teeth are numbered from the right maxillary third molar (#1) moving forward and across the arch to the left maxillary third molar (#16), then the mandibular left third molar (#17) and across to the right wisdom tooth (#32) (Fig. 20-1).
2. The pediatric dentition consists of 20 total deciduous teeth, including bilateral maxillary and mandibular central and lateral incisors, canines, and two molars (Fig. 20-1). The primary dentition is named by capital letters. Exfoliation of the deciduous teeth begins at approximately 6 years of age and the mixed dentition stage continues until 12 to 14 years of age. The teeth are attached to the alveolar processes of the maxilla and mandible by periodontal ligaments. Alveolar bone in younger age groups undergoes plastic deformation when subjected to trauma.

B. Evaluation
1. Clinical
   a. Account for all teeth. Count the teeth; attempt to locate any missing teeth at the location of the injury. With unaccounted or missing teeth, consider traumatic impaction into the local bone or surrounding soft tissues. Also, dislodged teeth can be aspirated or swallowed. Appropriate radiographs should be obtained to locate missing teeth.
   b. Evaluate the occlusion. Ask the patient if the bite feels normal. This is a simple yet sensitive screening tool to detect dentoalveolar and facial fractures. Occlusion should be evaluated for stability and symmetry. Occlusal discrepancies, traumatic gaps in the dental arches, and tears of the pink, firm attached gingiva should raise the suspicion of maxillary and mandibular fractures.

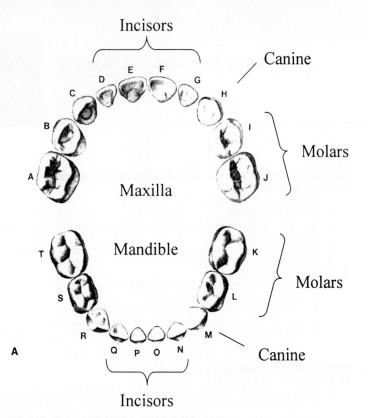

Figure 20-1. A: Pediatric dental arches. *(continued)*

    c. Evaluate damaged or displaced teeth. Fractured teeth can be classified to the depth and location of fracture (Fig. 20-2). Dislocated teeth can be totally avulsed or subluxed or an associated alveolar fracture may be present.

    2. Radiographs. A Panorex is a good screening radiograph for most dentoalveolar trauma. If not available, plain radiographs of the maxillofacial complex often suffice (posteroanterior, lateral, or oblique views). Isolated tooth fractures are best evaluated with intraoral dental radiographs. If these are not available, early dental referral should be sought.

C. Management

    1. Age of the patient, type of tooth (deciduous or permanent), status of tooth development, condition of tooth before trauma, patient motivation, time elapsed since injury, and associated injuries must be considered when deciding on management of dentoalveolar trauma.

    2. Intraoral soft-tissue lacerations are usually best treated by conservative debridement, irrigation, and primary repair with absorbable sutures after stabilization or definitive treatment of the dentoalveolar fracture.

    3. In general, isolated tooth crown fractures need emergent referral if the dental pulp (dark pink or red appearance) is exposed or if teeth are sensitive.

        a. Dislocated or subluxed teeth and dentoalveolar fractures need to be emergently reduced and stabilized with wire and composite resin bonding. Composite resins are opaque white filling material (similar to what

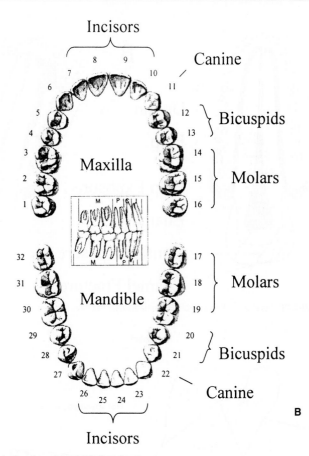

Incisors
8   9
Canine
7
6
10
11
5
12
Bicuspids
4
13
3
14
Maxilla
2
15
Molars
1
16

M   P   C

32
17
31
18
Molars
Mandible
30
19
29
20
28
21
Bicuspids
27
22
Canine
26
25   24   23
B
Incisors

Figure 20-1. (continued). **B:** Adult dental arches.

orthodontists use to bond brackets to teeth) that is either chemically or UV light activated.

b. Avulsed deciduous teeth should not be reimplanted because of low success rate and possibility of damage to the underlying developing permanent dentition.

c. Avulsed permanent teeth should be replaced into the tooth socket as soon as possible after the trauma. Immediate reimplantation is ideal. If this is not possible, the tooth should be stored in appropriate storage medium (avulsed tooth storage system → buccal vestibule → milk → saline → moist towel) and replaced as soon as possible. A delay of >2 hours or desiccation of the tooth root significantly affects the overall prognosis of the tooth. Once reimplanted, the tooth still requires composite resin splinting to the adjacent stable teeth and should not be in heavy contact with the opposing dentition during chewing motions.

III. MANDIBULAR FRACTURES. Aside from nasal fractures, mandibular fractures account for approximately two thirds of all bony maxillofacial trauma. The mechanism of injury is usually blunt trauma sustained from assault or motor vehicle accident.

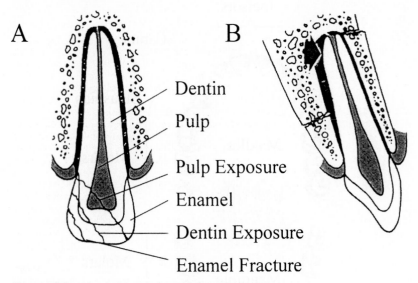

Figure 20-2. A: Level of tooth fractures. B: Dentoalveolar fracture.

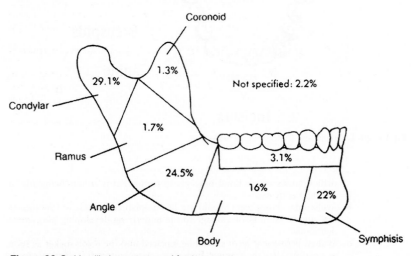

Figure 20-3. Mandibular anatomy and fracture zones.

A. Anatomy and location of injury. Fractures tend to occur at the local site of impact, areas of weakness, and are often multiple. The anatomic regions and associated incidence of fracture are shown in Figure 20-3. In edentulous patients, the incidence of subcondylar fractures accounts for 37% of all mandible fractures and is often paired with a contralateral body fracture. The inferior alveolar neurovascular bundle enters the mandible on the medial aspect of the mid ramus through the mandibular foramen and traverses an intrabony canal, exiting through the mental foramen located just inferior to the mandibular bicuspid root tips. It is strictly a sensory nerve (V_3) supplying the ipsilateral lower lip, teeth, and gingiva.

B. Evaluation
  1. Clinical
    a. Emergent situations
      i. Airway obstruction. Foreign bodies (e.g., dentures, avulsed teeth) can cause airway obstruction; remove them at the time of initial evaluation. In addition, airway obstruction can occur with bilateral mandibular parasymphyseal or body fractures. Manual anterior distraction of the flail anterior mandibular segment, allowing the patient to be semi-supine or to sit up, and oral suctioning can provide temporary relief, but a definitive airway should be secured urgently.
      ii. Hemorrhage is rarely a significant problem with mandibular fractures.
        a) The inferior alveolar artery traveling in the mandibular canal can be lacerated during the initial injury, but simple fracture reduction, direct pressure, or infiltration with epinephrine containing anesthetic solutions is usually adequate for hemostasis.
        b) Persistent or profuse bleeding is often associated with penetrating injuries and a secure airway must be the primary concern. Hemorrhage control should then be performed by direct surgical exploration or, on occasion, by interventional radiologic means. With mandibular bleeding, fracture reduction and temporary stabilization are preferable to local packing, which usually distracts and destabilizes the bony segments, allowing continued hemorrhage.
    b. Occlusion. Malocclusion is one of the first clinical signs detected in patients with mandibular fractures. If the fracture is in the tooth-bearing segment of the mandible, a noticeable step deformity or interdental gap may be detected. Floor of mouth ecchymosis is pathognomonic for a mandibular parasymphyseal or body fracture. If the fracture is located in the subcondylar region, a shift of the chin toward the affected side or an anterior or lateral open bite may be present (Fig. 20-4).
    c. Soft-tissue signs, such as ecchymosis, edema, pain, and gingival or mucosal lacerations, may be present at the fracture site.
    d. Sensation. Lower lip and chin paraesthesia or anesthesia is common in patients with mandibular fractures located between the mid ramus and canine region. Greater bony displacement increases the risk for inferior alveolar nerve injury or transection.
  2. Radiographs. Plain radiographs usually suffice for evaluation of mandibular fractures. At least two views at 90 degrees should be used to evaluate most injuries. This is especially important in the subcondylar region, where superimposition of other structures can mimic or obscure a fracture. The best initial radiograph is the Panorex, accompanied by an open mouth Towne's view. Other radiographs that can be used to evaluate mandibular fractures are the posteroanterior (PA) and lateral oblique views. Computed tomography (CT) can be helpful for the evaluation of patients with condylar or subcondylar fractures. This is particularly true in children because their condyles are developing and incompletely ossified, making plain radiology detection difficult. Patients (especially children) with a chin laceration and preauricular pain or swelling should be evaluated for a condylar or subcondylar fracture. Coronoid fractures account for <1% of all mandible fractures and are generally associated with an overlying zygomatic complex fracture that was displaced medially, creating the injury.
C. Management
  1. Cervical immobilization
    a. Depending on the force and mechanism of injury, cervical immobilization should be maintained until C-spine injury can be definitively ruled out.
  2. Management of emergent problems
    a. Initial management should be control of the airway and bleeding. Control of the airway is performed with distraction of flail bony segments, if possible. In the event of a compromised airway, endotracheal intubation

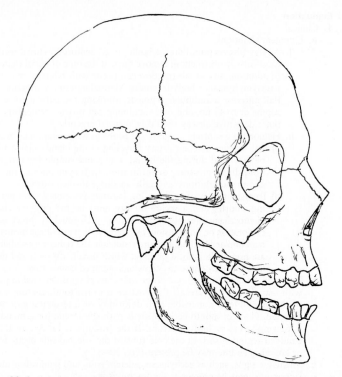

Figure 20-4. Anterior open bite caused by a condyle fracture with posterior vertical collapse.

or surgical airway should be established before surgical repair and stabilization of the mandibular fracture.

3. **Temporary immobilization**
   a. Temporary partial reduction and stabilization of the fracture segments can provide symptomatic relief, help control bleeding, and minimize damage to the inferior alveolar neurovascular bundle. This can be performed with a modified Barton's bandage (circumferential wrap from chin to skull vertex) or by placing a stainless steel bridal wire (24–26 gauge) around the necks of two teeth on either side of the line of fracture (Fig. 20-5).
4. **Definitive treatment.** Fractures should be reduced adequately, fixated, and immobilized for adequate healing to occur. This is typically accomplished via open reduction, with internal plate and screw fixation. Without immobilization, fracture segments usually become displaced by the attached muscle pull, leading to a malunion or nonunion. Isolated non- or minimally displaced fractures, particularly condylar and subcondylar, can be suitably treated by wiring the teeth together (maxillomandibular fixation [MMF]). The period of MMF is usually 6 to 8 weeks. The exception is for condylar fractures where, because of the risk of temporomandibular joint fibroosseous ankylosis, 2 weeks of MMF is the standard.
5. **Prophylactic antibiotics.** Mandibular fractures that include tooth-bearing segments are considered compound fractures because of the egress of saliva, bacteria, and other contaminants through the periodontal ligament or fracture site. Prophylactic antibiotics that cover most oral microorganisms (e.g., penicillin) or a first-generation cephalosporin are recommended, along with oral saline or antimicrobial rinses. In the penicillin-allergic patient, clindamycin is a good alternative.

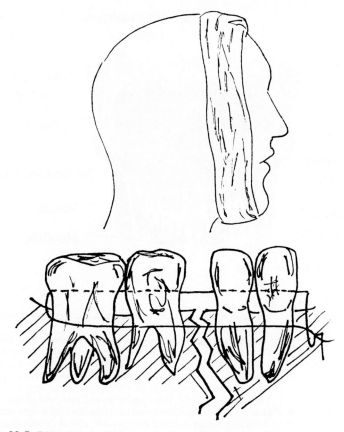

Figure 20-5. Bridal wiring to stabilize an anterior mandibular fracture site.

IV. **MIDFACE FRACTURES** can be defined as any fracture of the orbital-zygomatic-maxillary complex. The mechanism of injury is usually blunt from assault or motor vehicle accident.

   A. **General midfacial fracture management**

   1. **Anatomy and location of injury.** The midface is divided into the maxilla, the zygomatic complexes, and the nasal-orbital-ethmoid (NOE) complex (Fig. 20-6). Fractures tend to occur at the site of impact and inherently weak regions of the midfacial complex, including bony sutures, foramina, and apertures.

      a. The infraorbital neurovascular bundle enters the midfacial complex via the orbital region through the inferior orbital fissure and then traversing partially through a bony canal along the floor of the orbit to exit through the infraorbital foramen on the anterior surface of the maxilla. The infra-orbital nerve (V_2) supplies general sensation to the ipsilateral lower eyelid, lateral nose, upper lip, and anterior maxilla.

   2. **Evaluation**

      a. Clinical

         i. Emergent situations

            a) Airway obstruction. Foreign bodies (e.g., dentures, avulsed teeth) can cause airway obstruction and should be removed at the initial evaluation. In most clinical situations, airway obstruction occurs

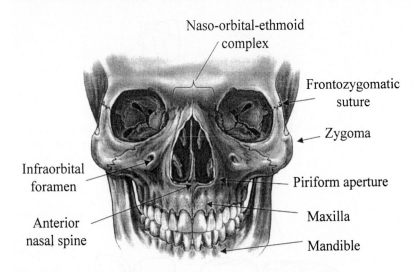

Figure 20-6. Midfacial anatomy.

in patients with panfacial trauma, including significant mandibular fractures.

b) Hemorrhage. Significant hemorrhage is more common with midfacial fractures than with mandibular fractures. The descending palatine arteries, which travel in a bony canal along the posterolateral surface of the nasal cavity within the palatine bone, can cause profuse posterior nasal hemorrhage. Other vessels that may be injured include nasal septal, sphenopalatine, and pterygoid plexus.

ii. Occlusion. Occlusal discrepancies are one of the first clinical signs detected in patients with certain midfacial fractures. Mobility of the maxillary dentition relative to other midfacial structures is indicative of a maxillary fracture. A posteriorly directed force of significant magnitude can cause a posteriorly impacted maxilla. Either an anterior or posterior open bite, or relative protrusion of the lower teeth, is indicative of a maxillary or midfacial fracture.

iii. Soft-tissue signs include ecchymosis, edema, pain, and mucosal lacerations.

iv. Palpation. Palpate all bones of the midface, including maxilla, orbital rims, zygomas, and nose; often, the patient is too sensitive to allow a complete examination. However, grasping the anterior maxillary teeth with the thumb and forefinger and attempting upward or side-to-side movement while stabilizing the entire forehead with the opposite hand is crucial in detection of a midfacial fracture.

v. Sensation. Upper lateral lip, nose, and cheek paraesthesia or anesthesia is common in patients with a fracture extending through the infraorbital foramen. Complete transection of the infraorbital nerve is uncommon in blunt trauma.

vi. Ophthalmologic examination. Any fracture involving the bony orbit or zygomatic complex can cause injuries to the globe or other orbital contents. Complete examination includes pupils, visual acuity, range of motion of the globe, globe position, and the globe itself, including a fundoscopic examination. Extraocular movements in multiple fields of gaze are often diminished in patients with significant orbital edema, but tend to be mild without a firm fixed sudden stop. Blowout fracture of one of the orbital walls (most commonly the medial orbital floor) can cause entrapment of the extraocular muscles (inferior rectus muscles or inferior oblique). A firm, fixed and reproducible point of limitation in upgaze or, more likely, downgaze should alert the practitioner to this possibility. An urgent specialist consultation is appropriate because prolonged muscle ischemia and resulting fibrosis can lead to long-term impairment of movement.

   vii. Nasal examination. Significant nasal trauma can be associated with nasal airway obstruction and significant epistaxis.

      a) Epistaxis from anterior vessels can be controlled with upright positioning, cold compresses, topical nasal vasoconstrictor sprays, local direct pressure, or, infrequently, anterior nasal packing.

      b) Posterior epistaxis may require compression tamponade.

      c) The nasal septum must be evaluated for the presence of a septal hematoma, which can lead to localized loss of septal support of the nasal dorsum and a "saddle nose" deformity.

  viii. Examination for cerebrospinal fluid (CSF) leak. CSF leaks most commonly occur with midfacial, frontal sinus, or basilar skull fractures.

      a) Fractures involving the NOE complex occasionally involve the cribriform plate in the superior aspect of the nasal cavity and floor of the anterior cranial fossa.

      b) Basilar skull fractures can involve the petrous temporal bone, resulting in leakage of CSF.

      c) Various tests, including the ring test and chloride or glucose sampling, have been described to establish a diagnosis of CSF leak, but contemporary testing for potential CSF leakage is with a *beta$_2$-transferrin* determination (positive with CSF leak) on the collected drainage sample.

   ix. Radiographs

      a) CT is the diagnostic modality of choice for the complete evaluation of midfacial trauma with thin sections (1.5 mm) in axial planes through the midface and the orbits. Direct coronal views are particularly helpful with orbital fractures but the patient's C-spine status may preclude obtaining them. Intravenous contrast is of no benefit to the CT scan evaluation of acute bony facial trauma.

      b) Plain radiographs sometimes can be used as an initial screening tool, but soft-tissue swelling and superimposition of other anatomic structures usually obscure some fracture lines. The best plain radiographic series includes the Water's view, the submental vertex view, and the lateral facial view.

      c) The panoramic radiograph is of little use in the evaluation of midfacial trauma, except in determining if a concomitant mandibular fracture exists.

3. Management

  a. With or severely displaced or multiple midfacial fractures, cervical immobilization is maintained until C-spine injury can be definitively excluded.

  b. Management of emergent problems

    i. Initial management should consist of control of the airway and bleeding.

   ii. Significant posterior nasal hemorrhage can be controlled with posterior nasopharynx occlusion with a Foley catheter that has been inserted transnasally into the nasopharynx, inflated with water or saline. Gentle anterior traction applied and then anterior nasal packing is performed.

  iii. Persistent deep hemorrhage can be problematic, and control may require surgical ligation of branches of the external carotid artery in the neck if bleeding is massive or, in the setting of less active bleeding, with interventional radiology.

    iv. Because of risk of inadvertent intracranial placement, blind (non-fiberoptic) nasal intubation with endotracheal tubes or nasogastric tubes are contraindicated in patients with suspected midfacial trauma involving the NOE complex.

  c. Treatment of ophthalmologic problems. Obtain ophthalmologic consultation for individuals with potential globe injuries. Fat herniation through an upper eyelid laceration or an irregular (not round) pointing pupil suggests a penetrating globe injury (Chapter 21).

  d. Decongestants. Spray decongestants should be used in patients with significant midfacial trauma to provide symptomatic relief for nasal airway obstruction and to minimize epistaxis.

    i. Phenylephrine

    ii. Oxymetazoline

  e. Edema prevention. Open surgical treatment of midfacial trauma can be difficult in an operative field with significant edema. Operative repair is usually delayed until edema has resolved. Prevention of facial edema can provide symptomatic relief for the patient as well as expedite definitive treatment.

    i. Steroids. Pharmacologic administration of glucocorticoids may hasten the resolution of facial edema in patients with maxillofacial trauma. Dexamethasone (4–8 mg) administered intravenously (IV) every 6 hours or methylprednisolone (125 mg) IV every 6 hours for 24 to 48 hours may be used. Administration of steroids is of questionable benefit after the edema is present. Caution should be used when administering high dose steroids in insulin-dependent diabetic patients. The steroids may acutely elevate the blood glucose and make regulation more difficult.

    ii. The head of bed. Elevate to at least 30 degrees for the first several days after sustaining facial trauma.

    iii. Intermittent application of cold compresses for the first 24 hours may be beneficial for the prevention of facial edema (20 minutes on and 20 minutes off).

  f. Definitive treatment of midfacial trauma fractures should be deferred until full clinical and radiographic evaluation and the patient is stabilized. Osseous healing can start as early as 7 days after the injury. Reduction and repair can be exceedingly difficult if surgery is delayed for more than 2 weeks. Contemporary treatment of midfacial fractures involves open reduction and internal fixation using titanium miniplates and screws. Minimally or nondisplaced nasal, orbital, zygomatic complex (tripod), and zygomatic arch fractures may not require surgical treatment. Nonunion of these isolated fractures is rare.

B. LeFort fractures are those of the midface that involve the maxillary dentoalveolar segment. The mechanism and location of impact usually determine the type of fracture sustained. Fractures tend to occur in certain patterns of the midface and are traditionally classified by the highest level of fracture (Fig. 20-7). Most LeFort fractures are not "pure" and can have comminution, additional levels or lines of fracture, and other associated facial fractures.

C. Zygomaticomaxillary complex fractures. Zygomaticomaxillary complex (ZMC, tripod or malar) fractures usually are sustained with direct blunt trauma to the zygomatic buttress of the face. The zygoma has four major stability points, with connections as follows: (*a*) the frontal bone at the frontozygomatic suture; (*b*) the maxilla at the medial inferior orbital rim; (*c*) at the zygomaticomaxillary buttress; and (*d*) the temporal bone at the zygomatic arch. A complete fracture of the complex usually involves all four of these major stability points (Fig. 20-8). Anteriorly, the fracture usually occurs in the maxilla obliquely through the infraorbital foramen because of the relatively weak nature of this bone resulting in a high incidence of V_2 sensory division paraesthesia. Other significant physical findings associated with ZMC fractures are depression of the zygomatic

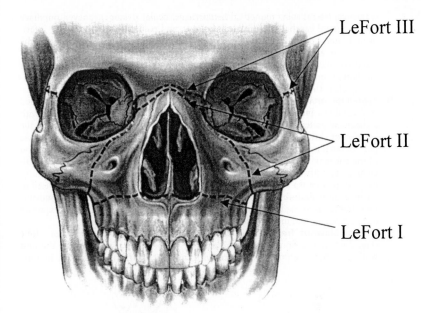

Figure 20-7. LeFort levels of fracture.

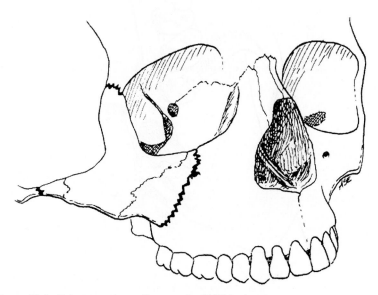

Figure 20-8. Right zygomaticomaxillary complex (ZMC) fracture.

eminence, lateral subconjunctival hemorrhage, ocular dystopia (uneven pupillary levels), lateral canthal ptosis, enophthalmos, and palpable fractures at the inferior and lateral orbital rims. With extreme medial and posterior displacement, the patient can exhibit limited mouth opening because of impingement of the fractured complex against the coronoid process of the mandible. For oral access or intubation, initial deviation of the mandible toward the uninjured side can sufficiently clear this mechanical obstruction.

  D. Zygomatic arch fractures. Isolated zygomatic arch fractures usually are sustained by focal direct blunt trauma to the zygomatic arch, creating three breakpoints with a classic W-pattern (Fig. 20-9). Common physical findings are a depression at the location of trauma and pain on mandibular opening caused by masseteric muscle pull. Limited mandibular opening can also exist because of mechanical obstruction of the coronoid process. A submental vertex or "jug-handle" view is usually sufficient to identify this fracture. Early (24–72 hours) surgical reduction without internal fixation via a lateral brow, temporal hairline (Gille's), or maxillary vestibular incision is desirable. Stability of the fracture reduction decreases beyond this time and tends to sag back inward, thus requiring a much more extensive exposure (e.g., a hemicoronal incision) for direct access and plating.

  E. Orbital blowout fractures occur from direct impact to the orbit or globe (Fig. 20-10). The floor of the orbit and the medial orbital wall are the thinnest walls and most commonly involved with this type of fracture. The surrounding

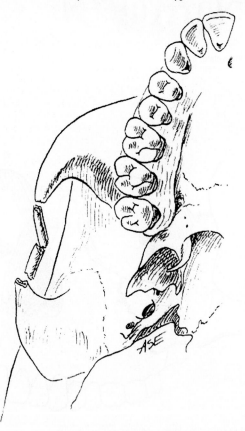

Figure 20-9. Right zygomatic arch fracture viewed from below.

maxillary sinus and ethmoid air cells act as "airbags of the orbit," cushioning the blow and absorbing the force, thus, protecting to some degree against globe rupture. The prolapse of some of the orbital contents into these spaces can produce enophthalmos or orbital dystopia because of a relative increase in the orbital volume. Additionally, suspensory fascia (Tenon's capsule) or extraocular muscles can be entrapped in the fracture line, leading to restricted eye movement and diplopia in certain fields of gaze. Coronal CT scans are invaluable when evaluating this injury and should be correlated with clinical findings. Indications for surgical correction include a significant cosmetic or functional deformity. A relative indication is >25% to 50% of the surface area of an orbital wall being involved in the fracture. If edema allows, optimal time for repair is within 24 hours. If significant edema exists, reevaluation and repair within 5 to 7 days is desirable. Systemic corticosteroids have limited usefulness in hastening resolution of this edema. Patients should be cautioned not to blow the nose, which can cause significant orbital emphysema. Repair usually entails open reduction or removal of the fractured segments, then reducing the orbital contents with possible autogenous or alloplastic implant reconstruction.

F. Nasal fracture is the most common fracture to the face. Complete examination should include evaluation for a septal hematoma. Epistaxis should be controlled. The diagnosis of a nasal fracture is primarily a clinical one. Nasal deformity, deviation, and bony crepitus with movement are the usual findings. Occasionally, radiographs can aid in the diagnosis. If edema allows, early reduction (within 24–48 hours) of isolated nasal and septal fractures affords the greatest stability. If not, repair should be performed within 5 to 7 days after sufficient resolution of the edema. Reduction of septal fractures and dislocations also should be performed at that time.

G. Fractures of the entire NOE complex occur after direct high impact to the region. Diagnosis usually can be made by clinical observation and direct palpation in the region of nasal dorsum and medial canthal tendons. Significant findings can include lateral displacement of the medial canthal tendons (telecanthus) causing an increased distance (normal medial intercanthal distance is 30–34 mm). Significant disruption in this region can lead to epiphora secondary to swelling or damage of the lacrimal drainage system. Primary surgical repair of significant fractures includes open reduction and plating of the bony segments, with direct repair of the canthal tendons. Repair should be done within the first 7 to 10 days, because secondary repair is exceedingly difficult and often leads to compromised results. Globe injuries and CSF leaks should be sought when a NOE injury is being evaluated.

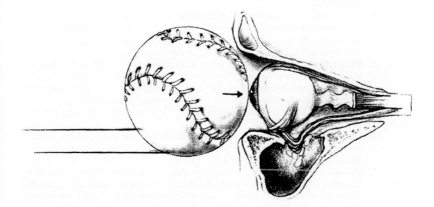

Figure 20-10.   Orbital floor blowout fracture.

V. FRONTAL SINUS FRACTURES

A. Anatomy and location of injury. The frontal sinus is usually divided into left and right halves by a midline septum; both sides drain into the middle meatus of the nose through their respective nasofrontal ducts or foramina. Of adults, 5% have no frontal sinus and 5% have only a unilateral sinus. Trauma to the forehead region can fracture the anterior or posterior walls of the frontal sinus or damage the nasofrontal ducts. With fracture of the posterior wall of the frontal sinus, consider the potential for a dural laceration or cerebral injury.

B. Evaluation

1. Clinical

    a. Emergent situations

        i. Open fracture of the anterior and posterior table of the frontal sinus are considered emergencies because of the high risk of meningitis from direct cerebral exposure. Emergent surgical intervention is indicated.

        ii. Cerebral contusions are common, with injuries to the frontal sinus.

    b. Local signs include ecchymosis, edema, pain, and cutaneous lacerations at the location of fracture, and fractures and deformity of the forehead and superior orbital rims.

    c. Sensation. Forehead and scalp paraesthesia or anesthesia. The supraorbital and supratrochlear nerves (V_1) supply this region.

    d. Nasal examination and CSF leaks. NOE complex trauma can be associated with frontal sinus fractures. CSF leaks can occur in patients with frontal sinus fractures. Questionable nasal discharge should be submitted for a β_2-transferrin level.

2. Radiographs. CT is the diagnostic modality of choice for the complete evaluation of frontal sinus trauma. Thin sections (1.5–3.0 mm) in the axial plane through the paranasal sinuses are usually adequate for most purposes. Both the anterior and posterior tables of the frontal sinus should be categorized as **fractured or noninvolved** and **displaced versus nondisplaced.** Displacement is defined as overlap by the amount of thickness of the adjacent cortical bone. Intermediate distinctions such as mild or moderate displacement are confusing and have no clinical relevance. A displaced posterior table (overlapped fracture margins) is often associated with dural tears or cerebral injury requiring neurosurgical intervention. Plain radiographs can be used as initial screening for bony injury but will not evaluate the underlying brain. The best plain radiographic series includes the Caldwell view and the lateral cephalogram.

C. Management

1. Cervical immobilization should be maintained until C-spine injury can be excluded.

2. Management of **emergent problems**. Open fractures of the anterior and posterior tables of the frontal sinus require emergent exploration and treatment. They can be treated with primary cutaneous repair and delayed treatment of the frontal sinus injury, as indicated.

3. Prophylactic antibiotics. Most frontal sinus fractures fill with blood and mucus early after trauma. Prophylactic antibiotics that cover most sinus microorganisms (e.g., ampicillin with clavulanate) or a first-generation cephalosporin usually are recommended in these situations. Posterior table involvement often is covered with a broader spectrum antibiotic that can cross the blood–brain barrier.

4. Decongestants. Because of mucosal edema and the potential for compromised frontal sinus drainage, decongestants should be used in patients with significant frontal sinus trauma.

5. Definitive treatment of frontal sinus fractures depends on the extent of the fracture. If the drainage system of the sinuses is significantly compromised, obliteration or cranialization is usually recommended. If only the anterior table is involved and nondisplaced, no surgical treatment is generally necessary. A displaced frontal sinus that is either extensive or creates a cosmetic deformity can be accessed directly through the fracture or via a liberal sinuso-tomy. The mucosal lining is then completely removed with curettage and drilling to deter formation of a mucocele at a usually much later date—such as years later. The nasofrontal ducts can then be obliterated with fascia or bone grafts and the frontal sinus can be obliterated with autologous fat, bone, pericranium, or alloplastic materials. If only the anterior table is displaced without involvement of the nasofrontal ducts, primary repair without obliter-ation can be performed. Significant involvement or displacement of the poste-rior table usually requires direct exploration, with repair or cranialization depending on the degree of damage. Smaller frontal sinuses in young patients can be cranialized by simply removing the posterior sinus wall, smoothing the edges, removing the mucosal lining, and obliterating the frontonasal ducts. This treatment in older patients and those with large frontal sinuses may predispose them to developing chronic subdural fluid accumulations. With displaced posterior table fractures, associated dural tears requiring neurosur-gical repair is the rule rather than the exception.

AXIOMS

- Control of both the airway and hemorrhage is the immediate goal in the management of bony injuries to the face.
- Assume that all patients with facial fractures have concomitant cervical spine injury.
- Malocclusion is an important clinical sign of mandibular or maxillary fractures.
- A nasal septal hematoma must be identified and evacuated to avoid saddle nose deformity.

Bibliography
Larsen PE, ed. Maxillofacial trauma. In: Miloro M, ed. *Peterson's Principles of Oral and Maxillofacial Surgery.* 2nd ed. Hamilton, Ontario: BC Decker; 2004:327–562.
Marciani RD, Hendler BH, eds. Trauma. In: Fonseca RJ, ed. *Oral and Maxillofacial Surgery.* Philadelphia, Pa: WB Saunders; 2000.
Ochs MW. Mandible fractures. In: Myers EN, Eibling DE, eds. *Operative Otolaryngology-Head and Neck Surgery.* 2nd ed. Philadelphia, Pa: Elsevier Science; 2005.
Ochs MW. Midfacial fractures. In: Myers EN, Eibling DE, eds. *Operative Otolaryngology-Head and Neck Surgery.* 2nd ed. Philadelphia, Pa: Elsevier Science; 2005.

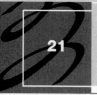

21

OPHTHALMIC INJURIES
S. TONYA STEFKO AND RANDALL L. BEATTY

I. INTRODUCTION

A. Eye injuries are common and require prompt evaluation and treatment to minimize the risk of loss of sight. These injuries may be obvious (as with penetrating trauma) or more subtle, yet still sight threatening. Additionally, competing injuries and altered responsiveness can hinder early ophthalmic assessment.

B. Prompt consultation with an ophthalmologist is recommended when either clear ocular injury exists or any suspicion of injury exists. Patients with periorbital or ocular trauma may have sight-threatening injuries with little superficial evidence, only to be discovered by an exam by an ophthalmologist.

II. HISTORY

A. Obtain as complete a history as possible of the injury. What type of object (e.g., ball, metal, etc.) hit the eye? Was it thrown or hit by a bat, and from how far away?

B. Obtain a history of preexisting ocular disease. Does the patient normally wear eyeglasses? Is there a history of ocular surgery or previous trauma?

C. Was the patient wearing eye/face protection?

D. What are the patient's complaints? Specifically, ask if there a change in vision, pain, photophobia, or other new visual symptom or change (such as floaters or sensation of a curtain obscuring the vision).

III. PHYSICAL EXAMINATION

A. Visual acuity is the "vital sign" of the eye. Regardless of how minor an injury may appear, documentation of visual acuity is the first step in evaluation of any patient with possible ocular trauma. In general, the ultimate visual outcome is directly related to the presenting visual acuity.

    1. Test each eye separately for vision by covering the opposite eye with either the palm of the patient's hand or an occlusive device.

        a. In the emergency setting, patients are often supine. A description of the ability to see letters on a card, a pen, or name tag is sufficient. In the case of a patient with reduced vision, the distance at which the patient can count fingers, see a hand wave, tell the direction of a light (light projection), or detect the presence of a light (light perception) provides an adequate preliminary assessment.

        b. If the patient has eyeglasses, check visual acuity with them in use. For older patients with bifocal glasses, test near vision with the patient looking through the bifocal portion at the bottom of the glasses.

            i. If the glasses have been lost or are not with the patient, a pinhole device (in a piece of paper or cardboard or a commercial device) may be used to approximate corrected vision.

            ii. Documentation in the medical record of "vision intact," "vision okay," "fine," or "the same" is inadequate.

    2. Test pupillary reactivity and compare one pupil to the other. Note the shape and reactivity. Documentation of the presence or absence of a relative afferent pupillary defect (RAPD) is important in characterization of injury.

    a. RAPD refers to a difference in reactivity of the pupils when a bright light is swung briskly from one eye to the other. The affected pupil will react less strongly, not at all, or perhaps even dilate when presented with the same light as produces a normal constriction of the unaffected pupil. **Presence of an RAPD indicates serious optic nerve or ophthalmic damage,** as it is a bulk response of the visual apparatus. Absence of an RAPD indicates no significant optic nerve damage or bilateral optic nerve damage (note, however, that in its absence severe eye injury may still be present).

3. Obtain visual field evaluation by confrontation testing (asking the patient to count fingers in all four quadrants of each eye separately) and document whether the patient is cooperative enough to undergo the test (Fig. 21-1 and Table 21-1).

4. Examine the extraocular movements and report any decrease or pain.

5. Document the gross appearance of the eye: Does it appear to be intact and quiet? If further evaluation is possible, assess the following:

    a. Eyelids. Assess for edema, laceration, ptosis, or other evidence of injury.

    b. Palpate the orbital rim for deformity or crepitus.

    c. Examine the globe without applying pressure. Assess the globe for possible displacement or entrapment, and describe the movement of the eye.

    d. Conjunctivae. Evaluate for subconjunctival hemorrhage, chemosis (swelling), or foreign bodies.

    e. Cornea. Assess for integrity, opacity, abrasions, foreign bodies, or contact lenses.

        i. Contacts should be removed from trauma patients. If unsure whether a patient wears contact lenses, a small amount of fluorescein will make the presence obvious. An unconscious patient can develop a perforating bacterial corneal ulcer from a contact lens left in the eye for several days.

        ii. Abrasions may be visualized with fluorescein instilled into the conjunctival sac. A cobalt blue light will cause bright yellow fluorescence of the injured area.

    f. Anterior chamber. Using a light directed at varying angles (direct and from side), assess for blood (hyphema) or abnormal depth. A shallow anterior chamber can result from an anterior penetrating wound, and a deep anterior chamber from injury to the posterior portion of the globe. A slit lamp exam is ideal for anterior chamber and corneal evaluation but can be impeded in immobilized or severely injured patients.

    g. Iris should be reactive and the pupil should be round.

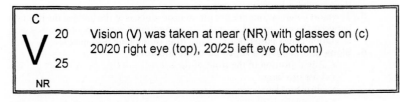

```
C
   20    Vision (V) was taken at near (NR) with glasses on (c)
V         20/20 right eye (top), 20/25 left eye (bottom)
   25
NR
```

Figure 21-1. Documentation of visual acuity.

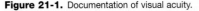

TABLE 21-1   **Documentation of Pupillary Responses**

PERRL–APD
Normal pupil responses to light, negative afferent pupillary defect

h. Lens should be in the normal location and transparent. A dislocated lens will often be apparent only because the edge will be visible in the pupil.

i. Vitreous should be transparent. Blood in the vitreous will obscure the normal red reflection of the slit lamp or ophthalmoscope light from the retina. Assess for foreign bodies.

j. Retina. Assess for hemorrhage or detachment. Use of an ophthalmoscope with papillary dilation limits the amount of retina visualized and ability to detect noncentral lesions. Again, a dilated exam using magnification performed by an ophthalmologist is ideal, but sometimes impractical in the severely injured patient. Dilating agents should be used only with ophthalmolic and neurosurgical input, given the potential impairment of the exam and potential complications in certain settings (e.g., open globe or elevated intraocular pressure).

IV. COMMON INJURIES

A. Chemical injury. Most ophthalmic injuries are unaffected by a short (minutes to an hour) delay in diagnosis. In contrast, **chemical injury is a true ocular emergency,** with care in the first minutes altering the outcome. A patient with chemical exposure to the eye must be irrigated copiously with saline (liters of normal saline connected to IV tubing with the needle end removed works well). Usually 15 minutes of constant irrigation is necessary before further exam should take place. The nature of the chemical is important in prognosis and further treatment. However, **the specific nature is irrelevant in the first 15 minutes and all injuries should be irrigated with saline or water.** Do not attempt to neutralize any acid or base by additions to the irrigating fluid.

B. Open globe. An open globe is the most serious sight-threatening ocular injury occurring in blunt maxillofacial trauma. It refers to a laceration or rupture of the eye wall with extrusion of intraocular contents.

1. With a suspected open globe, immediately place a rigid shield over but not touching the eye and consult an ophthalmologist. **Never place pressure or drops on the globe.** Even slight pressure can cause extrusion of intraocular contents and reduce the chance of restoring useful vision or avoiding enucleation. This includes the pressure exerted by the eyelids in a forced squeeze, local anesthesia injection into the periocular region, or inadvertent pressure while closing lacerations on the face.

2. Prehospital care of a suspected open globe involves protecting the eye with a plastic or metal shield taped from the forehead to the cheekbone.

3. Additional maneuvers that may help save sight include administration of pain medication and antiemetics if needed to avoid grimacing and Valsalva.

4. An ophthalmologist should perform ocular explorations under general anesthesia without local anesthetics.

5. The most common rupture site for an open globe is at the limbus, the junction between the cornea and sclera. The second most common site for a scleral laceration is just posterior to the insertion of the four recti muscles.

6. **Signs that suggest a ruptured globe include:**
   - Any distortion of the front of the eye
   - Loss of vision
   - Displaced lens
   - Traumatic hyphema
   - Hemorrhagic chemosis (hemorrhagic swelling of the conjunctivae, generalized or localized)
   - Shallow or deep anterior chamber

7. After the initial evaluation, obtain a computed tomographic (CT) scan of the orbit.

8. In the emergency department, prophylactic intravenous (IV) antibiotics, usually a cephalosporin, are started. Wounds contaminated with soil or dirt require clindamycin to prevent *Bacillus cereus* endophthalmitis.

C. **Traumatic hyphema.** This denotes blood in the anterior chamber of the eye, which can obscure the detail of the iris or lens. A hyphema may be associated with a more serious injury (e.g., a ruptured globe). The hemorrhage will be visible as a layer or wisps of red blood. A microhyphema is suspended red blood cells without layering, visible only with a slit lamp.

1. Any hyphema is treated with the following:
   a. Rigid shield to the affected eye
   b. Bed rest with the head elevated
   c. Avoidance of aspirin and other NSAIDs
   d. Dilation/cycloplegia (e.g., atropine 1% three times daily)
   e. Topical anti-inflammatory (e.g., prednisolone acetate 1% 4–6 times daily)
   f. Serial examinations with intraocular pressure checks by an ophthalmologist for at least the first 5 days postinjury
2. Order a sickle screen if the patient is African American.
3. Consider imaging studies to disclose associated injuries.
4. Most patients with microhyphemas and small hyphemas are treated as outpatients (Table 21-2). Patients with larger hyphemas, other periocular trauma, and sickle-cell trait usually are treated as inpatients (Table 21-3).

D. **Intraocular foreign bodies (IOFBs)** may be present despite excellent visual acuity. Small metallic fragments can enter the eye without the patient experiencing much discomfort. These metallic pieces are often <1 mm in diameter and can be multiple. Consider these in any eye injury, especially in a patient with a history of metal-on-metal hammering. The most useful imaging test is a high-resolution, thin-cut CT scan through the globe. Obtain axial and coronal views. Small IOFBs can indicate that other ocular injuries are present, and a detailed ophthalmologic examination must be performed. Surgical removal is usually accomplished by vitrectomy (Table 21-4).

E. **Corneal abrasions.** Abrasions are common and cause pain, tearing, a foreign body sensation, photophobia, and decreased visual acuity. Fluorescein will stain the corneal abrasion bright yellow when viewed with a cobalt blue filter.

1. Superficial corneal foreign bodies can be removed with irrigation. If the foreign bodies are embedded in the cornea, refer the patient to an ophthalmologist, after instilling ophthalmic ointment in the eye.
2. Patching the eye may be dangerous as it allows bacteria in dirty abrasions to multiply, and has not been shown to increase comfort.
3. Any abrasion should be treated with application of ophthalmic antibiotic ointment at least once daily until the epithelium is healed. Refer the patient to an

---

TABLE 21-2   **Outpatient Management of Hyphema**

Medications
- Atropine 1% three times daily
- Prednisolone acetate 1% one drop four times daily
- Topical antibiotics, if epithelial defects are present
- Acetaminophen—no aspirin or nonsteroidal anti-inflammatory drugs
- Acetazolamide or beta-blocker if intraocular pressure is elevated

Activities
- Bed rest with head elevated
- Limited activity—no bending, lifting (straining)
- Shield over injured eye

Follow-up
- Seen daily for 4–5 days

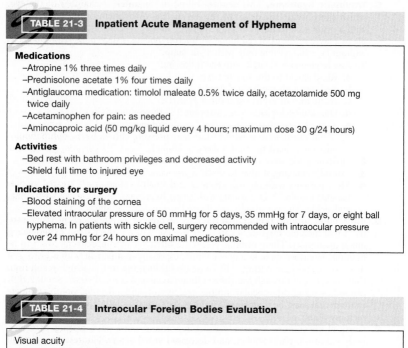

TABLE 21-3 Inpatient Acute Management of Hyphema

Medications
- Atropine 1% three times daily
- Prednisolone acetate 1% four times daily
- Antiglaucoma medication: timolol maleate 0.5% twice daily, acetazolamide 500 mg twice daily
- Acetaminophen for pain: as needed
- Aminocaproic acid (50 mg/kg liquid every 4 hours; maximum dose 30 g/24 hours)

Activities
- Bed rest with bathroom privileges and decreased activity
- Shield full time to injured eye

Indications for surgery
- Blood staining of the cornea
- Elevated intraocular pressure of 50 mmHg for 5 days, 35 mmHg for 7 days, or eight ball hyphema. In patients with sickle cell, surgery recommended with intraocular pressure over 24 mmHg for 24 hours on maximal medications.

TABLE 21-4 Intraocular Foreign Bodies Evaluation

Visual acuity
Dilated fundus examination
Shield
Computed tomography scan
Operating room

ophthalmologist for follow-up, and counsel the patient to seek immediate treatment if symptoms persist for more than 24 hours, or if a central abrasion or defect larger than 2 mm is detected.

F. Eyelid lacerations. Perform an ophthalmic examination on every patient with eyelid lacerations, and consider this for lacerations around the orbits (in general, the closer to eye, especially if any symptoms, the more detailed the exam). Soft-tissue injuries are repaired only after globe injuries are excluded and imaging studies performed. Even the most complex eyelid laceration repairs can be delayed for 24 to 48 hours with excellent surgical results.

  1. Specific eyelid complications include canthal tendon disinsertion, lacrimal drainage system (canalicular) lacerations, and levator aponeurosis laceration. These and transmarginal eyelid lacerations require special attention.

  2. Any laceration in the medial aspect of the eyelid, particularly if caused by a tearing injury, is likely to cause a canalicular laceration. Careful inspection, probing, and irrigation of the lacrimal apparatus are required to detect this injury. Irrigate and examine all wounds for the presence of foreign bodies.

  3. Complicated injuries and pediatric patients are best repaired in the operating room under monitored sedation or general anesthesia. Most superficial lacerations can be repaired with local eyelid blocks in the emergency department. In severe eyelid disruptions, the medial canthus should be addressed first with repair of the canalicular injury, silicone intubation of the lacrimal system, and repair of the deep head of the medial canthal tendon before closure of any other eyelid lacerations. These are best repaired by an ophthalmologist or plastic surgeon skilled in lid repair, in a procedure room or operating room.

4. Lacerations of the eyelid margin require a two-layered closure with 6-0 absorbable sutures in the deep tissue and nonabsorbable sutures in the eyelid margins (6-0 silk or 8-0 silk). Take care when closing deep eyelid tissue— **never place sutures in contact with the surface of the eyeball.**

5. Superficial skin closure is best accomplished with 7-0 or 8-0 monofilament or chromic gut sutures.

6. Ptosis secondary to the trauma is best observed for 6 to 12 months and then treated by a levator resection or advancement. Mechanical ptosis from hematoma or tissue edema usually improves slowly.

7. Topical antibiotic ointments offer bacterial prophylaxis and corneal protection in circumstances of poor eyelid closure. Ice packs and nondependent head positioning are important posttreatment maneuvers.

8. Avoid occluding the eye with pressure patching because of the risk of orbital hemorrhage. Check vision and pupils at regular intervals. The skin sutures usually are removed in 4 to 5 days. However, leave lid margin sutures in place 10 to 12 days.

G. **Hemorrhage and orbital bone fractures.** Orbital fractures can lead to acute, compressive orbital hemorrhage, an ophthalmologic emergency. The increasing intraorbital pressure resulting from an expanding hemorrhage can quickly lead to vascular compromise of the retina and optic nerve, resulting in permanent vision loss. Timely decompression with a lateral canthotomy and cantholysis can save vision in an eye with an expanding orbital hemorrhage.

1. Of orbital fractures, 40% are associated with serious ocular injuries, including retinal tears and detachments, retinal hemorrhage, vitreous hemorrhage, dislocation of the lens, hyphema, glaucoma, and traumatic cataract. Ocular injuries occur with midface, supraorbital, and frontal fractures. An open globe, retinal detachment, or traumatic optic neuropathy present contraindications to early bony repair. As a general guideline, fix the globe first. The bone can then be repaired in approximately 2 weeks.

2. Elevated intraocular pressure suggests increased orbital pressure, whereas lower intraocular pressure suggests a penetrating or perforating injury with globe disruption. Recognition of these ocular injuries is essential. Repair of isolated orbital fractures is almost never an operative emergency, and a complete ocular evaluation should be done before any orbital bone surgery.

3. Exception to this rule occurs in young patients who have greenstick fractures (trapdoors) of the orbital floor with inferior rectus entrapment. These patients often have a relatively white, quiet-looking eye, severe deficiency of upgaze, pain, and nausea. These must be repaired in the operating room as soon as safely possible, preferably within 24 hours.

H. **Traumatic optic neuropathies.** Traumatic vision loss with complete blindness occurs in approximately 3% of patients suffering blunt maxillofacial injuries. Of midface, supraorbital, or frontal sinus fractures, 4% are associated with severe optic nerve injuries. Early diagnosis and treatment of optic nerve injuries may minimize vision loss.

1. With a greater number of patients with closed head trauma surviving, more surviving patients have permanent loss of vision. Decreased visual acuity or visual fields with an afferent pupillary defect in the involved eye indicates optic nerve injury. It is sometimes difficult for the nonophthalmologist to make this determination because multiply injured trauma patients are often uncooperative or unconscious. Additionally, the optic disc may appear normal on ophthalmoscopy. It is necessary to carefully examine the pupils to make the diagnosis of an afferent pupillary defect.

2. Obtain thin-section CT scans through the orbit and optic canal to exclude the possibility of a bone fracture compromising the optic nerve.

3. Treatment of optic neuropathy in this setting is controversial. Very high-dose steroids are of unproven benefit but occasionally used. These may be given if

not otherwise contraindicated, then discontinued after 3 days if no response occurs. A surgical optic nerve decompression may be performed if bone fragments appear to be compromising the canal, but is realistic only in the hands of an experienced surgeon.

I. **Cataract.** A blunt injury to the eye can result in clouding (cataract) or displacement of the lens. A sharp injury to the lens capsule can also cause a cataract, but lens particles can also leak into the anterior chamber, resulting in severe uveitis, lens-induced glaucoma, and sometimes **lens anaphylaxis** (severe inflammation from exposure to lens proteins). A leaking lens must be removed.

J. **Retinal detachment.** Blunt trauma can cause retinal detachment, especially in patients who are nearsighted, have had previous ocular injury, or have had cataract surgery.

  1. Most retinal detachments caused by trauma do not occur at the time of injury, but occur weeks to months later. Although the risk never drops to zero, most detachments occur within 6 months of injury.

  2. The diagnosis is suspected when a patient presents with complaints of flashing lights and a curtain or shade interfering with some portion of the visual field. Confrontation visual fields may detect the field loss. The diagnosis is made by indirect ophthalmoscopy through a dilated pupil.

K. **Retina commotion.** A finger or other object directly hitting the eye or orbit can cause retinal damage that has the appearance of edema around the optic nerve or macula on ophthalmoscopy. This is caused by a shearing injury of the retina, and recovery is usually quick (weeks) and complete. Blood may also appear under the retina. Recovery can be complete or very limited.

AXIOMS

- Determination of visual acuity is essential for early detection of serious eye injury.
- Sutures are never placed in direct contact with the globe.
- If an open globe is suspected, put no pressure on the eye and use no drops in the eye.

Bibliography

Catalano R, Belin M. *Ocular Emergencies.* Philadelphia, Pa: WB Saunders; 1992.

Eagling E, Roper-Hall M. *Eye Injuries: An Illustrated Guide.* Philadelphia, Pa: JB Lippincott Co; 1986.

Kanitkar KD, Makar M, Kunimoto DY, eds. *The Wills Eye Manual: Office and Emergency Room Diagnosis and Treatment of Eye Disease.* 4th ed. Philadelphia, Pa: JB Lippincott Co; 1990.

Linberg J. *Oculoplastic and Orbital Emergencies.* Norwalk, Conn: Appleton & Lange; 1990.

Ocular trauma. In: *Advanced Trauma Life Support Manual.* Philadelphia, Pa: American College of Surgeons Committee on Trauma; 1993:385–390.

Spoor T, Nesi F. *Management of Ocular, Orbital and Adnexal Trauma.* New York, NY: Raven Press; 1988.

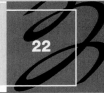

PENETRATING NECK TRAUMA

CAROL R. SCHERMER AND
KENNETH BOFFARD

22

I. INTRODUCTION. The evaluation and management of penetrating neck injuries has changed substantially over the past few decades, but the major challenges have not. The neck has a high density of vital structures that when injured can threaten both life and function. Although major vascular injuries may be readily recognized on presentation, aerodigestive and neurologic injuries may be more difficult to detect. Airway compromise may occur from either direct injury to the larynx or trachea or may result from an expanding hematoma due to vascular injury. As in the management of any injury, airway compromise is the primary concern and may be particularly challenging in the patient with a penetrating neck injury. In addition, a penetrating neck injury may violate the thorax, thus compromising a patient's ability to oxygenate and ventilate. The patient's chest and ability to breathe should be investigated promptly. Significant bleeding from the neck wound generally can be managed with direct pressure until operative exposure can be obtained.

II. MECHANISM OF INJURY. Gunshot wounds are generally more destructive than stab wounds and more likely to be associated with injuries requiring operation. Gunshot wounds are also more likely to be transcervical or extend through multiple zones. If possible, transcervical or transzone gunshot wounds should initially be evaluated with imaging or endoscopic/bronchoscopic studies to define the site of injury.

III. ANATOMY. Knowledge of neck anatomy is important due to the high density of structures and the morbidity that can occur when they are damaged. When the neck is in neutral position, the hyoid bone is at approximately the level of the third cervical vertebra, the notch of the thyroid cartilage at the fourth cervical vertebra. The cricoid cartilage is at approximately the sixth cervical vertebrae and also correlates with the beginning of the esophagus.

  A. Classically, the neck has been divided into anterior and posterior triangles and three zones from caudal to cranial. The borders of the anterior triangle of the neck are the sternocleidomastoid muscles laterally, the mandible superiorly, and the clavicles and sternal notch inferiorly. The posterior triangle is bounded by the sternocleidomastoid muscle anteriorly, the nuchal line of the occipital bone superiorly, and the trapezius muscle inferiorly.

  B. The zones of the neck are numbered in the caudocranial direction (Fig. 22-1).

  1. Zone I encompasses wounds from the clavicles and sternal notch to the cricoid cartilage. The trachea, great vessels including the subclavian arteries and veins, esophagus, thoracic duct, and lung apices may all be injured with a zone I penetrating injury.

  2. Zone II extends from the cricoid cartilage to the angle of the mandible. The common carotid and vertebral arteries, jugular veins, esophagus, pharynx, trachea, and larynx may be injured in a zone II injury.

  3. Zone III extends from the angle of the mandible superiorly to the base of the skull. Injuries to zone III may violate the external carotid artery or extracranial internal carotid artery, vertebral arteries, or jugular veins. Because zone III is above the esophageal inlet, aerodigestive injury involves the hypopharynx rather than esophagus at this level.

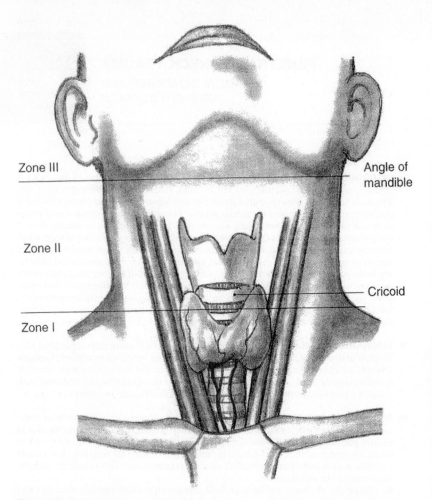

Figure 22-1. Zones of the neck. (Reprinted with permission from Borgstrom D, Weigelt JA. Neck: Aerodigestive tract. In: Ivatury RR, Cayten CG, eds. *The Textbook of Penetrating Trauma*. Philadelphia, Pa: Williams & Wilkins; 1996:482.)

IV. INITIAL ASSESSMENT AND MANAGEMENT. Only after the airway, breathing, and circulation portions of the resuscitation are complete should further neck examination be performed. Pertinent history that should be interrogated includes loss of consciousness, significant blood loss, hemoptysis, hematemesis, and voice changes.

A. If the patient has evidence of airway compromise, shock, or active hemorrhage; a large, expanding, or pulsatile neck hematoma; or massive subcutaneous air, the patient should be taken directly to the operating room for exploration.

B. If the patient is awake, alert, and hemodynamically stable, local wound exploration should be performed to determine if the injury violates the platysma. If the injury does not violate the platysma, no further evaluation is needed. Due to difficulty with operative exposure, and if possible based on hemodynamic status, patients with zone I or zone III injuries should undergo preoperative imaging to allow appropriate operative planning to assess the need for proximal and distal control via incisions other than an anterior neck incision.

V. EVALUATION OF PATIENTS WITHOUT INDICATIONS FOR EMERGENCY OPER-ATIVE INTERVENTION. In the hemodynamically stable patient without need for emergency operative intervention, evaluation of the patient includes physical exam followed by a number of options: observation, duplex ultrasonography, angiography, esophagography, tracheobronchoscopy, or CT angiography. The choices in evaluation and management depend on institutional resources and surgical capability.

A. Signs and symptoms that mandate further evaluation in the stable patient.
   1. hoarseness
   2. dysphonia or voice changes
   3. hemoptysis, dysphagia, or odynophagia
   4. hematemesis
   5. decreased radial pulse

B. Classic selective diagnosis. The high morbidity associated with nonoperative management of penetrating neck injuries in World War I led to a broad acceptance of routine exploration of zone II neck wounds during the last century. Because of the high negative exploration rate with mandatory exploration, selective management evolved. In the 1980s and 1990s, nonoperative evaluation routinely consisted of four-vessel angiography, laryngotracheo bronchoscopy, and esophagography or esophagoscopy. Four-vessel angiography is considered useful as a roadmap prior to surgery, particularly for zone I and zone III injuries. Although highly accurate, the low yield and potential morbidity of four-vessel angiography has led surgeons to investigate other options for evaluation of vascular injuries.

C. Observation alone. The accuracy of physical exam has been reported to range from 68% to 100%. Physical exam may be reliable to rule out vascular injuries in zone II. Patients with tracheal injuries tend to be symptomatic, hence their injuries are generally apparent on examination. Diagnosis of esophageal injuries from penetrating injury remain problematic.

D. Color flow Doppler imaging. In combination with physical exam, Doppler imaging is a safe and reliable alternative to contrast angiography for evaluating vascular injuries.

E. Esophagography and esopohagoscopy. Delay in detection of esophageal injuries increases morbidity and mortality. Although there is wide variability in the reported sensitivity and specificity of esophageal imaging, contrast esophagography performed under fluoroscopic supervision has a sensitivity near 90%. Rigid esophagoscopy, although technically difficult, has a sensitivity of approximately 85%. Some authors have recommended combining the two modalities. In the past, flexible esophagoscopy was reported as neither sensitive nor specific, but recent studies show it to have accuracy similar to the combination of esophagography and rigid endoscopy for detecting esophageal injuries.

F. Helical CT angiography (CTA). Use of CTA to evaluate penetrating neck injury has generally been reported in the context of its use to evaluate vascular injury. In cervical CTA, the contrast bolus and imaging are timed such that the carotid arteries are seen in the arterial phase; images need to be acquired from the top of the aortic arch through the base of the skull. A number of recent reports have demonstrated good sensitivity and specificity of CTA for the detection of vascular injuries and determination of missile trajectory. However, caution should be used in the use of CT for detecting esophageal injury, as no published data with adequate sample size support it as an isolated study for the evaluation of esophageal injuries.

VI. OPERATIVE EXPOSURE AND TECHNIQUE. The patient is generally positioned supine on the operating table with the arms tucked at the sides. Extension of the neck with rotation to the contralateral side is helpful if the cervical spine has been cleared.
   A. Active bleeding should be controlled with digital pressure until direct vascular control is achieved.
   B. Wounds should not be probed or locally explored; these maneuvers may lead to uncontrolled hemorrhage or embolism.

C. Skin preparation should include the entire neck and chin from the ears to midthighs (at least one groin prepared for potential saphenous vein harvest or vascular access) and to the table bilaterally (for access to both thoracic cavities and the mediastinum).

D. Most penetrating neck injuries are initially approached via an incision along the anterior border of the sternocleidomastoid muscle.

1. Operative exposure of zone I injury may require a supraclavicular incision with removal of the clavicular head or extension into a trapdoor type of incision where the medial end of the clavicular incision is extended onto the sternum and then to a left anterolateral thoracotomy.

2. Zone I injury on the right side of the neck can generally be managed by a median sternotomy with cephalad extension to an anterior sternocleidomastoid incision.

3. The most difficult exposure is zone III injury in which distal control of the vasculature is impeded by the base of the skull. At times subluxation, dislocation, or resection of the mandible is necessary to gain operative control. For zone II transcervical injury, both sides of the neck can be accessed via a transverse cervical collar incision that can be extended along the anterior borders of the sternocleidomastoid muscles. This incision is also useful for injuries that are known to be isolated to the larynx or trachea. Figure 22-2 demonstrates different incisions for exposure.

4. **Arterial injuries** can be managed by debridement and primary closure in cases without tension. Patch angioplasty and segmental resection with primary anastomosis are also viable options in the stable patient if not too time-consuming. Another option for a segmental defect is transposition of the external carotid to the internal carotid artery. Segmental interposition grafts do not have good patency rates.

5. In the neurologically intact patient, carotid arterial injuries should be repaired.

6. Carotid artery ligation should be reserved for patients who present obtunded or comatose, or when patients have uncontrollable hemorrhage and a temporary shunt is not possible.

7. Some also recommend carotid ligation in patients who do not demonstrate back-bleeding from the distal carotid artery.

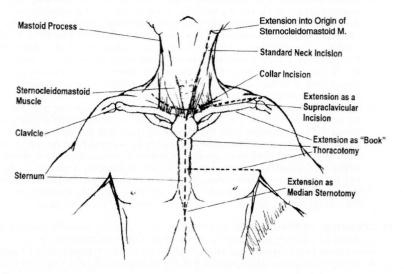

Figure 22-2. Incisions for exposure of penetrating neck injuries. (Reprinted with permission from Britt LD, Peyser MB. Penetrating and blunt neck trauma. In: Moore EE, Mattox KL, Feliciano DV, eds. *Trauma.* 4th ed. New York, NY: McGraw-Hill; 2000:444.)

8. Bleeding from an internal carotid artery that is at the base of the skull can be temporarily controlled with balloon occlusion.
9. Injury to the vertebral artery is infrequent due to its protected course within the bony foramina. If the contralateral vertebral artery is normal and the posterior inferior cerebellar artery is intact, unilateral ligation of the vertebral rarely results in a neurologic deficit. Because of difficulty in operative exposure and reports of injury managed angiographically, operative intervention of vertebral arteries should be reserved for life-threatening hemorrhage. Otherwise, endovascular techniques should be attempted.
E. For patients in shock, **venous injury** should be managed with ligation. Remember that air embolism may occur with venous injury, particularly if the patient is breathing spontaneously. The surgeon may notice on intubation of the patient and positive-pressure ventilation that there is increased bleeding from the neck wound due to the positive pressure transmitted to the large veins.
   1. In general, internal jugular venous injury can be managed with lateral venorrhaphy.
   2. Venous repair has high risk of thrombosis, hence patients should be systemically anticoagulated if are no other contraindications.
   3. External jugular venous injury can always be managed with ligation.
F. Delays in diagnosis and management of **esophageal injury** lead to increased morbidity and mortality. Esophageal injury should be debrided and closed in two layers, generally with an absorbable suture for the muscosal repair. Esophageal injury should be drained via a closed suction system to control possible anastomotic leak. Most authors recommend a contrast study and feeding prior to removal of the drain. Despite adequate repair, esophageal leaks occur in up to 6% of cases.
   1. A massively devitalized esophagus may require management with a cervical esophagostomy and feeding tube.
   2. For esophageal injuries combined with either vascular or tracheal injury, healthy tissue should be placed between the repairs. The strap muscles of the neck can be mobilized from their origin to provide this tissue layer.
   3. Penetrating hypopharyngeal wounds can be managed nonoperatively with NPO status and prophylactic antibiotics. Patients can be fed either parenterally or through a nasogastric tube.
   4. Unless dictated by a concomitant tracheal injury or emergency airway access, a surgical airway should be avoided in patients with esophageal injuries.
G. Definitive repair of **tracheal injury** should occur early; early repair is associated with lower complication rate when compared to late repair.
   1. Tracheal injury can generally be repaired in one layer with a monofilament absorbable suture.
   2. Extensive tracheal injury may require tracheostomy, but smaller injuries do not.

VII. **ANGIOGRAPHIC MANAGEMENT.** A number of case series of endovascular stenting and embolization of carotid and vertebral arterial injuries have been reported. This modality is particularly useful if the vessel is difficult to access surgically (such as a zone III injury) or if the vascular injury is not associated with injuries to other cervical structures that require operative management.

AXIOMS

- Immediate airway control, often difficult with penetrating neck injury, is the first priority.
- Active bleeding from the neck is best controlled in the trauma resuscitation area with direct digital pressure.
- If possible, injury to zone I or zone III should be imaged prior to operation; structures in these zones are difficult to access even with directed exploration.

Bibliography

Asensio JA, Chahwan S, Forno W, et al. Penetrating esophageal injuries: Multicenter study of the American Association for the Surgery of Trauma. *J Trauma* 2001;50(2):289–296.

Bynoe RP, Miles WS, Bell RM, et al. Non-invasive diagnosis of vascular trauma by duplex ultrasonography. *J Vasc Surg* 1991;14:346–352.

Demetriades D, Theodorou D, Cornwell E, et al. Evaluation of penetrating injuries of the neck: Prospective study of 223 patients. *World J Surg* 1997;21(1):41–47.

Fabian TC, George SM, Croce MA, et al. Carotid artery trauma: Management based on mechanism of injury. *J Trauma* 1990;30(8):953–961.

Gonzalez RP, Falimirski M, Holevar MR, Turk B. Penetrating zone II neck injury: Does dynamic computed tomographic scan contribute to the diagnostic sensitivity of physical examination for surgically significant injury? A prospective blinded study. *J Trauma* 2003;54(1):61–64; discussion 64–65.

Munera F, Cohn S, Rivas LA. Penetrating injuries of the neck: Use of helical computed tomographic angiography. *J Trauma* 2005;58(2):413–418.

Sclafani SJ, Panetta T, Goldstein AS, et al. The management of arterial injuries caused by penetration of zone III of the neck. *J Trauma* 1985;25:871–881.

Srinivasan R, Haywood T, Horwitz B, et al. Role of flexible endoscopy in the evaluation of possible esophageal trauma after penetrating injures. *Am J Gastroenterol* 2000;95(7):1725–1729.

Vassiliu P, Baker J, Henderson S, et al. Aerodigestive injuries of the neck. *Am Surg* 2001;67(1):75–79.

Winter RP, Weigelt JA. Cervical esophageal trauma: Incidence and cause of esophageal fistulas. *Arch Surg* 1990;125:849–852.

Yee LF, Olcott EW, Knudson MM, Lim RC Jr. Extraluminal, transluminal, and observational treatment for vertebral artery injuries. *J Trauma* 1995;39(3):480–484; discussion 484–486.

23

BLUNT NECK INJURY

TIFFANY K. BEE, JEFFREY A. CLARIDGE, AND MARTIN A. CROCE

I. INTRODUCTION. The surgeon frequently encounters blunt neck trauma, but significant injury (excluding that to the cervical spine) is relatively uncommon. Despite the infrequent occurrence, these injuries may be life threatening. The unrestrained driver hitting a steering wheel or a direct blow to the neck can provide a mechanism for this injury. Violent torsion, flexion, or extension of the neck also may result in blunt neck injury without any external signs of trauma. Patients with emergency airway control measure (intubation, etc.) have a higher degree of iatrogenic injury to the pharynx and upper esophagus. Often the signs and symptoms of blunt neck trauma are subtle. Give these injuries a high index of suspicion and be diligent in their diagnosis and management.

II. ANATOMY
- **A. Zones** (See Chapter 22 Penetrating Neck Injury)
    - **1.** Zone I—clavicle to cricoid
    - **2.** Zone II—cricoid to angle of mandible
    - **3.** Zone III—angle of mandible to skull base
- **B.** The neck contains a diversity of vital structures in a relatively small space. Vital portions of many organ systems are represented in the neck.
    - **1.** Respiratory
        - **a.** Trachea
        - **b.** Larynx
    - **2.** Cardiovascular
        - **a.** Carotid arteries
        - **b.** Jugular veins
        - **c.** Vertebral arteries
    - **3.** Neurologic
        - **a.** Cervical spinal cord
        - **b.** Vagus nerve
        - **c.** Phrenic nerve
        - **d.** recurrent Laryngeal nerves
    - **4.** Digestive
        - **a.** Pharynx
        - **b.** Esophagus
    - **5.** Endocrine
        - **a.** Thyroid
        - **b.** Parathyroids
    - **6.** Musculoskeletal
        - **a.** Spine and its ligaments

III. INITIAL EVALUATION
- **A.** All trauma patients should be systematically evaluated according to the Advanced Trauma Life Support (ATLS) protocols. Maintenance of cervical stability is important in the discussion and evaluation of patients with possible blunt cervical injury.
    - **1.** Airway
        - **a.** Patients having difficulty with oxygenation, ventilation, or decreased sensorium must be intubated, preferably orally. If unable to be intubated a

cricothyroidotomy should be performed. Care must be taken when obtaining a secure airway in patients with laryngotracheal injuries.

2. Breathing
   a. Pneumothorax may occur with laryngotracheal or esophageal trauma resulting in tension pneumothorax. If a tension pneumothorax is present, needle decompression followed by tube thoracostomy is indicated. Pneumomediastinum may be present, but it usually does not compromise breathing by itself.
   b. Tracheal or laryngeal disruption may lead to breathing difficulty.
3. Circulation
   a. Two large-bore peripheral IVs should be placed.
   b. Careful monitoring of peripheral pulses is necessary, evaluating for signs of deficit.
   c. Direct pressure should be applied to bleeding areas in the neck *without* probing or blind clamp placement.
4. Disability
   a. Spinal cord injury
   b. Neurologic finding not associated with head CT or spinal cord injury
5. Anisocoria or Horner's syndrome
   a. Weakness of extremity
   b. Change in mental status

B. Physical exam
   For adequate examination, removal of the cervical collar is necessary while maintaining inline immobilization.
   1. Inspection
      a. The neck should be evaluated for the presence of lacerations, abrasions, contusions, crepitance, jugular venous distension, asymmetry, "seat-belt sign," or other gross deformities.
   2. Auscultation
      a. A bruit over a carotid vessel may be a sign of vascular injury or chronic disease. If a bruit is heard in the presence of a hematoma, it should be assumed to be an acute injury.
      b. Stridor, hoarseness, odynophagia, and dysphagia are suggestive of laryngotracheal or aerodigestive injury.
   3. Palpation
      a. Presence of a pulse deficit, expanding pulsatile hematoma, or thrill is suggestive of vascular injury.
      b. Loss of the normal anatomic contours of the anterior neck, thyroid cartilage, or cricoid cartilage, is suggestive of laryngeal fracture.
      c. Assess that the trachea is in the midline. A defect in the tracheal wall ("step-off") is indicative of a tracheal disruption. Tracheal injury usually presents with subqutaneous emphysema.
      d. Subcutaneous emphysema is suggestive of pneumothorax or airway injury. It is unlikely that an esophageal injury will cause significant subcutaneous emphysema, but retropharyngeal air will likely be present.

C. Radiographic evaluation
   1. Cervical spine radiograph
      a. Tracheal deviation, increased soft tissue density and swelling are signs of hematoma.
      b. Pretracheal soft-tissue thickness greater than 5.0 mm is suggestive of cervical spine fracture, C1–3, greater than 10 mm, C4–7.
      c. Signs of subcutaneous emphysema or retropharyngeal air are suggestive of laryngotracheal or esophageal injury.
      d. Malalignment and or abnormal spacing of the vertebral bodies and their processes.
      e. Cervical immobilization should continue until radiographically and clinically cleared.

   2. Chest radiograph (See Chapter 24)
      a. Pneumothorax, subcutaneous emphysema, pneumomediastinum, and pneumopericardium may occur with upper airway injuries.
      b. Tube thoracostomy may be indicated, especially with positive pressure ventilation.
      c. Enlargement of the superior mediastinum and apical cap indicates great vessel injury at the thoracic outlet or base of the neck.

IV. DIAGNOSTIC MODALITIES. Patients with expanding hematomas or active hemorrhage should be taken immediately to the operating room. For hemodynamically stable patients, however, further diagnostic evaluation is necessary. Lateral cervical spine and chest radiographs should be obtained in the resuscitation area on all patients with blunt injury.
   A. CT and CT angiogram.
      1. Strengths
         a. Excellent for identifying injuries to the larynx, vertebral column, and vessels.
         b. May identify small collections of extraluminal air in the unusual case of blunt esophageal injury.
         c. Detection of soft-tissue injuries continues to improve.
         d. Multislice CT angiography can give valuable information.
         e. Excellent study for tracheal injury.
         f. Best single imaging study.
      2. Weaknesses
         a. Sensitivity for ligamentous is controversial (see MRI).
         b. Requires IV contrast.
   B. Laryngoscopy and bronchoscopy
      1. Strength
         a. Direct visualization of larynx and trachea.
      2. Weakness
         a. Injury to larynx or trachea may be obscured by endotracheal tube.
   C. Duplex ultrasound
      1. Strength
         a. Noninvasive test for occlusive carotid disease.
      2. Weaknesses
         a. Operator dependent.
         b. Difficult to visualize anatomy in the presence of a hematoma or subcutaneous emphysema.
         c. Unreliable for identification of acute blunt ICA dissection.
         d. Inadequate examination with cervical immobilization.
   D. Angiography
      1. Strengths
         a. Gold standard for diagnosis of carotid or vertebral artery injuries.
         b. May be able to perform therapeutic interventions at the same time.
         c. Provides information on intracerebral anatomy.
      2. Weaknesses
         a. Invasive.
         b. Requires IV contrast.
   E. Esophagram
      1. Strength
         a. Barium adequately distends the esophagus for easier identification of injury; water-soluble contrast is inadequate.
      2. Weakness
         a. Technically difficult in the intubated patient.
         b. Poor visualization of pharynx, and high esophagus.
   F. Flexible esophagoscopy
      1. Strengths
         a. Good visualization of esophagus, especially mid and distal portions.
         b. May safely be performed in patients with cervical immobilization (unlike rigid esophagoscopy).

2. Weakness
   a. May be difficult to adequately distend esophagus to identify small injuries.
   b. Poor visualization of pharynx, esophageal introitus and high esophagus.
G. MRI
   1. Strengths
      a. Good for evaluation of cervical spine ligamentous injury.
      b. Good for evaluation of spinal cord.
   2. Weaknesses
      a. Time-consuming.
      b. Difficult to perform in unstable acutely injured patient.

V. SPECIFIC INJURIES
A. Blunt cerebrovascular injuries (See Chapter 14)
   1. Incidence
      a. Increasing with awareness and screening.
      b. Estimate of incidence of blunt carotid injury is 0.5% of all blunt trauma admissions; the incidence of vertebral injuries is considered higher by a factor of 1.5–3.0.
   2. Mechanism best described by Crissey and Burnstein
      a. Crissey 1: Direct blow to the neck.
      b. Crissey 2: Blow to head with neck rotation and hyperextension causing the internal carotid to stretch.
      c. Crissey 3: Intraoral trauma.
      d. Crissey 4: Damage to intrapetrous portion of ICA.
B. Carotid artery
   1. Common carotid artery
      a. Usually due to direct blow to neck, with surrounding soft-tissue hematoma or contusion.
      b. May present with hemiparesis that is unexplained by brain CT findings.
      c. Associated facial (LeFort II and III) and cervical fractures are signs of severe trauma and should increase suspicion of vascular injury.
      d. Diagnosis is with angiography. A complete four-vessel angiogram is necessary to evaluate the presence or lack of cross filling, since only about one third of patients will have an intact circle of Willis. CT angiography may have an increased role in the diagnosis as the technology continues to improve.
      e. CT and CT angiogram are emerging as the screening procedure of choice.
      f. Injury grades of carotid injuries
         1. Grade I: Arteriographic appearance of irregularity of the vessel wall or dissection/intramural hematoma with less than 25% luminal narrowing.
         2. Grade II: Arteriographic appearance of an intimal flap or intramural hematoma with greater than 25% narrowing or dissection.
         3. Grade III: Arteriographic appearance of a pseudoaneurysm.
         4. Grade IV: Arteriographic appearance of occlusion.
         5. Grade V: Transection or hemodynamically significant injuries.
   2. Internal carotid artery
      a. Usually due to rapid deceleration with neck rotation and hyperextension. This causes the internal carotid to stretch usually over the second to third cervical transverse process, resulting in an intimal injury. Typically, there is dissection extending up to the skull base. There may be associated pseudoaneurysm.
      b. May present with hemiparesis or other neurologic deficit that is unexplained by brain CT findings. Horner's syndrome may be present due to associated injury to the sympathetic fibers, which are in close proximity to the distal ICA. The complete Horner's syndrome is not usually present, however, but miosis is typically present.
      c. Angiography is the gold standard of diagnosis. A complete four-vessel angiogram is necessary to evaluate the presence or lack of cross filling, since only about one third of patients will have an intact circle of Willis.

C. Vertebral artery
   1. Associated with flexion and rotation of the neck, also cervical spine fractures or subfixation. Fractures of the foramen transversarium are likewise associated with vascular injuries.
   2. With associated cervical injuries, angiography is indicated. Again, four-vessel study is indicated.
D. Larynx and trachea
   1. Usually due to direct blow to neck.
   2. Perforation of the upper aerodigestive tract is a result of the laryngeal cartilage being compressed by the vertebral bodies.
   3. Usually associated with subcutaneous emphysema and loss of the normal contour of the thyroid cartilage. A palpable defect may be felt in the tracheal wall.
   4. Awake patients with laryngotracheal injuries will assume a position in which they have a patent airway.
   5. **The airway *must* be secured.** The best option is a surgical airway (tracheostomy in this setting) using local anesthesia in the operating room.
   6. Nonobvious diagnosis is by direct laryngoscopy or bronchoscopy. However 3-D multislice CT diagnosis is excellent.
E. Esophagus
   1. Usually due to direct blow to neck; however, these injuries are uncommon.
   2. Diagnosis is by barium swallow.

VI. TREATMENT
   A. Carotid artery
   1. Operative management should be reserved for injuries to the common carotid or the proximal internal carotid. Blunt injuries, which are usually dissections (with or without associated pseudoaneurysm), typically extend distally, making primary repair impractical. Interposition grafting is usually necessary, and a long segment may be required.
   2. Nonoperative therapy, consisting of anticoagulation to prevent clot propagation or embolization, is the primary treatment for blunt traumatic ICA dissections. This remains controversial. Continuous heparin is the preferred treatment, although it must be used with extreme caution in patients with associated injuries, and may be relatively contraindicated in patients with cerebral intraparenchymal hemorrhage or contusion. The partial thromboplastin time (PTT) should be closely monitored, and the goal is 40 to 45 seconds. Follow-up angiography should be performed in approximately 14 days to assess for progression of injury. Therapy may be converted to warfarin or antiplatelet therapy with aspirin and should be continued for approximately 6 months. Follow-up study in 6 weeks should include angiography. However, magnetic resonance or CT angiography if practical at the institution may be used since they are less invasive than conventional angiography. Evidence of persistent injury should mandate continued antithrombotic treatment and possible operative intervention or stent placement. Treatment for pseudoaneurysms involves stent grafts with antiplatelet therapy until the stent has endothelialized—about 6 months. Aspirin is generally continued for the life of the stented patient.
   B. Vertebral artery
   1. Operative management is usually not necessary.
   2. Nonoperative management is similar to the anticoagulation and antiplatelet therapy for internal carotid injuries. Aspirin therapy may be substituted for occluded vessels.
   3. Radiologic embolization should be reserved arteriovenous fistula or active extravasation. Both proximal and distal segments need to be embolized.
   C. Larynx and trachea
   1. The first priority is to secure the airway, which may require emergent incision and intubation of the disrupted distal trachea.
   2. For destructive injuries, tracheal reconstruction may be necessary. Mathison and Grillo have established basic management principles.

    a. Avoid searching for recurrent laryngeal nerves.

    b. Separate tracheal and esophageal suture lines.

    c. Conserve viable trachea.

    d. Avoid tracheostomy through the repair.

    e. Flex the neck to avoid tension on the repair.

  3. Less destructive injuries (usually to the larynx) may be managed with tracheostomy distal to the injury and primary repair of the injury.

  4. Mild injuries with minimal swelling or nondisplaced cartilage may be treated with observation, voice rest, and humidified air.

  5. Hoarseness from bilateral vocal cord paralysis in laryngotracheal disruption may improve with time.

D. Esophagus

  1. Operative repair should be undertaken when the diagnosis is made. The esophagus should be repaired in two layers (inner mucosal, outer muscularis). The repair may be buttressed by surrounding strap muscles. If a drain is deemed necessary, it should be a closed suction drain.

VII. SUMMARY

A. The first priority is to obtain a secure airway, as with all trauma patients. This may be difficult in a patient with severe neck trauma.

B. Significant injuries to the larynx, trachea, carotid, or esophagus are not common, but are associated with relatively high morbidity and mortality.

C. A high index of suspicion for such injuries is necessary for early diagnosis and appropriate management to decrease the associated morbidity and mortality.

I. INTRODUCTION. Thoracic injuries account for approximately 25% of all trauma deaths and contribute to an additional 25% of deaths annually in the United States. Immediate deaths usually involve disruption of the heart or great vessel injury. Deaths within a few hours are frequently caused by airway obstruction, tension pneumothorax, hemorrhage, or cardiac tamponade. Pulmonary complications, sepsis, and missed injuries account for the late deaths. Although thoracic injuries are often life threatening, most patients with thoracic injuries are managed nonoperatively. Treatment options include analgesia, pulmonary hygiene, endotracheal intubation, and tube thoracostomy. Only 10% to 15% of patients with chest trauma will require thoracotomy or sternotomy.

II. IMMEDIATE EVALUATION
- **A. Physical examination** includes evaluation of upper airway, chest wall symmetry and stability, breath sounds, and heart tones. Findings of decreased breath sounds, subcutaneous emphysema, jugular venous distention (JVD), and tracheal deviation are specifically sought early in the evaluation.
- **B. Begin resuscitation** while performing concurrent diagnostic procedures. **Administer oxygen** by high-flow nonrebreathing mask. If the patient does not respond adequately to volume resuscitation (persistent hypotension, tachycardia, decreased mental status), consider ongoing blood loss, and reevaluate for cardiac tamponade, tension pneumothorax, and cardiogenic shock from blunt cardiac injury.
- **C.** Monitor pulse oxymetry and electrocardiogram (ECG) continuously.
- **D.** Obtain a **chest x-ray (CXR)** early in the evaluation of patients with thoracic injury. Sites of missile entry or penetration should be identified with radiopaque markers (e.g., metallic markers, paper clips).
- **E.** In patients with significant injury, an arterial blood gas (ABG) can be used to determine adequacy of ventilation and acid base status.
- **F.** Identify **indications for immediate operation.**
  1. Massive hemothorax (>1,500 mL blood returned on insertion of chest tube)
  2. Ongoing bleeding from chest (>200 mL/hour for ≥4 hours)
  3. Evidence of cardiac tamponade
  4. Penetrating transmediastinal chest wounds with unstable hemodynamics
  5. Chest wall disruption or impalement wounds to the chest
  6. Massive air leak from the chest tube or major tracheobronchial injury seen on bronchoscopy
  7. Mediastinal hematoma or radiographic evidence of great vessel injury with unstable hemodynamics
  8. Suspected air embolism

III. Immediate management of penetrating chest wounds
- **A.** Avoid probing the wound to determine depth or angle, which can produce pneumothorax or hemothorax.
- **B.** Obtain a **CXR** with metallic markers placed on all penetrating wounds.
  1. Attempt to **determine trajectory to estimate likely anatomic injury**.

2. Perform tube thoracostomy for pneumothorax or hemothorax.
   a. Administration of prophylactic antibiotics such as cefazolin, as a single dose before the start of the procedure, has been recommended to decrease the risk of empyema and pneumonia.
3. If initial CXR is negative, repeat film in 6 hours; 7% to 10% of this population will develop delayed pneumothorax.
C. Administer tetanus prophylaxis.
D. Routine antibiotics **are not** used for routine penetrating wounds treated without an operation or procedure.

IV. Immediate evaluation of transmediastinal penetrating wounds (Fig. 24-1)
   A. Diagnosis of transmediastinal penetration is based on clinical suspicion, trajectory of the bullet, or CXR findings. Perform a rapid assessment of patient to evaluate airway, hemodynamic status, and the need for hemorrhage control.
   B. Classify the patient, based on hemodynamics, as **extremis, unstable, or stable** (Fig. 24-2).
   C. The patient **in extremis** has agonal respirations without measurable blood pressure.

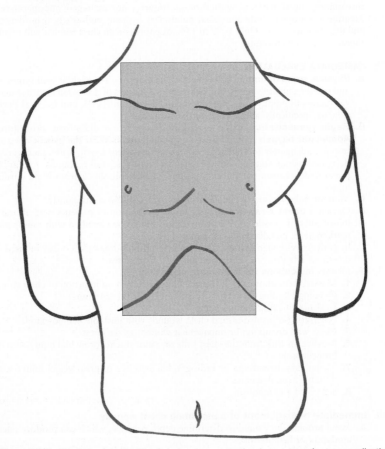

Figure 24-1. The box of death. *Shaded area* represents the danger zone for transmediastinal injury.

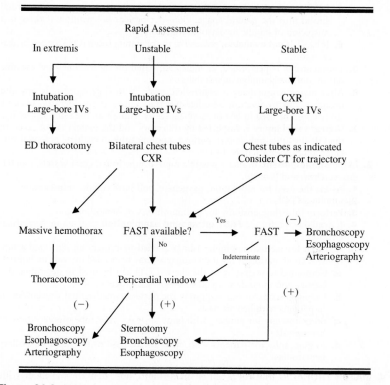

Figure 24-2. Diagnostic algorithm for transmediastinal penetrating trauma. FAST, focused abdominal sonography for trauma; CXR, chest x-ray; ED, emergency department; CT, computed tomography.

1. Intubate, oxygenate, and start volume resuscitation.
2. Perform immediate left anterolateral thoracotomy to control hemorrhage or relieve cardiac tamponade. Place a right chest tube to interrogate the right chest. If needed, extend across sternum to a right thoracotomy ("clamshell thoracotomy").
3. Control bleeding from pleural cavities or heart wound as necessary.

D. The **unstable patient** has a measurable blood pressure but is hypotensive, with a systolic blood pressure <90 mmHg. These patients, with associated transmediastinal trajectory, often have injuries to the following organs (in descending frequency): lung, heart, chest wall vessel, great vessels, esophagus, trachea or bronchi, and pulmonary artery or vein.

1. Assess the need for intubation, oxygenate, and start volume resuscitation.
2. Obtain a CXR.
3. Perform tube thoracostomy for pneumothorax or hemothorax.
4. Perform a **focused abdominal sonography for trauma (FAST) ultrasound examination** to diagnose pericardial effusion.
   a. A **positive** pericardial view on the FAST in an unstable patient is an indication to proceed with immediate median sternotomy.
   b. An **equivocal** pericardial view on the FAST examination necessitates either an operative pericardial window or an exploratory sternotomy.

    c. FAST can be **falsely negative** secondary to decompression of pericardial blood into the pleural space. Consider pericardial window if there is a suspicion of middle mediastinal trajectory.

    d. If FAST is **not available,** proceed to the operating room (OR) for pericardial window.

  5. Thoracotomy is performed, as indicated, based on the volume of chest tube return and the hemodynamic stability.

  6. After major hemorrhage is controlled, perform flexible esophagoscopy and bronchoscopy to diagnose aerodigestive tract injury. A gastrograffin swallow study could be used in lieu of esophagoscopy with about the same sensitivity.

  7. If great vessel injury is suspected by trajectory and the patient is not taken to the OR for other indications, perform **angiography** to evaluate potential vascular injury. (See Chapter 14.)

E. In the **stable patient**, evaluate possible injury to the heart, great vessels, esophagus, trachea, and bronchi.

  1. Assess the need for intubation, oxygenate, and start volume resuscitation.

  2. Obtain a CXR.

  3. Perform tube thoracostomy for pneumothorax or hemothorax.

  4. If available, perform a **FAST ultrasound examination** to diagnose pericardial effusion.

  5. A search for mediastinal injury can be guided by presenting signs and symptoms. A combination of the following tests may be needed to evaluate injuries.

    a. Computed tomography of the chest (CCT) can be used to determine trajectory and to guide subsequent diagnostic procedures.

    b. Esophagoscopy or esophagraphy for posterior mediastinal trajectories or in patients with hematemesis.

    c. Bronchoscopy for patients with large air leaks after tube thoracostomy or hemoptysis.

    d. Angiography for patients with mediastinal, base of the neck, or axillary hematomas.

V. **MAJOR THORACIC INJURIES** can be divided into those that are immediately life threatening and those that can be difficult to diagnose (Table 24-1).

A. Immediately life-threatening injuries

  1. Airway obstruction. Control of the airway is foremost in trauma resuscitation. The airway must be secured quickly, with attention to the possibility of associated cervical spine injury.

    a. Causes

      i. Relaxation of the tongue into the posterior pharynx in the unconscious patient

      ii. Loose dentures, avulsed teeth, lacerated tissue, secretions, and blood pooling in the mouth and hypopharynx

      iii. Bilateral mandibular fractures allowing the tongue to collapse into the hypopharynx

TABLE 24-1	Major Thoracic Injury
Lethal Seven	**Hidden Six**
Airway obstruction	Traumatic rupture of the aorta
Tension pneumothorax	Major tracheobronchial disruption
Cardiac tamponade	Blunt cardiac injury
Open pneumothorax	Diaphragmatic tear
Massive hemothorax	Esophageal perforation
Flail chest	Pulmonary contusion
Commotio Cordis	

    iv. Expanding neck hematomas producing deviation of the larynx and mechanical compression of the trachea

    v. Laryngeal trauma (e.g., thyroid cartilage or cricoid fractures) producing submucosal hemorrhage and edema

    vi. Tracheal tears or transections

  b. Physical findings include stridor, hoarseness, subcutaneous emphysema, altered mental status, accessory muscle use, air hunger, apnea, and cyanosis (sign of preterminal hypoxemia).

  c. Any suspicion of airway obstruction or inability to exchange air adequately mandates early intubation.

  d. Management (See Chapter 11.)

    i. When in doubt, intubate using a controlled rapid-sequence intubation (RSI). Oral intubation with direct view of the vocal cords and endotracheal tube is the standard.

    ii. Provide inline cervical spine immobilization during intubation.

    iii. Intubate early, especially in cases of neck hematoma or possible airway edema; airway edema can be insidious and progressive and can make delayed intubation more difficult.

    iv. Have equipment for emergency cricothyroidotomy readily available if endotracheal intubation fails.

    v. Rescue airway techniques such as the **Combitube** or **laryngeal mask airway (LMA)** should be used only by personnel who have had formal training in the use of these devices.

      a) These are **not definitive airways,** as defined as a cuffed tube passing through the vocal cords.

      b) If patients arrive with these airways in place, they should be changed out only by practitioners familiar with their design and use.

2. Tension pneumothorax occurs when air enters the pleural space from lung injury or through the chest wall without a means of exit. Pressure develops within the pleural space, compressing the superior and inferior vena cava, impairing venous return, and decreasing cardiac output.

  a. Most common causes

    i. Penetrating injury to the chest

    ii. Blunt trauma with parenchymal lung injury

    iii. Mechanical ventilation with high airway pressure

    iv. Spontaneous pneumothorax with blebs that failed to seal

  b. Diagnosis

    i. Tension pneumothorax **must** be a clinical diagnosis

      a) Severe respiratory distress

      b) Hypotension

      c) Unilateral absence of breath sounds

      d) Hyperresonance to percussion over affected hemithorax

      e) Neck vein distention (can be absent in hypovolemic patients)

      f) Tracheal deviation (late finding—not necessary to confirm clinical diagnosis)

    ii. If the tension pneumothorax has not been diagnosed on clinical findings (which it should be), **CXR** will usually show a pneumothorax large enough to cause tension. However, in a few cases a large anterior or posterior collapse will not be evident on plain film.

    iii. Bedside ultrasound is now being applied to the diagnosis of pneumothorax with good results.

  c. Treatment

    i. Immediately decompress by inserting a 12- or 14-gauge IV catheter into the second intercostal space in the midclavicular line. This converts the tension pneumothorax into a simple open pneumothorax.

    ii. Follow immediately with tube thoracostomy.

3. Pericardial tamponade is commonly the result of penetrating trauma, but it can also be seen in blunt chest trauma. The pericardial sac does not acutely distend; 75 to 100 mL of blood can produce tamponade physiology in the adult.

a. Diagnosis (Fig. 24-3)

    i. If awake, these patients are extremely anxious and even combative; they are reluctant to lie flat, and will often state that they sense "impending doom," and may appear "deathlike."

    ii. Suspect tamponade in those with persistent hypotension, acidosis, and base deficit, despite adequate blood and fluid resuscitation, especially if ongoing blood loss is not evident.

    iii. Classic signs. JVD, hypotension, and muffled heart tones (**Beck's triad**) are present in only 33% of patients with confirmed tamponade. JVD may not be present secondary to hypovolemia. **Pulsus paradoxus** is a decrease in systolic pressure of >10 mmHg during inspiration and suggests tamponade. **Kussmaul's sign** is a hard and true sign of tamponade; inspiration in a spontaneously breathing patient results in an increase of the JVD. The classic signs of cardiac tamponade are uncommon—**shock or ongoing hypotension without blood loss is the usual trigger to suggest this injury**.

    iv. If a pulmonary artery catheter is present, right- and left-side heart pressures will appear to equalize. Central venous pressure approaches the pulmonary arterial wedge pressure, and both will be elevated.

    v. If available, a **FAST ultrasound examination** should be performed to identify pericardial fluid.

        a) A **positive** pericardial view on the FAST in an **unstable** patient is an indication to proceed with median sternotomy or left anterolateral thoracotomy.

        b) An **equivocal** pericardial view on the FAST examination or a positive examination in a **stable** patient necessitates an operative pericardial window.

        c) A **negative** FAST in penetrating injury can be falsely negative secondary to decompression of pericardial fluid into the pleural space.

b. Treatment. Generally, the following multiple interventions occur simultaneously. These can be performed in either the emergency department (ED) or the OR, based on the clinical condition of the patient.

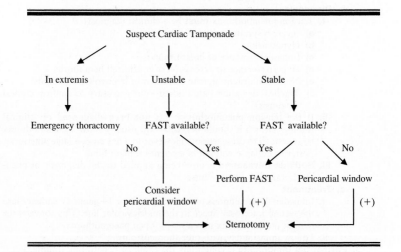

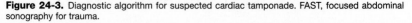

Figure 24-3. Diagnostic algorithm for suspected cardiac tamponade. FAST, focused abdominal sonography for trauma.

   i. Assess the need for intubation, oxygenate, and start volume resuscitation.

   ii. Pericardiocentesis can be used as a temporizing maneuver to relieve tamponade until definitive repair is possible. This is often difficult to successfully perform because of the "blind" nature of the procedure and relatively small blood volume in the sac.

   iii. If the patient is **in extremis**, an emergent left anterolateral thoracotomy should be performed to relieve the tamponade.

   iv. If the patient is **unstable**, urgent sternotomy should be performed in the OR.

   v. If the patient is **stable**, a diagnostic pericardial window can be performed in the OR to confirm the diagnosis. If this reveals blood in the sac, extend the incision to a sternotomy.

4. Open pneumothorax (sucking chest wound)

   a. Usually caused by impalement injury or destructive penetrating wound (shotgun)

   b. Large open defect in chest wall (>3 cm diameter) with equilibration between intrathoracic and atmospheric pressure

   i. If the opening is greater than two thirds the diameter of the trachea, air follows the path of least resistance through the chest wall with each inspiration, leading to profound hypoventilation and hypoxia. Signs and symptoms are usually proportional to the size of the defect.

   c. Management

   i. Intubate, if patient is unstable or in any respiratory distress.

   ii. Close the chest wall defect with a sterile occlusive dressing taped on three sides to act as a flutter-type valve. Avoid securing the dressing on all four sides in the absence of a chest tube, which can produce a tension pneumothorax.

   iii. Perform tube thoracostomy on the affected side. Avoid placing the tube near or through the traumatic wound.

   iv. Perform urgent thoracotomy to evacuate blood clot and treat associated intrathoracic injuries.

      a) Irrigate, debride, and close the chest wall defect in the OR. Leave a chest tube in place.

      b) Large defects may require flap closure.

5. Massive hemothorax

   a. Common in penetrating trauma with hilar or systemic vessel disruption

   i. Intercostal and internal mammary vessels are most commonly injured.

   ii. Each hemithorax can hold up to 3 L of blood.

   iii. Neck veins can be flat secondary to hypovolemia or distended because of the mechanical effects of intrathoracic blood.

   iv. Hilar or great vessel disruption will present with severe shock.

   b. Diagnosis

   i. Hemorrhagic shock.

   ii. Unilateral absence or diminution of breath sounds.

   iii. Unilateral dullness to percussion.

   iv. Flat neck veins.

   v. CXR will show unilateral "white out" (opacification).

   c. Treatment

   i. Intubate a patient in shock or with any respiratory difficulty.

   ii. Establish large-bore IV access and have blood available for infusion before decompression.

   iii. If available, have an autotransfusion setup for the chest tube collection system.

   iv. Perform tube thoracostomy with a large tube catheter (36 F or 40 F) in fifth intercostal space.

      a) A second chest tube may occasionally be necessary to adequately drain the hemothorax.

v. Thoracotomy is indicated for:
   a) Hemodynamic decompensation or ongoing instability because of chest bleeding
   b) ≥1,500 mL blood evacuated initially
   c) Ongoing bleeding of >200 mL/hour for ≥4 hours
   d) Failure to completely drain hemothorax, despite at least two functioning and appropriately positioned chest tubes
vi. Consider early video assisted thoracoscopy (VATS) for incompletely drained or clotted hemothorax.

6. Flail chest usually results from direct high-energy impact. The flail segment classically involves anterior (costochondral cartilage) or lateral rib fractures. Posterior rib fractures usually do not produce a flail segment because the heavy musculature provides stability.

a. Diagnosis
   i. Diagnosis is made when two or more ribs are fractured in two or more locations, which often may lead to paradoxical motion of that chest wall segment. Patients on positive pressure ventilation may not show this paradoxical motion.
   ii. Blunt force of injury typically produces an underlying pulmonary contusion. Morbidity and mortality are generally related to the lung parenchymal injury rather than the chest wall injury.
   iii. The patient is at high risk for pneumothorax or hemothorax, on both immediate and a delayed presentation.
   iv. The flail segment, underlying pulmonary contusion, and splinting caused by pain all exacerbate hypoxemia.
   v. Associated abdominal injuries occur in approximately 15% of patients with flail chest.

b. Management
   i. Immediately intubate for shock or signs of respiratory distress, such as:
      a) Labored breathing requiring use of accessory muscles of respiration
      b) Respiratory rate >35/minute or <8/minute
      c) Oxygen saturation <90%, PaO_2 <60 mmHg
      d) $PaCO_2$ >55 mmHg
   ii. Consider intubation for patients with a history of hemodynamic instability, the need for surgical repair of another problem, chronic obstructive pulmonary disease, cardiac disease, or advanced age.
   iii. Admit patient to the surgical intensive care unit (SICU). The natural progression of the injury is worsening hypoxemia and respiratory insufficiency.
   iv. Control pain (Chapter 40).
      a) Regional analgesia in the form of an epidural block is the most effective way to deliver pain relief for patients with chest wall trauma.
      b) Systemic opioids by continuous infusion or patient-controlled anesthesia (PCA).
      c) Intercostal nerve blocks.
   v. Monitor pulse oximetry and, if available, monitor continuous end-tidal CO_2.
   vi. Provide aggressive pulmonary hygiene, including incentive spirometry and cough-deep breathing. Adequate pain control and Continuous Positive Airway Pressure (CPAP) may preclude intubation.

7. Commotio cordis is sudden death after a blunt injury to the chest. The injury most often occurs during sporting events where a direct blow to the chest is caused by a fast-moving ball, such as a baseball or lacrosse ball.

a. Patients will not necessarily have a structural injury such as blunt cardiac injury (BCI).
b. The most common dysrhythmia is ventricular fibrillation, possibly caused by massive activation of potassium–ATP channels.

     c. Treatment consists of following advanced cardiac life support (ACLS) procedures and aggressive cardiopulmonary resuscitation. Despite prompt and skillful resuscitation, some patients will not be able to be revived.

B. Potentially life-threatening injuries

    1. Traumatic rupture of the aorta is defined as a tear in the wall of the aorta that is contained by the adventitia of artery and the parietal pleura.

       a. The mechanism of injury is rapid deceleration, such as falls from significant height, high-speed motor vehicle crashes, and ejected occupants. Thoracic aortic injury can also occur with significant lateral impact motor vehicle crash. Of these victims, 80% die at the scene. The remaining patients are at risk for delayed free rupture into the mediastinum or pleural space.

       b. Patients can be asymptomatic or complain of chest pain. Survivors have contained ruptures. Because free rupture of the transected aorta is rapidly fatal, persistent or recurring hypotension usually results from a secondary bleeding source, not the aortic injury.

       c. Laceration is usually located near the ligamentum arteriosum (85%). Less often, injury is situated in the ascending aorta, at the diaphragm, or in the mid descending thoracic aorta.

       d. Diagnosis (Fig. 24-4)

          i. Clinical signs

            a) Asymmetry in upper extremity blood pressures and upper extremity hypertension.

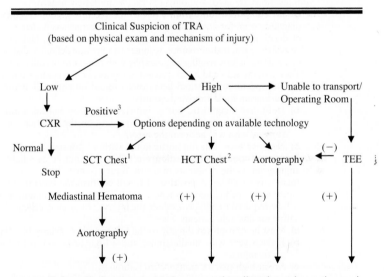

Early medical management to decrease aortic wall tension and operative repair

[1]Standard conventional computed tomography; [2]Helical computed tomography;
[3]Positive = findings listed in (IV.B.1.d.(2)). TEE = *Tranesophageal echocardiogram

Figure 24-4. Diagnostic algorithm for suspected traumatic rupture of the aorta (TRA). SCT, standard computed tomography; HCT, helical computed tomography.

b) Widened pulse pressure.

c) Chest wall contusion.

d) Posterior scapular pain, intrascapular murmur.

e) One half of patients with great vessel injury from blunt trauma have no external signs of blunt chest injury.

ii. Signs on **CXR**

a) Widened mediastinum (>8 cm); this is the most consistent finding.

b) Fracture of first three ribs, scapula, or sternum.

c) Obliteration of aortic knob.

d) Deviation of trachea to right.

e) Presence of pleural cap, usually on the left but occasionally bilaterally.

f) Elevation and rightward shift of the right mainstem bronchus.

g) Depression of the left mainstem bronchus >40 degrees from horizontal.

h) Obliteration of aortopulmonary window.

i) Deviation of nasogastric tube (esophagus) to right is an infrequent, matching but suggestive, sign.

j) Left pleural effusion.

k) No single sign reliably confirms or excludes aortic injury. However, a widened mediastinum is the most consistent finding on CXR and should prompt further evaluation.

1) Up to 15% of patients with traumatic rupture of the aorta will have a **normal CXR**.

iii. Historically, **aortography** was the gold standard for diagnosis. Approximately 10% of all angiograms are positive when liberal indications are used, and only 2% to 3% are falsely negative.

iv. Chest computed tomography (CCT) has recently become a valuable diagnostic tool for aortic injury. Standard CT scanners can characterize mediastinal hematomas that are suggestive of aortic injury. Helical and new high-speed, high-resolution scanners can provide definitive diagnosis of the aortic injury, rivaling angiography with respect to overall accuracy. Timing of the scan and bolus injection are critical for accurate studies.

a) Nonspecific mediastinal hematomas found on chest CT mandate aortogram for definitive diagnosis.

b) Definitive diagnostic aortic injuries found on helical scanners may also require aortography, depending on the practices of the surgeon who will perform the repair.

c) Negative scans rule out aortic injury with a 92% sensitivity.

v. Transesophageal echocardiogram (TEE) may not be as reliable as angiogram in the diagnosis of aortic injury (sensitivity of 63% and specificity of 84%). A positive TEE will confirm the location of the injury and expedite management. If the TEE is negative, an aortogram will be required to reliably exclude the injury. TEE is an excellent alternative for unstable patients who:

a) Must be transported directly to the OR for other cavitary bleeding.

b) Have a very wide mediastinum and a high suspicion of thoracic aortic injury.

c) Are at high risk for transport to radiology.

When stable, a negative TEE is followed by chest CT or aortography.

e. Management

i. Establish airway, as needed.

ii. Control and prevent hypertension. Maneuvers to decrease wall tension in the aorta preoperatively may decrease risk of rupture. Beta blockade should be instituted only after significant hemorrhage from other injuries has been ruled out. The goal for systolic blood pressure should be approximately 100 mmHg.

a) Esmolol is a short-acting beta-blocker that can be easily titrated to desired blood pressure. The loading dose is **500 μg/kg** followed by a continuous infusion of **50 μg/kg/min** titrated to a systolic blood pressure of 100 mmHg and a heart rate <100 beats/minute.

b) Labetolol is a longer acting beta- and alpha-blocker that can decrease wall tension. An initial IV dose of **20 mg** is given. Additional doses can be given to obtain parameters as already stated, up to **300 mg total.**

c) Nitroprusside can be added as a second agent if blood pressure is not controlled with beta blockade. It is administered as a continuous infusion at **0.1 μg/kg/min** titrated to effect up to a dose of 10 μg/kg/min.

iii. If the patient has a stable mediastinal hematoma and concomitant abdominal injury, perform a truncated laparotomy first. Take care not to pack the abdomen tightly or clamp the aorta, causing increased proximal aortic pressure. An intraoperative TEE can be used to evaluate the thoracic aorta.

iv. Several techniques are available for definitive repair.

a) Repair after full cardiac bypass often requires large doses of heparin and cannot be done in cases with many associated solid organ injuries, pelvic fractures, or traumatic brain injuries

b) Repair during passive bypass with heparin bonded shunts, or no bypass at all, is possible, although less often used. Paraplegia rates are reportedly lower with full or passive bypass.

b) Endovascular aortic stent grafts are now available at some centers and offer the advantage of avoiding a thoracotomy in patients who may have significant associated pulmonary compromise. Long-term patency and durability of stents in this setting are unknown.

2. Tracheobronchial injuries

a. Most patients with major airway injuries die at the scene as a result of asphyxia. Those who survive to reach the hospital are usually in extremis. More minor injuries can cause late sequelae such as granuloma formation with subsequent stenosis, persistent atelectasis, and recurring pneumonia.

b. Location

i. Cervical tracheal injuries

a) Usually present with upper airway obstruction and cyanosis unrelieved with O_2.

b) Symptoms include local pain, dysphagia, cough, and hemoptysis.

c) Subcutaneous emphysema.

d) Blunt transection is uncommon and tends to occur at the cricotracheal junction.

ii. Thoracic tracheal or bronchial injuries

a) Of major bronchial injuries, 80% occur within 2 cm of the carina.

b) Intrapleural laceration. The patient develops persistent dyspnea, massive air leak, and massive pneumothorax that does not reexpand with chest tube drainage. Intraparenchymal injuries usually seal spontaneously if the lung is adequately expanded.

c) Extrapleural rupture into the mediastinum. The patient will have pneumomediastinum and subcutaneous emphysema. Respiratory distress may be minimal, especially with partial bronchial transections. Of partial bronchial disruptions, 25% will go undetected for 2 to 4 weeks, but persistent atelectasis, recurrent pneumonia, and suppuration should prompt further investigation.

d) Radiographic signs on CXR

1) An abnormal admission CXR will be seen in 90% of cases; findings include pneumothorax, pleural effusion, subcutaneous emphysema, fractures of ipsilateral ribs 1 through 5, and mediastinal hematoma.

2) Specific findings
- Peribronchial air.
- Deep cervical emphysema; radiolucent line along prevertebral fascia (early and reliable sign).
- "Fallen lung," which refers to a pattern of lung collapse sometimes seen with these injuries. The lung collapses laterally with a medial pneumothorax.

e) Management

1) Endotracheal intubation is almost always indicated, although conversion to positive pressure often exacerbates the massive air leak.

2) Perform immediate bronchoscopy to localize the injury.

3) On occasion it may be possible during bronchoscopy to guide the endotracheal tube past a tracheal injury or into the uninjured mainstem bronchus to improve ventilation of the uninjured lung.

4) Definitive treatment includes primary repair with mucosa-to-mucosa closure using nonabsorbable, interrupted polypropylene sutures. Exposure of the injury depends on location:
- Median sternotomy provides access to the anterior or left lateral portion of the mediastinal trachea.
- Right posterolateral thoracotomy provides exposure of the right lateral or posterior aspect of the trachea or right lung bronchi or parenchymal injury.
- Left posterolateral thoracotomy provides access to the left lung bronchi or parenchymal laceration.

3. Blunt cardiac injury (BCI)

a. Definition. BCI is used to describe a spectrum of injury to the heart. It can range from asymptomatic myocardial muscle contusion to clinically significant dysrhythmia, acute heart failure, valvular injury, or cardiac rupture. Critical blunt cardiac injury, particularly that which causes hemodynamic instability, is rare.

i. The most common complication of blunt injury to the myocardium is dysrhythmias such as sinus tachycardia, premature atrial contractions, atrial fibrillation, and premature ventricular contractions. Other ECG changes that may be seen are right bundle branch block or acute current of injury with ST elevation and T-wave flattening.

b. Diagnosis. Debate is seen in the literature regarding the criteria for the diagnosis and significance of BCI (Fig. 24-5).

i. An admission 12-lead ECG should be performed as a screening test for all patients suspected of having BCI.

a) An ECG is considered positive if it demonstrates dysrhythmia, atrial or ventricular ectopy, S-T changes, bundle branch block, or hemifascicular blocks.

ii. Echocardiography (ECHO) can be used to assess wall motion and valvular competency. Transthoracic echocardiogram (TTE) is convenient and noninvasive although sometimes is technically limited. TEE is more invasive; however, it may be necessary when the TTE is inadequate.

iii. There is some new evidence that cardiac troponin I (cTnI) levels are correlated with subsequent risk of arrhythmias and complications from BCI. In one study by Rajan and Zellweger, levels of less than 1.05 µg/L within 6 hours after injury in asymptomatic patients has been shown to essentially rule out the risk of complications from BCI. These results have not been duplicated.

iv. The presence of a sternal fracture does not correlate with presence of BCI.

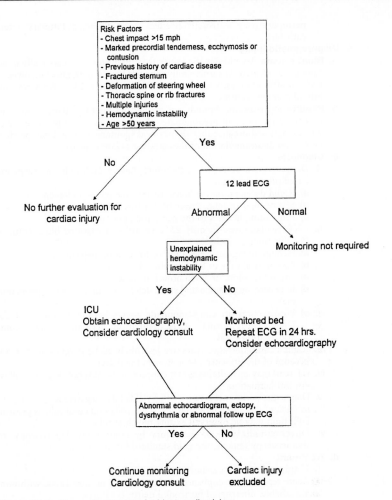

Figure 24-5. Diagnostic algorithm for blunt cardiac injury.

  c. **Treatment**
      i. Admit patients with suspected BCI to an ECG-monitored bed. Dysrhythmias are treated as necessary according to advanced cardiac life support (ACLS) protocol.
          a) Patients with ischemic changes on the ECG or elevated cardiac enzyme levels are treated similar to those with myocardial infarction.
          b) If echocardiographic-proved contusion (hypokinesis or abnormal wall movement) is seen, admit the patient to an ICU.
          c) If the patient develops signs and symptoms of acute heart failure, begin invasive monitoring with a pulmonary artery catheter.
      ii. Obtain follow-up ECG only for those with an abnormal tracing initially or new signs.
      iii. Blunt cardiac injury is not an absolute contraindication to surgery. If the patient with BCI requires noncardiac surgery, invasive monitoring

perioperatively is usually needed (arterial line, pulmonary artery catheter).

4. **Diaphragmatic injury**
   a. **Blunt trauma.** Diaphragmatic injury from blunt forces is classically large, radial, and located posterolaterally. The left hemidiaphragm is involved in 65% to 80% of cases. Diaphragmatic ruptures are markers for associated intraabdominal injuries.
   b. **Penetrating trauma.** Wounds are smaller but tend to enlarge over time. Left-sided injuries still predominate. These injuries need operative repair when diagnosed because they do not heal spontaneously and can produce herniation or strangulation of the intestine as late sequelae.
   c. **Diagnosis**
      i. Diagnosis can be difficult; therefore, have a high index of suspicion based on mechanism.
         a) Rapid deceleration or direct crush to the upper abdomen
         b) Severe chest trauma, lower rib fractures
         c) Penetrating injuries to the chest and upper abdomen
      ii. CXR is diagnostic in only 25% to 50% of cases of blunt trauma. Possible findings include:
         a) Hemidiaphragmatic elevation or lower lobe atelectasis.
         b) Nasogastric tube in left hemithorax.
         c) Stomach, colon, or small bowel in chest.
         d) In penetrating trauma and small defects, the diaphragm appears normal.
         e) Positive pressure can tamponade viscera herniation and make the CXR appear normal. After extubation, herniation may become apparent on CXR.
      iii. Right hemidiaphragm tears are less likely to be diagnosed by CXR because of the presence of the liver in the defect.
      iv. CT scan may miss diaphragmatic injury in the absence of gross hollow visceral herniation.
      v. Diagnostic peritoneal lavage (DPL) yields false negative results in 25% to 34% of diaphragmatic injuries. If an ipsilateral chest tube is present, DPL fluid may be observed exiting the chest tube.
      vi. Direct visualization of the injury by laparotomy, laparoscopy, or thoracoscopy remains the gold standard for diagnosis.
   d. **Treatment**
      i. Diaphragmatic tears require repair.
      ii. Acute repair is accomplished via laparotomy, in most cases, with nonabsorbable, interrupted horizontal mattress sutures.
      iii. Thoracotomy may be needed to reduce large defects in chronic herniation.
      iv. Prosthetic material or flaps are rarely needed to close the defect.
      v. The mortality rate is 25% to 40% because of the severity of associated injuries.

5. **Esophageal injury**
   a. Most injuries result from penetrating trauma. Blunt esophageal injury is rare (<0.1% incidence). Presentation varies according to location of injury:
      i. **Cervical esophagus:** subcutaneous emphysema, hematemesis (Chapters 22 and 23)
      ii. **Thoracic esophagus:** mediastinal emphysema, subcutaneous emphysema, pleural effusion, retroesophageal air, unexplained fever within 24 hours of injury
      iii. **Intraabdominal esophagus:** commonly asymptomatic initially; may have pneumoperitoneum, hemoperitoneum
   b. **Diagnosis**
      i. Penetrating trajectories involving the mediastinum or neck mandate diagnostic workup to exclude injury to the esophagus.

ii. Many penetrating injuries are detected at the time of emergency thoracotomy or laparotomy.

iii. **Esophagoscopy** and **esophagogram** are used with equal sensitivity (60%). Combining both studies will detect almost all esophageal injuries.

iv. CT scan may have a role in determining trajectory in stable patients.

c. Management

i. Operative exposure

a) **Cervical:** unilateral neck incision along the anterior border of the sternocleidomastoid muscle

b) **Proximal thoracic:** right posterolateral thoracotomy in fifth intercostal space

c) **Distal thoracic:** left posterolateral thoracotomy in sixth intercostal space

ii. Definitive repair

a) **Injury <6 hours old.** Close primarily in two layers with absorbable suture and cover with pleural or intercostal muscle flap. Distal esophageal repair can also be reinforced with Nissen wrap. Drain.

b) **Complex injury or >12 hours old.** Repair wound as above. Diverting cervical esophagostomy and oversewing of the distal esophagus should be considered with signs of mediastinitis. Wide drainage with chest tubes and feeding gastrostomy are both indicated.

c) **Injury 6 to 12 hours old.** Controversial; however, if there is shock with multiple injuries consider diversion as above.

6. Pulmonary contusion

a. The most common potentially lethal chest injury.

b. Caused by hemorrhage into lung parenchyma.

c. Commonly, this accompanies a flail segment or multiple fractured ribs. Pulmonary contusion can also accompany a penetrating injury.

d. Children may have a pulmonary contusion in the absence of rib fractures because of the resilience of the chest wall.

e. The natural progression is worsening hypoxemia for the first 24 to 48 hours.

i. Diagnosis. CXR findings are typically delayed in appearance and nonsegmental. If abnormalities are seen on the admission CXR, the pulmonary contusion is severe. Hemoptysis or blood in the endotracheal tube is a sign of pulmonary contusion.

ii. Treatment

a) Although excessive lung water can exacerbate pulmonary contusions, adequate volume resuscitation should not be withheld in patients with other injuries. The goal is euvolemia.

b) If the fluid status is in question, a pulmonary artery catheter may help facilitate fluid management.

c) Prophylactic antibiotics or steroids are **not** indicated.

d) **Mild contusion.** Give supplemental oxygen, monitor oxygen saturations, perform aggressive pulmonary toilet, and administer analgesia.

e) **Moderate to severe contusion.** In addition to above, intubate and mechanically ventilate with positive end-expiratory pressure.

f) **Catastrophic contusion.** If the patient is not responsive to conventional ventilation, consider pressure-limiting ventilatory modes, such as pressure control, airway pressure release ventilation (APRV), inverse ratio ventilation, or high-frequency jet ventilation. Extracorporeal membrane oxygenation (ECMO) is an option in centers with this expertise. For severe unilateral contusions, consider independent lung ventilation through a double-lumen tube.

VI. OTHER THORACIC INJURIES

A. Traumatic asphyxia

1. **Definition**
   a. Occurs with a severe crushing injury to the chest or upper abdomen. Intrathoracic and superior vena cava pressures increase and, together with reflux closure of the glottis, produce reversal of flow in the valveless veins of the head and neck with subsequent capillary disruption.
   b. Chest wall, intrathoracic, and intraabdominal injuries (heart, lung, liver) are frequently associated injuries.
   c. Increased intracranial pressure, cerebral edema, and hypoxic brain injury are rare sequelae.

2. **Diagnosis**
   a. Craniocervical cyanosis, followed by craniocervical rubor.
   b. Facial edema.
   c. Petechiae over the face, neck, and torso.
   d. Subconjunctival hemorrhage.
   e. Neurologic symptoms (e.g., loss of consciousness, seizures, confusion, and temporary or permanent blindness) occur occasionally.
   f. Hematuria, hematotympanum, or epistaxis occur rarely.

3. **Treatment**
   a. Elevate head of bed 30 degrees.
   b. Administer oxygen.
   c. Treat any underlying injuries.
   d. Perform adequate pulmonary hygiene.

B. Chest wall injury

1. **Fractures of the scapula** or first or second rib result from significant force. The risk of associated intrathoracic injury is >50%.
2. **Sternal fractures.** Of these, 40% will have associated rib fractures and 25% will have associated long bone injury.
3. **Fractures of ribs 3 through 8**
   a. The main clinical issues are pain and restriction of ventilation.
   b. Search for pulmonary contusion and blunt cardiac injury.
   c. Provide adequate pain relief by epidural anesthesia, PCA, or intercostal nerve blocks.
4. **Fractures of ribs 9 through 12.** A 10% risk exists of associated liver (right-sided fractures), and a 20% risk of spleen (left-sided fractures), or kidney injury.

VII. EMERGENCY THORACIC PROCEDURES

A. Tube thoracostomy (Fig. 24-6)

1. The usual insertion site is the fourth or fifth intercostal space just anterior to the midaxillary line. Identify the space between the pectoralis major anteriorly and the latissimus dorsi posteriorly (Fig. 24-6A). Do not insert tubes through traumatic wounds. Use a large caliber tube (≥32 F) to ensure adequate drainage of the pleural space.
2. Administer a single dose of prophylactic antibiotics such as cefazolin.
3. Prepare and drape the chest.
4. Anesthetize the site locally with 1% lidocaine (10–20 mL), including the skin, periosteum, subpleural space, and pleura. Except under the most life-threatening circumstances, proper local anesthesia must be used to minimize patient discomfort.
5. Make a 3- to 4-cm horizontal skin incision below the selected interspace and continue the incision down to the chest wall (Fig. 24-6B).
6. With a large curved Kelly clamp, carefully puncture the parietal pleura just above the rib, avoiding the neurovascular bundle running along the inferior border. Spread the intercostal muscles.
7. Remove the clamp and place a finger into the pleural space to confirm appropriate position and to clear any adhesions that may be present (Fig. 24-6C).

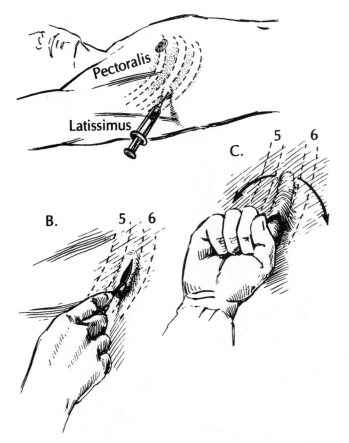

Figure 24-6. Steps for chest tube insertion. (From Trunkey DD, Guernsey JM. Surgical procedures. In: Blaisdell FW, Trunkey DD, eds. *Trauma Management—Cervicothoracic Trauma.* New York, NY: Thieme Medical Publishers; 1986:310, with permission.) (*continued*)

8. Use the clamp or a finger as a guide to advance the tube into the pleural space. Guide the tube posteriorly and toward the apex of the pleural space (Fig. 24.6D-F).

9. If correctly placed, the tube should "fog" with expiration. After placement, run a finger along the tube to confirm proper placement. Confirm that all of the holes are within the pleural space. Rotating the tube 360 degrees ensures that it is not kinked in the chest.

10. Connect the tube to an underwater-seal apparatus and place at 20 cm of water suction. For known hemothoraces, use an autotransfusion reservoir.

11. Secure tube with a heavy Prolene or silk suture. Tape all tube connections to prevent separation.

12. Obtain a CXR to confirm proper placement.

B. Pericardiocentesis (Fig. 24-7)

  1. Indications

  a. Acute distention of the pericardial sac with as little as 75 to 100 mL of blood can produce tamponade physiology. Withdrawal of this fluid is life-saving. However, it is difficult to tap this small pocket of fluid, especially if it accumulates posteriorly.

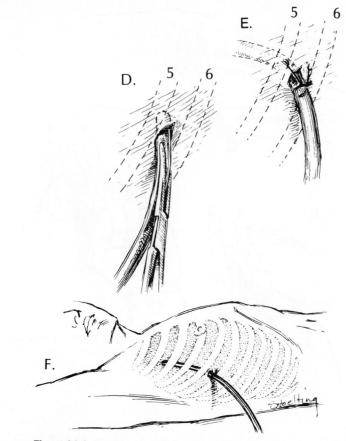

Figure 24-6. (continued)

    b. When used for diagnosis, pericardiocentesis can produce false negative results in 50% to 60% of cases because of pericardial blood clotting or needle misplacement.

    c. In acute cardiac tamponade, pericardiocentesis can be used as a temporizing maneuver until definitive pericardiotomy is possible.

    d. Pericardiocentesis is rarely indicated in a Level I trauma center.

2. Technique

    a. A 16- or 18-gauge long (6 inches) needle is connected to a 30-mL syringe. The needle is introduced at the left xiphosternal junction (Larrey's point) and directed toward the left shoulder and at a 45-degree angle to the skin. Back pressure is placed on the plunger of the syringe as the needle is advanced.

    b. Blood (30 mL) is withdrawn and the clinical situation is reassessed. If no improvement is noted, aspiration is repeated.

3. Complications

    a. Iatrogenic coronary artery injury, myocardial laceration, pneumothorax, hemothorax, and mediastinal hematoma can occur.

    b. False positive return can occur when the ventricle or a hemothorax is inadvertently tapped.

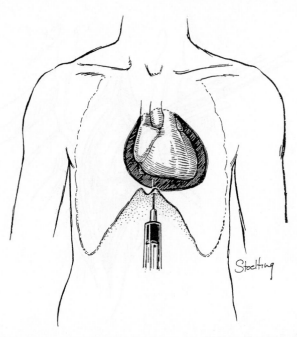

Figure 24-7. Pericardiocentesis. (From Rich NM, Spencer FC. *Vascular Trauma*. Philadelphia, Pa: WB Saunders; 1978:409, with permission.)

C. Pericardial window (Fig. 24-8)

   1. Pericardial window should be considered in the patient who is at risk of having cardiac injury but who has maintained adequate vital signs. As mentioned, pericardial tamponade is rapidly fatal. If the patient is in extremis or hypotensive, prompt left thoracotomy is indicated. However, in a more stable patient with a parasternal penetrating wound suggestive of possible cardiac injury, a pericardial window using a subxiphoid approach is safer and more definitive than pericardiocentesis.

   2. Technique

      a. Pericardial window is performed in the OR under general anesthesia.

      b. Prepare the patient from chin to midthighs before the induction of general anesthesia in anticipation of acute hemodynamic decompensation.

      c. An incision is made over the xiphoid process and in the upper midline of the abdomen.

      d. Excision of the xiphoid process may facilitate the procedure. The diaphragmatic attachments immediately deep to the sternum should be freed with finger dissection. The diaphragm can then be retracted toward the patient's feet with Kocher clamps. Reverse Trendelenburg's position helps expose the pericardium. A sponge stick can be used to mobilize the pericardial fat off the anterior surface of the pericardium. The tense, fibrous, white pericardium is then identified.

      e. An incision is made with scissors on the anterior surface of the pericardium using forceps to lift the pericardium away from the heart, and the incision is extended 1 to 2 cm.

         i. If blood is found in the pericardial sac, the procedure should be quickly converted to median sternotomy and the cardiac wound definitively

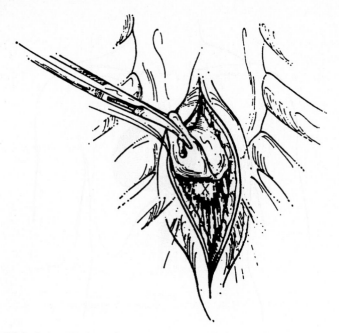

Figure 24-8. Pericardial window.

repaired. The sternal saw should always be in the OR during pericardial window for the possibility of need for prompt median sternotomy.

a) If no gross blood is aspirated, a red rubber tube is placed and the
pericardium is gently irrigated with warm saline to see if clots are
flushed from the pericardial space recesses.

Bibliography

Asensio JA, Berne JD, Demetriades D, et al. One hundred five penetrating cardiac injuries:
A 2-year prospective evaluation. *J Trauma* 1998;44:1073–1082.

Asensio JA, Berne JD, Demetriades D, et al. Penetrating esophageal injuries: Time interval
of safety for preoperative evaluation—How long is safe? *J Trauma* 1997;43:319–323.

Asensio JA, Demetriades D, Berne JD, et al. Stapled pulmonary tractotomy: A rapid way to control hemorrhage in penetrating pulmonary injuries. *J Am Coll Surg* 1997;185(5): 486–487.

Asensio JA, Stewart BM, Murray J, et al. Penetrating cardiac injuries. *Surg Clin North Am*
1996;76:685–724.

Fabian TC, Davis KA, Gavant ML, et al. Prospective study of blunt aortic injury: Helical
CT is diagnostic and anti-hypertensive therapy reduces rupture. *Ann Surg* 1998;227:
666–670.

Ferjani M, Droc G, Dreus S, et al. Circulating cardiac troponin T in myocardial contusion.
Chest 1997;111:427–433.

Flowers JL, Graham SM, Ugarte MA, et al. Flexible endoscopy for the diagnosis of
esophageal trauma. *J Trauma* 1996;40:261–265.

Gammie JS, Pham AS, Hattler BG, et al. Traumatic aortic rupture: Diagnosis and management. *Ann Thorac Surg* 1998;66:1295–1300.

Guth A, Pachter HL, Kim U. Pitfalls in the diagnosis of blunt diaphragmatic injury. *Am J
Surg* 1995;170:5–9.

Heniford BT, Carillo EH, Spain DA, et al. The role of thoracoscopy in the management of retained thoracic collections after trauma. *Ann Thorac Surg* 1997;63:940–943.

Link MS. Mechanically induced sudden death in chest wall impact (commotio cordis). *Prog Biophys Mol Biol* 2003;82:175–186.

Maenza RL, Seaberg D, DiAmico F. A meta-analysis of blunt cardiac trauma: Ending myocardial confusion. *Am J Emerg Med* 1996;14:237.

Moon RM, Luchette FA, Gibson SW, et al. Prospective, randomized comparison between epidural versus parenteral opioid analgesia in thoracic trauma. *Ann Surg* 1999;229: 684–692.

Ott MC, Stewart TC, Lawlor DK, et al. Management of blunt thoracic aortic injuries: Endovascular stents versus open repair. *J Trauma* 2004;56:565–570.

Rajan GP, Zellweger R. Cardiac troponin I as a predictor of arrhythmia and ventricular dysfunction in trauma patients with myocardial contusion. *J Trauma* 2004;57:801–808.

Richardson JD, Flint LM, Snow NJ, et al. Management of transmediastinal gunshot wounds. *Surgery* 1981;90:671–676.

Richardson JD, Miller FB, Carillo EH, et al. Complex thoracic injuries. *Surg Clin North Am* 1996;76:725–748.

Roszycki GS, Feliciano DV, Oschner MG, et al. The role of ultrasound in patients with possible penetrating cardiac wounds: A prospective multicenter study. *J Trauma* 1999;46:543–552.

Velhamos GC, Baker C, Demetriades D, et al. Lung-sparing surgery after penetrating trauma using tractotomy, partial lobectomy, and pneumonorrhaphy. *Arch Surg* 1999; 134:186–189.

Working group, ad hoc subcommittee on outcomes, American College of Surgeons committee on trauma. Practice management guidelines for emergency department thoracotomy. *J Am Coll Surg* 2001;193:303–308.

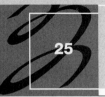

25

THORACIC VASCULAR INJURY
JOHN P. PRYOR AND JUAN A. ASENSIO

I. INTRODUCTION
   A. Hemodynamic instability from a chest wound indicates a major vascular or cardiac injury that mandates prompt control of bleeding. Ideally, emergency operations on the chest should be performed in the operating room (OR) after a brief resuscitation. However, cardiac tamponade or exsanguination will require definitive procedures in the trauma resuscitation area.
   B. The chest cavity is more compartmentalized than the abdomen. The bony chest wall, clavicles, and shoulders make operative exposure of injured viscera difficult. Large, relatively fixed structures limit exposure of the posterior mediastinum. *Thus, the choice of chest incision is determined by the expected anatomic injury, the urgency with which surgical access is required, and the patient's stability.*
   C. Patients with severe chest trauma are often initially evaluated by trauma surgeons and emergency physicians. All surgeons must be proficient in thoracic exposure and control of exsanguinating hemorrhage. After control of major bleeding, intraoperative consultation with a cardiothoracic surgeon may be considered. This is especially important with complex injuries to the pulmonary hilum, coronary arteries, or internal structures of the heart. The repair of these complex injuries is beyond the scope of this chapter.

II. MECHANISM OF INJURY
   A. Blunt thoracic injury is frequently associated with abdominal injuries, and patients requiring emergency operative control of a thoracic vascular injury can be assessed with FAST or DPL and may also need concurrent exploration of the abdomen to evaluate for injuries below the diaphragm.
   B. In **penetrating injury,** the trajectory of the weapon or bullet is the key to determining the anatomic structures at risk. In general, missile trajectories that pass the midline are at more risk for significant vascular and cardiac injury. Low-velocity injuries, such as stab wounds, more often cause problems such as pneumothorax and cardiac tamponade, whereas higher energy wounds, such as gunshot wounds, tend to cause extensive hemorrhage.

III. PRESENTATION AND DIAGNOSIS
   A. Presentation. Major thoracic or cardiac injuries will frequently present with hemodynamic instability. The goal is to quickly determine that a major injury exists and to prepare for emergent exploration and repair. Patients who arrive unresponsive without a measurable blood pressure are in extremis and should have immediate emergency thoracotomy (Section VI).
   B. Clinical signs of thoracic vascular or cardiac injury
      1. Hemodynamic instability (hypotension, altered sensorium, or other signs of shock) with a penetrating chest wound
      2. ↑CVP, JVD
      3. Restlessness
      4. Massive hemothorax (>1,500 mL on insertion of a chest tube, persistent hemothorax on chest x-ray (CXR), or >200 mL/hour for 4 hours)

  5. Cardiac tamponade
  6. Large mediastinal hematoma
C. Diagnosis
  1. Use **CXR** to diagnose a hemothorax or mediastinal hematoma. Penetrating wound sites should be marked with metallic clips to help determine trajectories. Anteroposterior and lateral views can help determine trajectory. The cardiac silhouette does not change appreciably in acute tamponade.
  2. Ultrasound. Focused abdominal sonography for trauma (FAST) examination, with special attention to the pericardial view, can detect the presence of fluid in the pericardium or abdomen.
  3. Tube thoracostomy can be both diagnostic and therapeutic. Pneumothorax or hemothorax can be confirmed by tube thoracostomy. For patients in shock, thoracostomy should be used as the initial diagnostic and therapeutic intervention, rather than CXR.
  4. CVP measurement.
D. Injury complexes. Certain thoracic vascular injuries can be predicted by the injury mechanism, trajectory, and findings on the initial CXR:
  1. Massive hemothorax involves injury to pulmonary hilum, proximal subclavian artery on the left, proximal innominate artery on the right, heart with a communication through the pericardium, intercostal artery, internal mammary artery, and azygous vein. For unstable patients who do not respond to chest tube drainage, the choice of incision is a **thoracotomy** on side of hemothorax.
  2. Superior mediastinal hematoma involves injury to innominate artery and vein, subclavian and carotid arteries bilaterally, superior vena cava, and heart. The best approach is through a median sternotomy with extensions into the neck at the anterior border of the sternocleidomastoid muscle.
  3. Middle mediastinal hematoma includes cardiac injuries with intact pericardium, aortic arch, proximal innominate artery, and left proximal carotid and subclavian arteries. It is best approached through a sternotomy or posterolateral thoracotomy.

IV. INITIAL EVALUATION AND RESUSCITATION. When a major thoracic vascular injury is suspected, initiate prompt resuscitation while searching for the cause.
A. Perform immediate endotracheal intubation.
B. Place two large-bore intravenous (IV) lines for volume infusion, ideally one above and one below the diaphragm. Avoid central lines on the side of injury.
C. Infuse prewarmed crystalloids. Consider transfusing warmed blood immediately, using other blood products as needed (Chapter 42) and initiate massive transfusion protocol.
D. Have rapid-infusion and cell-saver devices immediately available.
E. Administer tetanus prophylaxis and preoperative antibiotics.

V. THORACIC OPERATIONS (Table 25-1). Position the patient to allow maximal exposure to the chest, including the neck, abdomen, and groins in the operative field. If a median sternotomy is planned, the prepared area must include both lateral

---

| **TABLE 25-1** | **Conduct of Operations for Thoracic Vascular Injury** |

Preparation
   –Allow early notice to operating room staff to prepare for thoracic procedures
   –Maintain operating room temperature >80°F (27°C)
   –Have cell-saver and rapid-transfusion units available
   –Notify cardiopulmonary bypass (CPB) technicians of possible need for CPB
   –Have blood products immediately available, initiate massive transfusion protocol

(continued)

TABLE 25-1 **(Continued)**

Position
—Median sternotomy—supine with arms out at 90 degrees
  —Prepare from chin to midthighs, laterally to bed
—Emergency department thoracotomy—supine with left arm raised
  —Preparation is deferred
—Urgent left thoracotomy—taxi-hailing position with bump under left back
  —Prepare from chin to pubis and laterally to bed
  —Prepare out left arm
—Right thoracotomy—lateral decubitus position with bean bag

Anesthesia
—Place double-lumen tube, if indicated and stable
—Place arterial line in uninjured side
—Assure chest tubes in cavities not being explored are visible and connected to suction
—Assure access to peripheral and central intravenous lines
—Place urometer at patient's head to monitor urinary output
—Monitor central temperature via esophagus or bladder
—Warm the patient
  —Surface warming, where possible
  —Fluid warmer
  —Turn humidified heat on ventilator to maximum

Scrub Staff
—Open thoracotomy, sternotomy, and laparotomy sets
—Have long instruments available
—Have aortic clamp immediately available
—Assemble equipment for CPB in room for possible use
—Have GIA, endovascular GIA, and TA staplers available

GIA, gastrointestinal anastomosis; TA, thoracoabdominal.

chest walls to the bed posteriorly. It also helps to have a beanbag in position under the patient for a thoracotomy incision. If concurrent access to the abdomen is necessary, a modified "taxi hailing" position can be used (Fig. 25-1). Other preparations to consider:

A. Double-lumen endotracheal tube, if time and hemodynamics permit.
B. Large-bore central IV access with cell saver and rapid infusers if available.
C. Tube thoracostomy of the contralateral hemithorax, if any potential exists for contralateral injury. Have research visible to surgeon.
D. Appropriate padding of potential pressure areas and careful positioning to prevent nerve injury. The surgical team must actively participate in this process.
E. Internal defibrillation paddles and sternotomy scan on the field.
F. Vascular clamps to control pulmonary hilum and atrial appendage bleeding.
G. Staplers for lung parenchymal and hilar injury.
H. Hemostatic sealants available.

VI. THORACIC SURGERY APPROACHES

A. **Emergency department thoracotomy (EDT).** Enthusiasm for EDT has waned over the past several years since the overall mortality of patients receiving EDT is very high. Patients most likely to benefit from EDT are young and have isolated penetrating injury to the chest, preferably a cardiac wound (sw > qsw) with tamponade that can be easily released. Patients with blunt injury, exsanguination below the diaphragm, and associated head injuries do poorly.

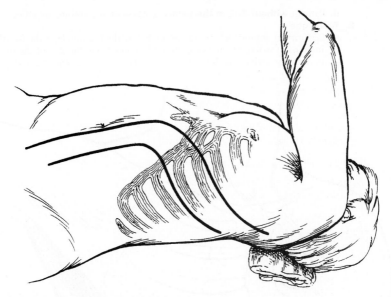

Figure 25-1. The "taxi-hailing" position that allows for access to the abdomen and left chest. (Adapted from Rutherford RB. *Atlas of Vascular Surgery: Basic Techniques and Exposures.* Philadelphia, Pa: WB Saunders; 1993:223, with permission.)

1. **Indications** (Table 25-2)
   a. EDT should be considered in patients who are in extremis or in cardiopulmonary arrest without **vitals signs**, which is defined as a measurable blood pressure or pulse. Patients should then be evaluated for when signs of life (SOL) were present and lost. SOL include:
      i. Spontaneous movements
      ii. Pupillary response, eye movement
      iii. Spontaneous respirations
      iv. Electrical complexes >40/minute on electrocardiogram (ECG)
   b. In patients with cardiopulmonary arrest from **blunt trauma**, EDT is indicated only if the patient has SOL **on arrival to the hospital**. Patients who have SOL in the field and lose them en route are considered dead on arrival (DOA).
   c. In **penetrating trauma arrest**, EDT is indicated if the patient had SOL in the field. Patients with penetrating injury should receive EDT even if SOL are lost en route. This expanded indication (compared with blunt trauma arrest) is specific because of the higher frequency of reparable lesions being present.

TABLE 25-2   Indications for Emergency Department Thoracotomy

No measurable blood pressure or pulse					
Blunt mechanism			Penetrating mechanism		
No SOL	SOL field only	SOL arrival	No SOL	SOL field only	SOL arrival
DOA	DOA	EDT	DOA	EDT	EDT

SOL, signs of life (eye movement, pupillary response, spontaneous respiration, electrical activity >40 complexes/min on electrogram); DOA, dead on arrival; EDT, emergency department thoracotomy.

      d. Patients **without SOL in the field**, regardless of mechanism, are DOA.
   2. Technique
      a. Perform an anterior left thoracotomy below the left nipple at the fourth intercostal space. The incision should be made from the edge of the sternum to the latissimus dorsi posteriorly (Fig. 25-2). In females, displace

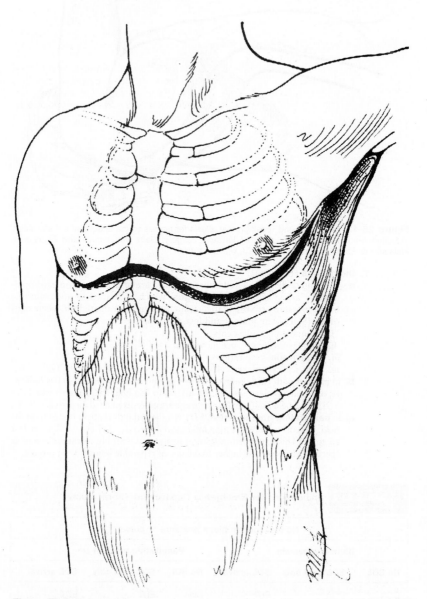

Figure 25-2. Emergency department thoracotomy. Extend the incision to the right side below the right nipple for easy access to the right chest. (Adapted from Moore EE, Eiseman B, Van Way CW. *Critical Decisions in Trauma*. St. Louis, Mo: Mosby; 1984:524, with permission.)

the breast cephalad and make the skin incision in the inframammary crease. Incise the intercostal muscle with scissors and insert a Finochietto or other large rib spreader. Take care to insert the rib spreader with the T-bar posteriorly near the bed; this will allow free access to extend the thoracotomy across the sternum to the right side if necessary (Fig. 25-3).

b. Open the pericardium anterior to the phrenic nerve. This relieves tamponade and allows more effective internal compressions. This should be done in the anterior portion of the pericardium in a caudal to cephalad plane, avoiding injury to the phrenic nerve. The opening should extend from the cardiac apex to the root of the aorta.

c. If the heart is not beating, perform internal massage with open hands spanning the left ventricle. Do not squeeze with one hand—this can lead to ventricular injury. If the heart is fibrillating, attempt internal cardioversion at 20 joules (J) followed by 30 J. If cardioversion fails, temporarily tamponade

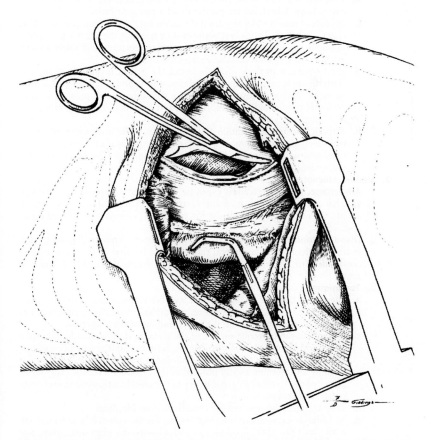

Figure 25-3. A view into the left chest during emergency department thoracotomy. A clamp is shown on the descending aorta and a sharp pericardiotomy is shown proceeding cephalad anterior to the phrenic vessels. (Adapted from Moore EE, Eiseman B, Van Way CW. *Critical Decisions in Trauma*. St. Louis, Mo: Mosby; 1984:529, with permission.)

the ascending aorta and perform gentle internal compression to perfuse the coronaries and reattempt cardioversion.

d. If the myocardium is ruptured or injured, compress the wound together gently or place a finger over the hole. Repair anterior wounds with a 2-0 to 4-0, nonabsorbable pledgeted suture placed in a horizontal mattress fashion. A larger needle is easier to use with active bleeding and beating for most physicians. Approximate but do not strangulate the myocardium as the suture is tied.

  i. Although some surgeons recommend placing a balloon catheter into a cardiac injury, this maneuver often enlarges the hole in the myocardium and may block ventricular outflow.

  ii. If the wound is adjacent to a coronary artery, the myocardial closure must not compromise the coronary artery. Pass a horizontal mattress suture under the coronary artery and "u" stitch and tie it to incorporate the cardiac wound.

  iii. Atrial wounds can be controlled with a partial occlusion clamp followed by repair with 2-0 to 4-0 pledgeted horizontal mattress suture.

e. If the thoracic aorta is bleeding, compress and clamp with a side-biting vascular clamp. Check for the possibility of a posterior hole.

f. In cases of massive bleeding from the pulmonary parenchyma or the hilum, clamp the hilum. This is best performed by releasing the inferior pulmonary ligament, passing a hand around the vascular structures, and safely guiding a Crawford-Debakey vascular clamp on the hilum.

g. If no reparable thoracic injury is found, the patient is unlikely to survive. With the chest open, compress the thoracic aorta and continue open cardiac massage. If this successfully restores a palpable carotid pulse in a short period of time, rapidly transport to the OR for repair of injuries below the diaphragm.

h. Although aortic mobilization and clamping is useful in experienced hands, it is safer to simply compress the thoracic aorta against the spine with a hand and without formal mobilization or clamping. This helps avoid the risk of injury to the esophagus or aorta.

B. Median sternotomy

1. Advantage. Provides excellent exposure of the heart and proximal great vessels, but not the posterior mediastinal structures. The incision can be extended into the neck or supraclavicular for more distal vascular control and repair (Fig. 25-4).

2. Disadvantages. Requires a sternal saw or Lebsche knife and usually takes more time than left anterolateral thoracotomy; because of this, it is not recommended for EDT. Also, access is limited to the esophagus and descending aorta.

3. Technique

a. The patient is supine on the OR table with both arms abducted to 90 degrees.

b. The skin and subcutaneous tissues are divided from the sternal notch to inferior to the xiphoid onto the upper midline of the abdomen.

c. A plane on the posterior surface of the sternum is developed bluntly from above and below before division of the sternum with the oscillating saw or Lebsche knife. Begin this at the caudal edge of the sternum, and lift the saw or knife and sternum as you proceed in the cephalad direction. Stay in the center of the sternum to avoid injury to the costal cartilages and entry into either hemithorax.

d. Bone wax may be required for cancellous bone bleeding.

e. To facilitate exposure of the great vessels, the incision can be extended laterally into the neck, dividing sternocleidomastoid, platysma, strap, and anterior scalene muscles (protecting the phrenic nerve).

f. Further exposure of the second and third portions of the subclavian vessels can be enhanced by resection or division of the clavicle.

g. Extension into the abdomen with a midline incision is easily accomplished.

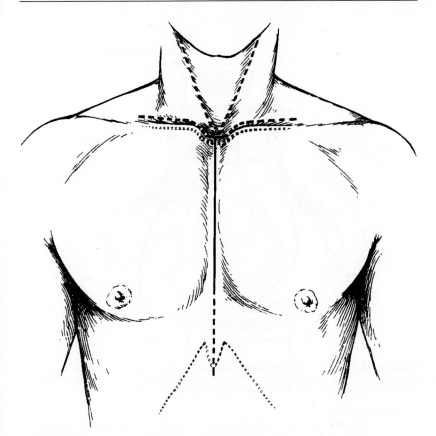

Figure 25-4. Extensions of the median sternotomy. Superclavicular and neck extensions are shown (*dotted lines*). (Adapted from Rutherford RB. *Atlas of Vascular Surgery: Basic Techniques and Exposures*. Philadelphia, Pa: WB Saunders; 1993:235, with permission.)

C. Left anterolateral thoracotomy

1. Advantage. Permits rapid access to the chest, especially for decompression of pericardial tamponade and for repair of the heart, left lung and hilum, and aorta. This can be extended across the sternum (bilateral or clamshell thoracotomy) to access the right chest (Fig. 25-5). Left anterolateral thoracotomy is the best initial operative approach for unstable patients or when the location of the intrathoracic injury is unclear.

2. Disadvantage. Poor access to the posterior mediastinum, distal subclavian vessels, and right chest.

3. Technique

    a. The patient should have a sandbag under the left chest to tilt the torso 30 degrees to the right. The left arm should be fully extended over the patient's head to provide extension of the incision on the posterior chest wall.

    b. An incision is made in the fourth or fifth intercostal space, from the sternal edge to the scapula.

    c. The muscles are divided with electrocautery and the intercostal muscles are divided or stripped from the rib below to avoid injury to the neurovascular bundle.

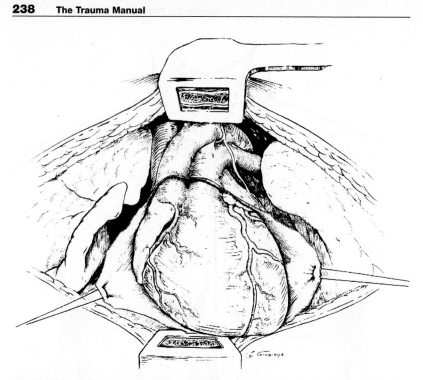

Figure 25-5. A view into the chest during a bilateral "clamshell" thoracotomy. Note the excellent exposure of the heart and great vessels. (Adapted from Moore EE, Eiseman B, Van Way CW. *Critical Decisions in Trauma.* St. Louis, Mo: Mosby; 1984:528, with permission.)

    d. A Finochietto rib spreader is inserted with the T-bar toward the back and opened widely.

    e. A thoracoabdominal incision can be accomplished by dividing the costal margin with heavy scissors or bone cutters and extending the incision into the abdomen.

D. Left or right posterolateral thoracotomy

  1. Advantages. Provides excellent access to the hemithorax. The left posterolateral thoracotomy permits access to the aorta and proximal left subclavian artery, the left lung, the left chest wall, and the distal esophagus. The right posterolateral thoracotomy provides access to the trachea, the right lung, the right chest wall, and the proximal esophagus.

  2. Disadvantages. The decubitus position for the posterior approach leaves little flexibility in gaining access to opposite chest or abdominal structures. Injuries elsewhere cannot be accessed.

  3. Technique

    a. Use the standard skin incision for elective thoracic surgery. By varying the interspace entered, all regions of the thoracic cavity can be exposed.

    b. The patient is placed in full lateral decubitus position with the upper arm supported over the head, the lower arm extended and padded with an axillary roll, the lower leg is flexed, and the upper leg extended with padding between the knees. The pelvis should be secured with tape and a sandbag (Fig. 25-6).

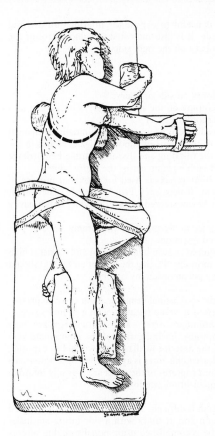

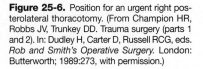

Figure 25-6. Position for an urgent right posterolateral thoracotomy. (From Champion HR, Robbs JV, Trunkey DD. Trauma surgery (parts 1 and 2). In: Dudley H, Carter D, Russell RCG, eds. *Rob and Smith's Operative Surgery.* London: Butterworth; 1989:273, with permission.)

    c. Using the tip of the scapula as a landmark, the muscles of the lateral chest wall are divided down to and including the intercostal muscles. In more stable patients requiring less exposure, sparing of the latissimus dorsi muscle is possible.

E. Bilateral thoracotomy (clamshell thoracotomy) (Fig. 25-5)

    1. Advantage. Permits wide exposure to all structures in the chest. Best incision for patients with multiple gunshot wounds that violate both pleural spaces, bilateral hemothoraces, and superior mediastinal hematomas.

    2. Disadvantage. Large incision, extensive heat loss from wound, both internal mammary arteries are ligated.

    3. Technique. After the anterolateral thoracotomy, the sternum is divided transversely with heavy scissors, Gigli saw, Lebsche knife, or sternal saw. The sternal incision is opened with the rib spreader. The incision is extended through the fourth interspace as far into the contralateral chest as possible.

        a. Care is taken to ligate the internal mammary arteries and veins on each side of the sternum. Often these arteries will start to bleed heavily with successful resuscitation and return of blood pressure.

F. Other approaches include:

    1. Right thoracotomy can be useful for isolated right hemothorax. It is also the incision of choice with high esophageal wounds and wounds to the trachea and tracheobronchial tree.

  2. **Thoracoabdominal incision** is useful to expose the inferior thoracic and supraceliac aorta on the left side. It is also indicated to gain control of the proximal thoracic inferior vena cava on the right side.

VII. SPECIFIC INJURIES
A. Pulmonary hilum
1. **Presentation.** Massive hemothorax on side of injury.
2. **Exposure.** Anterolateral thoracotomy on the side of injury. Control can also be gained through a median sternotomy.
3. **Technique.** Control of hilar bleeding can be accomplished initially by manual compression. Quick dissection of the inferior pulmonary ligament aids in the isolation and identification of the bleeding site. Exsanguinating hemorrhage can then be definitively stopped with a clamp across the entire hilum.
   a. Intrapericardial control of hilar vessels is used for proximal injuries to the pulmonary artery or vein, if necessary. Primary repair is desirable; however, lobectomy should be considered early if bleeding is not easily controlled.
   b. With the advent of stapled pneumonectomy and tractotomy, 85% of pulmonary injuries will be spared resection.
   c. Pneumonectomy is rarely required to stop hilar bleeding and carries a high postoperative morbidity and mortality. Placing the patient on ECMO should be considered if an emergency pneumonectomy is done.
B. Aorta and innominate artery
1. **Presentation.** Superior or middle mediastinal hematoma, but can also present with massive hemothorax if there is a communication with a pleural space.
2. **Exposure.** The proximal innominate artery and aortic arch are best approached by a median sternotomy. Early ligation of the innominate vein and associated thymic tissue in the anterior mediastinum will aid in exposing the aortic arch. The proximal descending aorta is approached by a posterolateral thoracotomy. Traumatic blunt ruptures of the aorta are typically found in this location just distal to the ligamentum arteriosum.
3. **Technique**
   a. Control of the aorta at the arch is difficult. Small injuries can be controlled initially with finger occlusion and at times with a side-biting Statinsky clamp. Primary repair can be accomplished using nonabsorbable sutures with or without pledgets. Treat proximal innominate artery injuries by ligating proximally and performing a bypass from the aortic to the distal innominate artery.
   b. Blunt, traumatic rupture of the aorta is repaired either primarily or with a short interposition graft. Options include direct repair without distal shunting, repair with passive shunting of blood distally using a Gott shunt, or repair using full or partial cardiopulmonary bypass. Our preference is to perform repair on bypass based on data suggesting that incidence of paraplegia following repair of the thoracic aorta is lower. The role of endovascular stents for repair, especially in a young population, is emerging.
C. Carotid artery
1. **Presentation.** Superior mediastinal hematoma or neck hematoma or hemothorax. Hemiplegia on physical examination is suggestive of a carotid injury.
2. **Exposure.** Median sternotomy with either a right or left cervical extension along the medial border of the sternocleidomastoid muscle (with proximal carotid artery injury).
3. **Technique.** Primary repair or interposition graft with vein or polytetrafluoroethylene (PTFE). Proximal internal carotid artery injuries can be treated by ligation and reconstitution by performing an end-to-end external to internal carotid artery bypass. Consider simple ligation without bypass for injuries that show no prograde flow preoperatively.

D. Subclavian artery
   1. **Presentation.** Superior mediastinal hematoma or neck hematoma or hemothorax. Proximal injuries on the left can present with massive left hemothorax.
   2. **Exposure.** The proximal right subclavian artery is accessed by a median sternotomy. An infra- or supraclavicular extension is used to gain distal control. The proximal left subclavian artery is best approached through a left lateral thoracotomy through the third intercostal space. Distal control on the left can be accomplished with an infraclavicular incision, with or without removal of the clavicle.
   3. **Technique.** Primary repair or interposition graft with PTFE or Dacron. Treat proximal injuries by ligation and end-to-side carotid-subclavian bypass.
   4. Placement of endovascular stents has been reported with success in the subclavian position. With difficult access to some of these injuries, stent placement may be an option.

E. Heart
   1. **Presentation.** Pericardial tamponade, mediastinal hematoma, or massive hemothorax with wounds that communicate through the pericardium.
   2. **Exposure.** Median sternotomy or left anterolateral thoracotomy. Extension of the left thoracotomy across to the right (clamshell) provides excellent exposure to the entire middle mediastinum.
   3. **Technique.** Wounds of the atria and auricles can be controlled with a partial occluding Statinsky clamp and repaired primarily with 3-0 or 4-0 polypropylene suture with or without pledgets. Wounds on the ventricles are repaired with individual mattress pledgeted sutures of 3-0 or 4-0 polypropylene, or nonpledgeted 2-0 polyproprolene sutures.

F. Intercostal arteries
   1. **Presentation.** Hemothorax or subcutaneous hematoma
   2. **Exposure.** Thoracotomy on side of injury
   3. **Technique.** Simple ligation proximal and distal to the injury

G. Internal mammary artery
   1. **Presentation.** Hemothorax, superior or middle mediastinal hematoma.
   2. **Exposure.** Median sternotomy or anterior thoracotomy.
   3. **Technique.** Simple ligation proximal and distal to the injury. Bilateral internal mammary artery ligation can be performed safely in most patients.

H. Azygous and hemiazygous veins
   1. **Presentation.** Hemothorax.
   2. **Exposure.** Thoracotomy on side of hemothorax.
   3. **Technique.** Suture ligation proximal and distal to injury. Take care to avoid inadvertent injury to the thoracic duct on the left.

Bibliography

Asensio JA, Arroyo H, Veloz W, et al. Penetrating thoracoabdominal injuries: Ongoing dilemma—Which cavity and when? *World J Surg* 2001;26:539–543.

Asensio JA, Berne JD, Demetriades D, et al. One hundred five penetrating cardiac injuries: A 2-year prospective evaluation. *J Trauma* 1998;44:1073–1082.

Asensio JA, Demetriades D, Berne JD, et al. Stapled pulmonary tractotomy: A rapid way to control hemorrhage in penetrating pulmonary injuries. *J Am Coll Surg* 1997;185(5):486–487.

Asensio JA, Demetriades D, Murray J, et al. Penetrating cardiac injuries: A prospective study of variables predicting outcomes. *J Am Coll Surg* 1997;186:24–34.

Asensio JA, Petrone P, Costa D, et al. An evidenced based critical appraisal of emergency department thoracotomy. *Evid Based Surg* 2003;1:11–21.

Blostein PA, Hodgman CG. Computed tomography of the chest in blunt thoracic trauma: Results of a prospective trial. *J Trauma* 1997;43:13–18.

Eisenberg HM, Middleton JD, Narayan RK. *Resources for the Optimal Care of the Injured Patient: 1993.* Committee on Trauma, American College of Surgeons, 1993.

Mitchell ME, Muakkassan FF, Poole GV, et al. Surgical approach of choice for penetrating cardiac wounds. *J Trauma* 1993;34:17–20.

Pate JW. Tracheobronchial and esophageal injuries. *Surg Clin North Am* 1989;69:111.

Richardson JD, Flint LM, Snow NJ. Management of transmediastinal gunshot wounds. *Surgery* 1981;90:671.

Richardson JD, Miller FB, Carrillo EH, et al. Complex thoracic injuries. *Surg Clin North Am* 1999;76:725–748.

Rozycki GS, Feliciano DV, Ochsner G, et al. The role of ultrasound in patients with possible penetrating cardiac wounds: A prospective multicenter study. *J Trauma* 1999;46:543–552.

Schwab CW, Adcock OT, Max MH. Emergency department thoracotomy (EDT): A 26-month experience using an "agonal" protocol. *Am Surg* 1986;52:20–29.

Wall MJ, Granchi T, Liscum K, et al. Penetrating thoracic vascular injuries. *Surg Clin North Am* 1999;76:749–762.

Working group, ad hoc subcommittee on outcomes, American College of Surgeons committee on trauma. Practice management guidelines for emergency department thoracotomy. *J Am Coll Surg* 2001;193:303–308.

26

ABDOMINAL INJURY

ALAN A. SIMEONE, HEIDI L. FRANKEL, AND GEORGE VELMAHOS

I. **OVERVIEW.** Abdominal injuries are divided into two broad categories, based on the mechanism of injury: **blunt** and **penetrating**. Expedient diagnosis and treatment of intraabdominal injuries are essential to avoid preventable morbidity and death. Because management guidelines are different for blunt and penetrating abdominal trauma, they will be discussed separately.

II. **BLUNT ABDOMINAL TRAUMA.** Motor vehicle crashes account for 75% of blunt abdominal injuries. Other mechanisms include falls, motorcycle or bicycle crashes, sporting mishaps, and assaults.
   A. **Intraabdominal injuries result from:**
      1. Compression causing a crush injury, such as direct impact against the steering wheel or a car's interior. A seat belt can also cause abdominal organ injuries, particularly in the presence of the "seat-belt sign," a skin contusion at the site that the lap seat belt was worn.
      2. An abrupt shearing force causing tears of organs or vascular pedicles, as it may occur in the liver or mesentery.
      3. A sudden rise in intraabdominal pressure causing rupture of an intraabdominal viscus, such as the bladder or small bowel.
   B. **Evaluation**
      1. Clinical. Information regarding the mechanism of injury is essential in determining the likelihood of an intraabdominal injury (Chapter 2). Abdominal examination after blunt trauma is often unreliable due to altered level of consciousness, spinal cord or other distracting injury, and medication or substance effects. However, careful clinical examination may uncover signs of hypoperfusion (e.g., obtundation, cool skin temperature, mottling, diminished pulse volume, and delayed capillary refill), which should initiate a search for a source of blood loss. Factors that have been associated with abdominal injury requiring laparotomy include chest injury, base deficit, pelvic fracture, and hypotension in the field or trauma resuscitation area.
         a. Evaluation of the abdomen may indicate distension or signs of peritoneal irritation (usually associated with injury to a hollow viscus). However, blood in the peritoneum often does not produce peritoneal signs, and massive hemoperitoneum may be present without abdominal distension.
         b. Commonly injured abdominal organs include the liver, spleen, bowel mesentery, and kidney. If the patient is a restrained victim in a motor vehicle crash, particularly with a visible contusion on the abdomen from a lap belt and/or a lumbar vertebral body fracture, suspect hollow viscus injury, an injury commonly missed.
      2. **Diagnostic tests.** The goal of the initial evaluation of the abdomen is to identify expeditiously those patients who require laparotomy. Although adjunctive tests are important in the evaluation of blunt abdominal trauma, **careful, repeated physical examination of the patient remains essential in the early diagnosis of abdominal injury**. The focused abdominal sonography for trauma (FAST) performed by emergency room physicians or surgeons has gained widespread popularity. FAST is associated with false negative and false

positive findings and its results should always be considered within the context of the clinical picture. The choice of adjunctive diagnostic tests depends, in part, on the hemodynamic stability of the patient, the associated injuries, and the patient volume at the treating institution (i.e., extremely busy centers may not have the personnel to perform serial physical examinations reliably) (Fig. 26-1).

a. **In hemodynamically unstable patients or patients with ongoing fluid requirements,** the abdomen should be first evaluated by FAST. If the FAST is positive the patient should be taken to the operating room (OR). If the FAST is negative and the hemodynamic instability cannot be explained by other injuries (massive hemothorax, unstable pelvis, multiple long bone fractures), the patient should have a diagnostic peritoneal lavage (DPL). The goal of the test is to identify major blood loss in the abdomen as the cause of the hemodynamic instability (discoverable by initial aspiration with placement of the catheter). If the DPL is positive, the patient should be taken to the OR; if negative, the patient should be evaluated further. In recent years, FAST and CT have diminished the role of DPL. The major role of DPL is currently in the small subgroup of patients who are hemodynamically unstable, have a negative FAST, and no other obvious injury that explains the hemodynamic instability.

b. **In the stable patient without immediate need for the OR,** abdominal computed tomography (CT) is the investigation of choice. For patients without an obvious indication for laparotomy, various modalities are available to evaluate the abdomen further. Ancillary evaluation above and beyond physical examination should be considered for patients with:
   - An abnormal or equivocal abdominal evaluation
   - Concurrent injury to the chest or pelvic ring
   - Gross hematuria
   - A diminished level of consciousness
   - Spinal cord injury
   - Other injuries requiring a long general anesthetic for management, rendering repeat abdominal examination impossible
   - Diminished capacity to tolerate a delay in diagnosis of abdominal injury (e.g., extremes of age)

c. The diagnostic test used depends on the mechanism of injury, associated injuries, and hemodynamic stability. **Remember that control of cavitary bleeding takes precedence over further diagnostic testing.**
   i. **Plain radiographs.** The chest radiograph may reveal a ruptured hemidiaphragm or pneumoperitoneum. Plain abdominal films are rarely productive, and unless there is a specific indication are not needed as part of the trauma evaluation.
   ii. **Laboratory evaluation.** Individual serum tests may not provide evidence of blunt abdominal injury. Patients with blunt injury received promptly from the scene may not be anemic or acidotic on presentation. Similarly, amylase levels can be normal with significant pancreatic or intestinal injury, and can be elevated from extraabdominal injury such as head and neck trauma.
   iii. **FAST** is designed for one primary goal: to identify the presence of free fluid in the abdominal cavity (Fig. 26-2). As such, it is used with increasing frequency as a screening test in essentially all blunt trauma patients with suspicion of abdominal trauma. A 3 to 5.0 megahertz (MHz) transducer is placed in the subxiphoid region in the sagittal plane to set the machine gain. Sagittal views of Morison's pouch and the splenorenal recess are performed, followed by a pelvic transverse view. Free fluid appears anechoic (black) compared with the surrounding structures.
      a) There is little contraindication to its use besides lack of expertise or obvious need for a laparotomy regardless of FAST results. The

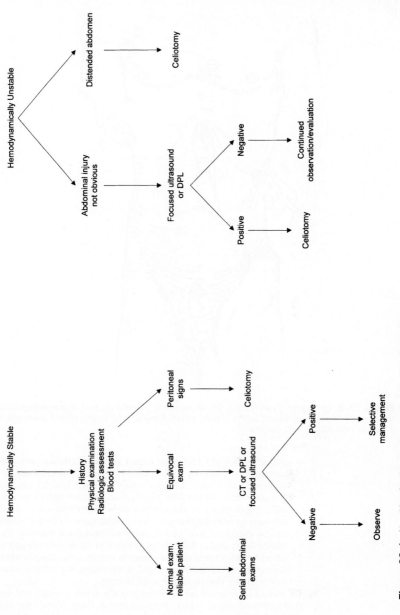

Figure 26-1. Algorithm for the management of blunt abdominal trauma.

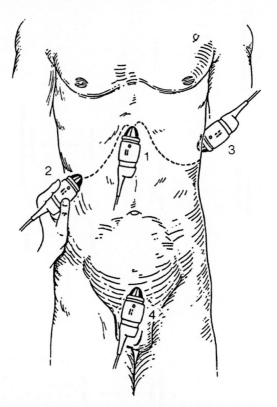

Figure 26-2. Ultrasound. (From Rozycki GS, Ochsner MG, Schmidt JA, et al. A prospective study of surgeon performed ultrasound as the primary adjuvant modality for injured patient assessment. *J Trauma* 1995;39:493, with permission.)

initial studies of FAST from expert teams reported a very high accuracy (in excess of 95%). Recent experience documents that such accuracy rates may not apply to most trauma centers. Accuracy rates around 80% may be more realistic. FAST may miss solid organ injury in the absence of hemoperitoneum or small amounts of hemoperitoneum; cannot distinguish between ascites, succus entericus, and blood; requires specialized training and competency; and is difficult to interpret in obese patients and in patients with extensive subcutaneous emphysema. Despite these limitations, FAST remains a rapid, noninvasive, cost-effective, and safe modality that should be used liberally.

iv. CT should be reserved for hemodynamically stable patients and can evaluate solid organ injury, intraabdominal fluid, blood, air, and retroperitoneal organ injuries. Intravenous contrast should be used routinely, unless there is a specific contraindication (renal failure, known reactions, etc.). The need for oral contrast is widely debated. Oral contrast may delay CT and lead to vomiting and aspiration. Many centers have stopped using it routinely, while other centers still adhere to its use.

a) CT is highly accurate for solid organ injuries. Hollow visceral, mesenteric, and pancreatic injuries may be missed, although the diagnostic ability is continuously improving with the newer generation multidetector scanners. Proximity between the trauma resuscitation bay and the CT suite is important. It should be remembered that **hemodynamically unstable patients do not belong in the CT suite.**

   v. DPL is a sensitive but not specific method for diagnosing intraabdominal free blood. Due to its invasive nature and potential for complications, it has been supplanted by ultrasound at most centers. As previously discussed, its best use at the current time is for the confirmation of the abdominal cavity as the source of significant bleeding in a hemodynamically unstable patient with a (false) negative FAST. In these scenarios, only an aspiration and not a full lavage is needed. For historical reasons we describe the full DPL in the following text. A catheter is placed infraumbilically (by an open or preferably a transcutaneous technique) into the peritoneal cavity for aspiration of blood or fluid. If this is negative, a liter of warmed normal saline solution is infused (or 10 mL/kg in children) into the abdomen and allowed to drain by gravity. The effluent is sent for laboratory analysis.

   a) Criteria for positive DPL
   - 10 mL gross blood on aspiration
   - >100,000 red blood cells/mm^3
   - >500 white blood cells/mm^3
   - Bacteria
   - Bile
   - Food particles

   In the presence of suspected pelvic fractures or pregnancy, DPL should be done above the umbilicus.

III. PENETRATING ABDOMINAL TRAUMA is usually caused by a gunshot wound (GSW) or stab wound. The likelihood of injury requiring operative repair is higher for abdominal GSW (70% to 90%) than for stab wounds (25% to 45%). Abdominal organs commonly injured with penetrating wounds include the small bowel, liver, stomach, colon, and vascular structures. Any penetrating wound from the nipple line anteriorly or scapular tip posteriorly to the buttocks inferiorly can produce an intraperitoneal injury (Fig. 26-3).

A. Gunshot injuries. Patients sustaining gunshot wounds to the abdomen that violate the peritoneal cavity require laparotomy as their diagnostic and therapeutic modality. Tangential GSW that do not violate the peritoneal cavity may be selectively observed.

   1. Physical examination. Carefully inspect the patient so as not to miss wounds. Bullets that do not strike bone or other solid objects generally travel in a straight line. **Trajectory determination is helpful to injury identification.** Nonetheless, hemodynamically unstable patients with abdominal GSW should not have extensive evaluation before celiotomy. Carefully examine the patient paying special attention to the body creases, perineum, and rectum. Bullet wounds should be counted and assessed. An odd number of wounds suggests a retained bullet; elongated wounds without penetration typify graze injuries. Palpate the abdomen for signs of tenderness. A neurologic examination should be performed to exclude spinal cord injury.

   2. Plain radiographs assist in determining trajectory. This is facilitated by marking cutaneous bullet wounds with radiopaque markers. In addition, the presence of pneumoperitoneum, spinal fractures, pneumo-, or hemothorax can be appreciated.

   3. CT scan has a questionable role in the evaluation of patients with abdominal GSW. Bullet trajectory can be estimated. Peritoneal penetration may be assessed and early discharge considered. However, false positives and negatives are also possible. The use of triple-contrast CT (IV, oral, and rectal) may increase its accuracy. A contrast may be adequate for most clinical scenarios.

   4. FAST has a limited role in evaluating gunshot injuries.

   5. Laparoscopy should also be considered with caution. There is a high potential for technical mishaps when used in the middle of the night and false

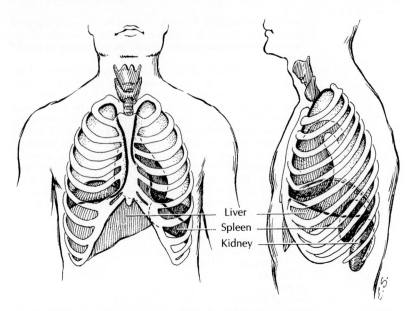

Figure 26-3. The intrathoracic abdomen. (From Blaisdell FW. Initial assessment. In: Blaisdell FW, Trunkey DD, eds. *Trauma Management—Cervicothoracic Trauma.* New York, NY: Thieme Medical Publishers; 1989:6, with permission.)

negatives are a reality when trying to explore the retroperitoneal space or "run" the bowel. However, laparoscopy is useful to detect possible diaphragmatic perforation in left thoracoabdominal penetrating injuries.

B. Stab wounds. Indications for immediate exploration include hypotension, peritoneal signs, and evisceration. If these are not present, a selective management approach is justified. Anterior stab wounds refer to those in front of the anterior axillary line. One third are extraperitoneal, one third are intraperitoneal requiring repair, and one third are intraperitoneal not requiring visceral repair. Flank stab wounds lie between the anterior and posterior axillary lines from the scapular tip to the iliac crest. Back stab wounds are posterior to the posterior axillary line. Abdominal organs are at risk with thoracic wounds inferior to the nipple line anteriorly (ICS 4) and scapular tip posteriorly (ICS 7) (Figs. 26-3 and 26-4).

1. **Serial examination** (selective management) can be used to detect the development of peritoneal signs in a hemodynamically stable patient with a reasonably reliable physical examination. The same surgeon should repeat abdominal examinations noting and documenting temperature, pulse rate, and white blood count. With this evaluation method, the delayed laparotomy rate is 4% with <3% mortality.

2. **Local wound exploration** can be performed in the trauma resuscitation area on patients without indications for operation after anterior abdominal stab. The skin is prepared and anesthetized and the original wound is enlarged. Exploration is considered positive if posterior fascial penetration is observed. Patients with positive local wound explorations progress to laparoscopy or laparotomy. Patients with wound exploration indicating no fascial penetration can be discharged from the emergency room. The risk of false negative local exploration is not negligible. We prefer to rely on physical symptoms rather than local exploration for ultimate decision making.

3. **CT scan with triple contrast** (oral, IV, and rectal) can be used to evaluate back and flank SW with a sensitivity of 89%, specificity of 98%, and

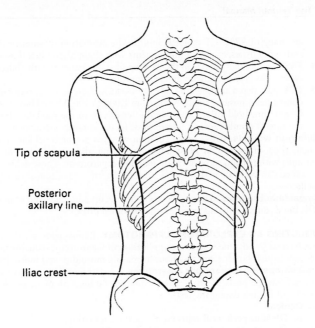

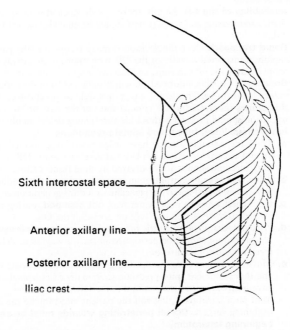

Figure 26-4. Posterior and flank zones of the abdomen. (From Champion HR, Robbs JV, Trunkey DD, eds. Trauma surgery [parts 1 and 2]. In: Dudley H, Carter D, Russell RCG, eds. *Rob and Smith's Operative Surgery.* London: Butterworth; 1989:102, with permission.)

accuracy of 97%. CT is not helpful in the evaluation of anterior abdominal stab wounds, especially in thin patients with slight abdominal musculature.

4. **FAST** is minimally useful in the workup of stable patients with abdominal stab wounds as is the case with gunshot injuries.

5. **DPL** has also a limited role, mostly because there is no agreement in what constitutes a positive test (ranging from 1,000 to 100,000 red blood cells/mm^3). Lower threshold values improve the sensitivity of the modality, but increase the rate of nontherapeutic laparotomy. Its use is rarely recommended.

C. **Shotgun wounds.** Close-range shotgun wounds are high-velocity injuries. As such, they can result in blast and penetrating abdominal wounds. Shotgun wounds with peritoneal penetration mandate laparotomy. Those delivered from a distance can be evaluated with CT scan to determine peritoneal penetration by pellets.

D. **Impalement injuries.** The impaled object is secured in place and removed in the OR under direct visualization with the abdomen open.

IV. **CONDUCTING AN EXPLORATORY LAPAROTOMY.** Refinements in diagnostic capabilities have allowed a more selective application of laparotomy, reducing the number of nontherapeutic laparotomies without increasing morbidity and mortality.

A. **Indications for exploratory laparotomy.** Laparotomy for trauma can be performed on the basis of physical examination findings alone or on the basis of results of further diagnostic tests.

1. **Clinical**
   a. Obvious peritoneal signs on physical examination
   b. Hypotension with a positive FAST or DPL after blunt trauma or hypotension after penetrating abdominal injury
   c. CT results consistent with hollow visceral injury
   d. Inability to evaluate clinically

B. **General setup**

1. **Availability of the OR.** An OR appropriately stocked with appropriate anesthetics and nursing and support staff should be immediately available 24 hours a day.

2. **Rapid transport.** Once the decision is made to operate, the patient must be rapidly transported directly to the OR with appropriate airway support personnel, trauma team surgeons, and trauma team nursing staff in attendance.

3. **Consent.** If possible, informed consent is obtained from the patient or relative before laparotomy. This is not always possible or practicable, depending on the injuries involved and the clinical state of the patient; in such cases, the operation should proceed without life-threatening delays to obtain consent.

4. **Intravenous lines, tubes, and spinal precautions**
   a. The patient should already have at least two large-bore IVs placed; other IV and arterial access can be placed as necessary in the OR. Control of cavitary bleeding should not be delayed by fluid resuscitation.
   b. Administer broad-spectrum, gram-negative, and anaerobic antibiotic coverage (e.g., an extended-spectrum penicillin or a third-generation cephalosporin).
   c. Place chest tubes to underwater seal, **not clamped**, during transport and immediately to suction drainage on arrival in the OR.
   d. Place nasogastric or orogastric tubes and a Foley catheter before laparotomy. No procedure should be performed in such a way as to delay control of bleeding and contamination.
   e. Move the patient onto the operating table with appropriate cervical spine and thoracolumbar spine precautions; in many cases, spinal injury will not have been excluded before arrival in the OR. If the patient is still immobilized on a backboard, log roll the patient and remove the board before beginning surgery. **Occult penetrating wounds must be sought before beginning laparotomy.**
   f. Sequential compression devices can be used for hemodynamically stable patients, if readily available.

5. **Rapid-infusion system.** Prime the infusion system to infuse blood products and "cell-saved blood" quickly via large-bore lines before the incision releases the tamponade. Ascertain that packed red blood cells (RBC) are in the OR and plasma and platelets are available for the patient with active hemorrhage.

6. **Preparation of the patient.** The patient is shaved, and then the entire antero-lateral neck (remove anterior portion of cervical collar and then sandbag to maintain cervical spine immobilization), chest to the table bilaterally, abdomen, groin, and thigh region (to the knees bilaterally) are prepared and draped in sterile fashion (Fig. 16.1 in Chapter 16).

C. **Initial goals. Stop bleeding and control gastrointestinal contamination.** The exploratory laparotomy for trauma is a sequential, consistently conducted, operative procedure.

1. **Incision.** For urgent laparotomy, a generous midline incision is preferred. Alternative abdominal incisions can be useful for known injuries in stable patients. Adequate exposure is critical. Self-retaining retractor systems and headlights are useful.

2. **Bleeding control.** Scoop free blood and rapidly pack all four quadrants to control bleeding as a first step. **With blunt injuries**, the likely sources of bleeding are the liver, spleen, and mesentery. Pack the liver and spleen, and quickly clamp the mesenteric bleeders. **With penetrating injuries**, the likely sources of significant bleeding are the liver, retroperitoneal vascular structures, and mesentery. Pack the liver and retroperitoneum, and quickly clamp mesenteric bleeding vessels. **If packing does not control a bleeding site, this source of hemorrhage must be controlled as the first priority.**

   a. **Recombinant activated Factor VII (Factor VIIa)** is being used as an adjunct for the correction of coagulopathy-induced severe hemorrhage in some centers. To date its role is not well defined and the existing evidence not confirmative. Additional study is ongoing, but it should be understood that Factor VIIa is not a replacement for the surgical control of surgical bleeding.

3. **Contamination control.** Quickly control bowel content contamination using Babcock clamps, Allis clamps, a stapler, rapid temporary sutures, or ligatures.

4. **Systematic exploration.** Systematically explore the entire abdomen, giving priority to areas of ongoing hemorrhage to definitively control bleeding:
   - Liver
   - Spleen
   - Stomach
   - Right colon, transverse colon, descending colon, sigmoid colon, rectum, and small bowel, from ligament of Treitz to terminal ileum, looking at the entire bowel wall and the mesentery
   - Pancreas, by opening lesser sac (visualize and palpate)
   - Kocher maneuver to visualize the duodenum, with evidence of possible injury
   - Left and right hemidiaphragms and retroperitoneum
   - Pelvic structures, including the bladder

   a. **With penetrating injuries**, exploration should focus on following the track of the weapon or missile.

5. Injury repair (Section V.A–H)

6. **Closure**
   a. Running nonabsorbable or absorbable monofilament suture (e.g., no. 1 nylon or no. 1 looped absorbable suture).
   b. Leave skin open with delayed secondary closure if there is contamination.
   c. If gross edema of abdominal contents precludes closure, absorbable mesh, sterile IV bags, or intestinal bags can be used with moist gauze and an impermeable dressing (e.g., Op-Site) to prevent possible abdominal compartment syndrome (Chapters 27, 28, and 29). Recognize the combination of complex injuries and physiologic signs (generally hypothermia, acidosis, and coagulopathy) that dictate abbreviated laparotomy (**damage control**).

V. SPECIFIC ORGAN INJURIES. Treatment of organ injuries is similar whether the injury mechanism is penetrating or blunt. An exception to the rule is a retroperitoneal hematoma. Explore all retroperitoneal hematomas caused by penetrating injuries.

A. Diaphragm

1. Incidence

  a. Injuries to the diaphragm account for 1% to 8% of blunt injuries; up to two thirds of ruptures occur on the left; 5% are central; and the heart will be seen through the defect.

  b. High-speed motor vehicle crashes account for 90% of injuries. Injuries from penetrating trauma are generally small.

  c. High incidence of associated intraabdominal injury (60% to 80%); the stomach has usually herniated through the defect, which may not be appreciated in the patient on positive pressure ventilation.

  d. High incidence in left thoracoabdominal penetrating trauma (40%) even in the absence of symptoms or radiographic findings (20%).

2. Anatomy. The anterior portion of the diaphragm attaches to the inferior portion of the sternum and the costal margin. Posteriorly, the diaphragm is attached to the 11th and 12th ribs. The central portion of the diaphragm is attached to the pericardium. Innervation is via the phrenic nerve (C3–C5).

3. Diagnosis. Clinical diagnosis of diaphragmatic injury is difficult.

  a. Findings can include diminished breath sounds on the affected side, bowel sounds audible in the hemithorax, or a scaphoid abdomen. The patient may complain of respiratory distress, chest pain, or abdominal pain.

  b. A chest radiograph may show hemopneumothorax and an elevated or indistinct hemidiaphragm with a stomach bubble or bowel gas pattern in the hemithorax. Of diaphragmatic ruptures, 40% present as an obvious finding on chest x-ray (CXR); in 40% the CXR is abnormal but not diagnostic; and in 20% the CXR is normal. Placement of a nasogastric tube with a follow-up chest radiograph may confirm displacement of the stomach through a torn diaphragm.

  c. DPL is not sensitive.

  d. Injuries to the diaphragm are easily missed on CT.

  e. Laparoscopy (or thoracoscopy) is the diagnostic method of choice if the diagnosis is not definitive by CXR.

4. Treatment

  a. Approach is via laparotomy or laparoscopy.

  b. Perform primary repair with simple, horizontal mattress, or a running suture of nonabsorbable material

  c. Irrigate the thoracic cavity (if repair is by laparotomy); generally, leave a chest tube in place.

  d. Perform repair via thoracotomy for delayed diagnosis (i.e., injuries presenting after many years); this facilitates lysis of adhesions between lung and abdominal contents.

  e. Selected isolated injuries to the right diaphragm from penetrating mechanisms can be managed expectantly, assuming the liver will prevent visceral herniation.

5. Outcome. If diaphragmatic injury is recognized and repaired early, the morbidity related to the diaphragmatic injury is usually related to ipsilateral pleural effusion or lower lobe pulmonary consolidation. If a diaphragmatic injury (whether from blunt or penetrating injury) is missed, morbidity is significant in the form of possible herniation and strangulation of abdominal viscera.

6. Organ injury scale (Appendix A)

B. Stomach

1. Incidence

  a. Blunt gastric injuries are rare, with an incidence of 0.9% to 1.8%. Gastric injury occurs in 10% to 15% of penetrating trauma.

2. Anatomy. The gastric wall has mucosal, submucosal, serosal, and three smooth muscle layers. The stomach has an extensive blood supply that includes the right gastric, left gastric, right gastroepiploic artery, and the left gastroepiploic and the short gastric arteries. The normal stomach contains few bacteria because of its high acid content.

3. **Diagnosis**
   a. Signs of chemical peritonitis (acid pH) on physical examination
   b. Blood in nasogastric aspirate (present in one third of patients with penetrating gastric wounds)
   c. Free subdiaphragmatic air on CXR in <50% of blunt gastric ruptures
   d. DPL or CT findings

4. **Treatment is operative**
   a. Administer preoperative antibiotics.
   b. Perform laparotomy through a midline incision. Because other intraperitoneal injuries are generally more immediately life threatening, address them first. Carefully visualize the gastric wall, including the posterior wall via the lesser sac, the gastroesophageal junction, and the greater and lesser curvatures (where injury may be obscured by the greater or lesser omentum).
   c. Debride and repair the stomach in two layers—the inner layer with running absorbable suture and the outer layer with nonabsorbable suture. Gastric resection is rarely required. Irrigate and remove gastric contents from the peritoneal cavity.

5. **Outcomes** are generally good. Morbidity and mortality are usually caused by associated injuries, which are common. On the other hand, recent papers have reported a high risk of abdominal infection with gastric injury.

6. Organ injury scale (Appendix A)

C. **Small bowel**

1. **Incidence**
   a. The small bowel is the most commonly injured intraabdominal organ in penetrating trauma; a blunt mechanism of injury is less common, but not rare (5% to 15%).
   b. Small isolated perforations probably result from blowouts of pseudo-closed loops (lap-belt injuries).
   c. Larger perforations, complete disruptions, and injuries associated with large mesenteric hematoma or lacerations are caused by direct blows or shearing injury.
   d. Perforation from blunt injury is most common at the ligament of Treitz, ileocecal valve, midjejunum, or in areas of adhesions.

2. **Anatomy.** The adult small bowel averages 6.5 m in length; the proximal 40% is jejunum. The proximal small bowel has few bacteria and is pH neutral; the bacterial content increases toward the distal small bowel. The blood supply is primarily from the superior mesenteric artery (SMA), with drainage via the superior mesenteric vein (SMV).

3. **Diagnosis**
   a. Suspect small-bowel injury with evidence of an abdominal wall lap-belt contusion; also, 30% to 60% risk of bowel injury with a Chance fracture of the lumbar spine.
   b. **Small-bowel injury is often not diagnosed on initial presentation**. This delay contributes significantly to morbidity and mortality. Small-bowel contents have a neutral pH, so the patient is less likely to have peritonitis on initial examination.
   c. **CT has a significant false negative rate in the diagnosis of small-bowel injury**. Findings suggestive of small-bowel injury include:
      i. Fluid collections without solid viscus injury
      ii. Bowel wall thickening
      iii. Mesenteric infiltration
      iv. Free intraperitoneal air
      v. Oral contrast extravasation

4. **Treatment is operative**
   a. Perform laparotomy and repair, and administer preoperative antibiotics.

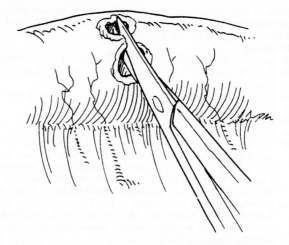

Figure 26-5. Adjacent small bowel lacerations are connected and closed. (From Champion HR, Robbs JV, Trunkey DD, eds. Trauma surgery [parts 1 and 2]. In: Dudley H, Carter D, Russell RCG, eds. *Rob and Smith's Operative Surgery*. London: Butterworth; 1989:406, with permission.)

    b. Imbricate antimesenteric wall hematomas or serosal injuries with Lembert stitches to reduce the risk of delayed perforation.

    c. Debride simple lacerations and close transversely in one layer to avoid stenosis.

    d. Similarly connect and close adjacent small lacerations (Fig. 26-5).

    e. Resect larger injuries and perform an end-to-end anastomosis.

    f. Injuries to the mesentery of the small bowel, which can bleed massively, must be rapidly controlled, with definitive repair of the small bowel delayed until later in the operation. Injury to the proximal SMA may require a saphenous vein interposition graft or shunting in a damage control scenario.

5. Outcome

    a. The outcome is generally good if the diagnosis is made quickly and the operation is promptly performed. The anastomotic leak rate is 1% to 2%, which can manifest as enterocutaneous fistula, peritonitis, or intraabdominal abscess.

    b. The incidence of subsequent bowel obstruction is 1% to 2%.

    6. Organ injury scale (Appendix A)

D. Colon and rectum

    1. Incidence. The colon is injured in 25% of GSW and 5% of stab wounds. Colonic injury occurs in 2% to 5% of blunt injuries. Rectal injuries represent up to 5% of all colon injuries. Blunt rectal perforation can be associated with pelvic fractures or concussion injuries (e.g., injuries from underwater explosions), or with devascularization from mesenteric injury. The morbidity and mortality rates are 5% to 10% with colonic injury and associated injuries.

    2. Anatomy. The colon is 1.5 m in length. Its major function is the absorption of water. The predominant organisms are anaerobes, gram-negative enteric organisms, and enterococci. The extraperitoneal rectum is 12 cm in length. The splenic flexure is the "watershed area" in terms of blood supply.

    3. Diagnosis

        a. Peritoneal signs on examination or free intraperitoneal air. At laparotomy, small injuries in the wall of the colon can be missed. Carefully explore all blood staining or hematomas of the colonic wall.

    b. Gross blood on rectal examination in the presence of a pelvic fracture should prompt proctoscopy in an effort to identify a rectal injury. Consider proctoscopy for any patient with a major pelvic fracture; devascularization of the sigmoid colon may result.

    c. Gross blood on rectal examination with a penetrating abdominal, buttock, or pelvic wound is pathognomonic of colorectal injury. If the patient is hemodynamically stable, perform rigid sigmoidoscopy in the OR to visualize the injury. The location of the injury can be important in planning the operation. **Even if the hole cannot be visualized on proctoscopy, assume the patient has a colorectal injury, if there is intraluminal blood.** In hemodynamically unstable patients, proceed with laparotomy first.

4. Treatment is operative

    a. Colon. In previous years colonic injury was treated by exteriorization or repair with a proximal diverting colostomy. (This was based on an extremely high pre-World War I [WWI] mortality with nonoperative treatment, a mortality >60% associated with suture closure of colon wounds during WWI, and a 35% mortality during World War II [WWII] when a policy of exteriorization or repair with proximal colostomy was adopted.)

        i. Current operative options include primary repair of the injury, resection and anastomosis, and colostomy. Recent data have indicated that primary repair (including resection and anastomosis, although this is more controversial) of selected injuries can be applied in most colonic injuries; anatomic location of the injury is not an absolute contraindication to this approach.

            a) The guidelines for primary repair include minimal fecal spillage, no shock (defined as systolic blood pressure <90 mmHg), minimal associated intraabdominal injuries, <8-hour delay in diagnosis and treatment, and <1-L blood loss.

            b) Traditional contraindications to primary repair include extensive intraperitoneal spillage of feces, extensive colonic injury requiring resection, and major loss of the abdominal wall or mesh repair of the abdominal wall; these contraindications have been challenged in recent papers. Primary repair is being applied with increasing frequency and in many centers with trauma expertise has almost entirely replaced fecal diversion.

            c) If a primary repair cannot be performed safely for anatomic reasons (bowel wall edema, vascular compromise), a colostomy may be a safer option.

    b. Rectum. Injuries to the rectum should be defined as intraperitoneal rectum or extraperitoneal rectal injuries. Often, intraperitoneal rectal injuries can be primarily repaired. Treat extraperitoneal rectal tears by diverting sigmoid colostomy. Acceptable options include Hartmann resection with end colostomy, end colostomy with a mucus fistula, or loop colostomy with a stapled distal end. If the defect is not readily identified on proctoscopy, do not extensively mobilize the rectum in attempting to identify the hole. Presacral drainage (closed suction or Penrose drains) and irrigation of the distal rectal stump have not shown to be of benefit and should not be used.

    c. If a colostomy is necessary in a patient with a pelvic fracture requiring fixation, place the colostomy in the left upper quadrant to facilitate the orthopedic procedure. This procedure can be delayed until the hemodynamically unstable patient is resuscitated.

    d. Perioperative broad-spectrum antibiotics should be administered for colon and rectal wounds.

5. Outcome

    a. Morbidity occurs in proportion to the magnitude of the original injury.

        i. 1% to 2% incidence of fecal fistula.

    ii. 5% incidence of intraabdominal abscess with primary repair.
   iii. 17% incidence of abscess formation in those requiring colostomy.
   iv. Most postoperative abscesses can be percutaneously drained.
    v. The mortality rate for pelvic fracture with rectal perforation is 20%.
   vi. Morbidity for the initial trauma laparotomy and subsequent colostomy takedown when colostomy was performed is higher than primary repair in a single procedure. The current approach is to avoid colostomy whenever possible. In the setting of colostomy, return to the OR within the first 10 days for colostomy reversal for selected cases is feasible and safe.
  6. Organ injury scale (Appendix A)
E. Duodenum and pancreas. Pancreatic and duodenal injuries are listed together because of their shared blood supply and incidence of concomitant injury (Fig. 26-6). Preoperative diagnosis of these injuries is often difficult; operative solutions can be complex.
  1. Pancreatic injury
    a. Incidence
      i. Relatively uncommon; most are caused by penetrating injury (70% to 75%); constitute <10% of abdominal trauma but represent a major diagnostic challenge, especially in blunt trauma cases. Blunt injury is more common in children. Blunt pancreatic injury generally occurs from a crushing injury of the pancreas between the spine and another object (e.g., steering wheel, handlebar, or blunt weapon).
     ii. Associated intraabdominal injury is found in >90% of pancreatic injuries, with vascular injury responsible for more than half of the morbidity and most of the immediate deaths. Major vascular injury (aorta, portal vein, or inferior vena cava [IVC]) is associated with 50% to 75% of penetrating pancreatic injuries and 12% of blunt pancreatic injuries. Intraabdominal organs most commonly injured in conjunction with pancreatic injury (whether blunt or penetrating) include the liver,

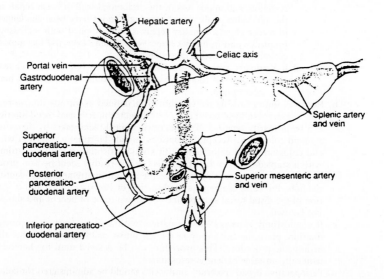

Figure 26-6. Anatomy of the pancreas. (From Frey W. Abdominal arterial trauma. In: Blaisdell FW, Trunkey DD, eds. *Trauma Management—Abdominal Trauma.* 2nd ed. New York, NY: Thieme Medical Publishers; 1993:346, with permission.)

spleen, duodenum, and small intestine. Early deaths are from hemorrhage and late deaths are from infection.

b. Anatomy. The pancreas is retroperitoneal. The head of the pancreas lies to the right of the midline originating at the level of L-2. The body crosses the midline with the pancreatic tail ending in the hilum of the spleen at the level of L-1. The SMA and SMV lie posteriorly in a groove in the neck of the pancreas.

  i. The main pancreatic duct of Wirsung usually runs the length of the pancreas. The accessory duct of Santorini usually branches from the pancreatic duct in the pancreas and empties separately into the duodenum; in 20%, the accessory duct drains into the main pancreatic duct and in 8% it is the sole drainage of the pancreas.

c. Diagnosis

  i. Pancreatic injury should be suspected, based on the mechanism of injury and the high incidence of associated intraabdominal injury. Physical examination, FAST, DPL, and CT findings consistent with other injuries may indicate the need for laparotomy in patients with preoperatively unrecognized pancreatic injuries. Isolated pancreatic injury is uncommon.

  ii. Generally, laparotomy is indicated for patients with pancreatic injury because of concomitant abdominal injuries. If not, the initial complaints with pancreatic injury may be vague and nonspecific; 6 to 24 hours after the injury, the patient will complain of midepigastric or back pain. Physical findings include nonspecific or midepigastric abdominal tenderness. Eventually, the patient will develop peritoneal signs.

  iii. Serum amylase levels are neither sensitive nor specific.

  iv. DPL is not reliable.

  v. CT may identify peripancreatic hematomas but may not identify pancreatic lacerations or even complete transections early in the postinjury period.

  vi. Endoscopic retrograde cholangiopancreatography (ERCP) or magnetic resonance cholangiopancreatogram (MRCP) can be used to diagnose pancreatic ductal injury in hemodynamically stable patients.

  vii. Intraoperative diagnosis depends on visual inspection and bimanual palpation of the pancreas by opening the gastrocolic ligament and entering the lesser sac, and by performing a Kocher maneuver. Mobilization of the spleen along with the tail of the pancreas and opening of the retroperitoneum to facilitate palpation of the substance of the gland may be necessary to determine transection versus contusion. **Identification of injury to the major duct is the critical issue in intraoperative management of pancreatic injury.**

    a) Intraoperative pancreatography may be useful for suspected pancreatic head ductal injuries but is rarely needed with **careful inspection and palpation of the pancreas**.

d. Treatment. Suspected pancreatic injuries should be surgically explored. Treatment principles include

  i. Control hemorrhage

  ii. Debride devitalized pancreas, which can require resection

  iii. Preserve maximal amount of viable pancreatic tissue

  iv. Wide drainage of pancreatic secretions with closed-suction drains

  v. Feeding jejunostomy for postoperative care with significant lesions

e. Treatment options

  i. Pancreatic contusion or capsular laceration without ductal injury → wide drainage.

  ii. Pancreatic transection distal to the SMA → distal pancreatectomy. Attempt splenic conservation in the stable patient. Control the resection line by stapling the pancreatic stump or closing with horizontal mattress sutures of nonabsorbable material. Attempt to visualize and directly oversew the pancreatic duct. Place closed suction drains.

   iii. Pancreatic transection to the right of the SMA (not involving the ampulla) → **no optimal operation.** The options include wide drainage of the area of injury to develop a controlled pancreatic fistula; ligation of both ends of the distal duct and wide drainage; and oversewing the proximal pancreas and performing a Roux-en-Y jejunostomy to the distal pancreas (indicated uncommonly). Generally, wide closed-suction drainage is sufficient acutely with injury to the head of the pancreas.

   iv. Severe injury to both the head of the pancreas and the duodenum may require pancreaticoduodenectomy; however, this is rarely indicated. It can be performed in staged, damage-control fashion.

  f. Outcome

   i. 7% to 35% incidence of pancreatic fistula; most spontaneously resolve.

   ii. Intraabdominal abscess or wound infection is also common.

   iii. 5% incidence of true pancreatic abscess.

   iv. Pancreatitis occurs in 8% to 18% of these patients.

   v. Pancreatic pseudocysts can occur.

  g. Organ injury scale (Appendix A)

2. Duodenal injury

  a. Incidence. Most injuries are from penetrating trauma, predominantly GSW. Blunt mechanisms account for 20% to 25% of duodenal injuries; the duodenum can be compressed between the spine and steering wheel, lap belt, or handlebars. The second portion of the duodenum is most commonly injured. Delays in diagnosis are common and significantly increase morbidity and mortality. Duodenal injury rarely is an isolated abdominal injury; up to 98% have associated abdominal injuries. Commonly associated injuries include (in order of decreasing frequency): liver, pancreas, small bowel, colon, IVC, portal vein, and aorta.

  b. Anatomy. The duodenum shares its blood supply with the pancreas. It extends from the pylorus to the ligament of Treitz (25 cm in length). There are four parts: the first portion (superior portion) of the duodenum is intraperitoneal; the second portion of the duodenum (descending portion) contains the orifices of the bile and pancreatic ducts; the third portion of the duodenum (transverse portion) extends from the ampulla of Vater to the mesenteric vessels, with the ureter, IVC, and aorta posteriorly and SMA anteriorly; the fourth portion of the duodenum (ascending portion) begins at the mesenteric vessels and ends at the jejunum, to the left of the lumbar column. Bile (1,000 mL/day), pancreatic juices (800–1,000 mL/day), and gastric juices (1,500–2,500 mL/day) mix in the duodenum.

  c. Diagnosis

   i. Clinical suspicion is based on the mechanism of injury. With blunt injury, the patient usually has midepigastric or right upper quadrant pain or tenderness and can have peritoneal signs. The symptoms and findings can be subtle. Retroperitoneal air or obliteration of the right psoas margin may be seen on abdominal x-ray study. The diagnosis is generally made at laparotomy for associated injuries. With penetrating mechanisms, duodenal injury is found at laparotomy, usually for GSW.

   ii. CT findings include paraduodenal hemorrhage and air or oral contrast leak.

   iii. With equivocal CT findings, an upper gastrointestinal (UGI) study may be essential. The contrast enhanced UGI study is first done with water-soluble contrast; if this is negative, barium is then used.

    a) Adequate intraoperative exposure is vital; duodenal injuries are among the most commonly missed at laparotomy. They should be exposed in a manner similar to that used for the pancreas, including a wide Kocher maneuver. Bile staining, air in the retroperitoneum, or a central retroperitoneal hematoma mandates thorough exploration of the duodenum.

d. Treatment

  i. Intramural duodenal hematoma is more common in children than in adults; may be a result of child abuse. A "coiled spring" appearance is seen on UGI series. Follow-up UGI with Gastrografin should be obtained every 7 days, if the obstruction persists clinically.

  a) Treated nonoperatively with nasogastric suction and IV alimentation. Operation is necessary to evacuate the hematoma if it does not resolve after 2 to 3 weeks.

  b) Treatment of an intramural hematoma found at early laparotomy is controversial.

  1) One option is to open serosa, evacuate the hematoma without violation of the mucosa, and repair the wall of the bowel. The concern is that this may convert a partial tear to a full-thickness tear of the duodenal wall.

  2) Another option is to explore the duodenum to exclude a perforation, leaving the intramural hematoma intact and planning nasogastric decompression postoperatively.

  3) Consider placement of a jejunal feeding tube for postoperative enteral feeding.

  ii. Duodenal perforation must be treated operatively. Many options are available, depending on injury severity.

  a) Transverse primary closure in one or two layers is applicable in 71% to 85% of duodenal injuries. This requires debridement of the edges of the duodenal wall and closure that avoids narrowing of the duodenal lumen. Longitudinal duodenal injuries can usually be closed transversely if the length of the duodenal injury is <50% of the circumference of the duodenum. More severe injuries may require repairs using pyloric exclusion, duodenal decompression, or more complex operations. The risk factors with duodenal injury include:
  • Associated vascular injury
  • Associated pancreatic injury
  • Blunt injury or missile injury
  • >75% of the wall involved
  • Injury in the first or second portion of the duodenum
  • >24 hours since injury
  • Associated common bile duct injury

  b) If the repair is considered to be tenuous, protect it by a retrograde jejunostomy drainage catheter. If more protection is required, divert the stomach contents by **pyloric exclusion** with gastrojejunostomy. Staple from the outside or oversew the pyloric outlet through a gastric incision (absorbable or nonabsorbable suture), using the incision as the gastrojejunostomy site (Fig. 26-7). Vagotomy is usually not performed; the pyloric closure generally reopens in 2 to 3 weeks.

  c) If primary closure would compromise the lumen of the duodenum, use a jejunal mucosal patch duodenoplasty (rarely used) or a jejunal serosal patch.

  d) A three-tube technique may also be used. This consists of a gastrostomy tube to decompress the stomach, a retrograde jejunostomy to decompress the duodenum, and an antegrade jejunostomy to feed the patient.

  e) If complete duodenal transection or long lacerations of the duodenal wall are found, perform debridement and primary closure. If this cannot be accomplished without tension, a Roux-en-Y jejunostomy over the defect or closure of the distal duodenum and Roux-en-Y duodenojejunostomy proximally may be required.

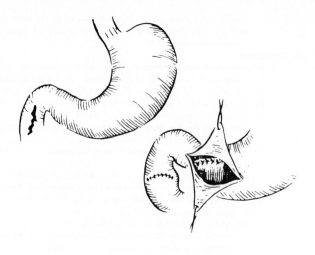

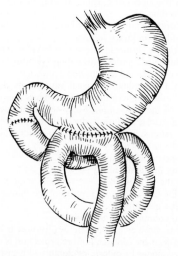

Figure 26-7. Pyloric exclusion. (From Frame SB, McSwain NE. *Retroperitoneal Trauma.* New York, NY: Thieme Medical Publishers; 1993:89, with permission.)

    f) The uncommon circumstance of destructive combined injuries to the duodenum and the head of the pancreas may necessitate pancreaticoduodenectomy (Whipple procedure). In this rare circumstance, experienced help is essential.

  e. Outcome

    i. The mortality rate reaches 40% if diagnosis is delayed >24 hours, but it is 2% to 11% if the patient has surgery within 24 hours of injury. Duodenal dehiscence with resultant sepsis accounts for nearly one half of the deaths. Complications occur in 64% of patients with duodenal injuries.

    ii. Retrograde tube decompression of the duodenum can be associated with a decreased mortality rate (9% with tube decompression vs. 19.4% without). The duodenal fistula rate was 2.3% with decompression versus 11.8% without decompression in the same review. Pyloric exclusion can also provide adequate decompression of the duodenal closure if the repair is tenuous or a concomitant pancreatic injury is found.

  f. Organ injury scale (Appendix A)

F. Liver

  1. Incidence. The liver is the most commonly injured intraabdominal organ; injury occurs more often in penetrating trauma than in blunt trauma. The mortality rate for liver injury is 10%.

  2. Anatomy. An understanding of hepatic anatomy is essential to manage complex liver injuries. A sagittal plane separates the right and left lobes of the liver from the IVC to the gallbladder fossa. The segmental anatomy of the liver is shown in Figure 26-8.

  a. The right and left hepatic veins have a short extrahepatic course before they empty directly in the IVC. The middle hepatic vein usually joins the left hepatic vein within the liver parenchyma. The retrohepatic IVC (8–10 cm in length) has multiple, small hepatic veins that enter the IVC directly; this area is exceedingly difficult to access and control.

  b. The portal vein delivers 75% of the hepatic blood flow and 50% of the oxygenated blood.

  c. The right and left hepatic arteries usually arise from the common hepatic artery. Anomalies are frequent and include the right hepatic artery originating from the SMA and the left hepatic artery originating from the left gastric artery.

  d. Adequate mobilization of the liver requires division of the ligamentous attachments.

  i. The falciform ligament divides the left lateral segment of the liver from the medial segment of the left lobe.

  ii. The coronary ligaments are the diaphragmatic attachments to the liver (anterior and posterior leaflets); they do not meet on the posterior surface of the liver (the bare area). The triangular ligaments (left and

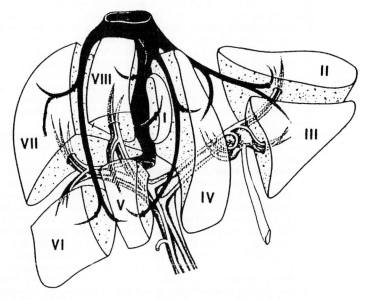

Figure 26-8. Hepatic anatomy. (From Bismuth H. Surgical anatomy and anatomical surgery of the liver. *World J Surg* 1982;6[1]:6, with permission.)

right) are the more lateral extensions of the coronary ligaments. Injury to the diaphragm, phrenic veins, and hepatic veins must be avoided when mobilizing the liver.

3. **Diagnosis**
   a. Physical examination is often unreliable in the blunt trauma victim.
   b. The appropriate diagnostic modality depends on the hemodynamic status of the patient on arrival in the trauma resuscitation area. If the patient is hemodynamically stable with a blunt mechanism of injury, CT is preferred. CT is sensitive and specific in stable patients with a clinical suspicion of injury. Most hemodynamically stable patients with liver injuries can be treated nonoperatively.

4. **Treatment**
   a. Management of blunt hepatic injuries has evolved substantially in the past several years. The hemodynamically stable patients with blunt injury of the liver, without other intraabdominal injury requiring laparotomy, can be treated nonoperatively, regardless of the grade of the liver injury. This may represent 50% to 80% of patients. The presence of hemoperitoneum on CT does not mandate laparotomy. **Arterial blush or pooling of contrast** on CT and high-grade (grade IV and V) hepatic injuries are most likely to fail nonoperative management. Nonetheless, embolization can circumvent the need for laparotomy; angioembolization has assumed an increasing role in the management of liver injury. The criteria for nonoperative management of blunt liver injuries include:
      i. Hemodynamic stability.
      ii. Absence of peritoneal signs.
      iii. Lack of continued need for transfusion for the hepatic injury; bleeding can be addressed with angioembolization.
   b. Posterior right lobe injuries (even if extensive) and the split-liver type of injuries (extensive injury along the relatively avascular plane between the left and right lobes) can generally be managed successfully nonoperatively.
   c. The details of nonoperative management are institution and provider specific. No support is seen for frequent hemoglobin sampling, bed rest, and prolonged intensive care unit (ICU) monitoring. Similarly, the need to reimage asymptomatic hepatic injuries by CT scan is not documented. Practitioners should tailor monitoring practices to their institutional resources. Follow-up CT scanning can be deferred, except to document healing (at ~8 weeks) in physically active patients (e.g., athletes) before resumption of normal activities.
   d. Immediate laparotomy or angiographic intervention is required for those patients who fail nonoperative therapy by demonstrating enlarging lesions on CT scan, hemodynamic instability, or continual blood product requirement (<10%).
   e. If the patient is hemodynamically unstable or has indications for laparotomy, operative management is required. Management principles include the following:
      i. **Adequate exposure of the injury is essential.** Exploration is through a long midline incision or bilateral subcostal incision. An extension to a median sternotomy or thoracotomy may be necessary for exposure of the injury. Use of a self-retaining retractor (Rochard, Thompson, or Upper Hand) to lift the upper edges of the wound cephalad and anteriorly facilitates exposure of the liver. Complete mobilization of the liver is performed, including division of the ligaments.
      ii. Most blunt and penetrating hepatic injuries are grade I and II (70% to 90%) and can be managed with simple techniques (e.g., electrocautery, simple suture, or hemostatic agents). Complex liver injuries can produce exsanguinating hemorrhage. Rapid, temporary tamponade of the bleeding by manual compression of the liver injury immediately after entering the abdomen allows the anesthesiologist to

resuscitate the patient. After resuscitation, the liver injury can be repaired.

iii. For complex hepatic injuries, occlude the portal triad with an atraumatic clamp (Pringle maneuver). This should reduce bleeding from the liver, except in retrohepatic venous injuries. Studies suggest that up to 60 to 90 minutes of warm hepatic ischemia can be tolerated.

iv. Hepatorrhaphy with individual vessel ligation is recommended but frequently large mass parenchymal suturing is necessary.

   a) Glisson's capsule is incised with the electrocautery.

   b) The injury within the liver is quickly approached by the finger fracture technique (Fig. 26-9) or by division of the liver tissue over a right-angled clamp with ligation of the hepatic tissue with 2-0 silk sutures.

   c) With gentle traction on the liver edges, expose the injury site. Blood vessels and bile ducts are directly visualized and ligated or repaired (Fig. 26-10).

   d) Debride nonviable liver tissue.

   e) Pack the defect in the liver with viable omentum.

v. Perform closed-suction drainage of grade III to V injuries. Drains are probably not necessary for grade I or II injuries if bleeding and bile leakage are controlled.

vi. Perform resectional debridement of nonviable tissue rather than formal anatomic resections.

vii. Perform perihepatic packing in cases of hemorrhage, hypothermia, and coagulopathy. Approximately 5% of patients with hepatic injury require perihepatic packing (i.e., damage control laparotomy). Indications

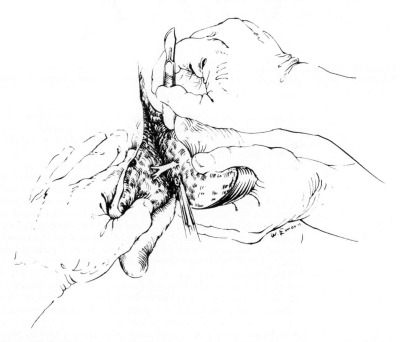

Figure 26-9. Finger fracture technique. (From Lim RC. Injuries to the liver and extra-hepatic ducts. In: Blaisdell FW, Trunkey DD, eds. *Trauma Management—Abdominal Trauma.* New York, NY: Thieme Medical Publishers; 1982:141, with permission.)

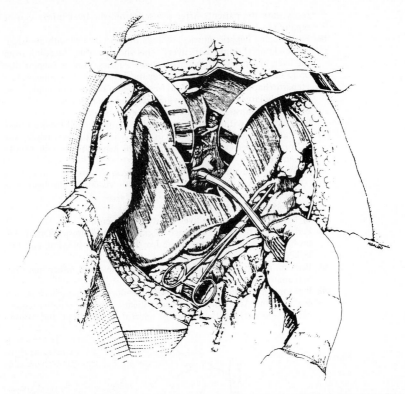

Figure 26-10. Blood vessels and bile ducts are directly visualized and ligated or repaired. (From Feliciano DV, Moore EE, Mattox KL. *Trauma.* 3rd ed. Stamford, Conn: Appleton & Lange; 1996:500, with permission.)

include coagulopathy, subcapsular hematomas, bilobar injuries, and hypothermia, or to allow transfer of the patient to a higher level of care. Pack the liver first by placing nonadhesive plastic on the liver, and placing laparotomy pads.

viii. Anatomic hepatic resection (segment or lobe) is not commonly required for liver injury; resectional debridement and direct suture control of the vessels and ducts can generally accomplish the same objectives, with lower mortality. Indications for formal hepatic resection include total destruction of a segment or lobe, an extensive injury that cannot be controlled with perihepatic packing and control of bleeding that can be achieved only by anatomic resection. Planned, delayed anatomic resection is also an approach for major hepatic injury, if packing sufficiently controls hemorrhage during the initial laparotomy.

ix. Selective hepatic artery ligation has been reported in 1% to 2% of hepatic injury cases. The liver will generally tolerate this because of the oxygen content of portal blood. Direct suture control of bleeding within the liver is preferable to hepatic artery ligation. Nonetheless, patients with significant central hepatic laceration who have damage control laparotomy may be candidates for arteriography with possible embolization postoperatively. Cholecystectomy may be required secondary to ischemic complications from interruption of the right hepatic artery.

f. Hepatic vascular isolation with occlusion of the suprahepatic and infrahepatic venae cavae, as well as application of the Pringle maneuver, may be required for major retrohepatic venous injury. If exposure is necessary, the midline incision can be extended to a median sternotomy, which will allow excellent exposure of the hepatic veins for retrohepatic venous injuries. Atrial-caval shunts have been recommended by some authors for retrohepatic caval injury. A 36 F chest tube or 9-mm endotracheal tube, each with extra side holes, is inserted through the right atrial appendage. The side holes allow flow from the shunt into the right atrium. The distal end of the tube is at the level of the renal veins. Survival with this technique is dismal. Alternatively, complex retrohepatic vascular injury in which tamponade does not achieve hemostasis can be repaired in an avascular field on venovenous bypass with total hepatic vascular isolation. Survival depends on prompt recognition of this anatomic site of injury.

g. Bleeding from penetrating wounds of the liver that are not easily accessed, at times, can be controlled with internal tamponade. This is accomplished by using Penrose drains tied at each end (as a balloon) over a red rubber catheter. The end of the Penrose drain is brought through the skin. Finally, in wounds where tamponade does not achieve hemostasis, consider repair under vascular isolation by experienced personnel.

5. Outcome. Mortality correlates with the degree of injury. Because most hepatic injuries are grade I or II, the overall mortality rate for liver injuries is 10%. However, the mortality rates for more severe liver injury are grade III, 25%; grade IV, 46%; grade V, 80%; and grade VI, fatal.

a. Complications

  i. With recurrent bleeding (occurs in 2% to 7% of patients) → return the patient to the OR or, in selected patients, obtain an angiogram and perform embolization. Recurrent bleeding is generally caused by inadequate initial hemostasis. Hypothermia and coagulopathy must be corrected. Preparations to control retrohepatic hemorrhage (i.e., vascular bypass) should be made.

  ii. Hemobilia is another complication of liver injury. The classic presentation is right upper quadrant pain, jaundice, and hemorrhage; one third of patients have all three components of the triad. The patient may present with hemobilia days or weeks after injury. Treatment is angiogram and embolization.

  iii. Intrahepatic or perihepatic abscess or biloma (occur in 7% to 40% of patients) can generally be drained percutaneously. Meticulous control of bleeding and repair of bile ducts, adequate debridement, and closed-suction drainage are essential to avoid abscess formation.

  iv. Biliary fistulas (>50 mL/day for >2 weeks) usually resolve nonoperatively if external drainage of the leak is adequate and distal obstruction is not present.

   a) If >300 mL of bile drains each day, further evaluation with a radionuclide scan, a fistulogram, ERCP, or a transhepatic cholangiogram may be necessary. Major ductal injury can be stented to facilitate healing of the injury or as a guide if operative repair is required. Endoscopic sphincterotomy or transampullary stenting may facilitate resolution of the biliary leak.

6. Organ injury scale (Appendix A)

G. Extrahepatic biliary tract injury is uncommon. The gallbladder is the most common site; cholecystectomy is the usual treatment. Injury to the extrahepatic bile ducts can be missed at laparotomy unless careful operative inspection of the porta hepatis is performed. A cholangiogram through the gallbladder or cystic duct stump helps define the injury. The location and severity of the injury will dictate the appropriate treatment. Simple bile duct injury (<50% of the circumference) can be repaired with primary suture repair. Complex bile duct injury (>50% of the circumference) may require Roux-en-Y choledochojejunostomy or hepaticojejunostomy.

Primary end-to-end anastomosis of the bile duct is not advised; the stricture rate approaches 50% (Appendix A).

H. Spleen

1. **Incidence.** Blunt splenic injury is produced by compression or deceleration force (e.g., from motor vehicle crashes, falls, or direct blows to the abdomen). Penetrating injury to the spleen is less common.

2. **Anatomy and function.** The spleen is bounded by the stomach, left hemidiaphragm, left kidney and adrenal gland, colon, and chest wall. These relationships define the attachment of the spleen: gastrosplenic ligament, splenorenal ligament, splenophrenic ligament, splenocolic ligament, and pancreaticosplenic attachments. The spleen receives 5% of the cardiac output, primarily through the splenic artery. The splenic artery usually bifurcates into superior and inferior polar arteries. Further division of the blood supply is along transverse planes. The spleen has an open microcirculation without endothelium. It filters blood-borne bacteria, particulate matter, and aged cells. The spleen produces antibodies, properdin, and tuftsin.

3. **Diagnosis**

   a. The patient may have signs of hypovolemia with tachycardia or hypotension, and complain of left upper quadrant tenderness or referred pain to the left shoulder (Kehr's sign).

   b. Physical examination is insensitive and nonspecific in the diagnosis of splenic injury. The patient may have signs of generalized peritoneal irritation or left upper quadrant tenderness or fullness.

   c. Of patients with left lower rib fractures (ribs 9 through 12), 25% will have a splenic injury.

   d. In the unstable trauma patient, ultrasound or DPL will provide the most rapid diagnosis of hemoperitoneum, the source of which is commonly the spleen.

   e. In the stable patient suffering from blunt injury, CT imaging of the abdomen allows delineation and grading of the splenic injury (Appendix A). The most common finding on CT in association with a splenic injury is hemoperitoneum.

   f. Angiography has been used as an adjunct in the management of splenic injury in highly selected patients, with therapeutic embolization of arterial bleeding.

4. **Treatment**

   a. The use of abdominal CT and an understanding of the importance of splenic function have resulted in the preservation of many injured spleens, by either nonoperative management or splenorrhaphy. Management of splenic injury depends primarily on the hemodynamic stability of the patient on presentation. Other factors include the age of the patient, associated injuries (which are the rule in adults), and the grade of the splenic injury.

      i. Nonoperative management of splenic injury is successful in >90% of children, irrespective of the grade of splenic injury.

      ii. Nonoperative management of blunt splenic injury in adults is becoming more routine, with approximately 65% to 75% of adults ultimately managed nonoperatively for blunt injury to the spleen.

   b. If hemodynamically stable, adult patients with grade I or II injury can often be treated nonoperatively (Fig. 26-11). Patients with grade IV or V splenic injuries are usually unstable. Grade III splenic injuries (certainly in children, and in selected adults) can be treated nonoperatively based on stability and reliable physical examination. The failure rate of nonoperative management of splenic injuries in adults increases with grade of splenic injury: grade I, 5%; grade II, 10%; grade III, 20%; grade IV, 33%; and grade V, 75%. In adults (but not children), risk of failure of nonoperative management of blunt splenic injury correlates with grade of splenic injury and quantity of hemoperitoneum. Most failures occur within 72 hours of injury.

MANAGEMENT GUIDELINES FOR BLUNT SPLENIC INJURY IN ADULTS

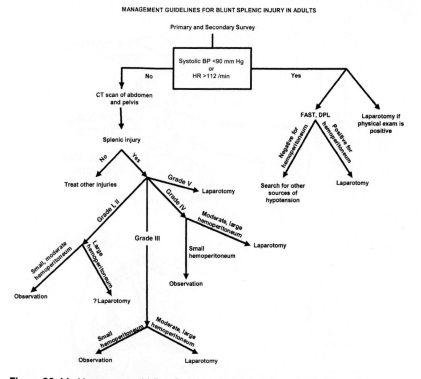

Figure 26-11. Management guidelines for blunt splenic injury. (BP, blood pressure; HR, heart rate; CT, computed tomography; DPL, diagnostic peritoneal lavage; Hcts, hematocrits.)

  c. Patients with significant splenic injuries treated nonoperatively should be observed in a monitored unit and have **immediate access to a CT scanner, a surgeon, and an OR**. Changes in physical examination, hemodynamic stability, ongoing blood, or fluid requirements indicate the need for laparotomy.
  d. Arteriography with embolization has been reported to increase the success rate.
  e. If the patient is hemodynamically unstable, operative treatment is required. Even if splenic conservation is desirable by splenorraphy, patients who require and operation due to splenic bleeding usually have complex enough injuries requiring splenectomy.
    i. Exploration is through a long midline incision. The abdomen is packed and explored. Exsanguinating hemorrhage and gastrointestinal soilage are controlled first.
    ii. Mobilize the spleen to visualize the injury. The operator's nondominant hand will provide medial traction on the spleen to facilitate the operation. The splenocolic ligament can be vascular and require ligation. The splenorenal and splenophrenic ligaments are avascular and should be divided sharply; avoid injury to the splenic capsule as this is performed (Fig. 26-12).
    iii. Further mobilize the spleen by bluntly freeing it from the retroperitoneum. It is important to stay in the plane posterior to the pancreas as the spleen and pancreas are mobilized. The hilum of the spleen can then be controlled with manual compression.

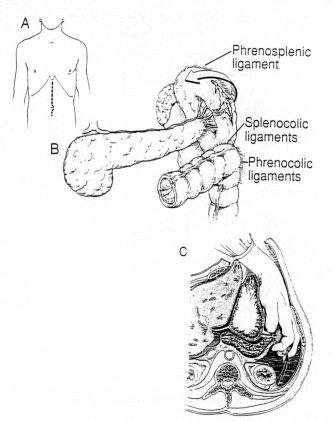

Figure 26-12. A: Midline incision. **B:** Phrenosplenic, splenocolic, and phrenocolic ligaments. **C:** Mobilization of spleen. (From Beal SL, Trunkey DD. Splenic injury. In: Blaisdell FW, Trunkey DD, eds. *Trauma Management—Abdominal Trauma.* 2nd ed. New York, NY: Thieme Medical Publishers; 1993:239, with permission.)

iv. The gastrosplenic ligament with the short gastric vessels is divided and ligated near the spleen to avoid injury or late necrosis of the gastric wall.

v. Then mobilize the spleen into the operative field. Splenectomy should be performed in unstable patients, and in those with associated life-threatening injury, multiple sources for postoperative blood loss (pelvic fracture, multiple long bone fractures, and so forth), and complex splenic injuries.

vi. Splenorrhaphy should be contemplated when circumstances permit. Because of the increased reliance on nonoperative management of splenic injury, splenorrhaphy is rarely possible. The technique is dictated by the magnitude of the splenic injury.

    a) Nonbleeding grade I splenic injury may require no further treatment. Topical hemostatic agents, an argon beam coagulator, or electrocautery may suffice.

    b) Grade II to III splenic injury may require the aforementioned interventions, suture repair, or mesh wrap of capsular defects. Suture repair in adults often requires Teflon pledgets to avoid tearing of the splenic capsule (Fig. 26-13).

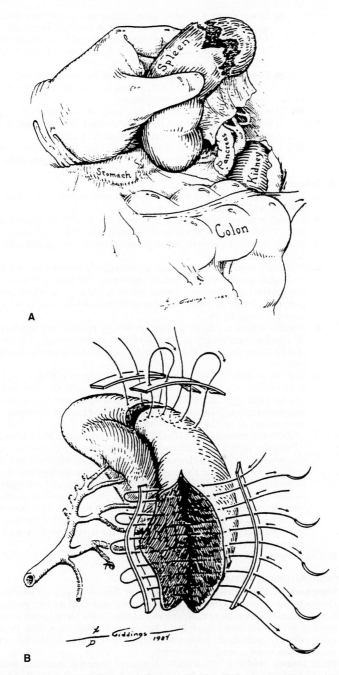

Figure 26-13. Splenic repair. **A:** The mobilized spleen in the operative field. **B:** Horizontal mattress sutures with pledgets for splenic repair. (From Champion HR, Robbs JV, Trunkey DD. Trauma surgery [parts 1 and 2]. In: Dudley H, Carter D, Russell RCG, eds. *Rob and Smith's Operative Surgery*. London: Butterworth, 1989:370, with permission.)

    c) Grade IV to V splenic injury may require anatomic resection, including ligation of the lobar artery. A small rim of capsule at the resection line may help reinforce the resection line. Pledgeted horizontal mattress sutures may also be necessary. Grade V splenic injury usually requires splenectomy.

    d) One third of the splenic mass must be functional to maintain immunocompetence. Thus, at least one half of the spleen must be preserved to justify splenorrhaphy.

  vii. Drainage of the splenic fossa is associated with an increased incidence of subphrenic abscess and should be avoided. The exception is when concern exists about injury to the tail of the pancreas.

  viii. Autotransplantation of the spleen has been reported and involves implanting multiple 1-mm slices of the spleen in the omentum after splenectomy. This technique remains experimental.

5. Outcome

  a. The outcome is generally good; rebleeding rates as low as 1% have been reported with splenorrhaphy.

  b. The failure rate of nonoperative therapy is 2% to 10% in children and as high as 18% in adults. It has been reported that adults >55 years of age are especially susceptible to failure of nonoperative therapy, although some question this.

  c. Pulmonary complications, which are common in patients treated operatively and nonoperatively, include atelectasis, left pleural effusion, and pneumonia. Left subphrenic abscess occurs in 3% to 13% of postoperative patients and may be more common with the use of drains or with concomitant bowel injury.

  d. Thrombocytosis occurs in as many as 50% of patients after splenectomy; the platelet count usually peaks 2 to 10 days postoperatively. The elevated platelet count generally abates in several weeks. Treatment is usually not required.

  e. The risk of overwhelming postsplenectomy infection (OPSI) is greater in children than in adults; the overall risk is less than 0.5%. The mortality rate for OPSI approaches 50%. The common organisms are encapsulated organisms: meningococcus, *Haemophilus influenzae,* and *Streptococcus pneumoniae,* as well as *Staphylococcus aureus* and *Escherichia coli.* After splenectomy, pneumococcal (Pneumovax), *H. influenzae,* and meningococcal vaccines should be administered. The timing of injection of the vaccine is controversial. Some authors recommend giving the vaccine 3 to 4 weeks postoperatively because the patient may be too immunosuppressed in the immediate postinjury period. Current recommendation is to repeat the pneumococcal vaccination at 5 years. The patient should be discharged from the hospital with a clear understanding of the concerns about OPSI, should wear a tag alerting health care providers of his or her asplenic state, and should begin penicillin therapy with the development of even mild infections.

6. Organ injury scale (Appendix A)

VI. RETROPERITONEAL HEMATOMAS

  A. Management of retroperitoneal hematomas depends largely on location and the mechanism of injury. Generally, all penetrating wounds of the retroperitoneum found at laparotomy require thorough exploration. Some simply observe nonexpanding perinephric hematomas. If the hematoma is large, expanding, or proximal to the retroperitoneal vessels (aorta, iliac artery, and so forth), first obtain proximal and distal control of the vessels.

  B. Blunt trauma produces 70% to 80% of retroperitoneal hematomas; most are caused by pelvic fracture. In general, nonexpanding lateral (zone II) or pelvic (zone III) hematomas secondary to blunt trauma do not require exploration. Be certain that the overlying bowel (i.e., colon or duodenum) is intact (Fig. 26-14).

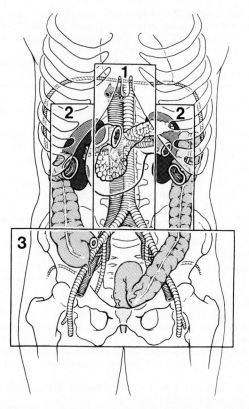

Figure 26-14. Zones of retroperitoneum. **1:** Central-medial retroperitoneal zone. **2:** Lateral retroperitoneal zone. **3:** Pelvic retroperitoneal zone. (From Kudsk KA, Sheldon GF. Retroperitoneal hematoma. In: Blaisdell FW, Trunkey DD, eds. *Trauma Management—Abdominal Trauma.* New York, NY: Thieme Medical Publishers; 1982:281, with permission.)

    1. Central hematomas (zone I) always require exploration to rule out a major vascular or visceral injury. In the case of ongoing hemorrhage, the aorta can be occluded at the diaphragmatic hiatus or above the diaphragm via a left thoracotomy, and the vascular structures approached by mobilizing the abdominal viscera from the retroperitoneum (right or left medial visceral rotation). Injury to the pancreas and duodenum must also be sought in exploration of a central hematoma.

  C. Most retroperitoneal vascular injuries can be repaired with a lateral arteriorrhaphy or venorrhaphy. If a patch is required, prosthetic material can be used, except in the setting of gross contamination with colon contents, in which case an autologous patch should be used.

Bibliography

Asensio JA, Feliciano DV, Britt LD, et al. Management of duodenal injuries. *Curr Probl Surg* 1993;30:1021–1100.

Blaisdell FW, Trunkey DD, eds. *Trauma Management—Abdominal Trauma.* New York, NY: Thieme Medical Publishers; 1993.

Boone DC, Federle M, Billiar TR, et al. Evolution of major hepatic trauma: Identification of patterns of injury. *J Trauma* 1995;39:344–350.

Buckman BF Jr, Miraliakbari R, Badellino MM. Juxtahepatic venous injuries: A critical review of reported management strategies. *J Trauma* 2000;48:978–984.

Cogbill T, Moore EE, Feliciano DV, et al. Conservative management of duodenal trauma: A multicenter perspective. *J Trauma* 1990;30:1469–1475.

Cogbill TH, Moore EE, Jurkovich J, et al. Nonoperative management of blunt splenic trauma: A multicenter experience. *J Trauma* 1989;29:1312–1317.

Demetriades D, Velmahos G. Indications for laparotomy. In: Feliciano DV, Moore EE, Mattox KL, eds. *Trauma*. 5th ed. New York, NY: McGraw-Hill; 2004:593–610.

Dutton RP, McCunn M, Hyder M, et al. Factor VIIa for correction of traumatic coagulopathy. *J Trauma* 2004;57:709–719.

Esposito TJ, Gamelli RL. Injury to the spleen. In: Feliciano DV, Moore EE, Mattox KL, eds. *Trauma*. Stamford, Conn: Appleton & Lange; 1996:525–550.

Fabian TC, Bee TK, Cagiano C, et al. Current issues in trauma. *Current Probl Surg* 2002;39:1160–1244.

Fabian TC, Croce MA. Abdominal trauma, including indications for celiotomy. In: Feliciano DV, Moore EE, Mattox KL, eds. *Trauma*. Stamford, Conn: Appleton & Lange; 1996:441–459.

Fealk M, Osipov R, Foster K, et al. The conundrum of traumatic colon injury. *Am J Surg* 2004;188:663–670.

Feliciano DV, Jordan GL, Bitondo CG, et al. Management of 1000 cases of hepatic trauma. *Ann Surg* 1986;294:438–445.

Grossman MD, Schwab CW, Reilly PR, et al. Determining anatomic injury with computed tomography in selected torso gunshot wounds. *J Trauma* 1998;45:446–456.

Haan JM, Biffl W, Knudson MM, et al. Splenic embolization revisited: A multicenter review. *J Trauma* 2003;56:542–547.

Hasson J, Stern D, Moss G. Penetrating duodenal trauma. *J Trauma* 1984;24:471–474.

Jurkovich GJ. Injury to the duodenum and pancreas. In: Feliciano DV, Moore EE, Mattox KL, eds. *Trauma*. Stamford, Conn: Appleton & Lange; 1996:573–594.

Mackersie RC, Tiwary AD, Shackford SR, et al. Intra-abdominal injury following blunt trauma—Identifying the high-risk patient using objective risk factors. *Arch Surg* 1989;124:809–813.

McGrath V, Fabian TC, Croce MA, et al. Rectal trauma: Management based on anatomic distinctions. *Am Surg* 1998;64:1136–1141.

Meyer AA, Kudsk KA, Sheldon GF. Retroperitoneal hematoma. In: Blaisdell FW, Trunkey DD, eds. *Trauma Management—Abdominal Trauma*. New York, NY: Thieme Medical Publishers; 1993:398–413.

Pachter HL, Knudson MM, Esrig B, et al. Status of nonoperative management of blunt hepatic injuries in 1995: A multicenter experience with 404 patients. *J Trauma* 1996;40:31–38.

Pachter HL, Liang HG, Hofstetter SR. Liver and biliary tract trauma. In: Feliciano DV, Moore EE, Mattox KL, eds. *Trauma*. Stamford, Conn: Appleton & Lange; 1996:487–523.

Patton JH Jr, Lyden SP, Croce MA, et al. Pancreatic trauma: A simplified management guideline. *J Trauma* 1997;43:234–241.

Peitzman AB, Heil B, Rivera L, et al. Blunt splenic injury in adults: Multi-institutional study of the Eastern Association for the Surgery of Trauma. *J Trauma* 2000;49:177–189.

Rozycki G, Ochsner M, Schmidt J, et al. A prospective study of surgeon-performed ultrasound as the primary adjunct modality for injured patient assessment. *J Trauma* 1995;39(3):492–500.

Singer DB. Post-splenectomy sepsis. In: Rosenburg HS, Bolande RP, eds. *Perspectives in Pediatric Pathology*. Chicago, Ill: Mosby—Year Book; 1973:285.

Snyder W, Weigelt J, Watkins WL, et al. The surgical management of duodenal trauma. *Arch Surg* 1980;115:422–429.

Stone HH, Fabian TC. Management of perforating colon trauma: Randomization between primary closure and exteriorization. *Am Surg* 1979;190:430–438.

Wilson RF, Walt AJ. General considerations in abdominal trauma. In: Wilson RF, Walt AJ, eds. *Management of Trauma: Pitfalls and Practices*. Baltimore, Md: Williams & Wilkins; 1996:411–431.

ABDOMINAL VASCULAR INJURY

MICHAEL B. SHAPIRO

27

I. **INTRODUCTION.** More than 90% of abdominal vascular injuries are caused by penetrating wounds. These injuries are found at laparotomy in 25% of patients with gunshot wounds and in 10% of patients with stab wounds. They are rarely isolated, and multiple associated intraabdominal injuries, including multiple hollow viscus injuries, should be expected. The availability of semiautomatic weapons has increased multiple shot assaults, and increased the incidence of these injuries.

II. **MECHANISM OF INJURY.** Abdominal vascular injury may result in a hematoma contained in the retroperitoneum or mesentery, or free intraperitoneal bleeding. This distinction is critical in defining a patient's status at initial presentation. Penetrating injuries cause through-and-through perforations or partial wall defects. Complete transection of abdominal vessels is likely to be immediately lethal and, therefore, uncommonly seen. Blast effect injuries from tangential high-power gunshot wounds are uncommon in abdominal vessels, but may present as an intimal flap. Blunt abdominal vascular injuries arise from a direct blow or rapid deceleration, often occurring in association with seatbelt injury, mesenteric avulsion, or pelvic fracture.

III. **PRESENTATION AND DIAGNOSIS.** Determination of missile trajectory is critical in establishing the diagnosis. A bullet that crosses the upper abdomen or violates the posterior abdomen or posterolateral pelvis frequently causes a vascular injury.
   A. **Normotensive patient.** With early presentation and contained hematoma, a patient may have normal blood pressure and little pain. This usually occurs with wounds to the flank or back. Evaluation may include chest and supine abdominal radiographs, which should include metallic markers (e.g., paper clips, x-ray markers, metallic buttons) at wound sites to help determine trajectory. Local wound exploration can also help define trajectory, especially for tangential wounds. Triple-contrast (oral, rectal, and intravenous [IV]) computerized tomography (CT) may define the extent of a contained hematoma, assess trajectory, and establish the presence of retroperitoneal colon injury in a patient with flank or posterior wounds. Angiographic evaluation with embolization can be definitive management for the patient with arterial bleeding after blunt pelvic injury, and may also be appropriate for the stable patient with isolated solid viscus injury. Endovascular repair of partial thickness aortic injury identified by CT in the stable, blunt-injured patient has been described.
   B. **Hypotensive patient.** A patient with a penetrating abdominal injury and hypotension should be presumed to have a vascular injury, which requires prompt laparotomy. Patients can also present with abdominal distention, gross hematuria, or loss of one or both lower extremity pulses. The patient with a contained hematoma can become normotensive with fluid resuscitation, whereas the patient with active hemorrhage will not. **The association of hypotension and a penetrating wound to the abdomen strongly suggests a major vascular injury in the abdomen or pelvis.**
   C. **Exsanguinated patient.** Some patients with abdominal injury present with profound hypotension, tachycardia or agonal rhythm, obtundation, or massive abdominal distention. Assume these patients have a major vascular injury with

free intraperitoneal hemorrhage and near total blood volume loss. They require **immediate laparotomy** for control of hemorrhage, resuscitation, and definitive injury management.

IV. INITIAL EVALUATION AND RESUSCITATION

A. Normotensive and hypotensive patients

1. Establish airway control early and definitively; administer 100% oxygen by face mask, bag-mask device, or endotracheal tube.

2. Intravenous access should be promptly established with multiple large-bore lines in the upper extremities, subclavian, or jugular veins. Avoid femoral lines if concern for abdominal vascular injury exists.

3. Prewarmed fluids and fluid warmers should be used to avoid hypothermia. All fluids should be warmed to 38°C to 40°C.

4. Use blood transfusion for patients who are actively bleeding. Blood is reconstituted with normal saline (250–500 mL) at 38°C to 40°C; this warms and dilutes the blood, decreasing viscosity and improving flow.

   a. Type O, universal donor blood, should be immediately available in the trauma room.

   b. Crossmatched blood may require 40 to 60 minutes to be available. **Do not delay transfusion in the unstable patient.**

   c. A massive transfusion protocols should be initiated.

5. Blood components (fresh frozen plasma and platelets) should be transfused early in the patient with a major vascular injury to avoid coagulopathy.

6. Blood bank notification is critical and a massive transfusion requirement should be expected. Request immediate delivery of 10 units of type O, universal donor packed red blood cells, to the operating room (OR). O-positive blood is given to male patients, O-negative to female patients. Also request immediate preparation of 10 units of fresh frozen plasma and 10 units of platelets for administration as soon as ready.

7. Use rapid-infusion and cell-saver devices in the OR.

8. Administer tetanus prophylaxis and antibiotics preoperatively, with coverage of aerobic and anaerobic organisms.

B. Exsanguinating patient

1. Immediately perform endotracheal intubation; administer 100% oxygen.

2. Begin blood transfusion immediately with type O, universal donor blood, and notify the blood bank of massive requirements, as previously stated.

3. **Immediate laparotomy with definitive control of injuries must be obtained promptly in the OR. Hemorrhage control and resuscitation occur simultaneously in the OR.**

4. Left anterolateral thoracotomy may be necessary to obtain aortic control. Consider this for the patient with agonal cardiac rhythm, systolic blood pressure <70 mmHg, and massive abdominal distension. This maneuver is rarely effective unless the abdominal source can be immediately controlled and the aorta unclamped.

5. **Damage control** operative procedures are necessary in this setting. The immediate goal with these patients is to prevent early death from exsanguination. This approach involves the following three phases.

   a. Rapid operative control of hemorrhage and contamination, followed by peritoneal packing and abdominal skin closure.

   b. Ongoing resuscitation in the intensive care unit (ICU) until rewarming and reversal of coagulopathy and hypothermia are achieved. **If hemorrhage from solid visceral injury is controlled with packing, consider immediate angiographic evaluation after the patient is physiologically resuscitated, both for anatomic clarification and**

therapeutic intervention, before returning to the OR for the definitive laparotomy.

c. Operative reexploration with definitive injury management and fascial closure.

V. Operation (Table 27-1)

A. Preparation. To avoid hypothermia, place the patient on a warming blanket with head and extremities wrapped in a Baer hugger, and maintain room temperature at >27°C. Skin should be prepared and the patient draped from the chin to the knees and to the table laterally, to enable access to the chest or groin, and saphenous vein harvesting.

B. Exploration

1. Explore the abdomen through a midline incision, extending from the xiphoid process to the symphysis pubis. A large retroperitoneal hematoma can cause significant distortion of normal anatomy and tissue planes.

TABLE 27-1 **Conduct of the Operation for Major Abdominal Vascular Injury**

Preparation
–Identify trauma operating room in advance, with anesthesia and operating equipment in place.
–Maintain operating room temperature >27°C.
–Have cell-saver and rapid-infusion devices in room.

Position
–Patient supine, both arms out
–Multiple, large-bore intravenous lines above the diaphragm
–Urinary catheter with collection bag beneath head of bed
–Chest tubes, if present, to suction and in view of nurses and anesthesiologists and surgeons
–Skin preparation from chin to knees, drape to expose torso and thighs, and laterally on the chest to allow thoracotomy
–Extra operating room help (i.e., scrub assistant or extra physician) to help operating surgeon

Incision
–Midline, xiphoid to symphysis pubis
–If patient is agonal and aortic control is needed, consider left thoracotomy with aortic occlusion first.

First Maneuvers: Assessment
–Use four-hand retraction, evacuate blood and clot, pack all four quadrants.
–Look for bleeding; if easy, control large bleeding sites.
–Note hematomas and sites of contamination.
–Place large, self-retaining retractor (e.g., Bookwalter, Thompson).

Second Maneuvers: Exposure
–With retroperitoneal hematoma, perform right or left medial visceral rotation, or other necessary maneuvers to expose retroperitoneal vascular structures.

Third Maneuvers: Control and Repair
–Control hemorrhage: decide on the "best" approach for proximal and distal control, or for control of an active bleeding site directly or through a hematoma.
–Control contamination: after arterial and venous control is obtained, control all hollow visceral injuries.
–Vascular repair: reestablish vascular continuity with repair or graft. If patient is in extremis; cold, coagulopathic, acidotic—consider damage control (with intravascular shunt) or vessel ligation.

2. Compress visible active arterial hemorrhage with digital pressure or packs. Control active hemorrhage from within or beneath a hematoma in the same fashion, after directly opening the hematoma. Proximal control can be obtained with occlusive clamps or tourniquets, or if the injury is visible, with side-biting vascular clamps that exclude the injury without occluding the vessel. Select a Fogarty or Foley balloon catheter, which can help control hemorrhage during local dissection, based on the size of the injured vessel. **When the patient's condition warrants a "damage control" strategy, continuity of critical vessels (e.g., superior mesenteric or common/external iliac arteries, etc.) can be maintained with a temporary vascular shunt.** The decision to utilize a damage control approach depends on the patient's complex of injuries and physiology (Chapter 28).

3. Venous hemorrhage may be controlled with finger or sponge stick compression while obtaining proximal and distal control. Allis or Babcock clamps can be used to approximate the edges of a venous injury to facilitate suture repair.

4. Use cell-saving techniques from the outset to ensure maximal blood salvage.

C. **Midline injury (zone 1)** is associated with injuries to the aorta, vena cava, their bifurcations, central branches, and tributaries. Operative approach is directed by findings of free hemorrhage versus hematoma, and its origin above or below the transverse mesocolon (Fig. 27-1).

1. **Exposure**

    a. If the hematoma is cephalad to the transverse mesocolon, obtain proximal control of the supraceliac aorta first. **Medial visceral rotation** of the left-sided viscera (spleen, tail of pancreas, colon, kidney) exposes the anterolateral

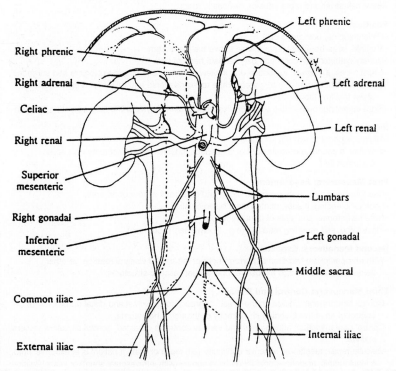

Figure 27-1. Abdominal vascular anatomy. (From Frey W. Abdominal arterial trauma. In: Blaisdell FW, Trunkey DD, eds. *Trauma Management—Abdominal Trauma.* 2nd ed. New York, NY: Thieme Medical Publishers; 1993:345, with permission.)

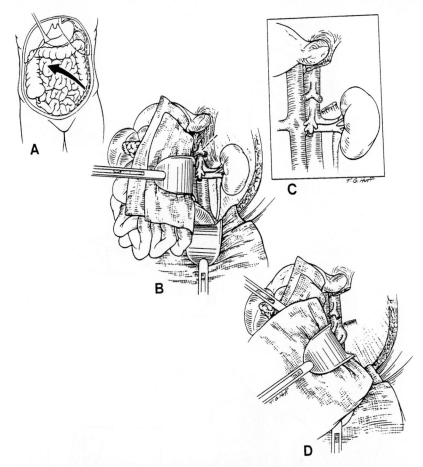

Figure 27-2. Left-sided medial visceral rotation. (From Frey W. Abdominal arterial trauma. In: Blaisdell FW, Trunkey DD, eds. *Trauma Management—Abdominal Trauma*. 2nd ed. New York, NY: Thieme Medical Publishers; 1993:345, with permission.)

aorta from the diaphragmatic hiatus to the bifurcation (Fig. 27-2). The distal descending thoracic aorta can be controlled in the posterior mediastinum by dividing the crural fibers of the diaphragm to the left of the aortic hiatus and the parasympathetic plexus surrounding it.

b. If hematoma is below the transverse mesocolon, reflection of the right colon with extensive mobilization of the duodenum and head of the pancreas (**right-sided medial visceral rotation**) is commonly used to expose the infrahepatic vena cava, and also effectively exposes the suprarenal aorta below the celiac axis and superior mesenteric artery, the distal aorta, and the right common iliac artery and vein (Fig. 27-3).

c. In contrast to the stable hematoma, when active hemorrhage cephalad to the transverse mesocolon is encountered, control the bleeding immediately by manual compression. The aorta can be controlled at the hiatus after dividing the gastrohepatic omentum by retraction of the stomach and esophagus to the left, finger dissection to the aorta on the vertebral column,

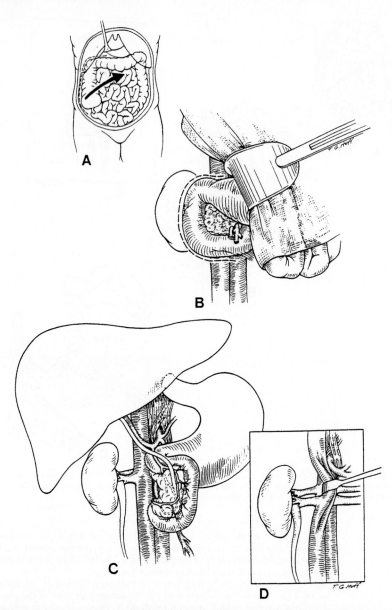

Figure 27-3. Right-sided medial visceral rotation. (From Frey W. Abdominal arterial trauma. In: Blaisdell FW, Trunkey DD, eds. *Trauma Management—Abdominal Trauma*. 2nd ed. New York, NY: Thieme Medical Publishers; 1993:345, with permission.)

and applying an aortic clamp or manual compression device. Exposure may require a thoracoabdominal incision into the left chest and takedown of the left hemidiaphragm.

d. If a central hematoma extending laterally into the flanks or active arterial hemorrhage is present caudal to the transverse mesocolon, control of the infrarenal aorta is obtained. The transverse colon and small intestine are reflected superiorly and to the right, respectively, and the midline retroperitoneum is divided to expose the aorta and vena cava from the renal vessels distally.

e. Hematoma or active venous bleeding from under the duodenum suggests a more proximal vena cava injury, which can be better visualized and controlled by the right-sided medial visceral rotation.

2. **The aorta.** Direct repair, in a transverse direction to limit narrowing, is performed with 4-0 polypropylene suture. In the event of a large lateral defect, narrowing may be avoided by a polytetrafluoroethylene (PTFE) patch. Extensive destruction may necessitate placement of a Dacron or PTFE graft. In desperate situations, the distal aorta, below the renal arteries, can be ligated, although lower extremity ischemia is likely and extraanatomic revascularization may be subsequently required (Table 27-2). Survival in this circumstance is unlikely.

3. **Celiac axis, superior mesenteric artery, and superior mesenteric vein.** The celiac axis is repaired with 5-0 or 6-0 polypropylene suture, but it can also be ligated without significant morbidity. Injury to the portal vein or proximal superior mesenteric artery or vein may require transection of the neck of the pancreas to visualize and control. Attempt primary repair with 5-0 or 6-0 polypropylene suture. Extensive injury to the superior mesenteric artery may require bypass with saphenous vein or PTFE graft to maintain midgut viability. Temporary shunting of the superior mesenteric artery with delayed reconstruction has been reported. In theory this artery can be ligated, but collateral flow in the trauma patient in shock is usually inadequate. If ligation is performed plan a second-look procedure within 24 hours. The superior mesenteric vein should be repaired, when possible; ligation is acceptable for the patient in extremis, but mesenteric viability will be jeopardized and a second-look operation is necessary within 24 hours.

TABLE 27-2   **Abdominal Vessel Ligation and Expected Complications***

Vessel	Complication	Recommendations
Celiac axis	None	
Splenic artery	None if short gastric vessels intact; possible splenic infarction	Consider splenectomy
Common hepatic artery	None if portal vein intact; possible gallbladder ischemia	Consider cholecystectomy
Superior mesenteric artery	Bowel ischemia	Second-look procedure
Superior mesenteric vein	Bowel ischemia	Second-look procedure
Portal vein	Bowel ischemia	Second-look procedure
Suprarenal inferior vena cava	Renal failure	
Infrarenal aorta	Lower extremity ischemia	Consider calf fasciotomies or extra-anatomic bypass
Infrarenal inferior vena cava	Lower extremity edema	Wrap and elevate legs
Left renal vein (proximal)	None	
Right renal vein	Renal ischemia	Nephrectomy
Common and external iliac artery	Lower extremity ischemia	Consider calf fasciotomies or extra-anatomic bypass
Common and external iliac vein	Lower extremity edema	Wrap and elevate legs
Internal iliac vein	None	

*Before ligation, consider arterial and venous temporary shunts.

4. **Mesenteric** injuries are usually visible on direct inspection. These can be controlled directly with local dissection and ligation; avoid blind clamping into the hematoma. It is imperative to reassess bowel viability after ligation. Close the mesenteric defect to prevent internal hernia.

5. **Inferior vena cava** injuries can be repaired with 5-0 polypropylene suture. The infrarenal vena cava can be ligated, although measures must be taken to minimize lower extremity edema postoperatively, and bilateral four-compartment calf fasciotomies are recommended. The suprarenal vena cava should be repaired or reconstructed to prevent possible renal failure, but it can be ligated in the patient in extremis.

D. **Lateral injury (zone 2)** is associated with injury to the renal artery and vein, and kidney. Penetrating injuries should be explored. In some centers with immediately available angioembolization capabilities, a selective approach is taken to exploration in which a stable hematoma is evaluated by angiography rather than operative examination. With blunt injury, a stable hematoma should not be disturbed if a hollow viscus injury can be excluded, especially if a preoperative study shows intact blood flow and urine excretion. This is true even if the study shows urinary extravasation, provided this is contained within Gerota's fascia.

1. **Exposure**

    a. With an expanding but contained perirenal hematoma, first obtain proximal control of the ipsilateral renal vessels through the midline retroperitoneum. Arterial control requires mobilization of the overlying left renal vein. Control of the right renal vein requires mobilization of right colon and duodenum (see Fig. 27.3). If hematoma extends from the lateral aspect to midline or beyond, then first obtain proximal and distal aortic control before disturbing the hematoma.

    b. Active bleeding from a renal injury and hemodynamic instability preclude proximal vessel control. The kidney is manually compressed and elevated through Gerota's fascia laterally, and a vascular clamp placed across the renal hilum.

2. **Renal artery** injuries should be repaired directly or with end-to-end anastomosis with 5-0 polypropylene suture. Interposition grafting with autogenous vein is appropriate only when the patient is stable and the kidney is believed salvageable. If palpation determines that the contralateral kidney is present and of normal size, then nephrectomy is advisable if the patient is unstable and the renal artery cannot be easily repaired.

3. **Renal vein.** Perform lateral venorrhaphy in a transverse direction with 5-0 polypropylene suture. Right renal vein ligation necessitates nephrectomy. The left renal vein can be ligated in the midline, proximal to patent adrenal and gonadal veins.

E. **Pelvic injury (zone 3)**

1. **Exposure.** Full exposure of pelvic vascular injuries may require mobilization of the colon from the pelvis.

    a. When an expanding pelvic hematoma is identified over the iliac vessels, obtain proximal control of the common iliac artery and vein through the midline retroperitoneum at the aortic and inferior vena cava bifurcation or, preferentially, proximal to the area of injury on the iliac vessels themselves. Temporary transection of the right common iliac artery may be necessary to enable control of the proximal right common iliac vein. Obtain distal control of the external iliac artery and vein just proximal to the inguinal ligament on the up-slope of the pelvic floor. Injuries to the distal iliac vessels may necessitate control of the common femoral vessels through a groin incision. Expose the internal iliac artery after gaining control of the common and external iliac vessels and opening the hematoma.

    b. Deep pelvic arterial bleeding and venous bleeding from deep pelvic, presacral veins is best handled by tamponade and arteriography with embolization.

2. **The iliac artery.** Repair common and external iliac artery injuries with 5-0 polypropylene suture or an autogenous vein or PTFE graft when direct repair

is not possible. Ligation of these vessels is associated with a 40% to 50% rate of subsequent amputation (ligation of the common iliac artery is better tolerated than the more distal external iliac artery). When ligation is necessary, consider a femoral-femoral, extra-anatomic bypass, or at minimum, a four-compartment calf fasciotomy. Internal iliac artery ligation is well-tolerated.

3. **The iliac vein** injuries should be repaired with 5-0 polypropylene suture, when possible, but ligation is well tolerated. Ligation of the external or common iliac vein can lead to significant lower extremity edema in the early postoperative period. Leg elevation and pressure wrapping from toes to high thighs is necessary. Anticoagulation after venous repair or ligation is controversial; the risk of iliofemoral thrombosis is nearly 30%.

F. Portal and retrohepatic injury

1. Exposure

a. **Hematoma or hemorrhage** in the porta hepatis is controlled with a vascular clamp across the portal structures just above the duodenum (Pringle maneuver); a second clamp at the liver edge may also be helpful. The hepatic artery and portal vein are dissected and isolated, and the injury identified.

b. Control of the retropancreatic portion of the portal vein may require transection of the neck of the pancreas.

c. An expanding retrohepatic hematoma or active hemorrhage is initially controlled with manual compression of the overlying liver. Although direct repair may be feasible, control can also require vascular isolation of the liver with occlusion of the hepatoduodenal ligament, and suprahepatic and infrahepatic vena cava.

i. Although some authors recommend an atriocaval shunt, necessitating median sternotomy, we generally do not. Expert help and exposure are essential in dealing with this injury.

ii. In some cases, when manual compression seems to control bleeding, firm packing may be appropriate (damage control) with subsequent angiographic embolization of bleeding arterial vessels or balloon control of the inferior vena cava.

iii. Veno-veno bypass with vascular isolation of the liver and direct repair of the liver is successful, when available.

2. **Hepatic artery.** Direct repair or end-to-end reanastomosis is performed with 5-0 polypropylene suture. Perform ligation in the presence of extensive injury or continued instability, which is well tolerated, but consider performing a cholecystectomy.

3. **Portal vein.** Perform direct transverse venorrhaphy with 5-0 polypropylene suture. The vein can be ligated in the presence of extensive injury, but hepatic and mesenteric viability can be compromised, and a second-look operation within 24 hours is necessary.

4. **Retrohepatic vena cava and Hepatic veins.** One attempt should be made to visualize the injury directly for control and repair. If this is impossible because of exsanguinating hemorrhage, resume compression of the overlying liver. Options for management include a direct transhepatic approach, vascular isolation of the liver, atriocaval shunt (usually performed with a 36 F chest tube or no. 8 or 9 endotracheal tube), or retrograde balloon catheter insertions through the femoral vein for occlusion above and below the injury or veno veno bypass and direct repair. Repair the vena cava transversely with 4-0 polypropylene suture. Branches of the hepatic veins can be ligated.

 AXIOMS

■ The patient with abdominal vascular injury can present normotensive, hypotensive, or in extremis from exsanguination.

■ In penetrating injury, determination of trajectory is the key to anatomic diagnosis in penetrating injury.

- A patient in shock with a penetrating injury and distended abdomen has a major vascular injury until proved otherwise.
- In cases of suspected abdominal vascular injury, anticipate massive transfusion requirements. Begin blood transfusion early, including replacement of plasma and platelets.
- Expect major distortion of anatomy by hemorrhage and hematoma.
- Direct pressure with fingers or packs is the first maneuver to control bleeding. Hemorrhage control may require a direct approach through the hematoma, with finger dissection and sponge stick or clamp control. Proximal and distal control are preferred for vascular repair, but may not always be possible initially.
- Patients who present in extremis with shock and exsanguinating injury benefit from a damage control approach, which emphasizes immediate control of hemorrhage and contamination, possible temporary vascular shunting and delayed definitive reconstruction.

Bibliography

Carrillo EH, Spain PA, Wilson MA, et al. Alternatives in the management of penetrating injuries to the iliac vessels. *J Trauma* 1998;44(6):1024–1030.

Feliciano DV. Abdominal vessels. In: Ivatury RR, Cayten CG, eds. *The Textbook of Penetrating Trauma*. Baltimore, Md: Williams & Wilkins; 1996:702–715.

Feliciano DV. Management of traumatic retroperitoneal hematoma. *Ann Surg* 1990; 211:109–123.

Fry WR, Fry RE, Fry WJ. Operative exposure of the abdominal arteries for trauma. *Arch Surg* 1991;126:289–291.

Reilly PM, Rotondo MF, Carpenter JC, et al. Temporary vascular continuity during damage control: Intraluminal shunting for proximal superior mesenteric artery injury. *J Trauma* 1995;39:757–760.

Rotondo MF, Schwab CW, McGonigal MD, et al. Damage control: An approach for improved survival in exsanguinating penetrating abdominal injury. *J Trauma* 1993; 35:375–383.

DAMAGE CONTROL

*ERIC A. TOSCHLOG, SCOTT G. SAGRAVES,
AND MICHAEL F. ROTONDO*

28

I. **INTRODUCTION.** The damage control approach arose out of the necessity to rapidly stop cavitary bleeding, stage physiologic resuscitation, and reverse the pathophysiological spiral leading to death. In select circumstances, the traditional approach to exsanguinating abdominal injury was often not effective. This appeared particularly true in physiologically unstable patients with multiple penetrating wounds or blunt high-energy transfer with massive blood loss. During the struggle for surgical control of bleeding, repeated bouts of hypotension and physiologic instability frequently resulted in a lethal "triad of death" comprised of metabolic acidosis, hypothermia, and coagulopathy. Historically, if the surgeon persisted with the traditional approach—completion of definitive laparotomy or thoracotomy—this vicious cycle of events invariably led to increased patient mortality.

Damage control surgery (DCS), an alternative to operating beyond the physiologic reserve of the patient, was first reported in the trauma literature in the early 1990s. For the trauma surgeon, damage control describes a technique of abbreviated laparotomy, with precise containment of bleeding and contamination, and temporary intraabdominal packing for initial injury control prompted by acidosis, hypothermia, and coagulopathy. Subsequently, the patient is transferred to the intensive care unit (ICU) for physiologic restoration and later definitive repair of all injuries in the operating room (OR). For the practicing general surgeon caring for trauma patients, this approach can be useful to stabilize and transfer the trauma patient to a Level I trauma center. For the general surgeon caring for the patient with an abdominal catastrophe, such as acute mesenteric ischemia or a ruptured abdominal aortic aneurysm, it may have important applicability in temporization and stabilization of the patient. In either case, damage control constitutes a premeditated, deliberate surgical exercise requiring careful judgment. Damage control is not surgical failure, but rather an aggressive and data-driven maneuver to break the pattern of physiologic failure and irreversible oxygen debt. In the decade following initial description, DCS has become the standard of care for the physiologically exhausted trauma patient, and has gained application in general, gynecologic, vascular, and orthopedic surgery.

A. **Definition.** Damage control is defined in three distinct phases.
   1. **Part I.** Application of simple techniques at initial exploratory laparotomy to control (1) hemorrhage and (2) contamination. Definitive reconstruction is delayed. Intraabdominal packing is applied to all dissected surfaces and injured organs and vascular injuries are ligated or shunted, followed by utilization of a temporary abdominal closure.
   2. **Part II.** Secondary and continued resuscitation in the ICU characterized by maximization of hemodynamics: aimed at optimization of oxygen delivery and consumption, lactate clearance, core rewarming, correction of coagulopathy, ventilatory support, monitoring for abdominal compartment syndrome, continued injury identification, and management of the open abdomen.
   3. **Part III.** Reoperation for removal of intraabdominal packing, definitive repair of abdominal injury, and attempted fascial closure, if possible. In addition, extraabdominal injury repair may ensue.

II. **PATIENT SELECTION.** Success of damage control is dependent on judicious selection of patients based on the development of abnormal physiology from profound hypoperfusion. Although multiple studies have attempted to identify objective elements in the selection process in an effort to define strict criteria, none have successfully done so. However, a number of important factors contributing to the identification of patients best served by DCS have been elucidated. The recognition of these factors is aided by the concurrent consideration of predictive (a) conditions, (b) injury complexes, and (c) critical physiologic factors.

A. Conditions. Pertinent mechanisms of injury and the presence of physiologic instability:

  1. High-energy blunt torso trauma
  2. Multiple torso penetrating injuries
  3. Profound hemodynamic instability and hypoperfusion
  4. Metabolic acidosis, hypothermia, and coagulopathy as a result of initial injury or comorbidity

B. Complexes. Recognition of injury patterns associated with the need for damage control:

  1. Major abdominal vascular injury with concomitant visceral injuries
  2. Multiregional exsanguination with concomitant visceral injuries
  3. Multiregional injury in the presence of intraabdominal injury with competing priorities, such as severe closed head injury, thoracic aortic injury, or pelvic fracture

C. Critical factors. Intraoperative considerations:

  1. Severe metabolic acidosis with pH <7.30
  2. Hypothermia with temperature <35°C
  3. Coagulopathy, as evidenced by the development of nonmechanical bleeding within the operative field, elevation of both prothrombin time (PT) and partial thromboplastin time (PTT), thrombocytopenia, hypofibrinogenemia, or massive transfusion (>10 units packed red blood cells [PRBCs]).
  4. Resuscitation and operative time >90 minutes

III. TECHNICAL CONSIDERATIONS. Elements of the damage control approach are contrary to traditional surgical teaching and, therefore, warrant special mention.

A. Damage control, part I. Critical elements in the first phase of damage control include recognition of the need for a truncated procedure and the need for establishing injury control. The foundation of injury control includes control of (a) hemorrhage and (b) contamination.

  1. Hemorrhage control

  a. Establish initial control of vascular injuries using vascular clamps and suture ligatures. Simple lateral repairs may be possible; however, complex reconstruction is not advised if critical factors identifying need for DCS are manifest. If complex reconstruction is required, temporary vascular shunting can be another useful adjunct.

  b. Complex repair of solid organ hemorrhage should also be avoided. Splenic and renal injuries should be managed by rapid resection. Hepatic injuries may require a variety of temporizing measures, including hepatic arterial and portal venous occlusion via the Pringle maneuver; manual pressure using the most experienced available surgical hands; packing with laparotomy pads; and plugging using procoagulant materials or balloon catheter tamponade. Complex anatomic resection or debridement, extended finger fracture techniques, and hepatorrhaphy should be avoided. Interventional radiology for complex hepatic, renal, pelvic, and muscle hemorrhage is of paramount importance and should immediately follow the abbreviated surgical procedure, when necessary.

  c. The operation should end when the patient is hypothermic, coagulopathic, and acidotic and only *nonsurgical* bleeding continues. It is critically important to understand that **leaving an abdomen with ongoing surgical bleeding is destined to continue bleeding.**

  2. Contamination control

  a. The goal of contamination control is to rapidly stop spillage of hollow viscus contents using the most simple technique available. Hollow viscus injuries are controlled by ligation, rapid oversewing of defects, rapid staple closure, or resection. Restoration of gastrointestinal continuity, stoma formation, and placement of gastrostomy or jejunostomy tubes should be deferred to damage control part III.

- **b.** Bile duct injuries are temporized by ligation, end choledochostomy, or simple drainage. Complex reconstructions should be avoided. A small catheter inserted into the proximal duct limb can be externalized to temporarily drain the biliary system.

- **c.** Pancreatic injuries must be drained, and if necessary, simple resection of the tail performed to control pancreatic secretions. Uncontrolled pancreatic secretions severely damages surrounding tissues and compromises later reconstruction efforts. Temporary drainage during damage control part I represents an opportunity to temporize the patient. Evaluation of pancreatic ductal integrity should be considered in damage control part II (ERCP) or III (Direct reinspection). **The most important principle in damage control of the pancreas is wide, closed suction drainage.**

3. **Packing.** Rapid packing of the abdominal cavity represents the first step in achieving hemorrhage control when significant hemoperitoneum is encountered. Laparotomy pads should be quickly placed in a sequential fashion into the four abdominal quadrants, beginning with the quadrant most suspicious for exsanguinating hemorrhage. Typically, packing is initiated in the right or left upper quadrants to tamponade hepatic or splenic hemorrhage. With effective packing, an interval for resuscitation with blood products by anesthesiology may ensue. If packing effectively stops hemorrhage, the packs should be left in place for rapid and complete examination of the abdomen. In general, laparotomy pads are applied over all dissected surfaces and any solid organ injuries. Of note, it is possible to "overpack" the abdominal cavity. Overzealous packing of liver injury may contribute to inferior vena caval compression and reductions in cardiac preload. Packing should be implemented in a manner that provides hemorrhage control without impeding venous return or arterial blood supply. *Fascial closure should be avoided due to the potential to increase operative time, contribute to the development of ACS, and promote fascial loss.*

4. **Abdominal closure.** The goal of abdominal closure as part of the damage control sequence is to provide rapid and temporary abdominal coverage while minimizing the potential for abdominal compartment syndrome (ACS) that plagues damage control part II. Myriad closure techniques have been described, ranging from towel clips applied to the skin to various materials sewn to skin edges. Closure techniques may be individualized provided they minimize the potential for ACS. Our preferred technique is the layered, vacuum-assisted closure (VAC) technique. In this technique, a plastic membrane (x-ray cassette or bowel bag) or an OR towel (covered with an adhesive membrane to prevent adherence to underlying viscera) is placed over the open abdominal wound and tucked beneath the fascial edges. The surface of this barrier is covered with laparotomy pads or gauze to maintain the bowel near the level of the fascia. Closed suction drains can be placed in the lateral subcutaneous gutters with an adhesive plastic membrane placed over the skin and dressing. Continuous suction is applied to the externalized drains, creating an effective seal and assisting with removal of blood and peritoneal resuscitative fluid.

5. **Pitfalls.** During the course of DCS, the surgeon must continually determine the appropriateness of damage control. At damage control part I, it is imperative to recognize bleeding or contamination that will **not** respond to packing. **Injury that is not adequately controlled will most certainly lead to death of the patient.** Conversely, damage control should not be applied in the absence of compelling clinical data. **Overapplication of damage control exposes the patient to the well-described morbidity and mortality** associated with the damage control sequence, including the separate but significant morbidity associated with abdominal wall reconstruction. In summary, constant attention to hemodynamic stability, pH, temperature, and presence of nonsurgical bleeding

are necessary; ongoing communication with anesthesiology is essential. Experience and sound judgment are essential in selection of the damage control patient.

B. Damage control, part II. Secondary resuscitation: breaking the vicious cycle. Damage control part II should be initiated in the ICU with a team-facilitated "horizontal resuscitation," utilizing all available personnel in a coordinated approach to reversal of oxygen debt. Monitoring is required; including CVP arterial vine, core temperature, bladder pressure and establishing laboratory baselines (Hgb, Hct, PT, PTT, INR, Platelets HCS, ABG, etc.) are a minimum. Rapid transfusion, and active and passive rewarming should proceed. ICU procedures should proceed with strict attention to maintenance of rewarming initiatives.

1. **Optimization of hemodynamics.** The foundation of damage control part II is restoration of adequate tissue perfusion, thereby reversing lactic metabolic acidosis and normalizing pH. Upon admission to the ICU, invasive monitoring including, at minimum, arterial catheterization no, is mandatory. The primary focus of treatment for the postdamage control patient in extremis is augmentation of cardiac preload. Pulmonary artery catheterization can be utilized to assess preload and ensure optimal oxygen delivery. Prominent contributors to oxygen delivery, including hemoglobin and cardiac index, should be optimized. Single endpoints of resuscitation may prove inaccurate during this resuscitative phase, therefore, resuscitation should be titrated to multiple complimentary endpoints, including lactate, base deficit, heart rate, blood pressure, urine output, pulmonary artery occlusion pressure, right ventricular end diastolic volume index, or venous oxygen saturation. Early in the posthemorrhage resuscitative phase, lactate and base deficit appear to be stoichiometrically related such that each may be used to guide resuscitation. Lactate clearance in critically ill trauma patients as typified at damage control part II predicts survivorship, therefore worsening lactate or base deficit levels should prompt (*a*) a reevaluation of the resuscitative strategy and (*b*) the potential for ongoing bleeding. Twenty percent of patients will require early reexploration for bleeding in this phase of damage control.

2. **Core rewarming.** Optimally, combined rewarming efforts should be employed on arrival at the emergency department and continued through damage control part I. On arrival at the ICU, immediate and aggressive core rewarming measures should be employed. A notable axiom of damage control part II relates to the acuity of rewarming; **neither coagulopathy nor hypoperfusion are reversible until the patient approaches normothermia.** Rewarming not only improves perfusion, but also helps reverse coagulopathy. At temperatures $<35°C$, hemoglobin releases oxygen less readily than normothermic hemoglobin. In addition, rewarming reverses hypothermia-induced thromboxane A_2 and serine protease dysfunction, critical to platelet aggregation and intrinsic/extrinsic clotting cascades.

   a. Rewarming techniques are categorized as active and passive. Active techniques include heating inspired air, body cavity lavage, cardiopulmonary bypass, and extracorporeal venovenous and arteriovenous bypass.

   b. Passive rewarming techniques include increasing ambient room temperature, using convective or insulating blankets, warming intravenous fluids using rapid transfusing devices, and removing the patient from wet surroundings.

   c. The most effective approach to rewarming in damage control part II includes a protocol-driven combination of active and passive methods. On arrival at the ICU, patients should be removed from wet conditions, convective blankets placed, ambient room temperature optimized, warming lamps applied if available, ventilator air warmed, and all resuscitative fluids warmed. The inability to rewarm a patient suggests of ongoing bleeding, and correlates with both morbidity and mortality.

3. **Correction of coagulopathy**

   a. The etiology of coagulopathy in damage control patients is multifactorial, and includes a number of mechanisms that are self-perpetuating. Hemorrhage with hemodilution initiates the interrelated mechanisms, inducing clotting abnormalities associated with hypothermia and acidosis. Concomitant brain injury, with release of neural tissue thromboplastin, can also contribute to coagulopathy in the damage control patient. Hemorrhage leads to a reduction in absolute numbers of both platelets and clotting factors. Resuscitation includes both crystalloid and PRBCs, which expand circulating volume but produce hemodilution. PRBCs are devoid of platelets and protein factors, and contribute 60 mL of citrate, which binds calcium integral to platelet and factor coagulation. Hypothermia induces both platelet and clotting factor dysfunction as described previously. Similarly, acidosis resulting from blood loss and hypoperfusion leads to changes in red blood cell–platelet interaction and microvascular sludging. Of the multiple and related coagulopathic mechanisms in the exsanguinating damage control patient, thrombocytopenia is the first and most common abnormality.

    b. The foundation of correcting coagulopathy in damage control part II includes effectively stopping hemorrhage, rewarming, and replacing deficient platelet and cellular factors. Repletion of platelet and clotting factors should be prompted by evidence of clinically overt bleeding, prior to laboratory assessment. After ICU admission, serial sampling of PT, PTT, platelet count, and fibrinogen levels should guide treatment. Factor loss is treated with fresh frozen plasma (FFP), which is rich in Factors V and VIII, and thrombocytopenia is treated with platelet administration accordingly. As an adjunct to FFP, recombinant Factor VIIa (rFVIIa), a potent prohemostatic agent, may be considered. Although few prospective controlled trials exist, rFVIIa has been demonstrated to have efficacy in patients with life-threatening hemorrhage without preexistent coagulation disorders. If fibrinogen levels are low, cryoprecipitate, with approximately 250 mg of fibrinogen per unit, should be administered. Due to thawing time necessary for factor preparation, it is imperative to be proactive in anticipating need. In addition, all components excluding platelets are amenable to transfusion with rapid transfusing devices.

4. Ventilatory support. During critical secondary resuscitation, most patients will require mandatory ventilatory support, the focus of which includes optimization of oxygenation and ventilation while minimizing alveolar volutrauma. Given the magnitude of the inflammatory response and requisite resuscitative volumes in damage control patients, with cytokine-induced activation of pulmonary neutrophils, this population is at high risk for development of acute lung injury and acute respiratory distress syndrome. As resuscitation proceeds, close attention to reduction in pulmonary compliance is warranted. Accordingly, ventilatory strategies should focus on minimizing pulmonary plateau pressures (P_{pl}). Reduction of P_{pl} and thus minimization of volutrauma can be accomplished through utilization of lower tidal volume (6–8 mL/kg) and pressure-regulated or pressure-controlled modes of ventilation. Judicious use of positive end expiratory pressure may be necessary to maintain oxygenation.

5. Sedation and analgesia. The open abdomen is frequently associated with multisystem trauma, therefore, vigilant attention to sedation and analgesia is required. Early in the damage control experience neuromuscular blockade was thought to be necessary for complete pharmacologic control. However, we now know this not to be the case, even for the management of the open abdomen, provided adequate sedation and analgesia are administered. The damage control patient is best suited to continuous infusions of both sedation and analgesia. We utilize bispectral analysis (BIS monitoring) during damage control part II, which provides a continuous assessment of sedation based on electroencephalogram data, to ensure adequate sedation, particularly if neuromuscular blockade is present.

6. Continued injury identification. Attempts at complete injury identification are essential during damage control part II. A tertiary survey, including a thorough repeat physical examination and review of radiology data, should be performed. Any further imaging obviated by damage control part I should be completed, provided the patient is stable for transport. Nonemergent imaging and transportation should always be deferred until the patient is normothermic and physiologically stable.

7. Pitfalls

a. Abdominal compartment syndrome (ACS). ACS is characterized by a constellation of clinical manifestations in combination with evidence of increased intraabdominal pressure (IAP) (Chapter 29). Clinical signs include increased pulmonary peak inspiratory pressure (PIP) with or without hypoxia and hypercarbia, oliguria (due to renal hypoperfusion and direct parenchymal compression), increased measures of cardiac preload (central venous or pulmonary artery occlusion pressures, right ventricular end diastolic volume index), reduced cardiac index, and abdominal distention.

  i. A more subtle presentation of ACS during damage control part II is exemplified by the patient who has resuscitated to normal endpoints and normothermia but begins to slowly exhibit loss of physiologic compliance. Such "physiologic drift," consisting of unexplained recurrence of acidosis or increased volume requirements, can be a harbinger of impending ACS.

  ii. Although diagnosis can be made based on clinical grounds alone, measurement of IAP assists in diagnosis. Bladder pressures exceeding 25 mmHg should raise the index of suspicion, and in combination with clinical manifestations, should prompt decompressive celiotomy. The temporizing abdominal closure should be opened immediately, with close attention to immediate changes in PIP. Decompression may be accomplished at the bedside in the ICU. However, if ongoing hemorrhage is suspected as a source of increased IAP, decompression is best undertaken in the OR. If instability precludes safe transport, further abdominal packing can be performed at the bedside.

  iii. In addition, at the time of abdominal decompression, a reperfusion syndrome secondary to accumulated lactic acid and potassium has been described, although we see this syndrome rarely. This potential complication should be anticipated. Some authors have recommended infusion of a solution of 2 L of 0.45% normal saline with 50 g of mannitol and 50 milliequivalent (mEq) sodium bicarbonate ($NaHCO_3$) prior to decompression to blunt reperfusion–induced circulatory collapse.

  iv. ACS in damage control part II should be largely preventable with application of a loose dressing as described previously. We avoid skin approximation of any type or application of a nonexpansible system when a large-volume resuscitation is anticipated. In addition, when hemodynamics, temperature, and coagulation have been restored, resuscitative volumes should be adjusted accordingly, as overresuscitation with crystalloid may select patients for ACS and contribute to multiple organ failure. In summary, early recognition and decompression are mainstays in the management of ACS in damage control part II.

b. Reoperation for hemorrhage. The need for immediate reoperation on the basis of ongoing uncontrolled hemorrhage must be continually assessed. The recognition of continued hemorrhage necessitating reoperation is challenging in the hypothermic and coagulopathic patient. Any rapid worsening of hemodynamics or acidosis should prompt reexploration. High abdominal drain output and/or dropping serial hemoglobin should raise an index of suspicion; however, in the context of relative hemodynamic stability, reexploration may be deferred until coagulopathy is reversed. Ongoing blood product requirements in the rewarmed patient should raise the index of suspicion that a surgical source of hemorrhage is ongoing. No established laboratory or transfusion criteria for reexploration exist, and the decision is based largely on judgment. Typically, when serial hemoglobin continues to fall or high abdominal drain output persists in the normothermic patient with reasonable clotting, reexploration is indicated.

8. **Timing of damage control, part III.** Timing for return to the OR for definitive laparotomy should be based on the reestablishment of normal physiology. Average time for restoration of normal physiology, although variable, is approximately 36 hours. Utilizing that time frame, we have encountered minimal difficulty with recurrent coagulopathy or electrolyte imbalance during definitive laparotomy. Furthermore, this duration of damage control part II allows ample time for a complete tertiary survey, additional radiographic examinations, and planning by consultants for definitive management of associated injuries. Although premature return to the OR may well end in coagulopathy and repacking, delayed return can lead to an increase in intraabdominal infection rate and missed opportunity for definitive repair of associated injuries. Aggressive efforts should be made to remove packing within 72 hours.

C. **Damage control, Part III. Second operation.**

1. **Reinspection and reconstruction**

   a. Preparations should be complete for anticipated definitive surgery. This may include arranging consultant assistance, imaging capabilities, or specialized instrumentation such as autotransfusion devices or argon beam coagulation. For Grade IV or V packed hepatic injury consideration of the need for venorenous bypass and vasculor isolation should be considered. Due to the potential for recurrent hemorrhage and instability, hypothermia prevention is critical. Transportation of the damage control patient is fraught with complication, and special attention should be directed at maintenance of positive end-expiratory pressure (PEEP), both during transport and intraoperatively.

   b. At reoperation, all areas previously packed must be carefully inspected and meticulous hemostasis obtained in areas with evidence of ongoing or recurrent hemorrhage. Solid organs, which have been packed, require the most care and attention. The packs should be carefully removed with copious amounts of irrigation and hemostasis obtained in a stepwise fashion. Coagulation can be achieved with electrocautery, argon beam coagulation, thrombin preparations, or other hemostatic materials. Uncontrolled hemorrhage may recur after pack removal, particularly when unpacking hepatic injuries. Based on the physiologic status of the patient, repacking is a viable option, with definitive resection or repair deferred to a third laparotomy. Consideration of angiographic embolization is warranted.

   c. All gastrointestinal repairs and anastamoses constructed at damage control part I should be meticulously inspected. Gastrointestinal continuity should be restored. If necessary, gastrostomy tubes, jejunostomy tubes, and end stomas can be completed, although all externalized tubes and stomas are best deferred until some form of abdominal closure is possible. If fascial closure has been unachievable, end stomas and enterostomy tubes should be avoided. In our experience with the open abdomen, these techniques are associated with an inordinately high complication rate as the relationship of the intraabdominal contents changes to the geometry of the anterior abdominal wall after damage control part III. Instead, primary anastomoses should be created for gastrointestinal continuity and both nasogastric tubes and nasoduodenal tubes should be placed and directed intraoperatively for proximal decompression and feeding respectively. Definitive colon management has shifted in recent years from diversion to anastomosis. If possible, anastomosis should be tucked deep inside fascial edges or covered with omentum to afford a natural habitat and promote sealing.

2. **Closure of the anterior abdominal wall and management of the open abdomen.** A number of choices exist for anterior abdominal wall closure. If a tension-free closure is possible, primary fascial closure followed by skin closure is optimal. After gross contamination during damage control part I, skin is best left open for delayed primary or secondary closure. To facilitate closure, separation of parts can mobilize the midline sufficiently to allow primary fascial closure. If fascial closure is not possible, skin closure only, with a planned ventral hernia repair, is an excellent choice. Given the morbidity associated with failure to close

the abdominal wall in some permanent or semipermanent fashion, and the component separation abdominal wall reconstruction later necessitated, a number of techniques to facilitate early permanent closure have been devised. Some have advocated immediate placement of prosthetic material, such as the Whitman patch, followed by sequential closure of the fascia and skin, although we have not found this to be efficacious. In addition, data are accumulating on the use of acellular human dermis to close fascial defects, although prospective controlled series are lacking.

   a. Others have advocated application of Vac-Pac dressing for several days after damage control part III in the patient who has persistent massive visceral edema and in whom abdominal closure is simply not possible. Meticulous reapplication of the Vac-Pac dressing is of utmost importance to minimize the risk of fistula formation. Fistula formation is difficult to manage in this setting. Remember, these are not enterocutaneous fistulas, but rather "enteroatmospheric" fistulas without a subcutaneous component and spontaneous closure without surgical intervention is impossible.

   b. Recent data suggest that prolonged application of vacuum-assisted dressings is safe, increases the rate of fascial closure at first hospitalization, and reduces need for later abdominal wall reconstruction. When it is clear that both bowel and anterior abdominal wall edema will not resolve in a reasonable time frame, application of a tension-free absorbable mesh fascial closure is indicated. After 7 to 14 days of local wound care over the absorbable mesh graft, a traditional split-thickness skin graft can be placed over an exuberant granulation bed.

   c. No single closure technique is applicable in all cases. The goals of individualized closure methods should focus on control of fluid and nutritional loss, maintenance of omentum, and minimization of the complication of gastrointestinal fistulization to the open abdominal wound. Interval repair of the subsequent abdominal wall hernia, considered by some authors to represent a separate part of the damage control sequence, can be done at 6 to 9 months when the patient has sufficiently recovered. At this point, reconstruction can be accomplished through excision of the split-thickness skin graft, complete adhesiolysis between the small-bowel mat and the parietal peritoneum, followed by anterior abdominal wall component separation technique.

3. Pitfalls. The second operation (damage control III) can be lengthy, on average 2 to 4 hours, but it is generally well tolerated. Some patients may redevelop metabolic acidosis and hypothermia and abrupt termination of operation and reapplication of packing may be necessary again. On average, blood product requirements can be as high as 6 to 8 units of PRBCs, with a corresponding amount of FFP or platelets. If the second operation must be terminated, the same principles of judgment applied in damage control part I should be used and the Vac-Pac reapplied to manage the open abdomen.

IV. MORBIDITY AND MORTALITY. The damage control principle is founded on the fact that decrease in mortality is achieved at a cost of increased morbidity.

   A. Mortality. Early literature following the advent of damage control surgery noted a mortality of approximately 50%. After over a decade of application, damage control has been demonstrated to improve survival, particularly when applied to penetrating injury. Recent reviews cite survival rates exceeding 50%, with select penetrating series that include stab wounds reporting rates as high as 90%.

   B. Morbidity. The incidence of abdominal complications is approximately 35%. These complications include abscess, intraabdominal abscess, biliary and gastrointestinal fistula, hepatic necrosis, obstruction, anastomotic leak, pancreatic fistula, and abdominal wall failure. Furthermore, other complications (e.g., fever, pneumonia, renal failure, sepsis, systemic inflammatory response syndrome, adult respiratory distress syndrome, and multiple organ dysfunction syndrome) are common in these severely injured patients.

AXIOMS

■ Damage control is a three-part approach to the exsanguinating trauma patient. It includes:

1. Abbreviated surgical control of hemorrhage and contamination
2. Continued and complete resuscitation in the ICU
3. Definitive repair and reconstruction

■ Damage control requires exquisite surgical judgment.
■ When attempting to resuscitate the patient in the ICU, recognition of failed surgical control of bleeding and the need for reexploration is essential.
■ Abdominal compartment syndrome can be avoided by managing the abdomen open.
■ Meticulous management of the open abdomen is warranted to avoid fistula formation.

Bibliography

Abou-Khalil B, Scalea T, Trooskin SZ, et al. Hemodynamic responses to shock in young trauma patients: Need for invasive monitoring. *Crit Care Med* 1994;22(4):633–639.

Asensio JA, Petrone P, Roldan G, et al. Has evolution in awareness of guidelines for institution of damage control improved outcome in the management of the posttraumatic open abdomen? *Arch Surg* 2004;139(2):209–214.

Barker DE, Kaufman HJ, Smith LA, et al. Vacuum pack technique of temporary abdominal closure: A 7-year experience with 112 patients. *J Trauma* 2000;8:201–207.

Burch JM, Denton JR, Noble RD. Physiologic rationale for abbreviated laparotomy. *Surg Clin North Am* 1997;77:779–782.

Burch JM, Moore EE, Moore FA, et al. The abdominal compartment syndrome. *Surg Clin North Am* 1996;76:833–842.

Burch JM, Ortiz VB, Richardson RJ, et al. Abbreviated laparotomy and planned reoperation for critically injured patients. *Ann Surg* 1992;215:476.

Carrillo EH, Spain DA, Wilson MA, et al. Alternatives in the management of penetrating injuries to the iliac vessels. *J Trauma* 1998;44(6):1024–1030.

Cosgriff N, Moore EE, Sauaia A, et al. Predicting life-threatening coagulopathy in the massively transfused trauma patient: Hypothermia and acidosis revisited. *J Trauma* 1997;42(5):857–862.

Cue JI, Cryer GH, Miller FB, et al. Packing and planned reexploration for hepatic and retroperitoneal hemorrhage: Critical refinements of a useful technique. *J Trauma* 1990;30:1007.

Cushman JG, Feliciano DV, Renz BM, et al. Iliac vessel injury: Operative physiology related to outcome. *J Trauma* 1997;2(6):1033–1040.

Eddy VA, Morris JA Jr, Cullinane DC. Hypothermia coagulopathy and acidosis. *Surg Clin North Am* 2000;80(3):845–854.

Fabian TC, Croce MA, Pritchard FE, et al. Planned ventral hernia, staged management for acute abdominal wall defects. *Ann Surg* 1994;219(6):643–653.

Gregory JS, Bergstein JM, Aprahamian C, et al. Comparison of three methods of rewarming from hypothermia: Advantages of extracorporeal blood warming. *J Trauma* 1991;31(9):1247–1252.

Gubler KD, Gentilello LM, Hassantash SA, et al. The impact of hypothermia on dilutional coagulopathy. *J Trauma* 1994;36(6):847–851.

Hirshberg A, Mattox KL. Planned reoperation for severe trauma. *Ann Surg* 1995;222(1):3–8.

Hirshberg A, Wall MJ, Mattox KL. Planned reoperation for trauma: A two year experience with 124 consecutive patients. *J Trauma* 1994;37(3):365–369.

Ivatury RR, Diebel L, Porter JM, et al. Intra-abdominal hypertension and the abdominal compartment syndrome. *Surg Clin North Am* 1997;77:783–800.

Johnson JW, Gracias VH, Schwab CW, et al. Evolution in damage control for exsanguinating penetrating abdominal injury. *J Trauma* 2001;51(2):261–271.

Jurkovich GJ, Greiser WB, Luterman A, et al. Hypothermia in trauma victims: An ominous predictor of survival. *J Trauma* 1987;27:1019.

Levi M, Peters M, Buller HR. Efficacy and safety of recombinant factor VIIa for treatment of severe bleeding: A systematic review. *Crit Care Med* 2005;33(4):883–890.

Lynn M, Jeroukhimov I, Klein Y, et al. Updates in the management of severe coagulopathy in trauma patients. *Intensive Care Med* 2002;28(suppl 2):S241–S247.

Mayberry JC, Mullins RJ, Crass RA, et al. Prevention of abdominal compartment syndrome by absorbable mesh prosthesis closure. *Arch Surg* 1997;132:957–962.

Moore EE, Burch JM, Franciose RJ, et al. Staged physiologic restoration and damage control surgery. *World J Surg* 1998;22:1184–1191.

Morris JA, Eddy VA, Rutherford EJ. The staged celiotomy: damage control. *Trauma Quarterly* 1993;10(1):60–70.

Nicholas JM, Rix EP, Easley KA, et al. Changing patterns in the management of penetrating abdominal trauma: The more things change, the more they stay the same. *J Trauma* 2003;55(6):1095–1110.

Patt A, McCroskey BL, Moore EE. Hypothermia-induced coagulopathies in trauma. *Surg Clin North Am* 1988;68:775.

Richardson JD, Polk HC. Reoperation for trauma. *Ann Surg* 1995;222(1):1–2.

Rotondo MF, Schwab CW, McGonigal MD, et al. Damage control: An approach for improved survival in exsanguinating penetrating abdominal injury. *J Trauma* 1993;35(3):375–383.

Rotondo MF, Zonies DH. The damage control sequence and underlying logic. *Surg Clin North Am* 1997;77:761–777.

Shapiro MB, Jenkins DH, Schwab CW, et al. Damage control: Collective review. *J Trauma* 2000;49:969–978.

Sherck J, Seiver A, Shatney C, et al. Covering the "open abdomen": A better technique. *Am Surg* 1998;64:854–857.

Smith LA, Barker DE, Chase CW, et al. Vacuum pack technique of temporary abdominal closure: A four year experience. *Am Surg* 1997;63:1102–1107.

Spiess BD. Traumatic coagulopathies. *Anesthesiol Clin North America* 1996;14(1):29–38.

Stewart TE, Meade MO, Cook DJ, et al. Evaluation of a ventilation strategy to prevent barotraumas in patients at high risk for acute respiratory distress syndrome. Pressure and volume-limited ventilation strategy group. *N Engl J Med* 1998;338:355–361.

The Acute Respiratory Distress Network. Ventilation with lower tidal volumes as compared with traditional tidal volumes for acute lung injury and the acute respiratory distress syndrome. The acute respiratory distress syndrome network. *N Engl J Med* 342:1301–1308.

ABDOMINAL COMPARTMENT SYNDROME

ROBERT A. MAXWELL AND RAO R. IVATURY

29

I. INTRODUCTION. Abdominal compartment syndrome (ACS) is a clinical condition in which elevated intraabdominal pressure (IAP) (intraabdominal hypertension [IAH]) leads to impaired end-organ perfusion of the viscera and kidneys causing gut ischemia and renal insufficiency. IAH also causes elevation of the diaphragm with resultant respiratory embarrassment and decreased cardiac return to the heart leading to decreased cardiac output and further deterioration in end-organ perfusion. The ultimate result is multiple system organ dysfunction and death if not appropriately diagnosed and treated. Onset can be insidious or fulminant; clinicians must be astute in making the diagnosis.

II. CLINICAL SCENARIOS. ACS has been reported after ruptured abdominal aortic aneurysm repair, intraperitoneal hemorrhage, pancreatitis, ileus, intestinal obstruction, postoperative bowel edema, pneumoperitoneum (e.g., secondary to barrotrauma), septic shock, overzealous resuscitation neoplasm, and liver transplantation. However, **the most common scenario is after major abdominal trauma**.

III. Two types of ACS have now been described, **primary** and **secondary. The following are the definitions from a consensus conference of the World Congress of Abdominal Compartment Syndrome:**
  A. Primary ACS is caused by a condition associated with injury or disease in the abdominopelvic region that frequently requires early surgical or angioradiological intervention, or a condition that develops following abdominal surgery (such as abdominal organ injuries that require surgical repair or damage control surgery, secondary peritonitis, bleeding pelvic fractures or other cause of massive retroperitoneal hematoma, liver transplantation). **Persistent hemorrhage**, can be either surgical (missed injury) or nonsurgical (coagulopathy/hypothermia) although visceral edema from third space losses are all important factors.
  B. Secondary ACS is caused by conditions that do not originate from the abdomen (such as sepsis and capillary leak, major burns, and other conditions requiring massive fluid resuscitation), yet result in the signs and symptoms commonly associated with primary ACS. The chief mechanism appears to be fluid sequestration within the viscera due to reperfusion injury and increased capillary permeability. Any patient with ongoing fluid **resuscitation >10 L crystalloid or 10 units of packed red blood cells (PRBCs)** in a 24-hour period should have bladder pressure monitoring.
  C. Recurrent ACS is caused by a condition in which ACS develops following prophylactic or therapeutic surgical or medical treatment of primary or secondary ACS (e.g., persistence of ACS after decompressive laparotomy) or development of a new ACS episode following definitive closure of the abdominal wall after the previous utilization of a temporary abdominal wall closure.

IV. CLINICAL MANIFESTATIONS. Diagnosis of ACS is purely clinical and should be considered in any trauma or ICU patient with oliguria and abdominal distention. Physical exam will generally reveal a distended, tight abdomen that is pathopneumonic for ACS.

A. **Pulmonary** effects occur via elevation of the diaphragm, which results in decreased thoracic compliance and elevated peak airway pressures (>40–60 cm H_2O). The end results are hypoxia, hypercapnia, and respiratory acidosis.

B. **Cardiac** manifestations occur due to elevated thoracic pressure, which causes **falsely elevated filling pressures (central venous pressure [CVP] and pulmonary capillary wedge pressure [PCWP])**, decreased cardiac return, and decreased cardiac compliance. The end result is low cardiac output and decreased end-organ perfusion.

C. **Renal** effects occur due to direct parynchemal and caval compression, and decreased cardiac output resulting in decreased **glomerular filtration rate (GFR)** and oliguria.

D. **Gastrointestinal (GI)** effects occur from hypoperfusion of the splanchnic beds (direct compression and decreased cardiac output) leading to bacterial translocation and increased septic complications.

V. **Diagnosis** of ACS is elementary once the idea is entertained.

A. **Bladder pressure** is the standard method for estimating intraabdominal pressure and can be performed at the bedside with the use of the arterial line pressure transducer.

1. **Cross-clamp** the Foley catheter drainage tubing just distal to the aspiration port.

2. **Inject** 50 to 100 cc of sterile saline into the bladder with a catheter-tipped syringe via the Foley catheter and reconnect to the drainage tubing.

3. **Connect** a 16-gauge needle to the arterial line pressure tubing; flush and insert into the aspiration port.

4. **Zero** the system at the symphysis pubis while the patient is supine.

B. **IAH** is defined by a sustained increase in IAP of 12 mmHg or more, recorded by a minimum of three standardized measurements conducted 4 to 6 hours apart, with or without an abdominal perfusion pressure (APP = MAP [mean arterial pressure] − IAP) <60 mmHg.

C. **ACS** is defined as a sustained increase in IAP of 20 mmHg or more with or without APP <60 mmHg **and** single or multiple organ system failure that was not previously present.

VI. **TREATMENT.** Intraabdominal pressure >20 mmHg is clearly an indication for abdominal decompression. Pressures between 15 and 20 should probably undergo decompression: with a new onset organ dysfunction.

A. **Decompressive celiotomy** for ACS is a surgical emergency and should be undertaken with the utmost urgency.

1. **Preoperative preparation.** In addition to ensuring that the patient is adequately resuscitated and the blood bank has additional blood products on hold, anesthesia should be carefully apprised of the situation.

2. **Operative facilities.** There may be temptation to perform decompression at the bedside, but this should be generally avoided in case ongoing bleeding or missed injury is discovered. Most ICUs are not the appropriate place to handle such problems.

3. **Reperfusion syndrome.** Decompression results in the release of numerous toxic metabolites and acids into the systemic circulation which can lead to profound cardiac depression and hypotension. Loading the patient with 2 to 4 amps of sodium bicarbonate just prior to or during decompression may prevent associated hemodynamic instability.

B. Management of concurrent bowel injury

1. Simple lacerations **of the small or large bowel can generally be repaired at the time of initial exploration rather than performing stapled resections that necessitate formal anastamosis at a later time**.

2. Destructive bowel injury **should generally be managed with the techniques of damage control laparotomy and undergo initial stapled resection. Definitive anastamosis or stoma formation may then be performed at secondary operations based on conditions of bowel edema and degree of peritoneal contamination.**

C. **Abdominal closure.** A variety of techniques have been employed for temporary abdominal closure and are usually institution specific.
   1. **Methods of temporary** closure
      a. **Towel clip** closure is a universal technique for rapidly completing a damage control procedure, but is generally inadequate for decompressing ACS.
      b. **Prosthetic coverage** with Bogata bags, Vac-Pacs, x-ray cassette covers, woven Vycril mesh, and fascial zippers have all been described **with the main risk being fistula formation**. Bogata bags and sterile x-ray cassette covers sewn to the skin are generally cheapest and usually adequate if early takeback is anticipated. Mesh sewn to the skin or fascia works well but can be a wound management problem when there are large volumes of ascites. The Vac-Pac works well under these circumstances.
   2. **Methods of permanent closure**
      a. **Primary closure of the fascia.** When visceral edema has sufficiently resolved, fascial closure should be performed. If primary closure cannot be performed by postop days 7 to 10, it will generally not occur because the abdomen becomes "socked-in" and stage reconstruction will be necessary. Delays up to 1 month may be achieved by a running skin closure over a vacuum sponge with incremental fascial approximation as edema subsides.
      b. **Split-thickness skin graft.** If primary fascial closure cannot be performed, the bowel will usually granulate enough to accept a skin graft by 3 to 4 weeks postop. This procedure will generally permit the bowel edema to resolve and adhesions to subside.
      c. **Skin mobilization and closure.** In patients with excessive skin, flaps can be mobilized on either side of the laparotomy wound and closed in the middle. This will avoid skin grafting and looks better cosmetically.
      d. **Delayed abdominal wall reconstruction.** When the skin graft can easily be lifted off the underlying bowel, generally 6 to 9 months following grafting, abdominal wall reconstruction can be performed. Rectus sheath advancement (components technique) or permanent prosthetic placement is usually necessary due to loss of abdominal domain.

VII. PREVENTION
   A. **Leave the abdomen open.** It is now widely accepted to use temporary closure techniques after laparotomy in face of significant visceral edema, especially when further fluid sequestration can be expected.
   B. **Correct coagulopathies and hypothermia.** Coagulopathies and hypothermia lead to nonsurgical bleeding, which causes increased intraabdominal pressure and further resuscitation requirements.

VIII. MORBIDITY AND MORTALITY
   A. **Morbidity.** Delayed diagnosis of ACS leads to multiple organ dysfunction.
   B. **Mortality** of ACS ranges from 42% to 68% after detection and treatment and 100% in those **not** undergoing decompression. Reduced rates of morbidity and mortality appear to hinge on early and aggressive detection and management.

 AXIOMS

- Abdominal compartment syndrome should be suspected in any trauma or burn patient with abdominal distention and oliguria despite normal or elevated filling pressures.
- As with any compartment syndrome, measurement of compartment (bladder) pressure is instrumental in establishing the diagnosis and should be routinely monitored in patients at risk.
- Patients with intraabdominal pressure >20 mmHg and signs of physiologic compromise should be decompressed.
- Forced fascial closure over swollen bowel or packs is generally contraindicated after trauma.

Bibliography

Balogh Z, McKinley BA, Cocanour CS, et al. Supranormal trauma resuscitation causes more cases of abdominal compartment syndrome. *Arch Surg* 2003;138:637–643.

Chavarria-Aguilar M, Maxwell RA, Cockerham WT, et al. Fate of bowel anastamosis following management of the open abdomen. *J Trauma* 2004;56:560–564.

Eddy V, Nunn C, Morris JA Jr. Abdominal compartment syndrome: The Nashville experience. *Surg Clin North Am* 1997;77:801–812.

Fabian TC, Croce MA, Pritchard FE, et al. Planned ventral hernia: Staged management for acute abdominal wall defects. *Ann Surg* 1994;219:643–650.

Ivatury R, Cheatham M, Malbrain M, Sugrue M. Abdominal compartment syndrome. Available at: http://www.eurekah.com/categories.php?catid=83&category=SURGERY.

Ivatury RR, Diebel LN, Porter JM, Simon RJ. Intra-abdominal hypertension and the abdominal compartment syndrome. *Surg Clin North Am* 1997;77:783–800.

Maxwell RA, Fabian TC, Croce MA, Davis KA. Secondary abdominal compartment syndrome: An underappreciated manifestation of severe hemorrhagic shock. *J Trauma* 1999;47:955–1003.

Meldrum DR, Moore FA, Moore EE, et al. Prospective characterization and selective management of the abdominal compartment syndrome. *Am J Surg* 1997;174:667–672.

Miller PR, Thompson JT, Faler BJ, et al. Late fascial closure in lieu of ventral hernia: The next step in open abdomen management. *J Trauma* 2002;53:843–849.

I. INTRODUCTION

A. Approximately 10% of trauma patients will sustain an injury to the genitourinary (GU) system, with the kidney most commonly involved. The mechanism of injury and physical exam findings can help alert the evaluating physician and guide the initial evaluation.

B. Hematuria is the hallmark of GU injury. However, substantial urologic injury can exist in the absence of blood in the urine. Hematuria can result from injury anywhere along the GU tract and multiple urologic injuries can coexist. The mechanism, location, and severity of injuries play an important role in determining the need and type of further diagnostic evaluation and/or therapeutic intervention.

II. Hematuria (Fig. 30-1)

A. Hematuria is either microscopic (presence of blood visible only with aid of microscope or urine dipstick) or macroscopic (presence of blood discernable with naked eye).

   1. Any degree of **macroscopic hematuria** warrants GU evaluation. Degree of hematuria **does not** correlate with degree of injury.

   2. **Microscopic** hematuria may indicate injury or infection. Testing of the initial aliquot of urine is important as hematuria can clear quickly and be missed.

     a. Guidelines have been developed to select which patients with microhematuria warrant further evaluation for GU injury based on mechanism of injury or physical exam findings. These include:

       i. Proximity of penetrating injuries

      ii. Children <15 years of age with **any** degree of hematuria

     iii. Adults with blunt trauma **and**

       a) Any recorded systolic blood pressure <90 mmHg

       b) Rapid deceleration injuries (e.g., motor vehicle crashes [MVCs], falls from heights)

       c) Mechanism of injury consistent with GU injury (e.g., straddle injury, flank blow)

       d) Multiple coexistent injuries

       e) Rib fractures/flank hematoma

III. IMAGING TECHNIQUES

A. Retrograde urethrogram (RUG)

   1. Performed mainly in male patients to evaluate for **urethral injury**.

   2. To perform: place patient in 30-degree oblique position with upper leg straight and lower leg flexed slightly forward. Insert Foley catheter into the meatus and inflate balloon with 2 to 3 cc of water to occlude urethra. Stretch penis to straighten anterior urethra. Slowly inject undiluted contrast with plain film images at 10-cc intervals.

   3. Evidence of contrast extravasation or occlusion of the urethra implies urethral injury. Urologic consultation should be sought **prior** to attempting Foley catheter placement.

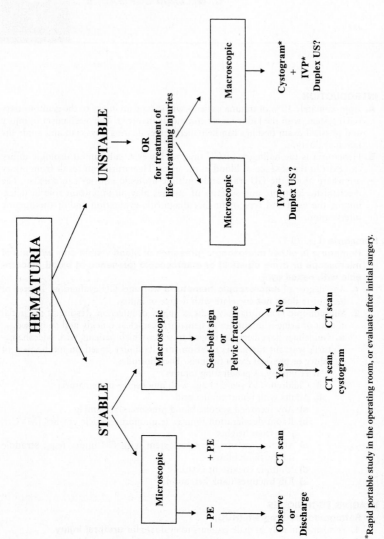

Figure 30-1. Hematuria workup. PE, flank mass, flank pain, lower rib fractures, spine fracture, hypotension (even transient).

*Rapid portable study in the operating room, or evaluate after initial surgery.

B. Cystography
1. **Plain-film cystogram.** With Foley catheter in bladder, obtain a **scout film**. Fill bladder with 350 cc of 30% dilute sterile contrast and obtain a **filled bladder AP film**. Drain the bladder entirely and obtain **postdrainage** AP film. Many small bladder injuries are appreciated **only** on postdrainage films. It is important to differentiate **intraperitoneal versus extraperitoneal** bladder rupture, as the management generally differs.
2. **CT cystography.** Alternative to traditional cystography in the stable patient. The study requires a Foley catheter and three scans: an **early filling** scan after gravity instillation of 100 cc of 30% contrast, a **complete fill** scan after gravity instillation of 350 cc of contrast, and a **postdrainage scan** after allowing the bladder to empty completely.
3. **CT** scans during the excretion phase following intravenous injection of contrast are generally **not sufficient** to rule out bladder injury.

C. CT scan
1. Rapidly performed and widely available, CT scanning allows simultaneous evaluation of the vascular and parenchymal integrity of the kidney.
2. The gold standard for the evaluation and staging of injury to the kidneys; useful in evaluation of the ureters and bladder.

D. Arteriography
1. The arteriogram is occasionally used in the setting of renal trauma to delineate the vascular integrity of the kidney, particularly in the setting of suspected renal arterial thrombosis or segmental renal arterial injury.
2. Arteriography followed by stenting or embolization may be therapeutic.

E. Intravenous pyelography (IVP)
1. Prior to CT technology, the IVP was the imaging study of choice for the investigation of renal trauma. Currently, its role is limited.

F. One-shot IVP
1. Rapidly obtainable on table x-ray. Can be useful in patients taken directly to the OR **prior** to radiologic investigations.
2. The purposes of the one-shot IVP are to assess for major renal injury or contrast extravasation, and to demonstrate and **document contralateral renal function**.
3. It has limited utility during the initial resuscitation and should not delay the transport of a patient to the operating room (OR). Its primary use is as an intraoperative study. Hypotension will limit the effectiveness of the study and is best performed when patient is normotensive.
4. To perform: 2 cc/kg (or 150 cc) of 50% contrast given as an IV bolus followed by a single-shot flat plate film 10 minutes later.

G. Ultrasound
1. Ultrasound can rapidly outline the kidney parenchyma and surrounding tissues and provide evidence that an additional study may be necessary.
2. The imaging study of choice in the evaluation of testicular injuries.
3. Useful in the evaluation of the transplanted kidney.

IV. Renal injuries (Fig. 30-2)
A. Mechanism and diagnosis
1. In the United States, approximately 80% of renal injuries are the result of blunt trauma and 20% penetrating trauma.
2. Renal injury should be suspected and evaluated in patients with hematuria, or a mechanism of injury or physical findings conducive to renal trauma (Section II).
3. Significant renal injury **can** exist in the absence of hematuria—specifically, major injuries to the renal pedicle or transection of the ureteropelvic junction (UPJ).
4. Staging of renal trauma is done either by CT or intraoperative findings.

B. Treatment
1. **Nonoperative management** is the standard of care for **hemodynamically stable** patients with grade I to III and nonvascular grade IV renal injuries.

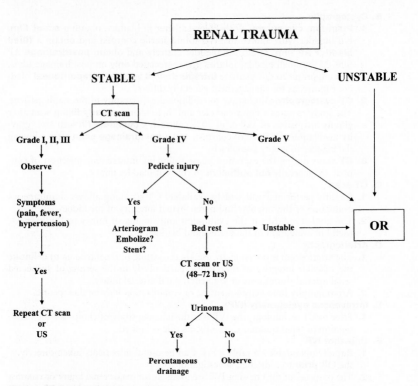

Figure 30-2. Renal trauma workup.

2. **Operative exploration** is indicated in unstable patients and those with renal hilar or pedicle injuries (vascular grade IV and V).

3. If the patient is explored for other reasons, prior to appropriate imaging evaluation, the retroperitoneum should be examined for evidence of expanding or pulsatile hematomas, the presence of which should prompt renal exploration. A **one-shot IVP** can be performed **prior** to renal exploration to document function of the contralateral side should nephrectomy become necessary.

4. The treatment of nonpulsatile, nonexpanding retroperitoneal hematomas found at the time of exploratory laparotomy is controversial. Generally, if such injuries are the result of blunt trauma, they may be safely watched. Stable retroperitoneal hematomas resulting from penetrating trauma should be explored. Again, evidence of contralateral renal function should be documented.

5. Early vascular control of the injured renal unit maximizes chances of renal unit salvage. This is best accomplished through a midline transperitoneal approach. Incision of the mesentery just medial and inferior to the inferior mesenteric vein allows exposure of the right- and left-sided renal vessels (Fig. 30-3).

6. Nephrectomy should be entertained when renal injuries are considered unreconstructable or when patients are clinically unstable from other injuries.

7. In stable patients with nonhilar vascular injuries or parenchymal injuries, renal reconstruction is frequently successful and should be considered. Principles include debridement of devascularized tissues, careful closure of collecting system injuries, and reinforcement of the site of repair with omentum or perinephric fat.

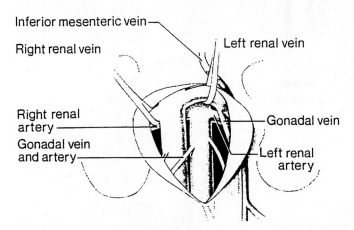

Figure 30-3. Incision of the mesentery just medial and inferior to the inferior mesenteric vein. (From Carroll PR, Dixon CM, McAninch JW. The management of renal and ureteral trauma. In: Blaisdell FW, Trunkey DD, eds. *Trauma.* 2nd ed. New York, NY: Thieme Medical Publishers; 1993:260, with permission.)

Use of fibrin glue may limit parenchymal bleeding. Postoperative drainage of the retroperitoneum is mandatory (Fig. 30-4).

C. Complications
1. Prolonged urine extravasation may be seen following renal reconstruction. Such drainage typically resolves spontaneously. Ureteric stent placement may be required to facilitate antegrade drainage.
2. Urinoma formation can occur days to weeks after repair. Retroperitoneal urinomas or perinephric abscesses may be treated with percutaneous drainage.
3. Postinjury hypertension can occur in up to 5% of patients following renal trauma and may occur up to 6 months after injury. This occasionally resolves spontaneously, but antihypertensive treatment is frequently required. Nephrectomy is the most common treatment if hypertension cannot be controlled.

V. URETERAL INJURIES
A. Mechanism and diagnosis
1. Ureteral injuries are rare. The majority occur from penetrating trauma; gunshots outnumber stab wounds. Blunt injuries to the ureter are rare and are usually seen at the level of the renal pelvis.
2. **Hematuria is not a consistent finding with ureteral injuries,** and as such, the absence of blood in the urine does not rule out ureteral injury. A high index of suspicion must be maintained as delayed diagnosis results in higher complication rates.
3. Stable patients able to undergo imaging studies are best evaluated with a CT with IV contrast and delayed views or an IVP. Retrograde pyelography is very sensitive and specific but can be logistically difficult in the setting of multiple injuries and/or active resuscitation or exploration.
4. Intraoperative exploration of retroperitoneal hematomas or periureteral injuries is mandatory if ureteral injury is suspected and retrograde ureteral study or stenting are not possible.

B. Treatment
1. Treatment options are largely guided by location and extent of injury. Frequently, injuries can be treated with stent placement and primary repair.
   a. Distal ureteral injuries may require ureteral reimplantation possibly along with psoas hitching to create a tension-free anastamosis.

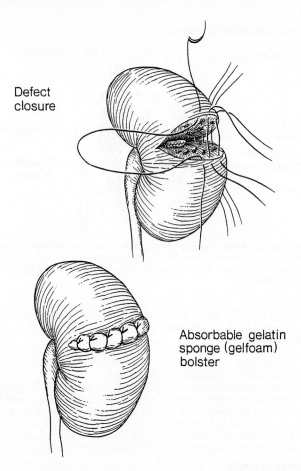

Defect
closure

Absorbable gelatin
sponge (gelfoam)
bolster

Figure 30-4. Repair of the renal parenchyma. (From Carroll PR, Dixon CM, McAninch JW. The management of renal and ureteral trauma. In: Blaisdell FW, Trunkey DD, eds. *Trauma*. 2nd ed. New York, NY: Thieme Medical Publishers; 1993:260, with permission.)

b. Midureteral injuries are often amenable to primary ureteroureterostomy. Injuries involving loss of long tissue segments may require formation of a Boari bladder flap.

c. Proximal ureteral injuries may be amenable to ureteroureterostomy. However, more complex reconstructive efforts may be required including ureteropyelostomy, ureterocalicostomy, transureteroureterostomy, or ileal segment interposition.

d. In the unstable patient with a high-grade ureteral injury, the establishment of temporary external drainage may be required until the patient is better suited for operative reconstruction. Options include creation of a cutaneous ureterostomy, or simple ureteral ligation with subsequent percutaneous nephrostomy tube (PCN) placement.

e. In the rare circumstance of long segment ureteral injury to a solitary kidney, successful autotransplantation has been reported.

2. Keys to successful repair include the adequate debridement of devitalized tissue, proximal and distal mobilization, spatulation allowing for a tension-free repair, use of an indwelling ureteral stent, creation of a watertight anastamosis using interrupted absorbable sutures, and postoperative retroperitoneal and bladder drainage.

C. Complications following repair of ureteral injuries include urine leak or fistula formation, abscess formation, and stricture formation.

VI. BLADDER INJURIES

A. Mechanism

1. The majority of bladder injuries are ruptures from blunt trauma; 80% are extraperitoneal and 20% are intraperitoneal.

2. 95% of bladder injuries are associated with gross hematuria.

3. Bladder injuries are highly associated with pelvic fractures.

B. Diagnosis

1. Plain-film or CT cystography is the study of choice (Section III.B).

2. Excretion or cystographic phase CT scanning is **NOT** sufficient as there is a high rate of false negative results.

3. The cystogram can be performed prior to a diagnostic peritoneal lavage (DPL) as identification of an intraperitoneal bladder rupture obviates the need for a DPL.

4. It is important to differentiate between intraperitoneal and extraperitoneal injuries as their management differs

  a. An **extraperitoneal** bladder rupture usually has a "sunburst" or "flame-shaped" appearance as contrast extravasates into the perivesical tissue. They are associated with fractures of the superior or inferior pubic rami.

  b. An **intraperitoneal** bladder rupture will reveal contrast outlining loops of bowel in the peritoneum. Such injuries are frequently associated with blunt trauma with a full bladder causing rupture at the dome or gunshot wounds.

C. Management

1. Contusions—injuries to the bladder causing **hematuria without obvious signs of contrast extravasation**—can be managed **conservatively** either with or without a bladder catheter.

2. Penetrating injuries to the bladder should be operatively explored and repaired.

3. Intraperitoneal ruptures require exploratory laparotomy and repair. Use of a large-caliber Foley catheter, closure of multiple layers over the injury, and postoperative perivesical drainage make for rare complications. Generally, bladder drainage is maintained for 7 to 10 days. A cystogram should be obtained prior to catheter removal to document healing. Continued contrast extravasation should prompt continued bladder drainage. Repeat imaging studies can be obtained at 7- to 14-day intervals. Perioperative antibiotics should be given. Antibiotic prophylaxis need only be maintained if the patient is at risk for seeding other sites (e.g., orthopedic hardware, cardiac valves, etc.).

4. Extraperitoneal ruptures can generally be managed nonoperatively with a catheter and repeated cystograpy in 7 to 10 days to confirm healing. Large defects with marked contrast extravasation may be best repaired operatively in a similar manner to that performed for intraperitoneal injuries.

5. Contraindications to the nonoperative management of extraperitoneal bladder ruptures include:

  a. Patients undergoing laparotomy for nonurologic injuries

  b. Active urinary tract infection

  c. Inadequate bladder drainage via urethral catheter

  d. Presence of bone fragments in the bladder

  e. Patients undergoing internal fixation of pelvic injuries (due to high infectious risk)

D. Complications include urinoma or pelvic abscess formation, fistula formation, incontinence, and neurogenic injury leading to voiding dysfunction.

VII. URETHRAL INJURIES
A. Mechanism
1. Urethral injuries are more common in males than females. The mechanism of urethral injury is usually blunt. They are frequently associated with significant concurrent injuries.
2. The **posterior urethra** is more commonly injured in males and is frequently **associated with pelvic fracture**. The anterior urethra may be injured in penetrating trauma or a straddle-type injury causing a crush of the bulbar urethra against the pubic ramus.
3. A straddle injury can cause urethral trauma in the absence of a pelvic fracture.
4. Injury to the female urethra is rare except in open pelvic fractures.

B. Diagnosis
1. **The gold standard of diagnosis is the retrograde urethrogram (RUG).**
2. A high index of suspicion is necessary in males sustaining blunt pelvic trauma with:
   a. An inability to void
   b. Blood at the urethral meatus
   c. A high-riding or indiscreet prostate on digital rectal examination
   d. Swelling or ecchymosis of the penis, scrotum, or perineum

C. Treatment
1. **Posterior urethral injury** management is controversial. Initial resuscitation, stabilization, and management of life-threatening injuries take initial priority. Immediate primary repair is generally associated with high rates of incontinence, impotence, and stricture formation. Typically such injuries are managed with placement of a large-caliber suprapubic tube followed by definitive repair 3 to 6 months later. Endoscopic urethral realignment may be attempted in the hemodynamically stable patient. When successful, this approach may reduce the incidence of urethral stricture and reduce the distance of the gap of urethra seen in complete disruptions. This approach also has the potential for significant morbidity.
2. **Anterior urethral injuries** can be also managed in a variety of ways. Partial disruptions can be managed with endoscopic catheter placement followed by a voiding cystourethrogram 10 to 14 days later to assess for healing prior to catheter removal. Injuries causing complete disruption or significant hematoma formation may be better served with suprapubic tube placement followed by endoscopic or radiologic assessment of the urethra weeks to months later. Immediate repair of a urethral injury can be challenging and should be limited to stable patients with penetrating injuries requiring simple closure.

D. Complications of urethral injuries are common and include urethral stricture formation, incontinence, and erectile dysfunction.

VIII. SCROTAL INJURIES
A. Mechanism
1. 85% of injuries to the scrotum are the result of blunt injuries—often sports-related injuries.
2. **Relationship of scrotum and urethra make concurrent injuries possible. Any suspicion should prompt performance of a RUG.**

B. Diagnosis
1. **Physical exam** may be difficult due to pain; however, a mechanism of injury and exam consistent with significant testicular injury warrants **prompt** surgical exploration.
2. Scrotal ultrasound is the single best study for evaluating scrotal injuries as it can evaluate testicular size, location, blood flow, and injury patterns.

C. Management
1. Except for superficial scrotal trauma, **all penetrating injuries warrant surgical exploration.**

2. Indications for scrotal exploration following **blunt** trauma include testicular rupture, torsion, presence of a large hematocele, and testicular dislocation.

3. Operative goals are evacuation of hematoma with copious irrigation, conservative debridement of nonviable tissue, closure of the tunica albuginea with absorbable suture, epididymal repair, and scrotal closure. A scrotal drain should be used.

4. Orchidectomy should be reserved for shattered testicles with limited remaining viable tissue.

5. Due to its extensibility, even large losses of scrotal skin can often be closed primarily. Exposed testicles following substantial scrotal skin loss are classically buried in the subcutaneous tissue of the thigh or abdomen. More recently, use of saline dressings to wrap the testicles has been used with good results. Following the development of healthy granulation tissue, split-thickness skin grafting can be performed with good cosmetic results.

IX. PENILE INJURIES
A. Mechanism
1. Penile injuries can be penetrating or blunt.
B. Penile fracture
1. Penile fracture is a rupture of the tunica albuginea surrounding the corpora cavernosa (erectile bodies) of the penis.
2. **This injury occurs almost exclusively to the erect penis** when a substantial angulation or blunt force is applied. Most frequently this results in the patient experiencing pain and hearing a loud "pop," followed by almost immediate detumescence.
3. Large penile hematomas, referred to as "**eggplant deformities**," are typical.
4. **Concurrent urethral injuries are frequent**, therefore a high level of suspicion must be maintained and RUG performed routinely.
5. **Management involves operative repair**—immediate urologic consultation should be obtained.
C. Penetrating injuries to the penis require exploration, copious irrigation, and repair.

X. VAGINAL INJURIES
A. Mechanism
1. Usually occurs through blunt trauma and is frequently associated with pelvic fracture.
B. Diagnosis
1. In females with pelvic fracture, a pelvic examination with speculum inspection of the vault **is mandatory** to avoid missing occult injuries.
2. Examination is best obtained with an anesthetized patient placed in lithotomy position.
C. Treatment
1. Most frequently, treatment is simple closure and, occasionally, drainage.

 AXIOMS

- Hematuria is the hallmark of injury to the genitourinary system; however, significant injury may exist in the absense of blood in the urine.
- All trauma patients with gross hematuria require further evaluation.
- The evaluation of trauma patients with microscopic hematuria is based on mechanism of injury and physical exam findings.
- CT scanning with IV contrast is essential in the evaluation and management decision making of stable patients with suspected renal injuries.
- Most ureteral injuries are from penetrating trauma.
- Extraperitoneal bladder ruptures can frequently be managed with catheter drainage.
- Maintain a low threshold for performing a retrograde urethrogram before attempting urethral catheter placement.

Bibliography
Brandes S, Coburn M, Armenakas N, et al. Diagnosis and management of ureteric injury: An evidence-based analysis. *BJU Int* 2004;94(3):277–289.
Chapple C, Barbagli G, Jordan G, et al. Consensus statement on urethral trauma. *BJU Int* 2004;93(9):1195–1202.
McAninch J, Santucci RA. Genitourinary trauma. In: Walsh PC, Retik AB, Vaughan ED Jr, et al., eds. *Campbell's Urology*. 8th ed. Philadelphia, Pa: WB Saunders; 2002: 3707–3744.
Santucci RA, Wessels H, Bartsch G, et al. Evaluation and management of renal injuries: Consensus statement of the renal trauma subcommittee. *BJU Int* 2004;93(7):937–954.

I. GENERAL PRINCIPLES OF DISLOCATIONS AND FRACTURES

A. Fractures and dislocations occur in a significant number of trauma patients, resulting from indirect or direct force. Evaluation of the trauma patient with a fracture or dislocation should always include a complete musculoskeletal evaluation. Pay careful attention to the mechanism of injury, which aids in the treatment of the patient and provides prognostic information.

1. Dislocation is defined as a complete loss of articular contact between two bones in a joint; this occurs with severe injury to ligamentous and capsular tissues. **Define the direction of the dislocation** with the distal piece described in relation to the proximal joint or bone. Most dislocations require urgent reduction to prevent complications. Dislocations should be identified during the secondary survey.

  a. Findings on examination with joint dislocation include pain, loss of motion, shortening of the extremity, and associated nerve or vascular injuries (Table 31-1).

  b. Relocation of major joint dislocation must occur as soon as possible after completion of a secondary survey. Relocation is performed generally with intravenous sedation and finesse rather than force. Occasionally, general anesthesia is necessary for relocation. Exception: A fracture dislocation of the proximal humerus may not be eligible for relocation and a proper diagnosis must be achieved prior to relocation.

2. Subluxation refers to the partial loss of articular congruity; sufficient capsular and ligamentous structures remain to prevent complete dislocation. On a continuum, subluxation represents less injury than dislocation, although a complete dislocation that has partially reduced from the elastic recoil of the soft tissue can deceptively appear to be a subluxation.

3. A fracture is a structural break in bone continuity. Clinical signs include pain, displacement, shortening, swelling, and loss of function. Fractures are classified as either **open** (communicates with the external environment) or **closed**. Clinical deformity should be described as well as the status of soft tissues and neurovascular structures. **Fractures are described according to a universal scheme.**

  a. The distal piece is described in relation to the proximal piece.

  b. Fractures are classified with respect to the following:

   i. Pattern: transverse, oblique, spiral, other

   ii. Morphology: simple (two parts) or comminuted (three or more parts)

   iii. Location: proximal, middle, or distal; extraarticular or intraarticular

   iv. Radiographic parameters: **displacement, angulation, rotation, shortening, apposition**

  c. Degree of soft-tissue injury in closed or open fractures is important. Extensive soft-tissue injury increases the risk of the development of compartment syndrome.

4. Pediatric fractures are further classified according to their **physeal (growth plate)** involvement (Salter-Harris classification).

TABLE 31-1	Neurovascular Injuries Associated with Fractures or Dislocations

Orthopedic injury	Neurovascular injury
Anterior shoulder dislocation	Axillary nerve injury, axillary artery injury
Humeral shaft fracture	Radial nerve injury
Supracondylar humeral fracture	Brachial artery
Distal radius fracture	Median nerve injury
Perilunate dislocation	Median nerve injury
Posterior hip dislocation	Sciatic nerve injury
Supracondylar femoral fracture/posterior knee dislocation/tibial plateau fracture	Popliteal artery injury/thrombosis
Proximal fibular fracture	Peroneal nerve
Mangled extremity/tibial fracture	All neurovascular structures of the lower leg, compartment syndrome

    a. Type I: displaced or nondisplaced through growth plate
    b. Type II: small metaphyseal fragment
    c. Type III: intraarticular through epiphysis
    d. Type IV: through metaphysis and epiphysis
    e. Type V: severe crush to growth plate (cannot be determined acutely, only after growth arrest)

B. The orthopedic **physical examination** focuses on the musculoskeletal system, but assessment for concomitant injuries is also necessary. Be familiar with the events surrounding the injury and with the patient's underlying medical conditions and current complaints. After obtaining a history, proceed systematically with the examination. In the multiply injured patient, 15% to 20% of minor fractures (hand, foot, clavicle) are missed initially.

    1. Visually **inspect** for obvious soft-tissue abnormalities, including breaks in the skin, and deformities or asymmetry of the extremities.

    2. Inspect the extremity throughout and turn the patient to the side (e.g., for spinal injuries, pelvic ring injuries extending to the anus).

    3. Palpate bone and soft tissues to evaluate tenderness, crepitus, and firmness of compartments.

    4. Test active and passive **range of motion** to detect bony injury, ligamentous injury, or weakness.

    5. A neurovascular examination records quality of peripheral pulses as well as sensory (pinprick, light touch), and motor function.

    6. Perform an additional **tertiary orthopedic survey** after the initial 24 to 48 hours or when the patient is more responsive (detect missed fractures of hand, foot, clavicle).

C. Radiographic evaluation

    1. At least two views at right angles (generally anteroposterior and lateral views) are obtained of the extremity. In periarticular fractures, proper views must be obtained to assess possible articular involvement. This may be overlooked if oblique views are taken (especially in the elbow). Oblique views used to define fractures of the tibial plateau have been replaced by computed tomography (CT). **Joints above and below the fracture or dislocation must always be visualized radiographically.** Other views (e.g., stress views of the ankle or knee) may be necessary to assess joint stability.

D. Tests designed for specific conditions or anatomic injuries conclude the examination: tomography, arthrography, CT, or magnetic resonance imaging (MRI). These should be ordered by the orthopedist.

E. Initial treatment of fractures or dislocations
1. **Reduce** the fracture or dislocation.
2. **Splint** the extremity.
3. **Irrigate** open fractures and cover with sterile saline-soaked gauze.
4. **Administer antibiotics** for open fractures or perioperatively in patients who require open reduction and internal fixation (ORIF).
5. **Administer tetanus prophylaxis** for open fractures or to patients who require ORIF.

F. Definitive treatment of fractures or dislocations. The goal in treatment of musculoskeletal injury is to restore normal anatomy and function and relieve pain as quickly as possible. The capability to perform early reduction and internal fixation in the multiply injured patient has significantly reduced morbidity and mortality. The method of fixation should be adapted to the general condition (i.e., external fixation in unstable patients). Stabilization of the spine, pelvis, and long bone fractures (femur, tibia) has allowed early mobilization of patients.
1. **Reduction** can be accomplished by either closed (external realignment) or open (direct operative approach).
2. **Immobilization of the extremity** by splint, cast, traction, orthosis, external fixation, or internal fixation.

G. Open fractures communicate externally through a break in the skin, vaginal wall, or rectum; they pose a threat for infection and amputation. **The most important measures in the care of open fractures are extensive and appropriate debridement followed by skeletal stabilization.** Prevention of infection is of paramount importance. Development of osteomyelitis because of inadequate debridement can be a devastating complication and will greatly increase the morbidity and potential for loss of function or limb. **Antibiotics cannot be a substitute for adequate debridement of necrotic and contaminated tissues.**
1. **Classification of open fractures (Gustilo and Anderson)**
   a. **Grade I:** low energy, <1-cm wound caused by protrusion of the bone through the skin or a low-velocity bullet
   b. **Grade II:** moderate energy, >1 cm with flap or avulsion wound in the skin with minimal devitalized soft tissue and minimal contamination
   c. **Grade III:** high energy, extensive soft-tissue injury (usually >10 cm), barnyard
      i. **IIIa:** adequate soft-tissue coverage
      ii. **IIIb:** significant soft-tissue loss with exposed bone that requires tissue transfer (muscle flap, rotation or free) for coverage
      iii. **IIIc:** vascular injury requiring repair for limb preservation; amputation rates reported from 25% to 50%. (Not all vascular injuries are limb threatening.)
2. **Management**
   a. Early irrigation of gross contamination in the trauma resuscitation area. Wounds should be managed using sterile saline-soaked gauze and covered with dry, sterile rolled gauze.
   b. Splint the extremity as soon as the wound is covered to reduce hemorrhage, prevent further injury, and alleviate pain.
   c. Antibiotic prophylaxis includes tetanus toxoid, first-generation cephalosporin, and aminoglycoside for contaminated wound or grade III fracture. Penicillin should be added for barnyard injury. Organisms may be gram-negative or gram-positive bacteria.
   d. Orthopedic consultation should be obtained early.
   e. Wounds require urgent operative irrigation and debridement; the orthopedic standard is within 6 to 8 hours if the patient is physiologically stable.
   f. Wounds require repeated irrigation and debridement in the operating room (OR) every 2 to 4 days, until definitive soft-tissue coverage can be achieved (usually, 5–10 days), which can require pedicle-based or free tissue flaps. **Minimize multiple inspections of the wound outside the OR, except**

by the surgeon making critical management decisions. Continue antibiotics until 48 hours after definitive coverage of soft tissue and wound.

g. Antibiotic-impregnated bone cement "beads" have been shown to benefit delivery of antibiotics to dead spaces that do not receive the systemic antibiotics. This local delivery has few systemic effects and is efficacious. The general mix dose is three vials of tobramycin (1.2 g each, 3.6 g total) per bag of cement. The beads are strung on a stainless-steel wire and, when hard, placed into the wound and covered with a liquid-sealed dressing (e.g., OpSite, Ioban). This "bead pouch" retains the fluid bathing the beads and is rich in antibiotic concentration. Tobramycin is used because in such high concentrations it provides coverage of both gram-positive and gram-negative organisms.

h. Internal fixation of grade I open fractures after adequate debridement and irrigation can be accomplished with infection rates of <2%. If soft-tissue loss is minimal and coverage is adequate, selected grade II open fractures can be treated with intramedullary fixation. External fixation may be necessary to stabilize grade III open fractures (infection rates of 10% to 50%). **A staged planned redebridement may be necessary in open fractures with severe soft-tissue damage.**

i. Wound closure may not be possible in all cases. Temporary closure with a vacuum system may be required and provides adequate coverage. At the end of the debridement, coverage of the bone should be attempted. If this cannot be achieved, a plastic surgeon should be consulted.

3. Gunshot wounds

a. **Low-velocity gunshot wounds** cause less soft-tissue destruction than high-velocity gunshot wounds. Because of the splintering effect of gunshot injuries, bone is often unstable and requires operative fixation. Debride the skin wounds and treat the bone as in closed injury. Prolonged antibiotic use is controversial; our practice is to administer oral antibiotics for 5 to 7 days.

b. **High-velocity gunshot wounds** and **close-range shotgun blasts** cause significant soft-tissue injury, and should be treated as severe grade III open fractures. These wounds often result in massive soft-tissue defects and require extensive reconstruction. Search for associated neural or vascular injuries.

II. SPECIFIC INJURIES

A. **Pelvis** (Chapter 32)

B. **Acetabular (hip socket) fractures** are complex, and can be associated with a hip dislocation. Acetabular fractures represent significant injury to the hip that can be associated with lifelong disability. Most acetabular fractures require temporary skeletal traction to maintain the reduction and prevent soft-tissue contracture. The acetabulum has anterior and posterior columns.

1. Types

a. **Central fracture** most often requires temporary skeletal traction.

b. **Posterior fracture or dislocation** requires urgent reduction under anesthesia. Sciatic nerve injuries have been reported in 10% to 30% of patients. A careful neurologic examination must be performed before and following reduction of the dislocation. Superior gluteal artery injuries can occur, usually presenting when the fracture exits into the greater sciatic notch. **Closed reduction may not be achieved if an associated fracture to the femoral head is present. In these cases, or if the fracture pattern causes redislocation, emergent definitive treatment may be required.**

c. **Anterior fracture or dislocation**, which is rare, is often associated with more severe acetabular fractures.

2. Radiographic evaluation includes anteroposterior, lateral, and obturator oblique and iliac oblique views (collectively called Judet views) of the pelvis. After reduction of the dislocation, CT scan of the acetabulum is performed with 3-mm cuts. The radiologist should provide reconstructions in multiple views.

3. Treatment
   a. Temporary skeletal traction
   b. Delayed ORIF is the treatment of choice for displaced fractures. Definitive operative intervention is usually from 2 to 7 days postinjury, which reduces the chance for bleeding complications at the operative site.
   c. Posttraumatic arthritis, chondrolysis, and heterotopic ossification are the common complications. **Meticulous intraoperative rinsing and careful muscular dissection is key to prevent heterotopic ossification.** Postoperatively, indomethacin (75 mg/day for 2 weeks) or radiation (single 700 [gray, or Gy] dose) can be used to prevent heterotopic ossification.
C. Hip dislocation, with or without associated acetabular fracture, occurs through the capsular area containing the blood supply to the femoral head (Fig. 31-1).
   1. Types (based on orientation of the femoral head to the acetabulum)
      a. Posterior dislocation is most common. Sciatic nerve injuries occur (10% to 30%). The leg is usually flexed and adducted.
      b. Anterior dislocation. The femoral head sits on top of the pubis or in the obturator foramen. The leg is generally abducted and externally rotated.
   2. Radiographic evaluation in the trauma resuscitation area includes anteroposterior, lateral, and Judet views. CT scan is required postreduction.
   3. Treatment. Dislocation of the hip requires urgent reduction because of the risk of avascular necrosis (AVN) of the femoral head. Delay in diagnosis and treatment increases the incidence of AVN, which can manifest years after injury. Reduction under intravenous sedation can be attempted (by an orthopedist) once the patient is in the trauma resuscitation area. If not achieved, perform urgent closed reduction under anesthesia. If closed reduction under anesthesia is unsuccessful after several attempts, open reduction is necessary.
      a. Postreduction CT scan (3-mm cuts) is obtained to exclude associated fracture or loose bodies.
      b. A careful neurologic examination testing femoral, posterior tibial, and peroneal nerve sensory and motor function is mandatory before and following reduction of the dislocation.
D. Lower extremity fractures play a significant role in the management of trauma patients. Early internal fixation has significantly reduced mortality and morbidity with these fractures. Stabilization of long bone fractures, including the femur and tibia, has allowed patients to mobilize early. Advances in orthopedic hardware, including the development of statically locked intramedullary nails, have significantly improved outcome. A variety of injuries or combination of injuries can be seen in the lower extremities. The most common injuries are discussed below.
   1. Femoral neck fractures in young patients are the result of high-energy impact. They commonly occur in the elderly, often from low-energy injuries (falls from a standing position). Femoral neck fractures are generally displaced. Femoral neck fractures occur concurrently with 15% of femoral diaphyseal fractures. For this reason, radiographic evaluation of the hip is essential before femoral shaft fracture fixation.
      a. Treatment. Displaced femoral neck fractures require immediate orthopedic consultation and urgent ORIF to reduce the complication rates of AVN and nonunion. Elderly patients with significant medical problems may have hemiarthroplasty in a delayed fashion. Morbidity and mortality of hip fractures in the elderly are related to preinjury cognitive function and associated medical illnesses.
   2. Peritrochanteric femur fractures are more common in elderly patients. If they occur in young patients high-energy trauma is present. Treatment is generally operative, but because the vascular supply is usually spared, ORIF is not as urgent as in femoral neck fractures; immediate or delayed ORIF is acceptable. Temporary skin traction is used for comfort before ORIF. Peritrochanteric femur fractures in the elderly have high morbidity and mortality because of comorbid diseases in this population.

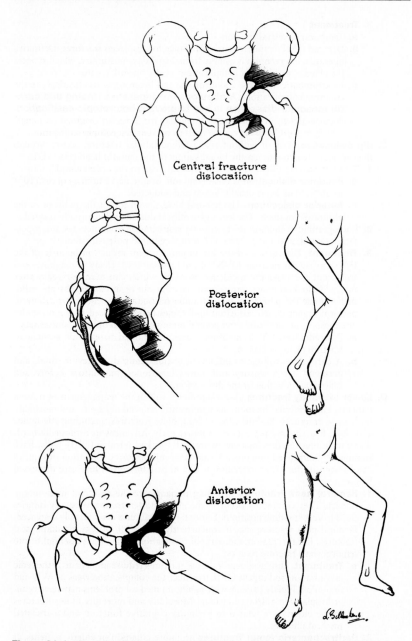

Figure 31-1. Hip dislocation. (From Mick CA. Initial management of fractures and joint injuries. In: Zuidema GD, Rutherford RB, Ballinger WF, eds. *The Management of Trauma*. Philadelphia, Pa: WB Saunders; 1985:673, with permission.)

a. **Treatment** has traditionally been with plates and screws. However, we have used newer intramedullary implants that permit immediate weight bearing in most cases, which allows more independence and more efficient care postoperatively. Preoperative planning is essential for these fractures. If operative intervention is delayed, skeletal traction should be employed. A high rate of nonunion and hardware failure is found in these fractures.

3. **Femoral shaft fractures** are defined as 5 cm distal to the lesser trochanter and 8 cm proximal to the knee joint. They result from high-energy forces. Hip or pelvis radiographs should be taken to rule out an associated femoral neck fracture. Describe fractures based on location, soft-tissue injury, comminution, and angulation.

    a. **Treatment.** Early intramedullary nailing is the treatment of choice. This is generally performed without actual exposure of the fracture site. This operative approach reduces the incidence of malrotation, shortening, and pulmonary complications.

4. **Supracondylar femur fractures** occur within 8 cm of the knee joint. They can be intraarticular or extraarticular, unicondylar or bicondylar. They can be associated with superficial femoral artery or popliteal artery injury.

    a. **Treatment.** Complex, intraarticular closed fracture requires careful preoperative planning and may be delayed. If delayed, use skeletal traction through the tibia or calcaneus.

5. **Knee dislocation** requires urgent reduction and immobilization. **Despite immediate reduction, important and significant complications can occur: compartment syndrome, arterial injury, and neurological complications (peroneal and tibial nerve injury).** Injury to the popliteal artery is common (20%) because the artery can be tethered between the adductor hiatus proximally and the interosseous membrane distally, and the symptoms from intimal tears may be secondary occlusion and/or embolus. Arteriography or immediate operation is essential if asymmetry is found in the neurovascular examination. Even in the absence of clear signs of arterial injury, consider arteriography for documented knee dislocation because of the risk of undetected intimal injury with late occlusion.

    a. **Types.** Anterior, posterior, medial, lateral, or rotatory.

    b. **Treatment.** Early reconstruction is not necessary but can be performed. Acute treatment can be achieved with a splint or hinged brace. Prompt evaluation of the arterial system is mandatory.

6. **Patellar fractures**

    a. Usually result from direct blow to the flexed knee. Displacement results in loss of continuity of the quadriceps mechanism.

    b. Nonoperative treatment for nondisplaced fractures. Operation is necessary to restore quadriceps function and articular surface integrity. Repair requires ORIF or partial patellectomy. Patellar retinacula must be repaired.

7. **Tibial plateau fractures** most frequently occur to the lateral tibial plateau. They involve the presence or absence of articular surface depression and fracture location. They can be nondisplaced or displaced (4 mm). Associated knee ligament injury or vascular injury occurs. Compartment syndrome is seen in up to 25% of patients with high-energy tibial plateau fractures.

    a. **Treatment.** ORIF is preferred for displaced fractures. Treat nondisplaced fractures nonoperatively or with percutaneous screw fixation. In the elderly, tibial plateau fractures are usually minimally displaced and can often be treated nonoperatively. In young adults with high-energy injury, the fracture often extends to the tibial diaphysis.

8. **Tibial shaft fractures** occur as high-energy injuries (e.g., motorcycle crashes, pedestrian–automobile impacts, crush injuries). Open tibial fractures occur commonly and are best treated by intramedullary nailing. Compartment syndrome occurs in 10% of tibia fractures, more commonly in proximal tibial fractures. Tibial fractures are described based on location (proximal one third,

middle one third, distal one third), displacement, comminution degree, and open versus closed.

a. Treatment

    i. Closed fractures can often be treated with closed reduction and casting. Open reduction and internal fixation with intramedullary nailing may be required for unstable fracture patterns, segmental fractures, or tibial fractures associated with ipsilateral femur fractures unless severe soft-tissue injury is present.

    ii. Open tibial fractures are treated based on the grade of the open fracture and degree of soft-tissue injury. Consider external fixation in fractures with significant soft-tissue injury because it provides adequate stability, minimizes the foreign body burden (metal implant), and allows access to the limb for soft-tissue reconstruction.

        a) Early soft-tissue coverage of open fractures has decreased the incidence of secondary infection. Flaps commonly used include (*a*) proximal one third fracture-gastrocnemius muscle, (*b*) middle one third fracture-soleus muscle, and (*c*) distal one third fracture-latissimus, gracilis, or rectus muscle.

        b) Early amputation may be indicated in severely crushed limbs or grade IIIc open fractures with anatomic disruption of the tibial nerve.

        c) Mangled extremity (Table 31-2). When the injured extremity has such severe injury that its salvageability is in question, decisions in management require input from the trauma surgeon and orthopedist; considerable judgment is necessary. Various scoring systems have been developed to help clinicians determine the benefit of early amputation versus attempts at limb salvage. The mangled extremity may be an open or closed fracture. Most scoring systems have been developed for the lower extremity; the most

---

TABLE 31-2   **Mangled Extremity Severity Scoring System**

Factor	Score
Skeletal/Soft-tissue Injury	
–Low energy (stab, fracture, civilian gunshot wound [GSW])	1
–Medium energy (open or multiple fracture)	2
–High energy (shotgun or high-velocity GSW, crush injury)	3
–Very high energy (above, combined with gross contamination)	4
Limb Ischemia (Double Value if Ischemia >6 Hours)	
–Pulse reduced or absent, but normal capillary fill	1
–Pulseless, diminished capillary fill	2
–Limb is cool, paralyzed, insensate	3
Shock	
–Systolic blood pressure consistently >90 mmHg	0
–Systolic blood pressure transiently <90 mmHg	1
–Systolic blood pressure persistently <90 mmHg	2
Age (Years)	
<30	0
30–50	1
>50	2

commonly used is the mangled extremity severity scoring (MESS) system. A limb with a MESS $\geq$7 is ultimately likely to undergo amputation of the extremity, whereas limbs with MESS <7 can generally be successfully salvaged. **The scoring system should be used as a guide, not as a rule of clinical practice.** The decision to perform a primary amputation as opposed to heroic attempts at limb salvage of the mangled extremity is difficult because of the psychological, functional, and morbid effects of this decision. Ability to salvage an extremity depends on the status of the skin, bone, muscles, vessels, and nerves. Prolonged attempts at limb salvage are inappropriate in the multiply injured patient with immediately life-threatening injuries of the chest, head, or abdomen.

   d) **Damage control** principles have been applied to the unstable, multiply injured patient with orthopedic injury. This approach involves rapid external fixation of extremity fractures to temporarily stabilize them. Certain clinical parameters predispose the patient to adverse outcome (Table 31-3). Intramedullary nailing is done when the patient is stabilized.

9. **Tibial plafond (pilon) fractures** occur in the distal tibia, usually involving the articular surface from an axial load. CT scan or tomograms can be useful in defining the character of the fracture. The fibula may be involved. Pilon fractures generally involve significant concomitant soft-tissue injury with high risk of associated soft-tissue loss and infection.

   a. **Treatment** should be dictated by the status of the soft-tissue envelope as wound complication rates are high. Temporary skeletal stabilization with an external fixator may be necessary until the soft-tissue edema decreases at which time ORIF can be performed safely. Posttraumatic arthritis usually requires late ankle arthrodesis.

10. **Ankle fractures** are produced by external rotation with a fracture to the fibula or an injury to the interosseous membrane (Maseoneuve injury). Ankle fractures are classified based on fracture location of the lateral malleolus (fibula) and the presence (or absence) of a medial malleolus fracture.

    a. Radiographic evaluation includes anteroposterior, lateral, and mortise views, both initially and after reduction.

    b. **Treatment** requires ORIF if any subluxation (>1 mm) or incongruity of the ankle joint is found. Perform this immediately, before soft-tissue swelling is significant, or on a delayed basis (7–14 days).

 TABLE 31-3   **Parameters Associated with Adverse Outcome in Polytrauma Patients**

Criteria

ISS $\geq$40 in the absence of additional thoracic injury

ISS >20 and additional thoracic trauma (AIS >2)

Multiple long bones + truncal injury AIS 2 or more

Polytrauma with abdom./pelvic trauma (> Moore 3) and hem. shock (initial RR <90 mmHg)

Bilateral lung contusions on first plain film

Presumed operation time >6 hours

Initial mean pulmonary arterial pressure >24 mmHg (if available)

(Adapted from Pape HC, Tscherne H. Early definitive fracture fixation, pulmonary function and systemic effects. In Baue AE, ed. *Multiple Organ Failure*. New York, NY: Springer-Verlag; 2000:279–290.)

11. **Calcaneus fractures** are usually the result of significant falls and are often bilateral. Associated spine injuries should be sought. Calcaneal fractures are disabling injuries and patients are often unable to return to labor.

   a. **Radiographic evaluation** includes anteroposterior, lateral, and axial views. Obtain CT scan (3-mm cuts) in two planes (axial and coronal) for adequate delineation of the fracture and joint.

   b. **Treatment.** Displaced intraarticular fractures require ORIF, which should be done when the soft-tissue swelling subsides (7–14 days). Use elevation and a foot pump to reduce swelling. For fractures that are not reconstructible, use primary arthrodesis. If the soft-tissue injury is extensive, external fixation or simple percutaneous pinning can also be used. Late subtalar arthrodesis should be performed for posttraumatic arthritis. The complication rate with ORIF is 15% to 30% and often results in the need for muscle flaps with risk of associated infection. This high risk of infection has prompted many to use only limited reductions and in situ pinning. This approach allows restoration of the hindfoot architecture and reconstructive procedures on a delayed basis, when less chance exists for soft-tissue complications.

12. **Talar neck fractures** are usually caused by forced hyperdorsiflexion of the foot on the ankle. Because of the precarious blood supply to the talar body, talar neck fractures require anatomic reduction. Associated subtalar or talar dislocations **should be reduced immediately** to minimize risk of AVN (as high as 85% to 100%), the incidence of which is related to fracture severity. Displaced fractures require ORIF and nondisplaced fractures can be treated with percutaneous screw fixation.

13. **Tarsometatarsal (Lisfranc) fractures** are usually associated with significant midfoot swelling, and are commonly missed at initial presentation. Foot compartment syndrome can occur and results in significant disability. ORIF is indicated for displaced fractures. These are devastating injuries and can be associated with significant injury to the plantar ligamentous structures, which can result in late deformity (e.g., planovalgus). Posttraumatic degenerative joint disease (DJD) is common and requires delayed arthrodesis.

14. **Metatarsal fractures** can usually be treated in a short leg walking cast. Open reduction is indicated for intraarticular displacement. Closed reduction and pin fixation is indicated for significant plantar displacement.

E. **Upper extremity fractures** also have an impact on the outcome of trauma patients. Upper extremities are necessary for activities of daily living and as weight-bearing structures when the lower extremities are compromised.

   1. **Sternoclavicular dislocation** can be anterior or posterior.

      a. Anterior dislocation is of minimal clinical significance. Perform a single attempt at closed reduction. However, reduction is usually unstable. Fixation and multiple attempts at relocation are contraindicated.

      b. Posterior dislocation of the clavicle can be associated with life-threatening mediastinal injuries. CT scan or arteriography may be necessary for evaluation. Closed reduction should be performed in the OR under general anesthesia. Open reduction is performed if closed reduction is unsuccessful. A general or thoracic surgeon should be on standby in the event complications arise.

   2. **Clavicle shaft fractures** are generally of minimal clinical significance. They are classified according to location of the fracture: medial one third, middle one third (most common), and distal one third. Associated injuries include brachial plexus injury, pneumothorax, and sternoclavicular or acromioclavicular joint injury.

      a. **Treatment.** These fractures are generally treated symptomatically with a sling; expect healing in 6 to 8 weeks. Figure-of-eight straps tend not to be well tolerated. ORIF is indicated for open fractures, neurovascular compromise, and skin compromise. Also, selected fractures of the distal one third of the clavicle may require ORIF.

3. **Acromioclavicular joint sprains (separated shoulder)** are usually treated symptomatically with a sling. ORIF is indicated for severe displacement with trapezoid ligament entrapment. Late distal clavicle excision may be necessary for symptomatic arthritis.

4. **Scapula fractures,** which are produced by high-energy impact, are frequently associated with intrathoracic injuries. Symptomatic treatment in a sling is usually sufficient with early motion. ORIF is indicated for the following:
   a. Large, displaced coracoid or acromial fragments
   b. Ipsilateral, displaced glenoid neck and displaced clavicle fracture (floating shoulder)
   c. Intraarticular glenoid (subluxation of the glenoid >25% surface)

5. **Glenohumeral dislocation (shoulder)** is usually anterior. Posterior dislocations can occur with seizures, electrocution, or dashboard injury. Careful neurovascular examination is needed to exclude axillary nerve or artery injury.
   a. **Radiographs** are obtained to assess concomitant fractures—anteroposterior and axillary lateral views.
   b. **Treatment.** Early closed reduction with adequate sedation followed by sling protection with supervised active range-of-motion when pain abates. Associated rotator cuff injuries are common in patients >40 years of age but do not change the initial management.

6. **Proximal humerus fractures** usually occur in elderly osteoporotic bone. When occurring in young patients, they are usually caused by high-energy trauma, and associated injuries are common.
   a. **Types.** Anatomic classification is based on four parts: head, greater tuberosity, lesser tuberosity, or metaphysis fractures. Displacement is defined as 1 cm of displacement or 45-degree angulation.
      i. One-part fracture: all undisplaced fractures, regardless of the number of fracture lines
      ii. Two-part fracture: fractures involving the anatomic neck, surgical neck, isolated lesser or greater tuberosity fractures
      iii. Three-part fracture: fracture of the neck and a tuberosity fracture
      iv. Four-part fracture: fracture of the neck, greater tuberosity fracture, and lesser tuberosity fracture
   b. **Treatment.** In young patients, efforts are aimed at accurate reduction of the fracture, often surgically, to maximize function. In the elderly or less active individuals, nonoperative management or hemiarthroplasty allows adequate pain relief and function.
      i. Stable, two-part impacted neck fractures → sling and swathe
      ii. Two-part neck or unstable → ORIF closed reduction, percutaneous pinning
      iii. Displaced greater tuberosity fracture → ORIF
      iv. Three-part in younger patients with good bone stock → ORIF
      v. Hemiarthroplasty for the following:
         a) Three-part in elderly patients
         b) Three-part with poor bone stock
         c) Four-part, except elderly debilitated patients or severe diabetics

7. **Humeral shaft fractures** have a high rate of union with nonoperative management using fracture braces. In the multiply injured patient, however, ORIF or intramedullary nailing may be indicated to facilitate nursing care or utilize the extremity for weight bearing and activities of daily living. Distal third fractures can be associated with radial nerve palsy (usually a neuropraxia).

8. **Distal humerus fractures** are more common in children than in adults. The classification scheme is as complex as the fractures themselves, based on intraarticular versus extraarticular, degree of comminution, and displacement. Intraarticular fractures mandate an anatomic reduction.
   a. **Pediatric distal humerus fractures** are associated with neurovascular injury and compartment syndrome. Urgent (not emergent) closed reduction should be performed in the OR. Percutaneous pinning is necessary for unstable fractures or those with significant soft-tissue swelling. Open

reduction is required if closed reduction is unsuccessful. Cubitus varus is a common complication.

b. Adult distal humerus fractures require ORIF in most cases. Heterotopic ossification can occur, especially in head-injured patients. Stiffness and ulnar neuropathy can occur.

c. Capitellum and trochlea fractures should be treated with ORIF for large, displaced fragments and excision for small, displaced fragments.

9. **Olecranon fractures** usually occur as traction injuries. ORIF with tension band techniques is indicated if displacement is >2 mm. For severely comminuted fractures, excise (<50% of the olecranon). With associated dislocation, early excision is contraindicated.

10. **Coronoid fractures** are treated with early motion if <50% and ORIF if >50%. They are common in elbow dislocations that remain unstable after closed reduction.

11. **Radial head fractures** occur from a fall on an outstretched hand.

   a. Treatment. Nondisplaced fractures should be treated with early motion. ORIF is performed if angulation is >30 degrees, 3-mm displacement, or depression greater than one third of the articular surface. Early excision can be performed for severely comminuted fractures. Manage associated dislocations first; suspect distal radioulnar injury.

12. **Elbow dislocations** are common and most often posterior. Dislocations and fractures of the elbow usually result from a fall on an outstretched arm or direct impact on the elbow. A careful neurovascular examination is performed to rule out injury to the ulnar, radial or median nerve, or the brachial artery; most nerve injuries are neuropraxia. Associated fractures of the coronoid, radial head, and medial epicondyle can occur; obtain radiographs to exclude an associated fracture. Treatment consists of immediate closed reduction and application of a posterior splint. Document median and ulnar nerve function before and after reduction; nerve entrapment can occur with reduction. The splint should be removed at 7 to 10 days and early active range of motion begun. In unstable cases, maintain suspicion of a coronoid or radial head fracture. A relocated elbow will demonstrate trochlear congruity on the anteroposterior radiograph, and congruence of the olecranon-humerus, and radius-capitellar articulations on the lateral radiograph.

13. **Combined radius and ulna fractures** in an adult should be treated with ORIF. Fractures of both bones in the forearm risk compartment syndrome. Posterior interosseous nerve injury is common with proximal third fractures. Severely contaminated open fractures may require external fixation.

14. **Ulnar shaft fractures** occur as a result of a direct blow. These fractures are generally treated with functional bracing, but delayed union is common. ORIF should be performed with angulation >10 degrees or displacement >50%. Associated injuries to the wrist and elbow should be suspected. **Monteggia's fracture-dislocation** is a proximal ulnar fracture with an associated radial head dislocation; this mandates ORIF.

15. **Radius fractures** are treated in a long arm cast in supination if they are nondisplaced and in the proximal one fifth. Fractures distal to this in the radial shaft should be treated by ORIF. **Galeazzi fracture** is a radial shaft fracture, at the junction of the middle and distal third of the radius, associated with dislocation of the distal radioulnar joint. Treatment is forearm immobilization in supination for 6 weeks.

16. **Distal radius fractures** usually occur from a fall on an outstretched arm. Associated median or ulnar nerve injury, distal radioulnar joint disruption, and carpal instability can occur. Extensor pollicis longus rupture can also occur and is usually seen 5 to 8 weeks after injury. **Colles fracture** is a fracture of the distal radius with displacement of the carpus. **Smith's fracture** is a reversed Colles fracture—a fracture of the distal radius with the distal fragment and accompanying carpal row displaced volarly. **Barton's fracture** is a distal radius fracture with displacement of a dorsally based triangular segment from

the radius. **Reversed Barton's fracture** is a distal radius fracture with displacement of a palmarly based triangular segment from the radius.

    a. Radiographic evaluation includes anteroposterior, lateral, and oblique views. Also obtain radiographs of the hand and elbow.

    b. Treatment is initially with closed reduction and casting. Fracture involving an intraarticular step-off, shortening, or severe comminution requires accurate reduction and fixation with pins or plates, with or without external fixation. ORIF is required with large, displaced articular fragments.

    17. Scaphoid fractures can be associated with other carpal injuries. For nondisplaced (<2 mm) fractures, treatment should consist of a long arm thumb spica. Treatment duration varies with fracture location, but ranges from 8 to 20 weeks. For displaced fractures, perform closed reduction and pinning or ORIF. An anatomic reduction is necessary to reduce the risk of nonunion and avascular necrosis. AVN and nonunion are more common with waist and proximal pole fractures.

    18. Perilunate dislocations are commonly missed at initial presentation. Careful radiologic evaluation is mandatory. Associated scaphoid fractures are common. Reduction and pinning are necessary, and dorsal ligament repair may also be required. Associated median nerve injury is also common and early carpal tunnel decompression may be required.

    19. Hand (Chapter 33)

III. AMPUTATION INJURIES can result in significant morbidity and potentially dysfunctional limbs. Therefore, amputation injuries should be handled only at institutions under the direction of a team whose care is directed by a microvascular surgeon. **Amputations are true limb- and life-threatening injuries and should be handled as such, with no delays in treatment.** Unsuccessful reimplantations can result in significant disability. Realistic expectations can be provided to the patient only after evaluation by the reimplantation surgeon.

    A. The physician responsible for replantation should be notified before acceptance. Acceptance is defined as evaluation for **possible** replantation.

    B. Necessary historical data on the patient includes the patient's name, age, occupation, handedness for upper extremity, **time of injury**, mechanism of injury, level of injury (bone, soft tissue), exact neurovascular status, concomitant injuries and associated medical conditions, and the location and telephone number of the nearest relative, especially if the patient is a minor.

    C. The OR should be prepared as soon as acceptance is made.

    D. Transport the patient expeditiously.

    E. Preserve amputated parts by wrapping in a sterile gauze moistened with sterile saline solution. Place in a watertight plastic container or resealable plastic bag, which should then be placed into an iced saline bath. **DO NOT use dry ice. DO NOT place the amputated part in direct contact with ice.** Clearly label the container with the patient's name and time placed.

        1. Administer tetanus and broad-spectrum antibiotics as for open fractures.

    F. The replantation team should be present at time of arrival to the emergency department; notify the OR. Perform primary and secondary surveys with resuscitation. Limbs and amputated parts should be evaluated and examined radiographically. Amputated parts are replaced in container (as previously discussed).

    G. Transfer the patient to the OR. A two-team approach is used if associated injuries require intervention.

    H. Factors associated with a poor outcome include crush injury, long ischemia time (>6 hours), proximal amputations, nerve injuries (axonotmesis), systemic hypotension, severe contamination, concomitant injuries or medical conditions, and whether the patient is elderly, has poor nutrition, or is psychologically compromised.

IV. BASIC SPLINTING. Splinting of extremity injuries is a practice about which all physicians should have some knowledge. Creativity is useful in constructing splints for various body parts and conditions. Splinting should never be harmful, and adequate knowledge of relevant anatomy and potential complications is necessary. Follow the principles of splinting described below.

A. The **purpose for splinting is immobilization.** This provides temporary stabilization of bone and soft tissue, aids in control of hemorrhage, and helps reduce pain and prevent further injury.

B. Principles of splinting include splinting open fractures as they lie. Gross angulation in closed fractures should be reduced by longitudinal traction. When commercial splints are unavailable, use your ingenuity. Neurovascular status must **always** be reassessed after the splint is applied. If neurovascular compromise is present, remove or loosen the splint. When splinting, include the joint above and joint below, and make sure the splint is rigid enough to provide immobilization. It should not be circumferentially compressive unless excessive hemorrhage is present.

C. Types of commercial splints
1. Military antishock trousers (MAST) can be used for pelvic fractures and lower extremity fractures. Be aware they can induce compartment syndrome. Rigid cervical orthosis should be used for cervical spine (C-spine), and backboard should be used for the spine.
   a. Air splints for extremity fractures can induce compartment syndrome.
   b. Structural aluminum malleable (SAM) splints consist of semirigid cardboard; they are useful for upper extremity, ankle, and foot fractures.
   c. Silicone splints function similar to air splints, but with less chance for compartment syndrome. They are useful for distal extremities.
   d. Hare and Thomas traction splints are useful for femur fractures, and they provide longitudinal traction from foot to ischial tuberosity. Other commercial splints include knee immobilizers, sling, or sling and swathe for shoulder and proximal humerus, and aluminum splints for fingers.

D. Other types of splints include plaster of paris, which is the gold standard for the orthopedist. It is readily available, relatively inexpensive, and easy to use. Newer premade fiberglass splints may be more rigid than the plaster counterpart and provide no added advantage. Pillow splints are easy to use, and they can be secured with ace wrap or roll gauze. They are effective, comfortable, and an excellent choice for distal extremities. Splints can also be fashioned with cardboard, blankets or towels, and aluminum.

E. Specific areas
1. C-spine may require a cervical collar and sandbags.
2. The spine may require a backboard and logroll.
3. The shoulder may require a sling, sling and swathe, and ace wrap arm to chest.
4. Splints for the humerus are the same as for the shoulder and also may include a SAM splint or plaster U-splint.
5. Elbows should be splinted at a 90-degree angle with a posterior plaster splint.
6. Splinting of the forearm, wrist, and hand should include the elbow at a 90-degree angle. Plaster U-splint or pillow splint can also be used.
7. MAST may be used initially to splint pelvic fractures.
8. Splinting of the proximal femur and femoral shaft should include Hare traction, posterior plaster splint, pillow splints, or MAST.
9. Splinting of the distal femur, knee, and proximal tibia may require a knee immobilizer, posterior plaster splint, pillow splints, or MAST.
10. Splinting of the tibial shaft should include posterior plaster or U-splint, pillow splints, silicone splints, or MAST.
11. Ankle and foot splinting can be performed with posterior plaster or U-splint, pillow splints, or silicone splints.

Bibliography
Hunt JP, Weintraub SL, Wang Y, et al. Kinematics of Trauma. In: Moore EE, Feliciano DV, Mattox KL, eds. *Trauma.* 5th ed. New York, NY: McGraw-Hill; 2004:141–158.
Gustilo RB, Anderson JT. Prevention of infection in the treatment of 1025 open fractures of long bones. *J Bone Joint Surg* 1976;58A:453–459.

Johansen K, Daines M, Howey T, et al. Objective criteria accurately predict amputation following lower extremity trauma. *J Trauma* 1990;30:568–573.

Pape HC, Tscherne H. Early definitive fracture fixation, pulmonary function and systemic effects. In: Baue AE, ed. *Multiple Organ Failure.* New York, NY: Springer-Verlag; 2000:279–290.

Pape HC, Giannoudis P, Rockwood C. *Rockwood and Green's Fractures in Adults.* 6th ed. Philadelphia, Pa: Lippincott Williams & Wilkins; 2005.

Poss R. *Orthopaedic Knowledge Update 3.* Rosemont, Ill: American Academy of Orthopaedic Surgeons; 1990.

32

PELVIC FRACTURES
BORIS A. ZELLE AND GARY S. GRUEN

I. INCIDENCE AND MECHANISM OF INJURY. Pelvic fractures may occur as a result of low-energy trauma (i.e., falls) or high-energy trauma. Pelvic fractures from low-energy trauma are often stable, and can be managed through nonoperative methods. Unstable pelvic ring disruptions are generally caused by high-energy events such as motor vehicle and motorcycle crashes, pedestrians struck by motor vehicles, and falls from heights. Between 3% and 5% of the traffic accidents are associated with pelvic injuries. More than 80% of the unstable pelvic ring disruptions occur as a result of traffic accidents; and more than 90% of the patients have associated injuries to the head, chest, abdomen, spine, or long bones. The most commonly associated intrapelvic injuries include urogenital injuries (bladder disruption, urethra disruption, and vagina tear), vascular injury, or bowel injury. In complex pelvic injuries, the mortality rate may be as high as 30%.

II. EXAMINATION. History and clinical examination of the pelvis, which are important for diagnosis of suspected injury, should be done concurrently with resuscitation, especially in the hypotensive patient. Early orthopedic consultation is important.

    A. The awake and communicative patient with a pelvic fracture may complain of pelvic pain, which guides further examination. Patients with urethral disruption may complain of an inability to void (urethral tears are uncommon in females).

    B. Inspection of the soft tissue around the pelvis is essential to identify a laceration or skin degloving. **Open fractures**, which occur in approximately 5% of pelvic fractures, contribute to 50% of the mortality. Patients with open pelvic fractures often require urgent exploratory laparotomy and a diverting colostomy. Temporarily cover open wounds with sterile compressive dressings. The posterior pelvis can be evaluated by logrolling the patient to inspect for lacerations or hematoma.

        1. In males, examine the scrotal contents for testicular displacement and inspect the urethral meatus for blood. The absence of blood does not exclude a urethral injury. Palpate the anterior pubic symphysis for diastasis and rami for crepitus.

        2. In females, appropriate evaluation of the external genitalia should include a visual and bimanual pelvic examination for lacerations that may involve the urethra, vagina, or rectum. If an adequate examination is not possible in the emergency department, thorough examination under anesthesia should be done as soon as possible. Vaginal lacerations should be irrigated and closed, if the tissues appear healthy. Perineal lacerations are generally managed open with serial debridement and delayed closure.

        3. Perform rectal examination before inserting the Foley catheter (check for a displaced prostate in males, which is indicative of urethral disruption). Urethral tears are more frequent in males and commonly occur below the urogenital diaphragm. Blood on the examining finger with rectal examination requires direct visualization of the anus and rectum; anoscopy and proctoscopy are indicated. A rectal tear in the setting of a pelvic fracture is a contaminated open fracture. Diverting colostomy and irrigation of the wound are indicated. Maintain a high suspicion for rectal injury in all cases of displaced pelvic fractures. Rectal tears can result from perforation by bony fragments, crush injury to the rectum, or ischemic injury to the rectum from mesenteric vessel injury. **Consider proctoscopy for all patients with significantly displaced pelvic fractures.**

4. **An open pelvic fracture with active bleeding** through a soft-tissue defect represents a difficult management problem. The fracture is no longer contained and the patient can rapidly exsanguinate (Fig. 32-1). Major vascular disruption occurs in only 1% of pelvic fractures, but has a 75% mortality rate. Management includes:

   a. Airway control and multiple-site, large-bore intravenous (IV) access; early blood transfusion.

   b. Pressure tamponade of soft-tissue bleeding in the trauma room.

   c. Transfer to the operating room (OR) for laparotomy, control of bleeding from extrapelvic sources, and simultaneous control and packing of pelvic bleeding. Control of pelvic bleeding may require suture ligation of obvious bleeding sites through both the abdomen and perineal wound.

   d. External fixation with diverting colostomy if the perineal wound involves the anus or rectum.

   e. Arteriogram with embolization if possible.

   f. Serial operative debridement with delayed definitive fracture management and wound closure.

C. The mechanical stability is often difficult to assess manually. Repetitive stressing of the pelvis is not advisable; this can exacerbate bleeding and increase patient discomfort. Direct manipulation of the pelvis in compression is a test of rotational stability, whereas the push-pull maneuver of the lower leg is a clinical sign of vertical displacement.

D. Perform a detailed motor and sensory examination of the lower extremities to evaluate for associated neurologic injury, particularly of the lumbosacral plexus. The examination should include sphincter tone, perineal sensation, as well as lower extremity function and sensation. The nerve roots may be injured through stretch

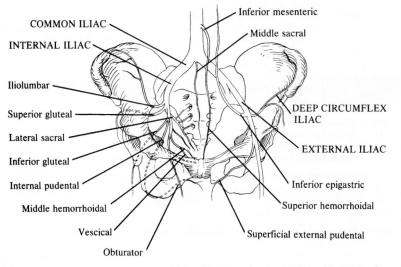

Figure 32-1. Arterial supply to the pelvis. (From Kudsk KA, Sheldon GF. Retroperitoneal hematoma. In: Blaisdell FW, Trunkey DD. *Trauma Management—Abdominal Trauma*. New York, NY: Thieme Medical Publishers; 1982:284, with permission.)

or laceration. Perform and document the examination both before and after fracture reduction.

III. **RADIOGRAPHIC EVALUATION.** All patients involved in high-energy trauma, and those complaining of pelvic pain after low-energy trauma, require an anteroposterior (AP) radiograph of the pelvis. It is important to note that displacement occurring at the time of injury can be greater than that visualized on the radiograph because of the elastic recoil of the pelvis.

A. If pelvis asymmetry or fracture is identified, obtain pelvic inlet and outlet views to determine AP and vertical displacement of the hemipelvis, respectively.

B. Obtain a **Judet** oblique radiograph in patients with suspicion of acetabular fractures.

C. Evidence of significant posterior or vertical instability includes displacement of the posterior pelvic complex by >5 mm.

1. Obtain a **computed tomography (CT)** scan of the pelvis, with 3-mm contiguous cuts, in patients with evidence of a pelvic fracture (when the patient is hemodynamically **stable**). The CT scan provides information on the extent of injury, magnitude of fracture or joint displacement, and foraminal compression of the sacrum. The CT scan is especially helpful in evaluating the posterior pelvic ring in comparison with plain radiographs. Information obtained from the CT defines the anatomic pattern in greater detail and may change what the orthopedic surgeon does operatively.

D. Evaluate the genitourinary tract in patients with hematuria, blood at the urethral meatus, or inability or urinate.

1. A retrograde urethrogram or cystogram is required to evaluate for potential urethral injury or bladder injury. Genitourinary injuries associated with pelvic fractures are missed 23% of the time on initial evaluation.

IV. **TYPES OF PELVIC FRACTURES.** Mechanisms of injury and force vectors involved determine the pelvic fracture pattern, as well as associated injuries. Numerous classification systems exist to describe the injured pelvis and deformity patterns. However, the most commonly used classification system is that of Tile, stratified on the instability of the bony injury (Table 32-1).

A. **Stable,** minimally displaced pelvic ring fractures are usually associated with low-energy trauma. These injuries are characterized by pubic rami fractures, avulsion fractures, or simple, transverse sacral or coccygeal fractures (Fig. 32-2A).

TABLE 32-1 Types of Pelvic Fractures

Type A: Stable
A1—Fractures not involving the ring; avulsion injuries
A2—Stable, minimal displacement
A3—Transverse fractures of the sacrum or coccyx

Type B: Rotationally Unstable; Vertically and Posteriorly Stable
B1—External rotation instability; open book injury
B2—Internal rotation instability; lateral compression injury
B3—Bilateral rotationally unstable injury

Type C: Rotationally, Posteriorly, and Vertically Unstable
C1—Unilateral injury
C2—Bilateral injury, with one side rotationally unstable and one side vertically unstable
C3—Bilateral injury, with both sides completely unstable

(From Tile M. Pelvic ring fractures: Should they be fixed? *J Bone Joint Surg* 1988;70:1, with permission.)

B. Rotationally unstable fractures consist of anterior and posterior pelvic ring injuries resulting in rotational laxity (through AP compression or lateral compression mechanisms) but vertical stability (Fig. 32-2B). The symphysis, rami, or both are involved anteriorly, whereas the sacrum, sacroiliac joint, or both are involved posteriorly. Both ipsilateral and contralateral injuries are represented (Fig. 32-2C).

C. Vertically and rotationally unstable fractures are characterized by disruptions in the anterior and posterior elements, with vertical displacement of either one or both hemipelves, either with or without associated acetabular fractures (Fig. 32-2D).

D. The mechanism of injury determines associated injuries, due to the vector of the force during injury:

    1. Lateral compression fractures: closed head injury, lung, spleen, liver

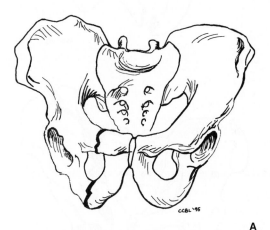

A

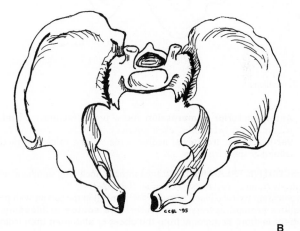

B

Figure 32-2. A: Stable, minimally displaced pelvic ring fracture. **B:** Rotationally unstable pubic symphysis diastasis. **C:** Rotationally unstable pubic ramus fracture and concomitant sacral injury. **D:** Vertically and rotationally unstable fracture with disruption of anterior and posterior elements and vertical displacement of the hemipelvis. (*continued*)

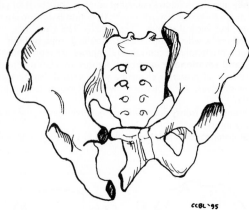

C

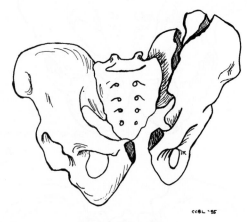

D

Figure 32-2. (continued)

    2. Anteroposterior compression (open book fractures): bladder, urethra, rectum, lower extremities, chest injuries

    3. Vertical shear fractures: neurovascular injury, calcaneal fractures, thoracolumbar spine fractures

V. RESUSCITATIVE TREATMENT. A team approach, including simultaneous evaluation by multiple trauma specialists, is essential (Fig. 32-3).

    A. Hypotension (systolic blood pressure <90 mmHg) in the patient with pelvic fracture requires prompt, aggressive treatment. **The source of bleeding in such a patient is more commonly from the chest or abdomen than from the pelvic fracture.** Major blood loss in the multiply injured patient with a displaced pelvic ring fracture can occur from the following five major areas:

        1. Intrathoracic bleeding may be detected on the screening chest radiograph obtained immediately on arrival to the emergency department (e.g., massive hemothorax).

Treatment of Pelvic Ring Fractures

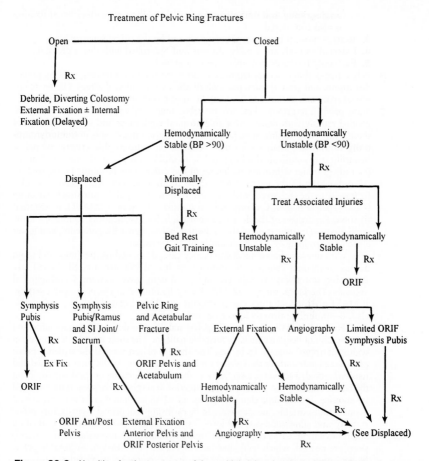

Figure 32-3. Algorithm for the treatment of the multiply injured patient with a pelvic ring fracture.

2. Intraperitoneal bleeding can be evaluated by **diagnostic peritoneal lavage (DPL) or ultrasound**, especially in the hemodynamically unstable patient. Assume hypotension is from an intraperitoneal injury rather than the pelvic fracture. Common abdominal injuries causing major bleeding include the spleen, liver, mesenteric tears, and lacerations to the iliac vessels. A **supraumbilical incision for DPL** decreases the rate of false-positive findings. If the patient requires laparotomy, or suprapubic tube, place the **incision as cephalad and central as possible** to avoid compromise of the surgical incisions required for open reduction and internal fixation (ORIF) of the pelvis. Assess peripheral pulses from the femoral artery to the dorsalis pedis.

   a. On rare occasion, the patient with a pelvic fracture presents with exsanguinating hemorrhage. The patient must be transferred immediately to the OR. The bleeding can be caused by major vascular injury (iliac or femoral arteries), intraperitoneal bleeding, or from the pelvis. Once in the abdomen, if the bleeding is from the pelvis and can be controlled with pressure, pack the pelvis and **transfer the patient promptly for pelvic**

angiography and embolization. Initial stabilization with external fixation is also considered.

3. Retroperitoneal bleeding, generally caused by the pelvic fracture.
4. External wounds are usually obvious and controlled with direct pressure.
5. Extremity fractures: multiple, open, or closed.

B. Pelvic hemorrhage occurs from exposed bone fracture surfaces, venous plexus disruption, and arterial tears, particularly the superior gluteal artery. The retroperitoneal space can accommodate many liters of blood before tamponade occurs.

C. Some pelvic fractures need immediate pelvic ring stabilization. This can be accomplished rapidly with readily available hospital equipment and supplies. Consider these temporary, noninvasive, pelvic immobilization maneuvers in **hemodynamically unstable** patients who meet clinical or radiographic criteria of pelvic instability: (*a*) clinical: the bony pelvis is mobile on physical examination, or (*b*) radiographic: significant widening of the anterior or posterior pelvic ring on AP radiograph of the pelvis. Under these conditions, temporary pelvic immobilization can be achieved with the circumferential pelvic antishock sheeting (CPAS), pelvic binder, C-clamp, military antishock trousers (MAST), or external fixation. Regardless of the device to be used, before application, complete a thorough physical examination of the abdomen, pelvis, buttocks, perineum, and lower extremities to identify all significant injuries or wounds.

With improved preclinical emergency care, decreased rescue times, and rapid access to trauma centers, the indications for MAST are limited. MAST are expensive, not always readily available, and deny lower extremity and inguinal accesses. Therefore, the role of MAST may be limited to the prehospital setting. If MAST are used, all three compartments should be inflated to low-pressure levels (30–40 mmHg; firm to squeezing, but not hard).

The use of CPAS plays a role in pelvic stabilization during the examination and resuscitation of hemodynamically unstable patients. The sheet is folded lengthwise in widths of approximately 18 inches. The sheet is placed around the patient's pelvis and crossed anteriorly at the level of the symphysis pubis. As the sheet is crossed and tension created, a second person "closes" the pelvis by pressing inward and firmly on the lateral buttocks just posterior to the anterior iliac spines. The sheet is then secured by knotting or with large clamps. The use of CPAS has found great acceptance as it is small, transportable, inexpensive, can be easily applied, provides satisfactory pelvic stability, and allows access to the lower extremities and abdomen during evaluation and resuscitation. CPAS can be used temporarily during the resuscitation and no incisions are needed, which facilitates later operative stabilization. Adjustable pelvic binders are now available for trauma patients for temporary stabilization.

External fixators are probably the most commonly used tools for rapid pelvic ring stabilizations. Various external fixation devices have been developed and the systems may be divided into anterior and posterior external fixation systems. Anterior pelvic external fixation is advocated for patients with unstable pelvic ring disruptions. The application of anterior external fixators requires the insertion of bilateral iliac crest pins that are attached to connecting rods to stabilize the unstable pelvic ring. Anterior pelvic external fixation stabilizes the anterior pelvis, but may actually increase the posterior pelvic deformity in some patients. The pelvic C-clamp has been advocated as a posterior pelvic external fixator, to stabilize displaced posterior pelvic injuries. The C-clamp consists of two pins that are applied to the posterior ilium in the region of the sacroiliac joint. This technique provides compression and stability to the posterior aspect of the pelvic ring. The application of the C-clamp may be technically challenging especially in patients with posterior pelvic deformities and a too posterior position of the device may not provide sufficient stabilization of the pelvic ring.

Regardless of the device selected, the application of these temporary immobilizers:

1. Must be done with the spine in the neutral position; logrolling, lifting the entire body without axial flexion or extension.
2. Used for a short period of time as a bridge to external fixation or angiographic control of hemorrhage.

D. Angiographic evaluation and embolization is indicated in patients with persistent hemodynamic instability who have had adequate volume resuscitation, correction of coagulopathy, treatment of extrapelvic sources of bleeding, and persistent bleeding, despite external or limited internal fixation. Hemodynamic instability from the pelvis is defined as ongoing resuscitation of >6 units of packed red blood cells (PRBCs) in a 4-hour time span. Broader indications for angiography include >6 units PRBCs in 48 hours because of pelvic bleeding; hemodynamic instability in a patient with a negative focused abdominal sonography for trauma (FAST) or DPL; large pelvic hematoma seen on CT or at laparotomy; and active extravasation noted on pelvic CT. Displaced pelvic fractures through the sciatic notch have a high incidence of associated vascular injury (superior gluteal artery). **Prompt recognition of patients who require angiography and embolization to control bleeding associated with pelvic fractures is essential**; minimizing time to definitive control of bleeding is as critical in this setting as with cavitary hemorrhage requiring operative control.

    1. Obvious bleeding is seen in <40% of pelvic angiograms (3% of all pelvic fractures).

VI. HEMODYNAMICALLY UNSTABLE PATIENTS. Acute stabilization of pelvic fractures in hemodynamically unstable trauma patients with associated extrapelvic injuries is controversial.

    A. Pneumatic antishock garment (PASG) or MAST is useful in the prehospital setting. The CPAS or adjustable pelvic binder also accomplishes the same goal.

    B. External fixation has certain advantages and disadvantages in the treatment of the patient with an unstable pelvic ring fracture.

        1. Advantages

            a. Restoration of the spherical bony anatomy of the disrupted pelvic ring is believed to tamponade and decrease hemorrhage, as well as stabilize the blood clot formed around the bleeding vessel or fractured bone.

            b. Transfusion requirements may be reduced as well as the duration of shock.

            c. The pelvic stability provided allows for easier intrahospital transport.

            d. Mobilization of the patient is facilitated, along with improved nursing care and diminished narcotic requirements.

            e. External fixation remains as the initial treatment of choice for open pelvic fractures (through skin, vagina, or rectum).

        2. Disadvantages

            a. Certain fracture patterns (e.g., fractures of the iliac wing) are not amenable to external fixation.

            b. Lateral compression fractures with disruption of the sacrum or sacroiliac joints are not adequately stabilized by standard anterior external fixation alone.

            c. Use of external fixation in osteopenic patients has been associated with additional comminution of the fracture.

            d. Potential complications include iatrogenic neurovascular injuries by the pin placement.

            e. External fixation for definitive care can be associated with loss of fracture reduction.

            f. The incisions used for pin placement, as well as pin tract infections, can preclude a surgical approach to the pelvis at the time of ORIF.

    C. Limited ORIF of the anterior pelvis (e.g., pubic symphysis disruption) can be performed acutely as part of the resuscitation effort, especially with laparotomy. Either extend the laparotomy incision or use a preferred Pfannenstiel incision. This same incision can be used to repair bladder and other genitourinary injuries.

    D. Open pelvic fracture may require vigorous packing as part of initial resuscitation for hemorrhage control.

VII. Definitive ORIF of the displaced pelvic ring fracture with posterior disruption is often necessary. Recent biomechanical studies indicate that internal fixation improves overall stability, particularly when all disrupted elements are stabilized.

A. ORIF of the anterior pelvis, including pubic symphysis or rami, with a plate can be done acutely, as previously noted, or on a delayed basis in the hemodynamically stable patient.

B. Posterior pelvic ring fractures of either the sacrum or sacroiliac joint are definitively treated with ORIF. Anterior and posterior approaches have been described. Iliosacral lag screws placed under fluoroscopic or CT guidance stabilize the posterior pelvis with minimal dissection. Displaced sacral fractures with nerve root impingement may require a posterior approach with foraminal decompression.

C. Acetabular fractures can be associated with pelvic ring fractures. Stabilization of the pelvic ring is the first priority, especially if the patient is in shock. If the iliac wing is fractured in association with the acetabular fracture, internal fixation is required. In stable patients, acetabular and pelvic ring fractures are often addressed simultaneously.

D. Internal stabilization of open fractures can be undertaken after serial irrigation and debridement produce a clean wound.

AXIOMS

■ Pelvic fractures have a high incidence of associated injuries that contribute significantly to morbidity and mortality.

■ The hypotensive patient with a pelvic fracture frequently has active bleeding from the abdomen or chest as the primary cause for hypotension.

■ The mechanism and vector of injury determine the pelvic fracture pattern, as well as associated injuries.

■ Carefully inspect the perineum, rectum, and vagina to detect open pelvic fractures.

■ Active bleeding in association with pelvic fracture requiring angiography and embolization must be recognized and controlled expeditiously.

Bibliography

Burgess AR, Eastridges BJ, Young JWR, et al. Pelvic ring disruptions: Effective classification system and treatment protocols. *J Trauma* 1990;30:848–856.

Flint L, Babikian G, Anders M, et al. Definitive control of mortality from severe pelvic fractures. *Ann Surg* 1990;211:703–706.

Gansslen A, Pohlemann T, Paul C, et al. Epidemiology of pelvic ring injuries. *Injury* 1996;27(suppl 1):S-A13–A20.

Ganz R, Krushell RJ, Jakob RP, et al. The antishock pelvic clamp. *Clin Orthop* 1991;267:71–78.

Giannoudis PV, Pape HC. Damage control orthopaedics in unstable pelvic ring injuries. *Injury* 2004;35:671–677.

Goldstein A, Phillips F, Scalfani SJA, et al. Early open reduction and internal fixation of the disrupted pelvic ring. *J Trauma* 1986;26:325–333.

Gruen GS, Leit ME, Gruen RJ, et al. The acute management of hemodynamically unstable multiple trauma patients with pelvic ring fractures. *J Trauma* 1994;36:706–711.

Kim WY, Hearn TC, Seleem O, et al. Effect of pin location on stability of pelvic external fixation. *Clin Orthop* 1999;361:237–244.

Panetta T, Scalfani SJ, Goldstein AS, et al. Percutaneous embolization for massive bleeding from pelvic fractures. *J Trauma* 1985;25:1021–1029.

Pohlemann T, Gansslen A, Stief CH. Complex injuries of the pelvis and acetabulum. *Orthopade* 1998;27:32–44.

Pohlemann T, Richter M, Otte D, et al. Mechanism of pelvic girdle injuries in street traffic. Medical-technical accident analysis. *Unfallchirurg* 2000;103:267–274.

Poole GV, Ward EF, Muakassa FF, et al. Pelvic fractures from major blunt trauma: Outcome is determined by associated injuries. *Ann Surg* 1991;213:532–538.

Richter M, Otte D, Gansslen A, et al. Injuries of the pelvic ring in road traffic accidents: A medical and technical analysis. *Injury* 2001;32:123–128.

Riemer BL, Butterfield SL, Diamond DL, et al. Acute mortality associated with injuries to the pelvis: The role of early patient mobilization and external fixation. *J Trauma* 1993;35:671–675.

Routt ML Jr, Falicov A, Woodhouse E, et al. Circumferential pelvic antishock sheeting: A temporary resuscitation aid. *J Orthop Trauma* 2002;16:45–48.

Routt ML Jr, Nork SE, Mills WJ. High-energy pelvic ring disruptions. *Orthop Clin North Am* 2002;33:59–72.

Shuler T, Boone DC, Gruen G, et al. Percutaneous iliosacral screw fixation: Optimal treatment for unstable posterior pelvic ring disruption. *J Trauma* 1995;38:453–458.

Tile M. Pelvic ring fractures: Should they be fixed? *J Bone Joint Surg* 1988;70:1–12.

33

HAND TRAUMA
KODI K. AZARI, RONIT WOLLSTEIN, AND W. P. ANDREW LEE

I. INTRODUCTION
   A. The upper extremity and the hand in particular are among the most commonly injured body parts due to their exposed position. Proper diagnosis and timely treatment are essential because upper extremity injuries are so common, the anatomy complex, and the consequences potentially serious. Fortunately, most hand injuries are minor; however, some may be life or limb threatening.
   B. Once the trauma patient is medically stabilized, the initial evaluation of the hand and upper extremity may begin. Accurate diagnosis of hand problems relies on a thorough history along with a careful and systematic physical examination. It is recommended that a practitioner trained in hand surgery assess and formulate an appropriate treatment plan so that permanent loss of function may be avoided.
   C. The purpose of this chapter is to provide information for the evaluation and treatment of patients with upper limb injuries and recommendation of when a hand specialist's intervention is appropriate.

II. EVALUATION
   A. History. Necessary components are:
   1. Patient's age, sex, occupation
   2. Handedness (which hand is dominant)
   3. Where and when the injury occurred
   4. Mechanism of injury (avulsion, crush, sharp cut, fall)
   5. Treatment prior to arrival
   6. Past medical history—focused
      a. Previous injuries to that hand/previous hand operations
      b. Tobacco product history
      c. Medications and allergies
      d. Diabetes, peripheral neuropathy, and other relevant systemic or congenital disease
      e. Concurrent injuries
   B. Physical examination
   1. **Observe**
      a. The whole patient
      b. The involved upper extremity
      c. Skin—edema, lacerations, open wounds, burns
      d. Neurovascular—vascularity (skin color), obvious bleeding
      e. Tendon—finger cascade, spontaneous movement, resting hand position
      f. Bones—swelling, discoloration, deformity, open fracture
   2. **Palpate** (most structures in the hand are not far from the skin)
      a. Temperature, pulses
      b. Crepitus, broken bones, instability
      c. Point tenderness (localize pathology)
   3. **Move** (passive and active range of motion)
   4. **Specific tests**
      a. Vascular
         i. Allen's test. Both the radial and the ulnar artery are occluded with the patient making a tight fist. The patient opens the fist and the examiner

releases one of the arteries. Return of color or vascularity is observed and should be brisk. The test is repeated with the second artery. Good refill demonstrates patency of the palmar arch and each artery. Slow or absent refill means the hand is dependent on one or both of the arteries for adequate inflow.

ii. Digital Allen's test. A handheld Doppler probe is placed on the lateral aspect of the digit to obtain a digital Doppler signal. Manual pressure is used to occlude the contralateral digital artery. If the Doppler signal disappears, the ipsilateral digital artery is occluded or lacerated.

b. Nerve (often these tests are not reliable in context of acute injury)

i. Sensory exam
- **a)** Light touch (subjective)
  - **1)** Compare to the other hand or other nerve distribution if possible.
- **b)** Moving two-point discrimination (objective)
  - **1)** Use a bent paperclip. Normal <6 mm; however, compare to contralateral side (Fig. 33-1).
- **c)** Pseudomotor function (objective)
  - **1)** Denervated skin is often dry and will not wrinkle when immersed in water.

ii. Motor
- **a) Cascade.** At rest with the wrist in neutral position the fingers assume a slightly flexed position with the nails pointing toward the scaphoid tubercle. The little finger will be flexed more than the ring and so on to the index. This is called the normal "cascade" of the fingers. This cascade will be disrupted if flexor tendons are injured or if there is motor nerve injury (Fig. 33-2).

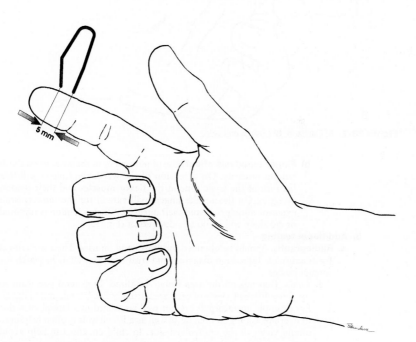

Figure 33-1. Two-point discrimination.

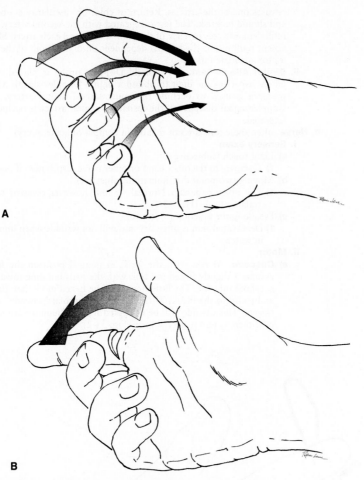

Figure 33-2. A: Cascade. **B:** Loss of cascade.

    b) Finger tenodesis effect. Use of movement in the wrist to establish tendon integrity. On extension of the wrist, the fingers will flex because of the basic tone in the flexor muscles and their tendon integrity. On flexion the fingers will extend for the same reason; extensor muscle tone and their integrity. When a tendon is ruptured or cut there will be no tenodesis effect (Fig. 33-3).

5. Additional testing
    a. Radiographs. Should be obtained for most hand injuries. These are critical for fracture or dislocation diagnosis and treatment as well as in search for foreign bodies.
        i. Views. Depends on the area being visualized. In general you want to see three different views of each area (usually PA, lateral, and oblique). For example, metacarpals are not well visualized in a lateral view due to overlap; ask for an oblique as well as a PA view. It is often helpful to obtain views of the uninvolved side. In children, this can help avoid confusion with epiphyseal plates.

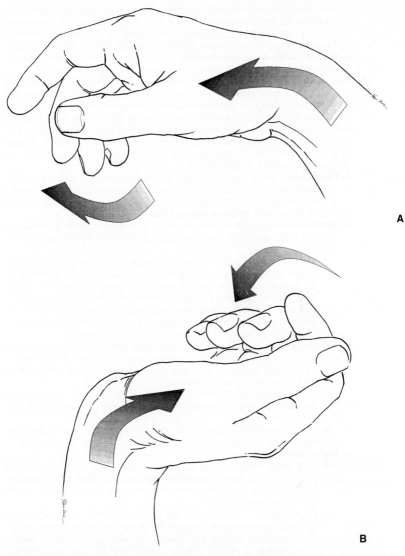

Figure 33-3. **A:** Tenodesis (volar flexion). **B:** Tenodesis (dorsal flexion).

    ii. Special views are obtained for specific joints or pathologies: clenched fist view for wrist ligamentous injury, better view for the thumb carpometacarpal (CMC) joint, and so on.

  b. Handheld pencil Doppler. Assessment of vascular patency.

  c. Compartment pressures. Measurement of compartment pressures in suspected compartment syndrome. In the forearm, measure the superficial and deep flexor compartments (most commonly involved), the radial compartment and, if necessary, the extensor compartments. In the hand, measure the thenar/hypothenar and interosseous compartments. Measurements are best done with commercially available compartment measuring kits or an 18-gauge IV catheter connected to a pressure transducer. Measurements that are considered elevated are >30 mmHg, or 20 mmHg difference between compartment pressure measurement and diastolic blood pressure.

d. Wound cultures. Cultures should be taken in any case of suspected infection. Do not be afraid to put a needle in a joint that you suspect is infected!

6. **Pain control** (Fig. 33-4). Adequate anesthesia is essential for the evaluation and management of hand injuries because only pain-free patients can make rational decisions about their care. Furthermore, the presence or fear of severe pain may cause limitations in range of motion, thus altering the physical exam findings. Prior to administration of anesthetic, a proper neurological exam should be performed and well documented. Thereafter, the type of anesthetic will be dictated by the anatomic level and severity of the injury. Generally, regional blocks are the preferred method of pain control.

a. Field block. When the exploration of deep structures is not anticipated, anesthetic agent can be directly infiltrated into tissue edges. Use a 25-gauge 1.5-inch needle, a 10-mL syringe, and a 50:50 mixture of 1% lidocaine and 0.25% Bupivicaine (**without epinephrine**).

b. Wrist block. The block of choice for most hand injuries. Four nerves can be blocked at the wrist; the nerves to be blocked depend on the region of the injury.

   i. Median nerve. Inject 5 mL of anesthetic just ulnar to the palmaris longus tendon and at a 45-degree angle. This places the anesthetic in the carpal canal. The flow of anesthetic should be easy and a slight bulge may be seen distal to the carpal tunnel. If the patient experiences an electrical shock, a sharp shooting pain, or parasthesias, the syringe needle is placed in the nerve and may cause permanent nerve damage if anesthetic is injected! Withdraw and redirect the needle.

   ii. Ulnar nerve. Inject 3 to 5 mL of anesthetic just ulnar to the flexor carpi ulnaris tendon. Draw back on the syringe to make sure there is not an intraarterial stick and, as with the median nerve, inject if there is no evidence of intraneural puncture.

   iii. Radial sensory nerve. Inject 5 to 10 mL of anesthetic 1 cm proximal to the radial styloid and around the dorsal radial wrist in the subcutaneous plain.

   iv. Ulnar sensory nerve. Inject 5 mL of anesthetic at the level of the ulnar styloid and around the dorsal ulnar wrist in the subcutaneous plain.

c. Digital block

   i. Web space. Using a 25- or 27-gauge needle, inject 3 mL of anesthetic 2 cm in the web space (less painful than palm) on both sides of the digit. Place 2 to 3 mL subcutaneously on the dorsal aspect of the digit to complete the block.

   ii. Digital sheath. At the level of the proximal palmar crease, advance a 25- or 27-gauge needle through the flexor tendon and to the bone. Then withdraw slightly, thus placing the needle in the digital sheath. Inject 3 mL of anesthetic solution. There should be minimal resistance and the finger may be observed to straighten slightly.

III. SPECIFIC INJURIES

A. Vascular injury. Vascular compromise is one of the true emergencies in hand injuries. The consequences of delayed treatment are necrosis with loss of limb/part and consequent loss of function.

1. **Arterial insufficiency.** The hand may:
   a. Feel cold
   b. Appear pale
   c. Exhibit decreased skin turgor
   d. Experience slow or absent capillary refill
   e. Be pulseless

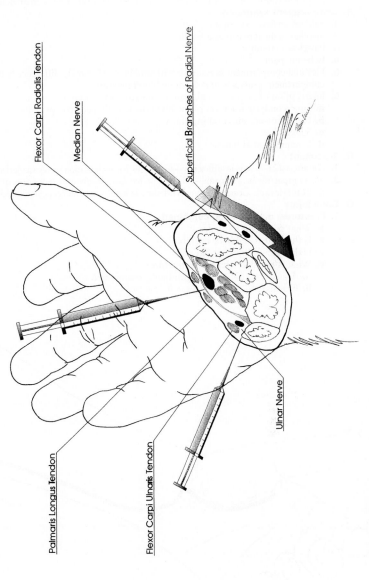

Figure 33-4. Nerve block.

2. Venous insufficiency
   a. Bluish, purplish color
   b. Brisk capillary refill
   c. Congested, swollen
   Often there will be a mixture of both arterial and venous insufficiency.

B. Compartment syndrome
1. Pain on passive extension
2. Swollen, tight forearm and hand
3. Pulseless extremity
4. Ischemic pain
5. Elevated compartment pressures: >30 mmHg, or 20 mmHg difference between compartment pressures and diastolic blood pressure
6. Interruption of arterial circulation to an extremity >4 hours
   a. Supracondylar fractures of the humerus (mostly pediatric patients)
   b. High-pressure injection injuries
   c. Snake bites
   d. Circumferential burns

C. Treatment
1. For arterial or venous insufficiency—to the OR for replantation or revascularization.
2. For compartment syndrome—to the OR for fasciotomy and reduction of fractures if relevant. Compartment syndrome is a surgical emergency (Fig. 33-5).

D. Bone injury
1. Fractures, dislocations, combined
   a. What bones are injured?
   b. Is the patient stable or unstable?
   c. Is the fracture open or closed?
   d. What is the character of the fracture?
      i. Transverse, oblique, longitudinal, comminuted
      ii. Translated angulated, rotated

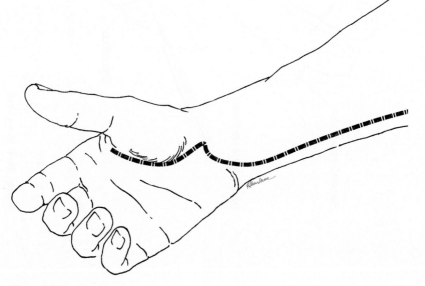

Figure 33-5. Fasciotomy.

  iii. Intraarticular, epiphyseal
  iv. Urgent treatment (usually in OR) for open fractures
  v. Operative treatment for unstable fractures, intraarticular fractures
2. Pediatric fracture classification (Fig. 33-6)
Pediatric growth plate fractures are divided into five catagories based on the Salter-Harris fracture classification:
Type I–There is complete epiphyseal separation from the metaphysis. The vital portion of the growth plate remains attached. Usually immobilization is sufficient treatment.
Type II–The most common growth plate fracture. There is a fracture of the metaphysis and partial separation from the epiphysis. May require reduction in addition to immobilization.
Type III–Rare in the upper extremity. The fracture completely traverses through the epiphysis and separates part of the epiphysis and growth plate from the metaphysis.
Type IV–This fracture traverses the epiphysis, across the growth plate, and into the metaphysis. Surgery may be needed to restore the joint surface to normal and to align the growth plate. Unless perfect alignment is achieved and maintained the prognosis for growth can be poor.
Type V–An uncommon injury that results in the crushing and compression of the growth plate. Prognosis can be poor, since premature stunting of growth is almost inevitable.
3. Phalangeal fractures
  a. Always look at the rotation or angulation of the finger. This will determine if the patient needs reduction and/or fixation (x-rays are not reliable for estimating rotation).
  b. Buddy taping is useful for fixation and for rotational control within a cast or splint.
4. Metacarpal fractures
  a. Tend to be unstable if more than one is fractured.
  b. Look at rotational deformity.

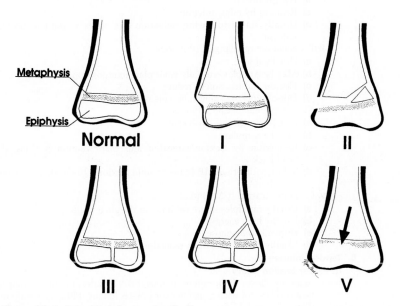

Figure 33-6. Salter-Harris fracture classification.

    c. Angulation is more of a problem in radial metacarpals (the CMC joint is less mobile).

    d. Specific: fracture of the metacarpal neck (Boxer's fracture); usually in the ulnar two metacarpals.

5. Thumb metacarpal fractures

    a. The CMC joint of the thumb has 360 degrees of motion compensating for angulation in the metacarpal shaft fracture without loss of function.

    b. Specific: intraarticular fractures of the base of the thumb (CMC joint).

        i. Bennett's fracture—volar-ulnar fragment held by the volar ligament, unstable because the APL pulls the shaft fragment. Usually needs fixation following reduction.

        ii. Rolando's fracture—comminuted intraarticular fracture of the metacarpal base. Needs ORIF unless nondisplaced.

6. Wrist fractures

    a. The wrist is composed of eight carpal bones with the associated joints as well as the distal radioulnar joint.

    b. Wrist injuries are usually difficult to diagnose and should be seen by a hand surgeon.

    c. The patient should be x-rayed and splinted in the position of safety.

7. Joint dislocations

    a. Closely linked to bony injury. Often both happen at once (avulsion of bone with a ligament injury and fracture dislocations).

    b. Simple dislocations can be easily reduced.

    c. Complex dislocations cannot be reduced closed or tend to dislocate again. This is usually because of interposed soft tissue or unstable bony fragments, therefore this must be treated by surgery.

    d. Cartilage in a dislocated joint suffers ischemia and damage, thus an effort should be made to reduce a joint expediently.

    e. When describing a dislocation, the direction describes the more distal part or fragment.

        i. Distal interphalangeal (DIP) joint

            a) Usually dorsal.

            b) Reduced by inline traction.

            c) Usually stable following reduction and needs a splint to protect reduction.

        ii. Proximal interphalangeal (PIP) joint

            a) Usually dorsal.

            b) May be complex—usually volar plate interposition.

            c) Flexion and traction to reduce.

            d) Dorsal blocking splint following reduction.

        iii. Metacarpophalangeal (MP) joint

            a) Usually dorsal but also volar.

            b) May be complex.

            c) Reduction by flexion/extension and then traction pushing the head back.

            d) Splint with other MP joints in mild flexion (20–30 degrees when dorsal).

        iv. Carpometacarpal (CMC) joint

            a) Usually multiple—more common in the ulnar digits.

            b) Usually high energy.

            c) Difficult to diagnose.

            d) Usually necessitates open reduction and fixation.

8. Tendon injuries

    a. Flexor tendon injury

        i. Anatomy. Flexor digitorum profundus (FDP) and flexor digitorum superficialis (FDS) for each finger. Flexor pollicis longus (FPL) for the thumb (Figs. 33-7 and 33-8).

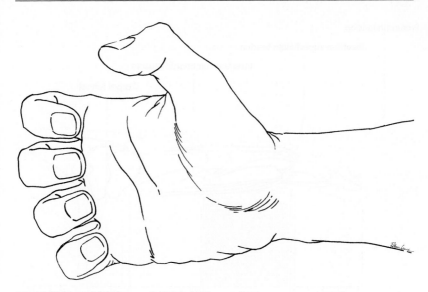

Figure 33-7. Flexor digitorum profundus (FDP).

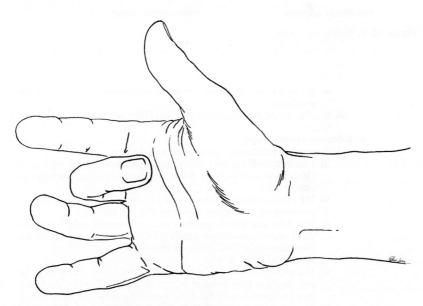

Figure 33-8. Flexor digitorum superficialis (FDS).

    ii. Zones of injury (Fig. 33-9)
        a) Remember that the zone of injury does not necessarily correlate with the laceration because it is also dependent on the position of the finger during injury.
        b) All flexor tendon injuries should be splinted in the emergency department (ED) in flexion of the fingers and then repaired in the OR.

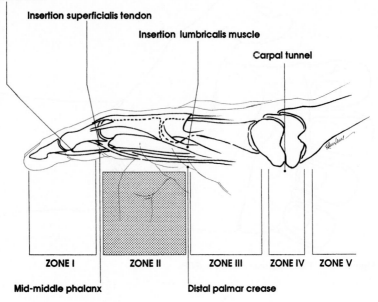

Figure 33-9. Tendon injury zone.

      c) Because of the proximity to the digital nerves, always check for sensation.

   iii. Specific: Jersey finger is avulsion of the FDP zone 1 usually to the ring finger.

b. Extensor tendon injury

    i. Anatomy. Xix extensor compartments at the wrist.

      a) Junctura tendinae may allow some extension of the digit even though the tendon is cut. Look for an extensor lag (inability to extend fully).

      b) MP joint extension is carried out by the extrinsic extensors; IP joint extension by the intrinsic extensors (Fig. 33-10).

      c) The index and little fingers have an extra extrinsic indices proprius (EIP) and extensor digiti quinti (EDQ). These are always on the ulnar side of the EDC tendon to that finger.

    ii. Zones of injury (Fig. 33.9)

      a) The extensor mechanism in the finger (zones 1–5/6) is difficult to fix and should usually be taken to the OR. Proximal to this, the injury may be repaired in the ED if the proximal end has not retracted.

      b) Always splint with the fingers (all) in extension and the wrist in mild extension (15–20 degrees).

         1) Mallet finger: tear of the extensor mechanism to the DIP joint.

         2) May be bony (with an avulsion fragment of variable size) or nonbony.

         3) Boutonnière deformity following an acute injury is injury to the extensor mechanism over the PIP joint.

         4) Splint in hyperextension of PIP joint and allow DIP joint flexion. Should be seen expediently by a hand surgeon.

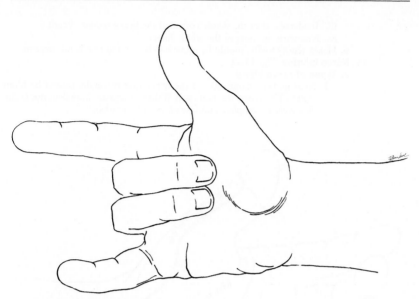

Figure 33-10. Independent extrinsic extensors.

9. **Combined injuries**
   a. Assess all involved tissues.
   b. Wash out or clean the wound.
   c. If it can all be repaired or reduced in the ED, then repair. If only some of the injuries can be repaired, splint, loosely close the wound, and send to the OR/hand surgeon.
   d. Administer antibiotics and tetanus prophylaxis.
10. **Infections** (for surgical drainage [abscess] versus antibiotic treatment only [cellulitis])
    a. Abscess
       i. Drain and wash out.
       ii. Allow for continuous drainage.
       iii. Splint in position of function.
       iv. Administer antibiotics.
    b. Specific
       i. Paronychia
       ii. Felon
       iii. Web space infections
       iv. Palmar infections
       v. Pyogenic flexor tenosynovitis
       vi. Ulnar and radial bursal infections
    c. Paronychia/Felon can often be treated in the ED. The other infections should be treated in the OR.
       i. Make incisions midaxially and not in the pulp if possible.
       ii. Drain by removing or partially removing the nail or lateral incisions.
       iii. Leave a small drain.
       iv. Splint for comfort.
    d. Pyogenic flexor tenosynovitis can be diagnosed by the existence of Kanavel's signs.
       i. Flexed position of the finger
       ii. Excruciating pain on passive extension

iii. Tenderness over the whole course of the flexor tendon sheath
iv. Symmetric swelling of the whole finger
e. Flexor tenosynovitis should be immediately referred to a hand surgeon.
11. Nerve injuries (Fig. 33-11)
    a. Types of nerve injury
        i. Neuropraxia. Contusion of the nerve that is usually caused by blunt injury. The axons are intact and Wallerian degeneration does not occur. Recovery is complete and fast (days to 3 months).

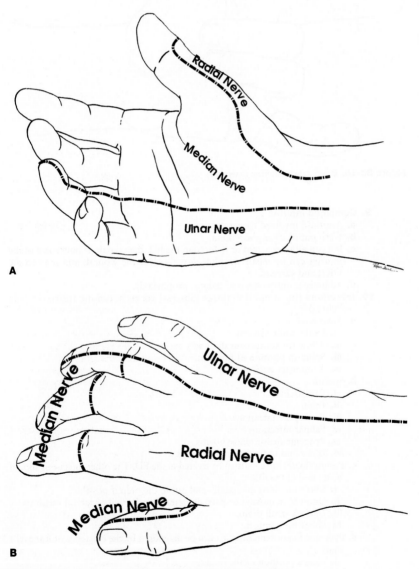

Figure 33-11. **A:** Sensory fields (volar). **B:** Sensory fields (dorsal).

ii. Axonotomesis. Axonal disruption or damage (epineurium remains intact) with Wallerian degeneration. Recovery is usually complete, but slow (approximately 1 inch per month).

iii. Neurotemesis. Transection of a peripheral nerve. Recovery is poor and nerve repair is necessary.

b. Repair of injured nerve. For the best chance of functional result, nerves should be primarily repaired if possible or nerve grafted. Repair should be done under the operative microscope for anatomical alignment. Optimally, nerves should be repaired as soon as possible (<10 days) and by a hand surgeon.

c. Median nerve injury
  i. Sensory. Sensation to thumb, index, middle, and radial ring finger, thenar eminence
  ii. Motor
    a) Median nerve proper. Flexor carpi radialis, pronator teres, palmaris longus, flexor digitorum superficialis, and flexor digitorum profundus to long finger.
    b) Anterior interosseous nerve. Flexor pollicis longus, flexor digitorum profundus to index, and pronator quadratus.
    c) Motor branch. Thenar musculature.
  iii. Tests
    a) The "OK sign." Patient is asked to touch the tip of the index to the tip of the thumb to make an OK sign. Tests the median nerve proximal to the carpal tunnel.
    b) Abductor pollicis brevis (APB) test. Patient is asked to abduct thumb from the plane of the hand and point toward the ceiling. The APB is a purely median innervated (motor branch) thenar muscle.

d. Ulnar nerve
  i. Sensory. Sensation to small finger, ulnar ring finger, hypothenar eminence, and ulnar dorsal hand.
  ii. Motor. Flexor carpi ulnaris, flexor digitorum profundus (ring and small finger), lumbricals, interosseous muscles, hypothenar muscles, deep head of flexor pollicis brevis, and adductor pollicis brevis.
  iii. Tests
    a) Intrinsic muscle weakness. Inability to cross fingers.
    b) Weakness of first dorsal interosseus muscle. Patient has weakness on radial abduction of index finger.
    c) Froment's sign. Patient is asked to forcibly hold a piece of paper between thumb and radial index finger proximal phalanx (key pinch). If the thumb interphalangeal joint flexes with this maneuver, the adductor pollicis muscle (ulnar innervated) is considered weak.
    d) Flexor digitorum profundus to the small finger. Weakness indicates ulnar nerve injury proximal to the wrist.

e. Radial nerve
  i. Sensory. Sensation to the dorsal and radial aspect of wrist and hand.
  ii. Motor. Brachioradialis, all extensors of wrist, and all extensors of the hand/digits.
  iii. Tests
    a) Sensation to radial dorsal hand.
    b) Extension of digits and wrist.

12. Amputations
  a. Amputations of the upper extremity are fairly common and can range from distal fingertip injuries (often seen in children) to major limb amputations. By definition, **replantation** is the reattachment of a completely amputated body part. **Revascularization** is the reattachment of an incompletely amputated body part. Any patient that has sustained an amputation-type injury and desires replantation or revascularization should be transferred to a replantation center. The transferring facility and accepting institution

must make no promises that reattachment is possible, and should inform the patients that they are being transferred **to evaluate for replantation**. The final decision to replant or revascularize must be made by the hand surgeon after thorough evaluation and individualized to the patients and their injuries.

b. Transport. The amputated segment should be properly retrieved from the field, wrapped in a saline-moistened gauze, and placed in a sealed plastic bag. The plastic bag is then placed on ice or slurry and particular care must be taken so that the amputated part does not come in direct contact with the ice (frostbite). When properly cooled, a digit can be successfully replanted up to 24 hours following amputation and up to 12 hours of ischemia time, if the amputated part has a significant amount of muscle attached (proximal to the forearm).

c. Assessment. In the field, actively bleeding vessels should be controlled with direct digital pressure. The use of tourniquets should be avoided if possible and a vessel should never be clamped. On arrival, a complete trauma assessment is necessary and life-threatening conditions must be addressed.

d. Indications for replantation
    i. Thumb amputations
    ii. Multiple finger amputations
    iii. Any part in a child
    iv. Isolated digit distal to the FDS insertion
    v. Partial or complete hand
    vi. Amputations proximal to wrist
    vii. Left ring finger in a woman (relative indication)

e. Relative contraindications
    i. Crush or avulsion injuries
    ii. Single digit in zone II (adults)
    iii. Heavy wound contamination
    iv. Proximal forearm and above with >6 hours of warm ischemia time
    v. Psychiatric disease
    vi. Patients older than 60 years of age

f. Contraindications
    i. Severe associated injuries (life threatening)
    ii. Multilevel amputations
    iii. Severe crush injuries and avulsion
    iv. Serious medical comorbidity

g. Sequence of surgery
    i. Two-team approach greatly facilitates a potentially lengthy operation.
        a) Amputation team. Prepares the amputated segment by isolating and tagging the digital arteries, nerves, veins, and tendons.
        b) Recipient team. Prepares the recipient site and harvests vein grafts (if needed).
    ii. Bone fixation
    iii. Tendon repair (flexor and extensor)
    iv. Arterial anastomosis
    v. Venous anastomosis
    vi. Nerve repair
    vii. Loose soft-tissue closure, skin graft, or allograft

13. High-pressure injection injuries
    a. Injury from high-pressure injection tools such as paint guns, grease guns, diesel guns, and spray guns. The fingertip and hands are the most commonly affected sites and injuries are potential surgical emergencies.
    b. Foreign material is injected under high pressures (2,000–10,000 psi) that cause tissue death and potentially severe inflammation. Patients need urgent operative intervention for decompression and debridement of foreign material and nonviable tissues.

14. Fingertip injuries (Fig. 33-12). Common (particularly in children) and in adults using sharp instruments and power tools.

   a. Subungual hematoma

      i. Isolated subungual hematomas can be drained with a heated paperclip.

      ii. If there is a distal phalanx fracture or obvious nailbed injury, the nailplate should be removed to repair the nailbed. The bed can be repaired with 6.0 chromic suture and the nailplate replaced to splint open the eponycheal fold.

   b. Amputations

      i. Injuries smaller than 1 cm² can be treated conservatively with wet to dry dressing changes.

      ii. Dorsal oblique injuries can be repaired with local advancement flap.

      iii. Volar oblique injuries can be reconstructed with cross finger flaps or a combination of local advancement flap and skin/allograft.

15. Soft-tissue injuries. Soft tissue injuries of the upper extremity are common and can vary from superficial lacerations to severe composite tissue loss.

   a. History and exam. A careful history should document mechanism of injury, time of injury, and pertinent associated medical conditions. Examination must include vascular, sensory, and motor functions. X-rays may be useful to exclude osseous injury and foreign objects.

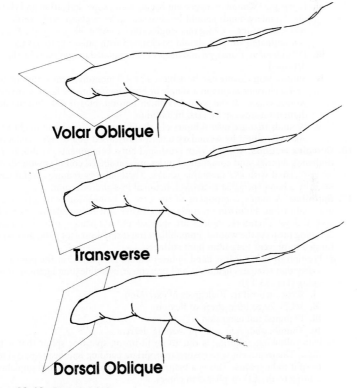

Volar Oblique

Transverse

Dorsal Oblique

Figure 33-12. Fingertip injuries.

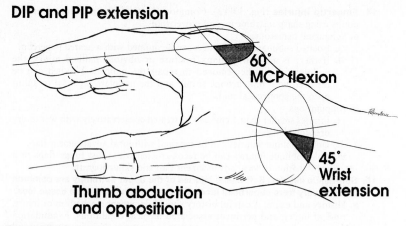

DIP and PIP extension

60° MCP flexion

45° Wrist extension

Thumb abduction and opposition

Figure 33-13. Position of safety.

  b. Treatment
      i. Anesthetic. For deeper wounds, local anesthetic is indicated.
      ii. Cleansing. Wound management begins with proper irrigation and cleansing. Simple wounds should be cleansed under pressure with sterile normal saline using an 18-gauge angiocatheter and a 30-cc syringe. Heavily contaminated wounds should be cleansed with pulsating jet lavage.
      iii. Debridement. Damaged and deeply contaminated tissues must be sharply debrided.
      iv. Suture. Skin closure can be achieved by 4.0 monofilament suture (nylon) or 4.0 chromic suture in a simple or horizontal mattress fashion (to evert wound edges). If the wound is under tension, buried 4.0 chromic deep dermal sutures can be used in addition.
      v. Wounds that are over 6 hours old should not be closed and ought to be allowed to heal by secondary intention or closed in a delayed fashion.
 16. **Complex wounds.** Wounds with crush and burst components, avulsions, and degloving injuries, and composite injuries are considered complex wounds and are associated with less favorable results. These injuries require careful treatment by a hand specialist to avoid functional loss and infection.
 17. **Splinting.** A major component of the care of hand injuries is appropriate immobilization. Following trauma, progressive soft-tissue edema ensues for several days. Therefore, injuries are splinted and not acutely placed in a cast. Splinting protects the wound, immobilizes fractures, decreases pain, and is performed to prevent long-term joint stiffness.
      a. Position of safety. Most hand injuries should be splinted in the position of safety that stretches ligaments and prevents irreversible joint ligament shortening (Fig. 33-13).
          i. Wrist: neutral to 30 degrees of extension
          ii. MCP: 70 to 90 degrees of flexion
          iii. IP joints: full extension
          iv. Thumb: abducted and opposed 45 degrees
      b. Pain following splinting is due to an ill-fitting splint or splint that is too tight. The treatment is to ensure appropriate padding had been applied and to split tight splints. This is a major reason for patient calls and unplanned returns to the ED or physician clinics.

COMPARTMENT SYNDROME
GREGORY A. WATSON AND JOHN C. LEE

34

I. **COMPARTMENT SYNDROME** occurs when increased tissue pressure within a limited anatomic space compromises perfusion. The forearm and lower leg are common locations encountered in trauma patients, most often following vascular or orthopedic injury. If left untreated, this syndrome leads to myoneural necrosis and permanent loss of function or amputation. The degree of damage depends on the degree of compartmental pressure elevation as well as the length of time that pressure is elevated. **Concomitant shock increases the degree of damage for any given pressure and time.**

A. **Etiology.** Any injury leading to severe tissue edema within the fascial compartments can cause compartment syndrome.

1. **Vascular injury** with limb **ischemia** leads to tissue edema. **Reperfusion** generates toxic oxygen metabolites and increases capillary permeability, which worsens the swelling. Bleeding within a closed space from disrupted vessels can also cause the syndrome.

2. **Crush injury.** Direct injury of tissues by crushing leads to edema and subsequent compartment syndrome.

3. **Fractures** account for 50% of compartment syndromes. Tibial fractures are the most common fracture causing the syndrome, but any extremity fracture can lead to increased compartment pressure. Open fractures do not preclude the development of compartment syndrome. Compartment syndrome can occur in the absence of fracture with soft-tissue injury, ischemia and reperfusion, prolonged compression (i.e., patients with altered level of consciousness), burns, and operative osteotomies.

4. Trauma situations with high risk for the development of compartment syndrome include reperfusion after >4 to 6 hours of ischemia, significant crush injury, and combined venous and arterial injury to a limb.

B. **Pathophysiology.** Tissue necrosis is the dreaded end result of untreated compartment syndrome. A vicious cycle is initiated when a progressive increase in compartment pressure exceeds venous capillary pressure, leading eventually to complete venous obstruction. Continued arterial inflow further elevates intracompartmental pressure, exacerbating the situation. Accompanying arterioles undergo reflex spasm as venous obstruction becomes more extensive, resulting in tissue ischemia. Progressive ischemia worsens tissue edema, contributing to further elevation of compartment pressure. If uninterrupted, this cycle continues until tissue necrosis occurs.

C. **Diagnosis.** Diagnosis of compartment syndrome can be difficult. It has no pathognomonic signs or symptoms, and a **high index of suspicion** must be present in the face of risk factors. Diagnosis is usually established by a collection of symptoms, serial physical examination, and measurement of compartment pressure.

1. **Symptoms. Pain out of proportion to physical findings** is a classic symptom and is usually elicited in conscious patients with compartment syndrome. **Paraesthesias** develop with continued hypoperfusion. **Paralysis is a late finding.**

2. **Signs** include a swollen, tense compartment and **pain on passive stretching.** Conscious patients may manifest sensory deficit and progressive motor weakness of the involved neuromuscular structures. **Loss of function may be the earliest sign. Loss of peripheral pulses is a late finding** usually

349

accompanied by irreversible damage. **A palpable distal pulse does not exclude compartment syndrome.**

a. Compartment syndrome occurs most frequently in the lower leg but can also occur in the forearm, thigh, foot, upper arm, and hand. The **lower leg** is composed of four compartments containing the following structures:

   i. **Anterior compartment:** tibialis anterior and great toe extensor muscles and the deep peroneal nerve

   ii. **Lateral (peroneal) compartment:** peroneus longus and brevis muscles and the superficial peroneal nerve

   iii. **Superficial posterior compartment:** gastrocnemius and soleus muscles and the sural nerve

   iv. **Deep posterior compartment:** tibialis posterior and great toe flexor muscles and the tibial nerve

b. The forearm is composed of three compartments containing the following structures:

   i. **Volar compartment:** wrist and finger flexor muscles and the ulnar and median nerves

   ii. **Dorsal compartment:** wrist and finger extensor muscles and the posterior interosseous nerve

   iii. **Mobile wad:** extensor carpi radialis longus, extensor carpi radialis brevis, and brachioradialis muscles

3. **Compartment pressures.** Elevation of compartment pressure precedes the development of symptoms. For this reason, pressure measurement is an important adjunct to diagnosis, particularly in patients with impaired consciousness in whom subjective information is limited and physical examination is unreliable. Although disagreement exists about the cutoff between normal and abnormal compartment pressure, **most clinicians consider compartment pressure >30 mmHg an indication for fasciotomy.** Compartment pressure between 20 and 30 mmHg in the symptomatic patient or in the face of prolonged hypotension also warrants fasciotomy. **Delay in performing fasciotomy worsens outcome. Therefore, if doubt exists regarding the diagnosis, fasciotomy should be performed.**

   a. Measurement devices commonly available include the needle catheter or Stryker handheld monitor. Needle catheters can produce falsely elevated pressures if used incorrectly, but are universally available. This type of measurement system can be constructed by attaching an 18-gauge needle to a length of saline-filled pressure tubing. This tubing is connected to a pressure transducer similar to that used for arterial pressure measurement. The Stryker monitor is portable and easy to use. Accuracy is comparable between the two devices when used correctly.

   b. Technique. The skin overlying the compartment to be measured is prepared in a sterile fashion and infiltrated with local anesthetic, if necessary. The needle is advanced through the skin until it pops through the fascia and into the muscular compartment. A small amount of saline is flushed to eliminate interference from catheter plugging, and the pressure is recorded. Correct needle position can be confirmed by noting a brief increase in pressure with compression of the compartment being measured. Measurements should be repeated to confirm elevated pressures.

D. **Treatment of compartment syndrome** is based on normalizing compartmental pressures to restore adequate tissue perfusion. It is accomplished through wide decompressive fasciotomy of the affected limb. At the time of fasciotomy, **debridement should be performed only for frankly necrotic tissue**. If tissue viability is questionable, the compartment should be reexamined to assess viability.

1. **Lower leg fasciotomy** (Fig. 34-1). Fasciotomy of the leg should release all four compartments (anterior, lateral, superficial, and deep posterior). This is easily accomplished with a double incision technique. Make an incision on the lateral leg from just below the head of the fibula to just above the ankle, approximately 1 cm anterior to the fibula. Identify the septum dividing the anterior and

lateral compartments and open the fascia on either side of this septum to release these compartments, taking care to avoid the superficial peroneal nerve located along the intercompartmental septum in the lateral compartment. Make a second incision of similar length on the medial side of the leg, 2 cm posterior to the tibia. Open the fascia here to release the superficial posterior compartment. Here, partially detach the proximal soleus from the back of the tibia and incise the fascia, which releases the deep posterior compartment.

2. **Thigh fasciotomy** involves the release of three compartments (quadriceps, hamstrings, and adductors). Access and release the quadriceps compartment through an anterolateral incision on the thigh. Then, decompress the hamstring compartment by dividing the intermuscular septum posteriorly. Release the adductor compartment through a separate incision medially along the length of the compartment.

3. **Forearm fasciotomy** (Fig. 34-2). Release the volar compartment through an incision along the volar aspect of the forearm, curving across joint spaces to avoid contracture with healing. Most authors advocate performing a carpal tunnel release with this procedure. At this point, measure the dorsal compartment pressures and, if they remain elevated, perform dorsal fasciotomy. Release the dorsal compartment through a single straight incision on the back of the forearm from the lateral epicondyle to the wrist.

4. **Closure.** These wounds are usually closed 5 to 10 days later with either primary closure or skin grafting. Alternatively, gradual closure with progressive tension using vessel loops has been described. The goal is to **avoid closing the wound under undue tension**.

E. **Complications.** The major complications of compartment syndrome include infection and rhabdomyolysis.

1. Infection occurs secondary to the presence of necrotic muscle. Control of sepsis requires aggressive debridement of all nonviable tissue, which can lead to significant limitation of function in the affected limb.

2. Rhabdomyolysis may be seen as the sequela of compartment syndrome and is discussed in detail in the following text.

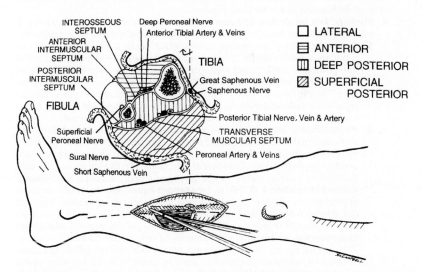

Figure 34-1. Technique for calf fasciotomy. (From Ombrellaro MP, Steven SL. Compartment syndrome: A collective review. In: Maull KI, Cleveland HC, Feliciano DV, et al., eds. *Advances in Trauma and Critical Care.* St. Louis, Mo: Mosby–Year Book; 1995;10:100, with permission.)

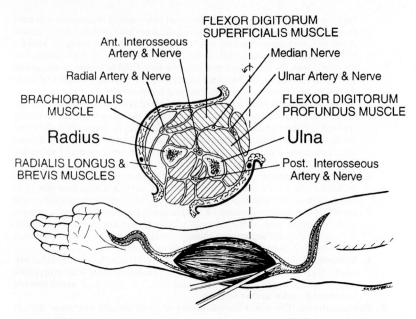

Figure 34-2. Technique for forearm fasciotomy. (From Ombrellaro MP, Steven SL. Compartment syndrome: A collective review. In: Maull KI, Cleveland HC, Feliciano DV, et al, eds. *Advances in Trauma and Critical Care.* St. Louis, Mo: Mosby—Year Book; 1995;10:100, with permission.)

II. **RHABDOMYOLYSIS** occurs when toxins are released from damaged muscle and enter the systemic circulation. Early recognition and treatment reduces the incidence of renal dysfunction and other complications.
   A. **Etiology. Any insult that damages skeletal muscle** can produce rhabdomyolysis. The causes are broadly divided into traumatic and nontraumatic categories.
      1. **Traumatic.** Direct compression of muscle leading to a local crush injury can result from blunt trauma, collapse with prolonged immobility (i.e., alcohol intoxication or stroke), and improper operative positioning. Epidemic forms of rhabdomyolysis have occurred following natural disasters (i.e., the Kobe, Japan earthquake of 1995). High-voltage electrical injury and ischemia-reperfusion following vascular injury can also damage muscle, leading to the release of myoglobin and other toxins into the systemic circulation.
      2. **Nontraumatic.** Several infectious agents, heritable conditions, and drugs can also cause rhabdomyolysis. Muscle damage may occur in the setting of certain viral (i.e., influenza, HIV, Epstein-Barr) and bacterial (*Legionella, Streptococcus, Staphylococcus, Salmonella*) infections. Hereditary causes of rhabdomyolysis include several of the glycogen storage diseases, **neuroleptic malignant syndrome (NMS)**, and **malignant hyperthermia**. NMS can occur in patients receiving any neuroleptic drug, commonly phenothiazine, haloperidol, dibenzoxepine, or dopamine-depleting drugs. NMS presents as fever, muscular rigidity, tachypnea, tachycardia, dystonia, or diaphoresis. **Malignant hyperthermia** is a hereditary hypermetabolic state of skeletal muscle resulting in high fever, rigidity, tachyarrhythmias, and rhabdomyolysis following administration of inhalation anesthetics. Steroids, neuromuscular blocking agents (i.e., vecuronium) and HMG-CoA Reductase inhibitors (statins), especially in combination with fibrate-derived lipid lowering agents such as niacin, have been implicated in the development of rhabdomyolysis.

B. Pathophysiology. Skeletal muscle ischemia leads to derangements in membrane ion flux, generation of reactive oxygen species, and cellular swelling which can cause cell lysis. Damaged muscle releases ions (i.e., potassium), reactive oxygen species, and **myoglobin,** which enter the systemic circulation and affect the function of other organs, such as the kidneys. **Acute renal failure occurs in 4% to 33% of patients with rhabdomyolysis** and results from decreased renal perfusion, tubular obstruction from cast formation, and direct effects of toxins. Myoglobin breakdown in the kidneys releases iron, which catalyzes the formation of additional reactive oxygen species (ROS) that directly damage tubular cells. Both hypovolemia (from skeletal muscle edema and "third spacing") and local release of vasoconstrictors (i.e., myoglobin stimulates platelet-activating factor release) contribute to decreased renal perfusion. Tubular obstruction results from the formation of myoglobin-protein casts, which is accelerated in an acid environment. Other systemic effects include cardiotoxicity (hyperkalemia), metastatic calcification (phosphate and calcium), and disseminated intravascular coagulation (thromboplastin release).

C. Diagnosis. Early diagnosis is critical and is suggested by a combination of signs, symptoms, and laboratory findings in the appropriate clinical setting. **A high index of suspicion is required.**

   1. Signs and symptoms. Identification of the patient at risk is the key to early diagnosis. Patients may have severe muscle pain and weakness and the urine may be dark and tea-colored. **Physical examination can be normal in up to 50% of patients.**

   2. Laboratory findings. Urinalysis that is dipstick positive for blood with few or no red blood cells on microscopic examination is highly suggestive of rhabdomyolysis. Urine myoglobin is usually positive and pigmented casts may be seen. **Elevated serum creatine phosphokinase is the most sensitive marker of muscle damage in rhabdomyolysis.** Muscle cell death also leads to hyperkalemia, hyperuricemia, and hyperphosphatemia. Hypocalcemia secondary to production of calcium phosphate salts commonly follows hyperphosphatemia.

D. Treatment of rhabdomyolysis centers on prevention of renal dysfunction, correction of electrolyte abnormalities, and identification and treatment of the underlying cause.

   1. Prevention of renal dysfunction

      a. Volume expansion. The cornerstone of treatment is expansion of intravascular volume. **Early and aggressive volume replacement** has been shown to prevent renal failure in both animals and humans. The optimal level of intravascular volume expansion to prevent renal failure is not known but should be enough to maintain urine flow of at least 1 to 2 mL/kg/h.

      b. Sodium bicarbonate. Some nonrandomized data suggest that **alkalinization of the urine** with sodium bicarbonate prevents the formation of pigmented casts and lessens the direct toxic effects of myoglobin, decreasing the incidence of renal failure. Sodium bicarbonate can be given as a bolus or as a continuous infusion with the goal of maintaining urine pH between 6 and 7.

      c. Diuretics. Although forced diuresis can be useful in maintaining urine flow, no prospective evidence proves that diuretics (e.g., mannitol or furosemide) are helpful in preventing renal failure in rhabdomyolysis. If diuretics are used, extreme care must be taken to avoid intravascular volume depletion, which has been conclusively shown to increase the incidence of renal failure.

      d. Experimental therapies. Free-radical scavengers (i.e., glutathione, vitamin E analogues), platelet-activating factor receptor blockers, and dantrolene are being investigated as adjunctive agents.

      e. Prognosis in renal failure associated with rhabdomyolysis. Even if patients develop renal failure and require dialysis, the prognosis is generally good. **Most patients regain baseline renal function within 3 to 4 weeks.**

2. **Correction of electrolyte abnormalities**
   a. **Hyperkalemia** is the most dangerous electrolyte abnormality seen and must be treated aggressively. Sodium bicarbonate and insulin administration along with dextrose help drive potassium into the intracellular compartment. Calcium stabilizes the myocardium and makes the heart more resistant to arrhythmias. Potassium binders should be used following these therapies. Emergency dialysis may be necessary for refractory hyperkalemia.
   b. Hyperphosphatemia responds to phosphate binding antacid administration. It can contribute to hypocalcemia and lead to **metastatic calcification**.
   c. Hypocalcemia. Although commonly seen in rhabdomyolysis, hypocalcemia is rarely associated with adverse clinical events and generally requires no specific therapy.

 AXIOMS

- Loss of function may be the earliest sign in the development of compartment syndrome.
- Loss of pulse or paralysis are late findings in the progression of compartment syndrome.
- Serum creatinine phosphokinase is the most sensitive marker for muscle injury.
- Whenever doubt exists regarding the presence of compartment syndrome, perform fasciotomy.

Bibliography

Better OS, Rubinstein I, Winaver J. Recent insights into the pathogenesis and early management of the crush syndrome. *Semin Nephrol* 1992;12:217–222.

Gulli B, Templeman D. Compartment syndrome of the lower extremity. *Orthop Clin North Am* 1994;25:677–684.

Kostler W, Strohm PC, Sudkamp NP. Acute compartment syndrome of the limb. *Injury* 2004;35:1221–1227.

Mabee JR. Compartment syndrome: A complication of acute extremity trauma. *J Emerg Med* 1994;12:651–656.

Mabee JR, Bostwick TL. Pathophysiology and mechanisms of compartment syndrome. *Orthopaed Rev* 1993;22:175–181.

Malinoski DJ, Slater MS, Mullins RJ. Crush injury and rhabdomyolysis. *Crit Care Clin* 2004;20:171–192.

Naidu SH, Heppenstall RB. Compartment syndrome of the forearm and hand. *Hand Clin* 1994;10:13–27.

Pina EM, Mehlman CT. Rhabdomyolysis: A primer for the orthopaedist. *Orthopaed Rev* 1994;23:28–32.

Poels PJ, Gabreels FJ. Rhabdomyolysis: A review of the literature. *Clin Neurol Neurosurg* 1993;95:175–192.

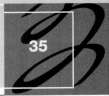

PERIPHERAL VASCULAR INJURIES
RYAN M. LEVY, LOUIS H. ALARCON, AND ERIC R. FRYKBERG

35

I. INTRODUCTION. Prompt diagnosis of peripheral vascular injury requiring operation is crucial to achieving optimal outcome. Delays in recognition and treatment are the leading causes of preventable limb loss. Vascular injuries result primarily from penetrating trauma, with injuries to the brachial vessels of the upper extremity and superficial femoral vessels of the lower extremity being the most common requiring surgical repair in civilians. Mandatory operative exploration is no longer the standard of care for all potential vascular injuries. The concept of "soft" signs is now largely obsolete since these signs do not correlate with vascular injury. Reliance on the physical examination findings of "hard" signs with selective use of arteriography has become a well-established paradigm. Unnecessary arteriography is a leading cause of treatment delay. Limb salvage is dependent on early diagnosis and timely reperfusion. Improving outcomes following vascular trauma requires strict attention to the factors associated with limb loss (Table 35-1).

II. ETIOLOGY

A. Penetrating vascular trauma can result from stab wounds, low-velocity firearms (including long-range shotgun wounds), or high-velocity projectiles from hunting rifles or close-range shotgun wounds (destructive wounds). The mechanism is critical to determine the risk of vascular injury from the knife, projectile, or blast effect. In combat series from the military, penetrating trauma comprises 95% to 100% of all peripheral vascular injuries, mainly from bomb and mine fragments and high-velocity gunshot wounds. In the civilian sector penetrating trauma accounts for 85% of peripheral vascular injuries, though only 6% of all penetrating extremity wounds result in vascular injury. Gunshot wounds constitute the majority of cases (50%), while stabs and lacerations are responsible for an additional 35%.

B. Blunt trauma accounts for only 10% to 15% of all civilian peripheral vascular injuries but results in a more extensive and wider application of kinetic energy. Delays in diagnosis and definitive therapy are more common. Consequently, this mechanism is associated with a higher amputation rate. Blunt vascular trauma is often associated with orthopedic injures as well (Table 35-2).

TABLE 35-1	Factors Associated with Higher Rates of Limb Loss in Vascular Trauma

Treatment delay >6 hours
Blunt mechanism of injury
Lower extremity injuries, especially of the popliteal artery
Associated injuries: nerve, vein, bone, soft-tissue loss
High-velocity gunshot wounds and close-range shotgun wounds
Preexisting chronic peripheral vascular disease and other comorbidities
Failure or delay in performing fasciotomy
Clinical presentation in shock or obvious limb ischemia

TABLE 35-2	Vascular Injuries Associated with Specific Orthopedic Injuries
Orthopedic injury	**Associated vascular injury**
Knee dislocation	Popliteal artery
Femur fracture	Superficial femoral artery
Supracondylar humerus fracture	Brachial artery
Clavicle fracture	Subclavian artery
Shoulder dislocation	Axillary artery

TABLE 35-3	Hard Signs of Arterial Injury

Absent distal pulses
Active hemorrhage
Large, expanding, or pulsatile hematoma
Palpable thrill or audible bruit
Signs of distal ischemia: 5 Ps—pain, pallor, paralysis, paresthesias, poikilothermia (coolness)

III. ARTERIAL INJURIES

A. Diagnosis. All injured extremities must be evaluated immediately for the presence of vascular trauma. Delays in diagnosis or therapy can be prevented through careful history and physical examination and appropriate use of diagnostic modalities. The clinical manifestations of major peripheral vascular injuries (hard signs) must be recognized promptly and addressed early (Table 35-3). A diagnostic algorithm for management of penetrating vascular trauma should be utilized (Fig. 35-1).

1. History. Details of the event, mechanism of injury, type of projectile, prehospital estimation of blood loss, and the vital signs during prehospital care are important clues in identification of major vascular injury. Eliciting a history of pulsatile blood loss before hospital arrival is also essential. As always, primary survey and stabilization of life-threatening injuries takes precedence over evaluation of the extremity. Active hemorrhage from an injured extremity is the only peripheral vascular injury that mandates intervention in the primary survey.

2. Physical examination. Important elements of the physical assessment are detailed vascular, neurologic, and soft-tissue or skeletal examinations. These findings will determine the potential for vascular injury and the risk for limb loss.

a. Vascular examination. Assess for the presence of any hard signs (Table 35-3) as these mandate immediate exclusion of vascular injury either by surgical exploration or diagnostic testing.

i. Palpate and document all pulses proximal and distal to the area of potential injury. Compare the injured extremity with the contralateral, uninjured extremity and note any pulse deficits.

ii. In uncomplicated penetrating extremity trauma, the presence of any hard sign mandates immediate surgical exploration, as virtually all of these patients will have injuries requiring operative repair. In general, evaluating such patients in the radiology department with formal arteriography should be avoided as it wastes time and consumes resources.

a) When the physical examination alone cannot answer the questions of whether a vascular injury exists or where it is located, diagnosis on the basis of hard signs becomes unreliable (Table 35-4). Diagnostic

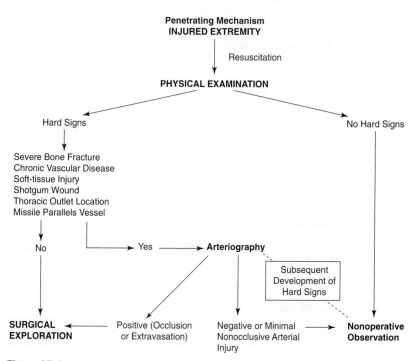

Figure 35-1. Algorithm for peripheral vascular trauma.

TABLE 35-4	Confounding Factors Requiring Imaging Following Penetrating Extremity Trauma with Hard Signs

Blunt mechanism
Associated skeletal trauma in same limb
Thoracic outlet or shoulder girdle location
Elderly patient with chronic vascular insufficiency
Shotgun or blast wounds (multiple potential sites of injury)
Missile path paralleling vessel over long distance
Delayed presentation

imaging with arteriography is indicated in this situation to confirm the presence and type of vascular injury and establish its location. In cases in which vascular injury is excluded, surgery may be avoided altogether.

  b) The absence of hard signs in an injured extremity excludes the presence of a major vascular injury as reliably as arteriography or any other imaging modality. This principle also applies to cases where concern exists for a proximal arterial injury due to a penetrating agent potentially crossing the anatomic path of a major artery.

  iii. Soft signs (small hematoma, injury to an adjacent nerve, unexplained hypotension, history of hemorrhage at the scene but no longer present in the hospital, proximity of wound to a major vessel) fail to correlate with the presence of extremity vascular injury and should not influence clinical decision making.

b. Neurologic evaluation. Perform and carefully record the details of the motor and sensory examination of the affected extremity and compare it with the uninjured extremity. Recall that vascular injury may initially manifest sensory and motor deficits due to peripheral nerve ischemia (Table 35-3). A nerve injury should never be assumed until either vascular perfusion is restored and sensorimotor deficits persist, or nerve injury is directly visualized.

c. Soft-tissue evaluation. Describe the associated soft-tissue injury and skeletal injury. In uncomplicated penetrating extremity trauma, the wound reveals the location of the vascular injury. Complete exposure of the patient and meticulous search for all bullet holes is critical. The presence of an odd number of sites of penetration implies that at least one projectile remains in the patient. The number of gunshot wounds plus the number of radiopaque foreign bodies on x-ray should equal an even number. If it does not, a search for other wounds or bullets should be undertaken.

3. Noninvasive tests. These adjuncts can be useful to evaluate intraoperative or postoperative vessel patency, but are inappropriate in the evaluation of patients with hard signs of arterial injury. They have not been shown to have advantage over physical examination in the initial diagnostic evaluation of injured extremities for vascular injury. Moreover, the information noninvasive tests yield in this setting can be misleading and falsely exclude a vascular injury on the basis of flow signals.

a. Ankle-brachial index (ABI). Measurement of systolic blood pressure with Doppler can be used to assess the ABI. Use a portable, handheld Doppler probe to identify the arterial signal proximal and distal to injury.

  i. Record the phase and, if appropriate, systolic pressure (use appropriate size cuff).

  ii. Compare ABI of injured versus uninjured extremity (ABI <0.9 has a reported accuracy of 95% for clinically significant arterial injury).

  iii. Injuries that do not obstruct flow, such as traumatic arteriovenous fistulae and pseudoaneurysms, may be associated with a normal ABI.

b. Duplex imaging can be a useful tool for intraoperative and postoperative evaluation of vessel patency in skilled hands, although the necessary expertise for reliable application and interpretation requires extensive training, not routinely available at all times in most hospitals. It is also inappropriate for use in patients with hard signs.

c. Plain radiography is useful in detecting fractures and location of retained projectiles.

4. Conventional contrast arteriography is the most accurate test in establishing the presence of vascular injury. Arteriography can exclude vascular trauma and help plan operative intervention if vascular injury exists. However, the price of this accuracy includes high costs, consumption of resources, potential delay of definitive therapy, and the small but constant rate of iatrogenic complications related to arterial puncture and intravenous contrast dye (1%–3%). In the absence of hard signs, suspicion of an arterial injury based on proximity of a wound to a major vessel is not an indication for arteriography unless a shotgun has caused the wound. Arteriogram in the face of hard signs of penetrating vascular injury is unnecessary unless the presence and site of injury cannot be determined on physical examination (Table 35-4).

Hemodynamically unstable patients should not be sent to the radiology department for diagnostic arteriography. An alternative to the formal arteriogram in the radiology suite is a surgeon-performed, on-table percutaneous arteriogram in the emergency department (ED) or operating room (OR). This should be done with the limb prepped and draped. Evidence shows that this approach conserves time and optimizes outcome in comparison to formal arteriography. The technique for this procedure is as follows:

    a. Use a short 16- to 20-gauge catheter in the proximal vessel.
    b. Just before and during hand injection of full-strength contrast, manually compress proximal inflow.
    c. Inject 20 to 30 mL of full-strength contrast.
    d. Image during injection with an x-ray plate beneath the extremity (one or two shots). Observe for evidence and location of occlusion or gross extravasation of contrast.
  B. Blunt and complex vascular injury involve concomitant injuries to extremity vessels, bone, soft tissue, and nerves. (Such injuries can be due to both blunt and destructive penetrating mechanisms as in shotgun and high-velocity firearm wounds.) These injuries have a higher probability of limb loss than simple penetrating trauma. A distinct management algorithm for combined arterial and skeletal trauma should be used (Fig. 35-2).

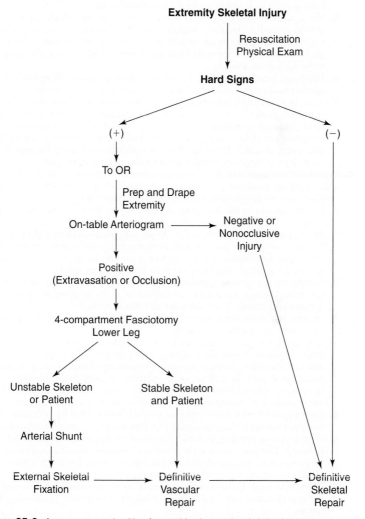

Figure 35-2. A management algorithm for combined artertal and skeletal trauma.

1. **History.** Examine the extremity, documenting change in examination over time. Obtain a full history from the prehospital providers (e.g., Was a joint dislocation relocated in the field?).

2. Delay in the diagnosis and treatment of complex extremity vascular injury is the single most common cause of limb loss in this setting. Maximizing limb salvage requires that reperfusion be the first priority after prompt diagnosis. Skeletal, nerve, or soft-tissue trauma should be addressed after revascularization has been accomplished.

3. Angulated fractures and joint dislocations can cause temporary vascular compromise. Perform careful vascular examination before and after fracture realignment or splinting and relocation of dislocated joints.

4. The presence of hard signs mandates immediate vascular evaluation by arteriography, as most hard signs are not due to vascular injury in the setting of blunt trauma (high false positive rate of physical exam). Adhering to this practice helps avoid a high rate of negative limb explorations.

5. The absence of hard signs excludes surgically significant vascular injury as reliably as any other diagnostic modality, thereby allowing the surgeon to bypass vascular imaging and direct immediate attention to other injuries. This principle holds true for all forms of blunt and complex limb trauma, including posterior knee dislocation.

6. Dressings, wraps, or splints can restrict venous or arterial flow. Swelling and edema can increase over time, leading to constriction by dressings.

7. There is a significant risk of compartment syndrome in the setting of blunt and complex vascular injury. Consequently, a high index of suspicion for compartment syndrome is necessary for early diagnosis either by direct measurement of compartment pressures, physical exam findings, or fasciotomy. Prophylactic fasciotomy should be encouraged and is preferable to delayed fasciotomy after overt signs of extremity compartment syndrome have developed.

C. **Operative management.** Arterial injuries should be repaired immediately, except when more life-threatening injuries are present. To maximize limb salvage, flow should be restored to the extremity within 6 hours of injury.

1. Do not attempt to blindly clamp bleeding vessels prior to obtaining adequate surgical exposure in the OR. Active hemorrhage should be controlled with direct pressure en route to the OR. In general, tourniquets should be avoided. Placement of a blood pressure cuff proximal to the injury may control hemorrhage during stabilization and transport to the OR. Inflation of the blood pressure cuff just above systolic blood pressure is recommended.

2. Administer perioperative antibiotics to cover gram-positive organisms. Broad spectrum therapy should be considered in cases of gross contamination. Tetanus prophylaxis is necessary for all open wounds.

3. Prepare and drape the uninjured extremity, anticipating the need to harvest a saphenous or cephalic vein conduit.

4. In general, fix vascular injuries before associated injuries in the extremity. Restoration of blood flow always takes priority. In combined skeletal and vascular injury, consider the use of temporary shunts to restore extremity perfusion in patients with unstable fractures or dislocations, life-threatening injuries, or ongoing hemodynamic instability. Temporary intraluminal shunts allow skeletal or patient stabilization before definitive arterial repair.

5. Gain proximal and distal vascular control before entering a hematoma or removing foreign bodies (e.g., knife) that may be tamponading the injured vessel.

6. Give systemic heparin, especially in cases of isolated injury with obvious ischemia. This may not be appropriate with massive blood loss, extensive soft-tissue injury, or multiple injuries. Local heparin can be flushed proximally and distally in the injured vessel in these settings.

7. Debride the injured vessel to remove areas of contused arterial wall or intimal flap.

8. Perform proximal and distal balloon catheter thrombectomy before completing repair.

9. Use primary repair, the preferred method for arterial repair. However, loss of vessel length from injury or appropriate debridement may make primary repair without undue tension impossible. Therefore, a reversed interposition saphenous vein graft harvested from the **contralateral** extremity is often necessary. Other conduit options include basilic or cephalic vein and polytetrafluoroethylene (PTFE) (avoid in heavily contaminated areas). Repair arterial injuries distal to the knee or elbow with interrupted sutures, at least on the anterior wall of the vessel.

10. Perform completion arteriography via cannulation with a small catheter proximal to the repair, proximal occlusion during the injection of full-strength contrast, and obtain the film during active injection. Image intensification provides superior images.

11. Consider fasciotomy in the presence of ischemic time exceeding 4 to 6 hours, uncertain limb viability, shock, popliteal artery injury, combined vascular and skeletal injury, or simultaneous arterial and venous injury. **Prophylactic rather than therapeutic fasciotomy offers the best opportunity for limb salvage and preservation of limb function.**

12. Immediately return the patient to the OR if vessel/graft thrombosis or compartment syndrome develop. Close intraoperative and postoperative monitoring with physical examination, Doppler pulse evaluation, and compartment pressure measurement (if immediate fasciotomy is not done) is critical to assess for these complications.

13. **Manage asymptomatic nonocclusive arterial injuries.** Selected extremity arterial injuries in the absence of hard signs and without extravasation or occlusion on arteriography are successfully managed nonoperatively in 90% of cases. These clinically occult, minimal arterial injuries include intimal flaps or other intraluminal irregularities, small pseudoaneurysms, and small arteriovenous fistulae The majority of these injuries have a benign natural history and may be safely observed with serial exam and close follow-up. The rare asymptomatic, nonocclusive arterial injury that worsens during follow-up is readily repaired without undue complications or increased risk of limb loss from the treatment delay. There is no need for prophylactic anticoagulation or antiplatelet therapy in the setting of nonocclusive arterial injury.

D. **Outcomes and complications**

1. Long-term outcome for successful arterial repair is good (>95% salvage rates under optimal conditions). Limb loss increases with delays in diagnosis and restoration of flow (>6 hours), high-velocity or destructive gunshot wounds with substantial tissue loss, injury to smaller (more distal) vessels, preexisting peripheral vascular disease, and in multiply injured or hemodynamically unstable patients.

2. Combined vascular and skeletal extremity injuries have higher rates of infection and amputation (70%) in some series (e.g., open tibia or fibula fractures with trifurcation injury are associated with high incidence of limb loss).

3. Peripheral nerve injuries are present in up to 50% of patients with extremity vascular trauma and are the most significant determinant of long-term disability.

4. Most **preventable** complications are associated with prolonged ischemic times or failure to perform fasciotomy. Complications include:

   a. **Early:** thrombosis, most often related to technical problems; bleeding; compartment syndrome; infection; limb loss; rhabdomyolysis with accompanying renal failure; venous thromboembolism related to immobility or venous injury; and death.

   b. **Late:** pseudoaneurysm, arteriovenous fistula, infection, and occlusion.

IV. **VENOUS INJURIES.** In general, venous injuries are most commonly recognized at the time of exploration for arterial injury. Management of venous injury is controversial and centers on the decision to repair or ligate. There is some benefit in repair of venous injury, especially if the popliteal vein is injured. Consider repair rather than ligation of the venous injury if the patient is stable and there is evidence of venous hypertension with excessive venous and soft tissue bleeding on completion of the arterial repair. Venous ligation is best considered if the patient is hemodynamically unstable, coagulopathic, acidotic, hypothermic, or has other life-threatening problems requiring urgent attention. Rarely will ligation cause chronic problems or adversely affect limb salvage. Should chronic sequelae develop, formal repair can be undertaken when the patient is in optimal condition.

A. Diagnosis

1. Clinical signs of venous injury include hemorrhage, venous engorgement, and swelling of the extremity. There is no rationale or proven role for the use of imaging to detect asymptomatic venous injury.

B. Treatment

1. Venous injury without active bleeding or hematoma does not require operation.
2. Venous injury found at the time of exploration can be repaired by lateral venorrhaphy if no pressing associated injuries exist. In some instances an interposition graft is necessary to repair venous injury. Lateral venorrhaphy is preferable, although long-term patency results are lower than arterial repair. Nonetheless, short-term patency reduces postoperative complications of swelling and edema.
3. In the extremities, ligation remains acceptable treatment of venous injury. If ligation is necessary, fasciotomy or leg elevation and compression stockings should be used.
4. There is no need to perform follow-up imaging of venous repairs unless clinically significant symptoms of venous insufficiency develop.

V. CONTROVERSIAL AREAS

A. Immediate amputation—the mangled extremity (Chapter 31). Indications for immediate amputation without attempting arterial repair include the following:

1. Nerve destruction, resulting in an insensate and paralyzed extremity, confirmed by direct examination of the nerve at exploration to exclude simple nerve contusion
2. Extensive concomitant bone and soft-tissue loss or destruction
3. Arterial injury in a patient with more immediately life-threatening injury
4. Open lower leg fractures with arterial injury (Gustilo III-C injuries)
5. Nonviable muscles in all compartments at fasciotomy
6. Severe comorbidities
7. Any setting in which arterial repair is deemed futile or has failed

B. Use of temporary conduits as a "damage control" bridge (i.e., shunts) combined with external fixation of skeletal injuries may allow rapid restoration of distal blood flow and provide the option to take the multiply injured patient to the intensive care unit (ICU) for further resuscitation. Definitive vascular repair may then be accomplished at a later time when the patient has been stabilized.

C. While the conduit of choice for vascular repair is the autogenous saphenous vein, associated injuries can preclude its use. Vein grafts have the highest long-term patency rates and lowest infection risk. PTFE may be necessary in contaminated fields and is better utilized in damage control circumstances when operative time must be minimized. Extraanatomic bypass is another option in this situation.

D. A damage control approach to vascular injury should be considered in all patients with multisystem trauma. This strategy includes the use of temporary shunts and synthetic materials for grafting. Although the risks of infection are significant with synthetic grafts, the long-term results are better in all patients who have rapid restoration of arterial blood supply.

E. Optimal sequence of repair: artery → vein → bone. Reestablishing distal perfusion is the first priority. Good surgical judgment is essential in the patient with combined skeletal and vascular injuries. At times, an arterial shunt is needed to temporarily restore flow while the fracture is realigned. Definitive vascular repair is the preferred method of immediate reperfusion in stable fractures with no anticipated need for extensive manipulation, subject to the judgment of the trauma or vascular surgeon. The trauma or vascular surgeon should be present during the orthopedic procedure to assist with any problems that may develop in the initially repaired or shunted vessels.

VI. MANAGEMENT OF SPECIFIC ARTERIAL INJURIES

A. Axillary artery

1. The axillary artery is a continuation of the subclavian artery that starts at the lateral border of the first rib and ends at the inferior border of the teres major muscle. The axillary artery has three segments from which six branches originate (Fig. 35-3). The axillary vein and brachial plexus course alongside the axillary artery.

2. From 3% to 9% of axillary artery injuries are from penetrating trauma. Associated nerve and venous injury occurs in 50% and 40% of cases, respectively.

3. The entire arm, neck, and chest should be included in the operative field. Expose the axillary artery via an S-shaped incision, starting at the midclavicle, following the deltopectoral groove and continuing to the groove between biceps and triceps muscles. Perform primary repair or resection with primary anastomosis, if possible. Do not sacrifice collaterals to complete primary repair; place an interposition graft in this setting.

B. Brachial artery

1. The brachial artery begins at the border of the teres major muscle and ends 1 cm below the antecubital fossa. Major branches include the profunda brachii, ulnar, and radial arteries (Fig. 35-4). The median nerve courses with the

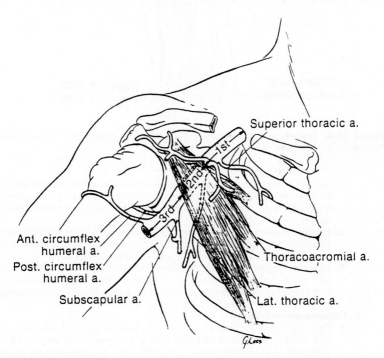

Figure 35-3. Anatomy of an axillary artery. (From Rich NM, Spencer FC. *Vascular Trauma.* Philadelphia, Pa: WB Saunders; 1978:331, with permission.)

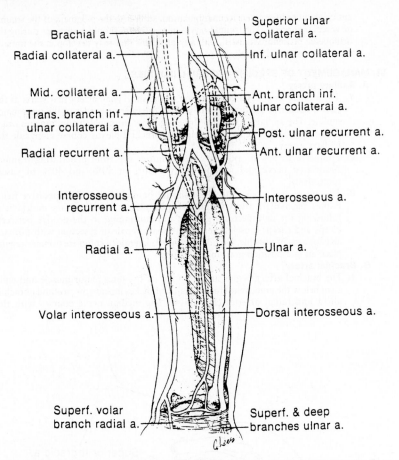

Figure 35-4. Anatomy of a brachial artery. (From Rich NM, Spencer FC. *Vascular Trauma.* Philadelphia, Pa: WB Saunders; 1978:331, with permission.)

brachial artery; radial and ulnar nerves are also in proximity. The degree of ischemia depends on whether injury is proximal or distal to the profunda brachii. Ischemia and ultimate amputation rate is higher for more proximal injuries.

2. Injuries are commonly due to penetrating trauma and include iatrogenic causes. Brachial artery injury comprises 20% of civilian vascular injury. Supracondylar humerus fracture can result in Volkmann's ischemic contracture.

3. Operative approach is along the groove between the triceps and biceps muscles, via an S-shaped extension if the incision crosses the antecubital fossa. End-to-end repair is generally possible, though a saphenous vein interposition graft is necessary on occasion.

C. **Forearm vascular injury**

1. One inch below the antecubital fossa, the brachial artery divides into radial and ulnar arteries (85% of hands have a dominant ulnar artery); 10% of patients have incomplete palmar arch; 60% have concomitant nerve injury.

2. Operative repair is through a longitudinal incision overlying the artery. If only the radial or ulnar artery is injured and distal neurologic function is intact,

perform ligation. Even with early successful repair, long-term patency of a repaired single vessel is only 50%.

D. Common, profunda, and superficial femoral arteries (Fig. 35-5)
   1. Commonly injured in civilians, comprise 20% of vascular injuries. Mechanism is usually penetrating, can be iatrogenic.
   2. Operative approach involves preparing the abdomen, entire injured leg, and proximal contralateral leg in case saphenous vein harvest is needed. Proximal control may require division of the inguinal ligament or retroperitoneal control of the external iliac artery. Begin with a longitudinal incision over the course of the femoral vessels. Approach to the superficial femoral artery involves a longitudinal incision along the anterior border of the sartorius muscle. Repair all arterial injuries except for distal injuries to the profunda femoris artery.

E. Popliteal artery
   1. The politeal artery starts at the adductor hiatus as a continuation of the superficial femoral artery. The proximal popliteal artery lies posterior to the femur while the distal aspect is situated behind the capsule of the knee joint (Fig. 35-6). Its fixation at the adductor hiatus proximally and soleus arch

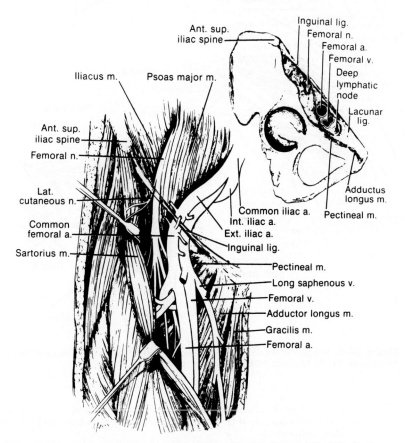

Figure 35-5. Anatomy of a femoral artery. (From Rich NM, Spencer FC. *Vascular Trauma.* Philadelphia, Pa: WB Saunders; 1978:331, with permission.)

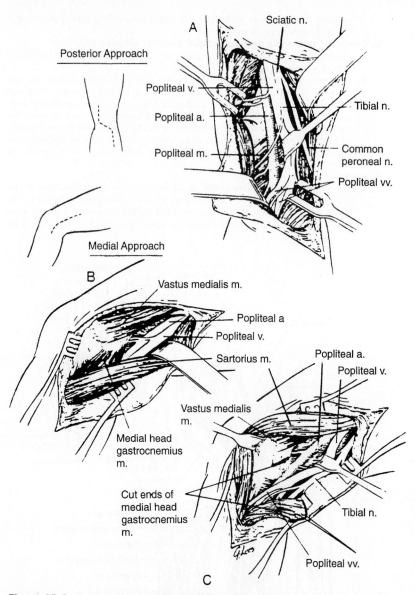

Figure 35-6. Anatomy of a popliteal artery. (From Rich NM, Spencer FC. *Vascular Trauma.* Philadelphia, Pa: WB Saunders; 1978:331, with permission.)

distally make it vulnerable to blunt injury. The popliteal vein courses from lateral to medial side of the artery in its midportion. Both artery and vein are commonly injured.

2. Popliteal injuries comprise 5% to 10% of civilian vascular trauma overall. Nearly 50% of popliteal trauma results from a blunt mechanism. Amputation

can be as high as 25% with blunt injury, whereas only 4% of popliteal gunshot wounds result in amputation. With blunt injury, the magnitude of the skeletal and soft tissue injuries often dictates the need for amputation.

3. Operative approach is generally via a medial exposure (Fig. 35-7). The contralateral leg must be prepared so that a saphenous vein can be harvested. Preserve the ipsilateral saphenous vein during the operation as this may be the only venous drainage from the injured extremity. The medial head of gastrocnemius muscle can be detached to improve distal exposure. Repair venous injuries if at all possible. Plan to perform fasciotomies as more than 60% of patients ultimately require fasciotomy. Completion arteriography is recommended after repair.

F. Anterior tibial, posterior tibial, and peroneal arteries

1. The anterior tibial artery is generally the first branch; tibioperoneal trunk bifurcates into the peroneal artery and posterior tibial artery.

2. Mechanism of injury is penetrating in two thirds of cases. Injury to the tibioperoneal trunk or all three vessels carries an amputation rate in excess of 50%. A single-vessel injury does not usually require repair. The presence of

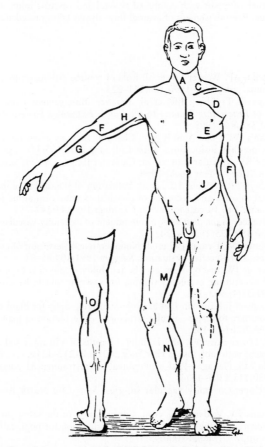

Figure 35-7. Operative approach to peripheral vascular trauma. (From Rich NM, Spencer FC. *Vascular Trauma*. Philadelphia, Pa: WB Saunders; 1978:331, with permission.)

limb ischemia, injury to the tibioperoneal trunk, or injury to multiple vessels requires restoration of flow through at least one vessel.

AXIOMS

- Physical examination is the cornerstone for the diagnosis of vascular injury. It is equivalent in accuracy and safety and superior in cost-effectiveness compared to other modalities.
- In uncomplicated penetrating trauma, hard signs of arterial injury mandate immediate operation; formal arteriography in the radiology department is dangerous and unnecessary in this setting.
- In blunt or complex extremity trauma, the presence of hard signs mandates arteriography.
- The absence of hard signs in any setting reliably excludes surgically significant arterial injury and eliminates the need for imaging. This applies to proximity injuries as well. The concept of soft signs of arterial injury does not have clinical relevance.
- Harvest saphenous vein from the contralateral, uninjured extremity.
- Most preventable amputations are associated with delayed diagnosis and treatment of arterial trauma or delayed or inadequate fasciotomy.
- Optimal sequence of repair with combined skeletal and vascular injury is artery, vein, bone, soft tissue. Reestablishment of arterial flow always takes precedence.

Bibliography

Applebaum R, Yellin AE, Weaver FA, et al. Role of routine arteriography in blunt lower extremity trauma. *Am J Surg* 1990;160:221–225.

Arrillaga A, Nagy K, Frykberg ER, et al. *Practice Management Guidelines for the Management of Penetrating Trauma to the Lower Extremity.* Eastern Association for the Surgery of Trauma; 1999.

Attebery LR, Dennis JW, Russo-Alesi F, et al. Changing patterns of arterial injuries associated with fractures and dislocations. *J Am Coll Surg* 1996;183:377–383.

Aucar JA, Mattox KL. Vascular trauma. In: Cameron JL, ed. *Current Surgical Therapy.* St. Louis, Mo: Mosby—Year Book; 1998.

Dennis JW, Frykberg ER, Veldenz HC, et al. Validation of nonoperative management of occult vascular injuries and accuracy of physical examination alone in penetrating extremity trauma: 5 to 10 year followup. *J Trauma* 1998;44:243–253.

Frykberg ER. Advances in the diagnosis and treatment of extremity vascular trauma. *Surg Clin North Am* 1995;75(2):207–224.

Frykberg ER, Crump JM, Dennis JW, et al. Nonoperative observation of clinically occult arterial injuries: A prospective evaluation. *Surgery* 1991;109:85–91.

Frykberg ER, Dennis JW, Bishop K, et al. The reliability of physical examination in the evaluation of penetrating extremity trauma for vascular injury: Results at one year. *J Trauma* 1991;31(4):502–511.

Gillespie DL, Woodson J, Kaufman J, et al. Role of arteriography for blunt or penetrating injuries in proximity to major vascular structures: An evolution in management. *Ann Vasc Surg* 1993;7(2):145–149.

Hafez HM, et al. Lower extremity arterial injury: Results of 550 cases and review of risk factors associated with limb loss. *J Vasc Surg* 2001;33:1212–1219.

Lim LT, Michuda MS, Flanagan P, et al. Popliteal artery trauma: 31 consecutive cases. *Arch Surg* 1980;115:1307–1313.

McCready RA. Upper-extremity vascular injuries. *Surg Clin North Am* 1988;68(4):725–740.

Miranda FE, Dennis JW, Veldenz HC, et al. Confirmation of the safety and accuracy of physical examination in the evaluation of knee dislocation for popliteal artery injury: A prospective study. *J Trauma* 2000;49:375.

Perry MO. Vascular trauma. *Adv Surg* 1995;28:59–70.

Rich NM. Management of venous trauma. *Surg Clin North Am* 1988;58(4):809–821.

Rutherford RB. Diagnostic evaluation of extremity vascular injuries. *Surg Clin North Am* 1988;68(4):683–691.

Schilling J. Extremity vascular trauma. In: Lopez-Viego MA, ed. *The Parkland Trauma Handbook*. St. Louis, Mo: Mosby—Year Book; 1994.

Thal ER, Snyder WH, Perry MO. Vascular injuries of the extremities. In: Rutherford RB, ed. *Vascular Surgery*. Philadelphia, Pa: WB Saunders; 1995.

SOFT-TISSUE TRAUMA
KIMBERLY A. DAVIS AND
AURELIO RODRIQUEZ

36

I. MECHANISM OF INJURY
A. Blunt
1. **Shear.** This is the most common mechanism of injury, resulting in laceration of tissues.
2. **Crush.** A result of compressive forces, this mechanism of injury creates wounds that are often stellate. Because of their devitalized nature, crush wounds are at high risk for complications and should be **debrided**.
B. Penetrating
1. Knife stab wounds are low velocity, and result in minimal tissue damage.
2. Gunshot wounds
   a. **Low-velocity** wounds are induced by most handguns (except .44 magnum). Damage to surrounding tissues ("cavitation") causes wound morbidity, including devitalization.
   b. **High-velocity** wounds are caused by missiles traveling at velocities >2,500 feet/second, and are associated with military weapons and some hunting rifles. These wounds have a large amount of associated soft-tissue injury and often require massive debridement in the operating room (OR). High-velocity wounds should rarely be closed primarily.
3. Shotgun wounds
   a. **Close-range** wounds are created when the shotgun is fired within 3 yards of the patient, and are considered high-velocity wounds. They are associated with significant devitalization of tissue. These are contaminated wounds because of retained wadding and clothing, and must be debrided aggressively.
   b. **Intermediate-range** wounds are created when the shotgun is fired within 3 to 7 yards of the patient, and can result in injuries to vital structures deep to fascia.
   c. **Far-range** wounds (shotgun blasts fired at >7 yards from the patient) result in multiple small, low-velocity wounds that rarely penetrate fascia, and that often do not require surgical intervention.

II. INITIAL MANAGEMENT
A. Assessment of tissue viability
1. **General examination.** Repeated examination is required as assessment of wound viability is difficult early after trauma.
2. **Skin** should be assessed by color, capillary refill, presence of dermal bleeding, and sensory examination.
3. **Subcutaneous tissues** are difficult to assess, as the viability of fat can be difficult to determine. However, subcutaneous tissue can readily be debrided, with care taken to avoid devascularization of the overlying skin.
4. **Muscle** is the most difficult tissue to assess, and should be examined for color, bleeding, and contractile response. Muscle of questionable viability can often be left in situ and reexamined at frequent intervals, while frankly necrotic muscle should be debrided. However, patients with muscle of questionable viability need close monitoring. Early reexploration with attention to the deeper muscle layers is indicated in any patient with sign of systemic sepsis.

5. **Nerve** viability is best assessed by visual inspection and electrical stimulation. If primary repair is not indicated (e.g., contaminated wound or other more important issues), tag nerves to ease later identification.

B. **Threats to wound healing**
   1. **Ischemia and necrosis.** Wound hypoxia results in decreased collagen deposition and impairs the functioning of immunocompetent cells.
   2. **Hemorrhage.** Inadequate hemostasis can result in wound hematomas. Hematomas are excellent culture media and reduce the quantity of bacterial contamination necessary to produce infection. If adequate hemostasis is not possible because of coagulopathy, delay wound closure.
   3. **Bacterial contamination.** Sources of contamination include both the patient's normal bacterial flora and external contamination at the time of the trauma. Frankly contaminated wounds should undergo sharp debridement, as well as with large-volume, pressurized (5–8 lb/in^2, produced by using ≤19-gauge needle tip) and pulsatile lavage.
   4. **Foreign material contamination.** A foreign body in the wound impairs phagocytosis and reduces the inoculum necessary to cause infection. In addition to "hand debridement" of materials, it is important to irrigate wounds with large-volume, pressurized (5–8 lb/in^2, produced by using ≤19-gauge needle tip) and pulsatile lavage for heavily contaminated wounds to decrease risk of wound infection.
   5. **Systemic factors.** Shock, malnutrition, and preexisting immunocompromise can impair wound healing and foster infection.

C. **Tetanus prophylaxis.** Assess the need for and type (active and passive vs. active alone) of tetanus prophylaxis for all wounds (Appendix B).

D. **Decision making.** Factors influencing the decision regarding management of a wound in the emergency department or the OR include the size of the wound, the degree of contamination, the presence of devitalized tissue, the anatomic location of the wound, and the presence of associated injuries. Patients in hemorrhagic shock should have obvious contamination and necrotic tissue debrided, but should have definitive wound management delayed until such time as the patient's hemodynamics have been stabilized (damage control approach is discussed in Chapter 28).

III. TREATMENT

A. **Anesthesia**
   1. **Local.** Lidocaine with epinephrine (0.5% to 1.0%) can be administered to a maximal dose of 4 to 7 mg/kg of body weight. Avoid epinephrine in wounds of the nose and digits, tissues with poor perfusion or recently grafted, and in extremity wounds of those patients with peripheral vascular disease. The maximal dose of lidocaine without epinephrine is 4 mg/kg of body weight. The addition of bicarbonate (1 mL from standard resuscitation ampule added to 10 mL anesthetic), warming to body temperature, and slow proximal to distal injections can minimize the pain of injection. Bupivacaine (0.25%, with or without epinephrine) is an alternative to lidocaine as it lasts longer, has a similar onset of action for infiltration or small nerve block, but causes less irritation.
   2. **Regional.** This is an extremely useful and underutilized technique for wounds of the distal extremities and the face.
   3. **Systemic analgesics.** These (especially opioids) can be powerful adjuncts or alternatives in complex cases (Chapter 40).

B. **Antibiotic prophylaxis.** Prophylactic antibiotics are not indicated in simple wounds (uncontaminated, noncrush, minimally devitalized, and of low depth) in a healthy patient because the underlying risk of infection is small. **Antibiotics are not a substitute for adequate debridement and local wound care.** Most surgeons recommend the use of preventive antibiotics in the following situations:
   1. Open fractures and joint spaces
   2. Wounds with heavy contamination or requiring extensive debridement
   3. Patients with immunocompromise, peripheral vascular disease, or cardiac valvular disease

C. Debridement

1. **Sharp** debridement remains the *sine qua non*, allowing the removal of dead skin, muscle, and fat.
2. **Mechanical** (pulsatile lavage). High-pressure irrigation (minimum 5–8 lb/in^2 using a $\leq$19-gauge needle or irrigation exit port) is the best method of clearing debris and bacteria, especially in wounds containing specialized tissues (nerves, tendons, and vessels) not amenable to sharp debridement.

D. Closure

1. **Primary closure** is appropriate for class I (simple, no contamination or devitalized tissue) and class II (minimal contamination or devitalized tissue) wounds, as long as the wound is closed within the first 8 hours of injury.
2. **Secondary closure** (also known as secondary intention) allows the wound to heal by granulation and subsequent contraction.
3. **Delayed primary closure** (also known as tertiary closure) is used for class III (contaminated) and class IV (infected) wounds. Wound edges are left open for up to 5 days, and packed with damp to dry sterile saline dressings. Thereafter, the wound is reapproximated with suture, staples, or sterile tapes.
4. **Vacuum-assisted wound closure** has been used successfully in a large variety of wounds, either to facilitate complex wound closure or to prepare a wound bed for subsequent skin grafting. The most popular device is the KCI V.A.C., which utilizes a reticulated foam dressing that is cut to conform to the wound. A vacuum tube is placed over the foam, and an occlusive dressing applied. The tube is then connected to a pump, which provides 50 to 125 mmHg of negative pressure to the wound bed. These dressings should be changed every 48 to 72 hours, and should not be utilized in frankly contaminated wounds. The device has been shown to enhance local blood flow, minimize edema, and accelerate granulation tissue formation in the wound.
5. **Skin grafting,** either split thickness or full thickness, can be used for the closure of traumatic wounds with tissue defects. In general, full-thickness grafts are used for the face and hands, with split-thickness grafts used elsewhere.
6. **Tissue transfer** involves the use of either myocutaneous rotational flaps (for truncal wounds) or free flaps, used predominantly in the reconstruction of lower extremity defects.
7. **Suture removal**
   a. Face: 3 to 5 days
   b. Abdominal wall: 7 to 10 days
   c. Scalp: 10 days
   d. Wounds crossing joints: 2 weeks
   e. Vertical torso wounds: 2 weeks

E. Difficult wounds

1. **Scalp.** The scalp can bleed extensively, and requires urgent hemostasis, using either Raney clips or temporary closure with heavy nylon sutures, incorporating the galea aponeurotica. Formal closure depends on the extent of the injury, but should always involve a layered closure, with careful approximation of the galea aponeurotica. For large lacerations, it may be beneficial to place a closed suction drain for 24 hours. Shaving or clipping hair around the wound edges is helpful to avoid entangling hair in the suture lines.
2. **Face.** Repair of facial lacerations can be delayed for up to 24 hours while the patient is stabilized. A good examination is necessary to identify facial fractures and intraoral lacerations. It is important to carefully reapproximate the vermillion border of the lip. Plastic surgical consultation for extensive lacerations may be warranted. Wounds with exposed cartilage should be treated with prophylactic antibiotics.
3. **Perineal degloving injuries** are complex injuries associated with mortality rates approaching 30%, usually secondary to hemorrhage or pelvic sepsis. Early sigmoidoscopy in search of rectal injury is mandatory. Should a rectal injury be identified, complete fecal diversion (with or without distal rectal washout) is indicated. For all perineal degloving injuries, early aggressive

debridement with subsequent daily debridement utilizing pulsatile lavage for at least 5 days postinjury has markedly reduced the incidence of late pelvic sepsis. The wounds should be allowed to heal by secondary intention; vacuum-assisted devices may be used in addition. These devastating wounds often require delayed split-thickness skin grafting or closure with myocutaneous flaps.

4. **Closed internal degloving injuries** are most commonly associated with pelvic and acetabular fractures (Morel-Lavallee lesions) in which the subcutaneous tissues tear away from the underlying fascia, resulting in a cavity filled with hematoma and liquefied fat. These injuries occur most commonly over the greater trochanter of the femur, but can also occur in the flank and lumbodorsal regions. These wounds require aggressive debridement either before or at the time of fracture fixation. The wounds should be left open, with repeated debridement, as indicated. As with any deep-tissue injury, repeated examination with attention to muscle viability is important. In patients with signs of systemic sepsis, early and aggressive reexploration with attention to the deep muscle layers and wide debridement of nonviable or infected material is necessary. Degloving wounds should be allowed to heal by secondary intention (vacuum-assisted devices may be used as well). These wounds often require delayed split-thickness skin grafting or closure with myocutaneous flaps.

IV. BITES AND STINGS

A. **Human bite** wounds are contaminated and devitalized, and at high risk for subsequent soft-tissue infection with *Streptococcus viridans, Staphylococcus* spp., *Eikenella corrodens, Bacteroides* spp., and microaerophilic *Streptococcus* spp. Human bites are treated using aggressive irrigation, debridement of devitalized tissue, systemic antibiotics (recommended is a β-lactam–β-lactamase inhibitor combination) and elevation. All wounds should be left open to heal by secondary intention, unless they are located on the face or other cosmetically sensitive area.

B. **Cat bite and scratch** wounds that penetrate the skin should also be considered heavily contaminated, with commonly infecting organisms including *Pasteurella multocida* and *Staphylococcus* spp. Management strategies are identical to those employed in the management of human bite wounds. The need for rabies and tetanus immunization should be considered.

C. **Dog bite** wounds are often associated with significant soft tissue damage because of the enormous force generated by the muscles of mastication. Infection is less common than in human and cat bites. Given the potential for tissue devitalization, aggressive debridement should be added to those management strategies employed in the management of human bites. The need for rabies and tetanus immunization should be considered.

D. **Snake bites** should initially be managed by immobilization, neutral positioning, and a lightly compressive dressing. The use of local suctioning and tourniquets are not currently recommended. Severe envenomations (severe or progressive extremity involvement, coagulopathy, or systemic signs) can be treated with antivenin. Supportive treatment with intensive care unit (ICU) monitoring and replacement of blood factors are the mainstays of therapy in extreme cases.

E. **Spider bites.** The two common species of poisonous spiders in the continental United States are the brown recluse and the black widow. The brown recluse (*Loxosceles reclusa*) is most common, and has a violin-shaped carapace on its body. Although initially painless, bites can progress to a hemorrhagic blister with subsequent necrosis. Treatment remains supportive and early debridement of dead tissue is helpful. The black widow (*Lactrodectus macrotans*) has a red hourglass on the ventral surface of the abdomen. Bites are characterized by a toxic systemic reaction, including pain, muscle rigidity, altered mental status, and seizures. Treatment is supportive, although an equine antivenin is available for severe cases.

Bibliography

Hak DJ, Olson SA, Matta JM. Diagnosis and management of closed internal degloving injuries associated with pelvic and acetabular fractures: The Morel-Lavallee lesion. *J Trauma* 1997;42(6):1046–1051.

Kudsk KA, McQueen MA, Voeller GR, et al. Management of complex perineal soft-tissue injuries. *J Trauma* 1990;30(9):1155–1160.

Morykwas MJ, Argenta LC, Shelton-Brown EI, et al. Vacuum-assisted closure: Method for wound control and treatment: Animal studies and basic foundation. *Ann Plast Surg* 1997;38:553–562.

Stewart RM, Page CP. Wounds, bites and stings. In: Feliciano DV, Moore EE, Mattox KL, eds. *Trauma*. 3rd ed. Stamford, Conn: Appleton & Lange; 1996:917–936.

PRIORITIES IN THE ICU CARE OF THE ADULT TRAUMA PATIENT

**PHILIP S. BARIE AND
SOUMITRA R. EACHEMPATI**

37

I. GOALS OF CARE

A. Fundamental goals of ICU management of the seriously injured patient include early restoration and maintenance of tissue oxygenation, diagnosis and treatment of occult injuries, and prevention and treatment of infection and organ dysfunction.

B. Most early deaths from trauma (in the first few days) occur from traumatic brain injury (TBI) or refractory shock, and are largely not preventable. Late deaths from multiple organ dysfunction syndrome (MODS) may be minimized by effective resuscitation, prevention of hospital-acquired infection, identification and treatment of all injuries, and avoidance of error. Errors of surgical technique and critical care management may contribute to one half of preventable trauma deaths.

C. Optimal trauma care in the ICU is provided by a multiprofessional team that consists of physicians, nurses, pharmacists, therapists, and others. An ICU environment where communication, patient safety, and infection control are part of the culture create conditions for the optimal care of the patient.

II. ICU ADMISSION CRITERIA.
The decision to admit the trauma patient to an ICU depends on the patient's age, injury severity, comorbid conditions, and availability of both ICU beds and intermediate-level care beds (Table 37-1).

III. PHASES OF ICU CARE

A. Early phase (<24 hours). Primary concerns in the early (<24 hours) care of the trauma patient in the ICU include shock, respiratory failure, intracranial hypertension, and the identification of occult injuries. The patient must often be diagnosed and treated simultaneously.

1. Repetition of the primary survey. Upon ICU admission it is possible for injuries to be as yet unidentified, or identified but as yet untreated. It is prudent to repeat the evaluation of the trauma patient, beginning with the primary survey to provide optimal diagnosis and treatment.

a. Airway. The airway should be secure and positioned appropriately.

b. Breathing. Ventilation of both lungs must be confirmed. Minute ventilation (V_E) must be adequate. The inspired oxygen concentration (FiO2) must be adequate to maintain arterial oxygen saturation (S_aO_2) above 90%. If the patient is on a mechanical ventilator, the mode and settings must meet the patient's physiologic requirements. Arterial blood gas determination provides important information about the status of resuscitation.

c. Circulation. Intravenous access must be sufficient for the administration of fluids, blood, and blood products adequate to support the circulation. If adequate peripheral venous access cannot be obtained, central venous access must be achieved. Heart rate, blood pressure, and urine output are monitored as dictated by the pattern and severity of injury. If the circulation cannot be monitored adequately by heart rate, blood pressure, and urine output, indices of acid status should be monitored and consideration should be given to invasive hemodynamic monitoring.

TABLE 37-1	Injuries and Postinjury Problems that Require ICU Admission

Injuries
- Multisystem trauma
- Severe traumatic brain injury (GCS ≤8)
  - Lesser traumatic brain injuries of anticoagulated patients (e.g., aspirin, warfarin)
- Cervical spinal cord injury
- Severe pulmonary contusion, flail chest
- Facial or neck trauma with threatened airway
- Repaired major vascular injuries
- Pelvic fracture with retroperitoneal hemorrhage or bony instability
- Blunt cardiac trauma with dysrhythmia or hypotension
- Crush injuries
- Severe burns (.20% TBSA, facial burns)
- Smoke inhalation
- Isolated high-grade solid-organ injuries (grade III–V liver or spleen)

Problems
- Respiratory failure requiring mechanical ventilation
- Ongoing shock or hemodynamic instability
- Massive blood or fluid resuscitation
- Base deficit (>5)
- Hypothermia
- Seizures
- Pregnancy

Posttraumatic Injuries or Problems Suitable for Intermediate Care Monitoring*
- Isolated liver or splenic injuries (especially grade I–II)
- Uncomplicated blunt anterior chest trauma
- Isolated multiple rib fractures or pulmonary contusion with adequate oxygenation and ventilation
- Isolated thoracic spinal cord injury with stable hemodynamics
- Lesser traumatic brain injury (GCS 9–14)
- Minor injuries with risk of alcohol withdrawal syndrome
- Isolated vascular injuries to the extremities

*Patients >65 years of age with comorbidity or any hemodynamic instability should be considered for ICU admission.
ICU, intensive care unit; GCS, Glasgow Coma Scale score; TBSA, total body surface area.

d. **Disability.** The Glasgow Coma Scale score is recalculated and compared with initial observations for signs of neurologic deterioration. All limbs are reinspected for deformity, abnormal or absent movement, and signs of vascular insufficiency. The level of sedation is assessed, and short-acting sedatives are given, if necessary, to protect the patient from self-harm.

e. **Environmental.** Core body temperature is obtained and hypothermia is treated or prevented.

2. **Repetition of the secondary survey.** The secondary survey is repeated. Laboratory and radiologic data obtained thus far are reviewed to identify missed injuries, particularly of the spinal column or spinal cord, bony or ligamentous injuries of the extremities, as well as possible injuries to the thoracic aorta, heart, or diaphragm. Abdominal compartment syndrome is possible from fluid resuscitation or abdominal packing, and may be confirmed by bladder pressure measurement in the appropriate clinical context.

B. **Intermediate phase (24–72 h).** From 24 to 72 hours postinjury, all injuries should be identified, but resuscitation may be ongoing. Management of respiratory failure and intracranial pressure following TBI may be particularly active during the first 72 hours.

C. **Late phase (>72 h).** Approximately one half of critically injured patients remain in the ICU for more than 72 hours. For these patients, the priorities are defined by injury severity, the prevention of complications, and management of complications that do arise. Patients who have improved may be weaned from mechanical ventilation and other forms of life support. Whereas continued ICU care defines a patient population needing multiple operations or prolonged life support, prolonged ICU care carries risks of hospital-acquired infection (Chapter 57), pressure ulcers, and organ dysfunction.

D. **Recovery phase.** In this phase (regardless of timing), patients are separated from life support and prepared for the transition to lower levels of care and eventual hospital discharge. At this time, disabilities may become apparent, and physical therapy, assessment of long-term rehabilitation needs and potential, and psychological support of patient and family are crucial. Approximately 4% of injured patients remain in the ICU for more than 28 days, but the chance of survival to hospital discharge is still >50%.

IV. **RESUSCITATION AND INITIAL MANAGEMENT.** To maximize chances for survival, treatment priorities must focus on resuscitation from shock (defined as inadequate tissue oxygenation to meet tissue O_2 requirements), including appropriate fluid resuscitation and rapid hemostasis. Inadequate oxygenation results in anaerobic metabolism and tissue acidosis. The depth and duration of shock leads to a cumulative oxygen debt. The traditional markers of "successful" resuscitation, including restoration of normal blood pressure, heart rate, and urine output, remain standard. However, occult ongoing hypoperfusion and tissue acidosis (i.e., compensated shock) often persists in the setting of normalization of vital signs. This unrecognized tissue hypoperfusion may lead to organ dysfunction and death.

A. **Endpoints of resuscitation.** When the traditional parameters remain abnormal (i.e., uncompensated shock), the need for additional resuscitation is clear. However, even after normalization of these parameters, up to 85% of severely injured patients have evidence of hypoperfusion, whether metabolic acidosis, a persistent base deficit, or an elevated blood lactate concentration. Recognition and rapid reversal of this state are crucial to minimize the risk of organ dysfunction or death. Resuscitation is complete when the oxygen debt has been repaid, and normal tissue pH and aerobic metabolism are restored in all tissue beds. Evidence-based guidelines for determining endpoints of resuscitation are provided in Table 37-2.

B. **Hemostasis in resuscitation.** Resuscitation from hemorrhagic shock is impossible without hemostasis. Fluid resuscitation strategies prior to obtaining hemostasis in patients with uncontrolled shock are controversial. Withholding of fluid resuscitation may lead to exsanguination, whereas aggressive fluid resuscitation may raise blood pressure excessively or dilute clotting factors, leading to increased bleeding. Limited, hypotensive, and/or delayed fluid resuscitation may be beneficial, but clinical trials have yielded conflicting results.

C. **Classification of shock** (Chapter 5)
1. **Hypovolemic shock.** Hypovolemia is the usual cause of hypotension or occult hypoperfusion in the early postinjury period, and may be caused by incomplete resuscitation, ongoing third-space fluid losses, or active hemorrhage. Cessation of hemorrhage must be the primary goal in patients who are bleeding. Volume replacement is titrated to accepted endpoints in hypovolemic patients. Failure to respond to volume replacement should stimulate search for ongoing hemorrhage (the most likely cause) or other causes of shock.
2. **Obstructive shock** is a possible cause (e.g., cardiac tamponade, tension pneumothorax, abdominal compartment syndrome [increased abdominal pressure from packing or overresuscitation leading to decreased venous return], ventilation with high levels of positive end-expiratory pressure [PEEP], or rarely tension pneumopericardium) that should be sought in the appropriate clinical context.
   a. Although cardiac chamber rupture producing tamponade is generally promptly lethal, the rare patient with chamber injury will survive to the trauma bay.

TABLE 37-2	Guidelines for Endpoints of Resuscitation by the Eastern Association for the Surgery of Trauma

A. Recommendations Regarding Stratification of Physiologic Derangement

Level 1

1. Standard hemodynamic parameters do not quantify adequately the degree of physiologic derangement in trauma patients. The initial base deficit or lactate concentration can be used to stratify patients with regard to the need for ongoing fluid resuscitation, including red blood cell concentrates and other blood products, and the risks of organ dysfunction and death.
2. The ability of a patient to attain supranormal O_2 delivery parameters correlates with an improved chance for survival.

Level 2

1. The time to normalization of base deficit and lactate concentration is predictive of survival.
2. Persistently high or worsening base deficit may be an early indicator of complications (e.g., ongoing hemorrhage, abdominal compartment syndrome).
3. The predictive value of the base deficit may be limited by ethanol intoxication or a hyper-chloremic metabolic acidosis, as well as administration of sodium bicarbonate.

Level 3

1. Right ventricular end diastolic volume index (RVEDVI) measurement may be a better indicator of adequate volume resuscitation (preload) than central venous pressure or pulmonary artery occlusion pressure (PAOP).
2. Measurements of tissue (subcutaneous or muscle) O_2 or CO_2 concentration may identify patients who require additional resuscitation and are at risk for organ dysfunction and death.
3. Serum bicarbonate concentration may be substituted for base deficit.

B. Recommendations Regarding Improved Patient Outcomes

Level 1

There are insufficient data to formulate a Level 1 recommendation.

Level 2

1. The optimal algorithms for fluid resuscitation, blood product replacement, and the use of inotropes and/or vasopressors have not been determined.

(From Tisherman SA, Barie P, Bokhari F, et al. Clinical practice guideline: Endpoints of resuscitation. *J Trauma* 2004;57:898–912.)

The diagnosis must be considered in the patient who fails to respond to seemingly adequate fluid resuscitation

3. **Cardiogenic shock.** Cardiogenic shock after trauma is usually caused by blunt myocardial injury, but the possibility of myocardial ischemia/infarction must be considered in elderly trauma patients. Blunt myocardial injury is excluded by an entirely normal electrocardiogram (ECG); with a normal ECG, cardiac enzyme determination is superfluous. Right ventricular function can be impaired by blunt myocardial injury, and is sensitive to volume repletion, followed by inotropic support if cardiac output is still inadequate. Valvular injury is uncommon in patients surviving severe chest trauma, but may require immediate surgical repair. Underlying valvular heart disease (e.g., aortic stenosis, mitral insufficiency) should be suspected in older trauma patients with cardiogenic shock.

4. **Neurogenic shock.** Neurogenic shock can occur with spinal cord injury (or rarely with brain death). Affected spinal cord injury patients are usually paraplegic or quadriplegic. Autonomic dysfunction (loss of sympathetic tone) leads to vasodilation, which is a form of distributive shock (defined in the next paragraph). Once euvolemia is ensured with volume replacement, the treatment is primarily with a vasoconstrictor (e.g., phenylephrine). Hemodynamic instability may be prolonged, and vasopressor therapy may be required for days to weeks.

5. **Vasogenic shock.** Vasogenic shock (distributive shock) is caused prototypically by severe sepsis and does not occur immediately after injury. However,

severely injured trauma patients can demonstrate an early hyperdynamic state, similar to systemic inflammatory response syndrome (SIRS), which is caused presumably by trauma-induced release of vasoactive mediators. A hyperdynamic circulation (cardiac index >3 L/minute/m^2), hypotension, and low systemic vascular resistance (<900 dyne/second/cm^{-5}) are characteristic. Occult blunt cardiac injury must be considered in the differential diagnosis.

V. MONITORING AND DATA INTERPRETATION. In the setting of normal blood pressure and heart rate, occult hypoperfusion may occur. Lactic acidemia or persistent acidosis indicate ongoing tissue hypoperfusion. Additional monitoring is necessary to optimize oxygen delivery to tissues when clinical uncertainty exists, or when refractory hemodynamic instability or other factors confound the clinical assessment of the response to therapy. **Remember that such instability is most commonly due to ongoing blood loss.**

  A. Blood testing. Collection of blood is essential for monitoring, but can be excessive. Blood removed for testing can easily exceed 70 mL/day. Because of the ease of sampling, an indwelling arterial catheter increases blood testing by up to one third. Blood is wasted each time blood is sampled via a catheter, and the risk of infection is increased both by catheter manipulation and the need to transfuse blood to treat iatrogenic anemia.

  1. Noninvasive hemodynamic monitoring, adoption of guidelines for diagnostic evaluation, and point-of-care (POC) testing can reduce blood testing while providing optimal patient care. Blood testing of critically ill surgical patients can be reduced by at least 50% without affecting patient care adversely. POC testing of blood at or near the bedside is accurate and advantageous.

  2. Glucose monitoring is the most prevalent example of POC testing, considering that "tight" glucose control reduces the risk of nosocomial infection, organ dysfunction, and death from critical illness. The value of POC testing of hemoglobin and blood gases have also been demonstrated in trauma resuscitation.

  B. Blood gas monitoring. Blood gas analyzers measure directly the partial pressures of oxygen (pO_2) and carbon dioxide (pCO_2), and blood pH. Arterial oxyhemoglobin saturation is calculated from the pO_2, assuming a normal P_{50} (SaO_2 is 50% at a pO_2 of 27 mmHg), and normal hemoglobin structure. Some analyzers incorporate cooximetry to measure hemoglobin concentration directly. Bicarbonate and base excess are calculated from the pH and pCO_2.

  1. A fresh, heparinized, bubble-free arterial blood sample is required. Heparin is acidic; if present to excess, pCO_2 and bicarbonate are reduced spuriously. Delay in measurement allows continued erythrocyte metabolism, reducing pH and pO_2 and increasing pCO_2. Icing the specimen allows an accurate assay for up to 1 hour. Air bubbles decrease pCO_2 and increase pO_2.

  C. Electrocardiography. Electrocardiography is standard; it is important for detection of tachycardia, which causes serious morbidity, especially in older patients. Tachycardia may be due to hypovolemia, hemorrhage, inadequate analgesia, or other causes. Tachycardia is inherently dangerous because of the risk of myocardial ischemia. However, routine ECG monitoring with four limb leads is insensitive for detection of acute ST or T wave changes, which may portend ischemia. A 12-lead ECG should be performed on patients suspected of myocardial ischemia, electrolyte abnormalities, blunt cardiac injury, or pericardial pathology. Continuous ECG monitoring is invaluable in ensuring heart rate control in patients at risk for myocardial ischemia.

  1. Perioperative mortality is decreased when beta-adrenergic blockade is started preoperatively before major elective general surgery, and recent data suggest the same to be true for elderly trauma patients. Even if beta-blockade cannot be started before an emergency operation (e.g., uncorrected hypovolemia), it should be started as soon as possible thereafter, provided underlying hypovolemia, pain, and sepsis are controlled.

  D. Pulse oximetry. Pulse oximetry can detect slight decreases in SaO_2 with a 60-second delay, by estimating the difference in signal intensity between oxygenated and deoxygenated blood from red (660 nanometer [nm]) and near-infrared (940 nm) light. Pulse oximetry is generally accurate ($\pm 2\%$) over the range of SaO_2 70% to 100%, but less accurate below 70%. Pulsatile blood flow is essential for accurate pulse oximetry; reliable data can be obtained from the finger, earlobe, or forehead.

1. Hypothermia, hypotension, hypovolemia, peripheral vascular disease, vasopressor therapy, ambient light, and motion artifact may cause inaccuracy.

2. An elevated carboxyhemoglobin concentration will elevate S_aO_2 falsely because reflected light is absorbed at the same wavelength as oxyhemoglobin.

E. **Temperature.** The most reliable temperature measurement is core temperature obtained by transoral esophageal probe, tympanic probe, or pulmonary artery catheter (PAC) thermistor. Hypothermia may contribute to metabolic acidosis, vasoconstriction, myocardial dysfunction, arrhythmia, electrolyte imbalances, altered pharmacokinetics and drug metabolism, platelet dysfunction, and an increased risk of surgical site infection. Hypothermia may develop from exposure in the field, from disease (e.g., sepsis, hypothalamic injury), or under anesthesia. Anesthesia-related hypothermia may be due to exposure, evaporative water loss, abolition of cutaneous vasoconstriction, or rapid infusion of ambient-temperature fluid or cold blood. Induced hypothermia is an adjunct to several heart, brain, and spinal procedures and after cardiac arrest, but is not beneficial after TBI.

1. **Fever.** Fever (temperature exceeding the hypothalamic "set point") or hyperthermia (a reset hypothalamic set point) will increase heart rate, oxygen consumption, and insensible fluid loss. Postoperative fever causes consternation, but is not invariably ominous. Fever has salutary effects on host defenses, and in nonneurologic patients should not be suppressed unless the patient has symptomatic myocardial ischemia or other serious manifestations.

   a. One half of episodes of postoperative fever are of noninfectious origin (Table 37-3); in the first 48 hours after surgery, the only consequential infectious causes of fever (other than an infection that prompted surgical intervention for source control) are surgical site infections caused by streptococci or clostridial organisms.

   b. Other than the physical examination, a laboratory evaluation of fever is not cost-effective until after the third postoperative day. Thereafter, the differential diagnosis of postoperative fever is extensive (Tables 37-3 and 37-4), and a specific cause should be sought.

2. **Hypothermia.** Hypothermia should be anticipated in injured patients who have suffered exposure or shock, had massive volume resuscitation, or prolonged surgery (Chapter 41). Patients who undergo damage control operations are by

TABLE 37-3   **Noninfectious Causes of Fever in the ICU**

Acute respiratory distress syndrome (ARDS)
Adrenal insufficiency
Atelectasis
Blood transfusion
Cardiac arrest
Ischemia
Hemorrhage/hematoma-parenchymal
    Brain
    Lung
    Retroperitoneum
    Soft tissue
    Solid organ (liver, spleen)
Multiple trauma
Venous thromboembolic disease

TABLE 37-4	Infectious Causes of Fever in the ICU

Bloodstream infection
    Bacteremia
    Catheter-related bloodstream infection
    Fungemia
Peritonitis/intraabdominal abscess
    Anastomotic or suture line dehiscence
    Abscess of solid organ (e.g., liver, spleen)
    Biliary tract
        Acalculous cholecystitis
        Cholangitis
Pneumonia
    Empyema
Retroperitoneum
    Iliopsoas abscess
    Pancreatic necrosis
Sinusitis
Skin/soft tissue
    Hematoma
    Suppurative phlebitis
    Surgical site infection
    Traumatic wound infection
Urinary tract
    Cystitis
    Perinephric abscess
    Pyelonephritis

definition hypothermic and coagulopathic. These patients are admitted to the ICU from a truncated operative procedure for secondary resuscitation, normalization of body temperature, and correction of coagulopathy. Return to the operating room (OR) for definitive repair of major injuries usually occurs at 24 to 48 hours. The crucial temperature of injured patients that influences mortality profoundly appears to be approximately 32°C, but substantial cardiac and hematologic morbidity is possible whenever the core body temperature is <35°C.

  a. Hypothermia is classified as mild (32°C to 35°C), moderate (28°C to 32°C), or severe (<28°C). The major complications of hypothermia are platelet dysfunction (decreased adhesion due to decreased thromboxane synthesis), impaired cardiac function (increased afterload due to systemic vasoconstriction), and dysrhythmias (altered myocardial sensitivity to endogenous catecholamines). Clotting factor function, which is temperature dependent, may also be reduced under hypothermic conditions.

  b. Methods used for rewarming (Chapter 41) depend on the severity of hypothermia, ongoing hemorrhage and coagulopathy, hemodynamic stability, and availability of equipment and technical support. Heightened awareness of possible core temperature loss should lead to preventive measures. It is easier to keep a patient warm than to rewarm a patient, as most methods are inefficient at transferring heat.

    i. Warmed resuscitation fluids and blood products are standard, as is topical warming with blankets or forced-air recirculating blankets. Active core rewarming may be achieved by several methods, most of which are invasive, including airway warming (warmed respiratory gases) peritoneal (via peritoneal lavage or dialysis catheter) or pleural lavage (via thoracostomy tube), continuous arteriovenous or venovenous rewarming, or partial cardiopulmonary bypass (Chapter 41).

F. Capnography. Capnography measures continuously the CO_2 concentration in expired gas, most reliably in ventilated patients. The peak CO_2 concentration occurs at end-exhalation [end-tidal CO_2 ($ETCO_2$)], at which time $ETCO_2$ approximates closely the alveolar gas concentration. Sidestream gas sampling is most common, but susceptible to accumulation of water vapor in the sampling line. In the ICU, humidified respiratory gases make mainstream (inline) sampling preferable.

  1. Capnography can confirm successful airway intubation and monitor resuscitation and weaning from mechanical ventilation. Use during ventilator weaning can diminish the need for blood gas analysis. Used with pulse oximetry, many patients can be weaned from mechanical ventilation without reliance on arterial blood gases or invasive hemodynamic monitoring.

  2. Capnography can provide other valuable information. Prognostically, an $ETCO_2$–$PaCO_2$ gradient ≥ 13 mmHg after resuscitation is associated with increased trauma-related mortality. Gradually decreasing $ETCO_2$ is associated with hypovolemia, whereas a sudden decrease or even disappearance of $ETCO_2$ is observed with a low cardiac output state, disconnection from the ventilator, or pulmonary thromboembolism (Table 37-5). A gradual increase of $ETCO_2$ occurs with hypoventilation; the converse is also true.

G. Near-infrared spectroscopy. Near-infrared spectroscopy (NIRS) is a noninvasive method to measure tissue oxygen tension in close to real time. Near-infrared light of four calibrated wavelengths (680 nm, 720 nm, 760 nm, and 800 nm) penetrates

---

TABLE 37-5   Changes in End-tidal CO_2 ($ETCO_2$)

Increased $ETCO_2$
Decreased alveolar ventilation
   Reduced respiratory rate
   Reduced tidal volume
   Increased equipment dead space
Increased CO_2 production
   Fever
   Hypercatabolism
   Excess carbohydrate intake
Increased inspired CO_2 concentration
   CO_2 absorber exhausted
   Increased CO_2 in inspired gas
   Rebreathing of expired gas

Decreased $ETCO_2$
Increased alveolar ventilation
   Increased respiratory rate
   Increased tidal volume
Decreased CO_2 production
   Hypothermia
   Hypocatabolic state
Increased alveolar dead space
   Decreased cardiac output
   Pulmonary embolism (clot, air, fat)
   High positive end-expiratory pressure (PEEP)
Sampling error
   Air in sample line (no or diminished signal)
   Water in sample line (no or diminished signal)
   Inadequate tidal volume (no or diminished signal)
   Disconnection of monitor from tubing (no signal)
   Airway not in trachea (e.g., esophageal intubation) (no signal)

tissue to a depth of approximately 15 mm below the sensor, which usually is placed on the thenar eminence. These wavelengths of light scatter in tissue and are absorbed differently. Light that is not absorbed is reflected back as an optical signal to the detector. Analysis of the reflected light is by conversion to a scaled 720-nm second derivative attenuation value, which produces an absolute measurement of tissue oxygenation (StO_2) in the skeletal muscle microcirculation. Skeletal muscle StO_2 correlates with $\dot{D}O_2I$, base deficit, and serum lactate concentration in experimental and clinical hemorrhagic shock. Detection is possible over a StO_2 range of 1% to 99%, but is most accurate for StO_2 >70%.

1. In a recent multicenter trial of 383 patients with major trauma who required blood transfusion, 50 of whom eventually developed MODS, NIRS monitoring was begun within 30 minutes of arrival in the emergency department (ED), and continued for 24 hours. A StO_2 >75% maintained during the first hour of monitoring indicated adequate tissue perfusion, with affected patients having an 88% MODS-free rate of survival. In contrast, StO_2 <75% in the first hour was manifested by 78% of patients who eventually developed MODS, and 91% of those who died. The results for minimum StO_2 within the first hour of arrival to the ED were comparable to the maximum base deficit collected within the first hour for both the MODS and mortality outcomes.

H. Noninvasive cardiac output determination

1. **Thoracic bioimpedance.** Thoracic bioimpedance derives information from electrodes placed on the anterior chest and neck to estimate Q (flow) by determining the left ventricular systolic time interval from time $1/\bar{\mu}$ derivative bioimpedance signals. The lag time for the system to provide data is approximately 2 to 5 minutes from initial lead placement and activation. The main drawback of thoracic bioimpedance is sensitivity to any alteration of the electrode contact or positioning on the patient.

2. **Esophageal Doppler monitor.** The esophageal Doppler monitor (EDM) device is a soft, 6-mm catheter that is placed noninvasively into the esophagus. A flow probe at the tip allows continuous monitoring of Q and stroke volume. A 4-MHz continuous wave ultrasound frequency is reflected to produce a waveform, representing the change in blood flow in the descending aorta (about 80% of Q) with each pulsation. An EDM may yield more accurate hemodynamic data than a PAC in patients with cardiac valvular lesions, septal defects, arrhythmias, or pulmonary hypertension. The primary disadvantage of the EDM is that the waveform may be lost with only a slight positional change and render damped, inaccurate readings.

VI. INVASIVE MONITORING

A. **Arterial catheterization.** Arterial blood pressure measurement is the simplest, most reproducible hemodynamic monitor. Although automated blood pressure cuffs are in common use in ORs and are suitable for periodic blood pressure measurement in stable patients (error, $\pm2\%$), low or fluctuating blood pressure may mandate continuous monitoring via an indwelling arterial catheter. Invasive blood pressure monitoring is indicated for prolonged operations (>4 hours), prolonged mechanical ventilation (>24–48 hours), unstable hemodynamics (e.g., shock), vasopressor therapy, substantial blood loss, frequent monitoring of blood samples, or when precise blood pressure control is needed (e.g., brain-injured patients with low cerebral perfusion pressure).

1. **Insertion technique.** Special-purpose thin-walled catheters are used to maintain fidelity of the waveform and minimize luminal obstruction. The radial artery at the wrist is the most common site; the ulnar artery is larger, but relatively inaccessible percutaneously. Patency of the collateral circulation to the hand should be confirmed before cannulation at the wrist to minimize the possibility of catastrophic tissue loss. Alternative sites are many. In neonates, the umbilical artery may be catheterized; intestinal ischemia is a rare complication. The axillary artery is relatively free of plaque, well collateralized at the shoulder, and easy to cannulate percutaneously. A risk with the axillary

arterial line is cerebral embolization when flushing the line. The superficial femoral artery is usable, but not preferred because of higher risks of distal embolization and infection. The dorsalis pedis artery is accessible, but should be avoided with peripheral vascular disease, hemodynamic instability, or lower extremity trauma. The brachial artery should be strictly avoided because collateral circulation at the elbow is poor; the risk of hand or forearm ischemia is high.

2. Peripheral vasoconstriction during vasopressor therapy may dampen the arterial waveform. A longer catheter placed at a more central location (e.g., axillary, femoral) may restore the fidelity of the tracing. Nosocomial infection of arterial catheters is unusual, provided basic tenets of infection control are honored and femoral artery catheterization is avoided.

B. Central venous pressure monitoring. The central venous pressure (CVP) is a function of circulating blood volume, venous tone, and right ventricular function. The CVP measures right ventricular filling pressure as an estimate of intravascular volume status. Strict adherence to asepsis, full barrier precautions, and adherence to the principles of infection control are crucial to avoid the potentially life-threatening complication of catheter-related bloodstream infection.

1. **Insertion technique.** Central venous access can be obtained using the basilic, femoral, external jugular, internal jugular, or subclavian veins.

    a. In the ICU, the internal jugular site is most popular because of ease of accessibility, a high success rate of cannulation, and relatively few complications.

    b. The subclavian site is the most technically demanding, having the highest rate of pneumothorax (1.5%–3.0%), but the lowest infection rate.

    c. The femoral vein site is least preferred in the ICU because of the highest complication rate, despite the relative ease of catheter placement. The risks of arterial puncture (9%–15%), infection, and venous thromboembolism are highest for femoral vein catheterization.

    d. Overall complications are comparable for internal jugular and subclavian vein cannulation (6%–12%), and much higher for femoral vein cannulation (13%–19%).

2. The operator dons cap, mask, eye protection, and a sterile gown and gloves before preparing the patient's skin (2% chlorhexidine gluconate is associated with fewer infections than 10% povidine-iodine) and draping the patient completely with a full-bed drape. After infiltration of a local anesthetic, a finder needle accesses the vein using the Seldinger technique. Once the tip is intraluminal and blood is aspirated freely, a flexible guidewire is introduced and the catheter is placed over the wire into the vein.

C. Pulmonary artery catheterization. Data from PACs are used mainly to determine Q (flow) and preload, which is most commonly estimated by the pulmonary artery occlusion pressure (PAOP). Other parameters calculated from Q include systemic and pulmonary vascular resistance (SVR, PVR) and right and left ventricular stroke work (RVSW, LVSW).

1. **Insertion technique.** The subclavian or internal jugular vein is accessed as for insertion of a CVP catheter, but instead of the catheter, an introducer sheath is placed through which the PAC is inserted with the balloon deflated. Once the catheter tip reaches the superior vena cava (~20 cm), partial inflation of the balloon (~0.5 mL) permits the catheter to advance with the flowing column of blood. The position of the catheter tip is usually determined by pressure monitoring. Entry into the right ventricle is indicated by a sudden increase in systolic pressure to at least 30 mmHg, whereas the diastolic pressure remains unchanged from right atrial pressure (0–5 mmHg). Catheter entry into the pulmonary artery is associated with constant systolic pressure, but diastolic pressure increases above right ventricular end-diastolic pressure or CVP. Catheter advancement with periodic inflation of the catheter "wedges" the balloon, occluding flow usually in a lobar pulmonary artery. Chest x-ray confirms proper placement and evaluates complications such as catheter malposition or pneumothorax. As a general rule, if the catheter tip

extends beyond the hilum, it must be withdrawn partially and repositioned to minimize the risk of usually fatal pulmonary artery rupture.

2. **Data interpretation.** Normally, PAOP (wedge pressure) approximates left atrial pressure, which in turn approximates left ventricular end-diastolic pressure (LVEDP), in theory, a reflection of left ventricular end-diastolic volume (LVEDV). The LVEDV represents preload, which is the actual target parameter.

    a. **Many factors cause PAOP to reflect LVEDV inaccurately,** including mitral stenosis, high levels of PEEP (>10 cm H_2O), and changes in left ventricular compliance (e.g., myocardial infarction, pericardial effusion, or increased afterload). Inaccurate readings may result from balloon overinflation, catheter malposition, alveolar pressure exceeding pulmonary venous pressure (PEEP ventilation), or pulmonary hypertension (which may make PAOP measurement difficult or, indeed, hazardous). Elevated PAOP occurs in left-sided heart failure. Decreased PAOP occurs with hypovolemia or decreased preload.

    b. Mixed venous oxygen saturation ($S_{mv}O_2$) may be measured, although superior vena cava S_vO_2 via a CVP catheter may provide data of comparable utility. Causes of low $S_{mv}O_2$ include anemia, pulmonary disease, carboxyhemoglobinemia, low Q, and increased tissue oxygen demand. The $S_aO_2:(S_aO_2$ minus $S_{mv}O_2)$ ratio determines the adequacy of O_2 delivery (DO_2). Ideally, the $P_{mv}O_2$ should be 35 to 40 mmHg, with a $S_{mv}O_2$ of about 70%. Values of $P_{mv}O_2$ <30 mmHg are critically low.

3. **Clinical use**

    a. Evidence is lacking that PAC use decreases morbidity or mortality. Some retrospective data even suggest that PAC use is associated with excess mortality. Monitoring by a less invasive method such as CVP monitoring or even by physical examination and clinical judgment may be equally useful in determining volume status. Data derived from the PAC can be difficult to interpret, and misinterpretation may have deleterious consequences.

    b. Ventilation of patients with acute respiratory distress syndrome (ARDS) on high levels of PEEP has been monitored commonly via PAC. The application of PEEP can decrease venous return markedly, and therefore Q, in a short time period; maintenance of Q is important to maintain ventilation-perfusion (V/Q) matching. However, the ARDSnet investigators demonstrated no difference in outcome of patients with acute lung injury (ALI)/ARDS when managed by PAC or CVP. Pulmonary artery catheters may still be useful in selected circumstances, such as cardiomyopathy, shock of various etiologies, oliguric acute renal failure, or an unpredicted poor response to fluid therapy. Critically ill patients who require inotropic agents despite large-volume fluid resuscitation may also benefit from monitoring by PAC.

4. **Complications.** Complications common to PACs include infection (2%–5%), hemo- or pneumothorax (2%–5%), migration (5%–10%), arrhythmia (10%–15%), and hemorrhage (0.2%). Less frequent complications include catheter knotting, pulmonary infarction, cardiac or pulmonary artery perforation, valvular injury, and endocarditis. A devastating complication is pulmonary artery rupture, which occurs in fewer than 0.1% of cases, during insertion or during routine determination of PAOP, and is usually fatal. Distal migration of the PAC within the pulmonary artery increases the risk dramatically of pulmonary artery rupture, and argues for routine daily bedside chest radiography for all patients with an indwelling PAC.

D. **Intracranial pressure monitoring.** Monitoring of intracranial pressure (ICP) is standard for monitoring patients with severe TBI (GCS <8). In TBI, these devices facilitate "optimized" cerebral perfusion pressure (CPP) (mean arterial pressure minus ICP) above 60 mmHg, although no class I data in human beings show an outcome benefit for ICP monitoring in patients with TBI.

1. Perhaps the most useful ICP monitor is the intraventricular or "ventriculostomy" catheter, because the catheter can also drain cerebrospinal fluid and thereby

decrease elevated ICP. However, ventriculostomy is the most invasive method of ICP monitoring, and poses the highest infection risk (~8%). Occasionally, the catheter may be impossible to place or may become occluded due to severe brain edema or extruding brain matter; an intraparenchymal monitor or the epidural "bolt" are alternatives. Despite the high risk of infection with ventriculostomy, neither prolonged antibiotic prophylaxis or regular replacement of the catheter at 5- to 7-day intervals serves to reduce the risk.

VII. MISSED INJURIES

A. However diligent the assessment in the ED, it is inevitable that some injuries will not be identified until the patient is in the ICU. An altered sensorium and the inability to make a complaint referable to the injury is a common reason, as is prior exigency of managing another life-threatening injury. Extremity fractures and dislocations are the most commonly missed injuries. The most serious missed injuries involve the spinal column, major cardiovascular structures, or aerodigestive hollow viscus.

B. Missed injuries are discussed in detail in Chapter 38. Many such injuries are discovered by vigilance in the ICU, at a time when stabilization and treatment can still result in a good outcome. For patients with multiple severe injuries, repetition of the secondary survey upon ICU admission may be a prudent and relatively high-yield strategy.

VIII. PROPHYLAXIS

A. Cardiovascular. Beta-adrenergic blockade, begun preoperatively and continued for approximately 7 days thereafter, reduces the risk of perioperative myocardial infarction and death among elderly patients undergoing major noncardiac surgery. Whether similar benefits may accrue to trauma patients is under active study. Trauma patients differ in that injury cannot be anticipated, therefore prophylaxis can be begun only after injury. Moreover, tachycardia is an important vital sign in the evaluation of the injured patient, particularly with respect to the presence of hypovolemia or pain, and may decrease cerebral perfusion pressure. Blunting the heart rate response could be deleterious if recognition of such underlying conditions is impaired. Preliminary reports of two retrospective studies of the administration of beta-blockers to patients with severe traumatic brain injury suggest that mortality from injury may be reduced by 50% to 70%. Additionally, beta-blockade has been shown to decrease catabolism in children with burns.

B. Stress-related gastric mucosal hemorrhage

1. Ischemia reperfusion injury of the stomach is associated with disruption of the mucosal blanket, back-diffusion of hydrogen ions, reduced buffering capacity, and ultimately gastric mucosal injury. Injury to the gastric mucosa may be exacerbated by lack of the trophic stimulus associated with enteral feeding. Mucosal injury has many manifestations, ranging from asymptomatic to overt upper gastrointestinal hemorrhage. The incidence has been reduced markedly by chemoprophylaxis and early nutritional support, and is now estimated to be approximately 4% in general critically ill patients. Patients at highest risk are those who receive mechanical ventilation for more than 24 hours, or who are coagulopathic. Trauma patients believed to be at increased risk include those with traumatic brain injury or burns.

2. Effective prophylaxis reduces the risk of hemorrhage by about one half. Agents in use for prophylaxis include H_2-histamine receptor antagonists, sucralfate, and increasingly, proton-pump inhibitors. Antacids are no longer recommended due to cumbersome administration and increased risk of pulmonary aspiration. Histamine receptor antagonists appear to have a lower incidence of overt bleeding (but not occult bleeding) than sucralfate. There are no class I data to support the use of proton-pump inhibitors for prophylaxis, despite widespread use.

a. Previously there was concern that acid-reduction strategies (e.g., histamine receptor antagonists) increased the risk of ventilator-associated pneumonia compared with the barrier protection strategy (i.e., sucralfate). Accumulated evidence indicates that this concern is unfounded, therefore the gastric cytoprotective strategy that is employed should be the one that is most effective for prevention of bleeding, however defined.

C. Prophylaxis of venous thromboembolism (VTE). The association between trauma and thromboembolism is well recognized. However, recent evidence suggests that the actual incidence if far lower than estimated historically, perhaps reflecting the aggressive and successful use of prophylaxis for VTE. Risk factors for VTE have recently been quantified from data on more than 450,000 patients in the National Trauma Data Bank (Table 37-6). Older age, major (Abbreviated Injury Score $\geq$3) lower extremity fracture or traumatic brain injury, and major operative procedures are all independent risk factors for VTE. However, the most powerful predictors of VTE are prolonged mechanical ventilation (>3 days) and major venous injury (Table 37-6). The association between VTE and prolonged ventilation (odds ratio >8) is striking and undoubtedly reflects prolonged bed rest, severity of injury, and a host of other factors. However, the strength of this association highlights the inclusion of VTE prophylaxis in the ventilator bundle (Section VIII.E) for prevention of complications in mechanically ventilated patients. Specific strategies for prevention, diagnosis, and therapy of VTE can be found elsewhere in this volume.

D. Metabolic prevention. Prevention of metabolic/nutritional complications is multifactorial, including glycemic control, early identification of adrenal insufficiency, and early nutritional support, preferably by the enteral route. These ostensible disparate aspects are linked through the hypophyseal-pituitary-adrenal (HPA) axis and other hormonal/metabolic pathways. For example, tight glycemic control by continuous infusion of insulin has been linked to a reduced incidence of surgical site infections and other nosocomial infections and also to reduced organ dysfunction and mortality in the ICU. However, both glucocorticoid therapy and nutritional support (especially via the parenteral route) can make glycemic control more difficult. Likewise, early enteral nutrition (e.g., within 36 hours after injury) has been estimated to reduce the incidence of infection by more than 50%.

TABLE 37-6	Risk Factor for Venous Thromboembolism after Trauma: Analysis of 1,602 Episodes for the National Trauma Data Bank	
Parameter	**Odds ratio**	**95% confidence interval**
Univariate Analysis		
Age >39 y	2.29	2.07–2.55
Pelvis fracture	2.93	2.01–4.27
Lower extremity fracture	3.16	2.85–3.51
Spinal cord injury with paralysis	3.39	2.41–4.77
Traumatic brain injury	2.59	2.31–2.90
Mechanical ventilation >3 d	10.62	9.32–12.11
Injury to major vein	7.93	5.83–10.78
Blood pressure <90 mmHg on admission	1.95	1.62–2.34
Major surgical procedure	4.32	3.91–4.77
Multivariate Analysis		
Age >39 y	2.01	1.74–2.32
Lower extremity fracture	1.92	1.64–2.26
Traumatic brain injury	1.24	1.05–1.46
Mechanical ventilation >3 d	8.08	6.86–9.52
Injury to major vein	3.56	2.22–5.72
Major surgical procedure	1.53	1.30–1.80

(From Knudson MM, Morabito D, Paiment GD, et al. Use of low molecular weight heparin in preventing thromboembolism in trauma patients. *J Trauma* 1996;41:446–459.)

1. **Glycemic control.** It has been assumed historically that the hyperglycemia associated with surgical stress or infection is obligatory, transitory, and inconsequential. However, class I data indicate that tight glycemic control following cardiac surgery is associated with a decreased incidence of surgical site infection and decreased mortality. An association with decreased infection and higher postoperative blood glucose concentrations has been made for major noncardiac surgery as well.

   a. The landmark trial of tight glucose control for surgical patients, published by Van den Berghe and colleagues in 2001, demonstrated a 40% reduction in mortality if blood glucose concentration was kept between 80 and 110 milligrams per deciliter (mg/dL) by continuous infusion of insulin, compared with 180 to 220 mg/dL. Debate has followed as to whether a more modest reduction of serum glucose concentration (e.g., ~145 mg/dL) would also be beneficial (probably yes).

   b. There has been debate as to whether acute or chronic (i.e., correlation with the hemoglobin A1c concentration) is most important (acute control), whether the same objectives can be obtained with subcutaneous insulin (no), whether diabetic and stressed nondiabetic patients benefit equally (they do), and whether glucose control per se or a putative anticatabolic effect of insulin effect is the mechanism in fact (it is glucose control).

   c. A meta-analysis of more than 30 trials suggests that surgical patients benefit in particular from tight glycemic control, whereas a similar benefit is elusive to demonstrate for critically ill medical patients, with an estimated odds ratio for mortality of 0.58 for the surgical patients. Moreover, diabetic patients and hyperglycemic nondiabetic patients appear to benefit equally, suggesting further that it is the magnitude of acute glucose control that is important. In trauma care, admission hyperglycemia and persistent hyperglycemia are both correlated with higher mortality after injury, and TBI patients may be at especially high risk. However, whether serum glucose concentration needs to be decreased to the same degree as for other critically ill surgical patients remains to be determined.

2. **Adrenal insufficiency.** Adrenal insufficiency can be occult, and can develop under stress in a patient with initially normal HPA-axis responsiveness. Adrenal insufficiency is in the differential diagnosis of fever, hyponatremia, unexplained hypotension, and a host of other ICU-related maladies. However, a host of controversies surround the diagnosis and therapy of adrenal insufficiency. Glucocorticoid therapy may also be indicated for severe sepsis/septic shock, refractory bronchospasm, subglottic airway edema (due usually to traumatic airway intubation), and other considerations. Among the controversies are the incidence of adrenal insufficiency in critical illness, the optimal method of diagnosis (random serum cortisol concentration vs. provocative testing), the dose of the corticotropin analogue cosyntropin to use for provocation (1 μg vs. 250 μg), and whether the presence of adrenal insufficiency is relevant to treatment decisions in severe sepsis/septic shock.

   a. The estimated incidence of adrenal insufficiency in critically ill patients varies widely up to 30% or more, which is a function of the vigor with which the diagnosis is sought, and the criteria used for diagnosis. The simplest diagnostic method is simply to determine a random serum cortisol concentration (diurnal variation is lost in critical illness), but accuracy is limited.

   b. Most authorities recommend provocative testing, comparing the difference between basal and 1-hour-stimulated cortisol concentrations in response to either 1 μg or 250 μg of cosyntropin (the former is probably more sensitive, but the latter dose is administered more widely). Consensus is lacking as to the interpretation of the cosyntropin stimulation test, as well, but a common strategy is that the diagnosis of adrenal insufficiency is confirmed with both basal and stimulated cortisol concentrations <15 μg/L, refuted when both are >35 μg/L, and indeterminate in between unless the stimulated cortisol concentration exceeds the basal concentration by ≥ 9 μg/L.

   c. Glucocorticoid therapy is now recommended as part of the therapy of severe sepsis/septic shock, but not in the massive doses of yesteryear. The dose of hydrocortisone for sepsis is not recommended to exceed 300 mg/day (or equivalent) for 7 days, but whether all patients, or only those found to have adrenal insufficiency by provocative testing, should be treated is a matter of debate.

E. **Ventilator "bundle."** Care of the patient who requires mechanical ventilation (MV) is more than just providing oxygen and a bellows. Such critically ill patients are at risk of numerous complications, not all of which are related directly to ARF or MV. The patient at prolonged bed rest is at risk for deconditioning, venous thromboembolic disease, and pressure ulcers. Sedatives and analgesics may impair the ability to protect the airway, increasing the risk of pulmonary aspiration of gastric contents. Oversedation may be one component of prolonged MV, which is a definite risk factor for development of ventilator-associated pneumonia. Prolonged MV (>48 hours) is itself a risk factor for development of stress-related gastric mucosal hemorrhage, a rare but serious complication (~50% mortality).

   1. Several "best practices" have been combined into a ventilator bundle of four maneuvers to optimize the outcomes of MV. Careful adherence can decrease the risk of prolonged MV.

      a. Keep the head of the patient's bed up at least 30 degrees from level at all times unless contraindicated medically.

      b. Administer prophylaxis against venous thromboembolic disease.

      c. Administer prophylaxis against stress-related gastric mucosal hemorrhage.

      d. Perform a daily "sedation holiday" to assess for readiness to liberate from MV.

IX. ORGAN SYSTEM SUPPORT

A. **Cardiovascular.** Cardiovascular support begins with adequate resuscitation and oxygen delivery, which relates to fluid resuscitation, blood transfusion, ventilatory support, and numerous other interventions. Specifically, cardiovascular support may consist of control of dysrhythmias, management of hypertensive urgencies and emergencies, and cardiopulmonary resuscitation.

   1. **Antiarrhythmic therapy**

      a. **Atrial and supraventricular rhythm disturbances.** The most common such arrhythmia in the trauma setting is atrial fibrillation, which is caused usually not by ischemia but rather by fluid overload (with atrial overdistention) or inflammation adjacent to the pericardium (e.g., pneumonia).

         i. New-onset atrial fibrillation can usually be converted to sinus rhythm once the precipitant can be controlled. Heart rate is controlled first, using a beta-blocker or calcium channel blocker (verapamil is preferred because of its particular effectiveness in slowing conduction through the atrioventricular node). Digoxin is an alternative, but seldom used now. The goal should be a heart rate <100 beats per minute (bpm), ideally <80 bpm if tolerated hemodynamically.

         ii. Many patients will revert to sinus rhythm with rate control only, but if atrial fibrillation persists, sinus rhythm may be restored with an infusion of either procainamide or amiodarone (the former is equally effective and less expensive, but difficult to dose with renal insufficiency). Long-term amiodarone toxicity (e.g., pulmonary, thyroid) is a nonissue with short-term control of dysrhythmias. Once sinus rhythm is restored, long-term therapy is seldom needed.

         iii. Failure to restore sinus rhythm is unusual with new-onset atrial fibrillation, but may require full heparin anticoagulation after 48 hours to reduce the risk of arterial embolism. The goal should be rate control and anticoagulation for paroxysmal or chronic atrial fibrillation, which are unlikely to convert.

iv. The usual causes of supraventricular tachycardia are the same as for atrial fibrillation in the trauma setting, with the addition of pulmonary embolism. The dysrhythmia can usually be terminated with a 5- to 15-mg bolus of verapamil, but repetitive episodes may require a continuous infusion, followed by oral therapy. The underlying cause must be treated.

v. With either atrial fibrillation or supraventricular tachycardia, a rapid ventricular rate (>140 bpm) may compromise diastolic filling to a degree that stroke volume is impaired, and decreased cardiac output may lead to hypotension. Synchronous electrical cardioversion should be considered for hemodynamically unstable atrial fibrillation or supraventricular tachycardia.

b. Ventricular dysrhythmias. Ventricular rhythm disturbances are more complex to diagnose and manage, and generally more dangerous to the patient. Ischemia, hypoxia, electrolyte abnormalities, and drug toxicity (the cause of the prolongation of the QT interval that precipitates the particular type of ventricular tachycardia called **torsades de pointes**). Unifocal ventricular premature contractions (VPCs) generally do not require antiarrhythmic therapy. Multifocal VPCs or couplet beats do, to avoid degeneration to ventricular tachycardia/fibrillation. Most complex ventricular arrhythmias can be suppressed with a bolus dose and infusion of lidocaine, or preferably amiodarone.

c. Hypertensive emergencies

i. The postoperative posttraumatic state is usually a hyperadrenergic, volume-overload state, in which some degree of hypertension is common. Aside from the autonomic hyperactivity and hypervolemia, pain, agitation, and intracranial hypertension are all in the differential diagnosis of hypertension. Fortunately, most episodes of hypertension in this setting are not dangerous, and do not require immediate specific antihypertensive therapy. Unfortunately, many cases of hypertension are overtreated as a consequence of "treating the number." Making a diagnosis of the cause of hypertension is important, as diuresis or analgesia may be the therapy that is really needed. Moreover, treating hypertension associated with intracranial hypertension is contraindicated if maintenance of CPP will be compromised.

ii. With the exception of fresh vascular suture lines, hemorrhage that is temporized by the use of temporary packing, or the aortic injury that is awaiting surgical repair, systolic blood pressure <160 to 180 mmHg may not require therapy to lower blood pressure immediately. In such cases as listed, systolic blood pressure as low as 100 mmHg may be the target. Otherwise, only when organ function is immediately threatened (e.g., hypertensive nephropathy, acute myocardial infarction with active ischemia) should blood pressure be lowered acutely.

iii. Antihypertensive agents that may be used to decrease blood pressure immediately include nitroprusside, labetalol, and nicardipine, all of which are given by a titrated continuous infusion and are relatively easy to titrate. Angiotensin converting enzyme inhibitors (e.g., enalaprilat) are relatively ineffective in states of volume overload, and not recommended for emergency blood pressure control. Although a potent vasodilator, hydralazine is also not recommended, as titration of the dose is difficult.

d. Cardiopulmonary resuscitation. Protocols for the conduct of cardiopulmonary resuscitation have changed recently (Table 37-7). The single rescuer should check the victim's responsiveness to voice and light touch; if no response, help should be summoned. To prepare for cardiopulmonary resuscitation (CPR), the patient should be placed supine on a hard surface. The airway should be opened with the head tilt/chin lift technique unless there is head or neck trauma. If a cervical spine injury is known or suspected (the risk is increased with maxillofacial trauma or a Glasgow

TABLE 37-7	New Developments in Recommendations for Cardiopulmonary Resuscitation (CPR) Relevant to the ICU

1. All breaths, by whatever method, should be given over 1 second with sufficient volume to achieve a visible chest rise.
2. A single, universal compression-to-ventilation ratio of 30:2 is recommended for single rescuers of victims of all ages (except newborn infants). The goal is to provide longer periods of uninterrupted chest compressions.
3. Increased emphasis on the importance of chest compressions: Rescuers should "push hard, push fast" at a rate of 100 compressions/minute, allow complete chest recoil, and minimize interruptions in chest compressions.
4. Provision of about five cycles (about 2 minutes) of CPR between rhythm checks during treatment of pulseless arrest. The rhythm should not be checked immediately after a shock; rather, CPR should be resumed immediately, beginning with chest compressions, after five cycles of CPR.
5. All rescue efforts (e.g., airway intubation, administration of medications, reassessment of the patient) should be performed in a way that minimizes interruption of chest compressions.
6. Only one shock (rather that the traditional three incremental shocks) should be followed immediately by CPR for treatment of ventricular fibrillation or pulseless ventricular tachycardia.

Coma Scale score of <8), a jaw thrust without head extension should be used. However, airway patency and adequate ventilation are a priority in CPR, therefore other steps should be taken, including consideration of the head tilt/chin lift maneuver. Manual spinal motion restriction is safer than immobilization devices in the CPR setting; a cervical collar may complicate airway management during CPR. Breathing is checked and two rescue breaths are given if the patient does not breathe within 10 seconds. If the pulse is restored but the patient remains apneic, one breath is given over 1 second every 5 seconds, and the pulse is rechecked every 2 minutes. If the patient is pulseless, chest compressions and breaths are given at a rate of 100 compressions/minute and a ratio of 30:2. When the defibrillator is ready, the cardiac rhythm is checked for a rhythm likely to respond to shock, which if present is treated with a single shock followed immediately by five additional cycles of CPR.

i. Electrical therapy. Early defibrillation is crucial for survival from sudden cardiac arrest (SCA) because ventricular fibrillation (VF) is the most common rhythm in witnessed CPR. Ventricular fibrillation is treated effectively by defibrillation, but the probability of successful defibrillation decrease rapidly over time, and VF tends to deteriorate to asystole, which does not respond to defibrillation.

a. Modern defibrillators may deliver current in either a monophasic or biphasic waveform, the latter characterizing almost all defibrillators being sold today. However, many monophasic defibrillators remain in use. Neither waveform is consistently associated with a higher success rate for defibrillation, and no direct comparison has been made. However, biphasic defibrillation is equally effective with lower energy discharge. Multiple prospective studies have failed to identify the optimum energy level for the initial or subsequent shocks from biphasic defibrillation. Given that biphasic defibrillators may use one of two waveforms (neither of which has been shown to be superior), the initial energy dose is device-specific (120 joules [J] for a rectilinear biphasic waveform; 150–200 J for a biphasic truncated exponential waveform). Subsequent shocks are at the same or higher dose, regardless of waveform. Likewise, there is no evidence that nonescalating or escalating energy shocks make any difference.

B. Acid-base and electrolyte disturbances. Disturbances in acid-base and electrolyte balance can be anticipated in patients in shock or after massive transfusion. Electrolyte abnormalities may be observed from dilution (e.g., hypomagnesemia, hyponatremia), diuresis (e.g., hypokalemia), therapeutic administration (e.g., hypernatremia), central nervous system injury (e.g., neurogenic diabetes insipidus causing hypernatremia, basilar skull fracture causing the syndrome of inappropriate antidiuretic hormone secretion and hyponatremia), acid-base disorders (acidosis-hyperkalemia, alkalosis-hypokalemia), or acute renal failure (e.g., hyperkalemia).

1. **Acid-base disorders.** Lactic acidosis, which is common and often multifactorial, is caused by shock, hypothermia, limb ischemia, or the metabolic response to trauma. Persistent lactic acidosis requires determination of the cause and consideration of invasive hemodynamic monitoring if impaired oxygen delivery is suspected. Lactic acidosis that fails to normalize within the first 24 hours of ICU admission portends a high risk of death. Most cases of persistent lactic acidosis in trauma are due to failure of resuscitation or ongoing bleeding, and the treatment is control of hemorrhage and ongoing fluid resuscitation with blood transfusions as indicated. Administration of sodium bicarbonate is controversial, but may be considered if the serum bicarbonate concentration is <15 milliequivalent per liter (mEq/L). Other metabolic acid-base disorders may occur acutely, including hyperchloremic metabolic acidosis caused by large-volume resuscitation with sodium chloride.

2. **Electrolyte disorders**

   a. **Hypokalemia.** The most common electrolyte disturbance of the injured patient is hypokalemia. Excessive renal losses of potassium occur as a result of diagnostic and therapeutic use of osmotic diuretics, high doses of glucocorticoids (e.g., methylprednisolone in spinal cord injury), or hyperaldosteronism due to hypovolemia. Alkalosis, high catecholamine concentrations, and hypothermia can also cause intracellular shifting of $K+$. Because transcellular shifts of potassium occur dynamically as acid-base status changes, and because total-body potassium depletion cannot be estimated from the serum potassium concentration, administration of potassium should be judicious and monitored closely.

   b. **Hyperkalemia.** Hyperkalemia may occur in patients with severe metabolic acidosis, large-volume blood transfusion, crush injury of skeletal muscle, rhabdomyolysis, or acute renal failure. Hyperkalemia (>6.0 mEq/L) requires aggressive treatment to prevent cardiac arrest. Coadministered dextrose (50% dextrose in water, 50 mL) and regular insulin (10 U) will cause an intracellular shift of potassium. Acidosis should be corrected by fluid resuscitation, sodium bicarbonate, or renal replacement therapy (RRT). However, only RRT or ion-exchange resin (sodium polystyrene sulfonate, which removes 1 mEq K/g administered by mouth or per rectum) remove potassium permanently from the body.

   c. **Hypocalcemia.** Hypocalcemia occurs frequently in the severely injured patient, and it is usually caused by a reduction in total calcium from dilutional hypoalbuminemia (~60% of total calcium is bound to albumin). Hypocalcemia can occur in patients with severe rhabdomyolysis. Despite the common occurrence of hypocalcemia, it is only clinically important when the physiologically active, ionized fraction (40%) is reduced. Clinical manifestations of true (ionized) hypocalcemia are generally not evident until ionized calcium concentration is <0.7 millimole per liter (mmol/L) (normal = 1.0−1.25 mmol/L) and include hypotension, impaired ventricular function, bradycardia, bronchospasm, laryngospasm, and impaired response to catecholamines. Ionized hypocalcemia may be caused by acute respiratory alkalosis. Hypocalcemia should be treated empirically with an IV calcium salt (calcium gluconate is preferred) if the ionized calcium concentration is low (<0.7 mmol/L) or when hemodynamic instability or other complications of hypocalcemia occur.

    d. Hypomagnesemia. Hypomagnesemia is also common in critically ill surgical patients, and is most commonly dilutional. Excessive renal or gastrointestinal losses and transcellular shifts (e.g., alkalosis) are other causes of hypomagnesemia. Complications of hypomagnesemia include hypocalcemia, refractory hypokalemia, skeletal muscle weakness, tetany, cardiac dysrhythmia, tremor, hyperreflexia, agitation, confusion, and seizures. Measurement of the serum magnesium concentration does not reflect the physiologically active ionized fraction (55%). A serum magnesium concentration <1 mEq/L is associated with hypokalemia and increased mortality and thus serves as a practical threshold for initiating aggressive therapy. Severe hypomagnesemia is treated with IV magnesium sulfate (2–5 g) (1 g = 8 mEq Mg^{+2}) administered slowly over 2 to 3 minutes with cardiac monitoring, followed by an optional continuous infusion (2 g/hour for 5 hours followed by 1 g/hour for 10 hours). Less severe degrees of hypomagnesemia can be treated as indicated by supplements added to intravenous fluid or parenteral nutrition solution, or by enteral administration of magnesium oxide.

C. Pulmonary support. The lung is the most common organ to fail in patients with severe injuries. Thus, acute respiratory failure (ARF) is the most common indication for care of the trauma patient in the ICU.

    1. Etiology of acute respiratory failure. The principal causes of ARF following injury are direct chest trauma, fluid overload, aspiration pneumonitis, ARDS, and cervical spinal cord injury. Pneumonia is the leading cause of ARF after the first 2 days.

        a. Chest trauma. Multiple rib fractures, or pulmonary contusion with or without flail chest, frequently causes ARF requiring MV. Rib fractures are challenging to manage because pain and splinting of the chest wall lead to hypoventilation; adequate analgesia may compromise spontaneous ventilation to the point that MV is required. Epidural analgesia can make management of the patient with multiple rib fractures simpler and safer, provided the torso does not need serial physical examinations to monitor injuries (e.g., splenic laceration) and that hemodynamics are stable.

            i. Rarely, a major airway injury makes adequate gas exchange difficult because of massive air leakage. Signs suggestive of a major airway injury include subcutaneous emphysema, bronchopleural fistula, pneumomediastinum, or hemoptysis. Most tracheal injuries in the neck occur at or above the fourth tracheal ring, whereas injuries in the mediastinum occur usually within 2.5 cm of the carina. The major airways are evaluated best by bronchoscopy. An air leak or pneumothorax that persists despite MV using minimal airway pressures is an indication for operative repair.

        b. Fluid overload. Massive fluid resuscitation sometimes results in acute pulmonary edema, particularly with concomitant ALI/ARDS. Care should be taken to provide sufficient fluid for resuscitation, but not to excess. At times, markedly positive fluid balance can be an unavoidable consequence of extensive resuscitation in some patients.

        c. Shock. Any form of shock can cause ARF indirectly, as the work of breathing becomes excessive because of severe metabolic acidosis or inadequate oxygen delivery to the respiratory muscles.

        d. Aspiration of gastric contents. Maxillofacial injury, impaired consciousness, and endotracheal intubation are factors that predispose to aspiration. Hypoxemia results both from airway obstruction from aspiration of large particulates and from ALI secondary to acid aspiration. Two thirds of patients develop only a sterile chemical pneumonitis, and do not progress to late bacterial pneumonia. Antibiotics should be reserved for patients with microbiological evidence of pneumonia.

        e. Acute respiratory distress syndrome

            i. Definition. In the setting of a precipitant, ARDS is characterized by severe hypoxemia (PaO_2:FiO_2 ≤200), diffuse bilateral pulmonary infiltrates, a PAOP <18 mmHg, and decreased lung compliance.

A less severe form of lung injury, acute lung injury (ALI), is defined by PaO_2:FiO_2 of 200 to 300.

ii. Causative factors. Common causative factors for ARDS include sepsis, multiple long bone or pelvis fractures, multiple transfusions, pulmonary contusion, near-drowning, and acute pancreatitis.

iii. Pathophysiology. Absent a direct lung injury, a systemic inflammatory response to the underlying precipitant activates circulating phagocytes, causing adherence to endothelial cells and invasion of the interstitial space, where their activation and degranulation amplify the inflammatory response. The lung is particularly susceptible because large numbers of phagocytes are marginated in the pulmonary circulation, and the pulmonary circulation is embolized by systemic particulates after hepatic reticuloendothelial host defenses are overwhelmed.

f. Spinal cord injury. Isolated high thoracic or cervical spinal cord injury can lead to ARF, as mechanical lung function is impaired consequent to denervation of respiratory muscles. Although overt respiratory failure may not be evident within the first 24 hours, these patients are at high risk for decompensation as a result of progression of the spinal injury (ascension) or poor pulmonary toilet.

2. Mechanical ventilation. Mechanical ventilation may be required to manage trauma, whether for airway protection, general anesthesia, or management of ARF. New technology now provides several modes of MV that provide improved gas exchange, better patient comfort, and more rapid liberation from the ventilator. Moreover, noninvasive positive-pressure ventilation (NIV) permits some cases of ARF to be managed without intubation.

Most patients require MV for management of ARF, during which the work of breathing increases four- to sixfold. The most common indication for MV is to decrease the work of breathing. Additional potential benefits of MV include improved gas exchange, enhanced coordination between MV and the patient's own efforts, resting of respiratory muscles, prevention of deconditioning, and prevention of iatrogenic (ventilator-induced) lung injury (VILI) while promoting healing. However, unless settings are chosen carefully to synchronize with the patient's own central respiratory drive, MV can cause an increase in work.

a. Indications for mechanical ventilation. Nearly all ventilators can be set to allow full support of the patient, or periods of exercise, thus the physician determines MV settings for most patients. Controlled ventilation with suppression of spontaneous breathing leads rapidly to respiratory muscle atrophy. Therefore, modes of assisted ventilation are preferred wherein machine-delivered breaths are triggered by the patient's own inspiratory efforts.

i. Basic modes of assisted ventilation include assist-control ventilation (ACV), synchronized intermittent mandatory ventilation (SIMV), and pressure support ventilation (PSV). More advanced modes include pressure control ventilation (PCV), inverse-ratio ventilation (IRV), and airway pressure release ventilation (APRV). Regardless of the mode, all MV applies positive pressure to the airway, and modulates the interplay of mechanical support and the patients' own efforts.

b. Ventilator-associated lung injury. Acute lung injury and ARDS affect the lungs heterogeneously. The distribution of edema fluid, ventilated versus flooded alveoli, and consequently V/Q matching vary among gas exchange units. Moreover, the lung has a brisk inflammatory response when injured or during MV, which may manifest locally or systemically. The ARDSnet trial demonstrated improved outcomes from ALI/ARDS after ventilation with lower V_T, resulting in lower airway pressures, less overdistention of recruitable alveoli, less shear stress on lung tissue, and lower mortality. If less ventilation is better, more may be injurious, leading to the concept of ventilator-induced lung injury (VILI).

    c. Ventilator-induced lung injury occurs from excessive mechanical stress to the lung, either from excessive V_T or high airway pressure. Mechanical ventilation induces a pulmonary and systemic cytokine response, which can be minimized by limiting overdistention and phasic recruitment/derecruitment of lung. The mechanism of VILI is the proinflammatory response in the lung and the periphery, and the response and injury are attenuated by lung protective ventilation strategies. New modes of ventilation and protective ventilation are designed to minimize the deleterious effects of MV.

3. Noninvasive ventilation. Ventilatory support delivered without establishing an endotracheal airway is NIV, which utilizes positive pressure ventilation delivered through a nasal mask or facemask. Benefits of NIV include avoidance of endotracheal intubation and preservation of swallowing, feeding, speech, cough, and nasooropharygeal air warming and humidification. Nonintubated patients communicate more effectively, require less sedation, are more comfortable, and can continue standard oral nutrition. Noninvasive ventilation eliminates complications such as trauma with tube insertion, mucosal ulceration, aspiration, infection (e.g., pneumonia, sinusitis), and dysphagia after extubation.

    a. Contraindications. Successful NIV requires an awake, cooperative, spontaneously breathing patient with an intact cough reflex and ability to clear secretions. Relative contraindications include inadequate seal of the mask to the face, inability to cough, or inability to remove the mask quickly. Morbid obesity is also a relative contraindication secondary to increased ventilatory pressure requirements arising from body habitus and the weight of the chest wall and abdominal viscera while the patient is supine.

    b. Complications. Focal skin necrosis may occur over the nasal bridge, or rarely over the zygoma. The incidence is 7% to 10% among patients receiving full-face mask NIV. Other complications (incidence, 1% to 2% each) include conjunctivitis, gastric distention, aspiration, and pneumothorax. Most serious is failure to recognize when NIV is not providing a patient with adequate ventilation, oxygenation, or airway patency. Delayed intubation may cause continued deterioration or death.

4. Pressure support ventilation. Pressure support can assist spontaneous breathing during MV, either partially or fully, or can be used as a stand-alone mode for patients not on MV. The patient triggers the ventilator, which responds by delivering a flow of gas up to a physician-preset pressure limit (for example, 10 cm H_2O) depending on the desired V_E. Gas flow cycles off when a certain percentage of peak inspiratory flow (usually 25%) has been reached. Tidal volume may vary, just as it does spontaneously.

    a. Positive end-expiratory pressure is added to restore functional residual capacity (FRC) to normal. When lung volumes are low, the work of breathing during early inhalation is reduced. Noncompliant lungs require higher intrapleural pressures to inflate to a normal V_T, even with PEEP. Addition of PS assists the patient to move up the pressure-volume curve (larger changes in volume for a given applied pressure [i.e., increased lung compliance]). PSV describes the combination of pressure support and PEEP. Weaning may be facilitated using this combination, as the backup (SIMV) rate is weaned initially, and then the PS.

5. Modes of mechanical ventilation

    a. Assist-control ventilation (ACV). The ACV mode is the most commonly used mode in surgical ICUs. Set parameters in ACV mode are inspiratory flow rate, frequency (f), and V_T. The ventilator delivers a set number of equal breaths per minute, each of a given V_T. Tidal volume and flow determine inspiratory (I) and expiratory (E) time and the I:E ratio. Plateau or alveolar pressure is related to V_T and respiratory system compliance. The patient has the ability to trigger extra breaths by exerting effort that exceeds a preset trigger level. Patient effort can be increased, if desired, by increasing triggering threshold or lowering V_T.

b. **Synchronized intermittent mandatory ventilation (SIMV).** In a passive patient, SIMV is indistinguishable from ACV. Minute ventilation is determined by f and V_T. However, the patient can perform work by spontaneous effort during mandatory breaths. If the triggering effort comes in a brief, defined interval before the next mandatory breath, the ventilator will deliver the mandatory breath ahead of schedule to synchronize with patient inspiratory effort. The SIMV mode is often used to augment patient work of breathing gradually by lowering the mandatory breath frequency or V_T, compelling the patient to breathe more rapidly in order to maintain adequate V_E. A useful combination is SIMV plus PSV as a means to add "sigh" breaths and decrease atelectasis, or as an adjunct to weaning from the ventilator.

c. **Positive end-expiratory pressure (PEEP).** Although ubiquitous in use, PEEP can be confusing because positive pressure is actually applied throughout the respiratory cycle. PEEP prevents alveolar derecruitment by restoring physiologic FRC, and protects against injury during phasic opening and closing of atelectatic units. Increasing FRC allows alveoli to deflate only to the point just above where inflation remains easy (the lower inflection point of the pressure-volume curve).

  i. Auto-PEEP is caused by gas trapped in alveoli at end-expiration. This gas is not in equilibrium with the atmosphere and is at positive pressure, increasing the work of breathing. Shortening of E (e.g., small airways disease, mucus plugging, pressure-controlled ventilation with inverted I:E) results in gas trapping at end-expiration, hyperinflation, and increased intrathoracic pressure, which abolishes the alveolar pressure gradient. Auto-PEEP can be minimized by lengthening E, shortening I, or decreasing the respiratory rate.

  ii. **Setting PEEP.** The ideal level of PEEP is controversial, perhaps being that which prevents derecruitment of the majority of alveoli while causing minimal overdistension. Alternatively, application of PEEP is a recruitment maneuver, arguing for higher pressures to be applied to overcome alveolar collapse. Applying PEEP to put more lung units on the favorable part of the pressure-volume curve maximizes gas exchange and minimizes overdistention, but is easier said than done because the lower inflection point is sometimes indistinct. Undoubtedly, the combination of some PEEP and low V_T prevents VILI, but the exact amount of PEEP to use is controversial.

d. **Pressure-controlled ventilation.** Pressure-controlled ventilation is controlled completely by the ventilator. Inspiratory airway pressure increases early in the respiratory cycle, and is maintained at that specified pressure throughout the remainder of the delivery phase. The major benefit of PCV is that inspiratory flow decreases exponentially during lung inflation in order to keep the airway pressure at the preselected value, which is beneficial for patients with suppressed respiratory efforts. The primary disadvantage of PCV is the tendency for inflation volumes to vary with changes in the mechanical properties of the lungs.

  i. **Inverse-ratio ventilation.** Inverse-ratio ventilation is a combination of PCV with a prolonged I (hence, PC-IRV), increasing I:E from the usual 1:4 to 2:1 (up to 4:1). Benefits of IRV include improved oxygenation and the prevention of alveolar collapse. The downside to PC-IRV is that is can lead to breath-stacking (auto-PEEP), with high airway pressures, hyperinflation and barotrauma, CO_2 retention, and metabolic acidosis. Also adverse is decreased Q due to auto-PEEP because increased transthoracic pressure decreases venous return.

e. **Airway pressure release ventilation.** Airway pressure release ventilation (APRV) allows for the unloading during exhalation of any positive pressure provided during inhalation, facilitating egress of the tidal breath. Technically, APRV is time-triggered, pressure-limited, time-cycled MV that can be conceptualized as continuous positive airway pressure (CPAP) with regular, brief, intermittent releases of airway pressure. It can augment ventilation in the patient breathing spontaneously, or provide full support to the apneic patient. Advantages of APRV include lower peak airway pressure, lower intrathoracic pressure, lower V_E, minimal effect on Q, and improved V/Q matching. Sedation requirements may be decreased, and spontaneous breathing is facilitated. Disadvantages of APRV include pressure control of ventilation, increased effects of airway and circuit resistance on ventilation, decreased transpulmonary pressure, and potential interference with spontaneous ventilation. Although increasingly popular, the advantage of APRV over other modes of ventilation is unproved.

  i. **Terminology of APRV.** The terminology of APRV differs from other modes of MV, and is not standardized. Four important terms include pressure high (P_{high}), pressure low (P_{low}), time high (T_{high}), and time low (T_{low}). The P_{high} term describes the baseline airway pressure (the higher of the two pressures), alternatively called CPAP, inflating pressure, or the P1 pressure. The P_{low} term describes the airway pressure resulting from the release of pressure (alternatively called PEEP, release pressure, or the P2 pressure). The T_{high} time refers to the time during which P_{high} is maintained (T1), whereas T_{low} refers to the duration of time when airway pressure is released (T2).

  ii. **Use of APRV.** Application of APRV must be individualized. Initial settings are deduced from an initial trial of conventional MV. The plateau airway pressure (P_{plat} [if not higher than 35 cm H_2O]) is converted to P_{high}, aiming for a V_E of 2 to 3 L/minute (lower than with conventional MV). The P_{low} pressure is set initially at 0 cm H_2O. The setting for T_{high} is a minimum of 4 seconds, and T_{low} is set at approximately 0.8 second (0.5–1.0 second). Spontaneous breathing is permitted. Rarely, a higher P_{high} (40–45 cm H_2O) is needed for patients with low compliance (e.g., morbid obesity, abdominal distention). For all patients, T_{high} is lengthened progressively to 12 to 15 seconds, usually in 1- to 2-second increments, as lung mechanics improve. Longer T_{high} prevents the cyclical opening and closing of small airways that is believed to be a cause of VILI. The T_{low} parameter is optimized when expiratory flow decreases to 25% to 50% of peak expiratory flow.

6. **Routine ventilator settings**

   a. Ventilator settings are based on the patient's ideal body mass and medical condition (Table 37-8). The normal lung (e.g., during general anesthesia) may be ventilated safely with V_T 8 to 10 mL/kg. Historically, critically ill patients with ALI/ARDS were ventilated with V_T 10 to 15 mL/kg, which is now considered excessive. Alveolar overdistention produces endothelial, epithelial, and basement membrane injuries associated with VILI.

   b. During MV, alveolar volume is estimated from peak alveolar pressure as obtained from the plateau pressure (P_{plat}), measured in a relaxed patient by occluding the ventilator circuit briefly at end-inspiration. In patients with ALI/ARDS, V_T is reduced to 4 to 6 mL/kg to achieve a P_{plat} <35 cm H_2O. Low V_T ventilation may lead to increased $PaCO_2$ which is termed **permissive hypercapnia.** If pH decreases below 7.25, V_E is increased or $NaHCO_3$ is administered.

   c. The set f depends on the mode. With ACV, the backup rate should be about 4 breaths/minute less than the patient's spontaneous rate to ensure that the ventilator will continue to supply adequate V_E, should the patient hypoventilate or become apneic. With SIMV, the rate is typically high at first and then decreased gradually in accordance with patient tolerance.

   d. An inspiratory flow rate of 60 L/minute is used with most patients during ACV and SIMV. With chronic airways obstruction, better gas exchange may be achieved at a flow rate of 100 L/minute because increased E allows more complete emptying of trapped gas. If flow is insufficient, the patient will strain against pulmonary impedance and that of the ventilator, with a

TABLE 37-8	Protocol Summary for the Institution of Mechanical Ventilation for ALI/ARDS

Initial Ventilator Settings

Use a volume-controlled mode initially to ensure that V_T is delivered.

Use initial V_T 8 mL/kg; reduce by 1 mL/kg/2 h until 6 mL/kg is reached. Minimum V_T 4 mL/kg.

Set ventilator rate at 12–20 breaths/min.

Set maximum ventilator rate at 35 breaths/min.

Adjust ventilator subsequently based on goals of arterial pH (7.25–7.45; ventilator rate) and end-inspiratory plateau pressure (P_{plat}) (<30 cm H_2O; V_T).

Measure arterial pH upon admission to the ICU, each morning, and 15 min after each change in respiratory rate or V_T.

Manage alkalemia by decreasing ventilator rate by at least 2 breaths/min.

Manage mild acidemia (pH 7.15–7.25) by increasing ventilator rate until pH >7.25 or $PaCO_2$ <25 mmHg up to 35 breaths/min. If ventilator rate = 35 or $PaCO_2$ <25 mmHg, give sodium bicarbonate.

Manage severe acidemia (pH <7.15) by increasing the ventilator rate up to 35 breaths/min. If ventilator rate = 35 and pH <7.15, and sodium bicarbonate has been given, increase V_T in increments of 1 mL/kg until pH >7.15. It may be necessary to exceed the target P_{plat} under these conditions.

Keep P_{plat} <30 cm H_2O. Measure P_{plat} at least every 8 h, and 5 min after each change in PEEP or V_T, and more frequently when changes in lung compliance are likely. Accurate measurement of P_{plat} requires a patient who is not moving or coughing.

If P_{plat} cannot be measured because of an air leak, substitute peak inspiratory pressure.

Set target ranges for PaO_2 at 55–80 mmHg, or SaO_2 >88%. The combination of PEEP and FiO_2 is discretionary, but FiO_2:PEEP should generally be <5 if FiO_2 >0.45.

When increasing PEEP above 10 cm H_2O, increase by 2–5 cm increments up to a maximum of 35 cm H_2O, until target ranges for PaO_2 are reached. Reduce PEEP to the previous level of PEEP if the change does not increase PaO_2 >5 mmHg or if decreased oxygen delivery results from a decrease of cardiac output.

Assess arterial oxygenation by blood gas determination or oximetry at least every 4 h.

If arterial oxygenation is below the target range, increase FiO_2 incrementally (up to 1.0), then PEEP (up to 35 cm H_2O within 30 min). Reassess every 15 min after each adjustment until target ranges for PaO_2 are regained. Brief periods of SaO_2 <88% (<5 min) may be tolerated. FiO_2 = 1.0 may be used transiently (<10 min) for arterial desaturation or during suctioning or bronchoscopy.

ALI, acute lung injury; ARDS, acute respiratory distress syndrome. (Adapted from Nathens AB, Johnson JL, Minei JP, et al, and the Inflammation and the Host Response to Injury Investigators. Inflammation and the Host Response to Injury, a large-scale collaborative project: Patient-oriented research core—Standard operating procedures for clinical care. I. Guidelines for mechanical ventilation of the trauma patient. *J Trauma* 2005;59:764–769.)

consequent increase in the work of breathing. In the ACV, SIMV, and PCV modes the patient must lower airway pressure below a preset threshold (usually minus 1–2 cm H_2O) in order to trigger the ventilator to deliver a tidal breath.

7. **Liberation from mechanical ventilation.** Objective measures and proactive strategies can hasten the liberation of the patient from the ventilator. Each day of MV increases the need for sedation and the risk of ventilator-associated pneumonia. Failure to separate readily from the ventilator may be due to disease- or therapy-related reasons (Table 37-9). Most clinical cases of failure are multifactorial, but respiratory muscle fatigue is a common denominator.

   a. Increased work of breathing results from increased airflow resistance (e.g., bronchospasm, tracheal stenosis, tracheomalacia, glottic edema or dysfunction, mucus plugging), or decreased thoracic compliance (muscle dysfunction, due to nutritional or electrolyte causes). Other potential causes

TABLE 37-9	Differential Diagnosis of Failure to Separate from Mechanical Ventilation

Increased load on the respiratory system
Demand for increased minute ventilation
Increased CO_2 production
  Catabolic state
  Excess carbohydrate administered during nutritional support
Increased work of breathing
  Increased airflow resistance (e.g., bronchospasm, tracheal stenosis, tracheomalacia,
    glottic edema or dysfunction, mucus plugging)
Decreased thoracic compliance (muscle dysfunction due to nutritional or electrolyte causes,
    hypoxemia, hypercarbia, or possibly anemia)
Increased dead space ventilation
  Decreased cardiac output
  Pulmonary embolism
  Pulmonary hypertension
  Severe acute lung injury
  Positive-pressure ventilation

Increased ventilatory drive
Muscle fatigue or failure
Stimulation of pulmonary J receptors
  Lung inflammation
  Lung parenchymal hemorrhage
  Central nervous system lesions
Psychological stress
  Inadequate analgesia or sedation
  Untreated agitation or delirium
  Acute alcohol or drug withdrawal

    of muscle failure include acidosis, hypoxemia, hypercarbia, hypophosphatemia, and possibly anemia.

b. The process of weaning begins by determining patient readiness. Patients should have hemodynamic stability, cooperative mental status, consistent and adequate wakefulness, ability to manage secretions, nutritional repletion, normalization of acid-base and electrolyte status, and an airway of adequate diameter. Patients who "fight" the ventilator are said to have patient-ventilator **dyssynchrony**. A systematic approach to evaluation is advocated; the problem may lie with the patient or the ventilator, anywhere on the continuum from the alveolus to the power outlet or the source of respiratory gases. The first step is always to ensure that the patient has a patent, properly positioned airway.

c. Up to 25% of patients become distressed during weaning from MV such that ventilation has to be reinstituted. Patients who cannot be weaned have a characteristic response to trials of spontaneous breathing: an almost-immediate increase in respiratory rate and decrease in V_T. As the trial of spontaneous breathing continues over 30 to 60 minutes, work of breathing increases substantially by four- to sevenfold. Pulmonary compliance decreases, and gas trapping from lengthened I:E increases auto-PEEP. Rapid, shallow breathing causes hypoxemia and CO_2 retention because of increased V_D ventilation despite increased V_E. There is also considerable cardiovascular stress.

d. Timing is important; if weaning is premature, failure may lead to cardiopulmonary decompensation and further prolonged MV. In general, MV should not be weaned with hemodynamic instability, or PaO_2 <60 mmHg with a $FiO2$ ≥0.60. However, satisfactory oxygenation does not predict success; more important is whether respiratory muscles can perform increased work. Clinical judgment alone is often erroneous. Parameters such as maximal negative inspiratory pressure, vital capacity, and V_E are inaccurate. Respiratory frequency during one minute of spontaneous breathing (the Rapid Shallow Breathing Index [f/V_T]) is more accurate (95% probability of success if f/V_T <80 after a 30-minute trial of spontaneous breathing). Calculation of f/V_T during PSV is considerably less accurate.

  e. There are four methods of weaning.

  i. Simplest is to perform spontaneous breathing trials each day with a T-piece circuit. Brief (5–10 minutes) trials can be increased in frequency and duration until the patient can breathe spontaneously for several hours.

  ii. An alternative is to perform a single daily T-piece trial of up to 2 hours; if successful, the patient is extubated; if not, the next attempt is the following day.

  iii. More common (and popular) are SIMV and PSV, which are often combined. Assistance is decreased gradually by decreasing f or the amount of PS. When combined, f is set to zero before the level of pressure is decreased. Patients who breathe comfortably at PS 5 to 8 cm H_2O should be extubated successfully. Approximately 10% to 20% of patients require reintubation; their mortality is sixfold higher. Use of NIV following extubation may improve the likelihood of successful extubation.

  iv. Weaning from APRV is accomplished by manipulation of P_{high} and T_{high}. High pressure is decreased in increments of 2 to 3 cm H_2O down to about 15 cm H_2O, and T_{high} is lengthened progressively to 12 to 15 seconds in 1- to 2-second increments. Patients must be monitored carefully for signs of hypoventilation during the transition. The goal is to switch the patient to pure CPAP of 6 to 12 cm H_2O, at which point the patient may be extubated.

D. Renal support. Acute renal failure affects 10% to 25% of critically ill patients. The most common cause is renal hypoperfusion and related parenchymal dysfunction, referred to as acute tubular necrosis (ATN). One third to one half of cases of ATN occur during sepsis/infection, with the rest related to hypovolemia or toxin exposure. Patients with preexisting renal failure or diabetes mellitus are at particularly high risk for iodinated radiologic contrast-induced nephropathy. Acute renal failure seldom develops in isolation; coexistent respiratory failure (~67%), cardiac failure (~50%), or hepatic failure (~30%) are manifestations of the multiple organ dysfunction syndrome. In many series, more than one half of patients who develop acute renal failure will require renal replacement therapy (RRT).

  In the critical care setting, the mortality rate for patients who require renal replacement therapy may exceed 50%. The systemic pathophysiology of acute renal failure (e.g., mental status changes, bleeding, pericarditis) increases the risk of developing nonrenal complications. Because acute renal failure is a systemic condition, there may be a limit to what can be achieved to improve organ dysfunction, and therefore acute renal failure–related morbidity and mortality, by even optimized RRT.

  1. Indications for renal replacement therapy in the critical care setting. Optimal management of the critically ill patient who requires RRT includes an understanding of problems that can be corrected effectively by RRT and the complications that may arise as a consequence.

  a. The established uses for dialysis as therapy are listed in Table 37-10, including removal of fluid, removal or addition of solutes, regulation of plasma composition and volume, correction of acid-base abnormalities, and treatment of uremia.

  b. The nonrenal indications for RRT are expanding, including some drug overdoses, rewarming of hypothermic patients (especially with peritoneal dialysis), treatment of congestive heart failure, and prevention of contrast-induced nephropathy (CIN).

TABLE 37-10	Indications for Initiation of Renal Replacement Therapy

Fluid and Electrolyte Abnormalities
Fluid overload
Hyperkalemia
Hypernatremia
Hyponatremia
Hypercalcemia
Hyperphosphatemia
Hyperuricemia
Metabolic acidosis
Metabolic alkalosis

Uremic Manifestations
Pericarditis
Uremic bleeding/platelet dysfunction
Encephalopathy
Nausea/vomiting

    c. Prior to initiation of RRT, less invasive therapeutic interventions (e.g., diuretics, ion exchange resins) should be considered. Renal replacement therapy is initiated and titrated typically to maintain a pretreatment blood urea nitrogen (BUN) concentration <100 mg/dL with optimized fluid and electrolyte balance. In the critical care setting, extrarenal, azotemia-related organ dysfunction (e.g., encephalopathy, bleeding) is a less common indication for RRT. By accepting a BUN concentration of 100 mg/dL for initiation of RRT, most of the clinical manifestations of uremia are of historical interest.

2. Principles of dialysis

    a. Two mechanisms govern solute transport: diffusion and convection. In diffusion, solutes and toxins pass (diffuse) through a semipermeable membrane by random molecular motion. Equilibration (i.e., dialysis) depends on the concentration gradient across the membrane. Clearance during intermittent hemodialysis is based largely on diffusion, which is affected by molecular weight, charge, protein binding, and membrane pore size. Convection (i.e., ultrafiltration) occurs when water is driven across a semipermeable membrane by either hydrostatic or osmotic pressure. Water brings with it dissolved solutes (i.e., "drag effect"), also based on molecular weight, charge, protein binding, and pore size. Convective clearance is an important contribution to overall clearance in both peritoneal dialysis and continuous RRT.

    b. Intermittent hemodialysis (HD) and peritoneal dialysis (PD) were the main RRTs used in the past, but longer-duration treatments such as sustained low efficiency dialysis (SLED) and continuous RRT (CRRT) are being utilized increasingly in the critical care setting. Slow removal of water and solutes over a prolonged period causes less hemodynamic instability and is more suitable for critically ill patients.

3. Peritoneal dialysis. Despite being technically simple and inexpensive, PD is now used seldom, but may be useful for patients with unstable hemodynamics, bleeding abnormalities, heparin allergy, or difficult vascular access. Patients with recent abdominal surgery, abdominal adhesions, abdominal hernia, diaphragmatic pleuroperitoneal defects, or severe liver failure are not candidates.

    To perform PD, specifically designed catheters are inserted into the lower abdomen. The dialysate solution is introduced into the peritoneal cavity, and after a prescribed "dwell" period is drained and discarded. A PD exchange starts with the drainage of fluid already in the abdominal cavity, followed by the infusion of fresh dialysate over 5 to 10 minutes. The fluid remains (dwells) in the abdomen for the prescribed dwell time in hours, after which it is drained over a 15- to 20-minute period.

The passage of uremic toxins and electrolytes across the peritoneal membrane occurs only during the dwell part of the cycle, and is driven by the concentration gradient established between the blood and the instilled dialysate. Acid-base status is corrected by the absorption of lactate from the dialysate that is metabolized by the liver to bicarbonate. Ultrafiltration and subsequent water removal is achieved by an osmotic gradient created by the high glucose content of the dialysate relative to the serum glucose concentration. The maximum gradient is present within the first 2 hours of any PD exchange. Over time, glucose from the dialysate is absorbed into the circulation, which has implications for glucose control.

a. **Dialysate selection for PD.** Peritoneal dialysate contains dextrose in various concentrations (1.5%, 2.5%, or 4.25%) to provide an osmotic gradient for ultrafiltration (i.e., higher concentrations stimulate more ultrafiltration). The amount of glucose absorbed during the dwell time may provide a patient with up to 1,000 kilocalories per day (kcal/day) and must be accounted for in the nutritional prescription. Several electrolytes are also present, including sodium, chloride, calcium, magnesium, and lactate (35–40 mEq/L). Solutions do not contain potassium, and can be used to lower the serum concentration, but clearance is low and PD is not preferred for management of severe hyperkalemia. However, hypokalemia can be corrected by adding 2 to 3 mEq/L potassium chloride (KCl) to the dialysate.

b. **Writing the PD prescription.** Solute clearance and ultrafiltration occur only during the dwell period of the cycle. Maximum ultrafiltration is achieved with short dwell times, whereas toxin clearance, especially for middle-sized or large uremic molecules, requires longer dwell times. Hypercatabolic states require prescriptions for higher urea and creatinine clearances. The PD prescription typically includes 5 to 12 exchanges per day to obtain the desired ultrafiltration and clearance. Brief exchanges (i.e., <1–2 hours) are unlikely to achieve either adequate ultrafiltration or clearance, but increase the chance of a breach of sterile technique and peritonitis.

  i. Depending on the patient's clinical condition, fluid status, blood pressure, and laboratory parameters, PD prescriptions (number of daily exchanges, dialysate electrolyte and dextrose concentrations, and volume of fluid infused per exchange) should be evaluated at least every 24 hours, or more frequently if necessary.

  ii. Several medications may be added to the dialysate solution, including heparin (200 to 500 international units per liter [IU/L]) for intraperitoneal infection or PD-related or other intraperitoneal nonsurgical bleeding (Figure 37-1). Heparin is added for bloody dialysate return to prevent fibrin or blood clot formation and catheter obstruction and malfunction. The aPTT does not require monitoring because heparin is not absorbed systemically. Regular insulin can be added for better blood glucose control, especially of diabetic patients. The recommended starting dose of regular insulin is 4 to 5 U/L (1.5% dextrose), 5 to 6 U/L (2.5% dextrose), or 7 to 10 U/L (4.25% dextrose). Close monitoring of the serum glucose concentration is mandatory. A wide array of antibiotics can be added, but systemic absorption after intraperitoneal administration is unpredictable, and therefore unreliable to treat a systemic infection. However, PD catheter-related peritonitis may respond better to intraperitoneal antibiotics. Antibiotics should be added to each PD exchange, but once-daily administration may be considered if the dwell time is at least 6 to 8 hours.

Quantifying a 7-day cycle of different renal replacement therapies

Peritoneal Dialysis	Intermittent Hemodialysis	Extracorporeal CRRT

Peritoneal Dialysis

Assumptions:
7 days
8L Infused Dialysate per day
10L Drained Dialysate per day
Urea [D] / [B] = .85

D_f	8000 mL/day
U_f	2000 mL/day
B_f	8500 mL/day

Urea clr	5.9 mL/min
UF	1.4 mL/min

Intermittent Hemodialysis

Assumptions:
Using 1.8 m^2 Polysulfone Dialyzer
3 day × 3.5 hr treatments (IHD)
5 days × 2.5 hr treatments (SDD)
5 days × 6.0 hr treatments (SLED)

IHD, SDD	B_f 400 mL/min
IHD, SDD	D_f 500 mL/min
IHD UF	1000 mL/hr
SDD UF	1000 mL/hr

IHD Urea clr	18 mL/min[1]
IHD UF	1.0 mL/min
SDD Urea clr	22 mL/min[1]
SDD UF	1.2 mL/min

SLED	B_f 300 mL/min
SLED	D_f 500 mL/min
SLED	U_F 300 mL/hr

SLED Urea clr	45 mL/min[2]
SLED UF	.89 mL/min

Extracorporeal CRRT

Assumptions:
7 days of continuous treatment
B_f = 180 mL/min
Urea [D] / [B] =1

SCUF
SCUF RF_f 0 mL/hr
SCUF D_f 0 mL/hr
SCUF UF 150 mL/hr

Urea clr	2.5 mL/min
UF	2.5 mL/min

CVVHHD

RF_f	1000 mL/hr
D_f	1000 mL/hr
UF	150 mL/hr

Urea clr	36 mL/min
UF	2.5 mL/min

Assumptions for urea clearance: (1) IHD, SDD 290 mL/min (2) SLED 250 mL/min.

Figure 37-1. A comparison of the clearance and ultrafiltration provided by prescriptions for different renal replacement therapies. As in practice, not all therapies are administered every day. To compare their effectiveness, calculations are based on a 7-day period during which treatments have been given for part or all of that time. For intermittent therapies these may be significantly less than intratreatment clearance and ultrafiltration.

c. PD-related complications

  i. Instilled dialysate causes abdominal distension, which may cause abdominal pain or respiratory distress. Smaller dialysate volumes or keeping the patient supine may improve symptoms. Dialysate may leak around the catheter or into the abdominal wall, especially when non-tunneled catheters are used immediately. Discontinuation of dialysis allows fluid reabsorption and sealing of the pericatheter area. Other potential complications include abdominal pain or hypothermia related to infusion of fluid that has not been warmed properly, inadequate drainage due to decreased bowel motility, adhesions, or migration of the catheter from the normal position in the pelvis. Rarely, perforation of a hollow viscus may occur.

  ii. Peritoneal dialysis-related infectious complications (peritonitis or exit site infection) may be avoided by following proper exchange and catheter care techniques. Peritonitis can be diagnosed by identifying cloudy fluid in a patient complaining of abdominal pain, nausea, or anorexia; fever is uncommon. More than 100 white blood cell/high-power field (WBC/hpf) with >50% neutrophils or the presence of bacteria on gram stain of peritoneal fluid is suggestive. Cultures identify coagulase-negative *Staphylococcus* or *S. aureus* commonly. Depending on susceptibility, a first-generation cephalosporin or vancomycin may be used for gram-positive infections, whereas gentamicin or a third-generation cephalosporin may be selected for gram-negative infections.

Fungal peritonitis is possible. During PD peritonitis, decreased ultrafiltration may require adjustment of the prescription. Unsuccessful antibiotic treatment requires catheter removal and conversion to RRT by vascular access.

4. **Intermittent hemodialysis (IHD).** Hemodialysis involves dialyzing the intravascular compartment. During IHD, intravascular refilling from the interstitial and intracellular compartments (spaces) provides solutes (e.g., urea, creatinine) and water for clearance and ultrafiltration. A dialysis prescription that attempts ultrafiltration more rapidly than water and solutes can be mobilized is likely to result in hypotension. Whereas a stable, end-stage renal disease patient may mobilize extravascular fluid at approximately 1 L/hour, the critically ill patient receiving dialysis often cannot.

   a. **Selecting the HD regimen.** The typical outpatient regimen for end-stage renal disease (thrice-weekly HD sessions for 3.0–4.5 hours/week) is insufficient for a critically ill patient with acute renal failure because of the higher degree of catabolism. Therapy should be individualized based on the patient's clinical condition and specific needs (e.g., fluid, electrolyte, and metabolic requirements), which may mean daily HD. Hemodynamic stability (i.e., normotension without vasopressor use) is generally the first consideration for selecting IHD. Peritoneal dialysis or CRRT may be more suited for patients with unstable hemodynamics. A second selection consideration is how much fluid a patient is receiving per day and how much needs to be removed. Intermittent HD is the superior choice when rapid clearance is required (i.e., hyperkalemia or dialyzable drug intoxication).

   b. **Hemodialysis access.** Several temporary access options allow effective IHD for acute renal failure. Catheters typically have two lumens, one for blood removal into the dialysis system ("arterial side," even though placed in a large vein) and the other for blood return to the patient ("venous side"). Catheters may be tunneled and have a subcutaneous cuff for fixation and to prevent infection (e.g., "perma-cath") or uncuffed ("vas-cath"), which are used for most acute HD treatments, at least initially. The latter are typically placed at the bedside in either the groin or neck area (i.e., external jugular, internal jugular [right side is preferred] or femoral vein). The subclavian vein is less desirable because of associated stenosis and thrombosis risk, which may compromise chronic access placement. Cuffed catheters generally are used chronically. Uncuffed catheters, especially in the femoral vein, need to be changed every 7 to 10 days. Cuffed catheters do not require changing and, if cared for properly, may be used for months. Blood flow through an uncuffed catheter may be positional, which may limit achievable blood flow. Between treatments, both types of catheters are filled with an anticoagulant (e.g., heparin, citrate) to prevent clotting. A patient who develops sepsis will require removal of either catheter, as the infection rate is high. On the other hand, IHD or CRRT of an infected patient should always begin via an uncuffed catheter, which may be removed and reinserted as necessary.

   c. **Selecting a dialyzer.** Two types of dialyzers are available for use, so-called high-flux and high-efficiency dialyzers. High-flux dialyzers, the dialyzers of choice, provide greater clearance for larger molecules at a given blood flow rate. Most high-flux dialyzers used in the ICU are made from a biocompatible polymer and no longer provoke much of an inflammatory reaction. The tendency to clot during treatment may also be an important selection consideration. Intermittent HD treatments can be performed without anticoagulation if the bleeding risk is high or the patient has had an adverse reaction to anticoagulants. However, clotting during IHD is not solely a function of biocompatibility, and may be influenced by other determinants of the dialyzer, including blood volume and surface area.

d. **Writing the IHD prescription.** Each prescription should be written with the goal of therapy in mind, whether clearance, ultrafiltration, or both. Most of the clearance achieved during IHD is via diffusion, which can be increased by longer treatments at higher blood flow rates. Dialysate solutions contain neither urea, creatinine, uric acid, nor phosphorus, to maximize their clearance. The potassium concentration is between 0 and 3 mEq/L depending on the urgency of potassium removal. Calcium-free dialysate may be used to treat hypercalcemia. The bicarbonate concentration can be varied (30–40 mEq/L) to correct metabolic acid-base disorders.

   i. If blood pressure is marginal or vasopressor-dependent, IHD can be prescribed for clearance only, omitting ultrafiltration. However, hypotensive patients sometimes need urgent ultrafiltration; blood pressure can be supported by increasing the sodium concentration in the dialysate, performing ultrafiltration earlier in the session when extracellular fluid volume is higher, decreasing the temperature to 35°C to promote vasoconstriction, administration of mannitol or 25% human albumin solution, or titrating vasopressor therapy.

   ii. Anticoagulation is usually required to prevent system clotting, usually heparin (20-IU/kg bolus, then 10 IU/kg/hour by infusion), which is a dose high enough to cause bleeding in a patient at risk. Anticoagulant-free treatments are prescribed commonly during the first 72 hours after surgery, when a patient is bleeding actively, or there is concern that bleeding may be precipitated (e.g., thrombocytopenia). If necessary, alternative anticoagulants (i.e., argatroban, citrate) can be used, but HD without anticoagulation is simpler and equally effective.

5. **Continuous renal replacement therapy (CRRT).** Extracorporeal CRRT developed because critically ill patients with acute renal failure often need ultrafiltration despite marginal hemodynamics, or a large ongoing large requirement for resuscitation, or to provide nutrition. Intolerance of the high ultrafiltration rates necessary to maintain fluid balance using IHD stimulated development of techniques to remove fluid more slowly over a prolonged period.

   a. Current systems can provide hemofiltration (convective clearance to produce a large-volume ultrafiltrate that can be replaced partially using pre- or postfilter replacement fluid, known as continuous venovenous hemofiltration [CVVH]); dialysis (use of dialysate to provide clearance in addition to the desired ultrafiltration, known as continuous venovenous hemodialysis [CVVHD]); production of relatively small amounts of ultrafiltrate (using no replacement fluid or dialysate, called slow continuous ultrafiltration [SCUF]); or all of these modalities combined, which is referred to as continuous venovenous hemodiafiltration [CVVHDF]. Selecting an ultrafiltration rate of 50 to 250 mL/hour provides up to 6 L/day of ultrafiltrate, which is equivalent to removal of 1.5 L/hour during a 4-hour IHD treatment.

   b. **Selecting the CRRT mode.** Treatments by CRRT are recommended for patients with marginal hemodynamics. Prefilter replacement fluid administration may be preferred for patients with a tendency to clot or in whom anticoagulant-free treatments are attempted. Prefilter fluid administration flushes the dialyzer with replacement fluid and facilitates ultrafiltration, but prefilter replacement fluid administration dilutes the blood pathway in the dialyzer and provides less efficient clearance. With postfilter replacement fluid administration, ultrafiltration rates are limited as blood viscosity increases in the dialyzer as fluid is removed.

   i. Patients with an adequate blood pressure who have a contraindication to anticoagulant use may be treated better with IHD. Hypotensive patients who cannot be anticoagulated, such as postoperative patients who require immediate treatment, may be considered for PD if they have not just had abdominal surgery.

    c. Writing the CRRT prescription. Selection of a specific dialyzer is generally not a consideration when initiating CRRT. Most systems include a high-flux dialyzer and tubing cartridge. Blood flow rate selection may vary, typically up to about 200 mL/minute; lower blood flow rates make little sense. Higher flow rates are associated with hypotension, whereas lower flow rates are associated with system clotting. Clearance and ultrafiltration rate are independent of blood flow rate at higher flows. Clearance, however, is highly dependent on both fluid replacement rate and dialysate flow rate.

        i. Replacement fluid is typically an isotonic sodium solution containing a supra-physiologic concentration of bicarbonate (30–40 mEq/L). Potassium (0–4 mEq/L), calcium (3 mEq/L), and magnesium (1 mEq/L) may be added as necessary. In severe metabolic acidosis, isotonic sodium bicarbonate (150 mEq/L) has been used as replacement fluid, but effectiveness is questionable if administered in a prefilter configuration. Replacement fluid rate contributes to overall clearance, therefore a fluid replacement rate <1 L/hour is unusual.

        ii. Anticoagulation with heparin is standard during CRRT, at the same starting dose for IHD. The dose is adjusted to maintain an aPTT approximately twice the upper limit of normal. Treatment with no anticoagulation is indicated for patients with active bleeding, thrombocytopenia, or another coagulopathy.

    d. Comparison of the continuous therapies and intermittent hemodialysis. Different forms of RRT appear to be better choices for different clinical situations. However, no best therapy has emerged clearly. Peritoneal dialysis provides the least amount of clearance compared with other therapies, but comparable ultrafiltration. Peritoneal dialysis perturbs hemodynamics minimally, and is suitable for hypotensive patients and for treatments when anticoagulation must be avoided. Low peritoneal dialysis clearance may make it unsuited for severely catabolic patients or patients with marked hyperkalemia or hypercalcemia. Peritoneal dialysais may not be the best choice for patients with recent abdominal surgery or marginal hepatic or pulmonary function.

        i. Intermittent HD provides high levels of clearance, and may be particularly useful to treat hyperkalemia. It is unlikely that critically ill patients will tolerate an ultrafiltration rate of 1,000 mL/hour. With the exception of the SLED model, IHD does not lend itself as well as CRRT to patients who require large amounts of fluid and concomitant ultrafiltration, especially with marginal blood pressure. Intermittent HD treatments may be most useful for "stable" patients in an ICU, to achieve a balance of clearance and ultrafiltration.

        ii. Extracorporeal CRRT variants provide excellent clearance and ultrafiltration and are particularly suitable for patients with borderline blood pressure who require substantial amounts of fluid as well as ultrafiltration, but are labor-intensive, especially without anticoagulation.

E. Support of coagulation. Clotting factor deficiency and thrombocytopenia occur commonly in trauma patients with hemorrhagic shock requiring large-volume resuscitation (from consumption due to blood loss, or dilution due to use of crystalloid fluids), or massive traumatic brain injury. Contributing factors include ongoing hemorrhage, shock, acidosis, hypothermia, and intraoperative blood salvage techniques. Coagulopathy may also occur with maternal-fetal hemorrhage, vitamin K deficiency, or due to drug therapy (e.g., aspirin, antiplatelet agents such as clopidogrel, warfarin, or heparinoids).

    Microvascular bleeding (also known as disseminated intravascular coagulation, DIC) refers to bleeding in the setting of massive consumption of clotting factors and platelets (once surgical bleeding is controlled). Microvascular bleeding is nonsurgical bleeding that appears as petechial hemorrhage, ecchymosis, or hematoma, and oozing from mucous membranes, puncture sites, and raw surfaces. It is not usually observed until the patient has received transfusion of red blood cell concentrates equal to 1 to 2 blood volumes.

1. **Management.** Normalization of body temperature (as previously discussed) in hypothermic patients is essential to ensure functional clotting factors and platelets.

Ongoing occult bleeding that requires operative intervention (surgical bleeding) must be sought if the patient remains in refractory shock. Blood component therapy (Chapter 42) is given based on identification of specific clotting defects in screening tests.

   a. Thrombocytopenia (most common) is treated with platelet concentrates, ideally to maintain the platelet count above 100,000/mm^3 until active bleeding has ceased. Platelet transfusions are often the first component therapy required in massive hemorrhage.

   b. Prolongation of the prothrombin time (common) or partial thromboplastin time (uncommon) is treated with fresh-frozen plasma, and hypofibrinogenemia (rare, except with obstetrical hemorrhage) is treated with cryoprecipitate. Determination of the activity of specific clotting factors is seldom necessary unless there is refractory coagulopathy. The role of recombinant Factor VII is still being defined, although anecdotes suggest that refractory coagulopathic hemorrhage can be stanched. Functional platelets are required for rFVII to exert its effect.

F. **Neurologic support**

1. **Increased intracranial pressure.** Traumatic brain injury (TBI) is a major cause of early mortality in blunt trauma patients admitted to the ICU. The fundamental goal in ICU management of the patient with severe TBI (after recognition and evacuation of intracranial mass lesions) is to prevent secondary brain injury from hypoperfusion, which may be due to increased ICP or decreased mean arterial blood pressure (MAP), either of which result in reduced cerebral perfusion pressure (CPP) (CPP = MAP − ICP). The uninjured brain can autoregulate cerebral perfusion and preserve cerebral blood flow across a wide range of blood pressures, but one of the cardinal features of TBI is loss of autoregulation. The injured brain is vulnerable to secondary injury with CPP <60 mmHg; as little as 5 minutes of hypoperfusion can double the risk of death from TBI. Therefore, monitoring and control of ICP and CPP in severe TBI (Glasgow Coma Scale (GCS) score ≤8 points) is a high priority of early postinjury care. Other insults that are known to worsen neurologic injury include hypoxia, hypercarbia (owing to cerebral vasodilation), and elevated body temperature (Chapter 17).

   a. **Control of elevated ICP.** The threshold for treatment of raised ICP is 20 to 25 mmHg. Increased ICP is controlled most simply and directly by the removal of cerebrospinal fluid (CSF) via an indwelling ventriculostomy. If a ventriculostomy is not used or venting of CSF is ineffective (e.g., massive brain swelling, obstructed catheter lumen), sequential use of sedation, hypertonic saline (usually 3% NaCl), neuromuscular blockade, mannitol, and barbiturates may be used to reduce refractory intracranial hypertension. Hypertonic saline has supplanted mannitol because mannitol crosses the blood-brain barrier and results in tachyphylaxis with repetitive use. Mannitol, 23.4% saline, or hyperventilation (PaCO$_2$ <25 mmHg) may be used to interdict transtentorial herniation that usually manifests by marked anisocoria and pupillary non-reactivity (the "blown" pupil). Marked hypocapnia (PaCO$_2$ <25 mmHg) should be avoided for more than a few minutes unless therapy is guided by cerebral blood flow measurements or other indices of brain oxygenation (e.g., jugular venous oximetry). Tachyphylaxis develops rapidly, but decreased cerebral blood flow from cerebral vasoconstriction may cause secondary brain injury. High-dose barbiturate therapy (barbiturate coma) is reserved for patients with refractory intracranial hypertension.

b. Prevention of other secondary insults. Mean arterial pressure, SaO_2, $ETCO_2$, and core body temperature are monitored closely to avoid secondary insults to the injured brain. The goal is to maintain CPP at least 60 mmHg, which is accomplished by a combination of low ICP and increased MAP. When ICP cannot be kept low, MAP must be supported to at least 90 mmHg (depending on the resulting CPP). When volume expansion is unsuccessful in maintaining CPP, a vasopressor (usually phenylephrine) is employed. Antipyretics and other cooling techniques are applied to keep core temperature $<38°C$ and reduce cerebral DO_2, but although fever is detrimental it is less clear whether avoidance or suppression of fever is salutary.

2. Sedation and analgesia. Almost every critically ill patient requires analgesia and sedation; some may require anesthesia administered at the bedside. Published guidelines describe in detail the sustained use of these agents for indications such as prolonged mechanical ventilation or control of increased ICP.

a. A panoply of agents is available for use during bedside procedures and operations (Table 37-11). The choice of agent is made on several factors.

TABLE 37-11	Selected Agents for Analgesia, Anesthesia, and Sedation in the ICU

Agent	Initial IV adult dose	Comments
Induction Agents		
Etomidate	6 mg or more	Maintains CO and BP. Reduces ICP but maintains CPP. Short $T_{1/2}$; use infusion for maintenance. Possible adrenal suppression.
Ketamine	1–2 mg/kg	Rapid-onset, short-duration agent. Can be given by continuous infusion for maintenance, and at lower dose for sedation without anesthesia. Transiently increases BP and HR. Raises ICP and intraocular pressure. Usually does not depress respiration. Generally safe in pregnancy and for neonates and children. Concurrent narcotics or barbiturates may prolong recovery. Anxiety, disorientation, dysphoria, and hallucinations during emergence, may be mitigated by a short-acting benzodiazepine. Atropine pretreatment can decrease secretions, but may increase incidence of dysphoria. Hepatic metabolism.
Propofol	1.5–2.5 mg/kg	Provides no analgesia. Potent amnestic effect. Causes apnea and loss of gag reflex. Can cause marked low BP. Infuse at 0.05–0.3 mg/kg/min for prolonged sedation. Minimal accumulation (hepatic insufficiency) facilitates rapid elimination. Account for 1 kcal/mL (lipid infusion) in nutrition prescription. Use of same vial >12 h associated with bacteremia. Safety for children still debated.
Thiopental	1–5 mg/kg	Used rarely, mostly for TBI management. Reduces BP and CPP. Accumulates with prolonged use or infusion, especially with hepatic insufficiency.
Intravenous Sedatives/Analgesics		
Midazolam	0.5–4.0 mg	Short $T_{1/2}$, but accumulates during infusion owing to active metabolites. Only benzodiazepine with potent amnestic effect. Can cause low BP and loss of airway. Primarily used for short-term sedation for ICU procedures. Renal elimination.

(continued)

TABLE 37.11	(Continued)

Agent	Initial IV adult dose	Comments
Diazepam	2.5–5.0 mg	Long $T_{1/2}$ limits use in ICU except for rare cases requiring very long-term sedation. Terminates seizure activity effectively. Hepatic elimination.
Lorazepam	1–4 mg	Effective anxiolytic. Preferred agent for continuous infusion of benzodiazepine (starting dose 1 mg/h). Can cause low BP, especially with hypovolemia, and paradoxical agitation. Hepatic elimination.
Morphine	2–10 mg	Analgesic and sedative effects. Can cause low BP, CO, and apnea. Tolerance and withdrawal possible after long-term use. Can be given as IV infusion or by PCA for analgesia or to facilitate prolonged mechanical ventilation or withdrawal of care. Hepatic elimination.
Hydromorphone	0.5–2.0 mg	Hydrated ketone of morphine with similar use and risk profiles. Approximately eightfold more potent than morphine. Hepatic elimination.
Fentanyl	50–100 µg	Approximately 50-fold potency compared with morphine, but less likely to cause low BP in appropriate dosage (less histamine release). Versatile for ICU use given IV or by epidural infusion or PCA. Less potent than local anesthetics for epidural analgesia or abrogation of surgical stress response. Can cause truncal rigidity and apnea with inability to ventilate by hand (use neuromuscular blockade to facilitate intubation in that setting). Hepatic elimination.
Neuromuscular Blocking Agents		
Atracurium	0.2–0.5 mg/kg	Short-acting nondepolarizing NMBAs (competitive inhibitors of Ach). Slow in onset compared with other agents in class. The drugs are similar, except atracurium causes histamine release and can cause high HR, low BP. Cisatracurium, now used preferentially, requires IV infusion for prolonged effect. Effect potentiated by hypokalemia. Many drug interactions. Elimination by Hoffman elimination and ester hydrolysis, thus can be used for patients with renal/hepatic insufficiency.
Cisatracurium	0.2–0.5 mg/kg	
Mivacurium	0.15 mg/kg	Nondepolarizing NMBA with slow onset and moderate duration of action. Can be given by continuous infusion. Releases histamine; causes bronchospasm. Can cause decreased or increased HR and cardiac dysrhythmias. Faster onset/recovery in children ages 2–12 years. Enhanced blockade in pregnant patients given magnesium for preeclampsia.
Pancuronium	0.05–0.1 mg	Rapid onset, prolonged effect. Causes increased BP and HR. Induces neuromuscular blockade, but should be converted, for example, to a maintenance cisatracurium infusion. Eliminated by kidneys and liver, accumulates in organ dysfunction with repeated doses.

(continued)

TABLE 37.11 (Continued)

Agent	Initial IV adult dose	Comments
Vecuronium	0.08–0.10 mg/kg	Nondepolarizing NMBA with rapid onset and short duration of action. Less potential for histamine release. Can cause malignant hyperthermia syndrome. Metabolized by liver.
Miscellaneous Agents		
Haloperidol	2–5 mg	Used for anxiolysis (often preferred to lorazepam), especially when respiratory depression is undesirable. Not FDA-approved for IV administration, but IV route is used commonly. Antidopaminergic properties contraindicate use in Parkinson disease. Can cause extrapyramidal effects. Hepatic elimination.
Ketorolac	0.5–1.0 mg/kg	Parenteral NSAID used in lieu of opioids or for opioid-sparing effect in combination. Interferes irreversibly with platelet function, and can cause incisional or GI hemorrhage and acute renal failure. Use strictly limited to <5 days in postoperative period.
Reversal Agents		
Flumazenil	0.1–0.2 mg	Benzodiazepine antagonist. Rapid onset and short duration. Adverse effect of benzodiazepine can persist after drug wears off. Repeated doses of up to 0.8 mg can be used. Abrupt antagonism of chronic benzodiazepine use can precipitate seizures.
Naloxone	up to 0.4 mg	Opioid antagonist. Rapid onset and short duration. Often diluted 0.4 mg/10 mL and titrated 0.04–0.08 mg at a time to reverse undesirable side effects while preserving analgesia. Repeated doses of up to 0.4 mg or continuous IV infusion can be used. Abrupt opioid antagonism can precipitate increased BP, increased HR, pulmonary edema, or myocardial infarction.
Edrophonium with Atropine	0.5–1.0 mg/kg 0.007–0.014 mg/kg	Edrophonium is a anticholinesterase inhibitor with antidysrhythmic properties. Rapid onset, short duration, therefore used usually with atropine, to counteract increased secretions, decreased HR, and bronchospasm. Does not reverse neuromuscular blockade caused by depolarizing agents. Renal and hepatic elimination (edrophonium). Atropine may cause fever.
Neostigmine with Glycopyrrolate	0.5–2.0 mg 0.1–0.2 mg	Cause salivation and severe low HR. May cause broncho- or laryngospasm. Renal metabolism. Does not reverse neuromuscular blockade caused by depolarizing agents. Give (same syringe) with glycopyrrolate (or atropine) to counteract low HR. May cause fever.

Ach, acetylcholine; BP, blood pressure; CO, cardiac output; CPP, cerebral perfusion pressure; ICP, intracranial pressure; FDA, U.S. Food and Drug Administration; GI, gastrointestinal; HR, heart rate; IV, intravenous; NMBA, neuromuscular blocking agent; NSAID, nonsteroidal antiinflammatory drug; PCA, patient-controlled analgesia; $T_{1/2}$, elimination half-life; TBI, traumatic brain injury; VO_2, oxygen consumption.

Is the patient intubated? Are the patient's hemodynamics stable and normal? Does the procedure require general anesthesia, or will local anesthesia suffice? For how long must the anesthesia be effective? Will neuromuscular blockade be needed? If sedation is planned, will it be conscious sedation, or maintained at a deeper level? Will repetitive administration be required for multiple procedures? Will the agents require reversal, or will they be allowed to "wear off"? Does the need for repetitive neurologic examinations require use of either a short-acting or reversible agent? Will metabolism of the agents be impaired by abnormal organ function? Will the personnel available be able to manage the agent(s) chosen?

X. SPECIAL CONSIDERATIONS IN ICU CARE

A. Transport.
The resources in personnel and portable monitoring equipment necessary for transport of a critically ill patient out of the ICU are substantial, and sometimes unjustifiable. However, every "roadtrip" must be assessed not only from a risk–benefit perspective, but also from a cost–benefit perspective. Those patients who should be transported are those who must, and no others.

1. Published guidelines for intrahospital transport indicate that, at a minimum, the ICU patient's respiratory therapist and nurse should accompany the patient out of the ICU for the duration of the transport, but to do so might require juggling the ICU staff to accommodate the departure, or it might be impossible if the patient does not have one-to-one nursing (a rarity). Physician accompaniment is a poor substitute, in that the physician is often a junior one with limited familiarity with the patient's case, and limited skills for troubleshooting the myriad things that can go wrong with infusion pumps, intravenous tubing, and the like. However, the putative lack of safety of the intrahospital roadtrip is probably overstated. The incidence of transport-related mishaps is only 5%, almost all of which are minor (e.g., tangled intravenous tubing, low battery). Even the sickest ICU patient can be transported safely if risk and benefits are weighed carefully, patients are stabilized insofar as possible before the transport is undertaken, and monitoring is continuous throughout. All transport team members must be educated in patient evaluation; potential risks, complications, and interventions; and equipment operation and troubleshooting. All team members must also understand their roles and responsibilities, and communicate effectively.

B. The ICU as operating room (OR)

1. **Preparation of the unit and staff.** The staff of the ICU must be familiar with the use of the ICU as an OR. Experienced staff reduce the chance of procedure-related complications. Detailed protocols that define roles and responsibilities, medications, monitoring equipment, disposable supplies, and surgical instruments needed for each procedure should be established. All needed equipment (and reasonably anticipated needs) must be at the bedside prior to the start of the procedure. Communication is essential so that if additional nursing personnel will need to be at the bedside for the procedure, adequate coverage for the other patients is assured. Consideration should also be given to whether an anesthesiologist or nurse anesthetist should be at the bedside for the procedure.

2. **Preparation of the patient.** Informed consent must be obtained unless the intervention is for an immediately life-threatening condition. Renal and hepatic function should be ascertained for proper dosing of medications. The risk of bleeding should also be assessed. Patients who have received aspirin or another nonsteroidal antiinflammatory agent should be considered for transfusion of platelets to "cover" the procedure, but specific guidelines do not exist. Patients with renal dysfunction (blood urea nitrogen concentration ≥ 70 mg/dL) also have platelet dysfunction, and can receive either cryoprecipitate or 1-desamino-8-D-arginine vasopressin to stabilize platelet function. Enteral feedings should be held for up to six hours prior to the procedure unless it is minor and positioning will not increase the risk of aspiration. Preoxygenation of all patients for about 15 minutes prior to the procedure may also be beneficial.

a. Coadministration of a narcotic, a benzodiazepine, and a neuromuscular blocking agent is essentially general anesthesia, depending on dosage. Monitoring and airway management skills must be equivalent to those standard in an operating room. Pulse oximetry, ECG, and blood pressure measurement represent a minimum standard of monitoring for even minor procedures. Invasive hemodynamic monitoring or end-tidal CO_2 monitoring may be required for more complex undertakings.

3. Operations performed in the ICU. Operations performed at the bedside will vary among ICUs based on specialty orientation and case mix. Among trauma patients, tracheostomy, thoracentesis and tube thoracostomy, paracentesis, cholecystostomy, and bedside laparotomy may be performed.

a. Tracheostomy. Tracheostomy is increasingly performed percutaneously, although some debate persists as to whether percutaneous tracheostomy is preferable. The most common indication for tracheostomy is acute respiratory failure with prolonged mechanical ventilation, followed by airway "protection" for the patient who is obtunded or whose gag reflex is impaired or absent. The third most common indication for tracheostomy is maxillofacial trauma.

  i. The timing of tracheostomy remains controversial. Proponents of early tracheostomy (generally within 7 days, as opposed to after 14 days) believe that pulmonary toilet is enhanced, leading to a lower incidence of pneumonia and shorter durations of mechanical ventilation and ICU length of stay. Detractors maintain that the putative benefits of early tracheostomy remain unproved, but recent comparative trials have found significantly lower incidences of unplanned extubation, pneumonia, and mortality following early tracheostomy, along with decreased length of stay in the ICU and duration of mechanical ventilation.

b. Thoracentesis and tube thoracostomy. Common bedside procedures on the thorax at the bedside include thoracentesis and tube thoracostomy. Thoracotomy is performed rarely and usually only for patients in extremis. Opening the pleural cavity has implications for oxygenation, ventilation, hemodynamics, and gas exchange that can be profound. Major thoracic surgery may require ventilatory support (e.g., split-lung ventilation) that is difficult to provide at the bedside.

c. Paracentesis. Ascites is common in critically ill patients, due to hepatic, renal, or cardiac failure, or anasarca with hypoalbuminemia. Occasionally, the presence of ascites warrants removal by paracentesis either for diagnosis or therapy. One therapeutic indication for paracentesis is decompression of abdominal compartment syndrome, with ascites due to massive fluid resuscitation. Rare but serious complications of paracentesis include local or intraperitoneal hemorrhage or bowel perforation. The abdominal examination and blood count should be monitored after the procedure. Hypotension may occur after large-volume paracentesis; restitution of intravascular fluid volume with crystalloid or colloid approximating the oncotic constitution of the removed fluid is restorative. Persistent drainage (ascitic fistula) may ensue after reaccumulation of tense ascites but is managed easily by placement of sutures in the abdominal wall.

d. Cholecystostomy. Acute acalculous cholecystitis is a manifestation of splanchnic ischemia-reperfusion injury relating to shock and resuscitation. Other risk factors include sepsis, diabetes mellitus, abdominal vasculitis, systemic lupus erythematous, congestive heart failure, renal disease, total parenteral nutrition, and hypovolemia. Abdominal pain (if the patient can communicate), fever, leukocytosis, jaundice from cholestasis, and gallbladder ischemia are characteristic.

  i. The diagnosis of acute acalculous cholecystitis may be difficult because most patients cannot communicate their symptoms. Additionally, the gallbladder may be only one of several sources of sepsis. Consequently, the diagnosis is most frequently accomplished by ultrasound imaging of the gallbladder. Gallbladder wall thickness of ≥3.5 mm with pericholecystic fluid is diagnostic. Computed tomography is equally accurate for the same findings.

ii. The usual treatment for acute acalculous cholecystitis is percutaneous cholecystostomy, either at the bedside or in the interventional radiology suite. Under local anesthesia and ultrasound guidance, the gallbladder is punctured, and an 8 F pigtail catheter is placed by the Seldinger technique. Complications of percutaneous cholecystostomy include bleeding and, rarely, visceral perforation. More common is spillage of infected bile into the peritoneum either during the procedure or alongside the indwelling tube. Consequently, if the patient worsens or fails to improve, the patient should be imaged to ensure that the catheter is patent, that bile has not leaked into the abdomen, and that no other diagnosis is possible. After the patient improves, a tube cholecystogram should confirm the absence of gallstones; if absent, the tube may be removed without interval cholecystectomy.

e. **Bedside laparotomy.** The OR is generally preferred for laparotomy, with optimized anesthetic adminstration, nursing, lighting, availability of instruments, and facilitated exposure. However, certain patients may be too unstable for transport or need immediate laparotomy in the ICU. The most urgent indication for bedside laparotomy may be decompression of abdominal compartment syndrome. Other reasons for bedside laparotomy include changing of abdominal dressings, or treatment of diffuse abdominal infection (tertiary peritonitis). Abdominal operations that require intestinal anastomoses, ostomy creation, or definitive control of hemorrhage are better performed in the OR. However, for patients who need a change of abdominal packing or a washout of infected fluid, bedside laparotomy is an option. Occasionally the open abdomen may also be closed at the bedside. Options include the vacuum pack, absorbable mesh, nonabsorbable mesh with a zipper, or other reclosable prosthetic devices.

XI. **REHABILITATION IN THE ICU.** Historically, bed rest and prolonged immobilization were commonplace as treatment, but are now understood to be detrimental. The deleterious effects of bed rest become apparent in several systems within 72 hours. Muscle strength decreases by as much as 1.5% per day during strict bed rest, with the greatest loss after the first week. Even when strength is only mildly decreased, poor endurance can still be a primary functional limitation. Both the central and peripheral cardiovascular systems are altered, with increased heart rate and decreased stroke volume and cardiac size. Osteoclysis also occurs, and on occasion can result in hypercalcemia. Pressure ulcers also occur with prolonged bed rest, with the incidence increasing dramatically after 7 days of critical illness.

A. Basic mobilization in the ICU can counteract the effects of prolonged bed rest, and maintain or improve strength, functional ability, and endurance. Patients who are unstable need to be turned every 2 hours around the clock to avoid prolonged pressure on the occiput, calacanei, trochanters, presacral tissue, and other pressure-sensitive areas. Particularly with prolonged ICU stays, initial interventions are passive, including an evaluation of positioning and the need for splinting devices to maintain joint integrity and to prevent skin breakdown. More stable patients are supported for their ability to roll, shift weight, grab, sit, and stand. The transition from a supine to sitting position can be especially challenging. Adequate pain control is mandatory to initiate mobilization.

1. Mechanical ventilation is not a contraindication to rehabilitation, assuming the patient is oxygenated adequately. If the patient is utilizing accessory muscles or is tachypneic (>35 breaths/minute), therapy may be inappropriate. For patients breathing spontaneously, therapy can promote improved lung aeration, rib cage expansion, diaphragm capacity, and decreased accessory muscle use. Participation of medically tenuous patients will fluctuate session to session, with respiratory rate, heart rate, and arterial oxygen saturation indicating how

well a patient is tolerating treatment. The impact of medications and pain on heart rate must also be considered.

2. Arousal level is also a frequent limitation. Elevating the head of the bed to stimulate the reticular activating system, repositioning, and olfactory and tactile stimulation are all used to enhance responsiveness. For the agitated patient, relaxation techniques, reorientation, and decreased environmental stimulation may be attempted before pharmacological treatment.

XII. END-OF-LIFE CARE. The mortality of blunt trauma is approximately 3%, whereas mortality is approximately 7% for penetrating trauma. Elderly patients have higher rates of mortality for a given degree of injury severity, sometimes bordering on the unsalvageable (e.g., TBI with a Glasgow Coma Score ≤8). Recognition that injuries or the complications thereof (e.g., sepsis and multiple organ dysfunction syndrome) may be nonsurvivable is crucial for effective and compassionate management. Consumerism in health care and the tenet of patient self-determinism are ending the era of paternalism in health care, in which the doctor "knows best." Patients (when they can participate) and their surrogates (when patients cannot participate) expect, and are entitled to, sufficient information about their diagnosis and prognosis to participate in decision making in a meaningful manner, including the right to forego additional treatment or to withdraw care, resulting in death.

A. Unfortunately, the majority of injured patients, young or old, have not made known their wishes for life-sustaining care, leaving trauma surgeons and surrogates to undertake what is believed to be in the best interests of the patient. The process is often laden with stress, given that the parties usually do not have a prior relationship, and surrogates may not be entirely reconciled (if not in denial) to the recent injury or newly acquired knowledge of the poor prognosis. In addition, caregivers may be struggling with the fact that the adverse outcome may sometimes be related to iatrogenesis, and a desire to "get the patient through."

B. Patients or surrogates should be asked if advance directives exist, whether living wills, durable powers of attorney for health care, or do-not-resuscitate (DNR) orders, depending on individual state laws. Patients with capacity must be offered the opportunity to designate a health care agent (proxy) by law in many states. Patients who lack capacity but who have executed an advance directive may have designated a health care agent; if so, that person should be identified and engaged in the dialogue as soon as possible.

1. The parameters under which limits on the provision of care may be set vary among jurisdictions, and clinicians must be aware of those applicable specifically to their practice locale. For example, not all jurisdictions use the same definition of "medical futility," or place the same weight on the living will. When end-of-life care planning is discussed, the patient's prognosis, religious preference, and functional limitations are all of paramount consideration. For example, some religious groups may refuse blood transfusion. It may be desired to arrange for hospital discharge so that the patient may die at home, or autopsy may be refused, even if mandated legally. Other religious groups may reject the concept of brain death as death in fact if cardiac electrical activity persists. Cardiopulmonary resuscitation may be refused in isolation (the classic DNR order), care may be limited ("no escalation"), or it may be withdrawn (although some jurisdictions do not distinguish between withholding and withdrawing of care). Most hospitals now have ethics committees that can assist in end-of-life care planning, particularly when there are varying opinions or frank disputes among clinicians or between clinicians and surrogates.

2. When care is withdrawn, the clinician should be the patient's advocate, seeking to eliminate suffering during the process. Often, mechanical ventilation is withdrawn. If the patient is brain dead by definition there will be no spontaneous breathing efforts, but in other circumstances there may be agonal respirations. It is permissible to relieve suffering with opioid medications, even if so doing may hasten demise by exacerbating hemodynamic instability.

3. However, palliative care is not just limited to the process of withdrawal of care, the dying patient only, or to just the patient himself or herself. Bereavement may accompany critical illness or injury regardless of the prognosis or outcome. Whereas the goals of critical care first and foremost are the saving of life, with the alleviation of suffering and improving the quality of life being secondary goals, for palliative care the hierarchy is reversed. Integration of critical care and palliative care brings these various (and sometimes conflicting) goals into concordance.

   a. Quality palliative care focus efforts in seven domains: patient/family-centered decision making, communication within the care team and with patients/families, continuity of care, emotional support for families, spiritual support for families, symptom management and comfort care, and emotional and organizational support for ICU clinicians. Psychosocial support should be offered to patients and families within 24 hours of admission, perhaps by formal assessment of an interdisciplinary team consisting of physicians, nurses, social workers, clergy, and others. Within 72 hours of admission, a family meeting is recommended with physician and nurse, to develop the comprehensive care plan, and to document the plan in the medical record.

XIII. IDENTIFICATION AND CARE OF THE POTENTIAL ORGAN DONOR (Chapter 44). Dying patients or their surrogates may be able to make the gift of life after death in the form of organ donation for orthotopic transplantation. The shortage of donor organs is so acute that to expand the donor pool, organs with marginal function may be considered for transplantation. For example, neither age nor bloodstream infection represent absolute contraindications to organ donation at the present time. In many jurisdictions, solicitation of potential organ donors is mandated legally. Recent initiatives by the Joint Commission on Accreditation of Healthcare Organizations (JCAHO) have added successful donor solicitation and organ procurement to its quality measures.

A. Potential organ donors may either be brain dead (in which case the organs are removed after declaration, before the patient is removed from life support) or neurologically devastated with no hope of recovery, but still with reflexive activity (in which case life support is removed, death ensues, and organs are removed thereafter in relative haste). The latter situation is facilitated by withdrawal of life support in the OR with the organ harvesting team at the ready. In all cases, the physicians assessing neurologic function and declaring death must not be involved with organ procurement or transplantation in any way. Criteria for the diagnosis of brain death are discussed elsewhere in Chapter 44. Regardless of the protocol, federal regulations require the local organ procurement organization to be notified in a timely manner of an impending death, so that the suitability of the donor can be assessed and donation can be discussed with the family. Increased rates of organ donation are achieved when trained individuals make the solicitation for donation.

B. Once donation has been agreed to, the donor maintenance phase supercedes. Hemodynamic instability is common and increases in proportion to the length of time between the declaration of brain death and organ procurement. Progression from brain death to somatic death can result in the ultimate medically unsuitability of up to 20% of initially suitable potential donors, so that careful management of the donor is crucial. Standardized algorithms and protocols are beneficial for donor maintenance in "stable" condition.

1. **Cardiovascular support.** Adverse effects of brain ischemia on the cardiovascular system include a sympathetic adrenergic diathesis to try to maintain CPP. Brain ischemia is associated with left ventricular subendocardial myonecrosis. Spinal cord ischemia coincides with transtentorial herniation and terminates the sympathetic response, adding to cardiac dysfunction and vasodilation.

   a. Management goals in the potential donor include maintenance of normovolemia, blood pressure, and optimization of cardiac output to promote organ perfusion while minimizing the use of vasoactive drugs. Hypotension is present initially in up to 80% of donors, and may persist despite vasoactive drug therapy in 20% of donors, and increases the risk of cardiac arrest and loss of the donor in the maintenance phase.

  b. Minimum thresholds include a mean arterial blood pressure >60 mmHg, maximal doses of dopamine (DA) or dobutamine (DOB) of 10 μg/kg/minute, urine output >1.0 mL/kg/hour, and echocardiographic left ventricular ejection fraction of ≥45%. If the parameters cannot be maintained, a PA catheter helps to assess volume status (treated with fluids or diuretics), pump status (treated with inotropes-DA, DOB, or epinephrine [EPI] ≤0.05 mg/kg/minute), and resistance (treated with EPI or norEPI ≤0.05 mg/kg/minute). If these goals are met with fluids or inotropes, monitoring is continued up to the time of procurement. If goals are not met, hormone replacement therapy is begun (albeit controversially), including thyroxine (20-μg bolus, then 3 μg/kg/hour), methylprednisolone (15 mg/kg bolus, then repeat at 24 hours), and insulin (10-U bolus [with 50% dextrose if necessary], insulin at least at 1 U/hour to maintain serum glucose concentration 80–150 mg/dL).

  c. Red blood cell concentrates are recommended to maintain hematocrit at 30%, and Ringer's lactate solution of 0.45% NaCl with $NaHCO_3$ 50 mmol/L (if the donor is acidemic) is administered rather than 0.9% NaCl, to minimize hypernatremia from neurogenic diabetes insipidus. Both hyperglycemia and hypernatremia induce an osmotic diuresis that induces hypovolemia. All infused fluids should be warmed to limit the risk of hypothermia. A more liberal fluid administration strategy is indicated if kidney harvesting is anticipated but procurement of the lungs is not.

  d. Cardiac dysrhythmias are common with brain herniation, institution of inotropic therapy, or preterminally, and are often refractory to antiarrhythmic therapy. Whenever possible, the cause of the cardiac rhythm disturbance should be corrected. Standard antiarrhythmic therapy for supraventricular (amiodarone) or ventricular (amiodarone or lidocaine) is indicated. Bradyarrhythmias due to brain stem compression will not respond to atropine, therefore isoproterenol or EPI will be needed. Cardiac arrest should be managed by standard Advanced Cardiac Life Support protocols, because recovery of cardiac function can result in successful transplantation.

2. Pulmonary support. Lung procurement is relatively rare (~20%), owing to VILI, pneumonia in patients with TBI, and neurogenic pulmonary edema accompanying brain death. The goals of mechanical ventilation of the potential organ donor include a FiO_2 of 0.40, PaO_2 >100 mmHg or SaO_2 >95%, $PaCO_2$ 35 to 40 mmHg, arterial pH 7.35 to 7.45, V_T 8 to 10 mL/kg, PEEP 5 cm H_2O, and static airway pressure <30 cm H_2O.

  a. Atelectasis and pulmonary edema are correctable causes of hypoxemia that preclude lung procurement. Bronchoscopy and targeted ventilatory maneuvers to promote lung expansion can increase procurement rates and organ quality. Fluid administration should be judicious (PWP = 12 mmHg, or CVP = 6 cm H_2O), including colloid administration rather than crystalloids, if lung harvesting is anticipated. Diuretic therapy may be necessary. Albuterol has been shown to promote the clearance of pulmonary edema, and may be coadministered with diuretic therapy.

3. Miscellaneous support

  a. Diabetes insipidus results from death of the posterior pituitary, and contributes to hyperosmolarity, hemodynamic instability, and electrolyte abnormalities due to excessive loss of free water. Diabetes insipidus must be distinguished from other causes of polyuria (e.g., mannitol, hyperglycemia, diuretics), but can be excluded quickly by a normal serum sodium concentration. Urine output should be matched mL/mL with 5% dextrose in water, up to 200 mL/hour, but higher levels of urine output require treatment with either arginine vasopressin or 1-desamino-8-D-arginine vasopressin.

b. Hyperglycemia is common, and must be controlled. Failure to control blood glucose leads to increased graft loss following liver transplantation, and hyperglycemic damage to pancreatic beta cells is also a risk factor for graft dysfunction after pancreas transplantation.

c. Coagulopathy is a common consequence of the release of thromboplastin cerebral gangliosides, and plasminogen-rich substrate from injured or necrotic brain. These factors can cause profound coagulopathy combined with other factors such as ongoing hemorrhage, transfusion, hypothermia, and acidosis, all of which may be present in the potential donor. Blood product therapy should aim to maintain hematocrit at 30%, international normalized ratio <2.0, and platelet count >80,000. The risk of sensitization may be minimized by using cytomegalovirus-seronegative blood.

d. Potential donors may become poikilothermic due to loss of the hypothalamus and the inability to shiver or vasoconstrict, exacerbated by environmental factors and administration of unwarmed fluids. Adverse effects of hypothermia include cardiac dysfunction, arrhythmias, coagulopathy, leftward shift of the oxyhemoglobin dissociation curve, and diuresis. Core temperature should be maintained >35°C using warmed fluids, heated humidification of inhaled gases, and liberal use of convective warming blankets. Hypothermia is easier to prevent than to treat, and temperatures lower than 35°C preclude or delay the declaration of brain death.

XIV. PATIENT SAFETY AND SYSTEM MANAGEMENT

A. The hazards of accidental injury by sharps (e.g., needles, scalpel blades) and the risks of bloodborne transmission of etiologic agents are real. Policies and procedures have been changed in all ORs to minimize the risk, which has been decreasing. In the OR, particular attention is paid to communication among team members, protocols for passing sharp instruments to and from the operative field and instrument table, and meticulous accounting of sharps throughout the operation. Similar attention to detail is mandatory if surgery at the bedside in the ICU will be made as safe as possible for the patient and the operating team. Sterile gowns, sterile double gloves, masks, caps, and eye protection should be used for any bedside procedure where the possibility exists of splashing blood or body fluids.

In particular, accounting for the whereabouts of sharps at the bedside remains an issue. The mattress must never be used as a "pincushion" for needles. The period of highest risk to practitioners appears to be during clean-up in the aftermath of minor procedures, during which the accounting process for sharps is informal and indeed, often haphazard. When drapes are collected for disposal at the end of the procedure (usually by the person who performed the procedure, who may have been working only with the patient's primary nurse), it is easy to overlook an unsecured sharp within the folds of the drape. Even if no injury occurs at the bedside, if a sharp is discarded inadvertently in the trash rather than the ubiquitous sharps containers, other hospital workers and sanitation workers are placed at risk.

B. Avoiding error

1. Most in-hospital trauma mortality occurs in the ICU during the first few days of admission because of closed head injury, respiratory failure, or refractory hemorrhagic shock; these deaths are largely not preventable. The remainder, many of which may be preventable, occur late, usually because of MODS. Technical, monitoring, and critical care management errors have been reported in up to one half of preventable trauma deaths.

a. Trauma care is high risk for medical errors. The patients are unstable, information (historical or laboratory data) may be incomplete, time-critical decisions must be made, and many medical and paramedical disciplines must be coordinated, making clear communication of paramount importance. Baseline mortality rates are high, the patient care is complex, and evidence-based management protocols inform only a portion of clinical decision making, especially for care after the initial resuscitation period. Recognizing this, trauma surgeons have been in the forefront of error reduction and quality improvement in medicine, long before interest became widespread.

2. Estimates of preventable death vary widely, indicating the variability of care inherent in trauma management and the need for standardized approaches. To reduce errors, institutions need effective means to identify errors and reduce error-associated deaths, which by their very infrequency may be difficult to characterize. Moreover, errors may occur for many reasons, including predisposing structural and systems factors, lack of knowledge, defective information processing, and errors of communication.

3. Trauma-related errors may be characterized in four domains: phase of trauma care, type of intervention, type of error, and cause of error.

   a. Errors characterized by the phase of trauma management may occur during initial assessment and resuscitation, secondary assessment, transport, initial intervention in the ED or OR, or in later phases of care in the ICU, on the ward, or even in the rehabilitation phase.

   b. Errors may occur in several clinical interventions in trauma care, including control of hemorrhage, airway management, hemodynamic resuscitation, management prioritization for unstable patients, performance of procedures, prophylaxis of potential complications, missed or delayed diagnoses, and several others.

   c. Errors of intervention may be characterized as to a relationship to diagnosis, treatment, or prevention, and further as to an input error (e.g., lack of data), intention error (e.g, lack of knowledge or skill, includng communication skill), or execution errors (e.g., technical flaw). Certain types of errors are characteristic of some domains, whereas other errors encompass multiple domains. For example, treatment-related errors (which are most common) are often intention errors, whereas prevention-related errors are most commonly related to execution. Diagnostic errors, which are less common than treatment and prevention errors, are most common during the secondary trauma survey and in the ICU. Errors of hemorrhage control (the most prevalent trauma-related errors) are common during initial assessment and in the ICU, whereas errors related to procedures and prophylaxis are far more common in the ICU.

   d. The initial assessment, resuscitation, and initial intervention phases of trauma care are particularly error-prone. Institutional policies regarding care in both the ED and ICU can reduce errors, but not prevent them entirely. The majority of error-related deaths are intention errors that affect treatment; these types of errors are most amenable to remediation with protocols and algorithms. However, protocols alone will be ineffective in reducing error when interactive approaches are used to facilitate learning through repetition and scenario management. In contrast, execution errors are addressed through technical training, and ensuring through appropriate supervision that those performing tasks are competent and credentialed for the task. Input errors require the proper use and interpretation of diagnostic tests. Attention to detail, checklists, and supervision can reduce both execution and input errors. Regardless of the type of error-related problem or its effective remediation, learning from errors must occur in an environment of trust and transparency, working to improve process rather than assign blame or exact retribution.

Bibliography

Abdeen O, Mehta RL. Dialysis modalities in the intensive care unit. *Crit Care Clin* 2002;18:223–247.

Annane D, Bellisant E, Bollaert PE, et al. Corticosteroids for severe sepsis and septic shock: A systematic review and meta-analysis. *BMJ* 2004;329:480–484.

Annane D, Bellisant E, Cavaillon JM. Septic shock. *Lancet* 2005;365:63–78.

Annane D, Maxime V, Ibrahim F, et al. Diagnosis of adrenal insufficiency in severe sepsis and septic shock. *Am J Respir Crit Care Med*. Published ahead of print September 14, 2006. Available at: http://ajrccm.atsjournals.org/cgi/content/abstract/174/12/1319.

Annane D, Sebille V, Charpentier C, et al. Effect of treatment with low doses of hydrocortisone and fludrocortisone on mortality in patients with septic shock. *JAMA* 2002; 288:862–871.

Arbabi S, Campion E, Ahrns KS, et al. *Beta-blocker Use Is Associated with Improved Outcomes in Adult Trauma Patients.* Proceedings of the Sixty-fifth Annual Meeting of the American Association for the Surgery of Trauma, New Orleans, LA, September 28–30, 2006. Abstract 42.

Balk RA. Optimum treatment of severe sepsis and septic shock: Evidence in support of the recommendations. *Dis Mon* 2004;50:163–213.

Barie PS, Hydo LJ, Eachempati SR. Causes and consequences of fever complicating critical surgical illness. *Surg Infect* 2004;5:145–159.

Barie PS, Eachempati SR. Acute acalculous cholecystitis. *Curr Gastroenterol Rep* 2003; 5:302–309.

Barie PS, Bacchetta MD, Eachempati SR. The contemporary surgical intensive care unit: Structure, staffing, and issues. *Surg Clin North Am* 2000;80:791–804.

Beilman GE, Groehler KE, Lazaron V, Ortner JP. Near-infrared spectroscopy measurement of regional tissue oxyhemoglobin saturation during hemorrhagic shock. *Shock* 1999;12:196–200.

Bochicchio GV, Sung J, Joshi M, et al. Persistent hyperglycemia is predictive of outcome in critically ill trauma patients. *J Trauma* 2005;58:921-924. Erratum in: *J Trauma* 2005;59:1277–1278.

Bouman CS, Oudemans-Van Straaten HM, Tijssen JG, et al. Effects of early high-volume continuous venovenous hemofiltration on survival and recovery of renal function in intensive care patients with acute renal failure: A prospective, randomized trial. *Crit Care Med* 2002;30:2205–2211.

Brasel KJ, Borgstrom CD, Weigelt JA. Cost-effective prevention of pulmonary embolus in high-risk trauma patients. *J Trauma* 1997;42:456–462.

Buchman TG, Cassell J, Ray SE, et al. Who should manage the dying patient? Rescue, shame, and the surgical ICU dilemma. *J Am Coll Surg* 2002;194:665–673.

Chang A, Schyve PM, Croteau RJ, et al. The JCAHO patient safety event taxonomy: A standardized terminology and classification schema for near misses and adverse events. *Int J Qual Health Care* 2005;17:95–105.

Clermont G, Acker CG, Angus DC, et al. Renal failure in the ICU: Comparison of the impact of acute renal failure and end-stage renal disease on ICU outcomes. *Kidney Int* 2002;62:986–996.

Cohn SM, Crookes BA, Proctor KG. Near-infrared spectroscopy in resuscitation. *J Trauma* 2003;54:S199–S202.

Cohn SM, Nathens AB, Moore FA, et al. Near infrared spectroscopy predicts organ dysfunction in trauma patients with shock: A prospective cohort study [abstract]. *J Trauma* 2006;61:509.

Cook DJ, Fuller HD, Guyatt GH, et al. Risk factors for gastrointestinal bleeding in critically ill patients. Canadian Critical Care Trials Group. *N Engl J Med* 1994; 330:377–381.

Cook DJ, Meade MO, Hand LE, McMullin JP. Toward understanding evidence uptake: Semirecumbency for pneumonia prevention. *Crit Care Med* 2002;30:1472–1477.

Cook DJ, Reeve BK, Guyatt GH, et al. Stress ulcer prophylaxis in critically ill patients: Resolving discordant meta-analyses. *JAMA* 1996;275:308–314.

Cook DJ, Rocker G, Giacommi M, et al. Understanding and changing attitudes toward withdrawal and withholding of life support in the intensive care unit. *Crit Care Med* 2006;34:S317–S323.

Cooper MS, Stewart PM. Corticosteroid insufficiency in acutely ill patients. *N Engl J Med* 2003;348:727–734.

Cotton BA, Snodgrass KB, Fleming SB, et al. *Beta-blocker Exposure Is Associated with Improved Survival Following Severe Traumatic Brain Injury.* Proceedings of the Sixty-fifth Annual Meeting of the American Association for the Surgery of Trauma, New Orleans, LA, September 28-30, 2006. Abstract 43.

Crookes BA, Cohn SM, Bloch S, et al. Can near-infrared spectroscopy identify the severity of shock in trauma patients? *J Trauma* 2005;58:806–813.

Davis JW, Hoyt DB, McArdle MS, et al. An analysis of errors causing morbidity and mortality in a trauma system: A guide for quality improvement. *J Trauma* 1992;32: 660–666.

De Backer D, Creteur J, Preiser JC, et al. Microvascular blood flow is altered in patients with sepsis. *Am J Respir Crit Care Med* 2002;166:98–104.

Deitch EA, Dayal SD. Intensive care unit management of the trauma patient. *Crit Care Med* 2006;34:2294–2301.

Dellinger RP, Carlet JM, Giannotti GD, et al. Surviving sepsis campaign guidelines for management of severe sepsis and septic chock. *Crit Care Med* 2004;32:858–873.

Dutton RP, Mackenzie CF, Scalea TM. Hypotensive resuscitation during active hemorrhage: Impact on in-hospital mortality. *J Trauma* 2002;52:1141–1146.

Eachempati SR, Barie PS, Reed RL II. Serum bicarbonate as an endpoint of resuscitation in critically ill patients. *Surg Infect* 2003;4:193–198.

Eachempati SR, Flomenbaum N, Seifert C, et al. Alterations of preliminary readings on radiographic examinations minimally affect outcomes of trauma patients discharged from the emergency department. *J Trauma* 2000;48:654–658.

Fong Y, Whalen GF, Hariri RH, Barie PS. Utility of daily chest radiographs in the surgical intensive care unit: A prospective study. *Arch Surg* 1995;130:764–768.

Fontes M. Progress in mechanical ventilation. *Curr Opin Anaesthesiol* 2002;15:45–51.

Freeman RB, Giatras I, Falagas ME, et al. Outcome of organs procured from bacteremic donors. *Transplantation* 1999;68:1107–1111.

Gasser M, Waaga AM, Laskowski IA, Tilney NL. Organ transplantation from brain-dead donors: Its impact on short and long term outcome revisited. *Transplant Rev* 2001;15:1–10.

Gattinoni L, Brazzi L, Pelosi P, et al. A trial of goal-oriented hemodynamic therapy in critically ill patients. *N Engl J Med* 1995;333:1025–1032.

Gearhart MM, Luchette FA, Proctor MC, et al. The risk assessment profile score identifies trauma patients at risk for deep vein thrombosis. *Surgery* 2000;128:631–640.

Geerts WH, Jay RM, Code KL, et al. A comparison of low-dose heparin with low moleculat weight heparin as prophylaxis against venous thromboembolism after major trauma. *N Engl J Med* 1996;335:701–707.

Gore DC, Chinkes D, Heggers J, et al. Association of hyperglycemia with increased mortality after severe burn injury. *J Trauma* 2001;51:540–544.

Gortmaker SL, Beasley CL, Sheehy E, et al. Improving the request process to increase family consent for organ donation. *J Transpl Coord* 1998;8:210–217.

Gruen RL, Jurkovich GJ, McIntyre LK, et al. Patterns of errors contributing to trauma mortality: Lessons learned from 2,594 deaths. *Ann Surg* 2006;244:371–380.

Helmreich RL, Musson DM, Sexton JB. Human factors and safety in surgery. In Manuel BN, Nora P, eds. *Surgical Patient Safety: Essential Information for Surgeons in Today's Environment.* Chicago, Ill: American College of Surgeons; 2004:5–18.

Herndon DN, Hart DW, Steven EW, et al. Reversal of catabolism by beta-blockade after severe burns. *N Engl J Med* 2001;345:1223–1229.

Hoste EA, De Waele JJ. Physiologic consequences of acute renal failure on the critically ill. *Crit Care Clin* 2005;21:251–260.

Inflammation and the Host Response to Injury, a large-scale collaborative project: Patient-oriented research core—Standard operating procedures for clinical care. II. Guidelines for prevention, diagnosis and treatment of ventilator-associated pneumonia (VAP) in the trauma patient. *J Trauma* 2006;60:1106–1113.

Jenkins DH, Reilly PM, Schwab CW. Improving the approach to organ donation: A review. *World J Surg* 1999;23:644–649.

Kincaid EH, Miller PR, Meredith JW, et al. Elevated arterial base deficit in trauma patients: A marker of impaired oxygen utilization. *J Am Coll Surg* 1998;187:873–877.

Knudson MM, Morabito D, Paiment GD, et al. Use of low molecular weight heparin in preventing thromboembolism in trauma patients. *J Trauma* 1996;41:446–459.

Levy MM, McBride DL. End-of-life care in the intensive care unit: State of the art in 2006. *Crit Care Med* 2006;34:S306–S308.

Lopez-Navidad A, Caballero F. Extended criteria for organ acceptance: Strategies for achieving organ safety and increasing organ pool. *Clin Transplant* 2003;17:308–324.

Maki DG, Crnich CJ. Line sepsis in the ICU: Prevention, diagnosis, and management. *Semin Respir Crit Care Med* 2003;24:23–36.

McGee DC, Gould MK. Preventing complications of central venous catheterization. *N Engl J Med* 2003;348:1123–1133.

McKinley BA, Marvin RG, Cocanour CS, Moore FA. Tissue hemoglobin O_2 saturation during resuscitation of hemorrhagic shock monitored using near infrared spectroscopy. *J Trauma* 2000;48:637–642.

Minei JP, Natrhens AB, West M, et al., and the Inflammation and the Host Response to Injury Large Scale Collaborative Research Program Investigators. Inflammation and the Host Response to Injury, a Large-Scale Collaborative Project: Patient-oriented research core—standard operating procedures for clinical care. II. Guidelines for prevention, diagnosis and treatment of ventilator-associated pneumonia (VAP) in the trauma patient. *J Trauma* 2006;60:1106–1113.

Mizock BA. Alterations in fuel metabolism in critical illness: Hyperglycaemia. *Best Pract Res Clin Endocrinol Metab* 2001;15:2140–2144.

Moore FA, McKinley BA, Moore EE, et al. Inflammation and the Host Response to Injury, a large-scale collaborative project: Patient-oriented research core—Standard operating procedures for clinical care. III. Guidelines for shock resuscitation. *J Trauma* 2006;61:82–89.

Morris RJ, Woodcock JP. Evidence-based compression-prevention of stasis and deep vein thrombosis. *Ann Surg* 2004;239:162–171.

Mosenthal AC, Murphy PA. Interdisciplinary model for palliative care in the trauma and surgical intensive care unit: Robert Wood Johnson Foundation Demonstration Project for Improving Palliative Care in the Intensive Care Unit. *Crit Care Med* 2006;34:S399–S403.

Mosenthal AC, Murphy PA. Trauma care and palliative care: Time to integrate the two? *J Am Coll Surg* 2003;197:509–516.

Mularski RA, Curtis JR, Billings JA, et al. Proposed quality measures for palliative care in the critically ill: A consensus from the Robert Wood Johnson Foundation Critical Care Workgroup. *Crit Care Med* 2006;34:S404–S411.

Myers DE. Noninvasive method for measuring local hemoglobin oxygen saturation in tissue using wide gap second derivative near-infrared spectroscopy. *J Biomed Optics* 2005;10:1–18.

Nathens AB, Johnson JL, Minei JP, et al., and the Inflammation and the Host Response to Injury Investigators. Inflammation and the Host Response to Injury, a large-scale collaborative project: Patient-oriented research core—Standard operating procedures for clinical care. I. Guidelines for mechanical ventilation of the trauma patient. *J Trauma* 2005;59:764–769.

National Heart, Lung, and Blood Institute Acute Respiratory Distress Syndrome (ARDS) Clinical Trials Network; Wheeler AP, Bernard GR, Thompson BT, et al. Pulmonary-artery versus central venous catheter to guide treatment of acute lung injury. *N Engl J Med* 2006;354:2213–2214.

Offner PJ, Hawkes A, Madayag R, et al. The role of temporary inferior vena cava filters in critically ill surgical patients. *Arch Surg* 2003;138:591–595.

Offner PJ, Moore EE, Biffl WL, et al. Increased rate of infection associated with transfusions of old blood after severe injury. *Arch Surg* 2002;137:711–717.

Phu NH, Hien TT, Mai NT, et al. Hemofiltration and peritoneal dialysis in infection-associated acute renal failure in Vietnam. *N Engl J Med* 2002;347:895–902.

Pittas AG, Siegel RD, Lau J. Insulin therapy for critically ill hospitalized patients. A meta-analysis of randomized controlled trials. *Arch Intern Med* 2004;164:2005–2011.

Polk HC Jr, Birkmeyer JD, Hunt D, et al. Quality and safety in surgical care. *Ann Surg* 2006;243:439–448.

Porter JM, Ivatury RR, Kavarana M, Verrier R. The surgical intensive care unit as a cost-efficient substitute for an operating room at a Level I trauma center. *Am Surg* 1999;65:328–330.

Prigent H, Maxime V, Annane D. Science review: Mechanisms of impaired adrenal function in sepsis and molecular actions of glucocorticoids. *Crit Care* 2004;8:243–252.

Reason J. Human error: Models and management. *BMJ* 2000;320:768–770.

Rebuck JA, Murry KR, Rhoney DH, et al. Infection related to intracranial pressure monitors in adults: Analysis of risk factors and antibiotic prophylaxis. *J Neurol Neurosurg Psychiatry* 2000;69:381–384.

Rivers E, Nguyen B, Havstad S, et al. Early goal-directed therapy in the treatment of severe sepsis and septic shock. *N Engl J Med* 2001;345:1368–1377.

Roberts I, Alderson P, Bunn F, et al. Colloids versus crystalloids for fluid resuscitation in critically ill patients. *Cochrane Database Syst Rev* 2004;4:CD000567.

Rogers FB. Venous thromboembolism in trauma patients: A review. *Surgery* 2001;130: 1–12.

Rosendale JD, Chabalewski FL, McBride MA, et al. Increased transplanted organs from the use of a standardized donor management protocol. *Am J Transplant* 2002;2:761–768.

Rumbak MJ, Newton M, Truncale T, et al. A prospective, randomized study comparing early percutaneous dilational tracheotomy to prolonged translaryngeal intubation (delayed tracheotomy) in critically ill medical patients. *Crit Care Med* 2004;32: 1689–1694. Erratum in: *Crit Care Med* 2004;32:256.

Salman M, Glantzounis GK, Yang W, et al. Measurement of critical lower limb tissue hypoxia by coupling chemical and optical techniques. *Clin Sci* 2005;108:159–165.

Schiffl H, Lang SM, Fischer R. Daily hemodialysis and the outcome of acute renal failure. *N Engl J Med* 2002;346:305–310.

Schnuelle P, Lorenz D, Mueller A, et al. Donor catecholamine use reduces acute allograft rejection and improves graft survival in solid organ transplantation. *Kidney Int* 1999;56:738–746.

Schrier RW, Wang W. Acute renal failure and sepsis. *N Engl J Med* 2004;351:159–169.

Shah MR, Hasselblad V, Stevenson LW, et al. Impact of the pulmonary artery catheter in critically ill patients: Meta-analysis of randomized clinical trials. *JAMA* 2005;294:1664–1670.

Spain DA, Richardson JD, Polk HC Jr, et al. Venous thromboembolism in the high-risk trauma patient: Do risks justify aggressive screening and prophylaxis? *J Trauma* 1997;42:463–469.

Streeten DHP, Anderson GH Jr, Bonaventura MM, et al. The potential for serious consequences from misinterpreting normal responses to the rapid adrenocorticotropin test. *J Clin Endocrinol Metab* 1996;81:285–290.

Sundaresan S, Semenkovich J, Ochoa L, et al. Successful outcome of lung transplantation is not compromised by the use of marginal donor lungs. *J Thorac Cardiovase Surg* 1995;109:1075–1079.

Sung J, Bochicchio GV, Joshi M, et al. Admission hyperglycemia is predictive of outcome in critically ill trauma patients. *J Trauma* 2005;59:80–83.

Szem JW, Hydo LJ, Fischer E, et al. High-risk intrahospital transport of critically ill patients: Safety and outcome of the necessary "road trip." *Crit Care Med* 1995; 23:1660-1666.

Talmor M, Hydo L, Barie PS. Relationship of systemic inflammatory response syndrome to organ dysfunction, length of stay, and mortality in critical surgical illness: Effect of intensive care unit resuscitation. *Arch Surg* 1999;134:81–87.

Taylor DE, Simonson SG. Use of near-infrared spectroscopy to monitor tissue oxygenation. *New Horiz* 1996;4:420–425.

Thomas EJ, Lipsitz SR, Studdert DM, et al. The reliability of medical record review for estimating adverse event rates. *Ann Intern Med* 2002;136:812–816.

Tisherman SA, Barie P, Bokhari F, et al. Clinical practice guideline: Endpoints of resuscitation. *J Trauma* 2004;57:898–912.

2005 American Heart Association Guidelines for Cardiopulmonary Resuscitation and Emergency Cardiovascular Care. Part 1. Introduction. *Circulation* 2005;112:IV-1–IV-5.

2005 American Heart Association Guidelines for Cardiopulmonary Resuscitation and Emergency Cardiovascular Care. Part 4. Adult basic life support. *Circulation* 2005; 112:IV-19–IV-33.

2005 American Heart Association Guidelines for Cardiopulmonary Resuscitation and Emergency Cardiovascular Care. Part 5. Electrical therapies. *Circulation* 2005;112: IV-35–IV-46.

Van Biesen W, Vanholder R, Lameire N. Dialysis strategies in critically ill acute renal failure patients. *Curr Opin Crit Care* 2003;9:491–495.

Van den Berghe G, Wouters PJ, Bouillon R, et al. Outcome benefit of intensive insulin therapy in the critically ill. *Crit Care Med* 2003;31:359–366.

Van den Berghe G, Wouters P, Weekers F, et al. Intensive insulin therapy in critically ill patients. *N Engl J Med* 2001;345:1359–1367.

Velmahos GC, Demetreiades D, Shoemaker WC, et al. Endpoints of resuscitation of critically injured patients: Normal or supranormal? A prospective randomized trial. *Ann Surg* 2000;232:409–418.

Ventilation with lower tidal volumes as compared with traditional tidal volumes for acute lung injury and the acute respiratory distress syndrome. The acute respiratory distress syndrome network. *N Engl J Med* 2000;342:1301–1308.

Vogelzang M, Nijboer JM, van der Horst IC, et al. Hyperglycemia has a stronger relation with outcome in trauma patients than in other critically ill patients. *J Trauma* 2006;60:873–877.

Warren J, Fromm RE Jr, Orr RA, et al, and the American College of Critical Care Medicine. Guidelines for the inter- and intrahospital transport of critically ill patients. *Crit Care Med* 2004;32:256–266.

West MA, Shapiro MB, Nathens AB, et al. Inflammation and the Host Response to Injury, a large-scale collaborative project: Patient-oriented research core—Standard operating procedures for clinical care. IV. Guidelines for transfusion in the trauma patient. *J Trauma* 2006;61:436–439.

Williams MA, Lipsett PA, Rushton CH, et al. The physician's role in discussing organ donation with families. *Crit Care Med* 2003;31:1568–1573.

Wood KE, Becker BN, McCartney JG, et al. Care of the potential organ donor. *N Engl J Med* 2004;351:2730–2739.

Yendamuri S, Fulda GJ, Tinkoff GH. Admission hyperglycemia as a prognostic indicator in trauma. *J Trauma* 2003;55:33–38.

Zallen G. Age of transfused blood is an independent risk factor for postinjury multiple organ failure. *Am J Surg* 1999;178:570–572.

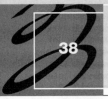

38 COMMONLY MISSED INJURIES AND PITFALLS
GERARD J. FULDA AND KIMBALL I. MAULL

I. INTRODUCTION. In caring for the injured, the clinician is often called on to make lifesaving decisions quickly and on an incomplete database. The first priority is to save the patient's life. Yet, missed injuries have the potential to convert the surgeon's best efforts into a calamity. It is important to recognize that missed injuries are not confined to the inexperienced or incompetent physician, that spectacular injuries can make less apparent injuries more likely to be overlooked, and that the incidence of missed injuries can be reduced but cannot be entirely eliminated. Missed injuries are a fact of life.

A. The **incidence** of missed injuries varies from 2% to 50%, depending on the definition of a missed injury. Most authors define a missed injury as one that is discovered either after completion of the initial assessment or more than 24 hours have elapsed since admission. All agree that the term "missed injury" applies to any patient who is discharged from the hospital with an undiagnosed injury. Therefore, the intent of this chapter is to provide the reader with information that will reduce the likelihood of a patient leaving the hospital with a missed injury.

B. Missed injuries can lead to an increased risk of complications and mortality and are a major cause of preventable trauma deaths and litigation. The greatest risk for missing injuries is in patients with brain injury or those undergoing emergent surgery.

C. The **tertiary survey** is an intentional reassessment of the patient, which is performed at a time when the patient can provide a history of the trauma incident, including a pertinent past history, and a reliable response to the physical examination. In many cases, this is on the second hospital day. In others, it may need to be delayed until after extubation or when the patient is ready to be ambulated. The tertiary survey follows the format of the secondary survey advocated by the Advanced Trauma Life Support Course sponsored by the American College of Surgeons (Chapter 10). In addition, all initial laboratory and radiographic studies are reviewed. It is particularly important when addressing initial unofficial x-ray results ("wet readings") to later confirm the radiologist's final report.

D. Patients and their families should be informed on admission of the potential for missed injuries. For example, this statement can go a long way in reducing later anxieties: **Our initial goal is to deal with the most obvious immediate threats to life and limb. It is not unusual to find additional injuries as time goes on.**

II. FACTORS THAT CONTRIBUTE TO MISSED INJURIES. The factors that contribute to a heightened incidence of missed injuries can be categorized as clinical factors, radiologic factors, and other factors.

A. Several **clinical factors** can lead to missed injuries. An intentional reassessment is always warranted under these conditions.

  1. Altered mental status (from head injury, alcohol, or medications) is the most common reason for missed injuries.

  2. Pain or distress from **multiple injuries** may distract the physician from detecting additional injuries.

  3. Unavailability for frequent evaluation. Patients who undergo prolonged operative procedures or lengthy diagnostic studies may develop manifestations of a missed injury while inaccessible to continued evaluation. Early reassessment is indicated. Further, if the patient arrived in shock and undergoes emergency operation, the patient likely had an incomplete workup at the time of presentation, and a tertiary survey should be completed after stabilization to detect additional injuries.

4. **Elderly patients** have little physiologic reserve and may deteriorate rapidly. Osteoporosis in elderly patients increases the risk of fractures occurring after apparently minor trauma. Conversely, children, athletes, and pregnant patients have well-developed compensatory mechanisms and injuries may not be initially apparent.

5. **Language barrier** prevents the clinician from being fully informed and interferes with obtaining a complete history. Injuries can be missed in this setting.

6. **Clinical omissions or misinterpretations** can interfere with early diagnosis of injury. Omission of aspects of the physical examination preclude the diagnosis of certain injuries. It is particularly important in the unresponsive patient to completely examine all joints and soft tissues, perform a rectal examination, and reassess the neurologic status of the patient. The inexperienced clinician may not fully appreciate findings on physical examination, which can also lead to delays in diagnosis.

7. **Information transfer.** Information is often lost when the care of a patient is transferred from one physician (or hospital) to another. Because the receiving physician is dependent on the medical record to guide the evaluation and therapy, documentation must be accurate and complete. When documentation is inadequate, the receiving physician must approach the patient as if the patient is being evaluated for the first time.

8. **Other clinical assessment pitfalls**
   a. **Incomplete history.** The initial history includes obtaining information on **a**llergies, **m**edications, past illness and **p**regnancy, **l**ast meal, and **e**vents of the injury (AMPLE). In some patients, no history may be initially available. A more complete history should be sought as part of the tertiary survey.
   b. **Lack of familiarity with injury patterns.** The clinician should be aware that certain injuries put the patient at risk for other associated injuries. In addition, certain insignificant physical signs may be tell-tale signs of more severe injuries. Soft-tissue contusions belie underlying trauma.
   c. **Failure or inability to perform a tertiary survey.** Failure to expose, inspect, auscultate, palpate, and percuss every major body region may result in missed injuries. Odor may be important in uncovering wounds, injuries, and preexisting medical conditions. In some cases, it is not physically possible to examine the patient completely (for example, facial swelling may prevent adequate examination of the eye), and a complete examination is delayed.

B. **Radiologic factors.** Injuries can be missed because the area of injury was simply not studied (not suspected), or it was not studied adequately, or because the study itself was misinterpreted. Failure to understand the limitations and sensitivity of diagnostic studies can result in injuries being overlooked.

1. **Radiographs taken in the trauma room** may be technically suboptimal. Although such films can exclude immediately life-threatening conditions, it may be wise to obtain repeat studies in the radiology department after the patient has been stabilized. Inadequate or incomplete views can obscure significant findings. In imaging extremities, injuries can be missed without the inclusion of at least two views and visualization of the joint above and below the suspected injury.

2. **Findings missed on initial review.** Many radiographic findings are subtle and may not be recognized on initial review. Follow-up films should be obtained for persistent complaints of pain. Joint radiology rounds consisting of both radiologist and trauma team members can reduce the incidence of missed injuries.

3. **Injuries missed with CT.** Despite high-resolution CT scanners and an experienced radiologist, small-bowel and some pancreatic injuries may not be detected by the initial CT scan. CT scans without oral contrast decrease the risk of patient aspiration but increases the risk of missing injuries to the bowel.

4. **Injuries missed with FAST.** Focused abdominal sonography for trauma (FAST) is operator dependent and is designed only to detect fluid in one of four spaces. Diagnostic limitations include the inability to diagnose bowel, mesenteric, pancreatic, diaphragmatic, and some solid organ injuries. Hemoperitoneum may not be present in some patients with proven abdominal injuries. Bowel gas may obstruct critical portions of the image or the study is limited in the morbidly obese. The accuracy of FAST is improved when combined with the clinical examination.

5. **Injuries missed with diagnostic peritoneal lavage (DPL).** DPL is sensitive but not specific for the detection of intraperitoneal hemorrhage requiring operative control. DPL does not allow direct evaluation of retroperitoneal structures and may be difficult to interpret in the presence of a major pelvic injury due to bleeding into the preperitoneal space. Diaphragmatic injuries are also difficult to detect with DPL unless effluent returns via the chest tube and its significance is recognized by the clinician.

6. **Injuries missed with laparoscopy.** Laparoscopy can be used to determine penetration of the peritoneal cavity and diaphragm. The presence or absence of blood or bile in the peritoneal cavity can easily be confirmed. Small perforations of the bowel can be difficult to diagnose even by an experienced laparoscopist.

C. **Other factors that lead to missed injuries**
   1. **Nonoperative management** relies on diagnostic studies and physical examination to exclude significant injuries. The major risk of nonoperative management is missed injury. Although most patients with full-thickness bowel injury complain of abdominal pain at presentation, their visceral injuries may not be appreciated until the perforation leads to obvious findings on physical examination.
   2. **The advertised "isolated injury"** patient is sent with an established diagnosis, which may be to a single organ system, often musculoskeletal. The pitfall is to assume the diagnosis of isolated injury is correct and to fail to pursue the possibility of other injuries.
   3. **Inappropriate service admission** results when the trauma patient is admitted to a nonsurgical service or, based on limited assessment, is admitted to a specialty service, surgical or nonsurgical. Under these conditions, the patient may not be fully assessed for injuries and missed injury is the result.

D. **Intraoperative missed injuries**
   1. Intraoperative missed injuries are the most lethal, with a mortality of 40%. Circumstances that lead to missing injuries intraoperatively include failure to fully explore the patient, the presence of adhesions, failure to explore the retroperitoneal space following penetrating trauma, failure to appreciate ischemia from vascular compromise, and surgical inexperience.
   2. Delay in appreciation of an intraoperative missed injury is the leading cause of adverse outcome. Delay may be based on overconfidence or failure to recognize that the patient is not improving as expected.
   3. The most common presentations of missed intraoperative injury in the postoperative period are hypotension, progressive multiorgan failure, persistent drain output, refractory acidosis, and peritonitis.

III. **COMMONLY MISSED INJURIES BY REGION**
   A. **Head and neck**
      1. **Occipital condyle and odontoid fractures** are usually associated with high-energy collisions. Their diagnosis can be enhanced with thin-slice CT images from C2 to the foramen magnum with three-dimensional reconstruction.

2. **Orbital floor fractures** are difficult to assess in the presence of significant soft-tissue swelling. Sagittal and coronal CT views are often necessary to detect these injuries.

3. **Carotid injury in blunt neck trauma.** The classic presentation for blunt carotid injury is a patient with a focal neurologic deficit with a normal initial CT scan of the head. A history of neck extension and rotation at the time of the impact is suggestive. A linear contusion, from seat-belt injury to the neck, should prompt either computed tomography angiography (CTA) or formal arteriography, even without a neurologic deficit.

4. **Cavernous sinus fistulas** may be occult until symptoms appear. Proptosis and an orbital bruit are suggestive. Although the lesion may be suspected with CT scan, the definitive diagnosis is made with angiography or magnetic resonance angiography (MRA).

5. **Hyoid/laryngeal injury** should be suspected when a patient with blunt trauma to the neck presents with hoarseness and subcutaneous emphysema. Cervical CT is usually diagnostic.

6. **Cervical spine fracture-dislocations**
   a. A cervical spine injury should be assumed in any patient with injury above the level of the clavicles. This includes maxillofacial trauma, head injury, and scalp lacerations. The lateral cervical spine radiograph is not totally reliable in detecting fractures and in patients at risk, additional studies are indicated.
   b. False negative radiographs may lead to missed cervical spine injuries, both stable and unstable.
   c. The three-view cervical spine series (lateral, anteroposterior, and odontoid views), combined with various combinations of flexion-extension plain films, CT, or MRI, improves accuracy.
   d. C1 to C2, C7 to T1, and unilateral facet fracture-dislocations are cervical injuries that are easily missed on initial radiographs. Even subtle abnormalities should prompt more complete radiologic assessment.
   e. MRI scans are less sensitive than CT in diagnosis of fractures through the posterior elements and injuries to the craniocervical junction.

7. **Cord syndromes.** Central or posterior cord syndromes can occur without a spinal fracture. The neurologic symptoms are often incorrectly attributed to hysteria, intoxication, head injury, or associated injuries.

B. **Thorax**

1. **Traumatic rupture of the diaphragm** is unrecognized on presentation in 50% to 69% of patients without visceral herniation. This injury may be missed on chest radiograph, CT, ultrasonography, or diagnostic peritoneal lavage. Diagnosis may be improved with placement of a nasogastric tube, GI contrast, repeat imaging, thoracoscopy, or laparoscopy.

2. **Esophageal injury.** Esophageal must not be excluded in any patient with a transmediastinal gunshot wound because symptoms may be delayed. Contrast study with dilute barium, combined with esophagoscopy, has a 97% diagnostic accuracy. Either study alone has 60% sensitivity.

3. **Thoracic aortic disruption** may be missed on plain chest radiograph because the mediastinum may be normal in 7% to 10% of patients. Rapid, high-resolution spiral CT of the chest in blunt chest injury will confirm an aortic injury or a demonstrate a mediastinal hematoma (which will require arteriography). Transesophageal echocardiography (TEE) may also be useful, especially for the patient in the operating room (OR) for other injuries. However, TEE is relatively insensitive (55%–75%).

4. **Pneumothorax on supine films** is subtle and requires careful review of the radiograph for air density over the diaphragm, an apparent depression and lucency of the lateral costophrenic angle (deep sulcus sign). If in doubt, obtain an erect chest x-ray as a follow-up radiograph. These injuries are easily identified on CT of the abdomen or chest.

5. **Cardiac wounds.** One third of patients with penetrating cardiac wounds may present without overt signs and symptoms of cardiac injury. Pericardial ultrasonography or a pericardial window may be required for diagnosis.

6. **Rib fractures** are frequently missed (50%) on conventional radiographs because they are simply not visible. In the elderly, even a single rib fracture increases the likelihood of ventilatory compromise.

7. **Scapular fractures and acromioclavicular (AC) separations** can be detected with careful attention to the physical examination and bony structure on the chest radiograph. Although early therapy may not be mandatory, early recognition is important as a determinant of high-energy trauma. CT scanning will not detect all of these injuries and the early use of MRI should be considered.

C. **Abdomen and pelvis**

1. **Traumatic abdominal wall hernias** are usually detected by CT; however, they may be missed during urgent laparotomy for other injuries.

2. **Hollow visceral injuries** of the duodenum, small bowel, and colon may be missed or delayed because abdominal CT is often nondiagnostic and physical findings may be delayed or masked. Unexplained fever, tachycardia, leukocytosis, abdominal distention, or abdominal tenderness when assessible require repeat or additional studies, including laparoscopy or laparotomy. Delay in the diagnosis of a small-bowel injury accounts for approximately 50% of deaths from these injuries.

3. **Pancreatic ductal injuries** can be missed on CT, DPL, FAST, or laparotomy. Serum chemistries are not sufficiently sensitive or specific. The mortality rate associated with missed pancreatic ductal injuries is approximately 50%. Complete inspection and bimanual palpation of the pancreas during laparotomy are mandatory in the presence of a peripancreatic hematoma or suspected injury. MRCP should be considered as an alternative to ERCP.

4. **Biliary duct disruption** can be missed in both blunt and penetrating trauma. When these injuries are missed, patients usually present with either biliary ascites or peritonitis. Diagnosis can be suspected on CT or ultrasonography and confirmed by HIDA scan, percutaneous transhepatic cholangiography (PTC), or endoscopic retrograde cholangiopancreatography (ERCP).

5. **Rectal injuries** should be suspected following proximity wounds to the buttocks and in all patients with unstable pelvic fractures. Proctoscopy or sigmoidoscopy is necessary to evaluate the rectum, even in the face of a negative exploratory laparotomy. Either devascularization or direct rectal wall trauma may result from the injury.

6. **Traumatic renal artery occlusion** may be occult because gross hematuria is commonly absent. High-resolution CT or angiography is required for diagnosis. At laparotomy, duplex ultrasonography or Doppler ultrasonography may be helpful. Repair is indicated if the injury is bilateral or in a patient with only one kidney, assuming warm ischemia time has not been prolonged.

7. **Ureteral injuries** from penetrating trauma may be missed unless completely visualized during exploratory laparotomy.

8. **Abdominal compartment syndrome (ACS)** requires a high index of suspicion for detection. The patient with multiple injuries who has undergone massive resuscitation should be assessed for ACS (Chapter 29).

9. **Adrenal insufficiency** may easily be missed. It may occur following resuscitation in elderly patients, steroid-dependent patients, and those unresponsive to pressor therapy. Hyponatremia, hyperkalemia, and unexplained eosinophilia are diagnostic clues. Diagnosis is made with a cosyntropin stimulation test.

D. **Extremities and spine**

1. **Fractures and dislocations.** The most commonly missed fractures in the emergency department (ED) include those of the wrist, elbow, calcaneus, ribs, and phalanges. Missed injuries to the femoral neck, scaphoid, and talus can lead to avascular necrosis of the bone and result in significant morbidity.

a. **Radioulnar dislocation.** Many of these injuries are missed initially because of inadequate radiographic views.

b. **Posterior dislocations of the shoulder** are uncommon but are associated with posterior glenoid rim fractures and anterior compression fractures of the humeral head. Compare the injured versus uninjured sides. If in doubt, immobilize the shoulder and obtain an MRI examination. Most are visible by 2 weeks.

c. **Carpal bone fractures or dislocations** are frequently missed on radiographs because of soft-tissue swelling, their irregular contour, bony overlap, and the presence of distracting fractures of the metacarpals and distal arm bones. When missed, these injuries frequently lead to nonunion. However, the fracture may not be visible on the initial x-ray. Special views and knowledge of fracture patterns increase the detection rate.

d. **Hand injuries** require a careful hand examination to determine the presence of nerve, ligamentous, or tendon injury. Common tendon injuries include flexor digitorum profundus, mallet fingers, central slip tendon, and extensor hood rupture.

e. **Lisfranc joint injuries** are complex fracture-dislocations of the tarsometatarsal apparatus that are frequently overlooked and can lead to chronic disability.

f. **Multilevel spinal fractures.** During evaluation of a patient with a spinal fracture, a second fracture will be discovered at another level in 15% to 25% of cases. This justifies the rule that **a spinal fracture found at any level requires radiologic assessment of the entire vertebral column**.

g. **Knee fractures.** Most fractures involving the knee are seen on anteroposterior and lateral films. Some types of knee fractures are more difficult to detect by standard views:

   i. **Tibial plateau fractures** can be seen on tangential or tunnel views.

   ii. **Fibular head dislocations** can be seen on the lateral view.

2. **Ligamentous injuries** surrounding the large joints will not be detected on radiographs. A complete examination and selected use of CT and/or MRI are required to confirm these injuries. Small chip fractures may be a clue to a significant ligamentous or tendon injury.

3. **Arterial injuries.** Color-flow duplex ultrasonography is highly specific (99%) but less sensitive (50% to 95%) compared with angiography for detection of arterial injuries. However, its sensitivity for detection of an arterial injury that requires surgical intervention is 90% to 100%. False aneurysms and arteriovenous fistulas are the most commonly missed injuries. Negative studies should be interpreted with caution, particularly in carotid, axillary, and brachial arteries. CT angiogram may miss small irregularities and, if in doubt, should be followed up with a formal angiogram. **The presence of distal pulses does not exclude significant arterial injury.**

4. **Lumbosacral root avulsions.** These injuries are usually missed on initial examination. Patients often have a neurologic deficit that involves varying degrees of lower extremity motor and sensory loss. MRI may assist in the diagnosis.

5. **Pelvic fractures.** Plain anteroposterior pelvic films typically underestimate the extent of pelvic boney injury. Sacral, pubic rami, and nondisplaced acetabular fractures frequently are not appreciated on plain films. Thin-slice pelvic CT scans can detect these injuries. A patient with pelvic pain with motion or ambulation has a fracture until proven otherwise by CT.

6. **Vaginal laceration** may be associated with pelvic fractures and may require speculum examination under anesthesia for diagnosis. All females with an anterior pelvic fracture mandate a careful visual and manual vaginal examination. Do not attribute vaginal bleeding to menses in a woman with pelvic fracture.

E. **Pediatrics.** The incidence of missed injuries in pediatric patients is about 16% overall with the majority occurring in head injured patients.

1. **Child abuse** patterns of injury may not be appreciated by the casual observer (Chapter 46).
2. **Spinal cord injury without radiologic abnormality (SCIWORA)** is more common in children. When it is attributed to head injury or masked by multiple injuries, delay in the initiation of steroid therapy and stabilization of the spine can increase morbidity.
3. **Hollow visceral injuries.** A delay in the diagnosis of small-bowel injuries may occur in children with blunt abdominal trauma. Early DPL and CT are not sensitive. On CT scan, pneumoperitoneum, bowel thickening, and unexplained free fluid may be indications of bowel injury. Unfortunately, these diagnostic radiologic signs are not always present. Delayed DPL may help diagnose bowel injury following a nondiagnostic CT scan.
4. **Monteggia fracture,** a fracture of the ulna with dislocation of the radial head at the elbow, may be subtle and easily missed.
5. **Nondisplaced lateral and supracondyler** elbow fractures are frequently missed. However, there is a high association of these fractures with elbow dislocation.

IV. COMMONLY ASSOCIATED INJURIES

A. **Head injury in patients with a Glasgow Coma Scale (GCS) score of 13 to 15.** Although most patients with minor head injury will not develop significant problems, a small percentage (2% to 9%) will have an intracranial lesion that requires neurosurgical intervention. About 10% to 35% will have posttraumatic findings on CT scan (Chapter 17). Soft-tissue injury, focal defects, basilar skull fracture, and advanced age all increase the likelihood of significant findings.

B. **Ocular injuries and orbital fractures.** Patients presenting with facial fractures, especially those involving the orbital bones, have an increased incidence of associated ocular injury and should undergo ophthalmologic evaluation. When an orbital injury is associated with impaired visual acuity, chance of ocular injury is high.

C. **Nerve root avulsions in traction injuries.** Motorcycle crashes often involve traction injuries to the upper extremities. When associated with head injury, the underlying traction injury to the cervical nerve roots or brachial plexus may go undetected. MRI or CT myelography assists in this diagnosis.

D. **Seat belts.** Patients who are wearing seat belts have an increased incidence of sternal fractures, hollow visceral injury, and hyperflexion fracture of the lumbar spine (Chance fracture). Most of these injuries occur with lap-belt only configuration or with an inappropriately applied seat belt.

E. The motorcycle/bicycle **straddle injury** is associated with pelvic fractures, urethral tears, bladder rupture, and dislocation of the testes.

F. **Calcaneal and spinal column fractures** are common in patients who fall from heights. The presence of either fracture should prompt an investigation for the other.

G. **Dislocation of the knee with popliteal artery injury** can exist in the presence of normal pulses. Failure to recognize this injury is a major cause of amputation. Because of the associated high morbidity, evaluation of the popliteal artery following posterior knee dislocation is required.

H. **Elbow dislocation** is an orthopedic emergency because it can compromise the **brachial artery**.

AXIOMS

- Musculoskeletal injuries are the most commonly missed injuries in trauma patients.
- A tertiary survey, including a careful review of all admitting imaging studies, is the best method to detect missed injuries.
- Central retroperitoneal hematomas require exploration.
- It is reasonable to tell patients and families on admission that other injuries may be discovered later during the patient's hospital course.

- Clear documentation and communication among members of the trauma team are essential in avoiding missed injuries.
- Normal blood pressure does not mean normal perfusion.
- Gastric and bladder distention may lead to vasovagal response and hypotension.
- Correct life-threatening problems as they are discovered.
- Do not wait for the chest radiograph to treat tension pneumothorax.
- Neck veins may not be distended in the hypovolemic patient with cardiac tamponade.
- Normal auscultation of the chest following penetrating trauma does not rule out hemoperitoneum or pneumothorax.
- The presence of free abdominal fluid on CT scan, without evidence of solid organ injury, may indicate hollow visceral injury.
- Doppler signals and palpable pulses do not exclude vascular injuries.
- Before discharge, personally observe the patient standing and ambulating.
- Do not rely on wet readings of radiologic studies without personal review or confirmation of the final written interpretation.
- If you hear phrases such as "I think so," "last I heard," "I was told," "I assume," "maybe," "sort of," or "kind of" used to describe patient information, go and check it out for yourself!
- The finding of a fracture at any level of the spinal column mandates radiologic assessment of the entire spine.
- Spectacular injuries cause less apparent injuries to go undetected.

Bibliography

Biffl WL, Harrington DT, Cioffi WG. Implementation of a tertiary trauma survey decreases missed injuries. *J Trauma* 2003;54:38–44.

Enderson BL, Maull, KI. Missed injuries. *Surg Clin North Am* 1991;71:399–418.

Enderson BL, Reath DB, Meadors J, et al. The tertiary trauma survey: A prospective study of missed injury. *J Trauma* 1990;30:666–669.

Hirshberg A, Wall MJ Jr, Allen MK, Mattox KL. Causes and patterns of missed injuries in trauma. *Am J Surg* 1994;168:299–303.

Janjua KJ, Sugrue M, Deane SA. Prospective evaluation of early missed injuries and the role of tertiary trauma survey. *J Trauma* 1998;44:1000–1006.

Robertson R, Mattox R, Collins T, et al. Missed injuries in a rural area trauma center. *Am J Surg* 1996;172:564–567.

Scalea TM, Phillips TF, Goldstein AD, et al. Injuries missed at operation: Nemesis of the trauma surgeon. *J Trauma* 1988;28:962–967.

Sung CK, Kim KH. Missed injuries in abdominal trauma. *J Trauma* 1996;41:276–282.

ANESTHESIA FOR THE TRAUMA PATIENT

JAMES W. KRUGH, MICHAEL RODRICKS, AND C. WILLIAM HANSON, III

I. **INTRODUCTION.** Anesthetic management of the trauma patient begins in the trauma resuscitation area and continues into the operating room (OR) and the intensive care unit (ICU). The specific role for the anesthesiologist varies according to local practice, but may include initial airway evaluation and management, assistance in the primary survey, intraoperative management, and postoperative intensive care management.

II. **EVALUATION**
   A. **Airway.** All patients arriving in the trauma resuscitation area are treated with supplemental oxygen by facemask. The patient's response to simple questions provides meaningful information about mentation and airway competence. The airway should be examined immediately for foreign bodies, vomitus or blood, and suctioned as needed. Continuous reassessment of the airway is mandatory.
   B. **Breathing.** Inspection and auscultation of the chest is an integral part of the primary assessment. Tracheal deviation, paradoxical chest wall motion, or chest wall injuries may be visualized. Immediately life-threatening injuries include tension pneumothorax, open pneumothorax, massive hemothorax, flail chest, pulmonary contusion, and cardiac tamponade; these injuries require immediate intervention.
   C. **All victims of blunt trauma** must be presumed to have a cervical spine injury. Cervical spine immobilization should be maintained with a cervical collar until the cervical spine is cleared.
   D. **If the airway** is patent and breathing is adequate, continue with the primary survey. If gas exchange is inadequate, support the patient with mask ventilation and prepare for endotracheal intubation.
   E. **Endotracheal intubation** (Chapter 11).
      1. If time permits, a quick evaluation of the patient's airway may alert the clinician to the possibility of a difficult airway.
         a. **Gross evaluation.** Evaluate dentition, jaw opening, micrognathia, or macrognathia. Temporomandibular joint disruption may make an otherwise routine airway very difficult because of limited jaw opening.
         b. **Thyromental distance.** A length of <6 cm (three finger breadths) from the lower edge of the mandible to the thyroid notch is predictive of difficult intubation.
         c. **Mallampati test.** Inability to visualize the uvula when a patient protrudes their tongue (Mallampati class III or IV) is a sensitive but nonspecific indicator of a difficult airway.
         d. **Atlantoaxial joint.** Movement of this joint is important in aligning the pharyngeal and laryngeal axes. However, cervical spine immobility must be maintained in the trauma patient making intubation more difficult.
      2. **All necessary equipment** should be ready prior to induction. A backup laryngoscope handle, several blades of varying size, endotracheal tube with stylet, and a functioning suction device with a Yankauer tip must be available.
      3. **As discussed** in Chapter 11, as many as three people are required for intubation: the individual intubating the patient, a person to hold cricoid pressure, and a third person to provide cervical spine immobilization. Cricoid

pressure (Sellick maneuver) is recommended because all trauma patients are assumed to have a full stomach. Cricoid pressure must be maintained until the endotracheal tube is placed, the cuff is inflated, and correct position is confirmed by auscultation of breath sounds and detection of carbon dioxide in the exhaled gas.

4. **A blind nasotracheal intubation** may be used in awake, spontaneously breathing patients only if performed by someone skilled in the technique. Due to its higher failure rate, more frequent complications (epistaxis), and longer average time to intubation, the nasotracheal route is not the preferred method to achieve a secure airway when alternative approaches are feasible. In certain situations, such as the entrapped patient, nasotracheal intubation may be the only possible approach, and therefore lifesaving.

5. **Fiberoptic intubation** is a useful alternative approach to the difficult airway. In an emergency setting this technique of airway management is not encouraged. Drawbacks include the time required to perform fiber-optic intubation, difficulty in visualizing anatomy in the presence of blood and secretions, possible precipitation of vomiting in the patient with a full stomach, and a high failure rate in uncooperative patients.

6. **Excessively** combative patients are best handled with orotracheal intubation after induction and paralysis. Ketamine and succinylcholine are readily absorbed after intramuscular administration and are quite useful in controlling patients in whom intravenous access cannot be obtained. After a definitive airway is established the patient may be more effectively evaluated.

7. **Laryngeal mask airways** (LMAs) may prove lifesaving in an emergency situation. An LMA is very quickly and easily placed in most patients, requires minimal training for use, and may be used as a bridge to a definitive airway. Its major drawback in the trauma patient is that **it does not protect against aspiration**; thus, the LMA represents a temporary airway.

F. **Intubated patients.** Endotracheal tubes placed prior to arrival in the trauma receiving area must be carefully checked for proper position. Determination of the presence of end-tidal carbon dioxide is essential. The most commonly malpositioned endotracheal tube is in the right mainstem bronchus, although esophageal intubation is not uncommon. The esophageal obturator airway (EOA) is not in common use, and should be converted promptly to an endotracheal tube.

G. **Surgical airway.** The inability to obtain a definitive airway using conventional techniques is a clear indication for a surgical airway. Severe maxillofacial injury may warrant a surgical airway as the initial means of airway control. In addition, multiple failed attempts at laryngoscopy may convert a patient who can be ventilated into a patient who cannot, creating the need for immediate surgical airway. The preferred method to obtain a surgical airway is a cricothyroidotomy. As access for an urgent airway, cricothyroidotomy is faster and easier to perform than tracheostomy.

III. CIRCULATION

A. **The unstable** trauma patient should have two large-bore intravenous (IV) lines (at least 16 gauge) secured in the trauma resuscitation area. If antecubital veins are not available, femoral, subclavian, or internal jugular veins may be used. Meticulous attention to aseptic technique is often not possible in the trauma resuscitation area; therefore, these lines should be changed within 24 hours.

B. **Intraosseous puncture** may be used for administration of volume and medications in children under six years of age in whom IV access cannot be obtained (Chapter 46).

C. **In the patient** with profound or persistent hypovolemia from bleeding, early blood transfusion is essential. Crossmatched blood is optimal, but type specific blood may be used if crossmatched blood is delayed. In the case of exsanguination, type O blood (Rh negative for females of childbearing age) may be used.

D. Hypothermia (Chapter 41). Many patients are hypothermic on arrival in the trauma resuscitation area. All IV fluids should be warmed to prevent further loss of body temperature. Techniques to warm fluids include the following:

1. **A supply** of prewarmed crystalloid should be kept on hand in the trauma resuscitation area.

2. **Standard blood** and fluid warmers. In the event of hypovolemic shock, these are of limited utility because of low flow rates.

3. **Level I warmer** (Level I Technologies, Rockland, Massachusetts). This device incorporates large-bore tubing to allow high flow rates. A wide-bore stopcock is positioned near the patient to allow for quick changes in the OR.

4. Active infusion units that provide rapid delivery of warmed fluids are commercially available. For example, the **Rapid Infusion System (RIS)** (Haemonetics Corporation, Braintree, Massachusetts) combines a 3-L reservoir, heater, pumps, and alarms. The reservoir allows mixing of nonsanguinous fluids, blood components, and drugs. The RIS allows up to 1.5 to 2.0 L/minute transfusion through two 8.5 F introducers with pressures <250 mmHg.

IV. HISTORY

A. Attempt to obtain a past medical history. This may be obtained from the patient or from accompanying family members. A medic alert bracelet or wallet card may also be invaluable in identifying premorbid disease processes. Past medical problems, drug allergies, medications, and time of last meal are all-important pieces of data. Beta-adrenergic blocker or calcium channel blocker agents may blunt the normal tachycardic response to hypovolemia.

B. Mechanism of injury. Paramedics can often provide a concise description of the mechanism of injury.

C. Street drugs. The trauma patient is frequently under the influence of intoxicants prior to the accident.

1. **Alcohol.** Acute intoxication reduces anesthetic drug requirements. Chronic alcohol use leads to a cross-tolerance among anesthetic agents and therefore a higher requirement. The cirrhotic patient may have decreased drug metabolism, an altered volume of distribution, and a preexisting coagulopathy.

2. **Cocaine.** Acute intoxication can induce volume contraction, metabolic acidosis, hypertension, myocardial ischemia or infarction, dysrhythmias, seizures, or stroke. Volume expansion will correct the metabolic acidosis. Chronic abuse has been associated with delusions and hypotension from depletion of catecholamines.

3. **Marijuana.** Acute intoxication can produce hypertension and tachycardia. Chronic use depletes catecholamines and leads to cardiovascular instability.

4. **Opioids.** Acute intoxication can produce hypertension and tachycardia. Chronic use will necessitate increased dosages of anesthetic agents. With chronic IV drug abuse vascular access is a problem, and there is a risk of bloodborne infections such as human immunodeficiency virus (HIV) or viral hepatitis. Opioid antagonists (i.e., naloxone) can cause acute withdrawal. Be prepared to treat withdrawal postoperatively.

5. **Ketamine.** Ketamine is a phencyclidine derivative that has recently gained popularity as a street drug. Acute intoxication is associated with graphic dreams and behavioral disturbances. Physiologic effects include hypertension, tachycardia, and an increase in cerebral blood flow.

V. LABORATORY

A. Trauma blood work. Laboratory work should be sent from the trauma resuscitation area. A complete blood count (CBC), chemistry panel, type and screen or type and cross, beta human chorionic gonadotropin (in all females of childbearing age), drug screen, and arterial blood gas may be useful.

B. Electrocardiogram (ECG) may be useful in evaluating blunt cardiac injuries as well as dysrhythmias and ischemia.

C. Radiographs (Chapter 13)

VI. OPERATING ROOM MANAGEMENT

A. Intraoperative monitoring is determined by the patient's condition. Insertion of invasive monitors should not delay definitive surgery.

1. **Standard monitors.** ECG, noninvasive blood pressure monitor, pulse oximetry, capnograph or multigas analyzer, oxygen analyzer, and temperature should be monitored in the OR.

2. **Arterial line.** An arterial line is useful in the hemodynamically unstable patient. It allows continuous monitoring of blood pressure as well as reliable access for serial blood gases and laboratory tests. The radial artery is the preferred site for placement of an arterial line.

3. **Central venous pressure** (CVP). Central veins provide reliable venous access and may be all that is available in a hemodynamically compromised, vasoconstricted patient. CVP may be helpful in assessing volume status in an ongoing resuscitation.

4. **Pulmonary artery catheter** (PAC). May prove useful in the patient with depressed ventricular function, valvular disease, persistent acidosis, or unclear volume status.

5. **Transesophageal echocardiography** (TEE). Can be used to evaluate the heart for tamponade, effusion, wall motion abnormalities, ejection fraction, intracardiac air, valve function, and volume status. The descending thoracic aorta may be visualized to diagnose aortic rupture or dissection.

6. **Temperature.** Trauma patients are often hypothermic because of exposure at the scene, open injuries, and ongoing resuscitation. Hypothermia causes decreased drug metabolism, impaired coagulation, increased incidence of wound infections, dehiscence, and increased oxygen consumption from postoperative shivering. Core temperature may be measured via the esophagus, bladder, or rectum. Measures to correct or minimize heat loss are as follows:

   a. **Warm OR.** Raising the OR temperature to 30°C minimizes convective heat losses and is essential to prevent hypothermia. After the patient is volume resuscitated and normothermic, the room temperature may be lowered for OR personnel comfort.

   b. **Warm preparation** and irrigation solutions.

   c. **Warm all IV fluids.**

   d. **Use a forced-air warmer** such as the Bair Hugger (Augustine Medical, Eden Prairie, Minnesota) on any area of the patient that is not prepped.

   e. **Wrap the head** or exposed limbs with blankets or plastic.

   f. **Heated** humidifier in the anesthetic circuit

7. **Neurological monitoring**

   a. **Intracranial pressure (ICP)** monitoring. An epidural or subarachnoid bolt or equivalent can be used to monitor ICP.

   b. A **ventriculostomy** can be used to monitor ICP as well as to drain cerebrospinal fluid (CSF) for ICP control.

   c. **Patients with head injuries** may be monitored with an electroencephalogram (EEG), brainstem auditory evoked responses, or somatosensory evoked potentials.

   d. **Bispectral analysis (BIS)** of the electroencephalogram (EEG) may be used to judge depth of anesthesia and to avoid intraoperative recall.

8. **Coagulation** can be monitored by prothrombin time (PT), partial thromboplastin time (PTT), activated coagulation time (ACT), platelet count, and thromboelastogram (TEG). Coagulation should be carefully monitored in patients with severe closed head injury, massive resuscitation, hypothermia, or liver dysfunction.

B. Anesthetic induction agents. Thiopental, etomidate, or ketamine are the drugs most commonly used for anesthesia induction. Tables 39-1 through 39-3 list induction dose, duration, respiratory, and cardiovascular side effects of these agents.

| TABLE 39-1 | Induction Doses and Characteristics |

Drug	Dose (mg/kg)	Onset (s)	Duration (min)	Excitation	Pain
Thiopental	3–5*	30	5–8+	+	+
Etomidate	0.2–0.4	15–45	3–12	+++	+++
Propofol	1.5–3.0	15–45	5–10	+	++
Midazolam	0.2–0.4	30–60	15–30	0	0
Ketamine	1–3	45	10–20	+	0

*Decrease for suspected hypovolemia.

+, minimal; +++, marked; ++, moderate; 0, none.

| TABLE 39-2 | Cardiovascular and Respiratory Effects of Induction Drugs |

Drug	Respiratory depression	MAP	HR	CO	Contractility	SVR	Venous dilatation
Thiopental	++	—	+	—	—	–	++
Etomidate	+	0	0	0	0	0	0
Propofol	++	—	–	–	–	—	++
Midazolam	+	0/–	–/+	0/–	0	–/0	+
Ketamine	0/+	++	++	+	+/–	+/–	0

++, marked increase; —, marked decrease; +, mild increase; –, mild decrease; 0, no change.

MAP, mean arterial pressure; HR, heart rate; CO, cardiac output; SVR, systemic vascular resistance.

| TABLE 39-3 | Central Nervous System Effects of Common Induction Drugs |

Drug	CMR O_2	CBF	CPP	ICP
Thiopental	—	—	–/0	—
Etomidate	—	—	0/+	—
Propofol	—	—	–/–	–
Midazolam	–	–/0	0	–
Ketamine	+	++	–/0/+	+

—, Marked decrease; –, mild decrease; 0, no change; +, mild increase; ++, marked increase.

CMR, cerebral metabolic rate; CBF, cerebral blood flow; CPP, cerebral perfusion pressure; ICP, intracranial pressure.

If the patient is brought to the OR still hypovolemic or in shock, small doses of an amnestic agent (scopolamine 0.2–0.4 mg, midazolam 1–2 mg, or a small dose of ketamine) are used to prevent recall until bleeding is controlled and the blood volume returns toward normal.

1. **Thiopental**
   a. **Dose:** 3–5 mg/kg IV (decrease for hypovolemic patients).
   b. **Respiratory:** moderate depression.
   c. **Cardiovascular:** decreases contractility, cardiac output, and mean arterial pressure (MAP); causes venous dilation.
   d. **Central nervous system** (CNS): cerebral protective by decreasing cerebral metabolic rate (CMR) O_2 and ICP.
   e. **Elimination:** action ends by redistribution in the body. It is then metabolized by the liver.
   f. **Duration of action:** 5–10 minutes.
   g. **Side effects:** hypotension in the hypovolemic patient. May precipitate acute intermittent porphyria.

2. **Etomidate**
   a. **Dose:** 0.2–0.4 mg/kg IV.
   b. **Respiratory:** mild depression.
   c. **Cardiovascular:** no significant change in cardiovascular parameters in a normovolemic patient.
   d. **CNS:** cerebral protective by decreasing cerebral metabolic rate (CMR) O_2 and ICP; probably not as protective as thiopental.
   e. **Elimination:** action ends by redistribution in the body, then metabolism by the liver.
   f. **Duration of action:** 5–10 minutes.
   g. **Side effects:** causes excitement on induction. Pain on injection may be decreased by IV lidocaine prior to injection. Inhibits adrenocortical functions.

3. **Propofol**
   a. **Dose:** 1.5–3.0 mg/kg.
   b. **Respiratory:** moderate depression.
   c. **Cardiovascular:** large decrease in systemic vascular resistance and increased venous dilatation; may have marked decrease in blood pressure with induction dose.
   d. **CNS:** Mild decrease in ICP.
   e. **Elimination:** action ends by redistribution in the body, then metabolism by the liver.
   f. **Duration of action:** 5–10 minutes.
   g. **Side effects:** causes mild excitement on induction. Pain on injection may be decreased by IV lidocaine prior to injection. Cardiovascular depression with resultant hypotension is common with propofol administration.

4. **Midazolam**
   a. **Dose:** 0.2–0.4 mg/kg.
   b. **Respiratory:** mild depression.
   c. **Cardiovascular:** little or no change in the cardiovascular system with normovolemic patient.
   d. **CNS:** mild decrease in ICP.
   e. **Elimination:** action ends by redistribution in the body, then metabolism by the liver.
   f. **Duration of action:** 15–30 minutes. Major problem in the head injured patient because a neurological examination may not be repeated readily.
   g. **Side effects:** minimal.

5. **Ketamine**
   a. **Dose:** 1–3 mg/kg IV, 5 mg/kg intramuscularly (IM).
   b. **Respiratory:** minimal depression, is a bronchodilator (useful in asthmatic patients).
   c. **Cardiovascular:** increased heart rate, contractility, cardiac output and MAP.
   d. **CNS:** increases CMR O_2, cerebral blood flow (CBF), and ICP. **Should not be used in head injured patients or in patients with coronary artery disease.**
   e. **Elimination:** action ends by redistribution in the body, then metabolism by the liver.

f. **Duration of action:** 10–20 minutes.

g. **Side effects:** good analgesic; excitement postoperatively, possible hallucinations (structurally related to phencyclidine).

h. **May be given IM** in the combative patient to provide safe contact with the patient.

C. **Neuromuscular blocking agents.** See Table 39-4 for doses and Table 39-5 for a summary of cardiovascular effects.

1. **Succinylcholine.** The only clinically used depolarizing agent.

   a. **Dose:** 1.0–2.0 mg/kg. If pretreated with a nondepolarizer, dose is increased to 1.5–2.0 mg/kg. Double the dose if given intramuscularly.

   b. **Duration:** excellent intubating conditions in 45 seconds, duration 5–10 minutes.

   c. **Elimination:** metabolized by plasma cholinesterase (pseudocholinesterase). Pseudocholinesterase levels may be abnormally low because of a genetic defect or liver dysfunction, either of which will prolong duration of action of succinylcholine.

   d. **Cardiovascular effects:** stimulates nicotinic receptors in sympathetic and parasympathetic ganglia, and muscarinic receptors in the sinoatrial node of the heart. Dysrhythmias such as bradycardia, sinus arrest, and junctional arrhythmias may follow succinylcholine administration, particularly after repeated doses.

   e. **Complications**

      i. **Hyperkalemia:** serum potassium rises 0.5 mEq/L in normal patients. A marked rise in serum potassium sufficient to cause cardiac arrest may be seen in burn patients (after 24 hours), massive crush injury (usually after several days), patients with neuromuscular diseases or upper motor neuron lesions, and in renal failure patients.

TABLE 39-4 Doses and Durations of Neuromuscular Drugs

Drug	Relaxant dose (mg/kg)	Intubation dose (mg/kg)	Duration in minutes (after intubating dose)
Succinylcholine		1.0–2.0	5–10
Rocuronium	0.3–0.4	0.6–1.0	45–75
Cisatracurium	0.1	0.15–0.2	45–90
Vecuronium	0.05	0.1–0.2	45–90
Pancuronium	0.05	0.08–0.12	60–120

TABLE 39-5 Autonomic Effects of Neuromuscular Agents

Drug	Autonomic ganglia	Cardiac muscarinic receptors	Histamine release
Succinylcholine	Stimulates	Stimulates	Slight
Rocuronium	None	None	None
Cisatracurium	None	None	None
Vecuronium	None	None	None
Pancuronium	None	Blocks moderately	None

      ii. Increased intraocular, intragastric, and intracranial pressures: may be due to fasiculations and may be partially attenuated by pretreatment with a nondepolarizer. Contraindicated in a patient with open globe injury.

      iii. Postoperative myalgias: associated with fasciculations.

      iv. Malignant hyperthermia: succinylcholine is a known trigger of malignant hyperthermia.

    f. Recommendations: 1.0–2.0 mg/kg intubating dose is the gold standard for a rapid sequence induction (if not contraindicated).

2. Rocuronium

    a. Dose: intubation dose 0.6–1.0 mg/kg.

    b. Onset: excellent intubating conditions in 60 seconds with a dose of 1.0 mg/kg.

    c. Duration: 30–45 minute duration of action.

    d. Elimination: eliminated in bile or stored in the liver.

    e. Cardiovascular effects: none.

    f. Complications: none.

    g. Recommendations: 1 mg/kg of rocuronium has been used with good results for a rapid sequence induction.

3. Cisatracurium

    a. Dose: 0.15–0.20 mg/kg intubation dose.

    b. Onset: excellent intubating conditions in 2–3 minutes.

    c. Duration: 60 minute duration of action.

    d. Elimination: degraded by Hoffman elimination in the plasma. Elimination is independent of hepatic and renal function.

    e. Cardiovascular effects: none.

    f. Complications: none.

4. Vecuronium

    a. Dose: intubation dose of 0.1–0.2 mg/kg.

    b. Onset: excellent intubating conditions in 2–3 minutes.

    c. Duration: 45–60 minute duration of action.

    d. Elimination: metabolized in the liver and excreted unchanged in the kidney.

    e. Complications: none.

    f. Recommendations: may be used for rapid sequence induction. To speed onset of adequate intubating conditions, 0.01 mg/kg followed after 3 minutes by 0.15 mg/kg will provide sufficient relaxation within 60–90 seconds.

5. Pancuronium

    a. Dose: intubation dose of 0.08–0.12 mg/kg.

    b. Onset: excellent intubating conditions in 3 minutes.

    c. Duration: 60+ minute duration of action.

    d. Elimination: eliminated by the kidneys with slight hepatic metabolism.

    e. Cardiovascular effects: mildly vagolytic.

    f. Complications: tachycardia.

D. Maintenance of anesthesia

1. Standard inhalation agents can be used after restoration of intravascular volume and correction of acidosis. Judicious doses of agents with minimal hemodynamic effects (scopolamine, benzodiazepines, ketamine) can be used in the unstable patient to prevent intraoperative awareness. Drugs are chosen based on the postoperative plan for the patient. Short-acting agents may be preferred if the patient is to be awakened rapidly postoperatively. If continued ventilator support is necessary because of associated injuries, a larger dose or longer acting opioids and neuromuscular agents should be used.

E. Common intraoperative problems. Continuous communication with the surgeon is essential in caring for the multiply injured patient. Sudden changes in vital signs must be communicated so that potentially occult injuries can be diagnosed. Similarly, the surgeon should be expected to give some notice when major bleeding can be expected to occur (i.e., before unclamping a vessel). In the event of persistent hypotension due to hypovolemia, the surgeon may pack off an area of uncontrolled bleeding or clamp a vessel until volume is restored.

1. **Hypothermia.** See the previous discussion on temperature monitoring and treatment. Mild hypothermia (34°C) has a cerebral protective effect in the event of cerebral ischemia. A damage control closure of the abdomen may be appropriate in the event of uncontrolled bleeding in a hypothermic patient.

2. **Massive transfusion** (Chapter 42)
   a. **Type O** and type specific blood must be available for immediate use in any trauma center. Crossmatched blood should be available within an hour of the patient's arrival at the trauma center. Rapid acquisition of fresh frozen plasma and platelets must be ensured. Close communication with the blood bank is essential.
   b. **Use** of intraoperative blood salvage techniques can markedly reduce the amount of banked blood required. Contamination with intestinal contents is a contraindication to blood salvage procedures.
   c. **Coagulation parameters** such as PT, PTT, and platelet count must be monitored. TEG and ACT may also be utilized.

3. **Hypoxemia** may develop because of pulmonary contusion, pulmonary edema, pneumothorax (simple or tension), or misplaced endotracheal tube. This may occur at any time during an operative procedure. Patients with displaced rib fractures, subcutaneous emphysema, or pneumothorax should have a chest tube inserted prior to receiving positive pressure ventilation.

4. **Hypotension:** even transient drops in blood pressure have been shown to have adverse effects on survival in patients with head injury.

5. **Abdominal hypertension.** Massive transfusion or significant abdominal injuries can result in intraabdominal hypertension and abdominal compartment syndrome. This may manifest as elevated peak inspiratory pressures, decreased urine output, hypotension, and decreased cardiac output. The condition is often observed on closure of the abdominal fascia. If abdominal compartment syndrome is suspected, a damage control closure should be employed (Chapter 28).

F. **Extubation.** Timing of extubation should be discussed with the surgeon.
   1. It may be appropriate to extubate the stable trauma patient in the OR at the end of the operation. All trauma patients are considered to have a full stomach, so extubation should not occur until the stomach is emptied and the patient is able to protect his or her airway.
   2. In the multiply injured patient, extubation may be delayed until the patient has been stabilized and ongoing issues have been resolved. With a history of substance abuse, comorbid conditions, or in the elderly, delayed extubation may be more appropriate. In the severely head injured patient or in the event of significant maxillofacial trauma, an early tracheostomy should be considered.

G. **Transfer to postoperative care.** At the completion of operative procedures the patient is taken to either the postanesthesia care unit (PACU) or an ICU. A complete report and plan should be communicated to the receiving caregiver. This report should include the following:
   1. **History:** A brief description of the mechanism of injury, allergies, medical problems, and preoperative medications should be given.
   2. **Procedure.** Describe the operative procedure and significant findings. Were there any surgical or anesthetic complications?
   3. **Airway.** If the patient is still intubated, discuss the plan for ventilation and extubation. A difficult intubation must be communicated to avoid a problem after extubation. Any difficulty with ventilation in the OR must be described.
   4. **Fluids.** Describe blood and fluid losses in the OR as well as all replacement fluids. Fresh frozen plasma, platelets, and any other coagulation products administered must be mentioned. Report how much blood is still available in the blood bank.
   5. **Medications.** Muscle relaxants, sedatives, and amnestic agents used as well as time of administration are important. Postoperative neurologic checks may be important and administration of certain medications may delay these examinations. Communicate when the next dose of antibiotics or steroids is due.

6. **Laboratory data.** Communicate the most recent hemoglobin, blood gas, and any other pertinent laboratory data.
7. **Lines.** Describe chest tubes, central lines, volume lines, etc. Were the lines placed in the OR or trauma resuscitation area? Were radiographs obtained after line placement?

Bibliography

American College of Surgeons Committee on Trauma. *Advanced Trauma Life Support for Doctors.* 6th ed. Chicago, Ill: American College of Surgeons Committee on Trauma; 1998.

Barash PG, Cullen BF, et al. *Clinical Anesthesia.* 4th ed. Philadelphia, Pa: JB Lippincott Co; 2000.

Miller RD, ed. *Anesthesia.* 6th ed. Philadelphia, Pa: Churchill Livingstone; 2004.

Rodricks MB, Deutschman CS. Emergent airway management. *Crit Care Clin*; July 2000.

40 TRAUMA PAIN MANAGEMENT
DONALD M. YEALY

I. **BASIC PRINCIPLES OF ANALGESIA.** Six basic principles of analgesia apply in all types of pain management.
   A. **Individualize the route and dose of analgesic.**
      1. Patients respond differently to painful stimuli based on the type and severity of injury, psychological makeup, and ethnic bias. In addition, individual analgesic requirements vary based on the time of day and previous use of analgesics or recreational substances. Although starting doses are offered (Table 40-1), the amount and timing should be altered based on the response.
      2. Patients may have expectations of being completely pain-free, or insensate; these expectations are often unrealistic. **Provide adequate analgesia, defined as enhancing comfort to a tolerable level without side effect.** The expected level of relief should be discussed with each patient to ensure understanding by both the provider and receiver.
      3. Intramuscular injection offers little analgesic advantage over oral or intravenous administration due to erratic absorption and pain on injection. The variable absorption with IM injection (due to hydration, sympathetic tone, muscle site and time of day factors) limits the ability to titrate analgesia to need in a timely fashion, forcing the physician to estimate the correct dose (which is inaccurate in up to two thirds of cases). This route should rarely be used and can be replaced with subcutaneous injections (which are less painful) in those who cannot tolerate oral medicines and without intravenous access.
   B. **Offer analgesics on a time-contingent basis during acute pain phases.**
      1. Time-contingent dosing affords steady blood levels of analgesia, avoiding the wide fluctuations with "prn" dosing. It also avoids making the patient request medication, still allowing for refusal if not needed; this increases the sense of empowerment and satisfaction, augmenting the perceived analgesia.
      2. Time-contingent dosing is best for all analgesic preparations, including NSAIDs, acetaminophen, and opioid analgesics. When providing oral analgesics, offer the medication based on the pharmacologic profile (e.g., hydrocodone or oxycodone every 4–6 hours around the clock) in the acute phase of injury. Parenteral opioids should be administered on a time-contingent basis as well, by hourly infusion (e.g., morphine, 1–2 mg/hour in opioid-naive patients) or via patient-controlled analgesia (PCA) device.
   C. **Opioids are the cornerstone of acute severe pain management.**
      1. Intravenous opioids offer the best opportunity to deliver rapid, titrated, adequate analgesia. Opioids, given in small increments every 5 to 10 minutes (e.g., morphine 2–5 mg, hydromorphone 0.5–1.0 mg, or fentanyl 50–100 μg for most opioid-naive adults), based on the pain and physiologic responses, remain the best agents for severe injury or initial postoperative pain. Oral opioids are inexpensive, effective, and tolerated well by patients with ongoing moderate to severe pain after the initial injury or postoperative period.
      2. PCA—using small patient-triggered boluses of an opioid (usually morphine) every 6 to 10 minutes maximum, with lockout intervals to prevent excess, allows safe and effective relief. PCA requires some initial loading—relief gained from bedside titration—before instituting patient maintenance. It can

TABLE 40-1	Opioid Analgesics			
	Equianalgesic dose (mg)		Starting oral dose	
	Oral	IV*	Adults	Children
Name	(mg and hour interval in adults)		(mg and hour interval)	(mg/kg)
Pure Agonists				
–Morphine	30 q3–4	5 q1–2	15–30 q3–4	0.3
–Meperidine (Demerol)	300 q2–3	75 q2–3	Not recommended	
–Hydromorphone (Dilaudid)	4–6 q3–4	1 q3–4	2–4 q4–6	0.06
–Codeine†	120–130 q3–4		30–60 q3–4	0.5–1.0
–Oxycodone (Roxicodone, Percocet, others)	30 q3–4		10–20 q3–4	0.3
–Hydrocodone (Lortab, Lorcet, Vicodin, others)	30 q3–4		10–20 q3–4	
–Methadone	20 q6–8	5 q6–8	5–10 q6–8	0.2
–Levorphanol (Levo-Dromoran)	4 q6–8	1 q6–8	2–4 q6–8	0.04
–Fentanyl		0.05 q0.5–1.0 (50 μg)		
Mixed Agonist-antagonists				
–Nalbuphine (Nubain)		5 q3–4		
–Butorphanol (Stadol)		1 q2–4		

*After initial titration, which is done using this dose at 10-minute intervals based on response; these are not recommended final doses but equipotent initial doses.
†Sedating and constipating in doses >60–90 mg; oxycodone and hydrocodone preferred.
q, every.

be combined with low-dose infusions to decrease needs safely and augment relief. PCA care paths or plans are best developed together with acute pain practitioners based on local resources.

D. Combination therapy affords the best analgesia, especially in mild to moderate pain syndromes and after acute severe pain is initially controlled.

1. Include an NSAID preparation with an opioid whenever possible to provide analgesia by two different and synergistic methods. All NSAIDs have similar effects when given in equipotent doses, and the least expensive drug and route should be used for most patients (Table 40-2).

a. Ketorolac (30–60 mg IM or 15–30 mg IV) is the only NSAID available for parenteral use. It is no more potent than oral ibuprofen (800 mg) or indomethacin (50 mg), although much more expensive than these NSAID and generic morphine or meperidine. Ketorolac should be reserved for short-term use (<3 days) in those patients who are unable to take an inexpensive NSAID orally.

b. Newer selective oral NSAID (termed **COX-2 inhibitors**) offer analgesic and antiinflammatory effects similar to traditional NSAID with a lower frequency of GI side effects and fewer antiplatelet effects. However, they are more expensive that traditional NSAID, and do not avoid GI or renal side effects; they should be reserved for those patients intolerant of traditional NSAID or at high risk for complications who need prolonged therapy.

TABLE 40-2	Nonopioid analgesics—NSAIDs		
Drug	**Usual adult dose**	**Usual pediatric dose**	**Comments**
Oral			
–Acetaminophen	650–1,000 mg q4h	10–15 mg/kg q4h	Acetaminophen lacks antiinflammatory activity.
–Aspirin	650–1,000 mg q4h	10–15 mg/kg q4h*	The standard against which other NSAIDs are compared. Inhibits platelet aggregation irreversibly (lasts 2 weeks); may cause postoperative bleeding.
–Ibuprofen (Motrin, others)	400–600 mg q4–6h	10 mg/kg q6–8h	Available as several brand names and as generic.
–Naproxen (Anaprox, Naprosyn others)	500–550 mg initial dose followed by 250–275 mg q6–8h		Available as several brand names and as generic.
Parenteral			
–Ketorolac tromethamine (Toradol)	30–60 mg IM or 15 mg IV initial dose followed by 15 or 30 mg q6h		Parenteral use should not exceed 5 days.

*Contraindicated in presence of fever or other evidence of viral illness.
†With the possible exception of trisalicylate and salsalate, all NSAIDs exhibit reversible antiplatelet effects. Also, these doses are associated with peak analgesic effects, although increased doses cause increased antiinflammatory effects along with more side effects.
NSAID, nonsteroidal antiinflammatory drug.

Finally, they may increase the risk of cardiovascular events; given the complex issues and limited need in acute pain (compared to other agents), these are not recommended currently for acute pain management.

2. Similarly, **acetaminophen** augments opioid and NSAID analgesia, allowing greater pain relief with less toxicity. When using acetaminophen–opioid combination preparations, attention to the daily acetaminophen dose is required to avoid toxicity, especially in patients with liver disease.

3. Antiemetics and phenothiazine/butyrophenones **do not augment analgesia and may increase side effects** (especially sedation and hypotension). These agents should be used to treat specific conditions but not routinely added to analgesic regimens.

4. **Benzodiazepines** (midazolam, diazepam, lorazepam) are pure sedatives. These drugs lessen anxiety, produce amnesia, and cause skeletal muscular relaxation, augmenting the *perceived* analgesia. However, pure sedatives should not be used alone to treat pain because of their lack of analgesia; **if used in combination with an opioid (e.g., during orthopedic manipulation), the dose of each should be lowered to avoid clinical respiratory depression or hypotension.**

E. **Recognize and treat side effects of analgesic therapy.**

1. NSAID drugs are associated with platelet aggregation inhibition, gastrointestinal dysfunction ranging from dyspepsia to gastrointestinal bleeding, renal insufficiency, and (rarely) mental status changes. These complications occur irrespective of the route (i.e., parenteral ketorolac causes similar side effects to an equipotent dose of an oral NSAID) and are treated by discontinuation of the drug.

2. Opioid analgesia is associated with nausea (up to 40% of patients), sedation, itching, constipation, urinary retention, and hypotension. Treatment of opioid-induced side effects includes decreasing the dose or changing the route of administration of the drug, as well as treating the side effect.

  a. Opioid-induced hypotension is the result of diminished peripheral sympathetic tone, histamine release, and vasodilation. This usually is mild and transient, but can be dramatic in the sympathetically depleted or hypovolemic patient. Hypotension is best avoided by optimizing volume status and delivering the drug in titrated, small doses. If hypotension occurs, further doses should be withheld and crystalloid bolus infusions given. Opioid antagonists do not reverse opioid-induced hypotension.

  b. Itching after an opioid is poorly understood but may be the result of histamine release or opioid receptor activity. Itching occurs with all agents to varying degrees, especially when given intravenously or in the epidural space. Antihistamines may be effective in relieving itching, with opioid antagonists (naloxone 0.1–0.2 mg) used for refractory or severe cases.

  c. Respiratory depression and sedation occur together, with sedation usually preceding clinical respiratory depression. Both can be reversed with incremental doses of an opioid antagonist. We recommend naloxone 0.04 mg every minute if lowered respiratory rate—prepared with 0.4 mg ampule diluted up to 10 cc with saline and given 1 cc at a time—to reverse the excessive effect but maintain analgesia. **For patients with profound coma or apnea, naloxone 0.4 mg IV should be given immediately.**

F. Pain is better treated early rather than later.

  1. There is evidence that "pain begets pain" probably secondary to peripheral and central neuromodulation that occurs after a prolonged painful stimulus such as injury.

  2. Early treatment of pain can decrease the overall need for analgesics and improve patient satisfaction. Similarly, avoiding periods of inadequate analgesia will also help avert up-regulation of pain receptors and thus improve pain relief.

  3. Early **titrated** pain therapy can alter the sympathetic responses to injury and improve regional blood flow, further aiding resuscitation. Overzealous analgesic administration can produce the opposite response.

II. OVERVIEW: PAIN MANAGEMENT IN THE TRAUMA PATIENT

  A. The principles of pain management in the trauma patient include the basic analgesic principles outlined and principles of acute postoperative pain management.

  B. Certain trauma patients present with special needs: patients with severe pain during resuscitation, those with substance abuse issues, and those with psychological issues either at the time of the injury or during the rehabilitation phase.

  C. A small number of trauma patients will require analgesia for a prolonged period of time, or may develop a chronic pain syndrome as a result of injury. These patients are best managed with a multidisciplinary approach that includes the trauma and primary care physicians, a physician pain specialist, physical therapists, and psychosocial clinicians.

III. ANALGESIA DURING RESUSCITATION

  A. Analgesia should not be withheld during the resuscitation unless one of three conditions exist:

  ■ Hemodynamic instability
  ■ Respiratory depression
  ■ Profound sedation or coma

  In patients without these contraindications, titrated intravenous opioids should be given to attenuate pain with close attention to the physiologic response (especially blood pressure and level of consciousness). **Any opioid or systemic sedative/induction agent can cause hypotension**, with the frequency and degree being the important difference between regimens.

B. Fentanyl causes the least hemodynamic effects and is the agent of choice for pain relief during resuscitation. In doses of 0.25 to 0.50 µg/kg (50–100 µg for average adults) every 5 to 10 minutes, it produces safe clinical analgesia up to 60 minutes in most patients. Side effects are treated as noted previously. Chest wall rigidity is a rare occurrence, seen mostly with larger doses (>6 µg/kg boluses). This can compromise ventilation, but is extremely rare in the doses recommended here. It is treated with positive pressure ventilation, opioid reversal agents and (in severe cases) neuromuscular blockade with endotracheal intubation.

C. Other inexpensive opioids (**morphine** 2–5 mg, **meperidine** 50–100 mg, **hydromorphone** 0.5- to 1.0-mg IV increments) produce longer analgesia but are associated with more hemodynamic effects. These drugs are best used in well-resuscitated patients. Other synthetic opioids (alfentanil, sufentanil, remifentanil) offer little advantage at a higher cost.

IV. PROCEDURAL SEDATION AND ANALGESIA

A. Patients usually require pharmacologic assistance when painful or anxiety-provoking procedures are planned. A continuum exists between mild sedation and systemic analgesia to general anesthesia. **In general, the deeper the intended or potential reflex and responsiveness change, the more closely the patient must be monitored by trained experts.**

B. Environmental and other adjuncts will ease the painful perceptions and anxiety. These include:

  1. Comfortable surroundings (dimmed lights, quiet area, music if possible)
  2. A calm, clear manner of communication, educating the patient of expected responses and asking for feedback to help improve care (e.g., "If you feel more pain, let me know and I will give more medicine.")
  3. Splinting and minimal or gentle handling of injured parts
  4. Family or friend presence (if possible, safe, and desired)
  5. Attempts to distract patient or help him or her think of other soothing or pleasing settings
  6. Local or topical anesthetics to ease nociceptive stimuli

C. Most procedures can be safely and comfortably performed with no pain involved and reduced anxiety for the patient (e.g., radiologic studies) or conscious sedation/systemic analgesia (e.g., wound debridement, joint or fracture care). Monitoring of responses, vital signs, and pulse oximetry can be performed by either a physician or a nurse with physician supervision.

  1. Opioids are the cornerstone of pain relief during procedures. Titrated fentanyl (0.25–0.5 µg/kg—often 50–100 µg in adults) every 2 to 3 minutes based on the response is a common method. Other opioids—morphine or meperidine—are alternatives, though the duration and hemodynamic effects differ from the limited amount seen with fentanyl.
  2. Benzodiazepines, especially midazolam (1–2 mg increments in adults) or diazepam (2.5- to 5-mg increments) are best for procedures requiring sedation or muscular relaxation. These drugs do not relieve pain, although patients may lack recall of the pain.
  3. Combination of opioids and benzodiazepines are often used for procedures that require pain and anxiety relief or pain relief and muscular relaxation. It is best to deliver the benzodiazepine first, and then add titrated doses of the opioid. Care to the effect is critical since an additive or synergistic effect can occur, risking airway or hemodynamic complications.
  4. Other agents can be used, including ketamine (0.25 mg/kg IV increments, creating a dissociative state with rare emergence reactions or laryngospasm) and etomidate (0.05–0.1 mg/kg increments, creating good sedation but a small risk of deep sedation).

D. General anesthesia is not sought in the trauma bay, emergency department, or floor outside of rapid intubation. Procedures requiring this are best performed in the OR.

E. In the rare instance **when deep sedation is planned** (e.g., for hip relocation or cardioversion), **it should be done where continuous monitoring equipment** (ECG, automated blood pressure and pulse oximeter mandatory, capnography) **are available, with a physician and nurse dedicated solely to delivering drugs and monitoring the patient.** Those two individuals must be expert in recognizing complications and treating them, from knowledge of reversal agents and cardiac drugs through airway support and endotracheal intubation. The physician performing the procedure cannot safely be responsible for this monitoring.

   1. Because of the needs for close monitoring, deep sedation is often carried out in the operating room (OR), although the emergency department (ED) and ICU are acceptable if the proper personnel (skilled in recognizing and treating complications, especially airway related) resources are available.

F. During procedural sedation/systemic analgesia of any level, create a record to document:

   1. Immediate preprocedural exam (including noting review of previous exam, allergies, medications, and last meal if after initial evaluation).

   2. Serial measurement of vital signs, responses to stimuli, oximetry reading, and any interventions. This is best done every 5 minutes.

   3. Complications, including (but not limited to) vomiting, loss of consciousness or respirations, rhythm changes, rashes, dyspnea, agitation, or any involuntary activity.

   4. Clear timing of drugs and doses, including route.

   5. Recovery period, including return to preprocedural state or age appropriate functioning and ability to sit up, walk (if permitted), and take oral liquids.

V. SPECIAL ANALGESIC NEEDS
A. Rib fractures and chest wall pain

   1. Rib fractures are in the category of severe pain syndromes; inadequate analgesia may lead to pulmonary compromise and pneumonia. Systemic opioids, especially via scheduled parenteral administration or PCA/continuous drip, are effective in most patients.

   2. These patients may benefit from **continuous epidural analgesia.**

   a. Indications: moderate to severe pain uncontrolled by systemic opioids, in those with preexisting or impending pulmonary compromise.

   b. Contraindications: coagulopathy, hypovolemia, spinal fracture or skin infection at site of intended placement, and dural tear. Low-molecular-weight heparin should not be used in patients with an epidural catheter because of increased risk of epidural hematoma.

   c. Methods: injection followed by continuous infusion of opioids (preservative free, usually morphine or fentanyl) and local anesthetics (lidocaine or bupivacaine), alone or together. These allow good pain relief at lower doses due to placement of the drug near the active site.

   d. Success is measured by adequate pain relief and improved pulmonary mechanics (or preservation of near normal in those without impairment). When a local anesthetic is infused, the dermatomal level of block can be estimated from a light touch/pin prick exam.

   e. Duration of therapy depends on the clinical response. Generally, catheters are removed after 3 to 5 days (although longer intervals are acceptable in the absence of complications or infection). Most patients can be converted to other systemic regimens within 48 hours.

   f. Epidural catheters should be removed immediately if signs of infection develop (erythema, drainage) or if they no longer function properly.

   g. Respiratory depression is rare compared to equipotent systemic doses, but can occur early (minutes from injection due to systemic absorption) or late (hours after injection from rostral spread).

   h. Itching is common with epidural opioids. Antihistamines or opioid antagonists (at low doses) can be used to reverse pruritus from epidural opioid administration, with the latter often added in low doses to the infusion.

3. Individual intercostal nerve blocks (using 0.25% to 0.5% bupivacaine with epinephrine) can also be effective in patients with three or fewer rib fractures.
4. Pleural administration of a local anesthetic (e.g., bupivacaine 10–15 mL of a 0.25% to 0.5% solution) can afford good pain relief for 6 to 12 hours. Although it can be instilled through a thoracostomy tube, this is not recommended in the initial phases of management since the tube must be clamped for 20 to 30 minutes to allow contact with the pleura. More commonly, a small-bore catheter can be placed in the extrapleural space during an open chest procedure and used postoperatively as a route for pleural anesthesia.

B. Nerve injury
   1. Any trauma may result in direct injury to nerves.
   2. Patients complaining of pain described as burning, electrical in nature, or pain complaints that seem out of proportion to the magnitude of traumatic injury may have neuropathic injury (pain from nerve injury).
   3. Opioid analgesia alone is often not beneficial for long-term treatment. The use of adjuvants are common, including antidepressants and membrane stabilizers (antiseizure medications).
      a. Cyclic antidepressants are best for those with this pain and sleep disturbance, taking advantage of their sedative effects. Amitriptyline (10–25 mg), nortriptyline (25–50 mg), and trazodone (25–50 mg) are the commonly used agents. These are usually started at bedtime and increased in dose and frequency based on the responses, with the lower doses used in the elderly.
      b. Selective serotonin reuptake inhibitor antidepressants can be used for others without sleep disturbance (e.g., fluoxetine 20 mg or sertraline 50 mg once daily initially).
      c. Carbamazepine (100–200 mg three times daily) and dilantin (1 g initially followed by 100–200 mg twice daily) are also useful, with doses adjusted upward as needed.
   4. Often, the advice of physicians that deal with advanced pain management is necessary to help with the analgesic plan and titration. Blood levels of these various agents generally do not predict success. Monitoring for side effects is necessary (e.g., serial blood counts and liver function studies in those on carbamazepine and ECG for elderly patients or those with conduction abnormalities in those on a cyclic antidepressant).

C. Long-term opioid therapy
   1. Those patients requiring multiple surgical procedures, or those with extensive orthopedic injuries (external fixators, pelvic fractures) may require opioid therapy for extended intervals, with the development of opioid tolerance.
   2. Patients receiving opioid therapy on a regular basis for more than 2 weeks are at risk for withdrawal if the opioid is abruptly discontinued. Mixed or partial opioid agonists/antagonists (e.g., butorphanol, pentacozine, nalbuphine) may produce withdrawal and should be avoided.
   3. Signs of opioid withdrawal include hypertension, tachycardia, tearing, salivation, piloerection, and anxiety.
   4. Opioid withdrawal may be avoided by ensuring that opioid therapy is discontinued according to a taper schedule that decreases the amount of opioid by 20% each 24 to 48 hours.

 AXIOMS

■ Pain is best treated early and continuously; do not require awake patients to ask for relief.
■ Intravenous opioids are the cornerstone of acute severe pain management. NSAIDs and acetaminophen are useful adjuncts in moderate to severe pain, and often adequate in mild to moderate pain syndromes. Morphine is inexpensive and predictable, while fentanyl offers limited hemodynamic effects at a higher (albeit still relatively low) cost and shorter duration of action.

- Intramuscular analgesics should be avoided.
- Analgesic regimens must be tailored to each individual, with variation of 5- to 10-fold seen in opioid-naive patients and even higher in those using these drugs or other sedatives chronically.
- The ideal dose of opioid is the one that creates analgesia without excessive sedation or hemodynamic effect, with ceiling doses based on side effects rather than absolute amounts. Switching between opioids before adequate titration offers little benefit.
- When providing procedural sedation and systemic analgesia, watch for excessive effects (especially respiratory drive and protective reflexes); mishaps are usually related to failure to seek, recognize, or quickly treat excessive sedation.

Bibliography

Acute Pain Management: Operative or Medical Procedures and Trauma. Rockville, Md: US Department of Health and Human Services, Agency for Health Care Policy and Research; February 1992.

Chudnofsky CR, Wright SW, Dronen SC, et al. The safety of fentanyl use in the emergency department. *Ann Emerg Med* 1989;18:635–639.

Grabinski PY, Kaiko RF, Rogers AG, et al. Plasma levels and analgesia following deltoid and gluteal injections of methadone and morphine. *J Clin Pharmacol* 1983;23:48–55.

Onghena P, Van Houdenhove B. Antidepressant-induced analgesia in chronic non-malignant pain: A meta-analysis of 39 placebo-controlled studies. *Pain* 1992;49:205–219.

Ward KR, Yealy DM. Systemic analgesia and sedation in managing orthopedic emergencies. *Emerg Med Clin North Am* 2000;18:141–166.

41

HYPOTHERMIA, COLD INJURY, AND DROWNING

SAMUEL A. TISHERMAN

I. **INTRODUCTION.** Hypothermia, defined as a body temperature of <35°C, occurs in up to half the victims of major trauma and is associated with significantly increased morbidity and mortality. Hypothermia in trauma patients, which occurs secondary to injury, environmental exposure, shock, fluid resuscitation, anesthesia, and alcohol or drug intoxication, must be differentiated from exposure hypothermia secondary to medical conditions (e.g., thyroid or adrenal insufficiency, alcohol intoxication). Uncontrolled, accidental hypothermia in these situations must also be differentiated from controlled, therapeutic hypothermia (as used in cardiac surgery and post-cardiac arrest) with induction of poikilothermia and prevention of shivering.

A. **Classification of hypothermia.** The severity of hypothermia is classified primarily by the patient's core temperature:
   1. **Mild:** 32°C to 35°C—physiologic findings subtle
   2. **Moderate:** 28°C to 32°C—signs and symptoms present, but variable
   3. **Severe:** Below 28°C—central nervous system (CNS) and hemodynamic alterations impending or present (often extreme)

B. **Core temperature must be measured.** This requires special probes that measure low temperatures. Rectal, bladder catheter, central venous, and esophageal thermistors offer the best temperature data. Rectal probes are preferred because of their safety and ease of insertion.

II. **PHYSIOLOGY OF HYPOTHERMIA**

A. **Maintenance of temperature** within a narrow range, despite widely varying environmental temperatures, is critical for homeothermic (warm-blooded) animals, such as humans. The normal response to a cold environment is to simultaneously minimize heat loss and increase heat production.
   1. **Heat loss** occurs via radiation, conduction, convection, and evaporation. Hypothermic patients can minimize heat loss by behavioral responses (moving to a warmer environment), use of warm clothing, and cutaneous vasoconstriction.
   2. **Increased physical activity, shivering, increased feeding, and nonshivering thermogenesis can increase heat production.** Shivering causes an increase in oxygen consumption for which the patient may not be able to physiologically compensate, vasodilation that may cause more heat loss, and metabolic acidosis. Thus, shivering may be detrimental and may not increase temperature. The need for pharmacologic (neuromuscular blockade) treatment of the shivering is controversial.

B. **Clinical effects of hypothermia.** A progression of changes occurs in all physiologic parameters as temperature decreases, with subtle and inconsistent findings seen in mild hypothermia and more predictable abnormalities seen in severe hypothermia.
   1. **Metabolic.** The body initially attempts to conserve body heat via increased metabolic activity and shivering during mild hypothermia. These responses are lost as hypothermia progresses, with an eventual decrease in metabolism (which may be protective).
   2. **Respiratory.** Tachypnea may be seen initially but with further cooling the respiratory rate slows, eventually leading to apnea. Arterial oxygenation is usually maintained, but tissue oxygenation may be impaired due to intense

vasoconstriction and leftward shift in the hemoglobin dissociation curve, leading to decreased release of oxygen. Hypothermia alters the measured arterial pH, PCO_2, and PO_2, tempting some to suggest "correcting" blood gas values for the patient's temperature before treating since all blood gas determinations are performed with the sample warmed to $37°C$. This is unnecessary as there is **no proven benefit in using the corrected values.**

3. **Hemodynamic.** Tachycardia is common in early or mild hypothermia, but bradycardia is seen with more severe hypothermia. On the electrocardiogram (ECG), prolonged PR, QRS, and QT intervals; J (Osborn) waves; sinus bradycardia; atrial flutter or fibrillation; and ventricular arrhythmias may be seen in moderate to severe hypothermia. Below $28°C$, there is a high risk of ventricular fibrillation (VF), heart block, or asystole. Pulses often are not palpable because of vasoconstriction, even if cardiac function continues and tissue perfusion is adequate for that temperature level. In addition to the changes in cardiac rhythm, vasodilation occurs with mild hypothermia and shivering, causing further heat loss and predisposing the patient to hypotension. Vasoconstriction occurs as the temperature decreases.

4. **Neurologic.** Changes with mild to moderate hypothermia may include apathy, confusion, or loss of coordination. An abnormal sensorium in a trauma patient at risk for hypothermia should not be attributed solely to hypothermia; closed head injuries, hypovolemia, and alcohol or drug intoxication need to be considered. With severe hypothermia, coma occurs, often with electroencephalogram silence, although normal neurologic recovery is still likely.

5. **Coagulation.** Hypothermia has important effects on coagulation parameters. One of the most frequent findings is thrombocytopenia due to platelet sequestration. This is further complicated by abnormal platelet function, leading to prolonged bleeding times. Impairment of the coagulation cascade occurs secondary to decreased enzyme function. Increased plasma fibrinolytic activity also may occur. In addition to hypothermia, massive transfusions with dilution of platelets and clotting factors, acidosis, and tissue trauma also play a role in coagulation changes that occur in trauma patients.

6. **Renal.** Hypothermia decreases the ability of the kidney to reabsorb fluid and electrolytes, leading to an inappropriate "cold" diuresis, which further increases the risk of hypotension. As temperature decreases further, urine output decreases. Consequently, urine output has limited utility as a marker of adequate organ perfusion in hypothermic patients.

III. HYPOTHERMIA IN TRAUMA

A. **Predisposition to hypothermia.** In trauma patients, the incidence and severity of hypothermia correlate directly with injury severity. Between 21% and 50% of severely injured trauma patients become hypothermic. This is due to:

1. **Exposure** in the field with inadequate or wet clothing.
2. **Blood loss** and shock.
3. **Common standard treatments**, including removal of all clothing, rapid infusion of cool fluids, and opening of body cavities.
4. **Limited ability to produce heat** because of trauma and hemorrhagic shock; analgesic, sedative, and anesthetic agents; or alcohol and other drugs taken by the patient. General anesthesia may decrease heat production by 20%.

B. **Clinical studies** often have shown higher mortality in trauma patients who become hypothermic, even when other factors that affect mortality are taken into account. Hypothermia may be the cause of, or contributor to complications, or may just be a marker of severe injury. As a result of severe trauma and resuscitation attempts, the patient is often hypothermic, coagulopathic, and acidotic. The "damage control" abbreviated laparotomy (rapid control of active arterial bleeding, rapid control of contamination, packing the abdomen, and rewarming in the intensive care unit [ICU], and delayed definitive procedures) has been used successfully to break the cycle of bleeding, transfusion, worsening coagulopathy, worsening hypothermia, and more bleeding.

C. **Animal studies** have shown a protective role for controlled hypothermia during hemorrhagic shock. In theory, hypothermia may protect organs that are ischemic or are vulnerable to ischemia (especially the brain and heart) and improve outcomes. The mechanisms of the beneficial effects of hypothermia include decreased metabolic demands and other poorly understood effects. Based on our current understanding of the effects of uncontrolled, exposure hypothermia, rapid rewarming of trauma patients is recommended, particularly if they are coagulopathic. Additional studies regarding therapeutic hypothermia are needed.

IV. TREATMENT

A. **Prevention.** Awareness of the potential for hypothermia in trauma patients is critical. Measures to prevent hypothermia should be initiated in the field and continued in the emergency department (ED), operating room (OR), and ICU. These include:

  1. **Warming the environment** in the transport vehicle, ED, OR, and ICU. Room temperature is a critical determinant of heat loss because it dictates the rate of heat loss by radiation, convection, and evaporation from skin and operative sites.
  2. Use of warm, humidified oxygen.
  3. Infusion of warmed intravenous fluids and blood. Countercurrent fluid warmers are particularly effective.
  4. Minimization of exposure. Radiant heat lights may help.
  5. Application of a heating blanket or other heat-conserving device.

B. **Standard treatment.** This begins with standard resuscitation efforts (outlined in Table 41-1 and Fig. 41-1).

TABLE 41-1 Treatment of Hypothermia

General
1. Handle the patient gently.
2. Prevent further heat loss.
3. Evaluate ABCs:
   A—Airway
   B—Breathing
   C—Circulation
4. For the patient in coma, consider empiric treatments:
   D50
   Naloxone
   Thiamine

Options for treatment
1. Passive external rewarming:
   Insulating blanket
   Warm room
2. Active external rewarming:
   Heating blankets (Bair Hugger)
   Heating lamps
   Immersion
3. Active internal rewarming:
   Warm IV fluids
   Warm, humidified oxygen
   Gastric, colonic, bladder lavage
   Peritoneal, pleural, mediastinal lavage
   Continuous arteriovenous rewarming
   Hemodialysis
   Cardiopulmonary bypass

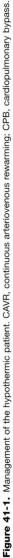

Figure 41-1. Management of the hypothermic patient. CAVR, continuous arteriovenous rewarming; CPB, cardiopulmonary bypass.

Hypothermic patient (core temp <35°C)
Start with ABCs
Rule out causes of secondary hypothermia

Intubate if:
Apneic
Reflexes absent

Core temp >28°C
Hemodynamically stable

Gently rewarm
Warm blankets +/– Bair Hugger
Warm IV fluids, O₂
Consider CAVR, peritoneal dialysis

Core temp <28°C
Hemodynamically unstable
or at risk

Core rewarming (CAVR, dialysis)
Consider CPB

Breathing spontaneously
Pulseless

Apneic
Pulseless

Start chest compressions
Rewarm/resuscitate with CPB
Dont stop until temp >30°C

1. **Airway and breathing.** Hypothermic patients who maintain a patent airway and have some spontaneous ventilation generally do not require urgent intubation. However, endotracheal intubation is indicated for the patient who is apneic or who has lost protective reflexes.

2. **Circulation.** External chest compressions should be initiated in all patients with ventricular fibrillation (VF) or asystole. If a severely hypothermic patient has no pulse but is breathing spontaneously and has evidence of an organized cardiac rhythm on the ECG, cardiac output should be sufficient to maintain the viability of vital organs. In these patients and those with a pulse but with hypotension or evidence of end-organ dysfunction, infusion of warm crystalloid solutions and blood (39°C–40°C) coupled with rapid rewarming is the primary treatment. For severely hypothermic patients in VF, up to three electrical countershocks should be attempted. If unsuccessful, the patient should have ongoing cardiopulmonary resuscitation (CPR) and be warmed prior to further defibrillation attempts. Antiarrhythmic agents tend to be ineffectual while the patient remains hypothermic. Hypovolemia, caused by capillary leak, cold diuresis, and injuries, needs to be corrected.

3. **Neurologic.** Other causes of coma, especially those which are easily reversed, such as head trauma, hypoglycemia, electrolyte abnormalities, or drug overdose, should be sought and treated (by dextrose 50%, naloxone, flumazenil, or thiamine). Additionally, spinal immobilization must be provided if any risk of torso or head injury exists.

C. **Procedures, patient handling, and VF.** As the core temperature decreases to 28°C and below, the risk of spontaneous VF increases. This risk may be enhanced by physical stimuli. It seems prudent to **handle all patients with moderate to severe hypothermia gently.** Only those procedures that are absolutely necessary should be performed. On the other hand, **intubation should not be withheld in apneic patients or those unable to maintain airway patency,** but it should be done with care. Topical anesthesia should be considered. Naso- and orogastric tubes, urinary bladder catheters, central venous catheters, and dramatic physical repositioning or movement of the patient are rarely lifesaving in the initial phases of resuscitation and should be withheld until the core temperature increases to mild to moderate hypothermia levels. Patients with mild hypothermia have a negligible risk of VF and should undergo procedures and transport in the usual fashion.

D. **Drug therapy.** Nonessential drugs should be avoided in hypothermic patients because of unpredictable metabolism, which may lead to toxicity as the patient rewarms.

E. **Signs of irreversibility.** Hypothermic patients may appear dead. Nonetheless, resuscitative efforts should start and not cease until moderate to severe hypothermia is completely reversed (i.e., the patient is nearly normothermic). The only exceptions are for those patients who have sustained other injuries incompatible with life or when hypothermia is the natural result of the poikilothermic state created with prolonged cardiac arrest in initially normothermic patients. Initial metabolic parameters such as a pH <6.8 or a potassium >7.0 mEq/L are relative markers of irreversibility.

V. **REWARMING.** In hypothermic trauma patients, after the primary survey has been completed and the ABCs have been addressed, rewarming should be initiated. The average warming rates of commonly used rewarming techniques are listed in Table 41-2.

A. **Mild hypothermia (32°C–35°C).** Patients with mild hypothermia can be treated with passive, external rewarming methods such as insulating blankets, or active, external rewarming methods such as heating blankets or convective air warmers (Bair Hugger, Augustine Medical, Inc., Eden Prairie, Minnesota)

B. **Moderate hypothermia (28°C–32°C).** External rewarming alone of moderately to severely hypothermic patients may lead to "afterdrop," a decrease in core temperature in part due to cold peripheral blood flowing to the core as peripheral vasodilation occurs. Patients with moderate hypothermia need more active, internal rewarming methods (e.g., warm IV fluids and warm inspired gas). Gastric,

TABLE 41-2	Rewarming Rates

Passive external rewarming	0.5–2.0°C/h
Shivering	3–4°C/h
Heated O_2	1.0–2.5°C/h
Peritoneal lavage/dialysis	1.0–2.5°C/h
Continuous arteriovenous rewarming	2–3°C/h
Cardiopulmonary bypass	10°C/h

colonic, or bladder lavage; peritoneal, pleural, or mediastinal lavage; or hemodialysis may be indicated. Continuous arteriovenous rewarming (CAVR) recently has been described for use in hypothermic patients. A heparin-bonded extracorporeal circuit with a countercurrent warming device is attached to cannulas placed in the femoral artery and vein. Venovenous rewarming also can be used in a similar fashion by adding a roller pump.

C. Severe hypothermia (<28°C). The severely hypothermic patient is at very high risk of cardiac arrest, particularly if dysrhythmias are already present. Use of cardiopulmonary bypass (CPB), initiated via the femoral vessels or the chest, is the treatment of choice since CPB is the most efficient rewarming method and CPB can support circulation in the event of cardiac arrest. If hemodynamics are adequate and dysrhythmias have not occurred, active, internal rewarming may be appropriate as long as CPB is available should the patient deteriorate.

VI. SPECIAL SITUATIONS

A. Exposure hypothermia (without trauma) causes approximately 100,000 deaths worldwide each year. To enhance survival, three things are essential: recognition of patients who are at risk, accurate identification of the condition using core temperature measurements, and early initiation of appropriate therapy.

1. Risk factors

  a. Extremes of age (the elderly and neonates/infants)

  b. Alcohol, sedative, or illicit drug use

  c. Concomitant neurologic disease or injury, especially stroke and spinal cord lesions

  d. Dermal disruption, including burns

  e. Certain medications, including adrenergic blockers, antipsychotics, and antidepressants

  f. Endocrinologic diseases such as hypothyroidism and hypoadrenalism

  g. Submersion and immersion

2. The cause of hypothermia may not be exposure alone. Clinical clues that there is an underlying cause of hypothermia include absence of bradycardia; inability to increase temperature with routine measures; and abnormal mental status, stupor, or coma after rewarming to >32°C in the absence of head trauma or a period of cardiac arrest.

B. Drowning, defined as suffocation from submersion in a liquid medium, is a common cause of accidental death, particularly in children. Risk factors for drowning and near-drowning (submersion with recovery) include hypothermia, inability to swim, diving accidents, alcohol and drug ingestion, and exhaustion. Submersion rapidly leads to hypothermia, which may increase risk of drowning, but may also provide critical cerebral protection if asphyxiation or cardiac arrest occur.

1. Pulmonary failure is common after drowning unless aspiration is prevented by laryngospasm, which occurs in 10% to 20% of victims. Freshwater aspiration causes pulmonary damage because of washout of surfactant and reflex mechanisms that cause increased airway resistance. Saltwater aspiration causes pulmonary damage via an osmotic gradient leading to shifts of protein-rich

fluid into the alveoli. The fluid shifts caused by both types of aspiration generally do not cause significant serum electrolyte imbalances. Water contaminants add to the damage from either type of aspiration.
2. **CNS damage** due to cerebral hypoxia is found in 12% to 27% of survivors. Cold water temperature can decrease brain temperature to protective levels before cardiac arrest occurs. Mild hypothermia for 12 to 24 hours can improve neurologic outcome and survival after normothermic cardiac arrest. It may be advantageous to continue mild hypothermia after resuscitation of the near-drowning victim if comatose.
3. **Cervical spine** injuries from diving accidents are common and need to be sought.
4. **Shock** is uncommon in near-drowning, and its presence should prompt a search for other causes.
5. **Treatment** is based on the standard ABCs. Attention should be paid to the possible need for ventilatory support, even if the initial chest x-ray is normal. There is no role for prophylactic antibiotics or steroids.
6. **Cold submersion victims** may appear dead. If the patient has been immersed for <1 hour, resuscitative efforts are indicated at least until the core temperature is >30°C.
C. **Frostbite**
1. **Pathophysiology.** The local complications of hypothermia to external organs (digits, appendages such as the nose or ear, etc.) is termed frostbite, which involves tissue freezing and microvascular occlusion leading to cellular ischemia and death. The extent of tissue injury varies from hyperemia and edema to vesicle formation to full-thickness necrosis.
2. **Treatment.** Limiting cold exposure is the best way to minimize progression of injury. Affected extremities should be rapidly rewarmed by immersion in warm water (38°C–41°C). The extremity should be elevated to minimize edema. Tetanus toxoid should be administered. Escharotomy may be needed if vascular compromise occurs. Surgical debridement or amputation should be delayed until clear demarcation has occurred, unless wound sepsis has intervened.

AXIOMS

- All trauma patients are at risk for developing hypothermia in the field, ED, OR, and ICU. The core temperature must be recorded early. A special thermometer for low temperatures may be needed.
- Prevention of secondary hypothermia during resuscitation is important. Using warmed fluids and blankets, removing wet clothing, and ensuring a warm treatment room are important in the management of all trauma patients.
- Moderately and severely hypothermic patients need active core rewarming.
- Severely hypothermic patients may present in cardiac arrest. Unless obvious injuries incompatible with life are present, patients should not be declared dead until they have been warmed.

Bibliography
Gentilello LM, Jurkovich GJ, Stark MS, et al. Is hypothermia in the victim of major trauma protective or harmful? *Ann Surg* 1997;226:439–447.
Gregory JS, Flancbaum L, Townsend MC, et al. Incidence and timing of hypothermia in trauma patients undergoing operations. *J Trauma* 1991;31:795–800.
Jurkovich GJ, Greiser WB, Luterman A, et al. Hypothermia in trauma victims: An ominous predictor of survival. *J Trauma* 1987;27:1019–1024.
Luna GK, Maier RV, Pavlin EG, et al. Incidence and effect of hypothermia in seriously injured patients. *J Trauma* 1987;27:1014–1018.
Martini WZ, Pusateri AE, Uscilowicz JM, et al. Independent contributions of hypothermia and acidosis to coagulopathy in swine. *J Trauma* 2005;58:1002–1010.

Splittgerber FH, Talbert JG, Sweezer WP, et al. Partial cardiopulmonary bypass for core rewarming in profound accidental hypothermia. *Am Surg* 1986;52:407–412.

Steinemann S, Shackford SR, Davis JW. Implications of admission hypothermia in trauma patients. *J Trauma* 1990;30:200–202.

Tisherman SA, Safar P, Rodriguez A. Therapeutic hypothermia in traumatology. *Surg Clin North Am* 1999;79:1269–1289.

Wang HE, Callaway CW, Peitzman AB, Tisherman SA. Admission hypothermia and outcome after major trauma. *Crit Care Med* 2005;33:1296–1301.

Wu X, Kochanek PM, Cochran K, et al. Mild hypothermia improves survival after prolonged, traumatic hemorrhagic shock in pigs. *J Trauma* 2005;59(2):291–299.

42

BLOOD TRANSFUSION
AJAI K. MALHOTRA

I. **INTRODUCTION.** Human blood is a complex suspension of cells—erythrocytes (red blood cells, RBCs), leukocytes (white blood cells, WBCs), and thrombocytes (platelets)—and proteins in an aqueous environment referred to as serum. Each of these elements has a distinct function: Erythrocytes provide oxygen transport, leukocytes are essential for immunity and healing, thrombocytes provide primary hemostasis, and the proteins have myriad functions including secondary hemostasis and immunity. Such a classification is an oversimplification since the various elements of blood work in conjunction with each other.

   A. There is active interaction between thrombocytes and coagulation proteins (factors) to produce a stable clot, and there is active collaboration between cellular immunity provided by leukocytes and humoral immunity provided by proteins (immunoglobulins). Not only that, there is extensive "crosstalk" among the hemostatic, inflammatory, and other plasma protein cascades. However, this simplified classification helps in understanding the foundation of modern blood component therapy.

   B. Whole blood after being obtained from healthy volunteers is collected in special bags with additives to prevent clotting and preservatives to allow storage. In modern blood banking whole blood is rarely if ever used for transfusion. Rather the blood is separated into various components—RBCs, platelets, and plasma—and stored. The plasma component, from a single donation or pooled plasma from multiple donors, may be further processed to produce other components, namely cryoprecipitate, individual clotting factors, and so on. Separating blood into such components helps in maximizing the utility of each donation.

   C. In the trauma patient, one or more of the essential life-sustaining functions of blood may be deficient due to either extensive blood loss and/or the inability of the body to manufacture enough of the specific component to maintain the essential function. In the past, either whole blood or component therapy was often utilized to not only support the essential function, but also to provide circulating volume. Currently, **the only indication for blood component therapy** is to replenish or temporarily support one or more of these essential life-sustaining functions. The most commonly utilized blood components on the trauma patient and the principal indication are given in Table 42-1. The mere presence of a deficiency is not an indication for blood component therapy; rather, the indication of blood component therapy is if the deficiency is causing a physiological derangement that can harm the patient.

II. **PACKED RBC (PRBC) TRANSFUSION.** Normal blood volume is 7% to 8% of ideal body weight. The normal hematocrit (percentage of blood volume constituted by cells) is 42% to 48% and the large majority of the cellular component is formed by RBC. The normal hemoglobin is 14 to 16 g/dL.

   A. **Indications. The only indication for PRBC therapy** is to improve tissue oxygen delivery when the cause of tissue hypoxia is poor oxygen-carrying capacity. One unit of PRBC usually increases the hemoglobin by ~1 g/dL and the hematocrit by 2% to 4%. The specific indications are:

      1. Acute blood loss resulting in class III or IV shock (loss of >30% blood volume). This degree of acute loss significantly decreases oxygen-carrying capacity and usually leads to tissue hypoxia.

TABLE 42-1	The Most Commonly Utilized Blood Components for the Trauma Patient, and Their Principal Indication	
Component	**Deficiency addressed**	**Principal indication**
Packed red blood cells	Lack of oxygen-carrying capacity	Tissue hypoxia secondary to lack of oxygen-carrying capacity
Platelets	Thrombocytopenia or thrombocytopathia	Diffuse nonsurgical bleeding secondary to deficiency in platelet numbers or function
Coagulation factors FFP, cryoprecipitate, individual factors	Lack of coagulation factors due to loss and/or consumption	Coagulopathy secondary to lack of coagulation factors

FFP, fresh frozen plasma.

2. Ongoing blood loss while measures to control the loss are being undertaken.
3. Low hematocrit (hemoglobin) affecting tissue oxygenation. The appropriate threshold for PRBC transfusion in the nonacute setting has not been established and is likely to vary for different patients. It will depend on other factors such as age, presence of coronary artery disease, and oxygen needs. A low hematocrit (15% to 18%) will be well tolerated in a young and healthy person who is not stressed or multiply injured. On the other hand, a higher hematocrit (24% to 30%) may be necessary in a critically ill older patient with coronary artery disease who is multiply injured or stressed due to an infection.

B. Administration

1. **Type and crossmatch.** Blood typing identifies ABO and Rh antigens present within the RBC membrane and also screens for antibodies to other minor surface antigens. Crossmatching involves actual mixing of the patient's plasma with donor red cells to lessen the risk of a transfusion reaction from undetected antibodies. Blood typing requires 5 to 10 minutes, and full crossmatching requires 20 to 30 minutes. Therefore, for emergent situations, 2 to 6 units of universal donor (type O) blood should be immediately available within the resuscitation area in all trauma centers at the time of patient arrival (O negative blood should be administered to females of childbearing age). On patient arrival, a blood sample is drawn (preferably before a large volume of type O blood has been administered), labeled, and sent to the blood bank for processing. In less urgent situations, type-specific blood can be administered before fully crossmatched blood becomes available.
    a. If no blood components are needed, the patient can have a "type and hold" performed so that the blood type is known, but the labor and cost of crossmatching are avoided.
    b. If massive transfusion (see the next paragraph) is required, 10 to 20 units of PRBCs and multiple units of platelets and fresh frozen plasma should be requested, prepared, and delivered promptly. If more than 4 units of type O blood are given to a patient of a non-O blood type, the patient should be recrossmatched before transfusion with blood of the original type (unless the change involved Rh incompatibility only).
2. **Infusion.** PRBCs may be infused without dilution or reconstitution, and can be administered extremely rapidly through a rapid infuser system that can at the same time warm the blood. In less urgent situations, to decrease the viscosity, PRBCs can be mixed with warm saline. Blood should never be warmed in a microwave.

III. PLATELETS. The normal platelet count is 150,000 to 500,000/mm^3. In nontrauma patients, spontaneous bleeding occurs with platelet counts of <20,000/mm^3. In an injured patient, especially with evidence of ongoing bleeding, the platelet count should be maintained above 50,000/mm^3. Bleeding time measures the interaction of platelets with injured vessel to form initial plug (normal <5 minutes—Ivy method). Abnormal bleeding time is usually due to decreased platelet count (thrombocytopenia) or function (thrombocytopathia). The most common cause for nonsurgical bleeding in the trauma patient is dilutional thrombocytopenia. There is a linear inverse relationship between the number of PRBC units infused and the platelet count. Fifty percent of patients have platelet counts of <50,000/mm^3 after a two-blood-volume (20 U of PRBCs) transfusion. Thrombocytopenia may also be caused by heparin. Thrombocytopathia may be seen in patients who are hypothermic, hypocalcemic, in renal failure, or are on certain medications. Thrombocytopathia due to hypothermia is not correctable by platelet transfusion. Platelets are stored at 4°C. One unit of platelets increases the platelet count by 5,000 to 10,000/mm^3 and contains approximately 70 mL of plasma.

A. Indications. The indication for platelet transfusion is when there is either ongoing, or risk of, diffuse nonsurgical bleeding due to low platelet numbers or poor platelet function (except when caused by hypothermia). The specific indications are:

1. Platelet count <20,000/mm^3.
2. Platelet count <50,000 in patients with
   a. Evidence of ongoing diffuse nonsurgical bleeding, or
   b. Severe risk of significant bleeding as in patients with solid organ injury being managed nonoperatively and patients with major pelvic fracture, or head, spine, or ophthalmic injury where a small amount of bleeding can be disastrous.
3. Diffuse nonsurgical bleeding with evidence of impaired platelet function in the form of increased bleeding time (except when the deranged function is due to hypothermia).
4. Platelet transfusion is usually required in patients receiving massive transfusion, especially after 15 units of PRBCs.
   a. Prophylactic administration of platelets has not been demonstrated to diminish transfusion requirements in the multiply transfused patient. However, hemostasis often is not possible once microvascular bleeding develops.

IV. COAGULATION FACTORS. Coagulation factors are essential for the formation of stable clot. Although a number of tests are available for measuring the various parts of the coagulation cascade, the two commonly used tests are prothrombin time (PT: measures the extrinsic system dependent on Factor VII activation by injured tissue—normal 10 to 14 seconds), and the activated partial thromboplastin time (aPTT: measures the intrinsic system dependent on sequential activation of multiple factors—normal 25 to 37 seconds). In the trauma patient these two tests and the direct measurement of fibrinogen level (normal 150–350 mg/100 mL plasma) are usually enough to establish the presence or absence of significant clotting abnormality and direct therapy. In the hypothermic patient, however, the extent of coagulopathy may be underestimated since PT and aPTT measurements are carried out in the laboratory at 37°C and not at the patient body temperature.

A. Coagulopathy can present as diffuse surgical bleeding, hematuria, mucosal bleeds, bleeding from minor wounds, venipuncture sites, and so on. The goal is to achieve normal hemostasis such that nonsurgical bleeding is rapidly stopped by the formation of stable clot. When there is generalized loss of factors due to bleeding, consumption, and/or dilution, the PT and aPTT are deranged, and the fibrinogen level may be low.

1. As for platelets, deficiency of clotting factors due to loss and dilution occurs in 70% of patients after 10 units of PRBC transfusion and in 100% after 12 units. If the degree of factor deficiency is such as to cause bleeding, factors must be provided to stop bleeding.

2. The PT, aPTT, and fibrinogen level in conjunction with the clinical scenario should be used as guides as to factor infusion. In almost all trauma patients (those without any specific factor deficiency), clotting factors are usually provided by one of two blood components, both derived from plasma: fresh frozen plasma (FFP) and cryoprecipitate.

B. **Fresh frozen plasma (FFP).** FFP is produced by separating plasma from fresh donated blood and rapidly freezing it. FFP requires 20 to 40 minutes to thaw and be ready for administration. Hence, it is imperative to anticipate need and start the process early before severe coagulopathy has developed.

1. **Indications**
   a. Ongoing diffuse nonsurgical bleeding caused by deficiency of clotting factors (documented or presumed)
   b. PT or aPTT prolongation in a patient with solid organ injury, major pelvic fracture, head, spine or ophthalmic injury
   c. Expected need of >10 to 15 units of PRBC transfusion
      i. **Dose.** In a coagulopathic patient with ongoing or eminent diffuse nonsurgical bleeding, 10 to 15 mL of FFP/kg ideal body weight should be administered initially. The decision to administer more should be based on a reevaluation of the clinical picture and repeat testing of the laboratory parameters.

C. **Cryoprecipitate.** Cryoprecipitate is produced by thawing FFP, removing the precipitate, and adding 10 mL of plasma. It is rich in fibrinogen (>150 mg/U), Factors VIII and XIII, and von Willebrand factor.

1. **Indications**
   a. Hypofibrinogenemia (<100 mg/100 mL) leading to diffuse nonsurgical bleeding.

V. MASSIVE TRANSFUSION (MT)

A. **Definition.** The transfusion of at least one blood volume (5 L of whole blood or 10 U of PRBCs in a 70-kg man) within 24 hours. With rapid transfusion devices and advances in blood banking, several times the patient's blood volume can safely be transfused rapidly.

B. Due to the mathematical properties of hemodilution, one-blood-volume transfusion replaces 70% to 75% of the patient's original blood. A two-volume transfusion replaces 90% of the patient's original blood.

C. Early identification of the patient who may require MT is important because this allows the best use of resources, alteration of resuscitation strategies, and recognition and treatment of the complications of MT. Common injuries requiring MT are a high-grade liver injury, torso vascular injury, unstable pelvic fracture, or multiple intra- and extracavitary blunt injuries.

D. **MT outcome.** Outcome is worsened by the following: preexisting systemic disease (particularly cirrhosis), advanced age, hypothermia, closed head injury, coagulopathy, prolonged shock, and a blunt mechanism of injury. Currently, penetrating trauma patients require MT more often than blunt trauma patients. The outcome in patients requiring MT is improved by shortening prehospital time, preventing hypothermia, minimizing resuscitation time, rapid surgical control of cavitary hemorrhage, and employing damage control techniques where appropriate (Chapter 28).

VI. DISSEMINATED INTRAVASCULAR COAGULOPATHY (DIC).

DIC occurs by activation of the coagulation cascade within the vasculature. It continues by ongoing, simultaneous thrombosis and thrombolysis within the vasculature. This results in rapid consumption of the available coagulation factors. It can be initiated by any situation in which tissue thromboplastinlike substances are released into the bloodstream. In the trauma patient, DIC may be seen after massive transfusion, hemolytic transfusion reaction, major soft-tissue injury, severe closed head injury, and in severe infections. DIC results in a fibrinogen level of <100 mg/dL, a platelet count <50,000/mm^3, and a D-dimer level >500 g/L. (Coagulopathy that develops with massive transfusion is rarely DIC.)

A. Treatment of DIC. Treatment consists of sequentially performing the following:
1. Treating the inciting event.
2. Supporting all failing organ systems (including the coagulation system).
3. **Heparin.** In case the process is not controlled by the first two measures, heparin therapy is used to break the cycle of ongoing intravascular coagulation.
4. **Epsilon aminocaprioic acid (EACA).** In rare situations where the process is dominated by thrombolysis rather than thrombosis, the antifibrinolytic agent, EACA, may be required.

VII. BLEEDING AND COAGULOPATHY IN THE PATIENT WITH PREMORBID DISEASE.
Coagulopathy may be due to certain disease states, or medications (Table 42-2).
A. Evaluation
1. Obtaining a good history is the most important initial step.
2. The laboratory tests will depend on the level of suspicion based on the history. Usually PT, PTT, and platelet count are all that are necessary. Sometimes the activity of individual factors, bleeding time, and platelet function tests are needed.
B. Treatment. Treatment will depend on the problem identified in the evaluation.
1. **Platelet deficiency.** Both thrombocytopenia and thrombocytopathia (except due to hypothermia) can be treated by platelet transfusions. Prolonged bleeding time in face of normal platelet count suggests thrombocytopathia. This is often seen with uremia, and may be treatable by infusion of desamino-8-D-arginine-vasopressin (DDAVP 0.3 μg/kg every 6–12 hours).

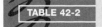

| TABLE 42-2 | Common Comorbid Conditions and Medications That Affect Bleeding and Coagulation |

Comorbid conditions	Medications and effect
Hypertension	Thrombocytopenia from thiazides, furosemide, alpha-methyldopa Thrombocytopathia from diltiazem, propanolol, verapamil
Atherosclerotic cardiovascular disease	Thrombocytopenia from quinidine Increased PT from warfarin Thrombocytopathia from aspirin, isosorbide
Congestive heart failure	Thrombocytopenia from furosemide
Alcoholism or liver disease	Thrombocytopenia Increased PT and aPTT Hypofibrinogenemia
Renal insufficiency	Thrombocytopathia
Malignancy	Thrombocytopenia in lymphoma, leukemia, myeloma, and from radiation therapy Increased PT and aPTT with liver metastasis Thrombocytopathia in polycythemia vera and from chemotherapy (daunorubicin, plicamycin, etc.)
Chronic diseases (e.g., CMV, TB, lupus)	Thrombocytopenia
Other medications	Thrombocytopenia by Methicillin, dilantin, heparin Thrombocytopathia by nonsteroidal antiinflammatory agents

PT, prothrombin time; aPTT, activated partial thromboplastin time; CMV, cytomegalovirus; TB, tuberculosis.

2. **Factor deficiency.** All factor deficiencies have been described. Deficiency of Factor VIII (hemophilia A) is the most common. The principles of treatment are similar for all individual factor deficiencies.
   a. **Hemophilia A.** An x-linked inherited abnormality resulting in >95% reduction in Factor VIII levels. Diagnosed by prolonged PTT (normal PT), and low level of Factor VIII activity. Treatment is by administering Factor VIII. Recombinant DNA Factor VIII has no infection risk but is expensive. Monoclonal Factor VIII has a small (<1%) infection risk but is less expensive; FFP and cryoprecipitate are also effective. Factor VIII has a short half-life; therefore, frequent infusions are needed. Levels should be brought to 30% of normal (50% or greater with major trauma) to ensure adequate hemostasis.
   b. **von Willebrand's disease.** An autosomal dominant inherited abnormality causing defective factor VIIIvWF production resulting in poor platelet adhesions. Diagnosed by special tests for platelet adhesiveness. Treated by administering cryoprecipitate or FFP. Some forms of the disease respond to DDAVP.
   c. **Liver disease and vitamin K deficiency.** Deficiency of vitamin K, seen in patients on prolonged or broad-spectrum antibiotics or warfarin therapy, can cause deficiency of vitamin K dependent factors (II, VII, IX, X). Treatment is by administration of vitamin K (intravenous), and discontinuation of warfarin. Intravenous vitamin K can reverse vitamin K deficiency–induced coagulopathy within six hours. In more urgent situations, FFP may be necessary to rapidly achieve normal hemostasis. The situation with liver disease can be much worse as the liver plays a central role in the production of most factors. In patients with advanced liver dysfunction, administration of vitamin K, FFP, cryoprecipitate, and platelets may all be required.
C. **Hypercoagulable states.** Deficiency of antithrombin III, protein C, and protein S can cause a hypercoagulable state. Protein C and S are vitamin K dependent. Treatment in acute situations is by administering FFP to provide the deficient factors.

VIII. **COMPLICATIONS OF BLOOD TRANSFUSIONS.** Blood transfusions are known to directly cause myriad complications. In addition, recent larger studies seem to suggest that blood transfusions may be an independent risk factor for adverse clinical outcome including death. The more common complications are discussed.
A. **Immunologic reactions**
   1. **Intravascular hemolytic transfusion reaction**
      a. **Pathophysiology.** This severe reaction is observed when the blood of wrong ABO type is transfused. The recipient's antibodies against RBC antigens cause extensive intravascular hemolysis of the donor RBCs resulting in an anaphylactic type of reaction (non-IgE mediated). Rarely it may be caused by incompatibility to the minor antigens. It is almost invariably caused by clerical error (misidentification or mislabeling of blood sample or unit).
      b. **Manifestations.** The clinical features are usually dramatic and seen within minutes of initiating the transfusion. Features include those of a generalized immunologic reaction (fever, nausea, vomiting, diarrhea, loin pain), vasomotor collapse (hypotension, angina, dyspnea), and coagulopathy (bleeding from operative sites, hematuria, etc). Coagulopathic features may be the first sign of such a reaction in a patient under general anesthesia. Mortality is about 10% and usually occurs in patients with vasomotor collapse.
      c. **Diagnosis.** The reaction is usually suspected in a patient with significant sudden change in clinical status occurring within a short period after initiation of transfusion. It may be confirmed by a direct Coombs test (evidence of hemolysis when a sample of the patient's blood is mixed with donor blood).

  d. Treatment. Stop transfusion, treat the vasomotor collapse (volume, vasopressors) and coagulopathy, and encourage vigorous alkaline diuresis (Mannitol, furesemide, sodium bicarbonate) to prevent pigment-induced (free hemoglobin) renal failure. A sample of the patient's blood along with the partially transfused unit should be returned to the blood bank.

2. **Other hemolytic transfusion reactions**
    a. **Pathophysiology.** These other reactions, not as serious as the intravascular hemolytic reaction, are due to sensitization to minor antigens (Duffy, Kell, Kidd, et al; rarely Rh) by prior transfusion or pregnancy. Sensitization risk from a single transfusion is 1.0% to 1.5%.
    b. **Manifestations.** Jaundice, fever, anemia, rarely hemoglobinuria, occurring weeks to months after transfusion.
    c. **Diagnosis.** Positive Coombs test (mentioned previously).
    d. **Treatment.** Only available recourse is prevention by avoiding unnecessary transfusions.

3. **Febrile transfusion reaction**
    a. **Pathophysiology.** Represents 75% of all transfusion reactions and is caused by preformed antibodies present in the recipient acting against donor leukocyte antigens.
    b. **Manifestations.** Fever, chills, urticaria, and headache. These reactions may be severe in some cases presenting with hypotension, tachycardia, dyspnea, and vomiting.
    c. **Diagnosis.** Is usually of exclusion.
    d. **Treatment.** Symptomatic with analgesics, antipyretics, and antihistamine agents. In case of severe reaction, future transfusions, if required, should use leukocyte-depleted blood.

4. **Allergic transfusion reaction**
    a. **Pathophysiology.** Usually caused by recipient antibodies against donor plasma proteins.
    b. **Manifestations.** Urticaria. Rarely, in patients with IgA deficiency, anaphylaxis may occur.
    c. **Diagnosis.** Is usually of exclusion.
    d. **Treatment.** Symptomatic only.

5. **Transfusion-related acute lung injury (TRALI)**
    a. **Pathophysiology.** TRALI is thought to be caused by complement activation resulting in neutrophil sequestration within the lung and injury to the alveolar membrane by activated neutrophils. Complement is probably activated by leukoagglutinating or human leukocyte antigen (HLA) specific antibodies in the plasma of the transfused blood component. Most patients who are well resuscitated usually improve within 24 to 48 hours. More recently, however, the concept of TRALI has been extended to include acute lung injury that may have been caused by other mechanisms (trauma, shock, other immunological mechanisms, etc.) and where transfusion may have played a part.
    b. **Manifestation.** Patients develop a diffusion deficit with a high A—a gradient similar to that seen in adult respiratory distress syndrome (ARDS) within 6 hours of transfusion. The patients generally are severely injured and in shock and have required large-volume transfusion of many blood components.
    c. **Diagnosis.** Acute lung injury occurring within 6 hours of transfusion, usually involving large-volume and multiple components.
    d. **Treatment.** Supportive ventilatory therapy with lung protective strategies as used in ARDS.

B. **Infectious complications.** Improvements in donor screening and routine testing of all donated blood has resulted in a steady decrease in the incidence of these complications.

1. **HIV/AIDS.** Although one of the most dreaded infectious complications, the actual risk of transmission of HIV from a single unit is low (1 in 4 million).

This decrease has come about by strict screening of donors and routine testing of all donated units. However, transmission of HIV is still possible since even the most sensitive serum tests do not become positive for 6 weeks to 6 months from the time of infection.

2. Transfusion-associated hepatitis

  a. Hepatitis B. Hepatitis B represents approximately 10% of transfusion-associated hepatitis. Incidence has been reduced by 90% by donor screening for hepatitis B surface antigen and the phasing out of professional donors. Current risk is 1 in 1 million units of transfusion.

  b. Hepatitis C. Formerly called non-A, non-B hepatitis. Risk is 1 in 3 million units of transfusion. Represents approximately 90% of transfusion-associated hepatitis. Results in chronic hepatitis in 50%, and cirrhosis in 20%. Hepatocellular carcinoma may develop. Risk has been decreased by donor screening with alanine aminotransferase (ALT) and core antigen.

  c. Type D (delta) hepatitis. This viral particle can exist only in conjunction with hepatitis B. No commercial screening test is available. Some donor units that are hepatitis B positive, but escape detection by HBsAg testing, are positive for hepatitis D.

3. Cytomegalovirus (CMV). Herpesvirus that may cause mononucleosislike symptoms. Most individuals are CMV Ab positive from environmental exposure. Severe illness can result in patients who are Ab negative, or immunocompromised, if they are given CMV positive blood. Hence, CMV negative blood should be given to neonates, pregnant women, and immunocompromised individuals.

4. Epstein-Barr virus (EBV). Readily transmissible through transfusion, yet rarely causes clinical symptoms.

5. Other nonviral infections and infestations

  a. Includes malaria, syphilis, brucellosis, and other organisms, all rare.

  b. Approximately 2.0% of all blood units may have bacterial contaminants; most are *Klebsiella* or *Pseudomonas*, resulting in fever, hypotension, and abdominal pain, but usually no long-term sequelae result if the patient has a normal immune system.

C. Complications of MT. Some complications of transfusion are unique to MT; the complications caused by the preservative solutions and the changes in blood associated with storage (Table 42-3) are significant only when large volumes of stored blood are transfused.

1. Hypothermia (Chapter 41)

  a. Occurs in the setting of severe injury or MT. Blood is stored at 4°C and, unless warmed to body temperature prior to transfusion, adds significantly to the heat loss.

TABLE 42-3	Characteristics of a PRBC Unit During Storage (4°C) Over Time (Average Storage Time of Transfused Blood)	
DAY 1	**DAY 14**	**DAY 30**
210 cc PRBC	210 cc PRBC	210 cc PRBC
40–90 cc plasma	40–90 cc plasma	40–90 cc plasma
pH = 6.6–7.0	pH = 6.6–7.0	pH = 6.6–7.0
K^+ = 10–40 mEq	K^+ = 20–40 mEq	K^+ = 30–40 mEq
Citrate = 2–5 mg/cc	Citrate = 2–5 mg/cc	Citrate = 2–5 mg/cc
2,3-DPG 100%	2,3-DPG 40%	2,3-DPG 5%
ATP 95%	ATP 90%	ATP 70%

PRBC, packed red blood cell(s); 2, 3-DPG, 2, 3 Diphosphoglycerate; ATP, adenosine triphosphate.

b. Results in decreased hepatic metabolism of citrate, impaired activity of thrombin and plasmin, decreased platelet function, diminished synthesis of clotting factors, and left shift of the oxygen dissociation curve.

2. Bleeding and coagulopathy. Results from dilution of platelets, consumption of coagulation factors, hypothermia, acidosis, and ongoing bleeding.

a. Citrate toxicity. Citrate is used as an anticoagulant (acts by chelating Ca^{2+}) in banked blood. If blood is given more rapidly than one unit every 5 minutes, citrate may reduce serum Ca^{2+} and Mg^{2+} levels affecting cardiac function and the coagulation cascade.

b. Manifestations. Decreased blood pressure, decreased cardiac contractility, QT interval prolongation, dysrhythmias.

c. Diagnosis. Diminished total and ionized serum calcium and magnesium. Ionized calcium and magnesium determinations can be made rapidly from microanalysis of whole blood. A 56% incidence of hypocalcemia was noted in a recent MT series of patients receiving one-blood-volume transfusion in 24 hours.

d. Treatment. Basing treatment on measured ionized calcium may be the safest approach. Some authors recommend prophylactic administration of 1.0 g calcium (as chloride solution) per 6 units of transfusion if PRBCs are given rapidly. Hypomagnesemia potentiates hypocalcemia. Hence, repletion of magnesium may be necessary (magnesium sulfate solution, 1.0 g = 8 mEq) to correct hypocalcemia.

3. Acidosis

a. Pathophysiology. The pH of stored blood is 6.6 to 7.0. The normal metabolic response to the transfusion of packed cells in the absence of shock is alkalosis, which favors hypokalemia. Acidosis with MT results from lactic acidosis due to inadequate tissue perfusion and inadequate clearance of citric acid by the hypoperfused liver.

b. Manifestations. Hypotension, decreased urine output, increased heart rate, and other signs of tissue hypoperfusion (shock).

c. Diagnosis. Presence of anion gap lactic acidosis.

d. Treatment. Maintenance of adequate tissue perfusion with fluids and inotropic agents, if indicated.

4. Potassium abnormalities

a. Pathophysiology. Hyperkalemia may occur, especially with very rapid transfusion (10–40 mEq of potassium may be present in each unit of PRBC depending on the age of the blood).

  i. This is rarely a clinical problem because the potassium load is cleared by renal excretion, red cell uptake, and the conversion of citrate to bicarbonate (favoring cellular uptake of potassium, thereby minimizing hyperkalemia and commonly resulting in hypokalemia).

  ii. In one series of patients receiving MT, 25% were hypokalemic, 15% hyperkalemic, and 60% had normal serum potassium measurement.

b. Manifestations. High-peaked T wave, widened QRS complex, and depressed ST segment are seen initially. Disappearance of T waves, heart block, and diastolic cardiac arrest may be seen with increasing potassium levels.

c. Diagnosis. Serum determination of potassium.

d. Treatment. Maintenance of adequate urine output and replacement of observed deficits for hypokalemia.

5. Decreased ATP

a. Pathophysiology. Decreased availability of phosphate secondary to volume shifts in MT is a feature of "old" blood (>50 days).

b. Manifestations. Diminished red cell deformability secondary to loss of biconcave shape.

c. Treatment. Usually none. In patients with hypophosphatemia, replete phosphate losses in intravenous fluids provide adequate FiO_2.

6. Decreased 2,3-DPG (2,3-Diphosphoglycerate). 2,3-DPG is a component of the red cell membrane that shifts the hemoglobin dissociation curve to the right (reduces P_{50}) thereby facilitating oxygen off-loading in the tissues.

  a. Pathophysiology. Citrate anticoagulation decreases 2,3-DPG levels over time (Table 42-3).

  b. Manifestations. Decreased oxygen delivery to the tissues.

  c. Treatment. In situations where oxygen delivery may be a problem, the freshest available blood should be used.

D. Transfusion as a risk factor for adverse outcome. Blood transfusion has been recognized as an independent risk factor contributing to poor outcomes in trauma patients, including: ARDS, multiple organ dysfunction syndrome (MODS), transfusion-related immunomodulation (TRIM; immunosuppression), and death. Since transfusion itself may contribute to the development of these adverse events, the clinician should carefully consider the risks and benefits involved before ordering any blood component therapy.

IX. ALTERNATIVES TO TRANSFUSION. In acute life-threatening emergencies caused by lack of one or more blood components, there is usually no alternative to blood transfusions. However, in less urgent situations, recognizing the dangers of transfusions, other therapies should be considered.

A. PRBCs

  1. Acute setting. In the patient with ongoing bleeding or class III or IV shock, there is no alternative to PRBC transfusion. However, low levels of hematocrit, even when caused by acute large-volume blood loss, may be tolerated in otherwise healthy individuals. Hence, the mere fact that a patient has a low hematocrit caused by blood loss should not prompt PRBC transfusions. Rather, PRBC transfusions should be ordered only if there is evidence that the low hematocrit (low oxygen-carrying capacity) is responsible for tissue hypoxia (shock) or the patient has ongoing bleeding.

  2. Nonacute setting. In the nonacute setting, usually encountered in the ICU, measures can be taken to minimize loss of blood and to encourage the body to produce more RBCs.

  a. Minimizing blood loss. Frequent "routine labs" significantly add to the volume of blood loss. Efforts should be made to minimize these routine and unnecessary blood tests that do not affect management of the patient.

  b. Encouraging body PRBC production. Recombinant erythropoietin has been shown to reduce the need for PRBC transfusion in ICU patients known to be at risk of anemia requiring transfusion therapy. It should be started early in such patients and the dosing should be appropriate (40,000 U intramuscularly every week).

  c. Coagulation factors. In a patient acutely hemorrhaging due to lack of coagulation factors, blood component therapy (FFP and/or cryoprecipitate) must be initiated to stem the hemorrhage. However, in less acute situations, consideration should be given to other measures that may help control the coagulopathy.

  i. Hypothermia. Hypothermia adversely affects all elements of coagulation. Prevention or reversal of hypothermia should be given high priority while managing any critically ill patient.

  ii. Vitamin K. In the past, vitamin K preparations could not be administered intravenously, and the time to effect following a subcutaneous or intramuscular injection was 24 to 48 hours. More recent formulations of the compound can be administered intravenously, and the effect of the injection seen in 6 hours. It should be considered in all coagulopathic patients. Intravenous administration (10 mg) must be under monitored conditions since hypotension is a known side effect of the intravenous formulation.

  iii. Platelets. In the nonacute setting platelet dysfunction, especially if caused by uremia, can be reversed by administering Desmopressin (DDAVP) at 0.3 µg/kg.

X. THE FUTURE

A. **Modified whole blood** as an option to whole blood. After sterile separation of PRBCs, platelets, plasma, and cryoprecipitate from the donor unit, the plasma and RBC components are recombined. The product lacks platelets and factors V and VIII, yet provides adequate levels of other factors. Its use can reduce the donor exposure in patients requiring multiple transfusions, and thus reduce the chances of disease transmission.

B. **Solvent and detergent (SD) treated plasma.** Pooled plasma is treated with TNBP and 1% Triton-100, followed by extraction to remove the SD agents. This eliminates the risk of viral disease transmission.

C. **Prolonging shelf life.** Attempts are being made to prolong shelf life by changing the anticoagulant mixture used. Also, technology is being developed to rapid freeze the blood, giving it an indefinite storage life. Indefinite storage life can be very helpful for rare blood types.

D. **Blood substitutes.** Solutions based on stroma-free Hgb or synthetic oxygen-carrying compounds such as perfluorocarbons are being developed. These will give all the advantages of blood without the risk of adverse effects.

Bibliography

Barnes A. Transfusion of universal donor and uncrossmatched blood. *Bibl Haematol* 1980;46:132–142.

Consensus Development Conference. Platelet transfusion therapy. *JAMA* 1987;257: 1777–1780.

Counts RB, Haisch C, Simon TL, et al. Hemostasis in massively transfused trauma patients. *Ann Surg* 1979;190:91–99.

Croce MA, Tolley FA, Claridge JA, et al. Transfusions result in pulmonary mortality and death after moderate degree of injury. *J Trauma* 2005;59:19–24.

Ferrara A, MacArthur JD, Wright HK, et al. Hypothermia and acidosis worsen coagulopathy in the patient requiring massive transfusion. *Am J Surg* 1990;160:515–518.

Harker LA, Slichter SJ. The bleeding time as a test for evaluation of platelet function. *N Eng J Med* 1972;287:155–159.

Harrigan C, Lucas CE, Ledgerwood AM, et al. Serial changes in primary hemostasis after massive transfusion. *Surgery* 1985;98:836–844.

Hebert PC, Wells G, Blajchman MA, et al. A multicenter, randomized, controlled clinical trial of transfusion requirements in critical care. *N Eng J Med* 1999;340:409–417.

Isbister JP. Decision making in perioperative transfusion. *Transfus Apheresis Sci* 2002; 27:19–28.

Kahn RC, Jaxcott D, Carlon GC, et al. Massive blood replacement: Correlation of ionized calcium, citrate and hydrogen ion concentration. *Anesth Analg* 1979;58:274–278.

Martin DJ, Lucas CE, Ledgerwood AM, et al. Fresh frozen plasma supplement to massive red blood cell transfusion. *Ann Surg* 1985;202:505–511.

Moore EE, Dunn E, Brstich DJ, et al. Platelet abnormalities associated with massive autotansfusion. *J Trauma* 1980;20:1052–1056.

Ness PM, Perkins HA. Cryoprecipitate as a reliable source of fibrinogen replacement. *JAMA* 1979;241:1690–1691.

Pantanowitz L, Kruskall MS, Uhl L. Cryoprecipitate—Patterns of use. *Am J Clin Pathol* 2003;119:874–881.

Practice guidelines for blood component therapy. *Anesthesiology* 1996;84:732–747.

Reed RL, Ciavarella D, Heimbach DM, et al. Prophylactic platelet administration during massive transfusion. *Ann Surg* 1986;203:40–48.

Schreiber GB, Busch MP, Kleinman SH, et al. The risk of transfusion-related viral infections. *N Engl J Med* 1996;122:130–138.

Silliman CC, Boshkov LK, Mehdizadehkashi Z, et al. Transfusion-related acute lung injury: Epidemiology and prospective analysis of etiologic factors. *Blood* 2003;101:454–462.

Sullivan MT, McCullough J, Schreiber GB, et al. Blood collection and transfusion in the United States in 1997. *Transfusion* 2002;42:1253–1260.

Wudel JH, Morris JA, Yates K, et al. Massive transfusion: Outcomes in blunt trauma patients. *J Trauma* 1991;13:1–7.

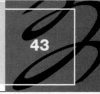

NUTRITIONAL INTERVENTION
JODIE A. BRYK AND JUAN B. OCHOA

43

I. **INTRODUCTION.** Nutrition intervention (NI) plays essential roles in benefiting clinical outcomes in trauma including a decrease in infections while improving organ function, including immune function and wound healing. The successful implementation of NI requires careful evaluation of the risks, benefits, and side effects.

NI is classically described as a "supportive therapy," while other treatments play the essential roles in the recovery of the traumatized patient. Far from being a supportive therapy, well-designed NI plays a central role in the management of the trauma patient.

A. **Nutritional balance under resting conditions.** Average adults and children in developed countries are able to consume a balanced diet that provides the necessary elements needed to maintain normal organ function.

1. **Starvation** occurs when an individual is unable to spontaneously take enough nutrients to provide for daily needs. The metabolic response to starvation is a defensive **physiologic** process. A successful adaptive starvation response in patients allows for normal organ function despite inadequate nutrient intake.

a. **Adaptation to starvation.** The starved (but otherwise healthy) individual sets forth metabolic mechanisms designed to protect muscle mass and energy stores while preserving normal organ function. The protective metabolic changes include:

i. Decreased nitrogen loss. The fed individual recycles approximately 15 to 20 g/d^2 of nitrogen daily. The lost amount matches the amount of nitrogen in the diet and thus maintains the nitrogen balance. Starved individuals go into negative nitrogen balance and utilize endogenous protein in their liver and muscles. However, the degree of protein recycling decreases by about two thirds compared to the fed state. Thus, the rate at which protein becomes depleted is ameliorated (Fig. 43-1).

ii. Protein-sparing effect of glucose. Endogenous protein destruction during starvation is necessary for the production of gluconeogenic amino acids (such as alanine) and the production of glucose. Nitrogen losses can be blocked by about 95% in the starved nonstressed individual by provision of small amounts of exogenous glucose (roughly 100 grams—<400 calories).

iii. Lipid metabolism. Lipid stores are mobilized and become the principal source of energy. An adequately nourished individual has enough lipid stores to provide energy for up to several months.

iv. Glucose metabolism. A normally fed 70-kg patient needs a minimum of 120 g/day of glucose to maintain proper CNS function. Glycogen stores are depleted within 24 hours. Protein catabolism begins to fulfill the baseline level of glucose following depletion of the carbohydrate stores.

v. Decreased basal metabolic rate. Starved individuals decrease their resting energy expenditures about 25%; thus, their energy stores are protected. Clinically decreased basal metabolic rates are translated into lower heart rates and temperature when compared to the fed individual.

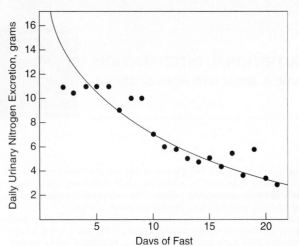

Figure 43-1. Daily urinary nitrogen excretion during prolonged fast. (From Freund E, Freund O. Beitrage zum Stoffwechsel im Hungerzustand. *Med Klin* 1901;15:69.)

vi. Through these adaptive mechanisms, the starved individual is able to preserve normal organ function for up to several weeks or months depending on the degree of starvation, the amount of metabolic stress, the age of the patient, and the preexisting nutritional state. Many trauma and critically ill patients are starved for varying amounts of time. **Nutritional intervention can be justified only if we can demonstrate the improvement of metabolic and clinical outcomes beyond those provided by starvation.**

B. Malnutrition. Eventually the starved individual exhausts adaptive responses and becomes malnourished if starvation continues unresolved. Malnourished patients exhibit significant and progressive deterioration of multiple organ functions, including that of decreased respiratory muscle function, wound breakdown, and severely impaired immune responses such as decreased T-cell function. The presence of malnutrition dramatically increases morbidity and mortality in trauma.

   1. Assessment of malnutrition. Traditional assessment of nutritional status is done through the evaluation of a clinical nutritional history (patient's basic nutritional habits), anthropometric measures such as fat-to-muscle ratios (i.e., midarm circumference), functional parameters (i.e., evaluation of the immune system), and biochemical parameters such as albumin, prealbumin, and retinol binding protein (Table 43-1).

   2. Traditional nutrition assessment parameters are dramatically altered by trauma so that their accuracy is lost. For example, patients who suffer severe trauma exhibit a decrease in T-lymphocyte counts and develop anergy. In addition, there is a significant drop in albumin and prealbumin levels within 24 to 48 hours of the injury. Thus, the traditional assessment of the nutritional status of a given trauma patient is often difficult or unreliable. More sophisticated nutritional assessment needs to be performed.

   3. Multiple calculated formulas have been designed to estimate caloric and protein requirements in traumatized patients. These formulas include the Harris-Benedict (Table 43-2) and the Ireton-Jones energy expenditure equations (Tables 43-3 and 43-4). Both of these formulas provide a rule of thumb to calculate initial goals of nutritional intervention. These formulas, however, may either overfeed or underfeed a significant proportion of patients. The inadequate therapy leads to increase in morbidity (and possibly mortality).

   4. Resting energy expenditure measured by evaluation of oxygen consumption and carbon dioxide production through indirect calorimetry provides the gold standard of calculating energy needs. This is done using metabolic carts. In

Guidelines for SGA Ranking

Well-nourished
No physical signs of muscle wasting
No or minimal subcutaneous fat loss
Dietary intake adequate or marginally inadequate for <2 weeks

Mild malnutrition
Mild muscle wasting
Mild subcutaneous fat loss
Inadequate dietary intake of 2–3 weeks
Functional capacity: working suboptimally

Moderate malnutrition
Moderate muscle wasting
Significant subcutaneous fat loss
Inadequate dietary intake 3–5 weeks
Functional capacity: semiambulatory, requiring assistance with activities of daily living

Severe malnutrition
Severe muscle wasting
Sever subcutaneous fat loss
Inadequate dietary intake >5 weeks
Functional capacity: minimally ambulatory, or bedridden

(From Pikul J. Degree of preoperative malnutrition is predictive of preoperative morbidity and mortality in liver transplant recipients. *Transplantation* 1994;57(3):469.)

Harris-Benedict Equation

EEE (males) = 66 + 13.7(wt in kg) + 5(ht in cm) − 6.8(age in y)
EEE (females) = 665 + 9.6(wt in kg) + 1.8(ht in cm) − 4.7(age in y)

Where EEE is estimated energy expenditure, wt is weight, and ht is height.

Ireton-Jones Equation for Ventilated Patients: Burn Patients

EEE = 1925 − 10(age in y) + 5(wt in kg) + 281(sex) + 292(trauma) + 851(burn)

Where sex is 0 for females and 1 for males, trauma is 1 for yes and 0 for no, and burn is 1 for yes and 0 for no.

Ireton-Jones Equation: Sepsis

EEE = −1000 + 100($\dot{V}_E$) + 1.3(Hb) + 300(sepsis)

Where $\dot{V}_E$ is expired minute ventilation and sepsis is 1 for yes and 0 for no.

addition, urine urea nitrogen excretion can be measured. This measurement helps calculate the amount of protein necessary to provide nitrogen balance. Despite better accuracy, the benefits of indirect calorimetry remain unproven.

II. METABOLIC DEMANDS OF TRAUMA. The trauma patient exhibits significant metabolic changes that profoundly affect the adaptive response to starvation. Trauma patients become significantly catabolic; the degree of catabolism is proportional to the degree of injury. Burn patients exhibit the highest degree of metabolic alterations among injured patients. Metabolic changes accompanying trauma include:

A. Increased protein breakdown. In addition to protein losses in wounds, blood, and other fluid loss, increased protein loss due to increased catabolism occurs following injury. Loss of protein can be high: Up to 15% of the lean body mass can be lost in 10 days. Severe protein malnutrition occurs when 25% to 30% of the lean body weight is lost. Thus, protein depletion (not calorie depletion) is a life-threatening condition in severe trauma. The high catabolic rate is resistant to nutrient supplementation including that of the provision of calories. However, protein synthetic rate does increase with amino acid infusions. Traditionally, traumatized patients are offered 1.5 to 2 g/k/day of protein. Higher amounts of protein supplementation have not been proven beneficial.

B. Hyperglycemia and resistance to insulin. Hyperglycemia is an independent predictor of poor prognosis. Hyperglycemia is due to complex factors. It is attributable primarily to excess hepatic gluconeogenesis due to the liver's increased avidity for gluconeogenic substrates (i.e., lactate, pyruvate, alanine). Hyperglycemia is also attributable to decreased glucose storage, increased circulating steroids, increased catecholamines, and increased glucagon.

  1. Insulin release is suppressed within a few hours after trauma and restored in the later phase. However, hyperglycemia persists since insulin resistance is also characteristic of severe trauma.

  2. Severe hyperglycemia is associated with decreased neutrophil chemotaxis, phagocytosis, oxidative bursts, and superoxide production. The condition of hyperglycemia is worsened by excessive provisions of glucose at high concentrations such as that given through total parenteral nutrition (TPN).

C. Lipid mobilization. Mobilization of lipid stores (lipolysis) is observed after trauma. This is a result of the activation of triglyceride lipases by elevation in the levels of catecholamines, thyroid hormones, cortisol, adrenocorticotropic hormone (ACTH), glucagon, and growth hormones. Lipids remain the main energy source.

D. Increased resting energy expenditure. Resting energy expenditure is increased after trauma and is proportional to the degree of severity of injury. Traditionally, physicians have been taught to provide increased amount of calories (beyond that of 25 kcal/kilo/day) to meet the metabolic demands of the patient. However, there is no clinical outcome evidence to demonstrate that provision of calories above baseline offers benefit. Indeed, data questioning the validity of feeding the patient at traditional caloric goals have started to accumulate. Some investigators even suggest that some critically ill patient populations should be fed "hypocaloric" diets (10 to 15 kcal/kg/day), a practice known as **permissive underfeeding**.

E. Vitamin deficiencies. Research on the development of specific nutrient deficiencies is in its infancy in the trauma patient. Therefore, there are no specific guidelines for the replacement of deficient vitamins beyond those advocated for normal individuals.

III. PUTTING IT ALL TOGETHER. Options for nutrition intervention fall into five categories:
- Oral intake at will
- Controlled starvation
- Enteral nutrition
- Parenteral nutrition
- Oral nutrition supplements

Inevitably, NI will fall into one or more of these categories. The option chosen will depend on a careful evaluation of the benefits and risks of a given choice, as well as a comparison with other alternative interventional options. The physician should consider the following factors in determining how to make this decision.

A. Oral intake at will. We interfere routinely with spontaneous oral intake in hospitalized patients. Dietary intake is altered at will for performance of different tests or procedures. The palatability of many in-hospital food preparations is often poor. In addition, disease frequently causes a significant degree of anorexia. As a result, patients who stay in the hospital for significant amounts of time may end up with poor oral intake and progression toward malnutrition. Careful evaluation of nutritional history on arrival of the trauma patient, followed by adequate monitoring of caloric/protein intake, is essential. It is also highly beneficial for the psychological well-being of the patient to be in charge of his or her own oral intake.

B. Controlled starvation. The decision to prevent oral intake in a patient occurs frequently in the hospitalized trauma patient. Virtually any member of the health care team can stop or prevent a patient from obtaining adequate oral intake. Careful consideration has to be given as to the risks versus benefits of maintaining a patient "nothing by mouth" (NPO). Physicians will often find that a more liberal approach toward permitting oral intake will benefit the patient. Examples of this include:

  1. Abandoning prolonged preoperative fasting. Fasting for 8 hours before surgery is still the norm in many hospitals despite clear data demonstrating that it is not necessary. In fact, patients who are allowed clear fluids until 2 hours before induction of anesthesia do just as well.

  2. Postoperative ileus. Despite multiple studies demonstrating the utility and the benefits of early oral or enteral intake, too frequently patients are kept NPO after surgery. In a meta-analysis, patients undergoing elective surgery who received oral or enteral intake exhibited a statistically significant decreased infection rate, a trend toward decreased mortality, and a decreased anastomotic breakdown.

C. Enteral nutrition (EN). Most trauma patients are able to tolerate oral or enteral intake within the first 24 hours following the injury. **The most important limiting factor for early EN is the presence of shock and poor gut perfusion.** Early EN is associated with easier tolerance to a diet and decreased infection rates. Enteral nutrition increases wound healing and decreases length of stay. Early EN has become the gold standard of nutrition interventions in the critically ill trauma patient to which all other forms of intervention must be compared.

  1. Enteral nutrition does have complications, including those stemming from the placement of feeding tubes, gastrostomies, or jejunostomies. In a recent report, up to 2% of the nasoenteral feeding tubes were misplaced within the trachea. Enteral nutrition is associated with diarrhea in up to 30% of patients. Enteral nutrition may also lead to vomiting and aspiration.

   a. A major complication of EN is that of bowel necrosis, which is observed when aggressive volumes of EN are delivered, especially in the presence of poor bowel perfusion and shock.

   b. The tip of the nasoenteral feeding tube can be left in the stomach or advanced into the duodenum or jejunum. Nasojejunal tube feeds appear better tolerated than nasogastric tube feeds and may be associated with a decreased incidence of aspiration.

D. Total parenteral nutrition (TPN). The advent of TPN in 1968 allowed for the provision of complete nutritional support in the absence of a functional gastrointestinal tract. TPN has undoubtedly saved innumerable patients from a certain death when the gastrointestinal tract is not available. Level 1 evidence of the benefit of TPN exists for the following indications:

  1. Severely malnourished patient who cannot eat and will be undergoing elective surgery. In this patient population, TPN decreases patient complications.

  2. Patients with short gut syndrome.

3. Inadequate use of TPN is associated with a significant increase in morbidity and mortality. Misuse of TPN is frequent. A careful policy of selective use of TPN has resulted in a >75% decrease in its utilization with a correspondent increase in enteral nutrition. **TPN is not indicated when the gastrointestinal tract is functional or during short periods of starvation.** TPN is inappropriately ordered when it is given to a patient "just in case" he or she will not have a functional GI tract within a reasonable amount of time. In these cases, TPN has been shown to increase morbidity and mortality even when compared to starvation alone.

E. Oral nutrition supplements. The use of oral nutritional supplements is advocated by many, and is strongly pressed commercially for indiscriminant use during illness. Nutritional supplements contain a source of protein and a high concentration of calories in the form of easily absorbed carbohydrates and long-chain fatty acids. There is no evidence to support the use of traditional bedside oral supplements after trauma. In fact, these can be associated with significant complications including hyperglycemia, and detract the patient from intake of a regular diet.

F. Immunonutrition. Preoperative nutritional supplements containing high concentrations of arginine, glutamine, and omega-3 fatty acids have been classified as **immune-enhancing diets (IEDs)**. Patients undergoing open cardiac surgery, colon resection, or pancreatic resection are candidates for receiving IEDs. There is **level 1 evidence** that preoperative nutritional supplementation with IEDs is associated with better organ perfusion, increased tolerance to surgical shock (including extracorporeal circulation), enhanced T-cell function, and improved nitrogen balance, and IEDs decrease infection rates. Currently, preoperative use of IEDs can be advocated for any high-risk surgery.

1. Studies have demonstrated that postoperative IEDs in the form of EN are also of benefit for elective surgical patients. However, because of the small size of the studies, the evidence advocating the use of IEDs in trauma is not as strong as that observed in high-risk surgery.

IV. NUTRIENT REQUIREMENTS

A. Meeting caloric goals. Traditional nutrition support states that meeting caloric requirements minimizes protein breakdown and lean body mass loss. As previously mentioned, multiple formulas have been designed to determine caloric requirements. In these formulas, a stress factor is often added so that the amount of calories provided to the patient are in excess of the basal energy expenditure. The American College of Chest Physicians (ACCP) and the American Society of Parental and Enteral Nutrition (ASPEN) have suggested in their guidelines that critically ill patients should receive approximately 25 kcal/kg/day.

1. There is no convincing clinical evidence demonstrating that meeting caloric goals in critically ill patients benefits clinical outcome. In fact, there is accumulating data to strongly suggest the contrary. For example, patients receiving enteral nutrition on average meet only 70% of their caloric goals, significantly less than those on TPN. However, the outcome is far better in patients receiving enteral nutrition, demonstrating that meeting caloric goals is not necessary to benefit outcome.

2. In addition, there is increased morbidity when patients receive excessive calories. Overfeeding increases length of stay on the ventilator and is associated with increased incidence of sepsis. Overfeeding occurs in up to one third of all patients when caloric requirements are calculated with the use of conventional formulas such as the Harris-Benedict equation. Indirect calorimetry, although a more elaborate and expensive approach, allows for more careful determination of energy requirements.

3. The Canadian Critical Care Nutrition Guidelines have refrained from suggesting a caloric goal because of the lack of evidence. Instead, they recommend (at least when using TPN) that the patient should receive approximately 50% of the traditional caloric goals. This new trend in **permissive underfeeding** has been tested in morbidly obese patients requiring TPN and appears to be associated with decreased length of stay, decreased antibiotic use, and decreased ventilator days. In a recent retrospective report in a medical ICU, patients who received 33% to 65% of their caloric goals (as determined by the ACCP) had decreased mortality, incidence of sepsis, and length of stay. It is currently unknown whether this new trend in permissive underfeeding will gain level 1 evidence in properly conducted prospective randomized trials.

B. Carbohydrate requirements. Several types of carbohydrates are commercially available and are classified according to their complexity. Complexity (the size of the individual carbohydrate polymers) determines the need for digestion prior to absorption. The complexity of carbohydrates is measured in dextrose equivalent (DE) units. The DE of dextrose is 100 and is readily absorbed. In contrast, unaltered cornstarch has a DE value of 1. Intermediate values are given for maltodextrin, corn syrup, and modified cornstarch.

C. Protein requirements. The provision of proteins to trauma patients is essential and may minimize loss of lean body mass. Protein intake should be 1.5 to 2.0 g/kg/day or 20% to 30% of the total caloric nutrient intake.

  1. Several types of protein are available commercially and are classified depending on their source. Sources of protein include casein, soy, and whey protein. To our knowledge, there are no data comparing the effect of the different type of protein on clinical outcome.

  2. Predigested protein presentations in the form of simple peptides or individual amino acids are also available. Peptide or amino acid–based diets are used in the disease states where there may be impaired digestion and absorption.

D. Lipid requirements. Lipids provide the most concentrated energy source of all macronutrients. Lipids have been essential in the formation of cell membranes and provide the substrate for the production of prostaglandins and leukotrienes.

  1. Traditionally, 30% of the calories delivered to a patient come from lipids. However, this percentage may vary significantly depending on the diet, ranging from 15% to up to 70% of the caloric goals.

  2. A diet free of lipids will result in the development of fatty acid deficiency (linoleic and linolenic acid) within a few weeks. Thus, the minimum amount of fat provided in the diet should be approximately 2% to 4% of the caloric goals to prevent essential fatty acid deficiency.

  3. The amount and type of lipid provided in the diet may play distinct physiologic roles affecting specific organ function, a fact that is being explored in different specialized diets.

   a. Long-chain fatty acids such as those provided in corn oil (omega-6 fatty acids) are traditional sources of lipids provided in many diets for critically ill patients. Intravenous lipid presentations in the United States are exclusively omega-6 fatty acids.

   b. Omega-3 fatty acids are contained in fish oil and are provided in significant concentrations in specialized enteral diets. Through inhibition of prostaglandin E2 in favor of prostaglandin E3, omega-3 fatty acids are said to be antiinflammatory. Fish oil and borage oil are mixed in specialized diets used in acute respiratory distress syndrome (ARDS). Omega-3 fatty acids are also provided in IEDs, which were discussed previously.

   c. Medium-chain triglycerides (containing 14 carbons) are absorbed directly into the bloodstream and can be used as energy sources in the absence of carnitine, which becomes deficient during critical illness. Carnitine is required for transport of long-chain triglycerides into the mitochondria.

   d. Short-chain fatty acids provide a main energy source for the colonic mucosa. Short-chain fatty acids are produced of broken-down digestible fibers.

E. Micronutrients. Little is known of dietary supplementation of micronutrients (vitamins and minerals) in trauma and critical illness. Therefore, under most circumstances micronutrients are provided in quantities sufficient to meet recommended dietary allowance (RDA). It is known that levels of vitamin C drop significantly after trauma or hemorrhagic shock. Preliminary trials suggest that the administration of supraphysiologic quantities of vitamin C as part of the resuscitation protocol may have a significant effect on overall outcome. Definitive trials are pending. Supplemental zinc, selenium, and vitamin C are traditionally used in patients with large wounds and decubitus ulcers.

V. SPECIAL PATIENT POPULATIONS

A. Burn patients. Nutritional needs for burn patients are far different from those observed in other populations. Most severe burn patients are taken care of in units where specialized nutritional support is available. Burn patients exhibit high metabolic rates, the need for provision of calories (in the form of carbohydrates) at significant rates, the need for provision of protein, and increased requirements for micronutrients such as zinc, vitamin C, and selenium.

B. Obese patients. An increase in the number of obese patients has been observed in the last 10 years. Obese patients have specific requirements for their care. Obese patients may exhibit occult but significant nutritional deficiencies. Accumulating evidence suggests that obese patients may benefit from the use of hypocaloric high-protein diets.

C. Elderly patients. There appears to be a significant increase in the incidence of trauma in the elderly population. Elderly patients have increased metabolic problems providing for significant challenges in nutritional intervention. They may be malnourished prior to injury, and they may also have chronic underlying diseases such as chronic renal insufficiency or diabetes. Hyperglycemia after trauma is common in these patients.

VI. CLINICAL GUIDELINES.

The Eastern Association for the Surgery of Trauma (EAST) has created guidelines to assist clinicians in the formulations of NI in trauma. Other associations have created guidelines for the management of NI in critical illness. These guidelines allow for formulating practical suggestions toward the approach of NI in trauma (Tables 43-5 and 43-6).

Consider the following:

A. Does the patient need nutritional intervention? If short periods of starvation are tolerated in a previously healthy patient, then NI is probably not warranted.

B. Nutrition intervention is indicated in patients that cannot eat by themselves. If the period of starvation is anticipated to be longer than 7 days, the patient is critically ill or the patient is hypercatabolic, then nutritional intervention should be considered.

TABLE 43-5	Formulations of NI in Critical Illness (EAST)						
	TraumaCal	**Replete**	**Jevity**	**Peptinex**	**Peptamen**	**Nepro**	**Nutri-hep**
Protein	22%	25%	16.7%	12%	16%	14.0%	11%
Carbohydrate	38%	45%	54.3%	55%	51%	43.0%	77%
Fat	40%	30%	29.0%	33%	33%	43.0%	12%
Calories per 8 fl oz	355	250	250	250	250	475	375

TABLE 43-6	Guidelines for the Management of NI in Critical Illness	
Name	**Type**	**Patient target**
Jevity	Standard polymeric	General-purpose formula
Replete	High protein	Severely traumatized
Peptinex	Peptide based	Malabsorption
Impact/Crucial/Pivot	Immune enhancing	High-risk surgical patient

C. Enteral nutrition is strongly favored over TPN. A functional GI tract is present in most patients. Starting TPN because you are not meeting caloric goals through EN is strongly discouraged. This practice is probably associated with increased morbidity.

D. Surgical manipulation of the gastrointestinal tract, including that of bowel resection, should not prevent the clinician from ordering enteral nutrition. Clinical exam alone (i.e., listening to bowel sounds) is not a sensitive mechanism to determine tolerance to enteral nutrition.

E. Enteral nutrition should be started early, ideally within the first 24 to 36 hours after the injury. It is not important to achieve caloric goals early. Rather, it is important to maintain a small rate of EN (i.e., **trickle feeds**) initially. An attempt to meet caloric goals should occur later in the hospital stay. **Feeding the gut when the patient is in shock (either related to resuscitation or sepsis), especially at high volume rates, is dangerous and associated with worsening of bowel ischemia and necrosis.**

F. **Do not overfeed** critically ill trauma patients. Overfeeding is associated with significant morbidity and possibly increased mortality.

G. Consider using a hypocaloric diet under some circumstances especially when ordering TPN. This is especially significant in obese patients and during sepsis.

H. Monitor nutritional interventions carefully. Avoid hyperglycemia and hyperlipidemia. A low albumin and prealbumin in trauma and critical illness is not necessarily an indication of malnutrition, but rather an indication of the severity of the disease. Overfeeding patients with low levels of albumin or prealbumin will not hasten the patient's recovery, especially if the patient has a septic focus or significant amounts of necrotic tissue.

I. Most patients can be fed a standard polymeric formula. Specialized nutritional formulas should be used in consultation with a nutritional support team. Diets containing omega-3 fatty acids, glutamine, and arginine (IEDs) can be used carefully and early for short periods of time (5 to 10 days). As previously noted, immune-enhancing diets should not be used if the patient becomes septic.

Bibliography

Bertolini G, Iapichino G, Radrizzani D, Facchini R. Early enteral immunonutrition in patients with severe sepsis: Results of an interim analysis of a randomized multicentre clinical trial. *Intens Care Med* 2003;29:671.

Bower RH, Cerra FB, Bershadsky B. Early enteral administration of a formula supplemented with arginine, nucleotides, and fish oil in intensive care unit patients: Results of a multicenter, prospective, randomized clinical trial. *Crit Care Med* 1995;23:436.

Brown R, Hunt H, Mowatt-Larssen C, Kudsk K. Comparison of specialized and standard enteral formulas in trauma patients. *Pharmacotherapy* 1994;14:314.

Cresci GA. Nutrition support in trauma. In: Gottschlich MM, ed. *The Science and Practice of Nutrition Support: A Case-Based Core Curriculum.* Dubuque, Iowa: Kendall/Hunt Publishing Co; 2001:445.

Dickerson RN, Boschert KJ, Kudsk KA, Brown RO. Hypocaloric enteral tube feeding in critically ill obese patients. *Nutrition* 2002;18:241.

Dickerson RN, Rosato EF, Mullen JL. Net protein anabolism with hypocaloric parenteral nutrition in obese stressed patients. *Am J Clin Nutr* 1986;44:747.

Frankenfield DC. Correlation between measured energy expenditure and clinically obtained variables in trauma and sepsis. *J Trauma* 1994;18:398.

Frankenfield D. Energy and macrosubstrate requirements. In: Gottschlich MM, ed. *The Science and Practice of Nutrition Support: A Case-Based Core Curriculum.* Dubuque, Iowa: Kendall/Hunt Publishing Co; 2001:31.

Freund E, Freund O. Beitrage zum Stoffwechsel im Hungerzustand. *Med Klin* 1901;15:69.

Fuhrman PM. Hepatic proteins and nutrition assessment. *J Am Diet Assoc* 2004;104:1258.

Hasselgren PO, Fisher JE. Counter-regulatory hormones and mechanisms in amino acid metabolism with special reference to the catabolic response in skeletal muscle. *Curr Opin Nutr Metab Care* 1999;2(1):9.

Hoffer LJ. Starvation. In: Shils ME, Olson JA, Shike M, eds. *Modern Nutrition in Health and Disease*. Philadelphia, Pa: Lea & Febiger; 1994:927.

Ireton-Jones CS. Equations for estimating energy expenditure in burn patients with special reference to ventilatory status. *J Burn Care Rehab* 1992;13(3):330–333.

Keys A. Basal metabolism. In: *The Biology of Human Starvation*. St. Paul, Minn: North Central Publishing Co; 1950:303.

Krishnan JA, Parce PB, Martinez A, et al. Caloric intake in medical ICU patients: Consistency of care with guidelines and relationship to clinical outcomes. *Chest* 2003;124:297.

Kudsk KA, Minard G, Croce MA, Brown RO. A randomized trial of isonitrogenous enteral diets after severe trauma: An immune-enhancing diet reduces septic complications. *Ann Surg* 1996;224:531.

Lewis SJ, Egger M, Sylvester PA, Thomas S. Early enteral feeding versus "nil by mouth" after gastrointestinal surgery: Systematic review and meta-analysis of controlled trials. *BMJ* 2001;323:773.

Lin E, Calvano SE, Lowry SF. Systemic response to injury and metabolic support. In: Brunicardi FC, Andersen DK, Billiar TR, et al. *Schwartz's Principles of Surgery*. New York, NY: McGraw-Hill Medical Publishing Div; 2005:3.

Long CL. Effect of amino acid infusion on glucose production in trauma patients. *J Trauma* 1996;40:335.

Long CL. Metabolic response to injury and illness: Estimation of energy and protein needs from indirect calorimetry and nitrogen balance. *J Parenter Enteral Nutr* 1979;3:452.

Marderstein EL, Simmons RL, Ochoa JB. Patient safety: Effect of institutional protocols on adverse events related to feeding tube placement in the critically ill. *J Am Coll Surg* 2004;199:39.

Marik PE, Pinsky M. Death by parenteral nutrition. *Intens Care Med* 2003;29:867.

McClave SA, Snider HL. Use of indirect calorimetry in clinical nutrition. *Nutr Clin Pract* 1992;7(5):207–221.

Moore FA, Moore EE, Kudsk KA. Clinical benefits of an immune enhancing diet for early postinjury enteral feeding. *J Trauma* 1994;37:607.

Piccione VA, LeVeen HH. Prehepatic hyperalimentation. *Surgery* 1987;87:263.

Pikul J. Degree of preoperative malnutrition is predictive of preoperative morbidity and mortality in liver transplant recipients. *Transplantation* 1994;57(3):469.

Sandstrom R, Drott C, Hyltander A, et al. The effect of postoperative intravenous feeding (TPN) on outcome following major surgery evaluated in a randomized study. *Ann Surg* 1993;217:185.

Tepaske R, Velthuis H. Effect of preoperative oral immune-enhancing nutritional supplement on patients at high risk of infection after cardiac surgery: A randomised placebo-controlled trial. *Lancet* 2001;358:696.

Zaloga GP. Permissive underfeeding. *New Horiz* 1994;2:257.

SUPPORT OF THE ORGAN DONOR

CARRIE SIMS, JUAN B. OCHOA, JUAN CARLOS PUYANA, AND PATRICK M. REILLY

44

I. **INTRODUCTION.** Organ availability remains the major limitation to the widespread use of organ transplantation in many diseases. In the past decade, the number of people awaiting organ transplantation has doubled, whereas the available organ supply has only increased by only one third. As a result, median waiting times for transplants have increased dramatically over the last decade. **More people die waiting for organs than ever receive an organ transplant.**

   A. Organs that can be transplanted include the heart, lung, liver, kidney, pancreas, and small bowel. Other tissues that can be transplanted include bone marrow, bone, fascia, cartilage, cornea, skin, and heart valves.

   B. Trauma patients with severe head injuries are common organ donors and currently provide over one third of the transplanted organs. The number of annual potential organ donors in the United States is estimated to be as high as 27,000. However, only 15% to 20% of these patients become actual donors. Therefore, strategies aimed at increasing the percentage of actual donors could result in an increase in organ availability.

   C. The failure to procure potential organs is multifactorial and includes family refusal, the lack of awareness by the treating physician, and the inadequate resuscitation of the brain-dead organ donor (Table 44-1). According to the Federal Conditions of Participation of the Centers for Medicare and Medicaid Services, hospitals are required to contact their local organ-procurement organization in a timely manner if a patient is expected to expire. The trauma physician plays a key role in identifying potential donors, contacting the organ procurement organization (OPO), and maintaining physiologic homeostasis in the brain-dead patient. The OPO should be notified early in the evaluation of *all* potential donors. The OPO and transplant surgeons, rather than the trauma staff, should assess the suitability of a potential donor. Additionally, the OPO is skilled in approaching the family of potential donors and is well versed in the diagnosis of brain death.

II. **THE CLINICAL DIAGNOSIS OF BRAIN DEATH**

   A. The definition of death has evolved from the cessation of cardiorespiratory functions to that of irreversible damage to the brain. An official change in the attitude toward the diagnosis of death was reflected in the publication of the Uniform Anatomical Gift Act in 1968. In 1981, the President's Commission for the Study of Ethical Problems in Medicine and Biomedical and Behavioral Research published the Uniform Determination of Death Act, which provides the legal basis for the declaration of death. It states: "An individual who has sustained either (1) irreversible cessation of circulatory and respiratory functions, *or* (2) irreversible cessation of all functions of the entire brain, including the brainstem, is dead." State statutes dictate the mechanism for determination of brain death.

   B. In trauma victims, the lethality of brain injury can often be determined soon after arrival of the patient (especially penetrating head injury). Once recognized, the OPO should be contacted to evaluate the patient as a potential organ donor. Inform the family of the severity of brain injury and the potential progression to brain death.

TABLE 44-1	Failure to Donate: Causes and Remedial Strategies

Causes	Remedial strategies
1. Failure to recognize potential organ donors	• Provide continuous education • Develop a hospital-based organ donation team (social workers, ministers, OPO, ICU staff)
2. Family refusal	
–Family approached about organ donation by the primary care team (perceived conflict of interest)	• Primary service informs family of death • OPO approaches family
–Family informed of death and approached about organ donation at the same time (perceived conflict of interest)	• Temporally separate the discussion of death and the request for donation • OPO should approach the family regarding donation
–Low acceptability of organ donation by minorities	• Understand cultural diversity
3. Failure to expedite diagnosis of brain death	• Create clear guidelines for the diagnosis of brain death
4. Failure to maintain organ homeostasis	• Optimize organ perfusion (volume first, followed by pressors as needed) • Use lung protective ventilatory strategies • Anticipate and treat endocrine abnormalities

OPO, organ procurement organization; ICU, intensive care unit.

   C. Failure to expedite the determination of brain death results in increased cost to families and the loss of organ donors because of irreversible deterioration of organ function (Table 44-2).

   D. Brain death is a clinical diagnosis. The practical determination of brain death varies among institutions. The usual criteria, largely determined by the state, are as follows:

     1. Documentation of coma

     2. No motor response to painful stimuli

     3. No brainstem reflexes

TABLE 44-2	Steps in the Organ Donation Process

1. Determine severity of head trauma.
2. Determine the likelihood of reversing the patient's disease process.
3. Notify the organ procurement organization (OPO).
4. Inform the family of the patient's condition and prognosis.
5. Optimize organ function, perfusion, and oxygen transport. Maintain homeostasis.
6. Determine irreversibility of brain injury. Perform first brain-death clinical examination.
7. Have OPO approach family regarding the possibility of organ donation.
8. Perform a second brain-death clinical examination, laboratory evaluations, and secondary investigational studies (e.g., nuclear medicine flow study).
9. Obtain consent.
10. Perform donation laboratory studies, echocardiogram, and bronchoscopy (if needed).
11. Procure the organ(s).

TABLE 44-3	Apnea Test

1. Meet the prerequisites:
   - Core temperature >36.5°C
   - Systolic blood pressure >90 mmHg
   - Euvolemia
   - Normal $PaCO_2$
   - Normal PaO_2
   - No paralytics, sedation, or drug intoxication
   - Normal electrolyte and acid-base status
2. Preoxygenate with 100% FiO_2 for 20 min.
3. Normalize $PaCO_2$ and draw a baseline ABG.
4. Connect pulse oximeter and disconnect ventilator.
5. Deliver 100% oxygen (8–12 L/min) into the trachea.
6. Look closely for respiratory movements.
7. Measure arterial PO_2, PCO_2, and pH after 5 and 10 min and reconnect to the ventilator.
   - If respiratory movements are absent and $PaCO_2$ increases to ≥60 mmHg, the apnea test is positive and supports the diagnosis of brain death.
   - If respiratory movements are seen, the apnea test is negative.
8. Abort the test if these occur:
   - Hemodynamic instability (i.e., decrease in SBP <90 mmHg) or ventricular arrhythmia
   - Oxygen desaturation (<90%)

SBP, systolic blood pressure; ABG, arterial blood gas.

---

  a. Pupils are nonreactive to a bright light.
  b. Ocular movements are absent; there is no response to head turning or tympanic caloric testing with ice water.
  c. Corneal reflexes are absent.
  d. Laryngeal and tracheal reflexes are absent.
  4. Apnea: The absence of respiratory movements with an increase in $PaCO_2$ >60 mmHg in the setting of normoxia (Table 44-3).
  5. No increase in heart rate following intravenous administration of 2 mg atropine.
E. The diagnosis of brain death also requires the exclusion of confounding factors, which include:
  1. Drug intoxication or poisoning (i.e., barbiturates)
  2. Hypothermia (core temperature must be at least 32°C)
  3. Severe electrolyte and acid-base abnormalities
  4. Severe endocrine disturbances
  5. Hemodynamic instability (systolic blood pressure <90 mmHg)
F. In addition to the clinical evaluation, an intracranial catastrophe must be documented. Most patients will undergo a neuroimaging procedure (computed tomography [CT] scan or magnetic resonance imaging [MRI]) to confirm the clinical impression.
G. A number of tests can aid in confirming the diagnosis of clinical brain death. They are particularly useful when a complete clinical evaluation cannot be done (i.e., in the setting of uremia or encephalopathy, the presence of central nervous system (CNS) depressants, or the inability to assess papillary response secondary to ocular trauma). The tests include:
  1. Electroencephalography (EEG)
  2. Cerebral angiography
  3. Transcranial Doppler ultrasonography
  4. Nuclear medicine flow study or xenon flow studies
  5. Somatosensory-evoked potentials

H. The clinical brain-death evaluation should be completed on at least two different occasions (traditionally 2 to 12 hours apart) and by two different qualified physicians who are not part of the transplant team.

III. THE ORGAN DONATION PROCESS

A. All patients identified to have a fatal or irreversible disease process should be considered potential organ donors. Contraindications to donation include:

1. Viral infections: human immunodeficiency virus (HIV) infection, human T-cell leukemia-lymphoma virus, systemic viral infections (e.g., measles, rabies, adenovirus, enterovirus, parvovirus), and herpetic meningoencephalitis.
2. Viral hepatitis: hepatitis-positive patients, however, can donate to hepatitis-positive recipients.
3. Tuberculosis.
4. Untreated septicemia: the presence of bacteremia or fungemia, however, are not absolute contraindications. Patients who receive organs from infected donors do not appear to do significantly worse than those who receive organs from noninfected donors.
5. Extracranial malignancies: exceptions include nonmelanoma skin cancers.
6. Intravenous drug abuse.
7. Known prior related disease.

B. After two clinical examinations, with additional confirmatory tests as needed, have corroborated lack of brain activity, the patient is declared dead. At many institutions, a single clinical examination and cerebral blood flow study may be sufficient to declare brain death in a patient with an obviously devastating brain injury. Two physicians who are not involved with the transplant team must sign the death certificate. The coroner's permission is required for removal of organs for transplantation, but he or she is not required to sign the death certificate. Permission for donation must be obtained from the patient's next of kin.

C. Referral to the local OPO is expedited if the following patient data are available: patient history, diagnosis and date of admission, patient height and weight, ABO group, hemodynamic data, urinalysis, laboratory data, current medications, and culture results.

D. A possible solution to the shortage of organ donors is the use of non-heart-beating cadaveric donors (NHBCD). These are patients who have been declared dead by the traditional cardiopulmonary parameters rather than by brain-death criteria. The limiting factor in this situation is warm ischemia time.

IV. CARE OF THE POTENTIAL ORGAN DONOR (Table 44-4). Physiologic derangements of multiple organ systems are common after brain death. Cardiopulmonary arrest generally follows brain death within hours. The main goal during this interim is to maintain organ function while preventing end-organ damage. Progression from brain death to somatic death results in the loss of 10% to 20% of potential donors. The use of standardized guidelines and algorithms improves the hemodynamic stability of potential donors and optimizes organ retrieval and graft outcome.

A systemic approach to hemodynamic support of the potential organ donor should achieve the goals of:

- Normovolemia
- Normal blood pressure
- Optimized cardiac output

Hypotension is associated with less successful organ retrieval and function and is commonly seen in patients with multifactorial hypovolemia. The overall goal is to maintain end-organ perfusion with the minimal use of vasoactive drugs.

If these goals cannot be met, then the patients should undergo invasive monitoring including pulmonary artery catheterization with the objective of maintaining a wedge pressure of 8 to 12 mmHg or a central venous pressure (CVP) of 6 to 8 mmHg. Cardiac index should ideally be maintained above 2.4 L/minute/m^2.

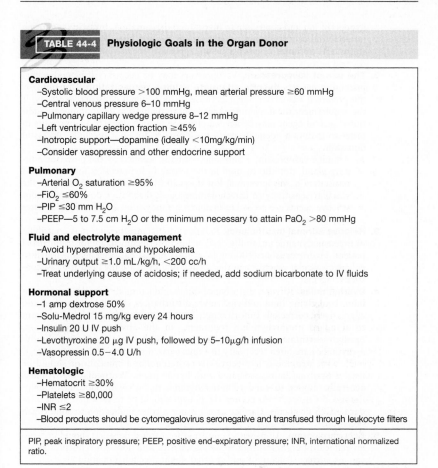

| **TABLE 44-4** | Physiologic Goals in the Organ Donor |

Cardiovascular
- Systolic blood pressure >100 mmHg, mean arterial pressure ≥60 mmHg
- Central venous pressure 6–10 mmHg
- Pulmonary capillary wedge pressure 8–12 mmHg
- Left ventricular ejection fraction ≥45%
- Inotropic support—dopamine (ideally <10mg/kg/min)
- Consider vasopressin and other endocrine support

Pulmonary
- Arterial O_2 saturation ≥95%
- FiO_2 ≤60%
- PIP ≤30 mm H_2O
- PEEP—5 to 7.5 cm H_2O or the minimum necessary to attain PaO_2 >80 mmHg

Fluid and electrolyte management
- Avoid hypernatremia and hypokalemia
- Urinary output ≥1.0 mL/kg/h, <200 cc/h
- Treat underlying cause of acidosis; if needed, add sodium bicarbonate to IV fluids

Hormonal support
- 1 amp dextrose 50%
- Solu-Medrol 15 mg/kg every 24 hours
- Insulin 20 U IV push
- Levothyroxine 20 µg IV push, followed by 5–10µg/h infusion
- Vasopressin 0.5–4.0 U/h

Hematologic
- Hematocrit ≥30%
- Platelets ≥80,000
- INR ≤2
- Blood products should be cytomegalovirus seronegative and transfused through leukocyte filters

PIP, peak inspiratory pressure; PEEP, positive end-expiratory pressure; INR, international normalized ratio.

A. Cardiovascular support. Brain death adversely affects the cardiovascular system. Prior to brain herniation, cerebral ischemia is associated with a robust sympathetic surge in an attempt to maintain cerebral perfusion pressure. As herniation ensues, the spinal cord becomes progressively ischemic and there is a deactivation of the sympathetic nervous system. A state of profound vasodilation develops and circulating levels of catecholamines plummet. Managing the cardiovascular status of the brain-dead patient requires anticipation of this hemodynamic instability.

1. Maintain euvolemia and adequate perfusion pressures. Approximately 30% of donor referrals for cardiac transplantation are refused secondary to poor hemodynamic function. Cardiac arrest in the donor is more common in the setting of hypotension. Adequate support can minimize cardiac dysfunction and improve the likelihood of successful donation. The goal is to maintain adequate systolic blood pressure and filling pressures to ensure organ perfusion. This is obtained initially by restoration of intravascular volume (see Table 44-4). Packed red blood cells should be transfused to a goal hematocrit of 30% in order to optimize oxygen delivery. Urine output should be maintained at >0.5 to 1.0 mL/kg/hour. Excessive use of vasoconstrictive drugs can exacerbate organ hypoperfusion and contribute to myocardial deterioration. Invasive monitoring (arterial and central venous access) should be used liberally to gauge volume status and optimize organ perfusion, especially when vasoactive support is deemed necessary.

2. **The use of vasopressors.** Vasopressors may be necessary if hemodynamic instability persists **despite adequate volume resuscitation**. Dopamine is the preferred vasoactive agent because of its minimal constrictive effects. If the requirement for dopamine exceeds more than 10 mg/kg/minute, an additional second agent may be needed. The use of high doses of vasopressors in order to maintain adequate perfusion pressure does not preclude successful donation.

   a. Arginine vasopressin, a hormone normally secreted by the posterior pituitary gland, can also be used in the setting of hypotension following fluid resuscitation. Vasopressin at low doses (0.01–0.04 U/minute) enhances the vascular sensitivity to catecholamines such that lower doses of vasoconstrictive agents are needed to maintain hemodynamic stability. Higher doses may be necessary if diabetes insipidus develops.

3. **Relative adrenal insufficiency.** Relative adrenal insufficiency may contribute to the hemodynamic instability observed in the critically ill and/or traumatized patient. Hydrocortisone (100 mg IV every 8 hours) has been demonstrated to enhance vascular reactivity in this setting and decrease the need for vasoconstictive agents.

4. **Dysrhythmias.** Rhythm disturbances and conduction abnormalities are common. Underlying fluid and electrolyte disturbances should be identified and aggressively corrected. Unfortunately, these arrhythmias are highly resistant to standard antiarrhythmic treatment. In the absence of hypotension, bradydysrhythmias require no treatment. With brain herniation, brady-arrhythmias are often secondary to vagus nerve disruption and standard treatment with atropine is ineffective. Isoproterenol and epinephrine should be used if bradycardia is associated with hypotension. Ventricular arrhythmias generally respond to standard antiarrhythmic therapy with lidocaine or amiodarone. If cardiac arrest occurs, the patient should be resuscitated using standard ACLS protocols. Cardiac arrest is not a contraindication to solid organ donation.

5. **Echocardiogram.** All patients considered for cardiac donation should undergo an echocardiogram in order to assess cardiac function. An echocardiogram can also detect structural problems that might preclude donation.

B. **Pulmonary support.** Lung procurement rates are relatively low (20%) and may be secondary to the initial lung injury, neurogenic pulmonary edema, the development of respiratory complications, and excessive fluid.

1. **"Pulmonary toilet."** Simple measures should be instituted to prevent accumulation of secretions and atelectasis. Frequent suctioning, bronchoscopy, and the use of inhaled albuterol may help.

2. **Ventilator settings.** Ventilator settings should minimize oxygen toxicity and barotrauma. Maneuvers directed at treating elevated intracranial pressure should be abandoned. Optimally, the ventilator settings should achieve a PaO_2 of 80 to 100 mmHg with the lowest possible FiO_2. Positive end-expiratory pressure (PEEP) of 5 to 7.5 should enhance alveolar recruitment without excessive barotraumas. The end inspiratory plateau pressure should be limited to <30 cm H_2O. A PaO_2/FiO_2 <250 and peak inspiratory pressures of >30 cm H_2O are indicative of poor lung function posttransplantation. Normocarbia and a normal pH should be maintained.

3. **Excessive volume resuscitation.** The use of excessive amounts of intravenous fluids can impair pulmonary function and affect the suitability of the lungs for organ donation. The use of a Swan-Ganz catheter can aid in guiding volume resuscitation with a goal pulmonary capillary wedge pressure of 8 to 12 mmHg. In the event of overresuscitation, judicious diuresis may help salvage potentially usable lungs.

C. **Fluid and electrolyte therapy**
   1. **Diabetes insipidus.** Diabetes insipidis (DI), with concomitant loss of free water, occurs frequently in brain-dead patients. The clinical diagnosis is confirmed by the presence of increased urinary output (>200 cc/hour), low urinary osmolality, and hypernatremia. Desmopressin acetate (DDAVP 0.3 mg/kg IV infusion) or vasopressin (0.5–4.0 U/hour) may be required. Adequate volume replacement is essential.
   2. **Hypernatremia.** Serum electrolytes should be monitored and aggressively corrected. Lactated Ringer's or half normal saline should be used to keep the sodium level <150 mmol/L. Failure to correct hypernatremia in the donor has been associated with poor graft outcome in liver transplantation.
   3. **Hyperglycemia.** Hyperglycemia, with its resultant osmotic diuresis, should be avoided. Tight glycemic control (80 to 150 mg/dL) can be achieved with the use of an insulin infusion and monitoring every 1 hour.
   4. **Acidosis.** Sodium bicarbonate (50 mmol/L) should be added to the maintenance IV fluid if the donor is acidotic.
   5. **Alternative colloids.** Hydroxyethyl starch has been associated with renal tubular cell injury and should be avoided.
D. **Endocrine support.** Hormone replacement therapy should be strongly considered in all potential donors who, despite goal-directed fluid resuscitation, remain hemodynamically unstable. Although controversial, several animal and human studies have demonstrated hypothalamic-pituitary-adrenal dysfunction in the setting of brain death. Low levels of thyroid hormone, cortisol, and vasopressin may contribute to cardiovascular lability. Exogenous hormonal replacement therapy appears to decrease the need for vasoactive support in unstable donors and is associated with an increase in the number of organs suitable for transplantation. Potential organ donors should receive 1 amp dextrose 50%, Solu-Medrol (15 mg/kg every 24 hours), insulin (20 U IV push), levothyroxine (20 μg IV push, followed by 5–10 μg/hour infusion), and vasopressin (0.5–4.0 U/hour).
E. **Hematologic support.** Disorders of blood coagulation are common in the setting of traumatized or necrotic brain tissue. Coagulopathy may be further exacerbated by ongoing hemorrhage, massive transfusion, acidosis, hypothermia, and consumption of coagulant factors. Blood products should be administered to achieve a hematocrit of >30%, to maintain a platelet count >80,000, and to correct an international normalized ratio (INR) to <2. Blood products should be cytomegalovirus seronegative and transfused through leukocyte filters.
F. **Maintain normothermia.** As a result of increased diuresis, donors require aggressive fluid resuscitation. This phenomenon generates many of the problems seen with donor management, including hypovolemia, hypotension, hypothermia, and electrolyte imbalances. Effective warming techniques must be implemented prior to infusion to avoid hypothermia.

AXIOMS

- Trauma victims constitute the largest population of potential organ donors.
- An extreme shortage of organs exists. Early recognition of potential donors, appropriate and timely diagnosis of brain death, and adequate physiologic care of the potential organ donor could increase the population of patients who actually donate.
- Brain death is diagnosed using a set of clinical criteria and confirmatory tests.
- Early involvement of the organ procurement coordinator increases the likelihood of organ donation.
- Preservation of organ homeostasis requires the understanding that physiologic changes are occurring in each organ after brain death ensues. Maintaining homeostasis increases the chances for a successful function of each transplanted organ.
- Potential organ donors should receive goal-directed fluid resuscitation. Vasoactive agents should be used only after the patient is appropriately fluid resuscitated.

- Hemodynamically unstable patients should receive hormonal supplementation.
- Lung protective strategies improve the likelihood of lung transplantation.
- Hypernatremia, hyperglycemia, and acidosis should be aggressively treated.

Bibliography

Evans RW, Orians CE, Ascher NL. The potential supply of organ donors. *JAMA* 1992;267(2):239–246.

Gram HJ, Meinhold H, Bickel U, et al. Acute endocrine failure after brain death? *Transplantation* 1992;54(5):851–857.

Grenvik A, Darby JM, Broznick BA. Organ transplantation: An overview of problems and concerns. In: Civetta JM, ed. *Critical Care*. Philadelphia, Pa: JB Lippincott Co; 1992:803–813.

Jenkins DH, Reilly PM, Schwab W. Improving the approach to organ donation: A review. *World J Surg* 1999;23:644–649.

Kauffman HM. Increased transplanted organs from the use of a standardized donor management protocol. *Am J Transplant* 2002;2(8):761–768.

Kennedy AP, West JC, Kelley SE, et al. Utilization of trauma-related deaths for organ and tissue harvesting. *J Trauma* 1992;33(4):516–520.

Klufas CI, Powner DJ, Darby JM, et al. Organ donor categories and management. In: Shoemaker WC, Ayres S, Grenvik A, et al., eds. *Textbook of Critical Care*. Philadelphia, Pa: WB Saunders; 1994:1604–1617.

Lee PP, Kissner P. Organ donation and the Uniform Anatomical Gift Act. *Surgery* 1986;100(5):867–875.

Marik PE, Zaloga GP. Adrenal insufficiency in the critically ill: A new look at an old problem. *Chest* 2002;122:1784–1796.

The Organ Donation Breakthrough Collaborative. Best practices final report. September 2003. Available at: http://www.organdonor.gov/bestpractice.htm. Accessed November 24, 2004.

Peitzman AB, Udekwu AO, Darby JM. Organ procurement and transplantation. In: Feliciano DV, Moore EE, Mattox KL, eds. *Trauma*. Norwalk, Conn: Appleton & Lange, 1996:989–997.

Pennefather SH, Bullock RE, Mantle D, et al. Use of low dose arginine vasopressin to support brain-dead organ donor. *Transplantation* 1995;59:58–62.

Pennefather SH, Dark JH, Bullock RE. Haemodynamic responses to surgery in brain-dead organ donors. *Anaesthesia* 1993;48:1034–1038.

Powner DJ, Darby JM, Grenvik A. Controversies in brain-death certification. In: Shoemaker W, ed. *Textbook of Critical Care*. 2nd ed. Philadelphia, Pa: WB Saunders; 1994:1579–1582.

Report of the Quality Standards Subcommittee of the American Academy of Neurology. Practice parameters for determining brain death in adults. *Neurology* 1995;45:1012–1014.

Rosendale JD, Kauffman HM, McBrideMA, et al. Aggressive pharmacologic donor management results in more transplanted organs. *Transplantation* 2003;75:482–487.

Salim A, Vassiliu P, Velmahos GC, et al. The role of thyroid hormone administration in potential organ donors. *Arch Surg* 2001;136:1377–1380.

Wheeldon DR, Potter CDO, Dunning J, et al. Hemodynamic correction in multiorgan donation. *Lancet* 1992;339:1175.

Wood KE, Becker BN, McCartney JG, et al. Care of the potential organ donor. *N Engl J Med* 2004;351(26):2730–2739.

BURNS/INHALATION INJURY

JAMES H. HOLMES AND
DAVID M. HEIMBACH

45

I. INTRODUCTION
A. Epidemiology
1. Annually, approximately 45,000 people in the United States require hospitalization for burn injuries, of which about 50% suffer concomitant inhalation injury.
2. Gross mortality rates exceed 5%, with a burn LD_{50} (50% lethal dose) for 70% total body surface area (TBSA).
3. Most burn deaths occur in residential fires, and nearly half are smoking related or due to substance abuse.
4. Child abuse must be suspected and reported for unusual burns in children, or when a given history doesn't match the injury.
5. Approximately 5% of burn patients have concomitant nonthermal injuries.

B. Transfer to burn center
1. **Prophylactic systemic antibiotics are *never* indicated for burns**
2. American Burn Association (ABA) criteria for transfer to a dedicated burn center:
   a. Partial-thickness burns >10% TBSA
   b. Burns involving the face, hands, feet, genitalia, perineum, or major joints
   c. Full-thickness burns of any size
   d. Electrical burns or injuries, including lightning
   e. Chemical burns
   f. Inhalation injury
   g. Burns in patients with preexisting medical conditions
   h. Burns associated with concomitant nonthermal trauma in which the burn injury poses the greatest risk of morbidity or mortality
   i. Burned children in hospitals without qualified personnel
   j. Burns in patients requiring special social, emotional, or long-term rehabilitation interventions

II. PREHOSPITAL
A. History
1. Time of injury (start time for calculating fluid resuscitation)
2. Open or closed space (inhalation injury more likely in closed space)
3. Source of burn: flame, liquid, steam, chemical, explosion, electrical
4. Duration of exposure
5. Presence of toxic materials: plastics, cyanide, petroleum products
6. Mechanism of any associated injury: motor vehicle crash (MVC), fall, and so on
7. Quantity of prehospital fluid

B. Care at scene
1. Burn victims are trauma patients and require trauma care.
2. Remove patient from source of injury.
3. Remove burning clothing.
4. Assess for immediate life-threatening injuries, as per Advanced Trauma Life Support (ATLS) and Advanced Burn Life Support (ABLS).
5. Provide supplemental oxygen and airway protection.
6. Apply dry dressings.
7. Initiate transport to hospital.

III. INITIAL ASSESSMENT AND RESUSCITATION

A. General

1. Burn injury can be dramatic and distract the resuscitation team from concomitant nonthermal injuries.
2. Patients with severe burn injury may appear **deceptively stable on arrival**. A patient may be talking (and even joking) on admission with stable blood pressure and mild tachycardia. Within 24 hours, the patient is frequently critically ill.
3. Provide early pain control with frequent small doses of intravenous (IV) opiates.
4. Elevate the ambient room temperature to avoid heat loss from the burn wound.
5. Burns are tetanus-prone and mandate prophylaxis.

B. Airway

1. **Note:** Although urgent endotracheal intubation is sometimes necessary, time usually exists to access the airway and provide a semielective intubation, when necessary.
2. Provide supplemental oxygen to all patients.
3. Criteria for intubation are the same as in all trauma patients. The following clinical conditions may require immediate or early intubation in a burn patient:
   a. Apnea, respiratory failure, or profound hypoxia.
   b. Patients with severe facial burns may appear initially stable. Consider semielective intubation because profound orofacial swelling over the next few hours can make intubation very difficult.
   c. Signs and symptoms of inhalation injury:
      - History of closed space fire
      - Carbon deposits in the naso/oropharynx
      - Expectorated, carbonaceous sputum
      - Wheezing
      - $PaO_2:FiO_2$ <300
      - Carbon monoxide levels estimated >10% at the scene
   d. Upper airway injury and obstruction frequently occur in patients with burns of the face and neck. Soft-tissue swelling of the face, oropharynx, glottis, and trachea can be dramatic, precluding safe intubation and making cricothyroidotomy/tracheostomy difficult. Any patient with phonation changes or stridor should be considered for intubation.

C. Breathing

1. If intubated, ventilate with 100% oxygen (generally with 5–10 cm H_2O of positive end-expiratory pressure [PEEP]) with a goal of avoiding high airway pressures while maintaining patient comfort. Perform arterial blood gases (ABG) to ensure adequate oxygenation, ventilation, and clearance of acidosis.
2. Perform a chest radiograph to look for associated trauma, early signs of inhalation injury, and position of tubes/lines.
3. Bronchoscopy may be necessary to assess inhalation injury.
4. Circumferential torso burns causing elevated airway pressures may require escharotomy. **Note:** Patients without complete circumferential torso burns may also require escharotomy to provide adequate ventilation.

D. Circulation

1. **Intravenous access** is ideally obtained with large-bore (14–16 gauge in adults) peripheral catheters placed through unburned tissue. In severe burns (>25% TBSA), it is optimal to obtain central venous access early before massive swelling and edema occur. Placement through burned tissue is acceptable if it is the only option.
2. **Initial fluid resuscitation**
   a. Typically, only burns >20% TBSA in adults require formal IV fluid resuscitation.
   b. Start with and use only **Lactated Ringer's (LR)**. Do not use normal saline (NS).
   c. The **Parkland/Baxter formula (4 mL LR/kg body weight/% TBSA burn)** is used to guide resuscitation.
   d. How to use the Parkland/Baxter formula:

- Hang 1,000 mL of LR wide open until time is available to calculate the rate.
- The formula is **only a guide** for fluid requirements in the **first 24 hours**. Fluid resuscitation should be adjusted based on the patient's physiologic response to treatment.
- Only **partial- and full-thickness burns** (second and third degree) are included in TBSA estimation.
- **TBSA** is determined by the **rule of nines** (Fig. 45-1) or age-appropriate burn diagrams.
- Give **one half of the calculated requirement** in the **first 8 hours** from the time of injury. The **second half** is given over subsequent **16 hours.**
- The **first 8 hours begins at the time of burn**, not at the time the patient is first seen.
- For example, 35% TBSA burn in a 70-kg person gets 9,800 mL LR over 24 hours, 4,900 mL over the first 8 hours (613 mL/hour), and 4,900 over subsequent 16 hours (306 mL/hour).

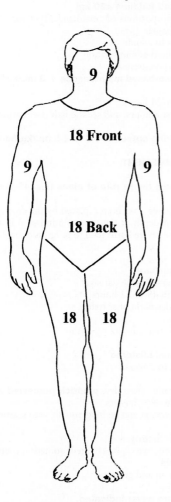

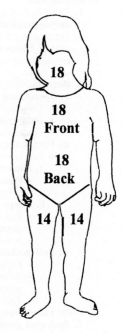

Figure 45-1. Rule of nines.

- Once started, use **urine output** to guide the fluid rate to obtain **~30 mL/hour** in an adult.
- In the second 24 hours postburn, a patient's maintenance fluid requirements are ~1.5 times normal. This volume should be given as crystalloid, with the composition of the fluid determined by serum electrolyte levels. Any colloid supplementation (i.e., albumin) should occur ⩾24 hours postburn.

  e. A subset of patients **(inhalation injury, high-voltage electrical, delayed resuscitation, massive deep burns)** may require additional fluid over that estimated by the Parkland/Baxter formula. Hemoconcentration (i.e., hematocrit >55%) may be an early clue to increased fluid requirements.

  f. Any patient who does not respond with adequate urine output during the first few hours of resuscitation, is elderly, or has a history of cardiopulmonary disease may require pulmonary artery catheter or ultrasound-guided fluid management.

  E. Pediatric fluid resuscitation (infants and toddlers <20 kg)
  1. The head and neck represent larger proportions of calculated TBSA than in adults (Fig. 45.1 and Table 46.1 in Chapter 46).
  2. Careful fluid resuscitation is necessary to avoid:
     a. Pulmonary edema from excessive fluid administration
     b. Cerebral edema associated with hyponatremia
  3. Formula for estimated fluid = **dextrose-based maintenance + 3 mL/kg/% TBSA LR over 24 hours**
     a. Maintenance volume prorated over 24 hours
     b. One half of burn component in first 8 hours, and second half over ensuing 16 hours
  4. Goal is a well-perfused child with a **urine output of 1.0 to 1.5 mL/kg/hour.**

IV. INITIAL WOUND ASSESSMENT AND MANAGEMENT
A. Assessment
1. The TBSA of any burn is best estimated by the **rule of nines** (Fig. 45-1) or **age-appropriate diagrams**.
2. Terminology for burn depth using "degree" has been replaced by the description of **"thickness."** Classification of depth at the time of admission is an estimate and may be inaccurate because severe burns tend to progress or evolve over time.
3. **Burn depth** (Fig. 45-2)
   a. Superficial (first degree, such as sunburn)
      - Confined to epidermis with minimal tissue damage.
      - **Mild erythema**, pain resolving in 48 to 72 hours.
      - Epidermis may peel in small scales without scarring.
   b. Partial thickness (second degree)
      - Involves entire epidermis with variable layers of dermis.
        i. Superficial
           - **Painful**, pink, edematous, and **blistered**
           - Spontaneous healing in <2 to 3 weeks
        ii. Deep
           - Red or mottled red and white, often dry, **pinprick perceived as pressure rather than pain**, +/− blisters
           - Prolonged healing without excision and grafting, usually with scarring
   c. Full thickness (third degree)
      - Entire epidermis and dermis destroyed
      - Relatively **painless**, leathery, waxy, or charred, sometimes with visible **thrombosed vessels**
      - Will not heal without excision and grafting

B. Initial burn wound management
1. **Systemic prophylactic antibiotics are never indicated.**
2. In the emergency department (ED) before transport to a burn center:

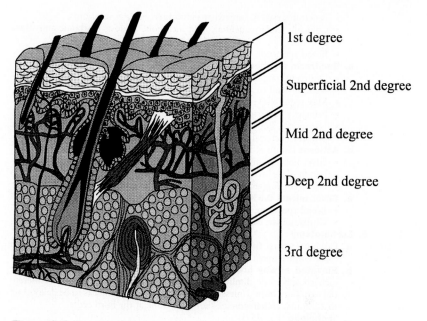

1st degree

Superficial 2nd degree

Mid 2nd degree

Deep 2nd degree

3rd degree

Figure 45-2. Burn wound depth.

    a. Wash gently with gauze soaked in saline.
    b. Remove any obviously loose skin.
    c. Apply **topical agents** (Section IV.B.4) **only** if anticipated **delay in transfer** because removal of the agent at the burn center can prolong the initial assessment.
    d. Irrigate debris from the eyes, as needed.
    e. Cover wounds with dry sterile dressings.
    f. Provide tetanus prophylaxis, as indicated.
  3. In the ED of the **burn center** or **definitive care hospital**:
    a. Burns <10% of the body surface area (BSA) can be cleansed, locally debrided, and covered with a topical agent.
    b. Treat **larger burns** by placing the patient in a special gurney (usually located in the burn unit), which allows for total exposure, overhead heating, rapid burn wound debridement by a specially trained team, cleansing using gentle hose spray, provision of adequate analgesia, and continuous monitoring of vital signs.
  4. Topical agents
    a. Silver sulfadiazine 1% cream (Silvadene, Hoechst Marion Roussel, Inc., Kansas City, Missouri)
      • Most common topical agent used on burn wounds.
      • Usually applied daily or twice daily in a thin layer, followed by wrapping loosely with sterile gauze.
      • Broad-spectrum, bacteriostatic, painless and usually soothing, antifungal activity.
      • Transient neutropenia (sulfa effect) can occur—of no clinical consequence.
      • Caution in pregnancy and very small infants (<2 months).
    b. Mafenide acetate cream or **5% solution** (Sulfamyalon, Bertek Pharmaceuticals, Triangle Park, North Carolina)

- Penetrates eschar, somewhat painful (cream >> solution)
- Clinically inconsequential, mild metabolic acidosis (carbonic anhydrase inhibitor)
- Broad-spectrum, bacteriostatic, no antifungal activity

c. Bacitracin ointment
- Ointment (not cream) usually applied to small superficial burns and surfaces difficult to cover with gauze (e.g., face)
- May require several applications per day
- Primarily bacteriostatic against gram-positive organisms
- Neosporin, Polysporin, or gentamicin ointments can be substituted for broader bacterial coverage.

d. Acticoat (Smith & Nephew, Largo, Florida)
- Silver impregnated membrane
- Left in place on the wound for 2 to 7 days depending on the formulation
- Useful for outpatient burn management and donor site dressings

e. Silver nitrate 0.5% solution
- Broad-spectrum, bacteriostatic, antifungal activity
- Costly, messy, electrolyte abnormalities (e.g., hyponatremia)

5. Escharotomy
a. Circumferential **full-thickness** burns of the **trunk** or **extremities** can cause compartment syndromes.
b. Elevated airway pressures in a circumferential torso burn mandate escharotomy as do **diminished or absent distal pulses** in a circumferential extremity burn. Unless transport to definitive center is to be delayed up to 12 hours, escharotomies should be done at the burn center.
c. Technique (Fig. 45-3)
- In theory, bloodless and painless (usually not the case).
- Provide adequate and appropriate analgesia and sedation.
- Perform with electrocautery, when available, or knife with topical hemostatic agents (e.g., Avitene).
- Divide the eschar only, not the subcutaneous tissues or fascia.
- Inadequate hemostasis with multiple escharotomies can result in significant blood loss, which can be troublesome if the patient is going to be transferred subsequent to the procedure.

V. INHALATION INJURY
A. Overview
1. Results from **direct thermal injury** (inhalation of superheated steam), **toxic chemicals** in inhaled smoke, or a combination of both.
2. Injury to the proximal airway can cause rapid edema and obstruction.
3. Chemical irritants stimulate an intense inflammatory response in the more distal airways. The history of the environment of injury may be predictive of the extent of injury.
4. Inhalation injury is the **most frequent cause of death** in thermal injuries.
B. Evaluation
1. Consider present in all patients in closed space fires, until ruled out.
2. Signs and symptoms are outlined in Section III.B.
3. Obtain a **carboxyhemoglobin (COHb)** level with initial laboratory studies.
a. Carbon monoxide (CO) has 200 times the affinity for Hb than does O_2.
b. Elimination half-life ($t_{1/2}$) of CO breathing 100% O_2 is ~1 hour, while breathing room air it is ~4 hours.
c. COHb levels and clinical findings of CO poisoning:
- <5%—normal
- <20%—usually asymptomatic
- 20% to 30%—headache, nausea/vomiting, loss of manual dexterity
- 30% to 40%—confusion, weakness, lethargy
- 40% to 60%—coma
- >60%—death

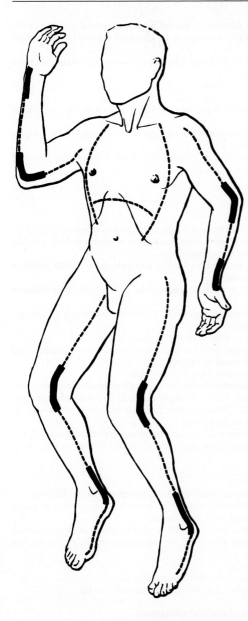

Figure 45-3. Preferred sites for escharotomy. (From Martin RR, Becker WK, Cioffi WG, et al. In: Wilson RF, ed. *Management of Trauma: Pitfalls and Practice.* Baltimore, Md: Williams & Wilkins, 1996; with permission.)

  d. Can occur as isolated CO poisoning. However, in the presence of thermal injury, an elevated COHb suggests an associated inhalation injury.
  e. A normal COHb level does not rule out inhalation injury.
  f. Note: Pulse oximetry (SpO_2) is grossly inaccurate with CO poisoning.
4. Initial chest radiograph may be normal.
5. Bronchoscopy
  a. An elective procedure that is delayed until the resuscitation is under way and the patient is hemodynamically stable.

    b. If the patient is not intubated, thread an endotracheal tube onto the scope so that a definitive airway can be obtained if bronchoscopic findings warrant.

    c. Positive findings include erythema, edema, ulcerations, carbonaceous material, and edematous cords.

    d. No material effect on outcome.

C. Treatment

    1. Administer **100% oxygen** to all patients until inhalation injury is excluded or the COHb is normal.

    2. Early **intubation and mechanical ventilation** is recommended for symptomatic patients, as previously described.

    3. Hyperbaric oxygen treatment is contraindicated in any burn patient requiring active IV fluid resuscitation or transfer.

VI. ELECTRICAL INJURY

A. Overview

    1. Electrical injuries are uncommon and frequently present a diagnostic challenge because of myriad clinical presentations. Small skin wounds can hide substantial underlying muscle and bony destruction.

    2. Generally, electrical injuries are classified as **low-voltage (<1,000 volts)** or **high-voltage (≥1,000 volts)**.

    3. Severity of injury depends on the **amperage** of the current and the **resistance** of the tissue (V = IR).

    4. The tissues with the greatest resistance tend to sustain the most heat damage. Tissue resistance in decreasing order is:

        a. Bone → fat → tendon → skin → muscle → vessel → nerve.

            i. However, high voltage does not necessarily respect this hierarchy and usually destroys all tissue in its path.

        b. Wet skin has much less resistance than dry skin.

    5. **Pathway of current is unpredictable,** but generally passes between two contact points: from the point of entry through the body to a grounded site (site with the lowest resistance). However, with high voltage, the pathway may be indiscriminate, exiting at multiple sites.

    6. In general, alternating current (AC) is more dangerous than direct current (DC).

    7. Electrical injuries may have associated serious traumatic injuries (e.g., fractures, dislocations, falls).

B. Low-voltage injury

    1. Usually occurs in the home.

    2. Cardiac **dysrhythmias** are common, particularly ventricular fibrillation.

    3. Tetanic skeletal muscle contractions (AC household current) can cause fractures or dislocations and respiratory arrest.

    4. Admit for telemetry monitoring if any EKG abnormalities are encountered. Otherwise analgesics and discharge are appropriate, unless burns are significant.

    5. **Oral burns in children**

        a. Small children sucking on an electrical cord or plug.

        b. Can involve all oral structures, but most commonly the **lip.**

        c. Treatment includes:

          • Hospitalize because of **feeding difficulties.**

          • Feed by straw or syringe; rarely is nasogastric access required.

          • Delayed debridement.

          • Intraoral splint may be necessary.

          • Tetanus prophylaxis.

C. High-voltage injury

    1. The extent of tissue damage is typically underestimated because of the unpredictable path of injury. These are usually **devastating** injuries.

2. An associated flash skin burn is not uncommon and can distract from the more devastating electrical injury to the deeper and remote tissues.
3. The deep injury is characterized by **myonecrosis**, especially along deeper tissues adjacent to bone (high resistance area). Vessel thrombosis and compartment syndrome (both early and delayed) are common sequelae.
4. Fluid management
    a. Anticipate need for **>4 mL/kg/% TBSA.**
    b. If **myoglobinuria** present, ensure urine output >100 mL/hour via fluid loading and mannitol (rarely) if fluids are inadequate.
5. Wound management
    a. Early, aggressive, and repetitive wound debridements.
    b. Extremity fasciotomy frequently required.
    c. Because of the variable tissue necrosis, amputation of a devitalized extremity may be necessary (even in the presence of adequate blood supply).
6. General management
    a. Tetanus prophylaxis
    b. Effective pain management
    c. Topical antimicrobials to thermal injury only
    d. Anticipate the need for ventilatory support and probable organ dysfunction.
7. After initial resuscitation started, all patients with high-voltage injury should be transferred to a burn center.

VII. CHEMICAL BURNS
A. Overview
1. Most burns are from **acids** or **alkalis.**
2. The extent of injury depends on the **concentration of agent** and **duration of contact.**
3. Tissue damage is frequently underestimated.
4. Alkali burns are generally more severe than acid burns.
B. Treatment
1. Remove all garments and brush off any dry powder.
2. In the field and on arrival, **copiously irrigate with tepid tap water** for at least 15 minutes (avoid hypothermia).
3. Irrigate the eyes and obtain an ophthalmology consult, as needed.
4. **No specific antidote** is available for most chemical burns, except hydrofluoric acid, and **neutralizers are contraindicated.**
C. Hydrofluoric acid burn
1. Highly toxic and painful
2. Can cause hypocalcemia and dysrhythmia with systemic absorption
3. Concentration >40% can be lethal if >2% TBSA is involved
4. Treatment
    a. Copious irrigation with water.
    b. Apply 2.5% **calcium gluconate** gel.
    c. Soft-tissue injection of calcium gluconate (1 g/10 mL) can be done in small areas in cases of persistent pain. Infuse calcium gluconate intraarterially for finger and hand burns with limited tissue space for injection.
    d. Indications for intraarterial infusion of calcium gluconate include severe pain, evidence of tissue necrosis, and pain not improving with calcium gluconate gel.
    e. Method for intraarterial calcium gluconate infusion:
        • Place a brachial artery catheter and perform angiogram to ensure adequacy of perfusion to involved fingers (a high brachial artery bifurcation is not uncommon).
        • Alternatively, a radial artery catheter can be used if only the thumb, index finger, or both are involved.
        • Infuse calcium gluconate (2 g) in D5W (100 mL) over 4 hours.
        • Repeat every 4 hours until pain is markedly decreased.
    f. Monitor serum electrolytes and aggressively treat abnormalities.

VIII. DEFINITIVE CARE OF THE BURN PATIENT

A. Burn wound

1. The depth of the burn wound may be obvious early. However, several days may be required to differentiate between superficial and deep partial-thickness wounds.
2. The best diagnostic tools are the eyes of a surgeon experienced in burn wound care.
3. **Superficial** (first degree) wounds require only cleansing and analgesia.
4. **Superficial partial-thickness** (second degree) wounds can heal spontaneously with cleansing, topical antibiotics (e.g., silver sulfadiazine), and analgesia.
   a. The appearance of epithelial "budding" is a useful predictor of primary healing, but is also associated with a transient increase in nosioception.
   b. Two or 3 weeks are usually required for epithelialization.
5. **Deep partial-thickness** (second degree) and full-thickness (third degree) wounds usually require excision and grafting to provide coverage and healing.
6. Topical creams and ointments are applied once or twice daily with dressing changes, whereas solutions are applied to dressings every 4 to 6 hours.

B. Excision

1. **Small wounds** (<5%–10% TBSA) typically can be excised and covered with a split-thickness skin graft (STSG) as soon as the patient is stable.
2. **Larger wounds** (>10%–20% TBSA) usually require staged excisions and placement of either temporary or permanent wound coverage.
3. A variety of dermatomes and free hand knives are available for excision.
4. **Tangential excision** (most common) attempts to remove only devitalized tissue and retain as many dermal elements as possible.
   a. Variable amounts of subcutaneous fat may be visible.
   b. Although fat can decrease the likelihood of graft success, it helps maintain cosmesis.
5. **Fascial excision** may be necessary in full-thickness burns with underlying fat necrosis.
   a. Although faster and with less blood loss than tangential excision, the cosmetic outcome is inferior.

C. Wound coverage

1. The best **permanent** coverage for most burn wounds is a **STSG**.
2. STSGs are harvested at 0.010- to 0.012-inch thickness and can be variably meshed to increase coverage.
3. The graft must be secured to the wound, covered with a nonadherent dressing, and further dressed to protect from mechanical injury.
4. Protective positioning and splinting of the patient may be necessary.
5. Subatmospheric dressings (V.A.C., KCI, San Antonio, Texas) work quite well on smaller burns.
6. The graft is usually inspected at 5 to 7 days (3–5 days with V.A.C.), unless signs of infection prompt an earlier evaluation.
7. **Temporary coverage** of the excised burn wound with **cadaver skin, pigskin,** or synthetic materials such as **Biobrane** (Dew Hickam, Inc., Sugarland, Texas) and **Trancyte** (Advanced Tissue Sciences, La Jolla, California) may be helpful in the following clinical circumstances:
   a. Inadequate autologous donor skin
   b. Uncertainty of the viability of the wound bed (i.e., potential need for further excisions)
   c. Need to reduce hypermetabolism resulting from the open wound
   d. To provide patient comfort
8. **Dermal substitutes,** which allow for the creation of a "neodermis" populated with autologous mesenchymal cells and ground substance, are commonly used for larger burns. **Integra** (Integra LifeSciences, Plainsboro, New Jersey), **Alloderm** (Lifecell, Branchburg, New Jersey), and **Dermagraft** (Advanced Tissue Sciences, La Jolla, California) are currently available, with Integra being most widely used.
   a. Allow for excision and coverage of the entire burn irrespective of available donor sites (except Alloderm).

   b. Employ ultra-thin STSG (0.006–0.008 in), which allows for earlier rehar-vesting of potentially limited donor sites and subsequently earlier perma-nent coverage for a given burn.

   c. Require additional, staged operation(s), except for Alloderm that is designed to be immediately grafted on application.

   d. Successful use is associated with a learning curve.

   e. Apparent improvements in functional and cosmetic outcomes are achieved with Integra.

   9. Cultured epithelial autografts, although fragile and very expensive, have been used to provide permanent coverage in massive burns where no autologous alternatives are available.

D. Critical care

   1. Most critical care management parallels that of the trauma patient (Chapter 37).

   2. Intensive care unit (ICU) issues specific to the burn patient include:

   a. Prophylactic antibiotics are not indicated, except perioperatively.

   b. The presence of inhalation injury and face/neck burns require a more con-servative approach to weaning and extubation than with most trauma patients.

   c. In large burns (>25% TBSA), the analgesia requirements for twice-daily dressing changes and sequential operative excisions may be significant, but should never be unduly limited. **Burns are painful.**

   d. A **warm environment** is needed to prevent heat loss from wounds.

   e. The burn patient has a **very high metabolic rate** until the wounds are fully covered, requiring ~2,000 kcal/m^2/day with a protein requirement of ≥2.0 g/kg/day.

   f. Enteral nutrition is vastly superior to parenteral support in improving outcome.

   g. Fever is common in burn patients, but does not necessarily mean an infec-tion exists.

   h. Ionized hypocalcemia is common in burn patients, especially during the initial resuscitation.

   i. Patients with major burns commonly develop an inability to concentrate their urine and may have an obligatory increased urine output. This usually occurs in the postresuscitation, critical care phase of their injury and can be misinterpreted as a parameter of adequate perfusion.

E. Burn wound sepsis

   1. In general, significant bacterial colonization of the wound does not occur prior to 72 hours following injury. However, soon thereafter, colonization occurs with endogenous and endemic organisms.

   2. The most common organisms recovered from burn wounds include *Staphylococcus* sp., B-hemolytic streptococcus, *Pseudomonas aeruginosa*, *Escherichia coli*, *Enterococcus* sp., and *Candida albicans*.

   3. Invasive infection (vs. colonization) is solely diagnosed by a burn wound biopsy and quantitative bacteriology demonstrating >10^5 organisms/gram of tissue.

   a. Early burn wound sepsis (first week) is usually caused by *Staphylococcus aureus* (mortality ~5%).

   b. Later burn wound sepsis (7–10 days) is usually caused by *P. aeruginosa* (mortality ~20% to 30%).

   c. *Candida albicans* is another cause of later burn wound sepsis with a more insidious onset (mortality ~30% to 50%).

   4. The best **prevention and treatment** is the application of topical antibiotics combined with early excision and grafting of the wound. Prophylactic, sys-temic antibiotics are not effective because of the poor blood flow to the burn wound. However, targeted antimicrobial therapy is indicated for burn wound sepsis suspected by clinical examination and diagnosed by wound biopsy with quantitative culture. Burn wound sepsis also mandates immediate excision, or even reexcision, if the patient is unstable.

F. Rehabilitation

1. Rehabilitation of the burn patient is one of the most challenging clinical issues in modern medicine because the process is lifelong and the scars are permanent.
2. Rehabilitation should begin with admission and include the following components:
   a. Early wound closure
   b. Exercise
   c. Positioning and splinting
   d. Skin care
   e. Thermoregulation
   f. Psychological support
   g. Restoration of function
3. Chapter 49 discusses rehabilitation after trauma.

AXIOMS

- After initial resuscitation is started, burn patients meeting ABA criteria should be transferred to a dedicated burn center.
- Burns often present as spectacular injuries; therefore, it is imperative to perform primary and secondary surveys as per ATLS and ABLS to assess for concomitant nonthermal trauma.
- Patients sustaining burns in a closed space (e.g., building, car) should be considered to have an inhalation injury until proven otherwise.
- Early intubation should be considered for patients with orofacial burns or possible inhalation injury.
- Document the time of burn injury and the amount of fluid infused before arrival at a hospital or burn center.
- Formulas for fluid requirements are only guides to resuscitation; adequate urine output in a responsive, normotensive patient is the best clinical measure of adequate volume resuscitation.
- Patients with associated inhalation injuries or electrical injuries usually require more resuscitation fluid than those without.
- The initial calculation of TBSA, using the rule of nines, is designed to be an estimate of only partial- and full-thickness burns.
- Inhalation injury is the most frequent cause of death in burn victims.
- The severity of high-voltage electrical injuries is often underestimated.
- Definitive care of the deep partial- and full-thickness burn wound usually requires excision and grafting with STSG. Apply temporary coverage with nonautologous skin, synthetic materials, or dermal templates during the process of permanent coverage.

Bibliography

Holmes JH IV, Heimbach DM. Burns. In: Brunicardi CF, Andersen DK, Billiar TR, et al., eds. *Schwartz's Principles of Surgery*. 8th ed. New York, NY: McGraw-Hill; 2005.
Sheridan, RL. Burns. *Crit Care Med* 2002;30(suppl.):S500–S514.

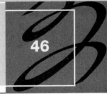

46

I. INCIDENCE
A. Trauma is the leading cause of mortality in children between the ages of 1 and 14 years in the United States; more children succumb to injuries and their sequelae than all other childhood diseases combined. Nearly 16,000,000 children visit emergency departments (EDs) for injuries each year. Of those, 15,000 die and 20,000 are temporarily disabled. The long-term disability is estimated to be more than three times the mortality rate, and is primarily the result of brain injury. As in adults, boys are more frequently injured than girls by a factor of 2:1.

II. MECHANISMS OF INJURY (Fig. 46-1)
A. Blunt trauma accounts for nearly 90% of pediatric injuries.
  1. Falls are the most frequent type of injury mechanism.
  2. Motor vehicle collisions are the most frequent cause of injury-related deaths.
B. Penetrating trauma accounts for less than 10% of pediatric injuries.

III. OVERVIEW: difference between children and adults
A. General body differences (Table 46-1)
B. Organ system differences

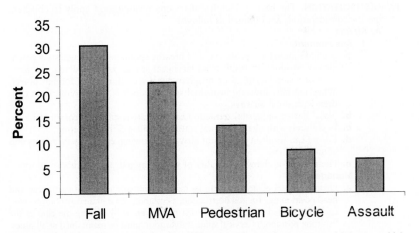

Figure 46-1. Distribution of the most common causes of pediatric trauma: fall, motor vehicle crash (MVC), pedestrian, bicycle-related, and assault as a percentage of all causes of pediatric trauma. Data supplied by the National Pediatric Trauma Registry, 1999.

TABLE 46-1	General Body Differences: Children Versus Adults

Factor	Difference
Size and shape	• Less fat and connective tissue available for protection. • Energy is transferred and dispersed over a smaller body surface area. • Internal organs are in relatively close proximity, which predisposes to multiple organ injuries. • Solid organs are larger compared with the rest of the abdomen. • Rib cage is higher, affording less protection to abdominal organs. • The infant's head is disproportionately larger compared with the adult and subjected to a high incidence of shear injuries.
Skeleton	• Incomplete ossification of bones causes them to be more pliable and thus less likely to fracture. As a result, pulmonary contusions and splenic lacerations often occur without rib fractures. • A different array of partial fractures (e.g., greenstick, torus, and buckle fractures). • Injuries to the growth plates during the various stages of childhood development result in a specific pattern of fractures.
Surface area	• Large surface-area-to-weight ratio results in a greater predisposition to heat loss (three times greater) and hypothermia.
Psychologic development	• Children often regress to a previous developmental stage during stressful and anxiety-provoking situations.
Long-term effects of injury	• Splenectomy in children places them at lifelong risk for overwhelming postsplenectomy infection (OPSI).

IV. RESUSCITATION. The basic principles of trauma resuscitation apply to children. Specific considerations are outlined as follows:

A. Airway

  1. Assessment

   a. A child's ability to speak, cry, and breathe spontaneously suggests a patent airway. Stridor can result from laryngeal spasm, airway edema, the presence of nasopharyngeal or oropharyngeal secretions, or a foreign object. Wheezing may indicate bronchial spasm, which is more common in children with small airways.

   b. Nasal flaring or sternal retraction can indicate respiratory compromise.

   c. In children with altered mental status, consider early intubation.

   d. Edema can result in significant airway narrowing, especially in infants and young children.

   e. Hoarseness or change in quality of voice may indicate an airway injury.

  2. Management

   a. Oropharyngeal obstruction can be managed initially with oral suctioning and head positioning. Tongue obstruction, a common cause of airway compromise, can be managed with the jaw thrust maneuver, or by placing the chin in the "sniffing position." Cervical spine stabilization must be maintained at all times.

   b. In most cases, bag-valve-mask (BVM) ventilation provides adequate oxygenation and ventilation for pediatric patients. Keep the neck in the neutral position to optimize airway diameter. Maintain cervical spine precautions at all times.

TABLE 46-2	Recommended Length of Insertion, Endotracheal Tube Size, and Blade Size		

Weight (kg)	Distance (cm) midtrachea to lip	Endotracheal tube (uncuffed)	Laryngoscope blade
Preemie (1–2)	8	2.5–3.0	0 straight
Newborn (3.5)	8.0–9.5	3.0–3.5	1 straight
6 mo (7)	9.5–11.0	3.5–4.0	1 straight
1 y (10)	11.0–12.5	4.0–4.5	2 straight
3 y (15)	12.5–14.0	4.5–5.0	2 straight
6 y (20)	14.0–15.5	5.0–5.5	2 straight
8 y (25)	17.0–18.5	6.0–6.5	2 straight/curved
10 y (30)	18.5–20.0	6.5–7.0	3 straight/curved
12 y (40)	20	7.0 (cuff)	3 straight/curved
15 y (50)	20.0–21.5	7.0–7.5 (cuff)	3 straight/curved
18 y (65)	20–23	7.0–8.0 (cuff)	3 straight/curved

(From the Children's Hospital of Pittsburgh, Benedum Pediatric Trauma Program, Pediatric Field Reference, October 2003, with permission.)

    c. Patients with compromised airway who do not respond to conservative measures (refer to the preceding a or b) or patients with severe head injury (Glasgow Coma Scale [GCS] score <8) require orotracheal intubation after adequate preoxygenation with BVM ventilation and cervical spine immobilization. This often requires two practitioners: one to secure the airway and a second to control the neck.

  3. Considerations during orotracheal intubation

    a. Preoxygenate, but do not hyperventilate.

    b. The larynx is more anterior and sits higher in the neck at the level of the third cervical vertebra.

    c. The epiglottis is omega shaped.

    d. The trachea is short, therefore right mainstem intubation occurs more frequently than in adults (Table 46-2).

    e. Right mainstem intubation is poorly tolerated in children, resulting in poor oxygenation and ventilation and potentially significant baro trauma.

  4. Nasotracheal intubation is **not** recommended because of the sharp angle between the nasopharynx and the oropharynx and the small diameter of endotracheal tube that can be placed through the child's nares.

  5. A surgical airway, which is rarely indicated, is associated with high complication rate, especially in younger children (<8 years). In older children (>12 years), options include surgical cricothyroidotomy or translaryngeal jet (needle) ventilation. **Remember, BVM ventilation is effective and, in most cases, allows sufficient time to perform tracheostomy under controlled conditions in the operating room (OR).**

  6. Pharmacologic management during endotracheal intubation (Fig. 46-2).

  7. Position of the endotracheal tube should be reassessed with each change in patient position, transfer, or if there are new ventilator alarms.

B. Breathing

  1. Auscultate in axillary area to reduce noise from opposite chest.

  2. Check for symmetric chest wall rise with every breath.

  3. Respiratory rate (RR) and tidal volume (TV) vary with age and weight (Table 46-3).

  4. Increased lung compliance permits easy lung expansion and ventilation. Therefore, vigorous assisted ventilation with large tidal volume can cause barotrauma, leading to bronchial rupture.

  5. Hypoventilation and hypoxia are common causes of cardiorespiratory arrest in pediatric trauma patients.

TABLE 46-3	Age-specific Vital Signs				
Age (y)	Weight (kg)	Pulse per min	Systolic blood pressure (mmHg)	Respiratory rate	Tidal volume (mL)
Newborn	3	160	70	60	240
1	9	130	85	40	700
3	15	120	89	30	1,200
6	24	110	94	25	2,000
10	35	90	100	20	2,800
Adults	75	70	120	15–20	5,000

(From the Children's Hospital of Pittsburgh, Benedum Pediatric Trauma Program, Pediatric Field Reference, October 1997, with permission.)

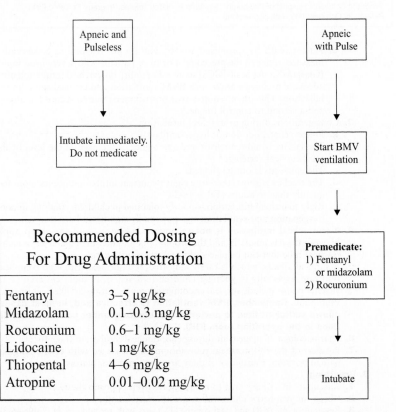

(continued)

Figure 46-2. Protocol for airway management for (**A**) apneic patients and (**B**) those breathing spontaneously with or without associated head trauma. Insert contains current recommendations for appropriate medication doses.

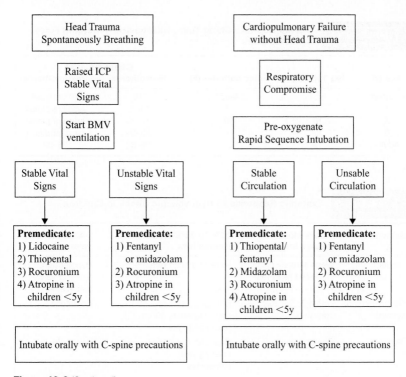

Figure 46-2 (Continued)

6. Inability to ventilate both lung fields after endotracheal intubation should raise concern about right mainstem intubation or pneumothorax. Assessment of endotracheal tube position and early chest x-ray study are recommended.
7. If tension pneumothorax is suspected, perform immediate needle decompression (Section V.C) followed by chest tube insertion. If hemothorax or pneumothorax is found on chest x-ray, insert chest tube (Table 46-4).

C. Circulation
1. Vital signs are age related and the response to shock differs in children (Table 46-5).
2. Elevated heart rate (HR) is the most important early indicator of hypovolemic shock in pediatric trauma patients.
3. Blood pressure is an inadequate measure of volume status or resuscitation endpoint. Children can maintain their blood pressure until significant volume loss ($\geq$45% of blood volume) has occurred. Stroke volume is relatively fixed in infants and young children and depends on venous return. Therefore, the response to hypovolemia is to increase HR to maintain blood pressure. Hypotension reflects loss of >45% of blood volume or failure of adaptive mechanisms. Bradycardia is an ominous sign of impending cardiovascular collapse.
4. Fluid resuscitation
   a. Blood volume is estimated at 80 mL/kg. Consider hypovolemic shock if:
      i. Heart rate is >10% of value calculated for age.
      ii. Blood pressure is <5th percentile ($70 + 2 \times$ age in years).

TABLE 46-4	Age-appropriate Chest Tube, Nasogastric Tube, and Foley Catheter Sizes

Age (y)	NG Tube (F)	Foley catheter (F)	Chest tube (F) Hemothorax	Chest tube (F) Pneumothorax
Newborn	5	5 feeding	10	10 or pigtail
1	10	8	10–12	small or pigtail
3	10	10	16–20	small or pigtail
6	12	10	20–24	small or pigtail
Adults	16	16	28–32	28–32

TABLE 46-5	Systemic Response to Hypovolemic Shock in Children

System	<25% blood volume loss	25% to 45% blood volume loss	>45% blood volume loss
Cardiac	Weak, thready pulse; increased heart rate	Increased heart rate	Hypotension, tachycardia to bradycardia
Central nervous system	Lethargic, irritable, confused	Change in level of consciousness, dulled response to pain	Comatose
Skin	Cool, clammy	Cyanotic, decreased capillary refill, cold extremities	Pale, cold
Kidneys	Minimal decrease in urinary output, increased specific gravity	Minimal urine output	No urinary output

    iii. Evidence of poor end-organ perfusion such as decreased capillary refill, mental status changes, and low urinary output.

    b. Begin fluid resuscitation with 20 mL/kg of Ringer's lactate, which can be repeated twice. If no improvement, transfuse O negative packed red blood cells (PRBCs) (10 mL/kg) and examine the patient for a source of ongoing bleeding.

    c. Basic fluid requirements (maintenance IVF) can be calculated using the following approaches:

        i. 100 mL/kg/day for the first 10 kg, plus 50 mL/kg/day for the next 5 kg, plus 20 mL/kg/day for each kg over 16 kg.

        ii. 4 mL/kg/hour for the first 10 kg; between 10 kg and 20 kg, 40 mL/hour plus 2 mL/kg/hour for every kilogram over 10; >20 kg, 60 mL/hour plus 1 mL/kg/hour for every kilogram over 20.

    d. The resuscitation fluid of choice is Ringer's lactate or normal saline. Dextrose-containing solutions are not indicated during the resuscitation period because of hyperglycemia from the elevated catecholamine response of stress response to injury.

    e. In infants, careful monitoring of blood glucose is essential as these patients have limited glycogen stores and can become profoundly hypoglycemic.

5. Intravenous access (IV)

    a. Place largest size IV possible, one on each side of the patient, in upper or lower extremities.

b. In the hypotensive child with difficult IV access, insert an intraosseous (IO) line before venous cutdown to initiate fluid resuscitation. The IO can be used for all resuscitative fluids and medications.

i. Place the IO line 1 cm inferior and medial to the tibial tuberosity.

ii. For children 0 to 1 year of age, use an 18- to 20-gauge spinal needle. A 13- to 16-gauge bone marrow needle is required for children >1 year of age.

iii. Contraindications include fracture in the same leg, pelvic fractures, or a conscious child.

iv. Remove the IO line within 4 hours to decrease risk of osteomyelitis.

c. If necessary, the preferred venous cutdown sites include:

i. Greater saphenous vein anterior to the medial malleolus at the ankle, or proximal thigh below junction with femoral vein

ii. Basilic and cephalic veins of the antecubital fossa

D. Disability: neurologic evaluation

1. Quick assessment

a. GCS score modified for pediatric patients (Table 46-6).

2. Goal is to minimize secondary brain injury. Secondary injuries can be prevented by maximizing cerebral perfusion pressure (mean arterial pressure [MAP] – intracranial pressure [ICP]) by adhering to basic principles of resuscitation. **Avoid the following:**

a. Hypoxemia: keep oxygen saturation >98%.

b. Hypercapnia or hypocapnia: maintain $PaCO_2$ between 32 and 35 mmHg.

c. Hypotension: maintain blood pressure around 50th percentile for age; $80 + 2 \times$ age in years.

3. Early uncontrasted CT scan of the head is critical to the diagnosis of surgically correctable lesions and obtaining prognostic information.

TABLE 46-6   **Glasgow Coma Scale Score**

Infant	Child
Eye opening	**Eye opening**
4 Spontaneously	4 Spontaneously
3 To speech	3 To command
2 To pain	2 To pain
1 No response	1 No response
Best verbal response	**Best verbal response**
5 Coos, babbles, smiles	5 Oriented
4 Irritable, crying	4 Confused
3 Cries, screams to pain	3 Inappropriate words
2 Moans, grunts	2 Incomprehensible
1 No response	1 No response
Best motor response	**Best motor response**
6 Spontaneously	6 Spontaneously
5 Withdraws from touch	5 Withdraws from touch
4 Withdraws from pain	4 Withdraws from pain
3 Flexion (decorticate)	3 Flexion (decorticate)
2 Extension (decerebrate)	2 Extension (decerebrate)
1 No response	1 No response

(From the Children's Hospital of Pittsburgh, Benedum Pediatric Trauma Program, Pediatric Field Reference, October 1997, with permission.)

4. Manifestation of head injuries in children
   a. Seizures. Use a short-acting benzodiazepine. Posttraumatic seizures are usually brief and treatment with anticonvulsants is unnecessary.
   b. Vomiting. Treat symptomatically, ensuring that significant intraabdominal injury has not occurred. During periods of emesis, maintain cervical spine precautions and avoid aspiration of vomitus.
5. Indications for ICP monitoring in the child with closed head injury:
   a. GCS <8
   b. Inability to monitor clinical examination (i.e., the patient requires general anesthesia for the treatment of other injuries)
E. Exposure. Infants and children are at significant risk for hypothermia secondary to their high body surface area.

V. SECONDARY SURVEY AND MANAGEMENT
A. Head
1. 75% of pediatric deaths due to trauma result from head injury.
2. Computed tomography (CT) is the most sensitive and specific modality to evaluate children with suspected head injury. Children with an altered mental status, or loss of consciousness, posttraumatic seizures, or emesis require an uncontrasted CT of the head. No role exists for skull films.
3. Scalp lacerations can cause significant blood loss, especially in a child. Examine lacerations for underlying skull fractures.
4. The fontanelle and sutures are open in children <18 months of age.
5. Intracranial lesions
   a. Diffuse are more common in children than adults.
      i. Concussion
      ii. Diffuse axonal injury
   b. Localized
      i. Epidural hematomas are more prevalent in children than subdural hematomas.
      ii. Intracranial hematomas can be managed nonoperatively when focal defects are absent and the child is awake and oriented. Operative intervention is required for expanding lesions or those that cause a mass effect or produce neurologic deficits.
      iii. Blood loss can be substantial with an intracranial hemorrhage in infants, and may necessitate blood transfusion. In older children, signs of continued blood loss require a thorough evaluation for other sites of bleeding.
      iv. Temporal bone fractures are in close proximity to the middle meningeal artery, which accounts for a high proportion of epidural bleeds with this fracture.
   c. Skull fractures
      i. Linear, complex, depressed
      ii. Skull fractures are relatively common, with most occurring in the parietal bone. A 10-fold increased risk of intracranial hematoma exists when a skull fracture is present.
      iii. Operative intervention is required in cases of an overlying scalp laceration; underlying intracranial lesion, which requires surgery; or depression greater than the thickness of the skull.
   d. Nonaccidental injury. A high index of suspicion regarding the possibility of head trauma must be maintained in infants with unexplained vomiting, excitability, or other injuries with an unclear etiology.
   e. Controversy exists regarding the long-term consequence of head injuries in children. In general, outcomes in pediatric patients are better than in adults.
B. Neck
1. Major anatomic differences in children
   a. Shorter neck with a proportionately heavy head promoting flexion of the neck

  b. Laxity of the ligaments and decreased muscle support
  c. Anterior wedging of the vertebral bodies
  d. Horizontally oriented facet joints of C1 to C4
  2. Cervical spine injuries
   a. **Cervical spine fractures.** Most (>85%) cervical spine fractures in children <8 years occur between C1 and C3. In children >10 years of age, the cervical spine is similar to, and the pattern of injury resembles, that seen in adults (C4–C7).
   b. **Pseudosubluxation** of C3 on C2 occurs in 40% of children <7 years as a normal variant.
   c. **Subluxations** occur in ~10% to 20% of cervical spine injuries alone or in conjunction with associated fractures.
   d. **Spinal cord injury without radiological abnormality (SCIWORA)** occurs predominantly in children and is responsible for 4% to 21% of cervical spine injuries. Transient or permanent neurologic defects occur without any radiologic abnormality on conventional imaging. MRI evaluation of the spine may demonstrate a cord contusion.
   e. **Altantoocciptal dislocation** (AOD) is the separation of the cranium from the cervical spinal column producing proximal spinal cord injury. This injury results predominately from the laxity of the transverse ligament in children. Mortality is nearly 100%.
   f. History of immediate arrest at the scene of the injury is highly suggestive of a high cervical spine injury.
 C. Chest injuries (85% blunt; 15% penetrating)
  1. Immediate life-threatening injuries
   a. **Tension pneumothorax.** Air trapped under pressure in the pleural space shifts the relatively mobile mediastinum in children to the opposite side of the chest, obstructing venous blood return to the heart.
    i. Midaxillary line (MAL) is the optimal place for needle decompression in infants and small children. Insertion via the second interspace, midclavicular line can injure the pulmonary artery.
    ii. For infants and young children, an 18- or 20-gauge needle is recommended for decompression.
   b. **Cardiac tamponade.** Treatment is similar to that for adults.
   c. **Hemothorax.** Initial drainage >20% of blood volume or continued bleeding of 1 to 2 mL/kg/hour are indications for thoracotomy.
   d. **Tracheobronchial injuries** are more common in children than in adults.
    i. Most laryngeal injuries occur at or above the fourth tracheal ring.
    ii. After securing the airway, early operative exploration and repair is indicated.
   e. **Penetrating injuries** to the chest are managed in similar manner as in adults.
    i. Children sustain many chest injuries by air-powered rifles (BB or pellet guns).
    ii. These potentially lethal injuries warrant a high index of suspicion, with 33% to 50% of patients requiring operative intervention.
  2. Potentially life-threatening injuries
   a. **Pneumothorax.** Air trapped in the pleural space.
    i. Requires urgent chest tube decompression.
    ii. Place all chest tubes laterally in the MAL.
    iii. Enter the pleural cavity with a hemostat, not a trocar, to avoid damage to the lung.
   b. **Rib fractures** are uncommon and indicate severe injury.
    i. Rib fractures represent significant transmission of energy and are associated with a 10% mortality rate from concomitant injuries.
    ii. Rib fractures are related to child abuse in 20% of the cases.
   c. **Pulmonary contusion**
    i. Pulmonary contusion is the most common injury to the chest.
    ii. Responds to conservative management with aggressive pulmonary physiotherapy and oxygenation.

iii. Fewer than 5% of all children with pulmonary contusion require intubation (Chapter 24).

d. Traumatic asphyxia

i. Sudden compression of the abdomen or chest against a closed glottis.

ii. A sudden increase in intrathoracic pressure that is transmitted to the superior vena cava.

iii. Seizures, mental status change, and respiratory failure may ensue and petechiae develop in the face.

e. Cardiac contusion

i. Cardiac contusion does not produce arrhythmias as in adults; however, cardiac monitoring is appropriate for 24 hours.

ii. Echocardiography may be helpful to define wall motion abnormalities.

D. Abdomen

1. Up to 60% of children with intraabdominal injuries have concomitant head injury.

2. Gastric distension from swallowing air during the act of crying is the most common cause of abdominal distension. If severe, abdominal distension can interfere with respiratory effort. In such cases, nasogastric decompression is indicated.

3. Upper abdominal organs are susceptible to injury from minimal forces because of the lack of protection from underdeveloped rib cage and musculature.

4. Evaluation

a. Inspect and palpate. Abdominal wall contusions, such as those from a seat belt, correlate with the presence of intraabdominal injuries.

b. Radiographic studies

i. CT with IV and enteral contrast is the most sensitive study to evaluate for the presence of intraabdominal injuries.

ii. The role of focused abdominal sonography for trauma (FAST) is still evolving in pediatric trauma and has not replaced contrasted CT for evaluation of blunt abdominal trauma in children. Hemoperitoneum is often not present with solid organ injury in children.

c. Laboratory tests

i. Amylase or lipase

ii. Aspartate aminotransferase (AST) and alanine aminotransferase (ALT). Elevations correlate with general intraabdominal injury as well as specific liver injury.

iii. Hemoglobin and hematocrit. Type and crossmatch or type and screen.

iv. Urinalysis greater than 50 RBCs per high power field correlates with intraabdominal injury.

v. Prothrombin time (PT) or partial thromboplastin time (PTT) in patients with suspected head injury

5. Specific injuries (Chapter 26)

a. Spleen

i. The most frequently injured abdominal organ in children (40%).

ii. Patients present with abdominal or shoulder pain (Kehr's sign) or shortness of breath.

iii. Of patients, 30% to 40% will have associated abdominal injuries, but **the vast majority of these do not require operative intervention**.

iv. Contrasted CT scan is 98% sensitive and the modality of choice for diagnosis.

v. Most pediatric patients are hemodynamically stable on presentation; 95% can be managed nonoperatively, most without blood transfusion.

vi. Hemodynamic instability, clinical deterioration, or associated hollow viscus or diaphragmatic injury mandates operation.

a) Fewer than 5% to 10% of patients will require blood transfusion.

vii. Overwhelming postsplenectomy infection (OPSI)

a) Lifetime risk is 0.026%.

b) Mortality rate for those who develop OPSI is 50%.

c) Prophylaxis with penicillin until the age of 18 years (controversial).

d) Vaccination against pneumococcus, *Haemophilus influenza*, and meningococcus.

viii. Long-term management

a) Repeat radiologic studies are not necessary.

b) Children may resume normal activity after a period of time that consists of CT grade plus 2 weeks. Return to contact sports may require a longer period of restriction.

b. Liver

i. Injuries to the liver are common (15% to 30%) and require operative repair more often than splenic injuries in children.

ii. Of patients, 10% will arrive in shock; 30% of children will have associated injuries.

iii. Most injuries (60% to 80%) occur in the right lobe.

iv. Indications for operative intervention are similar to splenic injuries.

a) Management in children is similar to adults, with major liver resection used sparingly.

b) Angiography and embolization of actively bleeding vessels may have a role in the management of children with these injuries if the appropriate expertise is available and the child is hemodynamically stable enough to tolerate the procedure.

v. Indications for "return to play" are similar to those for children with splenic injuries.

c. Intestinal injuries

i. Injuries occur at points of fixation of intestines with the jejunum, terminal ileum, and descending and sigmoid colon being most commonly injured.

ii. Seat-belt complex consists of abdominal wall ecchymosis above the anterior iliac spine and intestinal injury, and is associated with a transverse fracture of the lumbar vertebral body (Chance fracture).

a) Rapid deceleration results in flexion of the upper body around the seat belt, compression of the abdominal viscera, and a sudden increase in intraluminal pressure.

iii. Only 60% of radiographic studies will be diagnostic; delayed diagnosis occurs in 10% of cases. In patients with the appropriate mechanism and exam, the presence of free fluid in the absence of solid organ injury on CT scan is highly suggestive of an intestinal injury.

iv. A high index of suspicion must be maintained for the presence of these lesions.

v. Laparoscopic exploration may be beneficial in providing earlier diagnosis in equivocal cases and is less morbid than formal laparotomy.

d. Pancreas

i. Represents 1% to 3% of all blunt abdominal injuries in children; epigastric pain is the most common symptom.

ii. The classic mechanism for pancreatic injury involves blunt force to the abdomen from the handlebar of a bicycle.

iii. Pancreatic injuries include duct transection and contusion.

a) Pancreatic contusions can be treated nonoperatively.

b) Early operative intervention of major ductal injuries results in shorter hospitalization, earlier return to enteral feeding, and fewer complications than nonoperative management. Distal pancreatectomy with splenic preservation is the preferred operative technique.

iv. Differentiation between transection and contusion can be difficult.

a) Serum amylase <200 U/mL and lipase <1,800 U/mL combined with the physical examination (epigastric or abdominal tenderness) correlate with pancreatic transection or major ductal injury.

b) CT with IV contrast evaluation: 72% sensitive and 99% specific.

e. Duodenum
  i. Although uncommon, duodenal injuries are associated with serious complications.
  ii. Of duodenal injuries, 20% are related to child abuse. This number may be even higher in children <4 years of age.
  iii. Mortality (6% to 25%) and morbidity (33% to 60%) resulting from duodenal perforation is directly related to time of diagnosis and definitive treatment; **mortality increases fourfold when diagnosis is delayed by 24 hours**.
    a) Abdominal pain is the most common symptom (80% to 100%), followed by bilious vomiting (80%).
    b) CT is diagnostic in only 60% of the cases: extravasation of contrast or retroperitoneal air behind the duodenum and right colon are definitive findings.
    c) Upper GI can be helpful in evaluating for a duodenal hematoma.
  iv. Duodenal hematoma. Extrinsic compression of the lumen by a hematoma in the bowel wall causes partial or complete obstruction of the duodenum.
    a) Most will resolve with conservative treatment, including nasogastric tube decompression and hyperalimentation.
    b) Duodenal obstruction from hematoma can take 3 weeks to resolve. Failure to resolve can require operative evacuation.

E. Pelvic fractures
  1. Of children with pelvic fractures, 20% also sustain abdominal injuries. Unless displaced, these fractures are treated nonoperatively.
  2. Associated urethral injuries are rare.
  3. Hemodynamic instability resulting from a pelvic fracture is unusual in children.

F. Genitourinary (GU) tract injury (Chapter 30)
  1. The GU tract is injured in 10% of pediatric trauma patients; 98% from blunt trauma (85% from MVC).
  2. The degree of hematuria does not correlate with the severity of injury to the GU tract. Conversely, a normal urinalysis does not preclude the possibility of a GU tract injury.
  a. Renal injuries. Kidneys are relatively larger in children and assume a lower position in the abdomen.
    i. Renal injuries occur more frequently in children than in adults. The renal capsule (Gerota's fascia) is less developed in children than in adults.
    ii. Children typically present with abdominal pain and either microscopic or gross hematuria.
    iii. CT of the abdomen with IV contrast and delayed images is highly specific and sensitive. An angiogram is unnecessary in most cases.
    iv. Fewer than 5% of children with renal injuries require operative repair.
    v. Hypertension can develop 6 months to 15 years after injury to the renovascular pedicle; blood pressure must be monitored regularly following major renal injury.
    vi. Microscopic hematuria in a child after trauma that does not resolve warrants further investigation for possible congenital or neoplastic abnormalities of the urinary system.
  b. Bladder. The narrow and small pelvis of a child allows the bladder to assume an intraabdominal location.
    i. The dome of the bladder is mobile and distensible.
    ii. Of bladder injuries, 50% are associated with other abdominal injuries and 75% to 95% are associated with pelvic fractures.
    iii. Bladder size varies with age
      a) Children <2 years: bladder volume = 7 mL/kg.
      b) Children between the ages of 2 and 11 years: bladder volume = 2 (age in years) × 30 mL.

    c. Straddle injury. Compression of the soft tissue of the perineum against the bony pelvis in girls.

       i. Injuries are sustained from falls, bicycle-related crashes, and activities associated with playground equipment.

       ii. Patients present with a history of bleeding from the perineum (50%).

       iii. Examine under anesthesia with visualization of the vaginal vault.

       iv. Missed injuries can lead to late complications, including urethral and vaginal strictures.

G. Musculoskeletal injury

    1. Specific injuries in children

       a. Epiphyseal fractures

       b. Shaft fractures

       c. Dislocations

    2. Complications common after musculoskeletal injury in children

       a. Early ischemia

       b. Growth disturbances

       c. Vascular necrosis

       d. Joint instability

    3. Treatment

       a. Traction and splinting

       b. Reestablished circulation before fracture stabilization.

VI. BURNS (CHAPTER 45)

A. Burns resulting from house fires are the leading cause of accidental death in the home for children <14 years.

B. Of burned children, 20% are victims of abuse.

    1. Most burn injuries occur in children <4 years.

    2. Scald burns are the most common form of burn injury.

C. Ringer's lactate is the fluid of choice in the first 24 hours, with the quantity guided by the Parkland/Baxter formula:

    1. Resuscitate all patients with burns >15% to 20% body surface area (BSA) using the Parkland/Baxter formula as a guideline (Table 46-7).

    2. Estimated amount of fluid in first 24 hours = 4 mL × %BSA burn × wt (kg).

D. Fluids during the second 24 hours

    1. Compensates for evaporative loss and maintenance.

    2. Add colloid and D5-1/4 NS; prevent **hyponatremia** and **hypoglycemia**.

    3. The amount of albumin required can be calculated by the formula: 0.3 mL/kg of a 5% albumin solution for burns with a BSA of 30% to 50%.

TABLE 46-7	**Pediatric Burn Rule of Nines**				
			Age (y)		
	0	**1**	**5**	**10**	**Adult**
Head	19	17	13	11	7
Neck	2	2	2	2	2
Anterior trunk	13	13	13	13	13
Posterior trunk	13	13	13	13	13
Buttocks	2.5	2.5	2.5	2.5	2.5
Genitalia	1	1	1	1	1
Upper arm	2.5	2.5	2.5	2.5	2.5
Lower arm	3	3	3	3	3
Hand	2.5	2.5	2.5	2.5	2.5
Thigh	5.5	6.5	8	8.5	9.5
Leg	5	5	5.5	6	7
Foot	3.5	3.5	3.5	3.5	3.5

VII. CHILD ABUSE AND NONACCIDENTAL TRAUMA
   A. Legality
      1. Any professional is required to report suspected child abuse to civil authorities.
      2. This requirement supersedes doctor–patient relationships, carries penalties for failure to report, and provides immunity if reported in good faith.
      3. Abuse can consist of neglect, physical abuse, sexual abuse, or emotional abuse.
      4. Abuse occurs in all levels of society.
   B. Incidence
      1. Annually, 1 to 1.5 million children are abused; 60,000 with serious or life-threatening injuries; 1,000 to 2,000 die (usually <5 years of age).
      2. One of every 10 children treated in the emergency department for injury has sustained intentional injury.
   C. History
      1. Evasive parent or caregiver
      2. Changing story of the event
      3. Unwitnessed injury in young child
      4. Delay in seeking care for the child, often several hours or days
      5. Child endowed with physical powers beyond chronologic or physical development
      6. History of the incident and degree of injury do not agree
      7. Multiple ED or physician visits
   D. Patterns of injury associated with physical abuse
      1. Soft-tissue injuries: comprise most injuries.
         a. Bruising on normally nonbruised areas (behind the ear) or in various stages of healing
         b. Marks of objects (e.g., cigarettes, belt buckles, whips, fingers)
         c. Traumatic hair loss
      2. Musculoskeletal: second most common system affected.
         a. Spiral fractures attributed to a "fall"
         b. Subperiosteal calcification with no history of injury
         c. Multiple fractures in various stages of healing
         d. "Bucket-handle" or epiphyseal-metaphyseal separation from shaking or jerking
         e. Rib fractures in young children
      3. Intracranial: third most commonly injured area, but most common cause of death.
         a. Chronic or bilateral subdural hematoma
         b. "Shaken baby syndrome." Repetitive blunt force trauma to the head. Associated with cerebral edema, subdural hematomas (various ages), and retinal hemorrhages. Prognosis is poor.
      4. Visceral injuries: fourth most common area injured. Duodenal injuries in young children are often the result of physical abuse.
      5. Evaluation
         a. CT of head and abdomen, skeletal survey, optical examination for those <3 years of age, and laboratory studies (blood count, liver function, amylase, and lipase)

VIII. PEDIATRIC SCORING
   A. (PTS) (Table 46-8)
      1. The most common scoring system applied to pediatric trauma patients is the PTS.
      2. The PTS is an index used to predict outcome. It is based on anatomic and physiologic parameters and injuries sustained. Values are assigned to six components and range from −2 to +2. A combined score of ≤8 is associated with a poor outcome.
   B. Age-Specific Pediatric Trauma Score (Table 46-9)
      1. Current scoring systems used in pediatric trauma are not age specific.
      2. The Age-Specific Pediatric Trauma Score (ASPTS) incorporates age-specific values for systolic blood pressure, pulse, and respiratory rate in addition to the GCS.
      3. Values are assigned from 0 to 3 for each parameter.
   C. Other common scoring systems include the Injury Severity Score (ISS) and the Abbreviated Injury Score (AIS), both of which also correlate injury with outcome.

TABLE 46-8 Pediatric Trauma Score

Component	+2	+1	−1
Airway	Normal	Maintainable	Cannot be maintained
Central nervous system	Awake	Obtunded	Comatose
Weight	>20 kg	10–20 kg	<10 kg
Systolic blood pressure	>90 mmHg	50–90 mmHg	<50 mmHg
Open wounds	None	Minor	Major or penetrating
Fractures	None	Closed	Opened or multiple

(From the Children's Hospital of Pittsburgh, Benedum Pediatric Trauma Program, Pediatric Field Reference, October 1997, with permission.)

TABLE 46-9 Age-Specific Pediatric Trauma Score (ASPTS)

GCS	Systolic blood pressure (SBP)	Pulse	Respiratory rate (RR)	Coded score
14–15	Normal	Normal	Normal	3
10–13	Mild-moderate hypotension (SBP <Mean − 3 SD)	Tachycardia (Pulse >Mean − SD)	Tachypnea (RR >Mean + SD)	2
4–9	Severe hypotension (SBP <Mean − 3 SD)	Bradycardia (Pulse >Mean − SD)	Hypoventilation (RR >Mean − SD)	1
3	0	0	0 or intubated	0

Age-specific variables (SBP, pulse, and RR) and GCS were stratified by degree of severity, and coded values (0–3) were assigned to each variable. The ASPTS is the sum total of coded values for all four variables.

GCS, Glasgow Coma Scale score; SD, standard deviation.

Bibliography

Black TL, Snyder CL, Miller JP, et al. Significance of chest trauma in children. *South Med J* 1996;89(5):494–496.

Feliz A, Shultz B, McKenna C, Gaines BA. Diagnostic and therapeutic laparoscopy in pediatric abdominal trauma. *J Pediatr Surg* 2006;41(1):72–77.

Gaines BA, Ford HR. Abdominal and pelvic trauma in children. *Crit Care Med* 2002;30(11):S416–S423.

Gaines BA, Shultz BL, Morrison K, Ford HR. Duodenal injuries in children: Beware of child abuse. *J Pediatr Surg* 2004;39(4);600–602.

Kurkchubasche AG, Fendya DG, Tracy TF Jr., et al. Blunt intestinal injury in children: Diagnostic and therapeutic considerations. *Arch Surg* 1997;132(6):652–658.

Luerssen TG, Klauber MR, Marshall LF. Outcome from head injury related to patient's age: A longitudinal prospective study of adult and pediatric head injury. *J Neurosurg* 1988;68:409.

Mutabagani KH, Coley BD, Zumberge N, et al. Preliminary experience with focused abdominal sonography for trauma (FAST) in children: Is it useful? *J Pediatr Surg* 1999;34:48–52.

Nadler EP, Gardner M, Schall LC, et al. Management of blunt pancreatic injury in children. *J Trauma* 1999;47(6):1098–1103.

Nance ML, Lutz N, Carr MC, et al. Blunt renal injuries in children can be managed non-operatively: Outcome in a consecutive series of patients. *J Trauma* 2004;57(3):474–478; discussion 478.

Potoka DA, Schall LC, Ford HR. Development of a novel Age-Specific Pediatric Trauma Score. *J Pediatr Surg* 2001;36:106–112.

Sarihan H, Abes M, Akyazici R, et al. Traumatic asphyxia in children. *J Cardiovasc Surg* 1997;38:93–95.

Stylianos S. Compliance with evidence-based guidelines in children with isolated spleen or liver injury: A prospective study. *J Pediatr Surg* 2002;37(3):453–456.

Stylianos S. Evidence-based guidelines for resource utilization in children with isolated spleen or liver injury. The APSA Trauma Committee. *J Pediatr Surg* 2000;35:164.

Tso EL, Beaver BL, Haller A. Abdominal injuries in restrained pediatric passengers. *J Pediatr Surg* 1993;28(7):915–919.

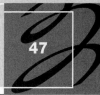

CARE OF THE PREGNANT TRAUMA PATIENT

GLEN TINKOFF

47

I. **INTRODUCTION.** Injury occurs in 6% to 7% of all pregnancies and is the leading nonobstetric cause of maternal death. Furthermore, maternal compromise and injury severity are the principal factors in trauma-related fetal demise. Accordingly, optimal early management of the pregnant trauma victim yields the best possible outcome for the fetus; thus the tenet "**save the mother, save the fetus**." Although initial treatment priorities remain the same, anatomic and physiologic changes that accompany pregnancy are important modifiers of trauma care in all settings.

II. **ANATOMIC CHANGES AND POTENTIAL CLINICAL CONSEQUENCES**
   A. Uterus
      1. Increased size (7 cm/70 g → 36 cm/1,100 g)
      2. Intraabdominal location after 12th week (Fig. 47-1)

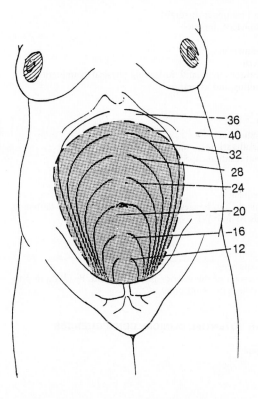

Figure 47-1. Uterine size. (From Knudson MM. Trauma in pregnancy. In: Blaisdell FW, Trunkey DD, eds. *Trauma Management—Abdominal Trauma.* 2nd ed. New York, NY: Thieme Medical Publishers; 1993: 326, with permission.)

515

3. Thinning of muscular wall
4. Increased blood flow (60 mL/minute → 600 mL/minute)
5. Potential clinical consequences
    a. Increased susceptibility to injury
    b. Increased bleeding
    c. Compression of inferior vena cava in supine position (supine hypotension syndrome)
B. Placenta
    1. Lack of elasticity
    2. Catecholamine sensitivity
    3. Potential clinical consequences
        a. Prone to separation from uterus wall (abruption)
        b. Decreased placental blood flow, with stress leading to fetal compromise
C. Pelvis
    1. Venous engorgement
    2. Ligamentous relaxation
    3. Potential clinical consequences
        a. Increased severity of hemorrhage
        b. Gait instability and increased risk of falls
        c. Altered radiologic appearance and misdiagnosis
D. Genitourinary
    1. Dilated collecting system
    2. Displaced bladder → intraabdominal
    3. Potential clinical consequences
        a. Altered radiologic appearance and misdiagnosis
        b. Increased risk for injury
E. Gastrointestinal
    1. Intestinal displacement into upper quadrant
    2. Alteration in gastroesophageal junction
    3. Peritoneal "stretching"
    4. Potential clinical consequences
        a. Altered injury pattern
        b. Decreased peritoneal sensitivity and misleading physical examination
        c. Increased risk for reflux and aspiration
F. Diaphragm
    1. Elevated (4 cm)
    2. Increased excursion (1–2 cm)
    3. Potential clinical consequences
        a. Altered anatomic landmark (e.g., misplaced chest tube)
        b. Decreased functional residual capacity (FRC)
G. Heart
    1. Displaced cephalad
    2. Potential clinical consequences
        a. Electrocardiographic (ECG) changes—left axis deviation; T-wave flattening, or inversion in leads III and AVF
H. Pituitary
    1. Enlarged by 135%
    2. Increased blood flow demands
    3. Potential clinical consequences
        a. Shock can cause necrosis of the interior pituitary gland, resulting in pituitary insufficiency (Sheehan's syndrome).

III. PHYSIOLOGIC CHANGES OR POTENTIAL CLINICAL CONSEQUENCES
A. Cardiovascular
    1. Increased cardiac output
    2. Increased heart rate

3. Increased blood pressure (second trimester)
4. Decreased central venous pressure
5. Decreased peripheral vascular resistance
6. Increased ectopy
7. Potential clinical consequences
    a. Altered vital signs
    b. Preexisting hyperdynamic condition
B. Hematologic
1. Increased blood volume predominantly caused by increased plasma volume
2. Decreased hematocrit (32% to 36%) caused by an increase in plasma greater than red blood cell (RBC) volume
3. Increased white blood cell (WBC) count (18–25 WBC/mm^3)
4. Increased Factor I, VII, VIII, IX, and X
5. Decreased plasminogen activator levels
6. Potential clinical consequences
    a. Altered hematologic parameters.
    b. Physiologic "anemia"; physiologic "hypervolemia."
    c. Signs of ongoing hemorrhage delayed; one third of the mother's blood volume can be lost without change in heart rate or blood pressure.
    d. Increased volume requirement with hemorrhage.
    e. Hypercoagulability; increased risk for venothromboembolism.
C. Respiratory
1. Increased minute ventilation
2. Increased tidal volume
3. Decreased functional residual capacity
4. Potential clinical consequences
    a. Chronic respiratory alkalosis
    b. Decreased respiratory buffering capacity
    c. Altered response to inhalation, anesthetics
    d. Propensity for rapid oxygen desaturation
    e. Decreased tolerance of hypoxemia
D. Renal
1. Increased renal blood flow
2. Increased creatinine clearance
3. Increased glomerular filtration rate
4. Decreased glucose resorption
5. Potential clinical consequences
    a. Decreased blood urea nitrogen
    b. Decreased serum creatinine
    c. Glucosuria
E. Gastrointestinal
1. Decreased gastric emptying
2. Increased gastric acid production
3. Impaired gallbladder contraction
4. Potential clinical consequences
    a. Increased risk for acid reflux or aspiration
    b. Bile stasis or increased gallstone formation
F. Endocrine
1. Increased placental lactogen
2. Increased progesterone
3. Increased estrogen
4. Increased parathormone
5. Increased calcitonin
    a. Insulin resistance or pregnancy-induced diabetes
    b. Lower esophageal sphincter relaxation
    c. Delayed gastric emptying
    d. Increased calcium absorption

G. Neurologic
    1. Pregnancy-induced hypertension (eclampsia)
        a. Increased risk for intracranial hemorrhage
        b. Increased risk for seizures
        c. Mimics head injury

IV. MECHANISMS OF INJURY
  A. Blunt
    1. Motor vehicle collisions (MVCs) >falls > assaults.
    2. MVCs are the leading nonobstetric cause of maternal and fetal mortality.
    3. Placental abruption is the most common cause of fetal death when the mother survives.
    4. Pelvic fractures are the most common maternal injury associated with fetal death.
    5. The most common fetal injury is skull fracture, with intracranial hemorrhage.
    6. Uterine rupture is associated with ejection from the vehicle and presents with maternal shock and uterine tenderness.
    7. Utilization and proper application of seatbelt is the most important factor in preventing maternal injury and associated fetal death.
    8. Pelvic ligamentous laxity and the protuberant abdomen contribute to gait instability and increased incidents of falls in pregnancy.
  B. Penetrating
    1. Gunshot wounds (GSWs) >stab wounds.
    2. Often associated with domestic violence.
    3. Risk of uterine injury is increased in the second and third trimester.
    4. Fetal injury associated with uterine injury is common and carries a high mortality rate (40% to 65%).
    5. Maternal mortality is rare.
    6. Upper abdominal penetrating injury is often associated with extensive gastrointestinal and vascular injuries.

V. MANAGEMENT
  A. General considerations
    1. Consider the potential for pregnancy in all female trauma victims of appropriate age. Routinely perform beta-human growth hormone (β-hCG) testing.
    2. Although two patients are being managed, the initial treatment priorities remain the same (i.e., Advanced Trauma Life Support [ATLS] protocol). **The best early treatment of the fetus is optimal resuscitation of the mother.**
    3. Early obstetric consultation and fetal assessment is mandatory. Subsequent care may require neonatal specialists.
  B. Prehospital
    1. As the fetus is exquisitely sensitive to hypoxia and hypovolemia, prehospital management of the pregnant trauma victim should include administration of supplemental oxygen and intravenous fluid as soon as possible.
    2. In late pregnancy, extrication, immobilization, and transport can be complicated by anatomic factors. Supine hypotension syndrome can be prevented by positioning the pregnant patient to avoid uterine compression of the inferior vena cava such as left lateral decubitus position, or with the right hip elevated and the uterus manually displaced. If a spinal injury is suspected, immobilize the gravid patient on a long backboard, which is tilted 15 degrees to the left.
    3. The pneumatic antishock garment (PASG) can be used to stabilize fractures or control hemorrhage. However, inflation of the abdominal compartment of the PASG is contraindicated because the increased intraabdominal pressure further compromises venous return.
    4. Field triage and interhospital transfer protocols must account for pregnancy. Assuming comparable transport times, transport pregnant patients to the facility best equipped to deal with the patient's injuries and simultaneously provide obstetric and neonatology expertise. Notify the receiving facility as early as possible to allow for timely preparation and response.

5. Do not attempt fetal assessment in the field. Rapid extrication, proper immobilization, and prompt transport are the best measures applied to safeguard mother and child.

C. Hospital

1. Primary survey
   a. Simultaneous resuscitation of vital signs and identification and management of life-threatening injuries are the same as for other trauma patients.
   b. Consider early intubation and mechanical ventilation in any pregnant trauma patient with marginal airway or ventilatory status to avoid fetal hypoxia.
   c. Because of "physiologic hypervolemia," the pregnant trauma patient can lose a significant amount of blood volume (1,500 mL) without manifesting any signs of hypovolemia. **Even if the mother's vital signs are normal, the fetus may be inadequately perfused.**
   d. Venous access in the upper extremities is preferred. Initiate prompt and vigorous volume resuscitation. Consider early RBC transfusion. Use type O, Rh-negative RBC transfusions to avoid Rh isoimmunization. Vasopressors reduce placental blood flow and should be avoided as an initial measure to correct maternal hypotension.

2. Secondary survey
   a. Obstetric history
      i. Date of last menstrual period
      ii. Expected date of delivery
      iii. First perception of fetal movement
      iv. Status of current and previous pregnancies
   b. Determine uterine size (Fig. 47-1) by assessing fundal height as measured in centimeters from the symphysis pubis, which provides a rapid measure of fetal age (1 cm = 1 week of gestational age).
   c. Examination of the gravid abdomen must include assessment of uterine tenderness and consistency, presence of contractions, and determination of fetal lie and movement. Perform internal pelvic examination with special attention to the presence of vaginal blood or amniotic fluid, and to cervical effacement, dilation, and fetal station. The presence of amniotic fluid (pH = 7) can be confirmed by the change in Nitrazine paper from blue-green to deep blue. (Normal amniotic fluid has a pH >7; normal vaginal fluid has a pH of 5.)

3. Fetal assessment
   a. Beyond 20 weeks gestation, fetal heart tones can be auscultated with a fetoscope or stethoscope to determine fetal heart rate. The normal range is from 120 to 160 beats/minute. Fetal bradycardia is indicative of fetal distress.
   b. Institute continuous electronic fetal monitoring for gravid patients at or beyond 20 to 24 weeks as the fetus may be viable if delivered. Obstetric personnel experienced in cardiotocography must be available to interpret fetal heart rate tracings for signs of fetal distress. These signs include an abnormal baseline rate; repetitive decelerations, especially after uterine contractions; and absence of accelerations or beat-to-beat variability.
   c. High-resolution, real-time ultrasonography is excellent for evaluating the fetus for gestational age, cardiac activity, and movement. As with cardiotocography, properly trained and credentialed personnel must be available to perform and interpret this study.

4. Diagnostic modalities
   a. Perform essential radiologic studies, including computed tomography. Whenever possible, shield the lower abdomen with a lead apron and avoid duplicating studies.
   b. Radiation exposure to the preimplantation embryo (<3 weeks) is lethal. During organogenesis (2–7 weeks), the embryo is most sensitive to the teratogenic, growth retarding, and postnatal neoplastic effects of radiation. Radiation exposure of <0.1 Gy is generally safe (Table 47-1).

TABLE 47-1	Absorbed Radiation Doses from Radiation Study

Radiographic study	Absorbed dose (rads)
Cervical spine series	0.0005
Anteroposterior chest	0.0025
Thoracic spine series	0.01
Anteroposterior pelvis	0.2
Lumbosacral spine series	0.75–1.0
Head CT scan	0.05
Chest CT scan	<1.0
Abdomen CT scan (including pelvis)	3.0–9.0
Limited upper abdomen CT scan	<3.0

CT, computed tomography.

    c. Indications for diagnostic peritoneal lavage (DPL) or focused abdominal sonography for trauma (FAST) are the same as for the nonpregnant patient. For patients in their second or third trimester, perform DPL above the umbilicus and in an open manner.

    d. FAST can be a helpful, noninvasive method of determining the presence of free fluid in the abdomen after trauma. Location of the transducer must be changed to allow for the anatomic displacement of structures.

5. Definitive care

    a. Proceed with urgent operative intervention as dictated by physical findings and diagnostic studies.

    b. Pregnant trauma patients who are critically ill should be managed in the appropriate surgical or trauma intensive care unit. On-site obstetric care and bedside fetal monitoring must be available.

    c. Stable gravid trauma patients requiring hospitalization should be obstetrically observed for 24 to 48 hours. Those patients whose fetus is beyond 20 to 24 weeks' gestation should have continuous cardiotocographic monitoring (CTM). A minimum of 24 hours is recommended for patients who present with frequent uterine activity (more than five contractions per hour), abdominal or uterine tenderness, vaginal bleeding, rupture of amniotic membranes, or hypotension.

    d. Asymptomatic gravid patients whose fetus is >20 to 24 weeks' gestation with minor injuries not requiring hospitalization with normal findings on CTM of at least 4 hours' duration can be released with appropriate instructions and follow-up care.

VI. CESAREAN SECTION AND TRAUMA

  A. Indications

    1. Fetal factors

      a. Risk of fetal distress exceeds risk of prematurity

      b. Placental abruption

      c. Uterine rupture

      d. Fetal malposition with premature labor

      e. Severe pelvic or lumbosacral spine fractures

    2. Maternal factors

      a. Inadequate exposure for control of other injuries

      b. Disseminated intravascular coagulation (DIC)

  B. Perimortem cesarean section can be considered in situations of fetal gestational age ≥26 weeks, and the interval between maternal death and delivery can be minimized (<15 minutes). Maternal cardiopulmonary resuscitation must be continued throughout cesarean section and neonatal intensive care support should be immediately available.

C. Technique
   1. Make a vertical midline abdominal incision.
   2. Incise the uterus vertically.
   3. Expose the infant's head, and suction oropharynx with a bulb syringe.
   4. Deliver the infant.
   5. Clamp and divide the umbilical cord.
   6. Manually remove the placenta.
   7. Inspect the endometrial surface to ensure removal of all membranes.
   8. Close the uterus in layers with absorbable suture.
   9. Administer oxytocin (usual dosage = 20 U intravenously) to treat postpartum uterine bleeding.

D. Cesarean section prolongs operative time and increases blood loss by at least 1,000 mL.

VII. SPECIFIC PROBLEMS UNIQUE TO PREGNANCY

A. Placental abruption (*abruptio placenta*) is the most common cause of fetal death with maternal survival. In late pregnancy, even minor injury can be associated with abruption. Placental separation from the uterine wall of >50% generally results in fetal death. Clinical findings include abdominal pain, vaginal bleeding, leakage of amniotic fluid, uterine tenderness and rigidity, expanding fundal height, and maternal shock. Minor degrees of placental separation are compatible with fetal survival in utero and should be carefully followed by serial ultrasound, external fetal monitoring, and observation for fetomaternal transfusion (Section VII.C).

B. Disseminated intravascular coagulation is caused by either the release of thromboplastic substances during placental abruption or amniotic fluid embolism. Maternal shock and death can occur precipitously. Treatment includes emergency evacuation of the uterus and blood component therapy to reverse the coagulopathy.

C. Fetomaternal transfusion, fetal hemorrhage into the maternal circulation, is common after trauma (~26%). Fetomaternal transfusion can result in fetal anemia and death, as well as isoimmunization of an Rh-negative mother. The Kleihauer-Betke (K-B) test measures fetomaternal hemorrhage. This test has been used to determine the need for Rh immunoglobulin in Rh-negative mothers and as an indicator of placental abruption. However, the amount of fetomaternal transfusion sufficient to sensitize Rh-negative mothers is far below the sensitivity of the K-B test. Therefore, it is recommended to treat all Rh-negative mothers who present with abdominal trauma with Rh immune globulin (50 μg if <16 weeks' gestation; 300 μg if >16 weeks). Furthermore, use cardiographic monitoring and high-resolution, real-time ultrasound in patients suspected of abruption, rather than relying on the K-B test.

D. Premature labor, defined as onset of uterine contractions before 36 weeks' gestation that are forceful enough to cause cervical dilation and effacement, is a common complication of maternal trauma. Most of these premature contractions stop without tocolysis. Tocolytics (usually β-adrenergic agonist or magnesium sulfate) are generally used to allow adequate time for complete evaluation of the preterm fetus. Administer these agents under the direction of an obstetrician and experienced personnel. Tocolysis is contraindicated with fetal distress, vaginal bleeding, suspected placental abruption, maternal shock or hypotension, cervical dilation >4 cm, or maternal comorbidities (e.g., diabetes, pregnancy-induced hypertension, cardiac disease, maternal hyperthyroidism).

E. Intrauterine fetal death does not necessitate immediate operative intervention. Labor usually ensues within 48 hours. Monitor coagulation studies closely if observation is entertained, as once DIC develops maternal shock and death can occur precipitously as previously mentioned.

VIII. MEDICATIONS IN PREGNANCY

A. Analgesics

1. Administer **opioids** (fetal respiratory depression) and nonsteroidal antiinflammatory drugs (NSAIDs; prostaglandin and platelet inhibition) with caution (lower dosing and appropriate monitoring).

B. Antibiotics

1. Penicillins, cephalosporins, erythromycin, and clindamycin are safe.

2. Administer aminoglycoside (fetal ototoxicity), sulfonamide (neonatal kernicterus), quinolone, and metronidazole with caution.

3. Chloramphenicol (maternal and fetal bone marrow toxicity), and tetracycline (inhibition of fetal bone growth) are contraindicated.

C. Anticoagulants (Chapter 50)

1. Heparin is indicated as it does not cross the placenta, has a short half-life, and is immediately reversible with protamine. Low-molecular-weight heparin is also considered safe for use in pregnancy.

2. Warfarin is contraindicated as it crosses the placenta, and has a long half-life and takes significant time to reverse.

D. Anticonvulsants

1. Administer **benzodiazepines and barbiturates** (fetal respiratory depression) with caution.

2. Phenytoin is contraindicated (teratogenic).

E. Antiemetics

1. Metoclopramide and prochlorperazine are safe.

F. Because local anesthetics cross the placenta, administer them with caution and avoid large doses.

G. General anesthesia and neuromuscular blockers are considered safe.

H. Stress prophylaxis

1. Sucralfate is safe.

2. Use H_2 blockers with caution.

I. Administer **tetanus prophylaxis** according to the standard guidelines.

AXIOMS

- "Save the mother, save the fetus."
- Perform a routine beta-HCG test on all women of childbearing age.
- In transporting trauma patients in late pregnancy, take measures to displace the uterus to the left side.
- The fetus can be in jeopardy, even with apparent minor maternal injury.
- Although two patients are being managed, the initial treatment priorities remain the same.
- The best early treatment of the fetus is optimal resuscitation of the mother.
- Significant blood loss can occur in the pregnant patient without change in vital signs.
- Placental abruption is the leading cause of fetal death in patients where the mother survives.
- Fetal death is not an indication for cesarean section.
- Under no circumstances should maintaining a pregnancy compromise the management of maternal wounds.

Bibliography

Knudson MH. Trauma in pregnancy. In: Blaisdell FW, Trunkey DD, eds. *Trauma Management: Abdominal Trauma*. New York, NY: Thieme Medical Publishers; 1993:324–339.

Rozyck GS, Knudson MM. Reproductive system trauma. In: Feliciano DV, Moore EE, Mattox KL, eds. *Trauma*. Stamford, Conn: Appleton & Lange; 1996:695–709.

Trauma in women. In: Committee on Trauma, American College of Surgeons. *Advanced Trauma Life Support for Doctors*. Chicago, Ill: American College of Surgeons; 1997:315–332.

Vaizey CJ, Jacobsen MJ, Cross FW. Trauma in pregnancy. *Br J Surg* 1994;81:1406–1415.

Wilson RF, Vincent C. Gynecologic and obstetric trauma. In: Wilson RF, Walt AS, eds. *Management of Trauma: Pitfalls and Practice*. Baltimore, Md: Williams & Wilkins; 1996:21–640.

48 GERIATRIC TRAUMA
DONALD R. KAUDER

I. DEMOGRAPHICS AND EPIDEMIOLOGY

A. In 1990, 30.9 million people in the United States were >65 years of age, accounting for 12.5% of the total population. By the year 2020, this segment of the population is projected to increase to 52 million, 6.7 million of whom will be >85 years of age. By the year 2040, persons >65 years of age will make up 20% of the populace.

B. The elderly are living longer and in better health than in past years partly because of advances in health care, improved social support, and heightened awareness of the complex medical and socioeconomic issues germane to this age group. These older adults continue to participate in many of the same pursuits as their younger counterparts and, therefore, are subject to a similar, and, in some instances, increased risk of injury. In 2001, over 3.2 million elderly patients who sustained unintentional injuries were evaluated in U.S. emergency departments (EDs); 2.2 million (68.7%) were admitted.

C. The 12.5% of our population >65 years of age accounts for almost one third of the deaths from injury. Furthermore, this group incurs higher population-based death rates than any other age group. In 2002 unintentional injury was the ninth leading cause of death in those age 65 and older, accounting for over 33,000 victims.

II. PHYSIOLOGY OF AGING

A. Cardiovascular system

1. Progressive stiffening of the myocardium is caused by increasing fibrosis and a progressive loss of myocytes. Accompanying this is a compensatory increase in myocyte volume in both ventricles along with fat cell infiltration in the interstitial space of the ventricular walls and septum. The myocardium progressively stiffens with resulting decreased diastolic relaxation and slowed ventricular filling.

2. The heart becomes less efficient with a progressive decrease in its ejection fraction. Stroke volume is diminished leading to an increased reliance on the atrial contribution to increase end-diastolic volume in order to maintain cardiac output. The heart can be extremely sensitive to both hypo- and hypervolemia, resulting in a very narrow therapeutic window.

3. Decreasing sensitivity to endogenous and exogenous catecholamines causes an inability to mount an appropriate tachycardia and, thus, a decreased ability to augment cardiac output in response to hypovolemia, pain, and stress.

4. Peripheral atherosclerotic disease predisposes to:
   a. Reduced flow to vital organs and diminished physiologic reserve
   b. Baseline diminution in peripheral pulses, potentially leading to a misinterpretation of the character of the pulse, thus, leading to the initiation of inappropriate therapy

5. The use of commonly prescribed medications (e.g., beta-blockers, calcium channel blockers, and digoxin) can mask or blunt the normal physiologic response to injury and stress. In some cases, the ingestion of prescription medications can directly exacerbate a patient's injuries (e.g., Coumadin).

B. Respiratory system
   1. Decreased lung elasticity and progressive stiffening of the chest wall lead to diminished pulmonary compliance and alteration in the ability to mount an effective cough.
   2. Coalescence of alveoli and reduction of small airways support lead to a decrease in surface area for gas exchange.
   3. Atrophy of pseudociliated epithelium lining the bronchi contributes to a decrease in clearance of particulate foreign matter and bacteria.
   4. Chronic colonization of the upper airway with enteric gram-negative bacteria and *Haemophilus* species predisposes to pneumonia.

C. Nervous system
   1. The brain undergoes progressive atrophy beginning in the fourth decade; by age 70 years, a 10% reduction in brain size occurs.
     a. The distance between the brain surface and the skull thus increases, putting the dural bridging veins on stretch and making them more susceptible to disruption and bleeding.
     b. The reduction in brain size results in increased intracranial "potential space." Thus, a significant amount of intracranial bleeding can be masked before symptoms of increased intracranial pressure occur. The initially asymptomatic elderly patient suffering a mechanism of injury that might predispose to an intracranial injury can suffer rapid deterioration from an insidious, progressive closed head injury.
   2. Functional deterioration occurs, increasing the predisposition to injury.
     a. Cognition
       i. Poor memory
       ii. Impaired judgment
       iii. Deficient data acquisition
     b. Hearing
       i. Decreased auditory acuity, especially to high-frequency sounds
       ii. Lack of adequate hearing aids because of financial constraints or limited access to health care
     c. Eyesight
       i. Decreased peripheral vision
       ii. Decreased visual acuity
       iii. Decreased tolerance to glare
       iv. Inadequate or inappropriate eyeglasses prescription
     d. Proprioception and coordination
       i. Tendency toward imbalance
       ii. Altered "righting" reflex

D. Renal
   1. A decline in renal mass occurs. By age 65 years, a 30% to 40% loss is common.
   2. The nephrons that remain show changes of aging and deterioration in the tubules and glomeruli.
   3. A normal serum creatinine does not imply normal renal function. An estimate of function can be calculated using the following formula for creatinine clearance (C_{cr}):
$$C_{cr} \text{ (mL/min)} = (140 - age) \times weight \text{ (kg)}/serum\ creatinine \times 72$$
   4. Exercise caution and good judgment in the use of potentially nephrotoxic agents, including:
     a. Iodinated contrast solutions
     b. Aminoglycosides
     c. Diuretics
     d. Vasopressors

E. Musculoskeletal system
   1. Osteoporosis predisposes to fractures with relatively minor energy transfer.
   2. Progressive erosion of cartilage and ligamentous stiffening especially in weight bearing joints affects mobility and can be a source of chronic pain.

3. Diminution in vertebral body height and osteoarthritis contribute to significant changes in the spine.
   a. Kyphoscoliosis leads to decreased mobility and difficulty looking upward, and in twisting and turning the head, predisposing to decreased obstacle avoidance and increased risk of injury.
   b. Spinal stenosis caused by osteoarthritis renders the spinal cord more susceptible to injury, especially with cervical extension. Central cord syndrome can occur in this setting.
4. Decrease in muscle mass and progressive fibrosis lead to diminished strength and agility. This predisposes to poor obstacle avoidance and the inability to avoid serious injury, especially when falling (the altered righting reflex).

III. INFLUENCE OF COMORBID CONDITIONS

A. In addition to the typical changes that occur with aging, the common development of significant disease states can have a profound impact on an elderly person's response to injury and stress. Knowledge of concurrent disease states is critical to the appropriate management of the injured elderly, and an aggressive search for such information is vital. This information will influence resuscitation strategies, as well as assist in planning care once the trauma patient is admitted to the hospital. A helpful listing of the more common conditions encountered and how to quantify them is found in Table 48-1.

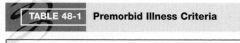

TABLE 48-1   **Premorbid Illness Criteria**

Cardiac disease
–History of cardiac surgery
–Any cardiac medication
–Myocardial infarction within 12 months of admission
–Myocardial infarction more that 12 months before admission

Diabetes mellitus
–Insulin-dependent
–Non-insulin-dependent

Liver disease
–Bilirubin >2 mg/dL (on admission)
–Cirrhosis

Malignancy
–Documented history

Pulmonary disease (chronic asthma, chronic obstructive pulmonary disease, others)
–Bronchodilator therapy
–No bronchodilator therapy

Obesity
–Female >200 lb
–Male >250 lb

Renal disease
–Serum creatinine >2 mg/dL (on admission)

Neurologic (cerebrovascular accident)
–Documented prior history

Hypertension
–Any antihypertensive medication
–Documented prior history

IV. MECHANISMS OF INJURY
A. Falls

1. Falls are the most frequent cause of accidental injury in people >75 years of age and the second most common cause of injury sustained by those between the ages of 65 and 74 years.

2. While frequently resulting in isolated orthopedic injury, falls in conjunction with significant energy transfer (e.g., down a flight of stairs or off a ladder or a roof) can be devastating.

3. The reason for the fall must be investigated carefully. Falls caused by the aging process are frequent, and postural instability, poor balance, altered gait, and decreased muscular strength and coordination can all be implicated. However, consider acute or chronic comorbid conditions (e.g., syncope, drop attacks, cardiac dysrhythmias, hypoglycemia, anemia, and transient cerebral ischemia) as possible causes. In the anticoagulated patient, a seemingly minor fall can have devastating consequences.

B. Motor vehicle crashes

1. People >65 years of age account for 13% of licensed drivers. As population demographics change, this percentage will increase. The elderly have a very high crash rate, second only to persons in the age group 16 to 25 years. Further, those aged ≥75 years have a higher rate of fatal crashes than any other age group.

2. Whereas falls are a more frequent mechanism of injury, a motor vehicle crash is the most common reason for an elderly individual to present to a trauma center. Most crashes take place in the daylight hours, in good weather, and close to home. Alcohol ingestion is encountered far less frequently than in younger populations. As in any mechanism of injury, the events leading to the incident must be elucidated. Physiologic decreases in musculoskeletal coordination and reaction time, visual impairment, alterations in auditory processing, and deficits in cognition function may contribute to the high incidence of crashes. Antecedent medical conditions also must be sought as a cause.

C. Pedestrian–automobile impacts

1. Pedestrian–automobile impacts seen in the elderly can produce devastating consequences. Those >65 years of age account for almost a quarter of fatalities caused by this mechanism in the United States each year. As in other mechanisms of injury, the effects of aging are frequently implicated as causative factors.

   a. Osteoarthritis of the spine and progressive kyphosis lead to a stooped posture, thus making it more difficult to lift the head so that traffic signals can be seen and onrushing vehicles identified and avoided.

   b. Changes in gait combined with a slower pace make it difficult to clear an intersection before the traffic signal changes, whereas decreased strength, agility, and reaction time make it difficult to effect a rapid change in direction critical to avoid a collision.

   c. Alterations in hearing and vision and poor judgment, cognition, and memory also may be implicated as contributing factors.

D. Injuries related to violence

1. Injuries resulting from shooting, stabbing, and blunt assault account for 4% to 14% of elderly trauma admissions. Those same changes of aging that predispose to falls and motor vehicle–related injury make older individuals easy prey for the criminal element. Decreased strength and agility alter the ability to fight or flee. Poor vision and hearing and cognitive changes leading to poor judgment also contribute to the potential for victimization. Suicide is the most common reason for gun-related deaths in older individuals. The elderly account for almost 25% of all deaths ascribed to suicide and <3% of homicides annually.

2. Domestic abuse of the elderly is a problem that is gaining more recognition. In excess of 240,000 cases are reported annually, but likely represent only 10% of cases that actually occur. As with young children, a high index of suspicion

must be maintained, and telltale signs must be sought. Frequent visits to the emergency department for "minor" injuries, multiple bruises in various stages of healing, poor nutrition, an unkempt appearance, and poor personal hygiene can all be warning signs for the physician to consult the appropriate social services agency to assist in an inquiry.

E. Burns

1. Burns account for ~8% of injury-related deaths in the elderly. When compared with a younger population, the elderly suffer larger and deeper burns and have a significantly higher mortality rate. The elderly are at risk for burn injury from a variety of factors.

    a. **Altered mobility.** Limitations in muscular strength and coordination, poor balance, and altered gait make escaping a fire more difficult.

    b. **Neurosensory changes.** Diminution of auditory and visual cues can make recognition of a fire less likely. Alterations in sensation because of peripheral neuropathy or ischemic peripheral vascular disease can lead to prolonged heat exposure (e.g., burns from scalding bath water). Further, poor judgment regarding safety issues (e.g., the unsupervised use of kerosene heaters) makes the elderly more likely to be involved in a fire.

    c. **Skin changes.** Thinning of the skin caused by decreased epidermal cell proliferation makes the elderly more likely to suffer a serious burn than a younger individual given the same thermal exposure.

V. RESUSCITATION AND INITIAL ASSESSMENT.

Initiate early, aggressive efforts to resuscitate the elderly trauma patient while efforts are being made to contact family members and to clearly delineate the patient's preinjury level of function, state of health, comorbid conditions, and presence of a living will or other predetermination documents.

A. ABCDEs.

The initial assessment of trauma victims, as outlined in earlier chapters, is the appropriate starting point for the evaluation of the geriatric trauma patient. However, an awareness of the physiology of aging and the presence of comorbid disease must be taken into account and the resuscitative effort modified as appropriate.

1. **Airway.** Early control of the airway is critical. A lack of pulmonary reserve, combined with a high likelihood that a patient may have underlying cardiovascular disease, can drastically alter the consequences of seemingly minimal hypoxemia. A patient who develops a significant tachycardia to compensate for injuries or hypoxia who then develops myocardial ischemia as a result may be better served with early intubation with careful control of oxygenation and ventilation.

2. **Breathing**

    a. A thorough search for serious chest injuries is vital in ensuring adequate levels of oxygenation. Initial assessment protocols for identification and treatment of immediately life-threatening injuries (e.g., tension pneumothorax, massive hemothorax) must be followed. Flail chest, particularly anterior flail chest, may not be obvious in the elderly patient. A hallmark of excellent treatment is adequate pain control. Although fractured ribs and chest wall contusions are not considered immediately life threatening, these exquisitely painful injuries in the setting of poor chest wall compliance, chronic obstructive pulmonary disease (COPD), and bacterial colonization of the oropharynx can be lethal if good pulmonary toilet is not ensured.

    b. Early use of epidural analgesia can be beneficial in this setting. Do not delay intubation and ventilatory support—another viable option. Delay in initiation of ventilatory support can result in an increased work of breathing and increased myocardial oxygen demand.

    c. The use of patient controlled analgesia can provide significant relief as well, but must be used with caution. Utilization of a basal rate of narcotic infusion should be avoided, as overnarcotization resulting in hypoventilation and hypoxemia can be deadly.

3. **Circulation**
   a. Restoring the elderly trauma victim to a normal volume status can present some unique challenges. Preexisting disease and senescence can lead to an inappropriate response to hypovolemia, depriving the physician of the usual signs (e.g., tachycardia and low blood pressure). Delayed capillary refill in the lower extremities secondary to peripheral vascular disease can be misinterpreted as a sign of volume contraction, leading to overzealous fluid administration, a significant problem in a patient with marginal cardiac reserve.
   b. Fluid resuscitation should be judicious. Give early consideration to transfusion with packed red blood cells to augment oxygen-carrying capacity and oxygen delivery, especially in those with known ischemic cardiovascular disease, thereby lessening the need for the compensatory tachycardia necessary to augment cardiac output. **Unrecognized hypoperfusion is common in the elderly and results in increased morbidity and mortality.**
   c. In many elderly patients, the volume status cannot be determined accurately. The use of invasive monitoring with pulmonary artery and intraarterial blood pressure catheters can be helpful and their early use, even during the initial resuscitation, should be considered. This information may uncover treatable and previously unrecognized hypovolemia or cardiac dysfunction.

4. **Disability**
   a. Early and accurate assessment of the neurologic status of the geriatric trauma patient is important and frequently difficult to accomplish. The history of preexisting mental dysfunction (e.g., senile dementia, Alzheimer's disease) or prior cerebrovascular accidents is frequently lacking or may be denied by the patient or family. If chronic disease states are misinterpreted as being acute, harmful overtreatment can occur. Conversely, a patient with a "normal" mental status following a blow to the head may be harboring a potentially lethal intracranial injury that simply has not had time to manifest itself because of the presence of extensive cerebral atrophy.
   b. Early, liberal use of head computed tomography (CT) scanning must be part of the evaluation of the elderly trauma victim with any suspicion of potentially serious head injury.
   c. A history of ingestion of anticoagulant therapy must be aggressively sought, particularly Coumadin or clopidogrel, both of which will exacerbate bleeding and can cause a minor cerebral contusion to transform into a catastrophic hemorrhage.

5. **Expose**
   a. As in any trauma patient, the elderly must be fully disrobed and carefully examined anteriorly as well as posteriorly. Large quantities of blood can be lost into the elastic soft tissues of elderly patients. Give special attention to the search for signs of prior surgical intervention, because this may provide a clue as to a patient's antecedent medical history. The presence of a median sternotomy incision or signs of peripheral vascular surgery should alert you to the presence of systemic arteriosclerotic disease. Failure to recognize a well-healed abdominal incision can lead to subsequent misinterpretation of abdominal CT scan or to a suboptimal therapeutic maneuver (e.g., diagnostic peritoneal lavage).

B. **Secondary survey**
   1. As in the initial assessment, examine the patient in a systematic fashion to search for serious injuries (Chapter 10). However, pay special attention to the history preceding the injury. Failure to do so can lead to inappropriate therapy or contribute to the recurrence of a potentially preventable event. Investigate the following issues:
      a. Did the crash involve a single vehicle during "normal" driving conditions? This scenario suggests that an antecedent medical condition may have been involved (e.g., a transient ischemic attack or cardiac dysrhythmia).

b. Is this one of several falls or motor vehicle crashes that have occurred in the last year? Clustering of events such as this also can be a clue that an untreated medical condition may be a contributing factor.

c. Has the trauma victim begun a new medication or had a recent change in dosage of an old prescription? A newly diagnosed diabetic can have difficulty regulating blood sugar, whereas some antihypertensive medications can cause dizziness or orthostatic hypotension.

VI. ISSUES UNIQUE TO THE SEVERELY INJURED GERIATRIC PATIENT

A. Outcome

1. Mortality rates are higher for comparable injuries and injury severity scores when comparing elderly patients with younger patients.

2. The presence of a preexisting medical illness increases the incidence of in-hospital morbidity and mortality, as well as mortality risk postdischarge.

3. Assessment of disability and functional outcome can be more meaningful measures of therapeutic success than mortality alone, but studies in these areas are lacking. It is clear that many elderly trauma victims can return to a preinjury level of function or at least return to some level of functional independence. To regard a patient's age as a sole determinant and predictor of return to the premorbid state would be naive. A multidisciplinary approach to the treatment and rehabilitation of the injured elderly that begins at the time of admission to the hospital is important. Home care agencies, spouses, and family members play an integral role in allowing patients to return home, and to a productive life.

4. Appropriateness of resuscitation

a. Moral and ethical issues surrounding the care of the injured elderly are difficult. It is appropriate to begin aggressive resuscitative efforts and to sustain them at least until some insight can be gained into the patient's and family's wishes. It is uncommon for people to have living wills or predetermination documents on their person at the time of a serious injury, but early contact with a family member or personal physician can yield crucial information that can influence medical decision making. It is equally important to help family members interpret such documents, especially with regard to the specifics of medical therapy. To illustrate, a well-meaning family can misinterpret mechanical ventilation that is being used as a bridge to recovery as being counter to a patient's request not to "end up on a ventilator."

B. Early involvement of social services, chaplaincy services, and, occasionally, an expert in medical ethics can be helpful. The need for frank and open discussion between the physician and the family regarding prognosis and expectations for meaningful recovery is essential. Only then can rational decisions be made regarding the appropriateness of care.

C. Family support

1. An assessment of the accident victim's family dynamics and early involvement of the family in discussions of acute care problems and long-term issues are paramount. It is not unusual for the children of the injured elderly to be elderly themselves. As such, they may not have the physical stamina or the economic resources to actively participate in the rehabilitation and final disposition of the patient. As mentioned, early involvement of the family can also serve to clarify issues of appropriateness of care.

VII. AN AGE-RELATED APPROACH TO PATIENT CARE

A. As the response to injury and illness changes with increasing age, a number of treatment axioms have been developed to serve as guidelines to the care of the injured elderly.

1. Age 55 through 64 years

a. Assume some mild decrease in physiologic reserve.

b. Suspect the presence of some common diseases of middle age (diabetes mellitus, arteriosclerotic cardiovascular disease, hypertension, previous surgery, history of transfusion).

   c. Suspect the use of prescription or nonprescription medications.
   d. Assume that the patient is competent to provide an accurate medical history.
   e. Look for subtle signs of organ dysfunction, especially cardiovascular and respiratory systems. Arterial blood gas measurement and an electrocardiogram (ECG) may be especially enlightening.
   f. With a history of loss of consciousness or abnormalities in cognitive function or personality, presume a serious brain injury is present. Liberal use of CT scan is essential; magnetic resonance imaging (MRI) can be a useful adjunct, especially in evaluating the nonbony components of the spine.
   g. Proceed with standard diagnostic and management schemes, unless contraindicated by information collected during history.

2. **Age 65 through 74 years**
   a. Accept the presence of age-related and acquired disease-induced physiologic alteration of organ systems.
   b. Accept the presence of acquired disease and medications to treat them. Assume a higher incidence of previous surgery and transfusion.
   c. Decide if the patient is competent to give a reliable medical history. Review the history as soon as possible with the patient's relatives or personal physician.
   d. Aggressively monitor the patient and control physiology to optimize cardiac performance and oxygen metabolism.
   e. Assume that any alteration in mental status or cognitive or sensory function indicates the presence of a brain injury. Imaging of the brain is mandatory in the patient with abnormal mental status.
   f. Proceed with standard diagnostic and management schemes, including early aggressive operative management.
   g. Be aware of poor outcome, especially with severe injury to the central nervous system (CNS) or marked physiologic deterioration secondary to injury. Check for advance directives.

3. **Age 75 years and older**
   a. Proceed as in 2a through f.
   b. Assume a poor outcome with moderately severe injury, especially with the CNS injury or any injury causing physiologic dysfunction.
   c. After aggressive initial resuscitation and diagnostic maneuvers, reassess the magnitude of the patient's injuries and discuss appropriateness of care with the patient (if competent) and family members.
   d. Be humane, and recognize the legal and ethical controversies involved. Consider early consultation with experts in ethics and social services to help the family and medical team with difficult decisions.

AXIOMS

- An accurate history is essential.
- Err on the side of early intubation.
- Epidural analgesia to relieve thoracic pain can be lifesaving.
- Early, open discussions with the family are critical.
- Early, proactive involvement by physical medicine and rehabilitation, physical therapy, occupational therapy, social services, and discharge planning is paramount.
- A normal serum creatinine is **not** normal renal function.
- Normal heart rate and blood pressure **do not** imply normovolemia.
- Never underestimate a chest injury.
- A "minor" head injury is a massive subdural hematoma in evolution until proven otherwise.
- Assume the elderly patient has an altered coagulation profile until proven otherwise.
- Geriatric trauma victims cannot tolerate any error; consider invasive monitoring.

Bibliography

Committee on Trauma, American College of Surgeons. *Advanced Trauma Life Support Student Manual.* Chicago, Ill: American College of Surgeons; 1997.

Grossman MD, Miller D, Scaff DW, Arcona S. When is an elder old? Effect of preexisting conditions on mortality in geriatric trauma. *J Trauma* 2002;52(2):242–246.

Inaba K, Goecke M, Sharkey P, et al. Long-term outcomes after injury in the elderly. *J Trauma* 2003;54(3):486–491.

Kauder DR, Schwab CW, Shapiro MB. Geriatric trauma: Patterns, care and outcomes. In: Moore EE, Feliciano DV, Mattox KL, eds. *Trauma.* 5th ed. New York, NY: McGraw-Hill; 2004:1041–1058.

McMahon DJ, Shapiro MB, Kauder DR. Geriatrics in the intensive care unit. *Surg Clin North Am* 2000;80(3):1005–1020.

Milzman DP, Boulanger BR, Rodriguez A, et al. Pre-existing disease in trauma patients: A predictor of fate independent of age and ISS. *J Trauma* 1992;32(2):236–244.

Scalea TM, Simon HM, Duncan AO, et al. Geriatric blunt multiple trauma: Improved survival with early invasive monitoring. *J Trauma* 1990;30(2):129–136.

Smith PC, Enderson BL, Maull KI. Trauma in the elderly: Determinants of outcome. *South Med J* 1990;78:171–177.

I. INTRODUCTION

A. Trauma results in an acute decrement in the ability of the individual to function. Spinal cord injury (SCI), traumatic brain injury (TBI), and general multiple trauma are typical examples of injuries that result in a need for rehabilitation services. Resulting pathology often leaves individuals with permanent impairments that affect their ability to care for themselves, to fulfill expected social roles, and to return to a pattern of daily activity associated with a meaningful and gratifying existence. Certain injuries (e.g., SCI or TBI) affect numerous physiologic, psychological, social, and vocational functions to the degree that the individual loses functional independence. The rehabilitation team is responsible for providing services that optimize function, maximize the return to independence, and enable the person to reestablish a meaningful existence. These services are optimal when begun in the acute care setting and carried into the postacute continuum. The rehabilitation team should be involved in the early stages of hospital care; such involvement has been shown to optimize outcome for the trauma patient as well as result in potential declines in cost and length of acute hospital stay.

B. Attention to the prevention of disabling complications during the acute phase of treatment can minimize required interventions during the rehabilitation phase of treatment. Secondary disabilities are decrements of function that follow the impairments that result from trauma, most often because of prolonged immobilization of the patient. Although rarely life threatening, they can limit eventual function and contribute greatly to total health care cost.

II. GENERAL EFFECTS OF NEUROTRAUMA AND IMMOBILIZATION AFTER INJURY

A. Cardiovascular deconditioning occurs rapidly with any period of inactivity when the heart and peripheral vascular mechanisms lose the capacity to respond to stressors. With certain types of trauma (e.g., SCI with its associated loss of sympathetic nervous system control), the inability to maintain perfusion pressure with changes in posture can limit attempts to mobilize the patient. The most important approach is to minimize immobility and begin to have the patient in an upright position as soon as possible. Additional benefits from this emphasis on early mobilization include improved respiratory functioning, with decreased atelectasis and attendant complications.

  1. Prolonged recumbency causes a progressive rise in the resting heart rate of 0.5 beats per minute per day. In addition, as the heart becomes deconditioned, it responds to demands by a greater rise in rate than preinjury. The combined effect of these changes is resting tachycardia and reduced ability to meet oxygen demands with activity; this persists for 26 to 72 days after return to activity.

  2. Peripheral factors, including decreases in vascular volume, loss of adaptive baroreceptor reflex responses to the upright posture, and increased pooling of blood in lower limb veins, contribute to the intolerance of the patient to an upright posture after immobility.

  a. In healthy individuals, the adaptation response to the upright position can be totally lost after 3 weeks of complete bed rest; it can take up to 72 days

533

to restore proper function of this response after remobilization. Estimates suggest that a loss of strength of 12% per week would occur in healthy individuals.

- **b. Older individuals** lose this capacity to respond even more quickly, and they return to baseline more slowly. Concomitant disease (e.g., cerebrovascular or cardiovascular lesions) makes older individuals less tolerant of this postural drop in blood pressure.
- **c. Minimization of immobility** is the single most important management technique. Increasing periods of sitting in a chair with the feet dependent helps reconditioning for those who are unable to stand.
  - **i. In severe cases,** a tilt table can be used to gradually place the person in an upright position while blood pressure is monitored.
  - **ii. Compressive garments,** full-length elastic stockings, and abdominal binders are also useful to limit venous pooling.
  - **iii. Proper nutrition** to maintain plasma protein levels, immune system function, and proper hydration are also important.
  - **iv. Orthostatic hypotension.** In severe cases where unresponsive to compression garments, increased salt intake and use of sympathomimetic agents (pseudoephedrine, ephedrine, midodrine, or phenylephrine) or mineralocorticoids (fludrocortisone) may assist.
  - **v.** Caution should exist in aggressive mobility among those persons with TBI who have known and unstable elevations in intracranial pressure.

B. Contractures and spasticity result when a joint is not subjected to frequent range of motion, either actively or passively. The formation of contractures is most often a consequence of untreated muscular spasticity because of upper motor neuron impairment, which causes sustained, uncontrolled muscle tension. Spasticity is classically seen as a response to velocity dependent stretch. Muscular tension becomes unbalanced across joints and, therefore, effectively reduces the mobility of the affected joint. The contracture produces a loss of joint range because of shortening and increased stiffness of the soft tissue around the joint. When the limitation of joint range persists, the soft tissues of the joint itself can also become contracted. Remodeling of the connective tissue around the joint contributes to decreased elasticity.

- **1. Contractures contribute to increased morbidity**
  - **a.** Difficulties in positioning the patient can lead to the formation of decubitus ulcers.
  - **b.** Hygiene, particularly in the perineum, palms of the hands, and axillae, can be difficult.
  - **c.** Contractures also can limit function as motor control is regained. This leads to prolonged rehabilitation, possible surgical intervention, and higher cost.
  - **d.** Contractures should be prevented.
- **2. Contractures may be prevented** in most cases by fully ranging all joints twice a day. Active ranging by the patient is preferred, if possible, because it also helps maintain strength and motor control. If weak but voluntary muscle power is present, use active assisted range of motion. In cases of paralysis or coma, passive range of motion must be used. This, however, may be made severe spasticity or rigidity induced by neurotrauma.
  - **a.** After ranging, positioning the patient can help reinforce the gains of therapy. Prone lying provides a prolonged stretch for hip flexion contractures. Splinting of the wrists, hands, and ankles is also useful. Use splints intermittently to avoid skin breakdown. Other physical modalities, in conjunction with range of motion, allow a greater stretch.
    - **i. Superficial heat** can cause reflex relaxation.
    - **ii. Deep heat** using ultrasound can increase the elasticity of collagen, but can be contraindicated in those with metallic implants.
    - **iii. Cooling** of the muscle decreases the activity of the muscle spindle mechanism, decreasing muscle tone.

b. Focal neurolysis. Motor point or peripheral nerve blocks using neurolytic agents (e.g., phenol) or neuromuscular blocking agents (e.g., botulinum toxin) are useful for temporarily reducing muscular tone in cases where abnormalities of muscle tone prevent maintenance of full range at a joint. These should be performed under EMG or stimulator guidance and may be a required step before splinting is effective or serial casting is tolerable. Phenol produces a direct neurolysis and its effect can last 6 to 12 months. Several serotypes of botulinum toxin have been described (A, B, C, D, and E), with only A and B commercially available in the United States.

c. Serial casting of an extremity is useful to provide a prolonged stretch. After adequate padding of bony prominences, a plaster or fiberglass cast is applied. Stretch is maintained as the cast solidifies. The cast is typically left in place for 3 to 5 days before removal. The cast can then be bivalved and used as a resting splint.

d. Antispasticity medication to reduce joint immobilization caused by tonic muscular contractions from hyperreactivity of the skeletal muscle. This phenomenon is common, although usually delayed in onset, in the head-injured patient as well as those patients with cerebral vascular accident or SCI. Common medications used include baclofen, tizanidine, diazepam, and dantrolene sodium. Baclofen and Valium are GABA analog agents. Both of these agents can produce sedation and baclofen can lower the seizure threshold. Rapid baclofen withdrawal can result in seizures, hyperthermia, and systemic collapse. In our opinion, baclofen appears most effective in those with SCI and perhaps less valuable in those with spasticity of cerebral origin. Dantrolene sodium is a peripheral acting agent that acts at the level of the sacroplasmic reticulum and appears to produce less cognitive disturbance among those with CNS injury. Caution should be taken in those with liver disturbance and careful monitoring is warranted as hepatic necrosis has been reported.

C. Decubitus ulcers are potentially preventable but common complications of injury. Pressure is the major factor in the development of an ulcer. Ulcers occur over bony prominences when the pressure of body weight is unrelieved for prolonged periods, causing ischemic damage to the skin and underlying soft tissues. Higher pressures cause breakdown in a shorter time than lower pressures.

1. Shear either between the skin and supporting surfaces or within the soft tissues causes ischemia at lower pressures than when shear is not present.

2. Anemia, excessive skin moisture from perspiration or urine, infection, poor nutrition, contractures, and lack of sensation contribute to development of pressure ulcers. An ulcer will not occur without prolonged, excessive pressure.

3. Prevention of ulceration should be the goal.

a. Carefully position the patient. Frequent turning, initially on a schedule of every 2 hours, is essential. Pay particular attention to the occiput, scapulae, sacrum, ischial tuberosities, greater trochanters, malleoli, and heels. Pillows and foam blocks can be used to relieve pressure or distribute it to other areas.

b. Inspect the skin regularly. If signs of breakdown are seen, avoid pressure to the area to the extent possible. The earliest sign of damage is an area of nonblanching erythema. Palpation may reveal induration of the underlying soft tissue.

c. Manage urinary and bowel incontinence to prevent prolonged contact between the skin and urine or feces, which is important in preventing skin irritation and infection.

d. For patients at high risk, consider use of specialized mattresses and seating surfaces, which have been shown to be a cost-effective component of a decubitus prevention program.

D. Heterotopic ossification is a pathologic process during which new bone is formed within periarticular soft tissue. It should be distinguished from **traumatic myositis** ossificans, in which bone is formed within traumatized muscles, often because of ossification of intramuscular hematoma. Populations at risk include those with burns, TBI, SCI, and those with prolonged immobilization.

1. Following SCI or TBI, incidence is from 11% to 79%.
2. The pathophysiology is not well understood. Its cause may be related to some form of trauma and disinhibition of factors allowing multipotential mesenchymal cells to be converted to osteoclastlike cells. Histologically normal bone develops in the soft tissues surrounding a joint.
3. Different distributions of ossification and time course occur in spinal cord versus brain injury. In both cases, the lesions develop below the level of the neurologic injury around major joints. The process appears to be more aggressive in limbs with greater spasticity-related muscular tone.
   a. **Upper extremity involvement is more common in brain injury.** Most patients with brain injury show a pattern of gradual neurologic recovery rather than the static picture following SCI. Heterotopic ossification tends to be more extensive and persistent following SCI.
   b. **Earliest manifestation of heterotopic ossification** is painful loss of range of motion. Otherwise, a striking similarity is seen to the clinical presentation of deep venous thrombosis, with a warm, swollen, erythematous limb.
   c. **Diagnostic tools.** Triple-phase bone scan, which can be useful to confirm the diagnosis, is the earliest, most specific test. The first and second phases are abnormal in heterotopic ossification. The level of alkaline phosphatase can be used to track the relative activity of new bone formation, although elevation of this enzyme tends to be nonspecific. Additional testing such as a c-reactive protein and creatine phosphokinase (CPK) have been suggested as useful in the diagnostic spectrum.
   d. **Consequences** of this process include painful loss of range of motion and compression of vascular or neurologic structures, which can lead to secondary venous thrombosis. When peripheral nerves are being actively damaged by compression, immediate surgical resection may be required. The bony mass also can lead to development of pressure ulceration of the overlying skin. Perhaps most important, it can simply result in a fixed and immobile joint, leading to an inability to sit or ambulate.
4. Mainstay of treatment is vigorous range of motion. When sensation is preserved (TBI, incomplete SCI), ranging can be painful, leading to increased agitation. Proper pharmacologic treatment and analgesia can permit appropriate physical therapy.
   a. **Heterotopic ossification** is treated with disodium etidronate (Didronel) 20 mg/kg enteral dose for 1 to 3 months, followed by 10 mg/kg for 3 months. While not widely practiced, one group has advocated the use of parenteral treatment early in the course of those with SCI and features of heterotopic ossification. Some have advocated higher dosing during this period; however, this agent has been labeled only for use in SCI. Heterotopic ossification prophylaxis and its utility in long-term treatment is not clear. Indomethacin and other NSAIDs have been used in treatment. Recent evidence suggests efficacy in SCI for its effectiveness is more convincing following total hip replacement than in trauma.
   b. **Radiation**, both as prophylaxis and as treatment, seems to be effective. When early surgical resection is required to reduce compressive phenomenon, radiation early after surgery is useful to prevent recurrence.
   c. **Surgical resection** to improve range of motion is useful, particularly when the joint has ankylosed. Surgery is usually delayed 12 to 18 months after injury, or until repeat three-phase bone scanning shows no active ossification. With good neurologic recovery, surgery usually provides a good result. Ossification tends to recur in cases of poor neurologic recovery or with resection while ossification is active. Postoperative radiation can be helpful in reducing the risk of recurrence.

E. **Musculoskeletal response to immobilization.** Just as exercise leads to strengthening, immobility leads to weakness of both muscles and bone.

Complete bed rest results in loss of 10% to 15% of muscle strength per week.

1. Particularly in type I (slow twitch) muscle fibers, which predominate in antigravity muscles. This reduction of type I capacity, combined with cardiovascular deconditioning, leads to poor endurance when the patient is eventually remobilized.

2. Relative sparing of type II (fast twitch) fibers and the anaerobic nature of strength-type tasks. The result is that in retraining, strength returns rapidly (weeks), whereas endurance requires much longer to return (months).

3. When a patient is immobilized for any length of time, maintain strength as much as possible through therapeutic exercise. Even when range of motion is not possible, isometric exercises can prevent weakness. When a patient is awake and cooperative, opportunities for regular upper and lower body exercise can be facilitated by an overhead trapeze and special color-coded bands made from elastic latex sheets with specific thickness (Thera-Band), which can provide controlled resistance exercise for the patient while in bed or sitting in a wheelchair.

   a. Daily contractions of 20% to 30% of maximal voluntary contraction for several seconds are sufficient to maintain strength. Use exercise that includes motion (isotonic or isokinetic), when possible, because joint motion and motor control can be maintained as well.

4. Skeletal strength is dependent on the forces of gravity and muscle pull acting on the bones. With inactivity, osteoclastic activity predominates with the breakdown of both cortical and trabecular bone. This breakdown can be particularly profound in acute tetraplegia of adolescent boys, resulting in markedly elevated calcium excretion with stone formation or hypercalcemia.

   a. Voluntary muscle activity and weight-bearing exercise are important in reversing this **disuse osteoporosis**. Once activity is resumed, it can take years to return to baseline bone density. Disuse osteoporosis is particularly problematic in individuals with preexisting osteoporosis from other reasons (postmenopausal women).

   b. Adequate hydration and vigilance for the clinical manifestations of immobilization hypercalcemia are important in preventing the adverse effects of this condition.

   c. Prophylactic use of agents that inhibit either osteoblastic or osteoclastic activity in at-risk patients is being investigated and shows promise in limiting the degree of disuse osteoporosis.

III. FREQUENT POSTINJURY PROBLEMS

A. **Agitation following recovery from TBI** can lead to further injury to the patient (e.g., self-extubation, falling out of bed, dislodgment of vascular catheters). In the acute care setting it can lead to significant pressure on the medical staff to stop this behavior. In the rehabilitation setting it can disrupt therapeutic intervention and impair progress. While no consensus definition exits, **we suggest that posttraumatic agitation be defined as a state of aggression during posttraumatic amnesia. This state occurs in the absence of other physical, medical, or psychiatric causes.**

B. The first management step is to attempt to understand the cause of the agitation and control the situation through the least intervention possible. First, exclude causes (e.g., hypoxemia, hypotension, hypoglycemia, seizures, pain, occult injury, neuroendocrine dysfunction, and new CNS dysfunction) as the etiology of the agitation.

   1. Assessment and behavioral management as a first step are key in the process. The Agitated Behavior Scale (ABS) is a 14-point scale that evaluates the frequency and intensity of agitated behaviors and provides an excellent reference for further therapy. ABS scores of 22 or greater suggest significant agitation. Agitation is often a response to a specific stimulus or inability of the individual to sort out overwhelming stimuli. Following brain injury, the individual is often presented with both external and internal stimuli that may

appear distorted by altered perception and difficult to interpret. Difficulty communicating may also lead to frustration and poorly controlled motor responses.

   a. Neuromedical issues. Seek and eliminate irritating internal stimuli such as pain (undiagnosed fractures, pressure ulcers, undertreatment of traumatically painful injuries); a full bowel or bladder; difficulty with breathing; and occult CNS dysfunction such as reoccurrence of a subdural hematoma, hydrocephalus, or seizures.

   b. Minimization of environmental stimuli should be the first approach. To the extent possible, present a single stimulus, allowing adequate time for cognitive processing and response. Noise should be reduced and lighting should be subdued. Verbal stimuli should be calm and simple in content. Careful observation usually detects when the patient is beginning to lose concentration. Perseveration and reduced accuracy of responses are typical clues to this problem. These factors are often difficult to accomplish practically in the acute care setting.

   i. Modification of the environment may be sufficient to control the situation and present minimal risk to the patient.

   ii. Defusing the emotional response of the staff to the patient's behavior is often part of the environmental control necessary.

   iii. Evaluation for signs of sleep dysregulation which can be a prominent source of agitation.

2. The goal of treatment when pharmacologic restraint is necessary is to minimize both the intervention so that the individual can participate in recovery as much as possible and the side effects of treatment.

   a. Short-acting benzodiazepines are useful for short-term episodic use when diagnostic testing is required or when the person represents a danger to self or others.

   b. If agitation occurs in a specific and reproducible daily pattern, attention to correcting the pattern of the proposed intervention or sleep–wake cycle disturbance may also help alleviate the concern. For example, a patient who becomes agitated in the evening and stays awake through the night would benefit from sedating medication such as trazodone given at bedtime to help induce sleep and limit nighttime agitation.

   c. Anticonvulsants (Valproic acid and Carbamazepine), antidepressants, beta-blockers, amantadine, and atypical antipsychotics have been used when agitation is frequent or persistent. A recent Cochrane database review suggested that, while data is limited, beta-blockers and anticonvulsants are among the most effective agents. Some of the newer serotonergic antidepressants can be particularly effective if the agitation is a manifestation of an underlying psychiatric disorder.

   d. Haloperidol, which is used frequently, is effective to control agitation and avoid respiratory depression; but avoid using it, if possible, in cases of TBI. Haloperidol may retard the rate of recovery from injury. Restrict its use to patients in whom all other measures fail. The use of neuroleptic antipsychotic agents in TBI is associated with an increased risk of posttraumatic seizures and neuroleptic malignant syndrome.

3. Physical restraints may be necessary, but caution is required. Cases of injury and death resulting from use of either vest or extremity restraints have been reported. In addition, the restraint is an irritating stimulus that can exacerbate agitation.

C. Autonomic dysreflexia, a life-threatening emergency that can occur following SCI, is the result of pathologic sympathetic reflex activity in response to a noxious stimulus below the level of injury. Interruption of descending pathways allows an uncontrolled sympathetic outflow, leading to a profound increase in blood pressure, piloerection, and diaphoresis.

1. Symptoms include severe pounding headache, nasal congestion, general malaise, sustained penile erection, and paresthesias, in addition to the diaphoresis and piloerection. The uncontrolled hypertension can lead to cardiac ischemia, stroke, or fatal intracerebral hemorrhage.

2. The baroreceptors of the great vessels and vagal outflow are still intact; associated bradycardia usually results.

3. Because reflex activity is necessary to cause autonomic dysreflexia, it is rarely seen early after injury when spinal shock is present. Typically, autonomic dysreflexia is seen in lesions above T6 and is more common at higher levels. With SCI at lower levels, the intact descending sympathetic control minimizes or prevents the syndrome.

4. **Treatment.** Because this syndrome occurs in response to a noxious stimulus, identify and remove the stimulus. Persons with autonomic dysreflexia should be sat up and immediately searched for the inciting stimulus. Most common causes include an overdistended bladder or overdistended bowel, decubitus ulcer, or ingrown toe nail. Relief of this distension is often the only treatment required, with rapid return of the blood pressure to normal.

   a. **Other causes** include fractures, infected decubiti, ingrown toenails, constricting clothing, intraabdominal emergencies, bowel program stimulation, dysmenorrhea, and onset of labor in pregnancy.

   b. In cases in which the cause is not readily identified and corrected, the blood pressure must be brought under control pharmacologically. Sublingual nifedipine (10 mg) is usually effective, but can cause a precipitous drop in blood pressure or cardiac arrhythmia. This is to be repeated in 15 to 20 minutes, if necessary. Nitroglycerine paste also has been used. Applied to the skin, it can also provide a more controlled reduction in blood pressure because removing the medication eliminates the effect of the transdermally absorbed nitroglycerine. This can be useful when elimination of the noxious-driving stimulus results in hypotension from the residual drug-related vasodilatation. In refractory cases, intravenous apresoline, nitroprusside, or spinal anesthesia can be used.

   c. In cases where the daily bowel or bladder management activities produce dysreflexia, use of topical anesthetic agents (lidocaine gel or alternatives) limits the cutaneous stimuli and, thus, the risk of developing these symptoms. Use lidocaine lubricating gel when attempting to disimpact a patient's bowel to minimize the noxious stimulus of this procedure. In recurrent cases (such as with bowel routines), prazosin in doses of 1 to 2 mg at night or oral guanethidine, starting with 5 mg daily, can be used prophylactically. Mecamylamine, starting with 2.5 mg twice daily and titrating up to a total dose of 25 mg daily, is an alternative agent.

   d. Monitor blood pressure closely. With concomitant relief of the noxious stimulus and the administration of a vasodilating agent, the danger exists of lowering the pressure too drastically.

D. **Neurogenic bladder** is one of the most serious alterations of physiologic function following neurologic trauma. In SCI, the most frequent cause of death (after initial survival) until recently was renal failure. Renal failure was caused by frequent infections combined with reflux and subsequent pyelonephritis. Renal failure is now rare, because of aggressive management of neurogenic bladder function. Coordinated function of sensory, reflex, and voluntary motor pathways allows normal elimination. The pathways include both autonomic (sympathetic and parasympathetic) and somatic motor tracts. Classification of the bladder dysfunction requires detailed knowledge of these pathways and is beyond the scope of this chapter. What is presented is a protocol of care for acute management of neurogenic bladder in SCI. This protocol allows safe management of the situation while other acute problems are addressed. For proper management of neurogenic bladder, further workup is necessary.

   1. Maintaining a high degree of suspicion is the single most important factor in diagnosis and management of neurogenic bladder. Any process that can affect balanced control of the bladder (TBI, SCI, lumbosacral plexus injury, stroke) has the potential to cause neurogenic bladder. Remember, the patient

with neurologic injury may maintain good urine output with a bladder that is operating at a very high residual volume, which induces a high risk of infection. Postvoid residual volumes must be checked to ensure that the bladder is emptying properly. Several postvoid volumes of >75 to 100 mL indicate that bladder function requires further attention. The protocol that follows for SCI also will suffice in the acute phase of management with other types of trauma.

a. **Discontinue Foley or suprapubic catheter** unless mandated by coexisting urethral or bladder injury, diabetes insipidus, pharmacologic diuresis, large fluid loads, or other conditions where a high urine volume is expected.

b. **Institute an intermittent catheterization program** as soon as possible after injury, unless contraindicated. Catheterization should be sterile when not performed by the patient. When performed by the patient, the technique can be "clean only." Use a 14 F Bard, Mentor, or MMG Nelaton–type PVC catheter. For intermittent self-catheterization, the catheter should be cleaned with warm water after use, dried, and stored dry in the package. It can be used for up to 1 month.

c. Urinary volumes obtained by catheterization should not exceed 300 mL. Adjust frequency of catheterization according to the patient's typical output pattern. Record all output volumes and incontinent episodes on a frequency and volume chart.

d. Restrict patient fluid intake when on intermittent catheterization so that the total urine output is <1,500 mL/24-hour period.

e. Perform a **fluorourodynamic study** when the patient's bladder is out of spinal shock or at least by 6 months after injury. With lower urinary tract dysfunction as evidenced by detrusor function (incontinence) or autonomic dysreflexia, perform this testing sooner. Repeat testing 1 to 3 months after the initiation of any intervention as a result of the initial urodynamic study, to evaluate the efficacy of the intervention. Conduct this examination on a yearly basis for the first 5 to 10 years after injury and continue on a biennial basis thereafter for optimal monitoring of the lower urinary tracts.

f. Perform a **baseline upper-tract radiologic evaluation** when the patient's bladder is out of spinal shock or at least by 6 months after injury. Renal ultrasound is recommended to evaluate structural abnormalities. Renal scans using intravenous radioisotopes evaluate function and can be quantified to provide an estimate of glomerular flow rate or effective renal plasma flow. Computerized tomography (CT) is essential in evaluating detected structural abnormalities. Plain abdominal x-ray (KUB) can be useful when renal or bladder stones are suspected. Intravenous pyelogram (IVP) does evaluate both function and structure. However, the attendant risks of adverse reaction to the contrast (allergic and nephrotoxic reactions), radiation exposure, and necessity for colonic bowel preparation all decrease the utility of this test as a screening examination for first-line evaluation. Carry out follow-up imaging at the urodynamic assessment intervals noted previously.

g. Carry out **baseline flexible cystoscopy** at the time of the initial urodynamic assessment and repeat at least yearly. With a suspicion of stones or anatomic anomalies, evaluate earlier.

h. Obtain **urine cultures** as a baseline and repeat only as suspicion of infection occurs or yearly in asymptomatic patients. Do not administer prophylactic antibiotics or urinary antiseptics unless a **complicated** urinary tract infection is documented. Complicated urinary tract infection is indicated by symptoms that can include:
   - Fever not attributable to other pathology
   - Increasing spasticity
   - Autonomic dysreflexia
   - Urinary retention or incontinence as a deviation from established patterns

- Hematuria
- More than 50 white blood cells per high-power field on microscopic evaluation
- Evidence of stone disease
- Bacteriuria—>10^2 colonies in specimen obtained by intermittent catheterization, or any growth in samples obtained from indwelling catheters

Existence of a "positive" bacterial culture alone is insufficient to prompt treatment in absence of any of the attendant symptoms described.

  i. Give **pharmacotherapy** to modify bladder function, as appropriate, **based on cystometrogram (CMG) findings.**

E. Neurogenic bowel usually coexists in patients in whom neurogenic bladder is present. Control of pathways for fecal elimination is similar to those for bladder control. The goal of a bowel program is to provide controlled fecal elimination with intervening periods of relative continence so that the individual can participate in daily activities. Because the individual with SCI usually has impaired or absent rectal and perineal sensation, symptoms are usually absent or vague. Lack of appetite or nonspecific malaise may be the only indication that the problem of retained feces exists.

  1. In the initial period after SCI, an ileus typically exists. Once the ileus subsides, the bowel program should be initiated on a routine basis. Initially this should be administered daily. Once the bowel program is producing predictable results, the schedule can be modified if desired. The patient's preinjury bowel pattern is the best guide to modification of timing. Individuals who had routine, daily bowel movements usually will continue with this pattern after injury. Individuals who had less frequent bowel movements may require a less frequent bowel program.

  2. Frequent liquid stools can indicate bowel motility is too great or inspissated feces are blocking the rectum or descending colon. Liquid stool from above passes around this blockage and leaks from the anus. It may be possible to detect a full colon on examination, but the most reliable method of detection is to obtain a KUB (flat plate x-ray study of the abdomen). The proper approach to this problem is to evacuate the colon and then institute a routine and reliable bowel program.

  3. Classify neurogenic bowel as either an upper motor neuron or lower motor neuron injury.

    a. In cases of upper motor neuron injury (tetraplegia), the sacral reflex arcs are intact. Presence of these reflexes is useful in initiating bowel evacuation. In some cases, the individual can initiate evacuation with digital stimulation (stretch) of the anal sphincter or use of a suppository.

    b. In lower motor neuron lesions (*conus medullaris* or *cauda equina* injuries), the local reflexes are lost. This situation is much more difficult to control, often requiring digital disimpaction on a routine basis.

  4. The following bowel program for individuals with SCI also can be initiated for other clinical entities in which bowel control is a problem.

    a. Start the bowel program once the postinjury ileus has resolved and the patient has resumed eating or tube feedings. The goal of the initial management is to start routine bowel management that leads to predictable continence.

    b. A typical bowel management protocol consists of a stool softener titrated to the patient's needs and a mild, orally administered stimulant laxative coordinated with a laxative enema (suppository in selected patients). Initially, this is done on a daily schedule so that evacuation occurs at a time convenient for the patient and nursing staff. Protocol for evening evacuation is Colace (100 mg) twice daily, two tablets of Senokot (Purdue Frederick, Norwalk, Connecticut) at noon, with a Fleet (Lynchburg, Virginia) bisacodyl enema or Dulcolax (Ciba, Woodbridge, New Jersey) suppository, in combination with digital stimulation of the rectum, in the evening. If morning evacuation is desired, the Senokot is given at bedtime.

IV. THE SCOPE OF REHABILITATION FOLLOWING TRAUMA

A. Rehabilitation of patients after trauma occurs in several stages, each with a corresponding venue.

1. **Inpatient rehabilitation** is required when patients, for either physical or cognitive reasons, are unable to manage their own basic self-care or mobility needs because of physical limitations. The goal of inpatient rehabilitation is to reestablish capability for basic routines of daily living so that the patient can function safely in the community, with a minimal amount of physical assistance or supervision. Ideally, patients are restored to the point where they are both physically and cognitively independent, although this is not always possible. Rehabilitation interventions are directed toward minimizing the amount of physical or cognitive assistance that a patient will require on return to the community.

2. Initial phases of **outpatient rehabilitation** are directed toward enhancing the ability of the patient to return to active participation in the community outside the home, and to improving the patient's ability to manage more complex instrumental activities of daily living (e.g., cooking, laundry, managing finances, home maintenance). These tasks involve more complex organizational and executive skills that are frequently affected in brain injury. Patients may also require assistance with behavioral problems that affect their interpersonal relationships. Residual deficits that limit mobility in the community can also be addressed along with continuing cognitive limitations. This phase of rehabilitation is sometimes referred to as "community reentry."

3. The final phase of rehabilitation involves helping the affected individual (now often referred to as a "client" rather than a "patient") return to some form of competitive employment. Referred to as **vocational rehabilitation**, this involves teaching training skills that enable an individual to return to the workplace. It can also involve providing some assistive services (e.g., job placement and job coaching) as well as trial placements in voluntary positions in the community.

Bibliography

Banovac K, Sherman AL, Estores IM, Banovac F. Prevention and treatment of heterotopic ossification after spinal cord injury. *J Spinal Cord Med* 2004;27(4):376–382.

Bar-Shai M, Carmeli E, Coleman R, Reznick AZ. Mechanisms in muscle atrophy in immobilization and aging. *Ann N Y Acad Sci* 2004;1019:475–478.

Kirschblum S, Campagnolo DI, Delisa JA, eds. *Spinal Cord Medicine.* Philadelphia, Pa: Lippincott Williams & Wilkins; 2002:261–274.

Lombard L, Zafonte R. Agitation after traumatic brain injury: Considerations and treatment options. *Am J Phys Med Rehabil* 2005;84(10):797–812.

Oleson CV, Burns AS, Ditunno JF, et al. Prognostic value of pinprick preservation in motor complete, sensory incomplete spinal cord injury. *Arch Phys Med Rehabil* 2005; 86(5):988–992.

Silver J, Yudofsky S, Anderson K. Aggressive disorders. In: Silver JM, McAllister TW, Yudofsky SC, eds. *Textbook of Traumatic Brain Injury.* Washington, DC: American Psychiatric Press; 2005.

Wagner AK, Fabio T, Zafonte RD, et al. Physical medicine and rehabilitation consultation: Relationships with acute functional outcome, length of stay and discharge planning after traumatic brain injury. *Am J Phys Med Rehabil* 2003;82(7):526–536.

Zafonte R, Lombard L, Elovic E. Antispasticity medications: Uses and limitations of enteral therapy. *Am J Phys Med Rehabil* 2004;83(10 suppl):S50–S58.

I. DEEP VENOUS THROMBOSIS (DVT)

A. Definition. DVT refers to any clot (obstructing or nonobstructing) in any deep venous system, including the upper extremity and the calf.

B. Pathophysiology. The mechanism behind clot development relates to **Virchow's Triad**: stasis, injury to the vessel wall, hypercoagulability.

1. Stasis causes interruption of normal laminar flow allowing platelets to come in contact with endothelium; interruption of endothelial integrity exposes the extracellular matrix to platelets.

2. Hypercoagulability relates to excess circulating procoagulant factors +/− diminished anticoagulant factors. In trauma, most evidence points to the intimal injury as the initial inciting event, followed by platelet adhesion, activation of the procoagulant system, and release of thrombin. Hence, direct thrombin inhibitors play a strong role in prevention.

C. Epidemiology

1. **Incidence.** DVT affects more than 2.5 million people each year in the United States. This is likely an underestimation, as many cases go unrecognized. Series have shown the incidence of DVT to be as high as 65% in the untreated major trauma patient.

2. **Risk factors** (Table 50-1). In general, these include age >75 years, immobilization, presence of an acute infectious disease, cancer, general anesthesia, major surgery, estrogen therapy, pregnancy, prior DVT, congestive heart failure, malignancy, hypercoagulable state, and tissue trauma. **Specific to trauma**, risk factors include advanced age, pelvic or lower extremity fracture, spinal cord injury (SCI), head injury (Abbreviated Injury Score [AIS] >3), ventilator days >3, shock, multiple blood transfusions, surgery, fracture of the femur or tibia, complex pelvic fracture, venous injury, immobility, and SCI. Scoring systems have been developed to assess risk factors and better estimate the risk of DVT or pulmonary embolism (PE).

3. **Location.** DVT can occur in any deep venous system.

   a. **Calf vein thrombosis.** Calf vein thrombosis is a clot localized to one or more of the three major named vessels below the knee. Untreated, these can propagate proximally in up to 23% of cases; however, they can also resolve without complications. Although treatment is controversial, follow-up duplex examination to rule out propagation should be performed.

   b. **Ileofemoral vein thrombosis.** Most common site in the trauma patient. Findings may be subtle. Classical presentation is phlegmasia cerulea dolens (PCD)—painful, swollen, bluish leg. More common on the left.

   c. **Upper extremity thrombosis.** The most common cause of upper extremity DVT is subclavian vein catheterization. The incidence of PE may be as high as 12%. Treatment is extrapolated from treatment regimens for lower extremity DVT as no good trials exist for this entity specifically.

   d. **Pelvic vein thrombosis.** Missed by commonly used screening modalities.

TABLE 50-1	DVT Risk Factor Categories

A. Risk factors
- Age >40 y
- Injury Severity Score (ISS) >9
- Blood transfusion
- Surgical procedure ≥2 h
- Lower extremity fracture
- Pelvis fracture
- Spinal cord injury (SCI)
- Immobilization
- Pregnancy
- Estrogen therapy
- History of DVT/PE
- Malignancy
- Hypercoaguable state (e.g., AT III deficiency)
- Extensive soft-tissue trauma
- Congestive heart failure (CHF)

B. High-risk factors
- Age >50 y
- ISS >15
- Femoral central venous catheter in trauma resuscitation
- Abbreviated Injury Score (AIS) ≥3 (any body region)
- Glasgow Coma Scale (GCS) score ≤8
- SCI
- Pelvis fracture
- Femur or tibia fracture
- Venous injury

C. Very high-risk factors
- SCI
- AIS head/neck ≥3 + long bone fracture (upper or lower)
- Severe pelvic fracture (posterior element) + long bone fracture (upper or lower)
- Multiple (≥3) long bone fractures

D. **Complications.** DVT is a major cause of morbidity and mortality.
   1. **Local complications.** Although rare, local ramifications of DVT include PCD (edematous bluish extremity) or phlegmasia alba dolens (PAD; blanching "milk leg") with potential ulceration, loss of arterial flow, or resultant venous gangrene.
   2. **Pulmonary embolism.** Incidence of pulmonary embolism (PE) after trauma varies with population, injury pattern, use of prophylaxis, and method of detection. Overall, 1% to 2% of patients with DVT after trauma will have a PE which carries a 30% to 50% mortality risk.
   3. **Postphlebitic syndrome.** Pathophysiologically, venous valves in the lower extremities are destroyed by clot formation when DVT occurs. After the clot dissolves, valvular competence is permanently lost in the affected segment of vein. As a result, nonpitting edema, swelling, discoloration, and pain frequently occur, which can progress to venous hypertension and venous stasis ulceration. The incidence of postphlebitic changes at 12 years post-DVT approximates 28%. Severe sequelae occur in less than 6%.

E. Diagnosis
   1. **Clinical manifestation.** Subjective complaints of pain or swelling of the affected extremity are rare; only 40% of patients have any clinical signs or symptoms. The classic syndrome of calf discomfort, edema, venous distension, and pain on dorsiflexion of the foot (Homans' sign) is seen in less than 30% of patients.
   2. **D-dimer.** D-dimers are a breakdown product of fibrin and should be elevated when venous thrombosis is present. However, fibrin degradation products are elevated in the first 48 hours after traumatic injury. This calls into question the utility of using admission D-dimer to diagnose DVT in the trauma patient.
   3. **Compression ultrasound.** Duplex ultrasound (DUS) combines real-time B-mode ultrasound with pulsed Doppler capability. In symptomatic patients, the sensitivity and specificity are greater than 95%; thus DUS is the most commonly performed test for the detection of infrainguinal DVT. The addition of color flow imaging reveals physiologic flow characteristics and may be useful in technically challenging examinations. Whether ultrasound is performed with flow assessment or not, **compression** of the vein along its length is the key aspect in evaluation for DVT. **Noncompressibility of the vein is the primary diagnostic criteria for acute DVT.** Other DUS findings include an echogenic thrombus within the vein lumen, venous distension, complete absence of spectral or color Doppler signal from the vein lumen, or loss of flow phasicity, response to Valsalva or augmentation. Limitations of DUS include patient characteristics (obesity, edema, or tenderness), inability to ultrasound through various devices (casts, etc.), or compression of a vein by perivenous pathology (tumor, hematoma). In addition, DUS is unreliable in evaluating iliac veins.
      a. **Surveillance ultrasound.** Routine weekly surveillance of patients at high risk for DVT has been demonstrated to help identify asymptomatic thrombi and may minimize PE rates. The cost-effectiveness of such an approach has not been demonstrated. Routine use of surveillance protocols remains controversial.
   4. **Contrast venography.** While contrast venography (CV) remains the gold standard for diagnosing DVT, it is rarely used due to the accuracy of noninvasive testing. CV is invasive and requires intravenous injection of contrast dye with all the risks associated; however, it is considered to be 100% sensitive and specific. Diagnosis requires a constant intraluminal filling defect in two views or an abrupt cutoff of a deep vein.
   5. **CT venography (CTV).** CTV uses venous phase contrast to directly visualize the inferior vena cava, pelvic, and lower extremity veins. It can be timed immediately after a CT pulmonary angiogram (CTPA) or used alone. However, when combined with CTPA, many series report a higher IV contrast dose necessary for accurate visualization of the vessels. CTV can be plagued by artifact, such as from orthopedic hardware or poor venous enhancement. The sensitivity and specificity are 89% to 100% and 94% to 100%, respectively. Some advantages of CTV are the ready availability of CT scan in most hospitals at off-hours and the ability to do one study to diagnose PE and DVT.
F. Prophylaxis (Fig. 50-1). As trauma patients are at high risk for developing VTE, many centers have developed standardized algorithms for prophylaxis. These forms include early ambulation, mechanical devices such as sequential compression devices (SCDs), and pharmacological therapy such as low-molecular-weight heparin.
   1. **Sequential compression devices (SCDs).** SCDs prevent VTE primarily by a mechanical mechanism. These devices expand intermittently to increase blood flow and expel blood from the lower extremities. They substitute for the calf muscle pumps that are inactive in the nonambulatory trauma patient. A second

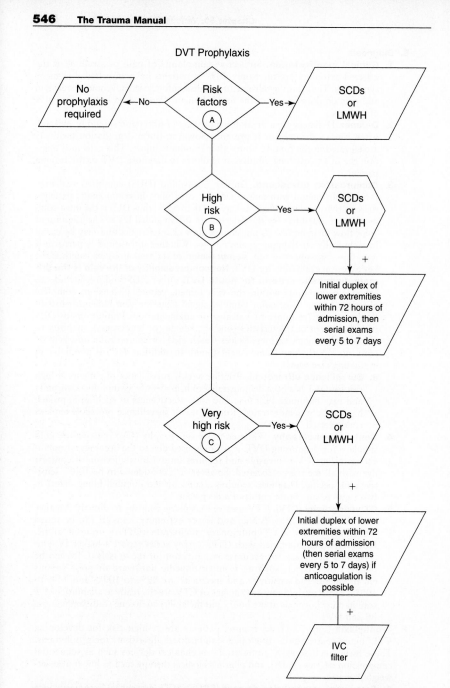

Figure 50-1. DVT prophylaxis. SCDs (sequential compression devices) are indicated when access to both lower extremities is available. Otherwise, LMWH (low-molecular-weight heparin) will be utilized. LMWH is contraindicated in patients with an epidural catheter in place. (Modified from *Clinical Management Guidelines, Deep Venous Thrombosis Prophylaxis*. Philadelphia: Division of Trauma and Surgical Care, Hospital of the University of Pennsylvania; 2000.)

mechanism of action of SCDs is their ability, albeit short-lived, to activate the fibrinolytic system. The intermittent venous compression results in release of plasminogen activators found in all venous walls. This is the means by which they are effective when placed on the upper extremities in cases where the lower extremities are unable to be used. Unfortunately, SCDs are unable to be used in up to 65% of trauma patients due to fractures or hardware. In addition, although the mechanism of action seems logical, randomized prospective trials in trauma patients have shown no benefit of SCDs over no prophylaxis in the prevention of DVT.

2. **AV foot pumps.** The discovery of a venous pump on the plantar aspect of the foot in 1983 led to the development of a device to reproduce this action. This device is attractive because it can often be used when SCDs cannot be placed or when they are ill-fitting. Also, similar to SCDs, they can be used when anticoagulant methods are contraindicated. Recent evidence suggests they may be even less effective than other traditional forms of DVT prophylaxis.

3. **Subcutaneous heparin (SCH).** Low-dose, unfractionated heparin (5,000 U by subcutaneous injection every 8–12 hours) primarily works by enhancing antithrombin III's ability to block Factor Xa, but does not induce a hypocoagulable state. Complications of heparin use primarily include bleeding risk and risk of heparin-induced thrombocytopenia (HIT) development. Although SCH is used regularly as prophylaxis in trauma patients, a meta-analysis of studies done in trauma patients reported no benefit of SCH over no prophylaxis. This among other studies has led to the recommendation to **not routinely use SCH** as prophylaxis in trauma patients.

4. **Low-molecular-weight heparins (LMWHs).** LMWHs are distillates of unfractionated heparin that have better bioavailability and longer plasma half-life. There is a low risk of hemorrhagic complications but not statistically different than SCH. LMWHs have now been widely studied in the trauma population and have been shown to reduce the incidence of DVT when compared to SCH, SCDs, and AV foot pumps. It is therefore recommended that **LMWHs be used for DVT prophylaxis when there is no contraindication to this form of prophylaxis**. Of note, the U.S. Food and Drug Administration has warned of potential bleeding complications in patients where placement of neuraxial anesthesia (epidural or spinal catheter) is to be initiated.

5. **Vitamin K antagonists (VKAs).** VKAs (e.g., warfarin) have been primarily studied in the pelvic and lower extremity fracture population as well as the total hip replacement population. The dosage must be monitored and an international normalized ratio (INR) of 2.5 is preferred. The risk of hemorrhagic complications is much higher than with LMWH or SCH and so it is not typically recommended in the general trauma population.

6. **Selective Factor Xa inhibitors.** This is a class of anticoagulant drugs that specifically provides antithrombin III inhibition of Factor Xa. Fondaparinux is the drug most studied to date and has been shown to reduce the relative risk of VTE by 50% compared to LMWH in large orthopedic trials. There is also preliminary evidence that it may have reduced immunomodulator properties when compared to heparin. Unfortunately, although Fondaparinux has many attractive properties, it has not been adequately studied in the major trauma population and so no recommendation for its use can be made at this time.

G. **Definitive treatment.** The goals of definitive DVT treatment include preventing clot propagation, reducing the risk of PE, facilitating clot lysis, preserving venous valve function, reducing extremity swelling, alleviating pain, and preventing recurrence.

1. **Anticoagulation.** Anticoagulation is the mainstay of DVT treatment, when no contraindication exists. As compared to a few years ago, several forms of anticoagulant therapy exist.

   a. **Heparin** (Table 50-2). Full-dose heparin by constant intravenous (IV) infusion is standard initial therapy for DVT treatment. The partial

TABLE 50-2	Heparin Dosing Guidelines

1. Initial order
Bolus: 70 U/kg
Infusion: 18 U/kg/h

2. Monitor efficacy (6–8 h after initial bolus or change in dosing)
Check PTT: Therapeutic range 51–68 s

3. Heparin adjustment

PTT	Adjustment
<41 s	Rebolus 35 U/kg
	Increase infusion 3 U/kg/h
41–50 s	Increase infusion 2 U/kg/h
51–68 s	No change
69–96 s	Decrease infusion 1 U/kg/h
96–120 s	Hold infusion 30 min
	Decrease infusion 2 U/kg/h
>120 s	Hold infusion 90 min
	Decrease infusion 3 U/kg/h

4. Concomitant orders
CBC with platelet count every other day while on heparin
No intramuscular injections
Check all stools for occult blood

PTT, partial thromboplastin time; CBC, complete blood count. Modified from *Heparin Dosing Protocol.*
Philadelphia: Hospital of the University of Pennsylvania; 2000.

thromboplastin time (PTT) is monitored and heparin is dose adjusted to keep the PTT at 60 to 80. The use of IV heparin is labor intensive and both over- and underanticoagulation can have devastating consequences. Once therapeutic range is reached and no contraindication to warfarin therapy exists, the initiation of warfarin is begun.

b. Direct thrombin inhibitors (DTIs). These are a class of compounds that directly bind with thrombin to prevent its interaction with enzyme substrates. They include lepirudin, argatroban, desirudin, and others. These compounds tend to be very expensive and are reserved to treating DVT or PE in settings where heparin is contraindicated. As of this time, there is no oral form available; therefore, the patient would need to be converted to warfarin just as with initial heparin therapy.

c. LMWH. LMWH at higher doses than for DVT prophylaxis has been proven to be an effective method for the treatment of DVT. Many centers use therapeutic doses of LMWH rather than IV heparin, until the INR is in the therapeutic range for warfarin. LMWH is much less labor intensive as PTT is not intensely monitored and the patient may be trained and discharged home on subcutaneous injections. Anti-Xa levels may be monitored to document therapeutic levels of LMWH compounds; however, this is not routinely done.

d. VKA (warfarin). Warfarin is started after therapeutic range for heparin or DTI is achieved or after 24 hours of LMWH, provided no need for anticoagulation reversal is foreseen. Patients are not started on warfarin as first-line anticoagulation because of the risk of warfarin-induced skin necrosis. The prothrombin time (PT) and INR are monitored and warfarin is dose adjusted to keep the INR at 2.0 to 3.0. The duration of therapy is 3 to 6 months.

2. **Other measures.** Ambulation is generally acceptable even after initial diagnosis. Elevation of the extremity when at rest helps reduce the swelling. Graded compression stockings also may be used to minimize swelling.

II. PULMONARY EMBOLISM (PE)

A. **Definition.** A clot in the main pulmonary artery or its branches that has embolized traditionally from a venous, noncardiac source.

B. **Incidence.** More than 500,000 cases of PE occur annually in the United States. The overall incidence of PE in the injured population is 0.3%; however, it increases to 1% to 2% in patients at risk. The mortality from PE in the severely injured patient may be as high as 20% to 50%.

C. **Diagnosis.** The diagnosis of PE in the trauma patient is often clouded by a number of other medical and surgical problems. In general, patients who have had a PE may have an "impending sense of doom." Dyspnea and pleuritic chest pain are the two most common symptoms. These are nonspecific symptoms frequently present in patients who have sustained thoracic trauma. In addition, signs and symptoms of PE often suggest a differential diagnosis that includes many common conditions and more sophisticated methods of diagnosis are necessary.

1. **Physical examination.** Tachypnea and tachycardia are the most frequently encountered physical signs associated with PE. With massive PE, cyanosis and hypotension may occur. Again, these are very nonspecific symptoms.

2. **Laboratory tests.** An **arterial blood gas (ABG)** is the most useful test to solidify a suspicion of PE. Ninety percent of patients with PE will have a room air PaO_2 <80 mmHg. Hypocarbia (from tachypnea) and hypoxemia are the initial abnormalities on ABG when PE is present. In the trauma patient, however, these abnormalities may be present for a variety of reasons. A **D-dimer** can be helpful as mentioned with DVT, although a positive result is largely unhelpful in the first few days after injury or surgical intervention.

3. **Chest x-ray (CXR).** Classic findings on CXR with PE present include atelectasis or pulmonary infiltrate and pleural effusion. These findings can be difficult to differentiate as cause for symptoms or as a result of PE or other pathology.

4. **Electrocardiogram (EKG).** EKG changes are common, as up to 70% of patients will have an abnormality. ST segment or T-wave changes are most common (up to 50%) and R-wave electrical abnormalities are uncommon (6%). An EKG is, of course, important as PE and myocardial infarction share much of the same symptomatology.

5. **Ventilation-perfusion scintigraphy (V/Q scan).** V/Q scans can be helpful in diagnosing PE; however, other pulmonary abnormalities limit its usefulness. The best chance of an accurate reading comes in the presence of a normal CXR (an uncommon finding in most trauma patients). Even with a normal CXR, a normal V/Q scan carries a 4% PE rate and a high-probability scan carries only an 88% PE rate.

6. **CT pulmonary angiography.** The recent generations of multislice spiral CT scanners have allowed CT pulmonary angiography to be performed as a diagnostic test. Advantages include the ready availability of CT imaging in most institutions, as well as the ability to diagnose other parenchymal or pleural processes that may be causing the physiologic abnormalities that have prompted the workup for a possible PE. Sensitivity and specificity are reported at greater than 90%, although some recent data suggest that the finding of small, peripheral emboli may be of unclear significance.

7. **Pulmonary angiography.** Formal pulmonary angiography remains the gold standard for diagnosis of pulmonary emboli. The test is invasive and involves a contrast load. Advantages include the ability for immediate invasive intervention (Section II.D.2) or placement of an inferior vena cava filter if indicated.

D. **Prophylaxis**

1. **DVT prophylaxis.** Preventing the initial source clot outright allows for the best prevention of PE, as previously stated.

2. **Inferior vena caval filters (IVCFs).** These are devices placed in the infrarenal IVC that prevent the embolic migration of pelvic or LE clots. Today, these are available as retrievable or permanent devices. Certain injury complexes that have historically been shown to be associated with high rates of PE may lend themselves to the placement of prophylactic IVCF. The ability to place retrievable filters may make them a more attractive option as a prophylactic therapy. Many patients at risk should be able to receive an anticoagulant or will have an acceptable mobility status 2 to 6 weeks from the initial injury, greatly reducing the risk of PE. Unfortunately, few data exist on the effectiveness of this approach to PE prevention. There are a number of documented complications from IVCF placement, including DVT, filter migration, and inferior vena caval thrombosis. These are rare, however.

E. **Treatment**

1. **Anticoagulation.** Anticoagulation with heparin, LMWH, or warfarin is the mainstay of therapy. If heparin is chosen, a PTT of 2× normal is the goal. If LMWH is chosen, therapeutic (not prophylactic) doses should be used. In cases where heparin or LMWH cannot be used (e.g., patients with HIT), DTIs may be used as the initial therapy. When Coumadin is started, an INR of 2 to 3 is the goal. Duration of therapy is usually at least 6 months.

2. **Thrombolysis.** This is a controversial method of PE treatment and is contraindicated with many injury profiles. Thrombolytics include streptokinase, urokinase, rTPA (alteplace, reteplace, and tenecteplace). In ICU patients, there seems to be no outcome difference in systemic or catheter-directed therapy. This therapy should be considered only in severely hemodynamically compromised patients, those with right ventricular hypokinesis, and where thrombolysis would not be contraindicated.

3. **Suction embolectomy.** Suction or catheter embolectomy may be warranted in severely compromised individuals with a central PE who have an unquestionable contraindication to thrombolytics. The procedure does require pulmonary angiography and by virtue of the procedure may lead to multiple more peripheral emboli, among other complications. There are scant data on this procedure in the trauma population.

4. **Surgical embolectomy.** The surgical extraction of central pulmonary artery thrombosis was largely abandoned and considered heroic but has recently been undertaken with better success rates than in past. It may be the only option in patients with impending cardiac arrest or severe right ventricular dysfunction/infarction. The procedure does require cardiopulmonary bypass.

AXIOMS

- The incidence of DVT after major trauma remains significant.
- Patients should be evaluated for risk of venous thromboembolism after injury and treated accordingly.
- Duplex ultrasound is a rapid, portable, and noninvasive technique to diagnose DVT.
- Pulmonary embolism should always be considered with unexplained hypoxia, hypocarbia, or an impending sense of doom.
- Prophylactic IVC filter placement may be indicated in the trauma patient with excessive risk.

Bibliography

Geerts WH, Code KI, Jay RM, et al. A prospective study of venous thromboembolism after major trauma. *N Engl J Med* 1994;331:1601–1606.

Geerts WH, Jay RM, Code KI, et al. A comparison of low-dose heparin with low molecular weight heparin as prophylaxis against venous thromboembolism after major trauma. *N Engl J Med* 1996;335:701–707.

Geerts WH, Pineo GF, Heit JH, et al. Prevention of Venous Thromboembolism: The Seventh ACCP Conference on Antithrombolytic Therapy. *Chest* 2004;126:338S–400S.

Knudson MM, Ikossi DG. Venous thromboembolism after trauma. *Curr Opin Crit Care* 2004;10:539–548.

Knudson MM, Morabito D, Paiemont GD, et al. Use of low molecular weight heparin in preventing thromboembolism in trauma patients. *J Trauma* 1996;41:446–459.

Patel S, Kazeerooni EA. Helical CT for the evaluation of acute pulmonary embolism. *Am J Roentgenol* 2005;1185:135–149.

Rosenthal D, Wellons ED, Levitt AB. Role of prophylactic temporary inferior vena cava filters placed at the ICU bedside under intravascular ultrasound guidance in patients with multiple trauma. *J Vasc Surg* 2004;40:958–964.

Winchell RJ, Hoyt DB, Walsh JC, et al. Risk factors associated with pulmonary embolism despite routine prophylaxis: Implications for improved protection. *J Trauma* 1994; 37:600–606.

II. INITIAL ASSESSMENT—TRIAGE AND INITIAL STABILIZATION

RESPONSE

51 DISASTERS/MULTICASUALTY ACCIDENTS
SUSAN M. BRIGGS

I. **INTRODUCTION.** Contemporary disasters follow no rules. The complexity, time, or location of the next disaster cannot be predicted. Disasters, both natural and human-made, including terrorism, encompass the spectrum of threats. Terrorism is the most challenging for medical providers. Weapons of mass destruction (WMDs) creating "contaminated" environments will be the greatest challenge of all. Traditionally, medical providers have held the erroneous belief that all disasters are different, especially those involving terrorism. **All disasters, regardless of etiology, have similar medical and public health concerns.** Disasters differ in the degree to which the medical and public health infrastructure of the affected community is disrupted and the degree to which outside assistance is needed to address these concerns. The severity and diversity of injuries, in addition to the number of victims, will be major factors in determining whether a mass casualty incident requires resources from outside the affected community.

A. **The key principle of disaster medical care is to do the greatest good for the greatest number of patients, while the objective of conventional medical care is to do the greatest good for the individual patient.** A consistent approach to disasters, based on an understanding of their common features and the response expertise they require, is becoming the accepted practice throughout the world. This strategy is called the **mass casualty incident (MCI) response**. MCI response has the primary objective of reducing the morbidity (injury/disease) and the mortality (death) associated with the disaster. All medical responders need to incorporate the key principles of the MCI response in their training given the complexity of today's disasters.

B. MCI management

1. Mass casualty incidents (MCIs) are events that cause casualties large enough to overwhelm the medical and public health services of the affected community. MCIs have traditionally implied a limited geographic location. Many of today's disasters, however, are complex disasters and often occur in austere environments. An austere environment is a setting where resources, transport, access, security, or other aspects of the physical, social, or economic environments impose severe constraints on the adequacy of immediate care for the population. The Asian tsunami (2005) and the Bam, Iran, earthquake (2004) are examples of complex natural disasters. WMDs that contaminate environments have the greatest potential to produce the ultimate austere environment.

2. Similar to the ABCs of trauma care, disaster response includes basic medical and public health concerns that are similar in all disasters. The difference is the degree to which certain responses are needed in a specific disaster, and the degree to which outside assistance, national or international, is needed to perform the ABCs of disaster care.

a. **ABCs of medical response to disasters**
   i. Search and rescue
   ii. Triage and initial stabilization
   iii. Definitive care
   iv. Evacuation

b. **ABCs of public health response to disasters**
   i. Water
   ii. Food
   iii. Shelter
   iv. Sanitation
   v. Safety/Security
   vi. Transportation
   vii. Communication
   viii. Disease surveillance
   ix. Endemic/epidemic diseases

II. **INCIDENT COMMAND SYSTEM.** Many different organizations participate in the response to disasters. The Incident Command System (ICS) was created to allow different agencies (fire, police, emergency medical services, hospitals) and/or multiple departments of organizations to work together effectively in response to a disaster. The ICS uses a common organizational structure and language to achieve this goal and is the accepted standard for all disaster response. ICS may expand or contract to meet needs in a specific disaster.

A. The organizational structure of ICS is built around five major management activities. Not all activities are used for every disaster. Functional requirements, not titles, determine ICS hierarchy.

1. **ICS hierarchy**
   a. **Incident Command**—maintains overall response for disaster response
   b. **Operations**—directs disaster resources
   c. **Planning**—develops action plans
   d. **Logistics**—provides personnel and supplies
   e. **Financial/Administrative**—monitors costs

2. Several principles are important for effective use of the ICS in disasters:
   a. The incident commander and other key positions must be identified and trained before a disaster occurs, not at the time of a disaster.
   b. ICS must be started early, before an incident gets out of control.
   c. Medical and public health responders, often used to working independently, must adhere to the structure of the ICS to avoid potentially negative consequences, including:
      i. Death of medical personnel due to lack of safety or training
      ii. Inadequate or inappropriate medical supplies to provide care
      iii. Staff working beyond their training or certification
   d. **The structure of the ICS is the same regardless of the nature of the disaster.** The only difference is in the particular expertise of key personnel and the extent of the ICS utilized in a particular disaster. For example, the safety officer will vary by the type of disaster:
      i. **Biological incident**—infection control expert
      ii. **Chemical incident**—hazardous material expert
      iii. **Radiation incident**—radiation detection expert

III. **MEDICAL RESPONSE TO DISASTERS**

A. **Search and rescue.** The local population near any disaster site is the immediate search and rescue resource. Many countries have developed specialized search and rescue teams as an integral part of their national disaster plans. Members of these teams receive specialized training in "confined space environments." Team members may be called on to provide critical care in the field, such as airway control, including intubation, vascular access, pain control, hypothermia care, and immobilization or amputation of injured extremities.

1. Search and rescue units generally include:
   a. A cadre of medical specialists
   b. Technical specialists knowledgeable in hazardous material, heavy equipment operation, structural engineering, and technical search and rescue techniques
   c. Trained canines and their handlers

B. **Triage and initial stabilization.** Triage is the most important, and often the most psychologically difficult, mission of any disaster medical response, regardless of the nature of the MCI. The objective of disaster triage (field triage) is to do the greatest good for the greatest number of people. Both undertriage and overtriage of victims limits the effectiveness of the disaster response.

1. **Field medical triage.** Field triage may be conducted at three levels, depending on the number of victims and available resources. Triage is a "dynamic" process.

   a. **On-site triage.** Victims are categorized at a casualty collection site into two categories, acute and nonacute. Simplified color coding may be done if resources permit. Personnel are typically first responders from the local population or local emergency medical personnel.

   b. **Medical triage.** Rapid categorization of victims at a casualty collection site is performed by experienced medical personnel with knowledge of the medical consequences of various injuries (e.g., burns; blast or crush injuries; or exposure to chemical, biological, or radioactive agents). Color coding may be used.

      i. Red = Casualties who require immediate lifesaving interventions

      ii. Yellow = Casualties for whom treatment can be delayed or casualties (expectant) who are not expected to survive due to severity of injuries or lack of resources

      iii. Green = Individuals who require minimal or no medical care

      iv. Black = Deceased victims

   c. **Evacuation triage.** Priorities for transfer to medical facilities are assigned to disaster victims. The casualty collection site for triage should be located in an upwind location from the contaminated environment and close to the disaster site but safe from hazards. The site should have easy visibility for disaster victims and convenient exit routes for air and land evacuation.

C. **Definitive medical care.** Definitive medical care refers to care that will improve, rather than simply stabilize, a casualty's condition. In some disasters, local hospitals may be destroyed, transportation to medical facilities may not be feasible, or the environment may be contaminated. In these situations, definitive care must be provided outside traditional medical facilities. Hospital teams with mobile equipment that can provide a graded, flexible response to the need for definitive medical care in disasters are key to a successful disaster response and have been developed by many countries and hospitals. Disaster medical assistance teams must be able to provide care for routine emergencies/diseases as well as disaster-related injuries.

1. **Evacuation.** Evacuation may be useful in a disaster to decompress the disaster area and provide specialized care for specific casualties, such as those with burns and crush injuries. Modes of evacuation include ground transport, helicopter transport, and transport by fixed-wing aircraft. Medical providers must take into account patient stresses of flight that may be encountered during evacuation and affect medical care. These include changes related to the hypobaric environment, decreased partial pressure of oxygen, turbulence, vibration, varying temperatures, and low humidity.

IV. **PUBLIC HEALTH RESPONSE TO DISASTERS.** Medical providers must understand the impact of disasters on the public health infrastructure in order to have an efficient medical response.

A. **Rapid needs assessment** provides timely evaluation of the impact of the disaster on the affected population. Rapid needs assessment includes (1) assessment of the magnitude of the disaster; (2) assessment of lifeline services (water, food, and emergency temporary shelter); and (3) assessment of the capacity of the affected community to respond to the disaster needs. Media reports can provide valuable information regarding the magnitude of the disaster, particularly in the area of greatest impact.

V. THE THREAT OF TERRORISM AND WMDs. Terrorism is the most challenging MCI for emergency responders. The spectrum of terrorist threats is limitless, ranging from suicide bombers (London attacks), conventional explosives, military weapons, and WMDs (nuclear, chemical, and biological).

A. One of the unique features of a terrorist threat, especially involving WMDs, is that psychogenic casualties predominate. Terrorists do not have to kill people to achieve their goals; creating a climate of fear and panic to overwhelm the medical infrastructure achieves their goals. In the March 1995 sarin attacks in Tokyo, 5,000 casualties were referred to hospitals. Fewer than 1,000 were suffering from the effects of the gas. The anthrax incidents in the United States dramatically increased the number of individuals presenting to emergency departments with nonspecific respiratory symptoms. WMDs have the greatest potential to generate casualties large enough to overwhelm most emergency medical systems and to produce "contaminated" environments. No longer will emergency responders be able to bring victims into hospitals for fear of contaminating medical facilities.

B. Blast injuries. Explosions and bombings related to terrorism continue to be a frequent cause of mass casualties in disasters. The majority of terrorist bombings consist of relatively small explosives that produce low casualty rates. The effects of the blast wave are increased in a closed space such as a building or bus and underwater. The high morbidity and mortality is related not only to the intensity of the blast, but also to the subsequent structural damage that leads to collapse of buildings, a common phenomena in large explosions.

1. Injuries caused by explosives and bombings can be divided into four categories:
   a. Primary blast injury
   b. Secondary blast injury
   c. Tertiary blast injury
   d. Miscellaneous injuries such as crush and burn injuries

2. Secondary blast injuries are the most common cause of death in explosions (flying debris, metal, and glass).

C. Biological agents. Biological terrorism is the use of microorganisms or toxins derived from living organisms to produce death or disease in humans, animals, or plants. The following disease agents are believed to have the greatest potential for bioterrorism:
   ■ Anthrax (bacteria)
   ■ Tularemia (bacteria)
   ■ Plague (bacteria)
   ■ Smallpox (virus)
   ■ Viral hemorrhagic fevers (virus)
   ■ Botulinum (toxin)

1. The route of exposure of greatest concern with biological terrorist attacks is inhalation of the agent. Oral routes of exposure for biological agents are less important, but still significant. Ensuring that food and water supply is free of contamination is an important function of public health after a biological attack. Dermal exposure is unusual but possible, especially if the skin is damaged.

2. The most effective and important prophylaxis against biological agents is physical protection. A full-face respirator prevents exposure of the respiratory and mucous membranes to infectious agents. Any dermal exposure should be treated immediately by washing with soap and water.

3. Early recognition of an MCI resulting from bioterrorism is the key to success. The following are indications of a possible biological attack:
   a. Disease entity that is unusual or does not occur naturally in a given geographic area
   b. Suspected aerosol route of exposure
   c. Massive point-source outbreak
   d. High morbidity and mortality

4. Chemical agents. Chemical agents are now terrorist weapons. Most chemical warfare agents are liquids. Chemical agents in liquid form must be dispersed in order to be maximally effective. This can be done in three general ways:

- Aerosolizing it with an aerial sprayer (such as done with pesticides)
- Aerosolizing it in an explosion
- Allowing it to evaporate and dispersing the vapor

a. The five principle classes of chemical agents are:
  i. Nerve agents
  ii. Vesicants (blistering agents)
  iii. Cyanide
  iv. Pulmonary agents
  v. Riot control agents
b. Personal protection (full protective equipment, including mask, gloves, and suit) and decontamination are the key priorities when responding to a chemical attack. The first thing responders should do is establish a clean treatment area ("cold zone") at least 300 yards upwind of the contaminated area ("hot zone").

5. **Radioactive agents. Nuclear material** use by terrorists would likely involve one of four scenarios:
  a. Detonation of a nuclear device
  b. Meltdown of a nuclear reactor
  c. Dispersal of material through use of conventional explosives: a radiation dispersal device (RDD) or "dirty bomb"
  d. Nonexplosive dispersal of nuclear material: placing radioactive materials in public places
  e. Casualties who have been irradiated are not radioactive themselves unless radioactive material ("fallout") has been deposited on or in their bodies. Since the clinical effects of all but the most severe radiation exposures are delayed, the clinical presentation of exposed casualties will be primarily related to conventional injuries, and normal trauma triage procedures should be employed.

VI. **DISASTER PREPAREDNESS. AN ALL-HAZARDS APPROACH IS THE KEY PRINCIPLE OF DISASTER PREPAREDNESS.** Medical treatment in disasters requires substantial modification in the content and application when compared with standard approaches used in everyday medical care. Training and supervision of medical professionals who aspire to work in these settings must pay explicit attention to these newly recognized challenges. Training of medical providers must include the basics of disaster care such as field triage, decontamination, and WMDs.

INJURY PREVENTION

CHARLES C. BRANAS

52

I. INTRODUCTION. Worldwide, injury is the leading cause of death for the first half of the human life span and a regular source of disability and disfigurement. Daily in the United States, more than 320,000 men, women, and children are injured severely enough to seek medical care. About 200 of these people will sustain a long-term disability due to their injuries and an additional 400 people will die.

Injury is among the top five causes of death in the United States. The composite of unintentional injury deaths, suicides, and homicides was the leading cause of death in those from 1 to 44 years of age. Unintentional injury alone is the fifth leading cause of death for all age groups and, when combined with suicide, is the fourth leading cause of death. In 2002, over 156,000 injury-related deaths were documented. The top five mechanisms of injury deaths in the United States were motor vehicles (45,579), firearms (30,242), poisonings (26,435), falls (17,116), and suffocation (12,791).

Around the world, about 16,000 individuals die each day, and nearly 6 million die each year from injuries. In all age groups, injury is a significant cause of death and 1 of 10 deaths globally is from an injury. In 1998, among high-income countries (including the United States), road traffic injuries were the leading cause of death for those aged 5 to 44 years. In these same countries, road traffic injuries, self-inflicted injuries, and interpersonal violence were the top three causes of death in the 15 to 44 years of age group.

Mortality alone does not characterize adequately the profound physical, psychosocial, and economic effects of injury. Over one third of all U.S. emergency department (ED) visits, an estimated 39 million, are related to injury. The most common injuries, accounting for 40% of injury-related ED visits, were from falls, nonvehicular strikes, and motor vehicle crashes (MVCs). It is estimated that nearly 1 in 6 Americans will require treatment for injuries and over 2 million Americans will be hospitalized for injuries each year. In 2000, total injury-attributable medical costs were estimated to be $117 billion, or about 10% of all medical costs in the United States. The estimated total cost of injury in the United States, based on direct medical care, rehabilitation, lost wages, lost productivity, and death and disability benefits, is estimated at $260 billion each year.

Injury most commonly affects individuals early in their productive life (i.e., young adults). The years of productive life lost from all injuries >3.5 million, outranking diseases such as cancer, heart disease, and human immunodeficiency virus (HIV) for which each has <2 million years of productive life lost. More recently, disability-adjusted life years (DALY) have been used to measure the burden of injury. DALYs combine the number of years of life loss from premature death with the loss of health and presence of disability in survivors of injury. Simplistically, one DALY is equivalent to one lost year of healthy and productive life. According to the World Health Organization (WHO), 16% of the world's burden of disease in 1998 was attributed to injury using the DALY methodology. The WHO projects that injuries will impose an even greater burden by the year 2020.

Physicians typically focus on the resuscitation and definitive treatment of injuries. However, recognizing the immense societal burden of injury, and the fact that as much as one half of all injury deaths take place at the scene of the injury or within minutes of the event itself, necessitates expansion of the medical mission to include prevention of injury before it occurs.

II. UNDERSTANDING INJURY PREVENTION

A. Injury deserves attention as a leading cause of death and disability around the world. Injury also deserves attention because it occurs as part of a unique disease process: violence, suicide attempts, falls, and MVCs are all disease-generating events that can suddenly kill or disable otherwise healthy people. This is in contrast to other leading diseases, which generally become noticeable after months or years of risk exposure and have relatively slow pathophysiologic processes. Thus, injury develops in a fraction of a second, often after a similarly sudden exposure to one or more risk factors, making its study and prevention especially challenging.

B. Injury occurs across a timeline or continuum: from early precursors to the defining disease event to immediate and long-term consequences. Opportunities to prevent or ameliorate injury correspondingly differ across this continuum: **primary prevention** seeks to completely avert injuries by altering susceptibility or reducing exposure; **secondary prevention** employs early detection and prompt treatment of injuries once they occur; and **tertiary prevention** focuses on limiting disability and restoring function for injured individuals.

Although the medical system is rooted in secondary and tertiary prevention, primary prevention is a potentially more efficient way to relieve the burden of injury. Thus, prevention of all types of injury is a priority and an expectation of personnel in hospitals, both trauma centers and those that are not. The Committee on Trauma (COT) of the American College of Surgeons mandates that trauma center personnel educate the public about injury as a major public health problem. Physicians are natural leaders in expanding trauma care to include the primary prevention of injury. The COT also suggests that physicians move beyond just public education to activities that include surveillance, epidemiology, intervention research, and the evaluation of prevention program effectiveness.

III. THE SCIENCE OF INJURY PREVENTION

A. The science of injury prevention has its roots in many fields including medicine, public health, criminology, engineering, and others. Among the earliest attempts to systematize the approach to injury prevention was put forth by Dr. William Haddon a quarter century ago in the form of 10 injury countermeasures:

1. Prevent the creation of the hazard in the first place.
2. Reduce the amount of the hazard brought into being.
3. Prevent the release of the hazard that already exists.
4. Modify the release of the hazard that already exists.
5. Separate, in time and space, the hazard and that which is to be protected.
6. Separate, by material barrier, the hazard and that which is to be protected.
7. Modify the relevant basic qualities of the hazard.
8. Make that to be protected more resistant to damage from the hazard.
9. Counter damage already done by the hazard.
10. Stabilize, repair, and rehabilitate the object of the hazard.

To the prevention strategist, these countermeasures gave basic guidance on when to intervene, what to intervene on, and how to intervene. More important, they offered a system whereby the prevention strategist would leave no stone unturned. That is, by considering all 10 countermeasures, he or she would ensure that no potentially effective intervention was overlooked.

B. Knowledge of successful strategies to reduce the burden of specific injuries has increased. The decline in incidence of motor vehicle injuries is a case in point. Although motor vehicle injuries continue to be the leading cause of injury death in the United States, their rates have declined considerably over the past 25 years (Fig. 52-1). This decrease is the result of systematic and multifaceted prevention efforts that include the implementation of adequate surveillance systems (for instance, the Fatality Analysis Reporting System at the National Highway

Mortality Rate, 1962–1997: *Firearm & Motor Vehicle-Related Death*

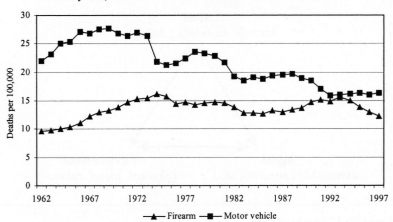

Figure 52-1. Firearm and motor vehicle–related death rates. (From National Center for Injury Prevention and Control, Centers for Disease Control and Prevention, with permission.)

Traffic Safety Administration), the enforcement of government regulations (such as through updated Federal Motor Vehicle Safety Standards), the introduction of active (such as seat belts) and passive (such as airbags) safety devices, improved roadway design (such as left-turn jughandles), advocacy for shifts in social norms (such as peer intolerance of drunk driving), and improved trauma care systems.

C. This success has, however, not extended to all mechanisms of injury, as can be seen in the concurrent increase in firearm injury fatality during the same time period that motor vehicle injury fatalities decreased (Fig. 52-1). Nevertheless, the successful injury prevention strategies used in reducing motor vehicle injuries can also be used to address other major injuries such as those related to firearms and falls. To ensure a high probability of success, these prevention strategies should always be multifaceted, essentially diversifying the prevention strategist's portfolio to defend against failure in any one particular intervention. Moreover, injury prevention strategists should always proceed scientifically, under the mantle of sound evidence, and with the understanding that injuries are not random events. The science of injury deterrence is best founded on epidemiologic surveillance followed by the implementation of prevention strategies that have been thoughtfully designed and systematically evaluated. The following four steps can be taken to more fully understand the epidemiology of specific injuries and mount prevention strategies:

1. Determine the magnitude, scope, and characteristics of the problem. National surveillance data provide a global indication of the scope of injury in the United States. Systems such as the Fatality Analysis Reporting System, a surveillance system for motor vehicle fatalities, and the National Electronic Injury Surveillance System (NEISS), a stratified sample of U.S. EDs, are illustrations of nationally available data that assist with prevention efforts. National- and state-level data can assist in identifying trends and allocating resources to address priority regional problems. However, it is most important to gain an understanding of injury in the local community. Electronic emergency medical services logs, hospital discharge databases, trauma registries,

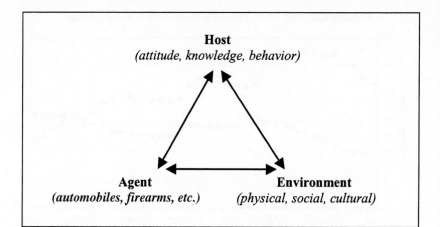

Figure 52-2. Public health model.

and electronic death certificate data can be used to study injury specific to a local community.

2. **Identify risk factors and determine which of those factors are potentially modifiable.** A traditional public health model is a helpful framework to identify and tackle modifiable risk factors for injury (Fig. 52.2). The components of this model are hosts (people and their risky behaviors), agents (automobiles, firearms, knives), and environments (physical [e.g., road design, throw rugs, poor lighting]; economic [e.g., high unemployment]; social [e.g., access to and use of drugs and alcohol]; and temporal [e.g., season or time of day]). By categorizing injury risks into host, agent, and environment, a comprehensive portfolio of interventions can be created that highlights the complexity of the etiologic chain of events leading to injury. Analysis of these events is an important step in identification of modifiable risk factors. Because the occurrence of injury is often the result of a series of complex, often nonmedical, processes, it is helpful to work with an interdisciplinary team that includes individuals such as other health care providers, epidemiologists, engineers, criminologists, political scientists, economists, and behavioral scientists.

3. **Consider a range of strategies to reduce injury.** All trauma centers are required to participate in trauma prevention. It is important for trauma centers to take the lead in examining the effectiveness of implementing interventions at the local level. In the absence of a program of prevention research, trauma centers can take interventions shown to be effective in other communities and examine if these same interventions can be transferred to their local community. A priori public support, commitment from community and political leaders, and media coverage are indicators that an intervention strategy might be successfully transplanted and implemented. In addition, strategies can best be judged if they are linked to specific, measurable outcomes (e.g., public feelings of safety, injury incidence, mortality) which should be discussed and decided on before actual implementation.
   a. **Implement and evaluate the most promising strategies.**

4. Some strategies, known to be effective, can form the foundation of a prevention program. Strategies such as seat-belt use, child restraints, separate storage and locking of ammunition and weapons, and designated driver programs are tested interventions that can be implemented in all communities.

IV. RESPONSIBILITIES OF PHYSICIANS

Primary prevention of injury is an important obligation, and physicians have two main roles: to spearhead trauma prevention at the community level and to incorporate patient-specific prevention in daily practice. These roles can manifest themselves as part of several day-to-day and long-term activities that physicians and other health care providers can participate in to begin reducing injury in their communities.

A. Educate the public that injuries are preventable, nonrandom events. Physicians are respected members of the community and can powerfully advocate for injury prevention. A vital first step is to overcome the fatalistic view of injuries as "accidents." Injuries are not random events and should be addressed accordingly. Asking trauma care providers to consider avoiding the word "accident" from their vocabulary is a key action that can help debunk public fatalism and more appropriately place injuries on solid public health footing with other diseases. Presenting unique profiles of individuals at risk for injury aids in identifying high-risk groups and the factors that contribute to the injury.

B. Recruit colleagues and collaborate with key players. Effective prevention efforts require a multitude of skills that extend beyond those typically held by physicians. As leaders of trauma centers and leaders in prevention, physicians can magnify their effectiveness by joining together with other interested parties. For example, involving the hospital media relations department can be key in helping establish contacts with local media and in framing any injury prevention messages that need to be communicated. Making connections with community leaders and elected officials will additionally bring new ideas, new contacts, and new people with nonmedical skills and resources to help solve the problem.

C. Identify priority injuries to address in the community. Defining the injury problem specific to the local community helps frame efforts and target resources to those injuries having the greatest impact on the local community. It is important to focus on a targeted at-risk population. A good first step is to use data that are retrievable from trauma center registries. This will provide information on the nature of injuries that reach the trauma center or centers in question. This can be supplemented by other sources of nonfatal and fatal injury data (e.g., hospital discharge data, morgue records, law enforcement, and emergency medical services run data) to create a community-specific profile. Local data analyses can then be placed in context by comparing them with state and national statistics. These data will highlight the injuries of importance to the community served by the trauma center. Injuries that should be prioritized for prevention activities are those that occur most frequently, have the highest mortality, or are most likely to result in prolonged disability. Data that are specific to the local community are the most persuasive in generating sustained interest and commitment from the public and community leaders.

D. Disseminate injury information of importance to the community. The general public has a general understanding of injury in their local community. In some cases this understanding of injury can be skewed and is often driven by the most recent high-profile event that received local or national media attention. These high profile cases, however, can be unusual and often do not adequately reflect the nature of the injury problem in a particular community. Furthermore, the general public is constantly exposed to messages that highlight their risks from a variety of threats, but have limited understanding or knowledge of how to weigh the importance of these various risks to their communities or their own lives. Trauma physicians are in a prime position to communicate the actual profile of injury risk in their specific communities and to inform the public of the relative risk of various activities or behaviors. In this way it is important to decide on the main injury prevention messages that will go to the community and to educate fellow professionals to be data-driven, objective spokespeople for these messages.

E. Secure funding and implement local projects. In today's health care environment, hospitals often cannot independently fund or implement prevention activities aimed at the community. Therefore, would-be injury prevention strategists would do well to promptly establish an advisory board, composed of community leaders, who can assist in obtaining funds to support community-based interventions. Moreover, although many trauma centers cannot undertake major research agendas in creating and testing injury prevention strategies, they can utilize established prevention programs. Using established programs that have already been shown to be effective is efficient and can secure interest and funding from local leaders. Efficient use of limited funds can also be accomplished by focusing on a specific mechanism of injury, a specific risk factor, or a specific target population. Choosing a specific prevention program is driven both by the data and by the interest and willingness of the community to support and participate. Together with colleagues, advisory board, and community partners, develop an implementation plan that will serve as a roadmap for what needs to be accomplished and who is responsible at what timeline milestones. Evaluate frequently to ensure that the planned activities are being carried out and that the program will produce results (including both proclamations of success as well as recognition of unsuccessful strategies that can be discontinued).

F. Help shape reasonable policy decisions.
   1. The most effective interventions are those that passively safeguard public health rather than those that require active behavioral change. In contrast to active interventions (most typically education campaigns), passive interventions, by definition, do not require individuals to do anything to protect themselves (e.g., better road design, air bags, padded floor in nursing homes). However, passive interventions do meet with public disapproval because they can sometimes limit personal liberties and burden the day-to-day lives of those they are intended to protect. Moreover, as with all interventions, they can have unintended consequences.
   2. Policymakers frequently look to experts in the field to secure information and help shape decisions. Physicians can be approached to present testimony before legislative bodies, giving them the opportunity to present relevant data combined with the human aspects of injury. Developing appropriate and reasonable injury prevention policies is an important function that trauma centers can perform in support of this. Physicians can also take a more proactive stance and spearhead efforts to enact legislation that is driven by their data. In this case, it is important to secure the support of one or more key legislators, and their staff, to sponsor the legislation. Injury data are more convincing when they are packaged in a way that presents an understandable, fair, and balanced portrayal of the problem at hand.

G. Work with industry to improve product design and safety. One strategy to reduce the burden of injury is to work directly with industry in creating safer products. Obviously, not all physicians will assume this role. However, this can be an effective intervention to reduce injury. Working with the Consumer Product Safety Commission, automobile manufacturers, child safety seat manufacturers, or firearm manufacturers to establish safety standards for their products are some examples of past industry involvements by health care providers.

H. Incorporate injury prevention into daily practice. Physicians can incorporate injury prevention as a core part of daily clinical practice. Trauma patients can be especially receptive to one-on-one prevention counseling from health care providers during the "teachable moment" that follows an injury. A helpful first step is to document risk factors that potentially contributed to the injury episode. Again, one consideration is to separate risk factors into host, agents, and environments. Documenting specific risk factors will guide potential interventions and might lead to appropriate strategies to reduce future injuries. These strategies can include counseling, teaching, and referrals to abuse counselors.

I. Systematize routine screens to identify patients at risk. Physicians should put systematic routine screens in place to identify patients at risk for recidivism. Screens to capture the presence of interpersonal violence (domestic and child abuse); use of illegal drugs (biological screens); elderly falls (physical surroundings, comorbid conditions, medications); and abuse of alcohol (CAGE, biological screens) can help identify patients at high risk. For example, the CAGE screen is one that has proved effective in identifying patients with an alcohol problem. CAGE is a mnemonic of the following four items: Have you ever felt you should **c**ut down on your drinking?; Have people **a**nnoyed you by criticizing your drinking?; Have you ever felt bad or **g**uilty about your drinking?; Have you ever had a drink first thing in the morning to steady your nerves or get rid of a hangover (**e**ye-opener)? A positive reply to any of these questions suggests the need for intervention and a positive response to two or more of these questions should prompt a referral for alcohol treatment.

J. Reduce recidivism by referring patients at high risk to appropriate services. Linking patients identified as high risk with established community services, either through positive routine screens or as indicated by the circumstances surrounding the injury event, allows the routine initiation of appropriate interventions to lessen the potential for recidivism. Such interventions include but are not limited to individual counseling of at-risk patients (e.g., seatbelt and helmet use, safe firearm storage); group counseling by capable professionals; referral to suitable in-hospital services (e.g., substance abuse, psychiatric follow-up); and linkages to community-based resources (e.g., domestic abuse hotlines and shelters). Although it will not be possible for all physicians, forays into the community, to visit front-line services and see the living conditions and actual risk factors that generate injuries for patients, are highly educational and will enhance any hospital-based injury prevention program.

V. SUMMARY

Physicians perform a key role in the prevention of injury. Individual physicians can focus on one aspect of prevention that is either clinically or research oriented. The prevention strategist who uses tested interventions in clinical practice is as pivotal as the research-based prevention strategist whose focus is largely in building generalizable knowledge about injury prevention. Prevention activities are a rewarding extension of the acute care trauma mission and hold the promise of greatly reducing the magnitude of injury morbidity and mortality.

Bibliography

Baker SP, O'Neill B, Ginsburg MJ, Li G. *The Injury Fact Book*. New York, NY: Oxford University Press; 1992:14–15.

Barss P, Smith GS, Baker SP, Mohan D. *Injury Prevention: An International Perspective*: *Epidemiology, Surveillance, and Policy*. New York, NY: Oxford University Press; 1998:1–11.

Bonnie RJ, Fulco CE, Liverman CT, eds. *Reducing the Burden of Injury: Advancing Prevention and Treatment*. Washington, DC: Institute of Medicine, National Academy Press; 1999.

Branas CC, Nance ML, Elliott MR, Richmond TS, Schwab CW. Urban-rural shifts in intentional firearm death: Different causes, same results. *Am J Public Health* 2004; 94(10):1750–1755.

Branas CC, Richmond TS, Schwab CW. Firearm homicide and firearm suicide: Opposite but equal. *Public Health Rep* 2004;119(2):114–124.

Centers for Disease Control and Prevention. Ten great public health achievements—United States, 1900–1999. *Morb Mortal Wkly Rep* 1999;48(12):241–243.

Cherpitel CJ. Screening for alcohol problems in the emergency department. *Ann Emerg Med* 1995;26(2):158–166.

Committee on Trauma, American College of Surgeons. *Resources for Optimal Care of the Injured Patient: 1999*. Chicago, Ill: American College of Surgeons; 1998.

Finkelstein EA, Fiebelkorn IC. Medical expenditures attributable to injuries—United States, 2000. *Morb Mortal Wkly Rep* 2004;53(1):1–4.

Haddon W. The basic strategies for reducing hazards of all kinds. *Hazard Prev* September/October 1980:8–12.

Haukeland JV. Welfare consequences of injuries due to traffic accidents. *Accident Analysis Prev* 1996;28:63–72.

Karlson TA, Hargarten SW. *Reducing Firearm Injury and Death.* New Brunswick, NJ: Rutgers University Press; 1997.

Kaufmann CR, Branas CC, Brawley ML. A population-based study of trauma recidivism. *J Trauma* 1998;45(2):325–331; discussion 331–332.

Krug EG, Sharma GK, Lozano R. The global burden of injuries. *Am J Public Health* 2000;90(4):523–526.

Meyer M. Death and disability from injury: A global challenge. *J Trauma* 1998; 44(1):1–12.

Murray C, Lopez AD. Alternative projections of mortality and disability by cause 1990–2020: Global burden of disease study. *Lancet* 1997;349(9064):1498–1504.

Murray C, Lopez AD. Mortality by cause for eight regions of the world: Global burden of disease study. *Lancet* 1997;349(9061):1269–1276.

National Center for Health Statistics. *Latest Final Mortality Statistics Available.* Available at: http://www.cdc.gov/nchs/releases/99facts/99sheets/97mortal.htm. Accessed January 2000.

National Center for Injury Prevention and Control. *Ten Leading Causes of Death, United States, 1997, All Races, Both Sexes.* Available at: http://www.cdc.gov/ncipc/osp/states/101c97.htm. Accessed January 2000.

National Center for Injury Prevention and Control. *Years of Potential Life Lost before Age 65 (YPLL) by Cause of Death, U.S. 1995.* Available at: http://www.cdc.gov/ncipc/images/ypll95.gif. Accessed January 2000.

Richmond TS, Schwab CW, Riely J, et al. Effective trauma center partnerships to address firearm injury: A new paradigm. *J Trauma* 2004;56(6):1197–1205.

Richmond TS, Thompson H, Deatrick J, Kauder DK. The journey towards recovery following physical trauma. *J Adv Nurs* 2000;32:1341–1347.

Rivera FP, Britt J. *You Can Do It: A Community Guide to Injury Prevention.* Available at: http://www.aast.org/YouCan.html. Accessed August 2000.

World Health Organization. *Injury: A Leading Cause of the Global Burden of Disease.* Geneva: World Health Report; 1999.

53

MISCELLANEOUS PROCEDURES
GLEN TINKOFF AND FORREST O. MOORE

I. URINARY CATHETER
A. Indications
1. Patient not following commands
2. Hemodynamic instability
3. Obvious indication for operative intervention (i.e., distended abdomen, open fractures)
4. External signs of major torso trauma
5. Spinal fractures

B. Contraindications
1. Stable patient with minimal evidence of trauma
2. High suspicion of urethral injury in the male
   a. Blood in urethral meatus
   b. Scrotal ecchymosis
   c. Boggy or high-riding prostate on rectal examination

C. Technique
1. **Insertion in the male patient**
   a. Prepare the glans of the penis with antiseptic solution.
   b. With the nondominant hand, stretch the shaft of the penis gently and extend upward.
   c. Hold the catheter close to the meatus and with the dominant hand gently insert the catheter with 1-cm advances.
   d. Resistance will be met at the posterior urethral sphincter. It is overcome by stopping the advancement temporarily and applying gentle, forward pressure on the catheter until the sphincter relaxes, which can take several seconds.
   e. Advance catheter until urine is obtained. (In a male patient, insert the catheter the entire length to avoid inflation of the balloon in the urethra.) Inflate the balloon, and then withdraw the catheter until gently tethered by the balloon.
   f. Discard the initial 5 mL of urine and test the second 5 mL for blood with a dipstick. Formal urinalysis is unnecessary in the male (Chapter 30).

2. **Insertion in the female patient**
   a. The anatomic position of the female urethra is variable and can be difficult to visualize. Use supplemental lighting and an assistant. Place the patient in a frogleg position, when possible, and have the assistant spread the labial folds.
   b. Prepare the urethra with antiseptic.
   c. Advance the catheter gently.
   d. Upon return of urine, inflate the balloon.
   e. Urethral injury is uncommon.

3. **Pediatric**
   a. Use an appropriately sized catheter (a small polyethylene feeding tube can be used in an infant) (Chapter 46).
   b. Gentle insertion is essential.
   c. During insertion, spontaneous voiding is common.
   d. Urethral injury is uncommon.

D. Complications
1. Urethral injury
2. Urinary tract infection

II. NASOGASTRIC TUBE
A. Indications
1. Gastric decompression
   a. Patient not following commands
   b. Obvious need for operative intervention
   c. Hemodynamic instability
   d. Positive pressure ventilation
   e. Any child with a distended abdomen
2. Gastric lavage
   a. Gastrointestinal bleeding
   b. Overdose
3. Enteral nutrition
B. Contraindications
1. Midface fractures or basilar skull fracture (an orogastric route is an alternative)
2. Obstruction of the nasopharynx
C. Technique
1. Explain the procedure to the patient if possible.
2. Consider placing the tube on ice to stiffen and preform a gentle curve.
3. Consider using topical anesthetic spray in the naso- and oropharynx.
4. Lubricate tube liberally with a water-soluble lubricant.
5. Elevate head of bed at least 30 degrees, if possible.
6. Insert tube gently into nostril, and slowly direct it posteriorly and caudad into the back of oropharynx by inserting 1- to 2-cm segments with hands and fingers close to the nostril.
7. Do not advance the tube while the patient is talking or actively inhaling. If the patient can cooperate, advance the tube in short segments as the patient swallows on command.
8. If the patient will not cooperate but can swallow spontaneously, the tube can be inserted by carefully observing the patient and with precise timing gently advancing the tube as the patient swallows.
9. If the patient can not swallow, gentle forward pressure should be applied in the posterior pharynx until the tube passes. Be aware of coiling or kinking of the tube in the pharynx.
10. Once in the esophagus, the tube should advance easily into the stomach. Gagging is common during insertion, but if the patient loses his or her voice, becomes hoarse, or has violent coughing, withdraw the tube as it is likely to be in the trachea.
11. Once inserted, air is injected into the tube and auscultated over the stomach.
12. Vigorously irrigate the tube to remove particulate gastric contents.
13. Postpyloric access:
    a. Use an 8, 10, or 12 F enteric feeding tube (length >100 cm) with Y adapter and stylet.
    b. A prokinetic agent (e.g., metoclopromide) can be administered prior to insertion to aide in pyloric passage.
    c. Once the tube is confirmed in intragastric position, roll the patient to the right lateral decubitus position, if possible.
    d. With the stylet still in place, rapidly insufflate the stomach with 500 to 1,000 mL of air, using the 60-mL regular tip syringe.
    e. Advance the feeding tube to a point such that only 10 cm of tubing remains externally.
    f. Return the patient to the supine position with stylet in place and secure the tube with tape.
    g. Assess tube position with chest or abdominal x-ray study.

       i. If tube is transpyloric, flush with 10 mL of sterile water and remove stylet before initiating tube feeds.

       ii. If tube is at the pylorus, wait 24 to 48 hours and reassess.

       iii. If the tube is looped around the stomach with the tip away from a pylorus, retract it to the centimeter mark estimating gastric placement. Consider administering a dose of a prokinetic agent and reattempt tube insertion.

    h. When properly positioned, secure tube to patient's nose and cheek and note centimeter marking on the tube at the tip of the patient's nose.

    i. If unsuccessful in transpyloric passage, arrange for a fluoroscopic or endoscopic manipulation.

  D. Complications

    1. Tracheobronchial insertion with resultant pneumothorax

    2. Intracranial insertion

    3. Alar necrosis

    4. Perforation (esophagogastroduodenal)

    5. Sinusitis

    6. Aspiration

III. CHEST TUBE (THORACOSTOMY)

  A. Refer to Chapters 24 and 25.

IV. NEEDLE DECOMPRESSION OF THORAX

  A. Refer to Chapter 6.

V. TRACTION SPLINT (HARE OR THOMAS)

  A. Indications

    1. Femur fracture—diaphyseal

  B. Contraindications

    1. Pelvic fracture

  C. Technique

    1. At a minimum, this is a two-person procedure.

    2. Prepare the splint before application (i.e., measure limb length and obtain straps).

    3. Administer intravenous (IV) analgesia.

    4. Assess the distal pulses before applying the splint.

    5. Apply manual traction via the foot strap while raising the leg.

    6. In a coordinated and precise effort, position the splint under the leg with the proximal covered rim of the splint against the ischial tuberosity.

    7. Slowly apply traction to the foot strap after affixing the traction hook to the foot strap sling.

    8. Apply leg straps (usually Velcro) to secure the leg in the splint; the straps do not need to be tight.

    9. Reassess distal pulses after the splint is applied.

  D. Complications

    1. Sloughing of skin at the ankle

    2. Loss of pulses

VI. SKELETAL TRACTION PIN

  A. Indications

    1. Femur fracture

  B. Contraindications

    1. Unstable knee injury

  C. Technique for tibial pin placement

    1. For short duration, insert 1 cm distal to anterior tibial tubercle.

    2. For more prolonged traction (i.e., >1 week) place in distal femur.

    3. Align leg in a straight line from the great toe, through the patella to the anterior iliac spine.

4. Elevate the leg on a pillow or blankets to allow the drill handle to turn without striking the bed.
5. Prepare and drape the knee and proximal tibia.
6. Infiltrate the lateral and medial skin and subcutaneous tissue with local anesthetic 2 cm distal and posterior to the anterior tibial tubercle.
7. Use a nonthreaded Steinman pin or Kirschner wire for tibial insertion (a threaded pin is used with femoral insertion). The pin is affixed to a hand or power drill using a chuck key.
8. Make a small skin incision laterally 2 cm distal and posterior to the anterior tibial tubercle.
9. Engage the pin against the bone and staying parallel to the ground drill through both cornices.
10. When the pin pushes against the medial skin, the skin is incised with the scalpel. The pin should extend beyond the skin 1 to 2 inches. A pin cutter is necessary to cut the pin length. The pin edges are usually capped with corks or rubber stoppers to avoid puncture injury to the caregivers.
11. Then place the pin in either the Steinman or Kirschner bow and attach to the appropriated traction. Dress the pin sites with povidone-iodine and a 2 × 2 gauze.
12. The most frequent error in placement is failure to get enough purchase on the bone (i.e., not posterior enough from the anterior tibial edge).

D. Complications
1. Bleeding
2. Pin site infection
3. Nerve injury

VII. BEDSIDE TRACHEOSTOMY

A. Indications
1. Airway protection
2. Pulmonary toilet
3. Prolonged ventilatory support
4. Decontamination of oropharynx
5. Extensive orofacial trauma

B. Contraindications
1. A cricothyroidotomy, not a tracheostomy, should be performed if an emergent surgical airway is needed.

C. Technique. A detailed description of open and percutaneous tracheostomy is beyond the scope of this manual.
1. Plan and time bedside tracheostomy for periods of optimal staffing. Have a checklist of supplies and have them available before the procedure.
2. Bedside tracheostomy can be done by the open or percutaneous dilational technique.
3. The patient should be intubated, except for emergency conditions.
4. Have resources for conscious sedation available, including continuous blood pressure, electrocardiography (ECG), and pulse oximetry monitoring.
5. Position the patient to extend the neck, if possible.
6. A person skilled at endotracheal intubation should be positioned at the head of the bed to control the endotracheal tube and reintubate, if necessary.
7. Have an instrument tray allowing for open tracheostomy available, even when using a percutaneous technique.
8. Have surgical lighting available over the patient's neck area. A portable headlight can be helpful.
9. The tracheostomy tube should be opened, tested, and prepared for insertion before beginning the procedure.
10. Bedside tracheostomy is a surgical procedure and the team should wear gown, gloves, cap, mask, and eye protection. The patient should be fully draped. Place equipment on tables, not directly on the bed.
11. Both the open and percutaneous technique should be considered a two-person technique. Have a scrubbed assistant available at the bedside.

12. The bedside nurse should direct full attention to this procedure during its performance.

13. The anterior neck skin is prepared, draped, and usually anesthetized with local anesthesia.

14. Many use routine bronchoscopic guidance in performing the percutaneous technique.

15. Have extra tracheostomy tubes, endotracheal tubes, and tracheostomy tray immediately available.

16. If a percutaneous endoscopic gastrostomy (PEG) is planned at the same time, it is usually preferable to follow the tracheostomy because the endotracheal tube will have been removed, facilitating endoscopy.

D. Complications

    1. Most serious complication during procedure—**loss of the airway**

        a. Hypoxia and bradycardia

        b. If uncertain about position of endotracheal or tracheostomy tube → reintubate

    2. Other complications

        a. Tube misplacement (e.g., pretracheal)

        b. Tracheal laceration

        c. Tube dislodgment

        d. Bleeding

        e. Pneumothorax

        f. Laryngeal nerve injury

        g. Tracheal stenosis

        h. Tracheoinnominate fistula

        i. Tracheoesophageal fistula

VIII. PERCUTANEOUS ENDOSCOPIC GASTROSTOMY (PEG)

A. Indication

    1. Long-term gastric access for either decompression or feeding. In general, if a patient is not expected to survive >30 days or will likely be eating within 30 days, a PEG may not be indicated.

B. Technical points

    1. Have the resources to provide and monitor conscious sedation available.

    2. If a PEG is to be combined with a tracheostomy, the PEG should be the second procedure.

    3. In general, plan the procedure at periods of optimal staffing to include the use of gastrointestinal endoscopy nurses, when practical.

    4. A remote monitor, in addition to the endoscope, facilitates coordination of the team performing the procedure.

    5. A PEG is a two-person procedure, in addition to the person monitoring the conscious sedation.

    6. Inspect the esophagus, stomach, and duodenum before beginning placement of the PEG tube.

    7. Gastric insufflation, transabdominal illumination, and endoscopic visualization of finger depression of the abdominal wall are essential for proper placement.

    8. Most endoscopists do not routinely reintroduce the endoscope to inspect the stomach after placement.

    9. Feeding can usually be started immediately.

C. Complications

    1. Pneumoperitoneum (common)

    2. Misplacement and inadvertent organ injury

    3. Early tube removal with gastric perforation

    4. Tube site cellulitis or hemorrhage

    5. Gastrocutaneous fistula

    6. Tube-related mechanical problems (e.g., clogging, breakage)

IX. FIBEROPTIC BRONCHOSCOPY (FOB)

A. Indications for the trauma patient

1. Adjunct to endotracheal intubation
2. Evaluation of posttraumatic hemoptysis, acute inhalation injury, suspected bronchial injury, and injury caused by prolonged intubation
3. Extraction of foreign bodies
4. Clearance of secretions and mucous plugs
5. Diagnosis of nosocomial pneumonia (Section IX.D)

B. Contraindications

1. Uncooperative patient
2. Persistent, marked hypoxemia or hypercarbia
3. Severe bronchospasm
4. Severe pulmonary hypertension
5. Cardiac ischemia
6. Coagulopathy (relative)

C. Procedure

1. Most trauma patients for whom FOB is indicated will have an endotracheal tube in place.
2. Consider those trauma patients not intubated and for whom FOB is indicated for endotracheal intubation before the procedure.
3. For patients not intubated, FOB should be performed by the most experienced bronchoscopist available.
4. Have cardiac and pulse oximetry monitoring and skilled assistance available.
5. Perform FOB only through a $\geq$8-mm internal diameter endotracheal or tracheostomy tube.
6. Maintain 100% FiO_2 throughout the procedure and minimize airway suctioning to avoid reduction in tidal volumes.
7. Make adjustments to mechanical ventilation before the procedure to maintain adequate minute ventilation and avoid increased inflation pressures.
8. Use local anesthetics judiciously; 200 to 300 mg of lidocaine (20–30 mL of 1% lidocaine solution).
9. Premedicate with IV analgesics and sedatives as indicated.
10. Use silicone spray rather than gel lubricant.
11. Consider use of a swivel adaptor, which minimizes air leak.

D. Diagnosis of nosocomial pneumonia

1. Cultures of sputum aspirates or traditional FOB specimens are unreliable because of contamination by upper airway secretions.
2. Use a protected brush catheter (PBC).
   a. A PBC is a telescoping double catheter with a recessed sterile brush.
   b. The inner catheter with brush can be advanced into subsegmental bronchi for sampling of focal infiltrates.
   c. Avoid proximal lidocaine administration and suctioning during the procedure.
   d. Postsampling. Retract the inner catheter and brush and remove from the bronchoscope. The brush is severed from the catheter for quantitative cultures ($>10^3$ colonies per milliliter).
3. Bronchoalveolar lavage (BAL)
   a. Bronchoscopic tip is wedged into a subsegmental bronchi.
   b. Instill sterile normal saline solution (NSS; 50–100 mL) and remove via suction.
   c. Take quantitative cultures of the sample ($>10^5$ colonies per milliliter).

X. INSERTION OF BEDSIDE INFERIOR VENA CAVAL FILTER (IVCF)

A. Indications

1. Recurrent pulmonary embolism despite anticoagulation.
2. Venous thromboembolic disease with contraindication to full anticoagulation.
3. Progression of ileofemoral clot, despite anticoagulation.
4. Large, free-floating thrombus in the iliac vein or IVC.

5. Massive pulmonary embolism (PE) in which recurrent emboli would prove fatal.

6. During or after surgical embolectomy.

7. Prophylaxis in patients who cannot receive anticoagulation because of increased bleeding risk and have high-risk injury pattern (e.g., severe closed head injury, spinal cord injury, complex pelvic fractures with associated long bone fracture, or multiple long bone fractures).

8. Bedside insertion of IVCFs can be performed with minimal complications and eliminate the risk associated with intrahospital transport; bedside application of this procedure reduces cost and operating room utilization.

B. Contraindications

1. Thrombus between access site and site of deployment (choose alternate access site)

C. Technique

1. Equipment

a. Fluoroscopic image intensifier and monitor (Cine-loop and subtraction capabilities preferred)

b. Fluoroscopic-ready bed

c. Lead aprons

d. Sterile barriers, gowns, masks, caps

e. Introducer kit with guidewire

f. Intravenous contrast material

g. Heparinized saline (10 U/mL NSS)

h. Radiopaque markers for measurements

Note: Be familiar with introducer system and size restrictions of individual vena cava filters.

2. Procedure

a. Prepare access site with povidone-iodine (solution or chlorhexidine gluconate, right internal jugular or femoral vein approach preferred).

b. Identify T-12 and all lumbar vertebrae under fluoroscopic guidance.

c. Gain venous access and advance guidewire under fluoroscopic guidance.

d. Insert introducer with dilator previously flushed with heparin solution.

e. Perform venogram (hand-injected or power-injected, if available) to assess for anomalies, venal caval size, and location of renal veins.

f. Flush introducer with heparinized saline solution and advance filter into infrarenal position.

g. Deploy filter under fluoroscopic guidance.

h. Remove introducer and hold pressure at site for 10 minutes or until bleeding stops.

i. Confirm placement of IVCF with abdominal x-ray.

D. Complications

1. Filter tilting, malposition, or migration

2. IVC erosion or obstruction

3. IVC thrombosis

4. Insertion site thrombosis

5. Bleeding

6. Pulmonary embolism

AXIOMS

■ Remember—even minor procedures can have associated complications.

■ A urinary catheter should be placed by an experienced member of the trauma team if a urethral injury is suspected.

■ Nasogastric tube placement should be avoided in patients with midface and basilar skull fractures.

■ Always reassess distal pulses after placement of a traction splint or pin.

■ For bedside procedures such as tracheostomy, PEG, FOB, and IVCF insertion, have resources and monitoring available to provide conscious sedation.

Bibliography

Croce MA, Fabian TC, Schurr MJ, et al. Using bronchoalveolar lavage to distinguish nosocomial pneumonia from systemic inflammatory response syndrome: A prospective analysis. *J Trauma* 1995;39:1134–1138.

Dellinger PR. Fiberoptic bronchoscopy in critical care medicine. In: Shoemaker WC, Ayers SH, Grenvig A, et al., eds. *Textbook of Critical Care.* Philadelphia, Pa: WB Saunders; 1995:761–769.

Lord LM, Weiser-Maimone A, Pulhamus M, et al. Comparison of weighted vs nonweighted enteral feeding tubes for efficiency of transpyloric intubation. *JPEN* 1993;17:271–273.

Rogers FB, Cipolle MD, Velmahos G, et al. Practice management guidelines for the management of venous thromboembolism in trauma patients. Available at: http://www.east.org.

Schultz MD, Santatello SA, Monk J, et al. An improved method for transpyloric placement of nasoenteric feeding tubes. *Int Surg* 1993;78:79–82.

Shoemaker WC, Velmahos GC, Demetriades Demetrios, eds. *Procedures and Monitoring for the Critically Ill.* Philadelphia, Pa: WB Saunders; 2002.

Sing RF, Smith CH, Miles WS, Messick WJ. Preliminary results of bedside inferior vena cava filter placement: Safe and cost-effective. *Chest* 1998;114(1):315–316.

INTRODUCTION TO EMERGENCY SURGERY

54

MICHAEL RHODES

$\mathcal{T}$here are at least four imperatives that have driven the addition of emergency surgery to the third edition of *The Trauma Manual*. First, there are many common pathophysiologic and treatment principles in the management of trauma and other non-injury-related surgical emergencies. Second, most trauma team leaders in hospitals throughout the United States are general surgeons who also manage emergency general (and many times vascular) surgeries as part of their practice. Third, emergency medicine physicians have always been essential to the early identification and initial management of surgical emergencies and are now full partners with surgeons in the management of traumatic injuries. Fourth, the specialty of **acute care surgery** has been conceived by the leaders of American surgery and will likely be born and consummated within the next decade.

Acute care surgery includes the clinical areas of trauma, surgical critical care, and emergency surgery. This clinical function already exists in many hospitals in the United States and these surgeons are sometimes perceived as the "surgical hospitalists." The scope of emergency surgery may range from general surgery to vascular surgery to initial surgical stabilization of orthopedic and neurosurgical injuries as is practiced in some European countries.

Therefore, it seems logical to combine the educational offerings in this manual in recognition of the changing clinical practice models and to reflect the common physiologic and anatomic underpinnings between traumatic injury and, particularly, emergency general surgery. Accordingly, new chapters discuss surgical emergencies that are managed by attendings and residents in surgery and emergency medicine.

EVALUATION OF ACUTE ABDOMINAL PAIN
55
ROHIT K. SAHAI AND RAQUEL M. FORSYTHE

I. INTRODUCTION
   A. Definition. Although there is no standardized definition, an "acute abdomen" refers to abdominal symptoms and signs secondary to nontraumatic pathology that began recently (<72 hours). It usually refers to disease that may, but not necessarily, require an operation, and thus a surgical consult is often obtained.
   B. Incidence. Five percent to 10% of all emergency visits in the United States are secondary to abdominal pain.
   C. Pathophysiology. Abdominal pathology can cause visceral, parietal pain, or referred pain.
   1. Visceral pain/sensation
      a. Occurs from innervation of the autonomic and visceral afferent type C fibers. Innervation is bilateral.
      b. Pain is sensed secondary to stretch but also distension, contraction, traction, compression, and torsion. In addition, mucosal pain receptors respond to chemical stimuli including ischemia and inflammation.
      c. The pain perceived is usually dull, not well localized, midline and corresponds to the embryologic origin of the affected organ.
      d. Epigastric pain usually indicates a foregut etiology as visceral afferents from the foregut travel with the celiac trunk.
      e. Periumbilical pain, on the other hand, indicates a midgut etiology as these afferents travel with superior mesenteric artery branches.
      f. Lower midline pain indicates hindgut or pelvic pathology as these fibers travel with the inferior mesenteric artery branches.
   2. Parietal pain
      a. Occurs secondary to irritation of the parietal peritoneum leading to somatic nerve activation (type C and A delta fibers).
      b. Chemical peritonitis can occur from irritation by blood, urine, or gastrointestinal secretions. Blood, however, causes very little inflammation by itself. Secondary infection of blood leads to chemical peritonitis.
      c. In contrast to visceral pain, parietal pain is sharp and well localized.
      d. **Appendicitis** demonstrates both visceral and parietal pain. The inflammation and distension of the appendix (part of the midgut) classically results in poorly localized, dull periumbilical pain. As the inflammation progresses and irritates the parietal peritoneum, the pain becomes sharper and better localized to the right lower quadrant (RLQ).
   3. Referred pain
      a. Pain that is sensed on the superficial surface but is due to a visceral process. There are common patterns associated with certain abdominal processes (Fig. 55-1).
      b. Occurs secondary to nerves carrying both autonomic and somatic innervation and both being activated. For example, the phrenic nerve and other afferents (derived from C3 to C5 dermatomes) innervate the diaphragm and the associated peritoneum. Somatic C3 to C5 dermatomes innervate the shoulder. Thus, the pain from intraabdominal pathology irritating the upper peritoneum is referred to the shoulder via the common C3 to C5 dermatome.

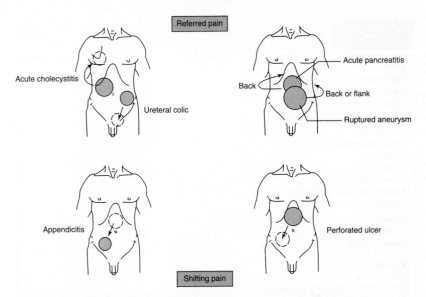

Figure 55-1. Referred pain and shifting pain in the acute abdomen. Solid circles indicate the site of maximum pain; dashed circles indicate sites of lesser pain. (From Doherty GM, Boey JH. The acute abdomen. In: Way LW, Doherty GM. *Current Surgical Diagnosis and Treatment.* 11th ed. New York, NY: McGraw-Hill; 2003:505, with permission.)

    D. Differential diagnosis. The differential diagnosis is large for acute abdominal pain. It can be divided into gastrointestinal, vascular, gynecological, urological, and nonabdominal causes (Table 55-1).

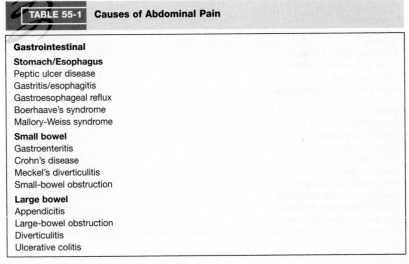

TABLE 55-1	Causes of Abdominal Pain

Gastrointestinal

Stomach/Esophagus
Peptic ulcer disease
Gastritis/esophagitis
Gastroesophageal reflux
Boerhaave's syndrome
Mallory-Weiss syndrome

Small bowel
Gastroenteritis
Crohn's disease
Meckel's diverticulitis
Small-bowel obstruction

Large bowel
Appendicitis
Large-bowel obstruction
Diverticulitis
Ulcerative colitis

(continued)

TABLE 55-1 Continued

Other
Perforated viscus
Hernia
Cancer

Hepatobiliary/Pancreatic
Cholecystitis
Acute pancreatitis
Cholangitis
Hepatitis
Hepatic abscess
Sphincter of Oddi dysfunction
Hepatic tumor

Splenic
Splenic infarct
Splenic rupture

Urological
Kidney stone
Urinary tract infection/acute cystitis
Acute pyelonephritis
Ruptured bladder
Acute epididymitis
Testicular torsion
Renal infact

Gynecological
Ovarian torsion
Ectopic pregnancy
Ovulation
Ovarian cyst
Pelvic inflammatory disease
Tuboovarian abscess
Endometriosis

Vascular
Abdominal aortic aneurysm
Acute mesenteric ischemia
Aortic dissection
Mesenteric venous thrombosis

Other
Pneumonia
Myocardial infarction
Diabetes mellitus
Porphyria
Sickle-cell anemia
Henoch-Schonlein purpura
Muscular contusion/hematoma
Familial Mediterranean Fever
Retroperitoneal hemorrhage

II. HISTORY
  A. A careful and detailed history is the most helpful factor in leading to the correct diagnosis.
  B. Location
    1. Identifying the location of pain aids significantly in narrowing the differential (Fig. 55-2).
    2. At times this can be deceptive. For example, in perforated peptic ulcer disease, the source is the stomach, but pain may be perceived along the RLQ secondary to gastric and pancreatic/biliary fluid tracking down the right paracolic gutter.
    3. In addition, pain can be referred to a site away from the process (i.e., left shoulder pain after a ruptured spleen).
  C. Radiation of pain. There are classic radiation patterns that strengthen a diagnosis (Fig. 55-1).
    1. Periumbilical pain radiating to the back is associated with pancreatitis, perforated peptic ulcer disease, or aortic dissection.
    2. Subcostal left-sided abdominal pain with radiation to the shoulder may indicate an evolving myocardial infarction (MI), splenic pathology, or left subdiaphragmatic abscess.
    3. Pain from the flank radiating to the groin may indicate the presence of a ureteral stone.
  D. Onset of pain
    1. Acute or abrupt onset of pain can be associated with a vascular etiology (acute mesenteric embolism, abdominal aortic aneurysm rupture) or a perforated viscus.
    2. On the other hand, a gradual onset of pain is more characteristic of peptic ulcer disease, cholecystitis, pancreatitis, diverticulitis, and appendicitis.

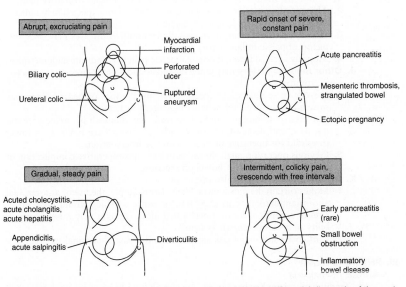

Figure 55-2. The location and character of pain are helpful in the differential diagnosis of the acute abdomen. (From Doherty GM, Boey JH. The acute abdomen. In: Way LW, Doherty GM. *Current Surgical Diagnosis and Treatment.* 11th ed. New York, NY: McGraw-Hill; 2003:506, with permission.)

E. Character. Taken together with location, the character of pain can give further clues as to the abdominal process responsible for it (Fig 55-2).

1. Cramping pain (colicky) is characteristic of bowel obstruction and gastroenteritis.
2. Steadily increasing constant pain indicates inflammatory and infectious etiologies, such as appendicitis, pancreatitis, cholecystitis, and diverticulitis.
3. Burning pain occurs with peptic ulcer disease.
4. Colicky pain, or sharp intermittent pain with periods of less severe pain, is often used to refer to pain from a biliary or renal source. However, "biliary colic" is a misnomer as most biliary pain is constant and lasts a few hours.

F. Severity

1. Usually the greater the severity, the higher the likelihood of abdominal pathology requiring operation.
2. However, patient characteristics—personality, medications, age, comorbidities—can all influence the perceived severity.
3. Serially following the severity of abdominal pain is often useful. This should be performed by the same examiner whenever possible to avoid interobserver variability. Pain scales can also help by reducing this variability.

G. Aggravating/Alleviating factors can be helpful.

1. Sitting up and leaning forward classically decreases pain in patients with pancreatitis.
2. Movement aggravates pain in patients with peritonitis.
3. Eating fatty foods may precipitate an attack of right upper quadrant (RUQ) pain secondary to gallbladder pathology.

H. Associated symptoms. Associated symptoms help narrow a differential diagnosis. For example, bloody diarrhea, fever, and abdominal pain may indicate acute mesenteric ischemia or inflammatory bowel disease. Nausea and vomiting with diarrhea prior to the onset of pain helps in the diagnosis of gastroenteritis when other intraabdominal pathology has been ruled out.

I. Gynecological/Menstrual history. This history should be obtained in all women.

1. Pain in the middle of the menstrual cycle may indicate ovulatory pain.
2. Absence of menses or unusually light menses when expected may indicate the possibility of an ectopic pregnancy.
3. Previous pelvic infections or sexually transmitted diseases may raise suspicion of pelvic inflammatory disease.
4. Monthly cyclical lower abdominal/pelvic pain may indicate endometriosis.

J. Other medical history may guide diagnosis and raise awareness to nonclassical symptoms.

1. History of recent heart surgery, atrial fibrillation, or heart failure may raise a higher suspicion of acute mesenteric ischemia.
2. Diabetes or an immunosuppressed state may diminish perceived abdominal pain and decrease physical findings. Also, there might be a lower threshold for operative or other definitive intervention.
3. Previous operation might be indicative of a postoperative complication or adhesions as a cause of bowel obstruction.

K. A medication history is also important.

1. Makes certain diagnoses more likely. For example, the use of nonsteroidal antiinflammatory drugs (NSAIDs) or corticosteroids would raise suspicion of a peptic ulcer or a perforated ulcer. Digoxin may raise the possibility of acute mesenteric ischemia.
2. Corticosteroids may mask significant underlying abdominal pathology.

III. PHYSICAL EXAM

A. Role of analgesia

1. Traditionally there has been much concern about administering analgesia prior to surgical evaluation. However, recent studies have shown this be to a safe practice. In general, physical findings and diagnostic accuracy were not significantly changed in patients receiving analgesia compared to those not receiving it.

2. Good communication with the surgical team as to the medications given prior to consultation is essential.

B. Appearance. The general appearance of a patient helps not only with diagnosis but also with determining the urgency for treatment.

1. Patients with jaundice usually have a hepatobiliary source of their pain.
2. A patient who is restless points to renal colic, as opposed to the patient with peritonitis who tries to lie motionless.
3. Findings such as lethargy, sunken eyes, and poor skin turgor may indicate dehydration, seen in cases of bowel obstruction, pancreatitis, and colitis with prolonged diarrhea.

C. Vital signs

1. Many patients with an inflammatory or infectious process will have low-grade fevers. However, fever may be absent.
2. A hypotensive patient with acute abdominal pain usually indicates concomitant septic shock or rupture of an abdominal aortic aneurysm (AAA).

D. Peritonitis. In most cases, peritonitis defines an acute abdomen. Peritonitis refers to findings of rebound or percussion tenderness, or involuntary guarding.

1. Involuntary guarding, as opposed to voluntary guarding, is continued nonrelaxation of the abdominal muscles with pressure.
2. A patient with rebound tenderness has aggravation or onset of pain immediately after removing pressure from the abdomen. The presence of peritonitis is not tested by this method to avoid the extreme pain it can cause.
3. Instead, peritonitis can be assessed effectively by percussion, rocking the patient's bed, or tapping the patient's heel. In a child, this can be assessed by having the child hop on one foot.
4. Furthermore, the diffuseness of peritonitis dictates management. Diffuse peritonitis usually indicates an abdominal catastrophe and mandates surgical exploration, with minor exceptions. However, some causes of local peritonitis (e.g., noncomplicated diverticulitis or pelvic inflammatory disease) may resolve with nonoperative treatment and usually require more investigation or observation.

E. Examination

1. Inspection. The presence of masses, bulges, scars, discolorations, or hematomas can help identify the cause of abdominal pain. For example, a bulge in the groin or umbilicus may be secondary to an incarcerated hernia. A flank hematoma (Grey-Turner's sign) or periumbilical hematoma (Cullen's sign) could indicate severe hemorrhagic pancreatitis. Incisions indicate previous operations, raising the possibility of bowel obstruction or perioperative complications.
2. Auscultation. The presence of active, high-pitched bowel sounds may indicate a mechanical small bowel obstruction. However, absence of bowel sounds often are not as helpful. A good auscultatory exam requires several minutes. Sometimes, bruits over the renal veins or over visceral aneurysms may also be heard.
3. Percussion. Percussion can be used to determine the presence of peritonitis (see above), ascites, distended bowel, and liver span.
4. Palpation. Palpation should generally start from the opposite quadrant from the maximum point of pain. Localizing the pain to a specific area often helps limit the differential and aids in determining what, if any, investigational study needs to be performed. The costovertebral areas should also be palpated or lightly tapped. Tenderness may indicate acute pyelonephritis.
5. Special maneuvers/signs
   a. **Rovsig's sign.** Pain in the RLQ when pressure is applied to the LLQ (seen in cases of appendicitis)
   b. **Psoas sign.** Pain with flexion or extension of the hip (seen in patients with appendicitis or psoas abscess)
   c. **Obturator sign.** Pain with internal/external rotation of the hip (seen in patients with appendicitis)
   d. **Murphy's sign.** Abrupt stop in inspiration during palpation over the right subcostal area (seen in patients with acute cholecystitis)

6. Rectal exam. The rectal exam with stool guaiac is an important part of a complete physical exam. Findings of fecal impaction may diagnose the cause of the patient's abdominal pain. Tenderness along the right rectal vault may support appendicitis or an abscess. A guaiac-positive study may point to colitis, GI bleeding (i.e., peptic ulcer or colitis), or cancer causing or contributing to the pain.

7. Pelvic exam. In women with lower abdominal pain, a pelvic exam is essential in helping differentiate gynecological from other abdominal causes of pain.
   a. Discharge is consistent with pelvic infection and pelvic inflammatory disease.
   b. A bimanual exam should be performed and can help in diagnosis of pelvic inflammatory disease, ovarian mass, or tuboovarian abscess.

8. Other important parts of an exam. A **thorough exam** should be done as it may identify a source other than the abdomen as the cause of the abdominal pain or help in diagnosis of an abdominal source. For example, rhonchi/crackles with dullness to percussion may indicate a lower lobe pneumonia masquerading as upper abdominal pain. A heart murmur or an irregular heart rhythm might heighten the suspicion of intestinal ischemia from an embolic source.

F. **Miscellaneous.** The physical exam, even if it reveals few physical findings, nevertheless remains important. In fact, a high index of suspicion with a good history despite minimal physical exam findings remain the most important factors in early diagnosis of mesenteric ischemia.

IV. LABORATORY STUDIES
A. CBC with differential
1. An elevated white blood cell (WBC) count is not always seen in the acute abdomen. However, it raises suspicion of an infectious or inflammatory event if present.
2. A "left shift" or "bandemia" can occur even if the WBC count is normal and is indicative of an infective process.
3. An elevated hemoglobin and hematocrit are often seen in a patient with dehydration (i.e., after excessive vomiting, third spacing, or diarrhea). Anemia can be seen in a ruptured abdominal aortic aneurysm (AAA) or a retroperitoneal hematoma.

B. Electrolytes, urea nitrogen, and creatinine
1. Hypochloremic, hypokalemic, metabolic alkalosis is often seen after prolonged vomiting.
2. An anion gap metabolic acidosis (serum [Na] – serum [Cl] – serum [HCO_3] ≥ 12) indicates uremia, diabetic ketoacidosis, or lactic acidosis as concomitant processes.
3. An increased BUN/Cr ratio (>20:1) is indicative of dehydration.
4. Creatinine is often needed prior to a contrast computed tomography (CT) scan to determine risk versus benefit.

C. Liver function tests
1. Transaminases (AST, ALT). These can be elevated from many hepatobiliary disease states. Significant elevations indicating a hepatic process (i.e., viral hepatitis, abscess, ischemia, acetaminophen poisoning) usually occur with levels greater than three times normal levels. Lower levels can be nonspecific and due to a variety of causes including common bile duct stones, pancreatitis, steatohepatitis, and medications (i.e., statins).
2. Alkaline Phosphatase/GGTP. Alkaline phosphatase is produced by the cells lining the biliary tree. Elevation in its levels usually points to a biliary process such as common bile duct stone, cholangitis, primary biliary sclerosis, or primary sclerosing cholangitis. However, alkaline phosphatase is produced by other organs including the gut, placenta, and bone. Therefore, obtaining a GGTP level can be useful as it isolates the increased alkaline phosphatase as originating from the biliary tree.
3. Others. Often the prothrombin time (PT) and albumin level are forgotten as part of liver function tests. They are actually the best test to determine **function**

of the liver. An elevated PT and/or decreased albumin level can indicate long-standing liver disease such as cirrhosis, important in the event a patient needs an operation.

D. Amylase/Lipase

1. Amylase
   a. Elevated in pancreatitis with rise within 2 to 12 hours of symptoms and return to normal over next 3 to 5 days. Peak levels occur within the first 48 hours of symptoms.
   b. Also elevated in inflammation of the gastrointestinal tract, many gynecological diseases, renal failure, and salivary gland inflammation. Specificity for pancreatitis can be increased by using cutoff of three times the upper limit of normal.
   c. Because of pancreas "burnout" in chronic pancreatitis, levels can be normal despite an episode of acute pancreatitis.
   d. **Levels do not correlate with etiology or severity.**

2. Lipase
   a. Elevated in pancreatitis with rise slightly later (4–8 hours), peak earlier (24 hours), and return to normal longer (8–14 days) than amylase.
   b. Similar to amylase, can be elevated in other intraabdominal pathology and renal insufficiency.
   c. Considered more specific than serum amylase for acute pancreatitis, especially in alcoholic pancreatitis.
   d. **Levels do not correlate with etiology or severity.**

E. Urinanalysis (UA)

1. Microscopic hematuria raises the possibility of a kidney stone or urological cancer.
2. Pyuria, positive nitrite, and leukoesterase indicate acute pyelonephritis or cystitis.
3. However, a "positive" UA (i.e., with positive leukoesterase and few WBCs) could be secondary to an inflammatory process in the abdomen such as appendicitis rather than a urinary tract infection.

F. Pregnancy test

1. This test is mandatory in women of childbearing age.
2. It is able to identify possible etiologies of pain and/or help with further management of the patient. For example, a patient with lower pelvic pain and a positive pregnancy test may lead to a diagnosis of an ectopic pregnancy.

G. Lactate level

1. D (−) lactate is sensitive but nonspecific for acute mesenteric ischemia.
2. Elevated in many patients who are dehydrated.

V. RADIOGRAPHIC STUDIES.
The approach to obtaining further radiographic investigation should be methodical and thoughtful.

A. Acute abdominal series.
Often the initial start of imaging.

1. A series usually consists of an upright chest x-ray, flat plate, and an upright abdominal x-ray or lateral decubitus film.
2. Advantages of plain films include inexpensiveness, speed, noninvasiveness, and accessibility.
3. Disadvantages include poor resolution and difficulty in diagnosing most causes of acute abdomen.
4. Findings
   a. "Air"
      i. A primary reason to obtain plain films in a patient with an acute abdomen is to identify the presence of pneumoperitoneum quickly. Pneumoperitoneum would indicate a likely perforated viscous mandating operative intervention.
      ii. Air in the portovenous system usually indicates intestinal ischemia or an infectious process as the air is really gas produced by bacteria.
      iii. Pneumointestinalis, air in the bowel wall, may also be present indicating ischemia.

b. Bowel gas pattern/air fluid levels
   i. The other major indication for plain films is to help rule out bowel obstruction. Plain films have 50% to 60% sensitivity in diagnosing bowel obstructions.
   ii. A "sentinel loop" or single dilated loop of bowel may also be seen next to an inflamed organ.
c. Bowel wall thickness. Thickened bowel wall is difficult to see on plain films unless two loops of bowel are in contact with each other.
   i. If the colonic wall seems thick, it could indicate colitis (*C. difficile*, ischemic, inflammatory bowel disease, infectious).
   ii. If the walls of the small bowel are thick, a diagnosis of acute mesenteric ischemia might be entertained. However, "thumbprinting" or thickening of bowel loops occur in less than 40% of patients with acute mesenteric ischemia.
d. Calcifications. Calcifications can appear in the pancreas, gallbladder, or aorta.
   i. Only 15% of gallstones are radiopaque, but 90% of kidney stones are opaque.
   ii. The finding of a fecolith, occurring in ~50% cases of appendicitis, can be helpful.
   iii. An AAA may be visible on x-ray by a rim of calcium.
   iv. Calcifications in the area of the pancreas indicate chronic pancreatitis and raise the possibility of acute pancreatitis.
B. **CT.** Most sensitive study in determining cause of vague abdominal pain.
   1. Noncontrast versus contrast
      a. Oral contrast is helpful in most cases as it helps differentiate bowel from other abdominal organs.
      b. In most causes of acute abdominal pain, a nonintravenous contrast CT scan is sufficient. However, a contrast-enhanced scan is able to provide better resolution and is required when a vascular cause is being considered.
   2. Advantages of CT include high resolution, relative speed, noninvasiveness, and the ability to diagnose many causes of acute abdominal pain. It is extremely helpful in vague or unexplained abdominal pain and for looking at the retroperitoneum.
   3. Disadvantages to CT are relatively few and include radiation use, rare cases of anaphylaxis, potential for nephrotoxicity if intravenous contrast is used, and delay in treatment especially in critically ill patients. In addition, CT misses 20% to 25% of gallstones and is of limited value in looking at pelvic pathology.
   4. Specific diseases
      a. Appendicitis. CT has an overall sensitivity of ~95% and specificity of ~90%.
      b. Mesenteric venous thrombosis. Contrast-enhanced CT is the investigation of choice.
      c. Acute mesenteric ischemia. Contrast-enhanced CT and CT angiograph may help in the diagnosis of acute mesenteric ischemia. Sensitivities of 64% and higher and specificities of 92% and higher have been reported. Findings in acute mesenteric ischemia include bowel lumen dilatation, bowel wall thickening, abnormal bowel wall enhancement, arterial occlusion, venous thrombosis, pneumatosis (gas in the bowel wall), portal venous gas, ascites, and other areas of infarcts in other organs.
      d. Ruptured AAA. The study of choice in a **hemodynamically stable patient** with suspected ruptured AAA.
C. **Ultrasound (US).** Often ordered as the initial test for RUQ pain.
   1. Advantages of US include its noninvasiveness, lack of radiation, low cost, portability, and access.
   2. Disadvantages include operator variability and poor resolution. Also bone and bowel gas can interfere with the study.
   3. Specific diseases

   a. Cholelithiasis/Cholecystitis. US is the study of choice to diagnose these diseases.

     i. Gallstones can be detected in most (>95%) patients with cholelithiasis.

     ii. Positive findings of cholecystit is include gallbladder wall thickening (>3 mm), pericholecystic fluid, and sonographic Murphy's sign, in addition to the presence of stones.

     iii. Dilation of the common bile duct (CBD; variable according to age but >7–8 mm) may indicate biliary obstruction secondary to a stone, stricture, or mass.

   b. Appendicitis. A sensitivity of ~85% and specificity of ~80% have been reported. Positive findings include a distended (>6 mm) and incompressible appendix.

   c. Gynecological/Obstetrical disease. Pelvic US and transvaginal US are also useful and are probably the initial diagnostic study of choice in these diseases (i.e., ovarian cyst, torsion, ectopic pregnancy).

D. Magnetic resonance imaging (MRI) and magnetic resonance cholangiopancreatography (MRCP)

   1. MRI, because it is time intensive, is rarely used in the setting of acute abdominal pain.

   2. MRCP, however, can be used to diagnose CBD stones often not seen on US or CT scans.

E. Radionuclide imaging studies

   1. Hepatobiliary imaging (HIDA). Nonfilling of the gallbladder 60 minutes after administration of an intravenous biliary radiopharmaceutical can be used to diagnose cholecystitis with equivocal US results or in acalculous cholecystitis. The specificity can be increased by giving morphine. False positives do occur in critically ill, malnourished, or patients on total parental nutrition.

   2. Technetium-99m pertechnetate scans are used to diagnose Meckel's diverticulum as this compound is taken up by ectopic gastric mucosa often found in the diverticulum.

   3. Radioisotope-labeled red blood cell (RBC) scans can be used to detect GI bleeding.

F. Angiography

   1. Disadvantages of angiography include its invasiveness, cost, difficult accessibility, use of contrast, and time constraint.

   2. Angiography is the investigation of choice in acute mesenteric ischemia.

   3. Should be biplanar—anteroposterior and lateral views—to help identify distal and proximal blood flow respectively.

   4. It also has the potential of being therapeutic. A papaverine infusion can be started in cases of ischemia. Embolization can be performed in cases of GI bleeding.

VI. PROCEDURES

A. Colonoscopy/Sigmoidoscopy. May be helpful in diagnosing or excluding certain pathology.

   1. Flexible sigmoidoscopy or colonoscopy is often used to diagnose colonic ischemia, especially in the setting of abdominal pain and diarrhea after abdominal aorta surgery.

   2. Used in the evaluation of possible inflammatory bowel disease, infectious colitis (e.g., presence of pseudomembranes), and volvulus.

   3. A relative contraindication for colonoscopy is in the setting of diverticulitis or toxic megacolon because of the concern for perforation.

B. Laparoscopy. May be helpful in the diagnosis of acute abdominal pain.

   1. It is especially useful in the setting of continued acute abdominal pain when non-invasive tests do not help identify an etiology or the diagnosis is uncertain.

   2. It may be especially useful in ruling out ischemic bowel.

C. Laparotomy. In the setting of diffuse peritonitis or an unstable patient it can be diagnostic and therapeutic.

VII. OBSERVATION. A patient with abdominal pain for longer than 6 hours without a clearly identifiable etiology and without peritoneal signs should be admitted and observed, often with repeat physical exams, laboratory studies, and radiographic workup. Patients with significant pathology will declare themselves while others will often improve without treatment (i.e., gastroenteritis). A common example occurs in the setting of questionable appendicitis.

References

Balthazar EJ, Birnbaum BA, Yee J, et al. Acute appendicitis: CT and ultrasound correlation in one hundred patients. *Radiology* 1994;190:31–35.

David V. Radiology of abdominal pain. *Lippincotts Prim Care Pract* 1999;3:498–513.

Desai SR, Cox MR, Martin CJ. Superior mesenteric vein thrombosis: Computed tomography diagnosis. *Aust N Z J Surg* 1998;68:811–812.

Graff LG, Robinson D. Abdominal pain and emergency department evaluation. *Emerg Med Clin North Am* 2001;19:123–136.

Maglinte DT, Balthazar EJ, Kelvin FM, et al. The role of radiography in diagnosis of SBO. *Am J Roentgenol* 1997;168:1171–1180.

Rao PM, Rhea JT, Novelline RA, et al. Helical CT technique for the diagnosis of appendicitis: Prospective evaluation of a focused appendix CT examination. *Radiology* 1997;202:139–144.

Smotkin J, Tenner S. Laboratory diagnostic tests in acute pancreatitis. *J Clin Gastroenterol* 2002;34(4):459–462.

Taourel PG, Deneuville M, Pradel JA, et al. Acute mesenteric ischemia: Diagnosis with contrast–enhanced CT. *Radiology* 1996;199:632–636.

Terasawa T, Blackmore CC, Bent S, Kohlwes RJ. Systematic review: Computed tomography and ultrasonography to detect acute appendicitis in adults and adolescents. *Ann Intern Med* 2004;141(7):537–546.

Thomas SH, Silen W, Cheema F, et al. Effects of morphine analgesia on diagnostic accuracy in emergency department patients with abdominal pain: A prospective, randomized trial. *J Am Coll Surg* 2003;196(1):18–31.

Wolf EL, Sprayregen S, Bakal CW. Radiology in intestinal ischemia: Plain film, contrast, and other imaging studies. *Surg Clin North Am* 1992;72(1):107–124.

THE APPROACH AND RESUSCITATION OF THE GENERAL SURGERY PATIENT
VISHAL BANSAL AND LOUIS ALARCON

I. INTRODUCTION
   A. General surgical emergencies can be divided into five broad categories:
   1. Infection
   2. Hemorrhage
   3. Obstruction
   4. Ischemia
   5. Injury

   These patients often present as consultations through the emergency department (ED) or from medical services where patients are hospitalized and evaluated for varying acute, preexisting, and chronic disease. They may have confusing medical histories with varying ages and complex medical comorbidities. Often, these patients are obtunded, in acute physiologic distress or agonal states where complete history and information cannot be ascertained. The physiologic parameters of blood pressure, pulse, respiratory rate, and temperature help immediately stratify patients based on the severity of illness and hence the tempo of evaluation and resuscitation necessary.

   B. The etiology of specific emergencies can arise from single pathology, such as a ruptured aortic aneurysm, or multiple factors, such as trauma.
   1. **Sepsis.** Perforated viscus, gangrenous organs or limbs, necrotizing fasciitis or cellulitis, an undrained abscess, or empyema.
   2. **Hemorrhage.** Ruptured aneurysm, gastrointestinal bleeding, iatrogenic either from medical procedures or hypocoagulability, and traumatic.
   3. **Obstruction.** Bowel obstructions, incarcerated hernias, pseudoobstructions.
   4. **Ischemia.** Arterial emboli (i.e., mesenteric or limb), thrombosis, or compartment syndromes.
   5. **Injury.** Localized or global trauma/burns affecting part or all major organ systems resulting in hemorrhage, hyperinflammatory states, and specific organ injury and dysfunction.
      a. Great differences may exist in the definitive operative management phase of these patients; however, the initial assessment and approach varies little with the goal of physiologic stability being paramount.

II. INITIAL MANAGEMENT
   A. Unlike the usual paradigm of medical practice, where a definitive diagnosis is made and directed treatment implemented, the acute surgical patient must be resuscitated quickly and aggressively before complete information can be sorted and reviewed. The resuscitation is dynamic, often ongoing as the patient enters the operating room (OR), and requires the presence of adequate nursing support. The sequential approach to patient resuscitation by the Advanced Trauma Life Support Course (ATLS) can be applied to all critically ill patients, emergency surgery, or trauma. Rarely do these events transpire sequentially; rather, rapid assessment should happen in a coordinated all-at-once manner. An important tenet to surgical assessment is prompt and judicious physiologic monitoring which serves as both diagnostic clues and resuscitative evaluation.

1. **Airway.** Assessment and control of a patient's airway is of foremost importance. Lack of airway control results in quick asphyxiation, leading to global hypoxia and rapid cardiovascular collapse. Indications for endotracheal intubation include the following:
   a. Inability to phonate
   b. Stridor
   c. Profound hypotension
   d. Somnolence
   e. Mechanical obstruction (secretions, traumatic or edematous oropharynx)
      i. Rapid-sequence induction (RIS) and endotracheal intubation is our preferred method. However, in an acute situation if the airway cannot be established, one must be prepared to execute a cricothyrotomy. Endotracheal intubation is verified by direct visualization of the endotracheal tube passing through the vocal cords. The use of expiratory capnography and auscultation of the lungs can be useful for successful intubation but is not definitive. A chest x-ray following intubation confirms position of the endotracheal tube but may not distinguish tracheal versus esophageal intubation.

2. **Breathing.** The inability to ventilate adequately leads to cardiac arrest. Assessment of patient breathing gives diagnostic clues and helps evaluate the degree of physiologic extremis. The immediate approach includes:
   a. Auscultation of the chest
   b. Pulse oximetery
   c. Arterial blood gas (ABG)
   d. Chest x-ray
      i. Auscultation and x-ray images may detect a pneumothorax, hemothorax, edema, or lobar collapse and serves as an overall guide toward immediate management. A tension pneumothorax classically presents with decreased breath sounds, hypotension, and tracheal deviation away from the affected side. Radiography is unnecessary. The diagnosis is clinical and treatment should be rendered without delay. Immediate pleural decompression in the most expeditious manner, usually with a large-bore needle, should be performed followed by placement of a thoracostomy tube, relieving high intrathoracic pressure from a pneumothrax and restoring adequate ventilation and hemodynamic instability.
      ii. Evacuation of over 1,500 mL of blood upon insertion of a chest tube or chest tube outputs of 200 cc/hour over 2 hours sequentially are indications for a thoracotomy. Except for the rare trauma patient, a thoracotomy should be done in an OR in a controlled environment.

         Lobar collapse is best treated by aggressive bronchoscopy which removes mucus plugging of the bronchial tree, allowing air movement and expansion of the lung. Pulse oximetry can be very useful in guiding real-time oxygenation. However, it may need to be supplemented with ABG to assess arterial CO_2 and O_2 partial pressures. If there is inability to adequately oxygenate, mechanical ventilation may be necessary.

3. **Circulation.** Pulse and blood pressure must be assessed through rapidly cycled brachial cuff measurements, arterial lines, cardiac electrical monitoring, and the immediate insertion of adequate vascular access (14–16 F brachial venous catheters). If peripheral access cannot be achieved then central access using an 8 F introducer, preferably in the femoral vein, is mandatory. Hypovolemia is common and life threatening in almost all surgical emergencies, leading to lack of end-organ perfusion and shock. The degree and class of shock varies according to percentage loss of intravascular volume. Viscus perforation, small-bowel obstructions, and severe sepsis also have massive fluid deficits.
   a. Crystalloid fluid resuscitation should be initiated immediately, and can be titrated after further management decisions have been made. An ABG with base deficit measurement may help determine degree of systemic hypoperfusion, especially in the immediate posttrauma period. However, if patients

have been hospitalized for a lengthy interval of time and have received exogenous bicarbonate infusions, the base deficit will be inaccurate in determining hypoperfusion. Serum lactate is an indication of anaerobic metabolism which may reflect organ ischemia.

b. A Foley catheter should be inserted to monitor urine output, which is a good indication of overall body fluid deficits.

c. The determination must be made quickly as to the cause of ongoing patient hypovolemia (i.e., hemorrhage, sepsis). If the patient is bleeding, determining the source and control of the hemorrhage is imperative. Packed red blood cells (PRBCs), fresh frozen plasma (FFP), and platelets may be necessary for resuscitation and resultant coagulopathy. Ultimately, most serious bleeding is controlled with surgical correction of the problem, not with transfusion of blood products.

i. Once initial circulatory access and monitoring is established, further history and laboratory values are useful for definitive planning.

III. OTHER PHYSIOLOGIC ABNORMALITIES. Once airway stabilization, adequate ventilation, and access and volume resuscitation are initiated, other physiologic abnormalities must be managed. This phase is not exclusive of initial resuscitative efforts since cardiac monitoring, early laboratory values, radiology results, and urine output help guide further management.

A. Cardiovascular. Cardiac electrical tracing can suggest ischemia or life-threatening dysrhythmias (rapid atrial fibrillation or supraventricular tachycardias [SVT], ventricular ectopy, fibrillation, severe bradycardia, or juntional rhythms). These abnormalities may be secondary to severe electrolyte abnormalities, shock, myocardial ischemia, or a hyperdynamic cardiac response secondary to a generalized hyperinflammatory state. Correction of these abnormalities depends largely on the cause. Ventricular fibrillation and hemodynamically significant SVT should follow Advanced Cardiac Life Support (ACLS) guidelines with electric cardioversion and medications. Cardiac ischemia is common, but the cause of ischemia must be evaluated promptly. If ischemia is a result of ongoing tachycardia and dehydration from sepsis, fluid resuscitation and beta-blockade may be a useful preoperative measure. However, for new ischemic changes secondary to acute hemorrhage (i.e., trauma or GI bleeding) operative control coupled with intraoperative PRBC resuscitation is the ultimate solution for ongoing ischemia and should not be delayed.

B. Pulmonary. As mentioned previously, the inability to ventilate can stem from a pneumothorax, hemothorax, lobar collapse, or flash pulmonary edema. Constant vigilance must be given to changes in ventilatory status. The establishment of a secure airway does not indicate adequate ventilation as iatrogenic barotrauma or an unappreciated pneumo- or hemothorax may exist. If any suspicion of ventilatory comprise does exists, patients should be intubated and mechanical ventilation established. Pulse oximetry is helpful to assess oxygenation once endotracheal intubation is complete. Pulmonary edema can be problematic, since diuresis in the acute patient may lead to hemodynamic compromise. Most life-threatening pulmonary complications can be dealt with using appropriately placed tubes: endotracheal or intrapleural.

C. Electrolyte abnormalities. Acute bowel obstruction, massive injury, and limb ischemia can lead to significant electrolyte imbalance, most commonly acidosis and hyper- or hypokalemia. Acidosis results most often from significant volume depletion and is readily determined by measuring ABG and base deficit. Infusion of crystalloid or possible PRBCs with an improving base deficit helps determine resuscitation endpoints. Hyperkalemia can be fatal if unrecognized, especially under the induction of a general anesthetic. Administration of calcium stabilizes myocardial cell membranes and reduces the risk of fatal ventricular arrhythmias. Its correction is most rapid by intravenous administration of insulin and glucose followed by a bicarbonate infusion. Ultimate correction with hemodialysis may be necessary but is rare. Other electrolyte abnormalities, specifically hypocalcemia and hypomagnesemia, may warrant correction.

D. Endocrine. Certain patients on chronic steroids for rheumatologic disorders or immunosuppression may suffer an Addisonian crisis manifested by severe hypotension when physiologically stressed. A 1-mg/kg stress dose of a glucocorticoid may be preventative and curative.

E. Coagulopathy. Overwhelming sepsis, anticoagulant medications, substantial transfusions of PRBCs, and hypothermia can lead to significant coagulopathies. Transfusion of FFP, intravenous (IV) calcium, and rewarming may help with correction. Emergency operative intervention should not be delayed, especially since ongoing bleeding only worsens coagulopathy.

IV. DEFINITIVE MANAGEMENT. The decision for operative intervention must be swift and based on the primary patient problem, physiologic parameters, and objectives. A concise yet complete physical exam combined with radiologic imaging and laboratory values help guide the definitive management stage of the emergency surgical patient. There are several preoperative maneuvers that serve as crucial adjuncts. As mentioned, decisions and operative interventions can occur without complete or adequate information or diagnosis (Table 56A-1).

V. REASSESSMENT AND REEVALUATION. Once resuscitation has commenced and a plan for operative or nonoperative management has been initiated, constant reassessment and reevaluation is vital to deem whether the patient is responding to resuscitation efforts or is in need of further diagnostic or therapeutic approaches. The security of the airway must constantly be monitored. Blood pressure, pulse, urine output, serial ABGs, hematocrits, and radiologic images are helpful for continual physiologic supervision and correction of metabolic abnormalities.

VI. SUMMARY. The acute surgical patient must be approached aggressively and without delay. Operation may be the definitive management but the initial approach should focus on establishing an airway, confirming ventilation, adequate vascular access and circulation coupled with physiologic monitoring and, secondarily, laboratory and radiology. A definitive diagnosis often comes after resuscitative measures have commenced. Preoperative evaluation and stabilization should be expeditious and thorough, but unnecessary delay may only worsen the patient's physiologic condition.

TABLE 56A-1

Operative emergency	Associated physical exam	Associated radiology findings	Associated laboratory values	Preoperative management
Peritonitis	Fever, tachycardia, guarding, rebound tenderness	Pneumoperitoneum, abdominal fluid	Leukocytosis with bandemia, elevated serum lactate	Broad-spectrum antibiotics, fluid resuscitation
Hemorrhage	Tachycardia, hypotension, hypothermia, clamminess	Hemoperitoneum, hemothorax, retroperitnoeal hemorrhage	Decreased hematocrit (late finding), coagulopathy	PRBCs, FFP, platelets (uncrossmatched or type specific), large-bore IV access

(continued)

TABLE 56A-1   Continued

Operative emergency	Associated physical exam	Associated radiology findings	Associated laboratory values	Preoperative management
Bowel obstruction	Abdominal distention, tenderness	Dilated stomach, small bowel, colon; transition point or hernia visible on CT imaging	Hypochloremic, hypokalemic metabolic alkalosis with prolonged vomiting; leukocytosis with bandemia, elevated serum lactate	Nasogastric decompression, fluid resuscitation, correction of electrolytes
Trauma	External tissue loss, limb fractures, abdominal distention, tenderness, hypotension, tachycardia, dyspnea	Hemoperitoneum, pneumothorax or hemothorax, retroperitoneal hemorrhage, skeletal fractures, neurologic trauma	Decreased hematocrit (late), coagulopathy, severe base deficit	Fluid resuscitation; possible transfusion of PRBCs, FFP, and platelets
Ischemia	Abdominal pain out of proportion to exam; limb pallor, cool extremity, limb compartment tension and edema, decreased pulses	Skeletal fractures or dislocation, vascular occlusion on angiography	Elevated serum lactates, CPK, hemoglobinuria	Fluid resuscitation

PREOPERATIVE ASSESSMENT OF THE SURGICAL PATIENT

FRANCIS X. SOLANO, JR. AND
ANTHONY B. FIORILLO

I. **INTRODUCTION.** The critically ill general surgical or trauma patient on presentation poses challenges to the surgeon, anesthesiologist, and medical consultant. For patients who need immediate lifesaving surgery a rapid preoperative evaluation includes age, gender, existing medical conditions, medication and allergy history, the correction of intravascular volume, and the establishment of airway. On the other hand, patients with less urgent surgical need may be more fully assessed prior to operation. This chapter outlines the general principles in the evaluation of risk for surgery as it relates to patients with concurrent medical issues.

II. **PREOPERATIVE CLEARANCE FOR FURTHER OPERATIVE INTERVENTION**

A. **History and fitness.** The most crucial aspects of preoperative assessment are the history and physical exam. Fitness can be assessed by historical information in 96% of patients. Functional status is also critical; the American Heart Association/American College of Cardiology guidelines provide detailed information on functional assessment as a perioperative and long-term predictor of risk. Patients who can perform less than 4 METs of activity (inability to walk four blocks or climb two flights of stairs) are considered high risk and should be subjected to further preoperative assessment.

B. **Assessing patients 50 years and older.** Patients at age 50 years or older may have comorbid medical conditions that place them at risk for cardiovascular and pulmonary complications. Assessment of pretrauma functional capacity with evaluation of the patient's level of daily activity has predictive value for perioperative complications. Attention to the presence of underlying coronary artery disease (CAD), congestive heart failure (CHF), emphysema, cerebrovascular disease, diabetes, and hypertension allows the consultant to risk assess and optimize those conditions.

C. **Key elements in risk assessment.** In making such an assessment the patient's medical problems must be optimally managed. Based on how well stabilized those conditions are, the medical consultant gives a risk assessment to the surgeon and the patient. The risk assessment includes consideration of the type of surgery and the potential duration of surgery.

D. **Tools for risk assessment.** Goldman, Detsky, and Eagle have all developed preoperative risk assessment tools that will facilitate preoperative assessment. Independent risk factors include a history of a myocardial infarction (MI) within 6 months, angina or unstable angina, a history of or current pulmonary edema, valvular heart disease—particularly aortic stenosis, presence of premature ventricular contractions (PVCs) and premature atrial contractions (PACs), poor medical status with respect to renal function, liver disease or nutritional issues, retention of carbon dioxide >45 mmHg, and age >70 years. Finally, the emergency surgery the patient faces is another factor that increases the risk of perioperative complications. A Goldman index or a Detsky "score," while useful in clinical studies, is time-consuming in clinical practice. Their principal utilities for the clinician are to give structure to the preoperative assessment and to direct attention to and correct the identified risks.

E. **Laboratory assessment.** The literature supports selective directed preoperative laboratory testing. Testing should reflect an assessment of the underlying conditions of the patient. Broad nonspecific preoperative screening tests contribute little value to the perioperative care, particularly in the healthy population.

III. SPECIFIC RISK FACTORS

A. Cardiovascular risk. The risk of cardiovascular disease (coronary and carotid atherosclerosis) increases with age. For patients over the age of 45 years, consider the existence of such disease. Increased severity of cardiovascular disease increases the risk of a vascular perioperative event: an acute MI, CHF, or death. Patients with low-level angina or an angina equivalent should undergo a noninvasive pharmacological stress test, if time permits and exercise stress testing is not possible. Eagle has validated a clinical index in combination with pharmacological stress. If a patient has one area of territory at risk for ischemia, that patient can be treated medically. A patient with global ischemia should undergo catherization and revascularization. The use of preoperative beta-blocker improves outcome for surgical patients that have CAD or have major risk factors for CAD. Such patients, as well as patients for which no assessment is possible, should start preoperative beta blockade (oral atenolol 50 mg daily or intravenous [IV] metoprolol 5 mg every 6 hours) to reduce heart rate to <60 beats per minute (bpm).

1. Preop electrocardiogram (ECG). The ECG has been a poor predictor of cardiovascular risk when using ST and T wave segments. A left bundle branch block on ECG is a marker for potential left ventricular dysfunction and can be helpful for identifying patients at risk for CHF. The finding of a silent MI is rare, yet approximately 0.3% of patients may be identified as at risk.

2. Recent myocardial infarction. An MI within 6 months of planned surgery has been a historical benchmark to indicate a patient at risk for perioperative MI. More recent information suggests that these patients have a lower risk of MI than previously reported. Rao, Jacobs, and El Etr demonstrated a 5.7% risk of perioperative MI within 3 months of recent MI and a 2.3% risk in the 3- to 6-month post-MI period. This risk may be even lower with the use of thrombolytics and percutaneous angioplasty/stents, but data are lacking. For elective surgery, post-MI patients who remain angina free should wait 4 to 6 weeks before surgery. This is usually not an option in the patient requiring urgent operation. We recommend initiating beta-blocker therapy as previously outlined.

3. Congestive heart failure. CHF has consistently been shown to increase perioperative morbidity and mortality. Patients with a history of CHF have a 6% risk of recurrent CHF and a 5% mortality. Patients with active CHF with an S3 gallop, jugular venous distention (JVD), or rales can have 20% mortality. Patients with CHF who do not require urgent surgery should be managed with diuretics to reduce intravascular and intrapulmonary volume. Adequate beta blockade and the use of angiotensin converting enzyme (ACE) inhibitors or angiotensin receptor blockers should be encouraged. All of these agents have been shown to improve survival, morbidity, and quality of life. Instrumentation with a Swan-Ganz catheter may be helpful for volume management up to 3 days postoperatively when fluid shifts are likely to occur.

4. Valvular heart disease. In patients with moderate to severe mitral and aortic stenosis, small changes in intravascular volume may result in CHF due to the presence of a fixed obstructive cardiac output. Too little volume results in hypotension and poor organ perfusion. Large volume expansion results in pulmonary edema. In the past, this valve disease was primarily caused by rheumatic heart disease, but calcific aortic stenosis has displaced this as the primary cause in our aging population. Patients with regurgitant aortic or mitral valve lesions and preserved left ventricular function tend to do well with surgery since many anesthetic agents reduce afterload. Patients should be given antibiotics as endocarditis prophylaxis if there is trauma or manipulation of the gastrointestinal or genitourinary tracts. Patients who are on Coumadin (warfarin) can be reversed with vitamin K and fresh frozen plasma urgently, and can be restarted on either unfractionated heparin or low-molecular-weight heparin within 24 hours of surgery if there are no other contraindications.

5. **Atrial fibrillation.** Patients with controlled atrial fibrillation (ventricular rate of 80 bpm) pose no increased risk for cardiac complications. Decompensated atrial fibrillation with a rapid ventricular rate and associated CHF must be managed prior to surgery. Risk assessment must include consideration of the underlying disease that resulted in the atrial fibrillation (i.e., CAD, valvular disease, thyroid disease, or decompensated heart failure). Most management issues revolve around anticoagulation issues and rate control. Anticoagulants can be managed in a similar manner as outlined previously for the patient with valvular disease. Intravenous calcium channel blockers such as diltiazem (5 to 10 mg per hour) or intravenous beta-blockers (lopressor 5 mg per hour) can be used for rate control in the perioperative period.

B. **Hypertension.** Hypertension has been poorly studied as a risk factor for surgery despite its prevalence in the population; 59 million Americans are affected with hypertension. The standard has been that patients with diastolic pressure >110 mmHg or systolic pressure >200 mmHg should not undergo surgery. Most of these data are from the 1950s and 1960s and are based on the fact that autoregulation of central nervous system blood flow is impaired at these levels. Due to this bias, it is difficult to find data on patients with severe hypertension who have undergone surgical treatment. Most of the risk of mild or moderate hypertension is related to the risk of increased peri- and postoperative exacerbation of hypertension. About 25% of patients will exhibit an increase in blood pressure independent of their preoperative control. It is important to remember that patients with hypertension often have concomitant medical problems that place them at higher risk for cardiovascular complications. Antihypertensive oral medication should be given preoperatively and postoperatively with a sip of water. For patients who are unable to take oral medication, there are several intravenous medications available (calcium channel blockers and beta-blockers) as well as transdermal delivery mechanisms for clonidine.

C. **Cerebrovascular disease.** Patients with asymptomatic significant (>70%) carotid stenosis are at low risk for stroke (1%–2%) following anesthesia and this condition is not a contraindication to surgery. Patients with recent transient ischemic attacks are at increased risk for stroke within 6 weeks of the event.

D. **Pulmonary issues.** Trauma patients with thoracic and extremity injuries are at increased risk for postoperative pulmonary complications such as atelectasis, pulmonary embolism, or pneumonia. Attention should be paid to trauma-related injuries to the lungs, pleura, pericardium, myocardium, and renal system as these are important risk factors for surgery. Indolent pulmonary embolism, pulmonary contusion, pneumonia, and pleural effusion can be causes of hypoxemia that may be noted at the time of preoperative assessment for surgery. In our experience, fat emboli are uncommon since long bone injuries are aggressively treated early in the management of the trauma patient.

1. Patients with chronic obstructive lung disease should be optimally managed before proceeding with surgery if possible. There is no clear-cut level of forced expiratory volume in 1 second (FEV1) which can be used as a cutoff for risk. The maximum voluntary minute ventilation (MVMV) is helpful since this is a measure of respiratory drive. If MVMV >50% the patient is at risk for pulmonary complications. PCO_2 >45 mm is a risk factor for pulmonary complications.

E. **Diabetes.** Diabetes affects almost 8% of the population. Diabetes is not an independent risk factor for surgery. However, patients with Type II diabetes mellitus have been identified as coronary disease risk equivalents. Predictors of complications are the presence of cardiac, renal, and diabetic end-organ damage. Particular attention should be paid to assessment of renal function as critically ill surgical patients may be exposed to intravascular volume shifts, radiocontrast agents, and nephrotoxic antibiotics. Tight glucose control perioperatively has been shown to reduce complications.

F. **Thyroid disease.** Hypothyroidism poses no special risks for patients on replacement therapy. Patients with undiagnosed hypothyroidism are at risk for myxedema postoperatively. Patients can be given intravenous thyroid hormone replacement if they develop symptomatic myxedema postoperatively. Patients with untreated hyperthyroidism are at risk for thyroid storm and should be aggressively treated with beta-blockers and either propylthiouracil or methimazole preoperatively to avoid this complication.

G. Special issues for trauma patients

1. **Renal issues.** Rhabdomyolysis and renal failure can often be overlooked in the acute setting. Ureteral injuries secondary to visceral injuries or surgery and antibiotic usage are other causes of late renal insufficiency in trauma patients. Renal failure secondary to acute tubular necrosis from hypotension is a problem that can be detected late in the course of the trauma patient. Nephrotoxic drugs such as antibiotics and NSAIDs can also cause renal injury.

2. **Indolent pulmonary embolism, pulmonary contusion, pneumonia, and pleural effusion** can be causes of silent hypoxemia that may be noted at the time of preoperative assessment for surgery.

3. **Indolent pancreatitis** secondary to trauma or hypotension should also be a diagnosis of awareness preoperatively.

4. **Liver injury abnormalities** are not uncommon in the setting of visceral injury and generally pose no serious risk if there is no evidence of obstruction to the biliary tree. Laceration of the liver will often cause transaminasemia.

5. **Fever** late in the course of the trauma patient's hospitalization is a common cause of consultation. In most instances blood, urine cultures, white blood cell (WBC) counts, and chest x-ray (CXR) have been obtained and are normal. Indolent infections with *Clostridium difficile,* pulmonary embolism, and atelectasis (seen on CT scan) with normal CXR can cause fever. Long bone injuries, hip fractures, and pelvic fractures with hematoma can cause fever as well. In our experience, septic thrombophlebitis in pelvic trauma is a most uncommon cause of fever. Wound infection must also be excluded, as should osteomyelitis. These are generally uncommon since the trauma service has typically done surveillance in this area.

6. **Hematology issues.** Postoperative anemia or anemia secondary to bone or visceral injuries is common. Hemolytic anemia is very uncommon. Thrombocytosis as a reactive phenomenon is common; we have seen platelet counts in excess of 1 million in patients who sustained multiple injuries with and without splenectomy. Thrombocytopenia secondary to consumption is also a common event. Thrombocytopenias developing 3 to 5 days postinstitution of heparin can also occur in 1% to 3% of patients who receive heparin or LMW heparin. Consumptive coagulopathy has been discussed in other chapters. Posttransfusion purpura is a rare complication of red blood cell transfusion occurring 3 to 10 days posttransfusion. Leukopenia secondary to antibiotics is also seen on rare occasion; Vancomycin and semisynthetic penicillins are associated with this phenomenon. Significant leukocytosis with leukemoid reaction has also been seen in the trauma patient with multiple injuries. WBC counts of up to 50,000 can be seen on occasion. Generally the white cell differential is normal, but on occasion one can see immature WBC forms. Infection and bacteremia need to be excluded in these patients.

7. **Gastrointestinal issues.** Gastroesophageal reflux disease (GERD) remains a major pre- and posttrauma phenomenon. Gastric motility issues are other complications commonly seen in general surgical and trauma patients, particularly prolonged ileus. It is important to exclude mechanical causes of obstruction in these patients. Diarrhea secondary to antibiotics and antibiotic-associated *C. difficile* are also common problems posthospitalization.

Bibliography

Alberti KG, Thomas DJB. The management of diabetes during surgery. *Br J Anaesth* 1979;51:693–708.

Auerbach AD, Goldman L. Beta blockers and reduction of cardiac events in noncardiac surgery: Scientific review. *JAMA* 2002;287:1435–1444.

Barnes RW, Marszalek PB, Rittgers SE. Asymptomatic carotid disease in preoperative patients. *Stroke* 1980;11:136.

Brodsky JB, Bravo JJ. Acute postoperative clonidine withdrawal syndrome. *Anesthesiology* 1976;44:519.

Celli BR. What is the value of preoperative pulmonary function testing? *Med Clin North Am* 1993;77:309–325.

Cleland JGF. Beta blockers for heart failure: Why, which, when and where. *Med Clin North Am* 2003;87:339–371.

Detsky AS, Abrams HB, McLaughlin JR, et al. Predicting cardiac complications in patients undergoing non-cardiac surgery. *J Gen Intern Med* 1986;1:211–219.

Eagle KA, Berger PB, Calkins H, et al. *Perioperative Cardiovascular Evaluation for Noncardiac Surgery Update.* American College of Cardiology Foundation Web site. Available at: http://www.acc.org/clinical/guidelines/perio/update/periupdate_index.htm.

Eagle KA, Coley CM, Newell JB, et al. Combining clinical and thallium data optimizes preoperative assessment of cardiac risk before major vascular surgery. *Ann Intern Med* 1989;110:859–866.

Executive Committee for the Asymptomatic Carotid Atherosclerosis Study. Endarterectomy for asymptomatic carotid artery stenosis. *JAMA* 1995;273:1421–1428.

Ferguson B, Coombs LP, Peterson ED. Preoperative β blocker use and mortality and morbidity following CABG surgery in North America. *JAMA* 2002;287:2221–2227.

Ferguson GG. Extracranial carotid artery surgery. *Clin Neurosurg* 1982;29:543–574.

Ford GT, Guenter CA. Toward prevention of postoperative pulmonary complications. *Am Rev Respir Dis* 1984;130:4–5.

Furnary AP, Zerr KJ, Grunkemeier GL, et al. Continuous intravenous insulin infusion reduces the incidence of deep sternal wound infection in diabetic patients after cardiac surgical procedures. *Ann Thorac Surg* 1999;67:352–360.

Gass GD, Olsen GN. Preoperative pulmonary function testing to predict postoperative morbidity and mortality. *Chest* 1986;89:127–135.

Goldman L. Cardiac risks and complications of noncardiac surgery. *Ann Intern Med* 1983;98:504–513.

Goldman L. Noncardiac surgery in patients receiving propranolol: Case reports and a recommended approach. *Arch Intern Med* 1981;141:193.

Goldman L, Caldera DL. Risks of general anesthesia and elective operation in the hypertensive patient. *Anesthesiology* 1979;50:285–292.

Goldman L, Caldera DL, Nussbaum SR, et al. Multifactorial index of cardiac risk in noncardiac surgical procedures. *N Engl J Med* 1977;297:845–850.

Grundy SM, Cleeman JI, Bairey Merz CN. Implications of recent trials for the National Cholesterol Education Program Adult Treatment Panel III Guidelines. *Circulation* 2004;110:227–239.

Guarnieri KM, Mekeon BP. *Perioperative Medicine.* New York, NY: McGraw-Hill; 1994:479.

Hollenberg M, Mangano DT, Browner WS, et al. Predictors of postoperative myocardial ischemia in patients undergoing noncardiac surgery. The Study of Perioperative Ischemia Research Group. *JAMA* 1992;268(2):205–209.

Kaplan EB, Sheiner LB, Boeckman AJ, et al. The usefulness of preoperative laboratory screening. *JAMA* 1985;253:3576–3581.

Lette J, Waters D, Lapointe J, et al. Usefulness of the severity and extent of reversible perfusion defects during thallium-dipyridamole imaging for cardiac risk assessment before noncardiac surgery. *Am J Cardiol* 1989;64:276–281.

London MJ, Tubau JF, Wong MG, et al. The natural history of segmental wall motion abnormalities in patients undergoing noncardiac surgery. *Anesthesiology* 1990;73:644–655.

Macpherson DS. Preoperative laboratory testing: Should any tests be routine before surgery? *Med Clin North Am* 1993;77(2):289–308.

Mangano DT, Goldman L. Current concepts: Preoperative assessment of patients with known or suspected coronary disease. *N Engl J Med* 1995;333:1750–1756.

Mangano DT, Layug EL, Wallace A, et al. Effect of atenolol on mortality and cardiovascular morbidity after noncardiac surgery. Multicenter Study of Perioperative Ischemia

Research Group (published erratum appears in *N Engl J Med* 1997;336[14]:1039). *N Engl J Med* 1996;335:1713–1720.

McMurry J. Wound healing with diabetes mellitus. *Surg Clin North Am* 1984;64:769–778.

Moore WS, Barnet HJM, Beebe HG, et al. Guidelines for carotid endarterectomy. *Stroke* 1995;26:188–201.

Myers J, Do D, Herbert W, et al. A nomogram to predict exercise capacity from a specific activity questionnaire and clinical data. *Am J Cardiol* 1994;73:591–596.

Nolan CM, Beaty HN, Bagdade JD. Further characterization of the impaired bactericidal function of granulocytes in patients with poorly controlled diabetes. *Diabetes* 1978;27:889–894.

North American Symptomatic Carotid Endarterectomy trial collaborators. Beneficial effects of carotid endarterectomy in symptomatic patients with high grade stenosis. *N Engl J Med* 1991;325:445–453.

Nunn DB. Carotid endarterectomy in patients with territorial transient ischemic attacks. *J Vasc Surg* 1988;8:447–452.

Poe RH, Kally MC, Dass T, et al. Can postoperative pulmonary complications after elective cholecystectomy be predicted? *Am J Med Sci* 1988;295:29–34.

Poldermans D, Boersma E, Bax JJ, et al. The effect of bisoprolol on perioperative mortality and myocardial infarction in high-risk patients undergoing vascular surgery. Dutch Echocardiographic Cardiac Risk Evaluation Applying Stress Echocardiography Study Group. *N Engl J Med* 1999;341:1789–1794.

Poole-Wilson PA. ACE inhibitors and ARBs in chronic heart failure: The established, the expected and the pragmatic. *Med Clin N Am* 2003;87:373–389.

Presley AP, Alexander-Williams J. Postoperative chest infection. *Br J Surg* 1974;61:448.

Prys-Roberts C. Hypertension and anesthesia: Fifty years on. *Anesthesiology* 1979;50:281.

Rao TL, Jacobs KH, El Etr AA. Reinfarction following anesthesia in patients with myocardial infarction. *Anesthesiology* 1983;59:499–505.

Reilly DF, McNeely MJ, Doerner D, et al. Self-reported exercise tolerance and the risk of serious perioperative complications. *Arch Intern Med* 1999;159:2185–2192.

Seeger JM, Rosenthal GR, Self SB, et al. Does routine stress thallium cardiac scanning reduce postoperative cardiac complications? *Ann Surg* 1994;219:654–663.

Steen PA, Tinker JH, Tarhan S. Myocardial re-infarction after anesthesia and surgery. *JAMA* 1978;239:2566–2570.

Symonds JM, George RH, Dimock F, et al. Identification of *Clostridium difficile* as a cause of pseudomembranous colitis. *Br Med J* 1978;1:695.

Tahran S, Moffitt EA, Taylor WF, et al. Myocardial infarction after general anesthesia. *JAMA* 1972;220:1451–1454.

Tisi GM. Preoperative evaluation of pulmonary function. *Am Rev Respir Dis* 1979;119:293–310.

Toole JF, Yuson CP, Janeway R, et al. Transient ischmic attacks: A prospective study of 225 patients. *Neurology* 1988;18:746–753.

Turnbull JM, Buck C. The value of preoperative screening investigations in otherwise healthy individuals. *Arch Intern Med* 1987;147:1101–1105.

Wallace A, Layug B, Tateo I, et al. Prophylactic atenolol reduces postoperative myocardial ischemia. McSPI Research Group. *Anesthesiology* 1998;88:7–17.

Warkentin AU, Greinacher TA. Heparin-induced thrombocytopenia: Recognition, treatment, and prevention: The Seventh ACCP Conference on Antithrombotic and Thrombolytic Therapy. *Chest* 2004;126(3 suppl):311S–337S.

Whisnant JP, Sandok BA, Sundt TM. Carotid endarterectomy for unilateral carotid system transient cerebral ischemia. *Mayo Clin Proc* 1983;56:171–175.

Willians CD, Brenowitz JB. Prohibitive lung function and major surgical procedures. *Am J Surg* 1976;132:763–766.

Wilson ME, Williams NB, Baskett PJF, et al. Assessment of fitness for surgical procedures and the variability of anesthetists' judgements. *Br Med J* 1980;1:509–513.

INFECTIONS OF TRAUMA PATIENTS
PHILIP S. BARIE AND
SOUMITRA R. EACHEMPATI

57

I. EPIDEMIOLOGY
A. Incidence.
The incidence of infection following injury approaches 25%. Although most trauma-related deaths occur within the first 24 hours after injury, from exsanguination or massive injury to the central nervous system, the leading cause of posttraumatic death after the initial 24 hours is infection, usually manifesting as the multiple organ dysfunction syndrome (MODS). The high risk of infection is due to the host immune response to injury and stress; inadequate attention to the principles of infection control under emergency conditions; direct inoculation of wounds by clothing, dirt, or debris; blood transfusions; and poor glycemic control. Appropriate antibiotic prophylaxis reduces the risk, but inappropriate prophylaxis may increase the risk of infection.

B. Patterns of injury.
Infections following injury occur in the injured tissue, the surgical site (incision), or as a health care–associated (nosocomial) infection (HAI) such as pneumonia or catheter-related bloodstream infection (CR-BSI) (Table 57-1). Considered together, HAIs are as common as infections of the injured tissues. The likelihood of infection is higher with increasing injury severity score (ISS), increasing number of abdominal organs injured, traumatic brain injury, colon injury, shock, number of blood transfusions, and creation of an ostomy. Traumatic wounds are characterized by devitalized, ischemic tissue, with increased risk of infection if contaminated by enteric contents (e.g., penetrating abdominal trauma), fragments of clothing fabric (e.g., gunshot wounds), dirt or gravel (e.g., motor vehicle or farm injuries), or vegetation (e.g., fall from

TABLE 57-1	Rates of Health Care–Associated Pneumonia and Catheter-Related Bacteremia Among Various ICU Types			
ICU type	**CVC use* infection rate mean/median**		**TT use† infection rate mean/median**	
Medical	0.52	5.0/3.9	0.46	4.9/3.7
Pediatric	0.46	6.6/5.2	0.39	2.9/2.3
Surgical	0.61	4.6/3.4	0.44	9.3/8.3
Cardiovascular	0.79	2.7/1.8	0.43	7.2/6.3
Neurosurgical	0.48	4.6/3.1	0.39	11.2/6.2
Trauma	0.61	7.4/5.2	0.56	15.2/11.4

*Number of days of catheter placement /1,000 patient-days in ICU.
†Number of days of indwelling endotracheal tube or tracheostomy/1,000 patient-days in ICU.
Infection rates are indexed per 1,000 patient-days.
(Based on the National Nosocomial Infection Surveillance System, U.S. Centers for Disease Control and Prevention. From Bercker S, Weber-Carstens S, Deja M, et al. Critical illness polyneuropathy and myopathy in patients with acute respiratory distress syndrome. *Crit Care Med* 2005;33:711–715.)

height into a tree). More wound contamination increases the risk of infection of injured tissue.

C. **Comparison with critically ill surgical patients (nontrauma).** The epidemiology of HAI is changing among critically ill patients, with higher incidences of pneumonia and CR-BSI, and stable or fewer urinary tract infections and surgical site infections. The epidemiology of infection following trauma appears to differ from other critically ill surgical patients. Trauma patients are both more likely to become infected (Table 57-1) and develop infection earlier postinjury. Pneumonia is the most common HAI following injury. The timing of onset of infection influences the choice of antimicrobial therapy.

II. **RISK FACTORS.** The host is put at risk of invasion by microbial pathogens whenever a natural epithelial barrier (e.g., skin, respiratory tract mucosa, gastrointestinal mucosa) is breached. Colonization of the epithelial barriers occurs even in healthy hosts. However, invasion does not occur unless injury or some other mechanism of inoculation occurs. Injury, catheterization, or incision breach an epithelial barrier and create a portal for tissue invasion by pathogens. Potential pathogens are ubiquitous in the environment. Innate immunity provides continuous surveillance against invasion by foreign antigens, and stimulates a repair response (inflammation), which may result in counterproductive augmentation of the inflammatory response that is destructive to the host. Prolonged or severe inflammation (e.g., the systemic inflammatory response syndrome, SIRS) (Table 57-2) is associated with the multiple organ dysfunction syndrome (MODS).

A. **Injury severity.** Severity of injury is directly related to the risk of infection. Shock and higher Injury Severity Score (ISS) increase the risk of infection globally. Thoracoabdominal penetrating injury is associated with a higher risk of infection than either abdominal or thoracic injury alone. The risk of intraabdominal infection is higher with increasing numbers of abdominal organs injured. Several "local" injuries induce systemic immune, inflammatory, and coagulation responses, including pulmonary contusion and traumatic brain injury, the latter being the injury most associated with infection, especially pneumonia.

TABLE 57-2   **Immune Dysfunction after Trauma**

Specific Immunity
- Lymphopenia
- Helper: Suppressor T-cell ratio <1
- Downregulated:
  - –T, B cell proliferation
  - –NK cell activity
  - –IL-2 receptor expression
  - –IL-4, -10 production
  - –HLA-DR expression
  - –DTH skin test response

Nonspecific immunity
- Monocytosis
- Upregulated:
  - –Acute-phase proteins
  - –TNF, IL-6 production
  - –Eicosanoid production
- Downregulated:
  - –Neutrophil function

NK, natural killer cell; IL, interleukin; HLA-DR, human leukocyte antigen; DTH, delayed topical hypersensitivity; TNF, tumor necrosis factor.

TABLE 57-3	Systemic Inflammatory Response Syndrome (SIRS)

Temperature >38°C or <36°C
Heart rate >90 bpm
Respiratory rate >20 breaths/min or $PaCO_2$ <32 mmHg
White blood cell count >12.0 × 10⁹/L or <4.0 × 10⁹/L*

*In the absence of another explanation (e.g., antineoplastic therapy). SIRS is present if two or more criteria are met. Sepsis is diagnosed when SIRS is caused by infection.

TABLE 57-4	Overview of the Stress Response to Injury

Activation of the sympathetic nervous system
Activation of hypophyseal-pituitary-adrenal axis
Peripheral insulin resistance
Production of pro- and antiinflammatory cytokines
Acute-phase changes of hepatic protein synthesis
Recruitment and activation of neutrophils, monocyte/macrophages, and lymphocytes
Upregulation of procoagulant activity

B. Immune dysfunction
   1. The immune response to injury is immediate and complex (Table 57-3). The consequences are immediate activation of:
      a. Coagulation as a result of endothelial dysfunction and activation of platelets
      b. Mononuclear and polymorphonuclear leukocytes causing release of both pro- and antiinflammatory cytokines and activation of host defenses against microbial invasion
      c. Depression of humoral and cell-mediated immunity with predisposition to later HAI
   2. Inflammation and the stress response. The stress hormone response that characterizes the "fight or flight" response:
      a. Augments cardiovascular function through the sympathetic nervous system
      b. Enhances glycogenolysis
      c. Mobilizes peripheral lean muscle and fat as fuel
      d. Enhances coagulation to stanch hemorrhage
      e. Stimulates a proinflammatory cytokine response to begin the process of tissue repair (Table 57-4). Humoral and cellular immunity are depressed in large part by the actions of cortisol (Table 57-5).
C. Medical comorbidity. Both very young and elderly patients are at increased risk of infection (Table 57-6). Obesity, malnutrition, diabetes mellitus, hypocholesterolemia, hypothermia, and chronic renal insufficiency pose an increased risk of infection. Perioperative hypoxemia and male gender may be risk factors for infection, but the data are conflicting.
D. Transfusion
   1. Blood transfusion cannot be avoided in the bleeding trauma patient. However, hemodynamically stable patients who are not bleeding may tolerate anemia and may not require transfusion. Trauma patients are more than fivefold more likely to develop infection if a blood transfusion is administered; red cell transfusion should be given only when necessary. Several theories exist as to why transfusion predisposes to infection:

TABLE 57-5	Principal Hormonal Responses to Surgical Stress	
Endocrine gland	**Hormones**	**Change in secretion**
Anterior pituitary		
	ACTH	Increased
	Growth hormone	Increased
	TSH	Variable
	FSH/LH	Variable
Posterior pituitary		
	AVP	Increased
Adrenal cortex		
	Cortisol	Increased
	Aldosterone	Increased
Pancreas		
	Insulin	Decreased
	Glucagon	Increased
Thyroid		
	Thyroxine	Decreased
	Triiodothyronine	Decreased

ACTH, adrenocorticotropic hormone; TSH, thyroid-stimulating hormone; FSH, follicle-stimulating hormone; LH, luteinizing hormone; AVP, arginine vasopressin.

TABLE 57-6	Conditions Known to Increase the Risk of Infection

- Extremes of age
- Malnutrition
- Obesity
- Diabetes
- Prior site irradiation
- Hypothermia
- Hypoxemia
- Remote infection
- Corticosteroid therapy
- Recent operation, especially of the chest or abdomen
- Chronic inflammation
- Hypocholesterolemia

  a. Transfusion may be immunosuppressive through leukocyte antigen–mediated decreases in cell-mediated immunity, specifically a shift to the Th2 (immunosuppressive) response phenotype.
  b. Augmentation of the SIRS response.
  c. Mechanically, the "storage lesion" that develops after 2 weeks of storage in the blood bank depletes erythrocyte 2,3-diphosphoglycerate and cell membrane stores of adenosine triphosphate, decreasing oxygen delivery and red blood cell deformability, respectively. The latter lesion impairs the ability of the red blood cell to transit the microcirculation, resulting in rouleaux formation and obstruction of the microcirculation.
  d. Moreover, each unit of red blood cell concentrate results in the administration of about 200 mg free iron, which is vital for microbial growth.

2. Critically ill patients who are not bleeding and without active coronary artery disease tolerate a hemoglobin concentration as low as 7 g/dL. It may be reasonable to extrapolate these data to trauma patients, who are generally younger with a lower incidence of coronary disease than general surgical intensive care unit (ICU) populations.

E. Hyperglycemia

1. Hyperglycemia was viewed as inevitable following critical illness and injury as a consequence of the counterregulatory stress hormone response, the mobilization of glucose through glycogenolysis, and the subsequent mobilization of amino acids for glucose synthesis through catabolism of lean tissue. This was despite evidence that hyperglycemia (>200 mg/dL) was associated with an increased incidence of surgical site infection following cardiac or major general surgery.

2. Despite these observations, little priority was assigned to prevention of hyperglycemia until the publication in 2001 by van den Berghe et al. of a prospective trial of tight glucose control (80–110 mg/dL) in critically ill surgical patients (mostly cardiac surgery) by continuous infusion of insulin.

   a. Mortality was reduced by 40%. Bloodstream infections and several manifestations of MODS were reduced.

   b. Meta-analysis of recent trials confirmed that tight glucose control reduces the risk of death of critically ill surgical patients by more than 40%. The effect appears to be related to control of serum glucose concentration directly, not to any anabolic effects of insulin administration. The benefit is equivalent for diabetic and nondiabetic patients. Administration of subcutaneous insulin for glucose control does not have similar benefit. It is unknown whether lesser degrees of glucose control (e.g., 140–150 mg/dL) will provide similar benefit.

3. Glucose dyshomeostasis has several manifestations during stress (Table 57-7).

   a. Peripheral glucose uptake and utilization are increased.

   b. Glycogenolysis is depressed after initial, short-term mobilization of hepatic glycogen stores.

   c. Increased gluconeogenesis.

   d. Peripheral insulin resistance.

   e. Importantly, hyperglycemia impairs immune cell function.

      i. Neutrophils may activate spontaneously, with increased generation of adhesion molecules, impairing microcirculatory flow.

      ii. Insulin-stimulated chemokinesis is decreased.

      iii. Phagocytes manifest decreased respiratory burst and thus impaired microbial killing.

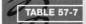

TABLE 57-7 Glucose Dyshomeostasis During Stress and Effects on Cellular Immunity

Effects of stress response on carbohydrate metabolism
- Enhanced peripheral glucose uptake/utilization
- Hyperlactatemia
- Increased gluconeogenesis
- Depressed glycogenolysis
- Peripheral insulin resistance

Effects of hyperglycemia on immune cell function
- Decreased respiratory burst of alveolar macrophages
- Decreased insulin-stimulated chemokinesis
    –Glucose-induced protein kinase C activation
- Increased adherence
    –Increased adhesion molecule generation
- Spontaneous activation of neutrophils

4. Given that the stress response is stereotypical and pervasive among critically ill and injured surgical patients, it is reasonable to expect that tight glucose control is as important for trauma patients as it is for surgical patients, but limited data are available.

III. PREVENTION OF INFECTION

A. **Principles.** Infection is morbid, costly, and potentially a lethal complication in trauma patients. Infection can be prevented in part. However, no single method of prophylaxis is universally effective, and each patient presents a unique challenge; all available modalities must be utilized for every case. Infection control is paramount, but often underemphasized. Traumatic wounds must be cleansed thoroughly and debrided to remove devitalized tissue. Surgical incisions must be handled gently, inspected daily, and dressed if necessary using aseptic technique. Drains and catheters must be avoided if possible, and if utilized, removed as soon as possible. Antibiotics should be used sparingly so as to minimize antibiotic selection pressure on the emergence of antibiotic-resistant pathogens.

B. **Infection control**

1. Infection control is an individual responsibility as well as a responsibility of the trauma team and trauma unit. **Hand hygiene is the single most effective means to reduce the spread of infection.** Yet, if adherence to handwashing is studied, it is invariably found to be lacking. To be effective, hand cleansing with soap and water requires a minimum of 30 to 45 seconds. Alcohol gel hand cleansers are equally effective as soap and water, and compliance is higher. Universal precautions (i.e., cap, mask, gown, gloves, and protective eyewear) must be observed whenever there is a risk of splashing of body fluids (at all times in the trauma bay, and commonly in the ICU).

2. The source of the bacteria causing infection are the patients' endogenous flora, and skin surfaces, airways, gut lumen, wounds, catheters, and inanimate surfaces within the patient's room (e.g., bed rails, and computer terminals do become colonized). Any break in natural epithelial barriers (e.g., incisions, percutaneous catheters, airway or urinary catheters) provides a portal of entry for invasion of the host by pathogenic organisms.

3. Whether infection develops is determined primarily by the response of host defenses, as many organisms that cause infection following injury are inherently avirulent (e.g., *Candida, Enterococcus, Pseudomonas*). The fecal-oral route is the most common manner by which autoinfection develops, but health care workers can hasten the transmission of pathogens around a unit.

4. Contact isolation is an important part of infection control, and should be used selectively to prevent the spread of pathogens such as methicillin-resistant *Staphylococcus aureus* and vancomycin-resistant enterococci, or multi-drug-resistant gram-negative bacilli. However, contact isolation may decrease the amount of time that caregivers have direct patient contact, because donning protective garb is time-consuming. By guarding against this phenomenon, an appropriate balance can be struck between attention and protection.

C. **Appropriate catheter care includes:**

1. Avoidance of insertion when nonessential.

2. Appropriate skin cleansing and barrier protection during insertion.

3. Selection of the proper catheter.

4. Proper dressings while catheters are indwelling.

5. Removal as soon as possible when no longer needed, or if inserted under less than ideal circumstances. **The benefit of the information gained by catheterization must always be weighed against the risk of infection.**

6. Any indwelling catheter carries a risk of infection, but nontunneled central venous catheters (and pulmonary artery catheters) pose the highest risk, including local site infections and bloodstream infections (Table 57-1). Other catheters that have a significant risk of infection include:

   a. Thoracostomy catheters (particularly if inserted as an emergency procedure).

   b. Ventriculostomy catheters for monitoring of intracranial pressure.

   c. Urinary bladder catheters.
   d. Each day of endotracheal intubation and mechanical ventilation increases the risk of pneumonia. It is controversial whether tracheostomy with facilitation of pulmonary toilet decreases the risk.
   e. In terms of preventing infection, abdominal drains are the most superfluous.
7. Whenever possible, skin preparation should be with chlorhexidine solution, which is viricidal and fungicidal as well as bacteridal. Extensive evidence-based guidelines exist for prevention of catheter-related infection.
   a. Chlorhexidine is superior to povidone-iodine solution for skin preparation prior to central venous catheter insertion. When povidone-iodine solution is used, it must be allowed to dry; it is not bactericidal when wet.
   b. Full barrier precautions (i.e., cap, mask, sterile gown, sterile gloves, eye protection, and a large field drape) are mandatory for all bedside catheterization procedures except arterial and urinary bladder catheterization, for which sterile gloves and a sterile field suffice.
   c. Anytime a deep catheter is inserted under less than ideal conditions as described (e.g., a central venous catheter placed hastily during a trauma or cardiac resuscitation) it must be removed (and replaced at a different site if still needed) as soon as permitted by the patient's hemodynamic status, but no longer than 24 hours after insertion.
   d. A single dose but no more of a first-generation cephalosporin (e.g., cefazolin) may prevent some infections following emergency tube thoracostomy or all ventriculostomy placements, but is not indicated for vascular or bladder catheterizations. Topical antiseptics placed postprocedure at the insertion site are of no benefit.
8. The choice of catheter may play a role in decreasing the risk of infection with endotracheal tubes, central venous catheters, and urinary catheters.
   a. An endotracheal tube with an extra lumen that opens to the airway just above the balloon, to facilitate the aspiration of secretions that accumulate in an area that cannot be reached by routine suctioning, below the vocal cords but above the balloon on the endotracheal tube (subglottic secretions), can decrease the incidence of ventilator-associated pneumonia by one half.
   b. Antibiotic- (e.g., minocycline/rifampin) or antiseptic-coated central venous catheters (e.g., chlorhexidine/silver sulfadiazine) are effective in reducing the incidence of catheter-related bloodstream infection; the catheter coated with minocycline/rifampin appears to be most effective.
   c. Urinary bladder catheters coated with ionic silver reduce the incidence of catheter-related bacterial cystitis.
9. Dressings must be maintained clean, dry, and intact. Maintaining an intact dressing may be difficult when the patient is agitated or the body surface is irregular (e.g., the neck [internal jugular vein catheterization] as opposed to the chest wall [subclavian vein catheterization]), but its importance must be emphasized.
   a. A simple gauze dressing is best. Occlusive transparent dressings can accumulate moisture beneath that is a usable growth medium for residual skin flora, which recolonize the skin anyway within a few hours.
   b. Mark the dressing clearly with the date and time of each change.
   c. Dressing carts or similar apparatus should not be brought from patient to patient; rather, sufficient supplies should be kept in each patient's room. Be cognizant of the possibility for inanimate objects (e.g., stethoscopes, scissors) to be transmission vectors if not cleansed thoroughly after contact with each patient.
10. Every indwelling catheter must be evaluated daily for its continued utility; catheters must be removed as soon as possible.
   a. Protocolized ventilator weaning facilitated by daily sedation holidays and spontaneous breathing trials allow earlier endotracheal extubation and decrease the risk of pneumonia. An even better strategy may be avoidance

of catheterization (intubation) entirely. Some episodes of respiratory failure can be managed with noninvasive positive-pressure ventilation delivered by mask (e.g., continuous positive airway pressure [CPAP], bilevel positive airway pressure [BiPAP]).

b. Improved resuscitation techniques and noninvasive monitoring techniques have decreased the utilization of pulmonary artery flotation catheters (which pose an especially high risk of infection).

c. Most abdominal drains do not decrease the risk of infection. On the contrary, the risk is probably increased because the catheters hold open a portal for invasion by bacteria and soon become a "two-way street." Other than for hepatic or pancreatic injuries, abdominal drains are seldom useful. Closed suction drains should not be left in proximity to intestinal suture lines; the negative pressures generated, particularly when such drains are "stripped," may cause disruption.

D. Antibiotic prophylaxis

1. Pharmacokinetics. Shock, hypoperfusion, and hemorrhage complicate the pharmacokinetics of prophylactic antibiotic administration immediately following trauma. Shock, hypovolemia, and hypoperfusion may also increase the risk of organ dysfunction caused by antibiotics (e.g., aminoglycosides and renal injury). Young injured patients also have higher glomerular filtration rates than older patients, which will result in more rapid clearance of antibiotics excreted in the urine. Historic recommendations, based paradoxically on the administration of aminoglycosides after trauma, recommended higher doses for prophylaxis that are given conventionally for therapy. Tissue edema associated with resuscitation will change volume of distribution of drugs, and hypoalbuminemia associated with hemodilution, plasma loss, and down-regulation of albumin synthesis (negative acute-phase reactant) can affect tissue antibiotic concentrations. However, there is little documented correlation between measured tissue concentrations and efficacy of prophylaxis. Aminoglycosides are no longer used in this indication for the most part.

2. It may be reasonable to increase the dose of drug administered to patients in shock. However, with modern beta-lactam antibiotics, what is necessary is for the drug to be in the tissues in a concentration above the minimum inhibitory concentration (MIC) for the likely pathogens that may cause surgical site infection (e.g., *S. aureus, Escherichia coli*). Conventional prophylactic doses (e.g., cefazolin 1 g, cefoxitin 1–2 g) probably suffice unless the patient is morbidly obese or bleeding briskly.

IV. DURATION

A. It is important that antibiotics with short elimination half-lives (e.g., cefazolin and cefoxitin) are redosed intraoperatively to ensure that tissue concentrations remain adequate during the vulnerable period when the incision is open. **Surgical site infection and only surgical site infection is prevented by antibiotic prophylaxis.** Antibiotic prophylaxis more than 24 hours beyond injury increases the risk of nosocomial infection. Thus, antibiotic prophylaxis in trauma must not extend beyond 24 hours except *perhaps* for grade III open fractures.

B. Numerous randomized prospective trials have shown that 12 to 24 hours of antibiotic prophylaxis for penetrating abdominal trauma is equivalent to 5 days of prophylaxis, even when a colon injury is present, provided surgery is performed within 12 hours of injury. Penetrating abdominal trauma with no intestinal injury probably requires only a single dose of antibiotic prophylaxis.

C. Catheter insertion procedures require only a single dose of prophylactic antibiotics, except *perhaps* for emergency tube thoracostomy. Indwelling catheters otherwise should *never* receive prolonged antibiotic prophylaxis. There is no benefit, and the risk is that, should infection develop, it is more likely to be because of multi-drug-resistant pathogen.

V. SPECIFIC INJURIES
A. Abdominal injury

1. The data are unequivocal that prophylaxis of no more than 24 hours of a second-generation cephalosporin (e.g., cefoxitin) is equivalent to a longer course (e.g., 5 days) for penetrating abdominal trauma with injury to a hollow viscus, provided the surgery is performed within 12 hours of injury. Penetrating trauma that does not injure a hollow viscus needs only a single dose of antibiotics given prior to operation.

2. Although not as well studied, the principle is similar for blunt abdominal trauma; if managed nonoperatively no antibiotics are required. If surgery is performed, the duration of prophylaxis (a single dose or 24 hours of prophylaxis) is determined by the pattern of injury.

3. The abdomen may be left open temporarily as part of **damage control** or to prevent or manage the abdominal compartment syndrome. There is no evidence that the open abdomen requires prolonged antibiotic prophylaxis, even if a prosthesis is employed as part of the temporary closure. Another dose of prophylactic antibiotic aimed against skin flora (e.g., gram-positive cocci) is appropriate when the abdominal wall is closed or reconstructed.

4. Neither is there evidence that prophylactic antibiotics are required if the liver and spleen are embolized as part of the nonoperative management of blunt trauma to those organs. Although suppuration of devitalized tissue is a risk following therapeutic interventional radiology for liver or spleen injury, there are no data regarding antibiotic prophylaxis.

5. The infection risk associated with the late postsplenectomy period (bacteremia from encapsulated gram-positive cocci, for the most part, or "postsplenectomy sepsis"), is genuine for children but low for adults. Expert opinion often recommends prophylaxis with oral penicillin until age 18 years for splenectomized children. Adults do not require long-term antibiotic prophylaxis.

6. All individuals who undergo splenectomy should receive the polyvalent pneumococcal vaccine, with booster doses at 5-year intervals. We coadminister vaccines against *Haemophilus influenzae* and *Neisseria meningitidis;* timing of booster doses, if any, is unknown. Also unknown is whether patients who have undergone splenic embolization or the increasingly rare splenorrhaphy procedure should be vaccinated against postsplenectomy sepsis. Splenocyte immune function cannot be assessed in vivo, and the degree of devitalization of the spleen varies from patient to patient. Vaccination of the embolized patient following splenic injury is our practice, especially for children.

B. Chest injuries.
Little data exist to guide antibiotic prophylaxis of chest trauma. For blunt chest trauma, no antibiotic prophylaxis is indicated, even in the presence of pulmonary contusion.

1. For suspected aspiration of gastric contents, clinical judgment must be exercised. Two thirds of patients who aspirate do not develop pneumonia, so withholding of antibiotics (technically empiric therapy, not prophylaxis in this case) is reasonable until objective evidence of pneumonia is obtained. If antibiotics are started they should be discontinued within 48 hours if the development of pneumonia is unproved (Section VII.A).

2. Penetrating trauma to the chest should be governed by the decision of whether to administer antibiotic prophylaxis for trauma chest tubes (next point). With a thoracoabdominal injury (and corresponding increased incidence of empyema thoracis), the principles governing antibiotic prophylaxis for penetrating abdominal trauma should govern the situation.

3. Prophylaxis of chest tubes is controversial. The guidelines of the Eastern Association for the Surgery of Trauma recommend 24 hours of prophylaxis of emergency trauma chest tubes only as a Level III recommendation (based on expert opinion).

C. Fractures.
Prolonged antibiotic prophylaxis of open fractures is popular among orthopedic surgeons despite the fact that current practices are supported only by

retrospective data from the 1970s. A meta-analysis of 22 studies including more than 8,000 patients with **closed** long bone fractures showed that the incidence of infection (superficial or deep incisional surgical site infection, urinary tract infection, respiratory tract infection) was reduced by 60% by a single dose of antibiotic prophylaxis. Multidose prophylaxis did not protect against urinary or respiratory infections in that study. One recent trial of single-dose versus 5 days of prophylaxis of grade I to II open tibial fractures with a fluoroquinolone showed equivalence for single-dose prophylaxis. The guidelines of the Eastern Association for the Surgery of Trauma recommend 24 hours of prophylaxis of grade I to II open long bone fractures with an agent active against gram-positive cocci. For grade III open fractures, the addition of an agent active against gram-negative bacilli is recommended, but for 72 hours.

D. Skin and soft-tissue injuries. Few studies have examined the antibiotic management of infected traumatic wounds specifically, but inclusion of small numbers of such wounds in larger trials of therapy for complicated skin and skin structure infections (cSSSI) suggests that the principles of management are similar. Infected traumatic wounds may comprise as many as 13% of all infections after injury. The likelihood of infection is influenced foremost by the degree of contamination of the wound, ranging from approximately 3% for clean wounds to about 25% for wounds that are grossly contaminated. Wounds must be inspected carefully for the removal of foreign material (e.g., clothing, gravel, vegetable matter, wadding from shotgun shells), irrigation with physiologic saline, and debridement of devitalized tissue.

1. Risk factors for infection of traumatic lacerations repaired in the emergency department include diabetes mellitus, age (increased risk per year), foreign body, and the width of the incision. Lacerations of the head/neck region are less likely to become infected. Despite a high risk of infection posed by some wounds, there is scant evidence that traumatic injuries should receive antibiotic prophylaxis; administration is generally not recommended. The most common pathogens of infected traumatic wounds are aerobic gram-positive cocci (e.g., *S. aureus*), with aerobic gram-negative bacilli (e.g., *E. coli, P. aeruginosa*) being less common; antibiotic therapy when indicated (for overt infection) should be directed against likely pathogens. Numerous antibiotics of several classes are approved for therapy of cSSSI.

2. Animal and human bites should be presumed to be infected because of the large bacterial inoculum that is deposited in deep tissues and the resulting challenges inherent in local wound care.

   a. The pathogens differ in bite wounds, with dog and cat bites showing a predilection for *Eikenella corrodens* and *Pasturella multocida*, respectively. A meta-analysis of eight randomized, placebo-controlled clinical trials of penicillin or macrolide prophylaxis of dog bite wounds revealed that the rate of infection was reduced by more than 40% from the control infection rate of 16%, and to an even greater degree for bites of the hand. However, the duration of prophylaxis was not defined.

   b. Human bites are likely to cause infection with oral anaerobes (e.g., anaerobic streptococci, rarely *Bacteroides fragilis*).

E. Nutrition (Chapter 43). There is still much debate as to the ideal formula, route, and rate of feeding for injured patients. However, the effect of early enteral feeding to reduce the risk of infection following trauma or burn injury is well established.

VI. MICROBIOLOGY

A. Principles of resistance. Bacteria use four different mechanisms to develop resistance to antibiotics.

1. Cell wall permeability to antibiotics is decreased by changes in porin channels (especially important for gram-negative bacteria with complex cell walls, affecting aminoglycosides, β-lactam drugs, chloramphenicol, sulfonamides, tetracyclines, and possibly quinolones).

2. Production of specific antibiotic inactivating-enzymes by either plasmid-mediated or chromosomally mediated mechanisms affects aminoglycosides, β-lactam drugs, chloramphenicol, and macrolides.

3. Alteration of the target for antibiotic binding in the cell wall affects β-lactam drugs and vancomycin, whereas alteration of target enzymes can affect β-lactam drugs, sulfonamides, quinolones, and rifampin.

4. Drugs that bind to the bacterial ribosome (aminoglycosides, chloramphenicol, macrolides, lincosamides, streptogramins, and tetracyclines) are also susceptible to alteration of the receptor on the ribosome.

5. Antibiotics may be extruded actively once entry to the cell is achieved in the case of macrolides, lincosamines, streptogramins, quinolones, and tetracyclines.

B. **Gram-positive cocci.** Gram-positive cocci are collectively the most common causes of infection following injury. Infections most likely caused by gram-positive cocci include infections following neurosurgery (e.g., ventriculitis following invasive monitoring of intracranial pressure), sinusitis, CR-BSI, device/implant-associated infections, and cSSSI. Respiratory tract and urinary tract infections may also be caused by gram-positive cocci.

1. *S. aureus* is the most important pathogen among the gram-positive cocci. Sixty percent of hospital-acquired isolates of *S. aureus* are resistant to methicillin (MRSA), whereas 25% of community-acquired strains are now resistant (CA-MRSA). Staphylococcal resistance to vancomycin is reported but remains rare and is induced only after prolonged exposure to vancomycin among debilitated patients (e.g., dialysis patients). *S. aureus* is a major pathogen in sinusitis, CR-BSI, cSSSI, and pneumonia.

2. *S. epidermidis* is almost invariably resistant to methicillin (MRSE, 85%), and is the major pathogen in CR-BSI and device/implant-associated infections. *Enterococcus* spp. can cause cSSSI, CR-BSI, and infections of the urinary tract. About 30% of enterococci are resistant to vancomycin (VRE), but the pattern is species specific. Whereas 70% of *E. faecium* isolated are VRE, the same is true for only 3% of *E. faecalis* isolates. The incidence of VRE may be reaching a plateau, but VRE poses a threat only to debilitated patients after prolonged hospitalization. Colonization of the feces with VRE usually precedes invasive infection, and cannot be eradicated pharmacologically. Risk factors for the acquisition of VRE include prolonged hospitalization, readmission to the ICU, and therapy with vancomycin or third-generation cephalosporins.

3. Because of the high prevalence of MRSA, vancomycin remains the most-prescribed antibiotic for resistant gram-positive cocci despite poor tissue penetration and the risk of toxicity.

4. Alternatives for therapy include linezolid, tigecycline, daptomycin (but **not** for pneumonia) and quinupristin/dalfopristin (used seldom because of multiple toxicities). Some retrospective analyses suggest that outcomes for pneumonia and soft tissue infection may be improved when linezolid is used compared to vancomycin, but prospective corroboration is required.

C. **Gram-negative bacilli.** Gram-negative bacilli are less common as pathogens than gram-positive cocci, but are important in the pathogenesis of skin/skin structure infection (particularly after inoculation of a wound), lower respiratory tract infection, and intraabdominal infection. Although *Enterobacteriaceae* such as *E. coli* or *Klebsiella* spp. predominate in intraabdominal infection, *P. aeruginosa* is the second most common ICU pathogen overall and the bacterium most closely associated with death from HAI. *P. aeruginosa* can infect virtually any tissue, including synovium and vitreous humor. *P. aeruginosa* bacteremia can cause or complicate pneumonia, and other metastatic infections can follow. Antimicrobial resistance is a major problem with *P. aeruginosa*, *Acinetobacter* sp., and *Klebsiella* sp., and increasing among *Enterobacteriaceae* other than *Klebsiella*.

1. Cephalosporin resistance among gram-negative bacilli can be the result of induction of chromosomal β-lactamases after prolonged or repeated exposure to the antibiotic. The extended-spectrum cephalosporins are rendered ineffective when

bacteria such as enteric gram-negative bacilli mutate to produce constitutively a β-lactamase that is normally an inducible enzyme. Although resistance to cephalosporins can occur by several mechanisms, the appearance of chromosomally mediated β-lactamases has been identified as a consequence of the use of third-generation cephalosporins. Resistance rates decline when use is restricted. The mutant bacteria develop resistance rapidly to both cephalosporins and entire other classes of β-lactam antibiotics. It is justifiable therefore to restrict the use of ceftazidime, especially in institutions grappling with an ESBL-producing bacterium.

2. The carbapenems and aminoglycosides generally retain useful microbicidal activity against ESBL-producing strains, but ESBL-producing strains can cause fatal infections because of delayed recognition and consequent delayed empiric antimicrobial therapy. Unfortunately, routine antimicrobial susceptibility testing does not detect ESBL-producing strains. Therefore, heightened clinical suspicion must be followed by confirmatory laboratory testing of the suspicious organism.

3. The resistance problem in gram-negative bacteria is not limited to cephalosporin resistance. Metalloproteinases and carbapenemases threaten the utility of carbapenems to treat infections caused by *Pseudomonas* and *Acinetobacter*.

4. The fastest-growing resistance problem for gram-negative bacilli in the United States is quinolone resistance, particularly against *Pseudomonas*. Quinolone resistance is chromosomally mediated for the most part, primarily by changes in the target sites (DNA gyrase or topoisomerase IV) for the antibiotic. Changes in permeability or efflux may cause resistance to quinolones as well.

5. Quinolone resistance is easy to induce if a less-than-maximally effective drug or dose is chosen for initial therapy. Resistance to one quinolone may also increase the MIC for other quinolones against the organism, so a highly active agent given in adequate dosage is essential for empiric therapy with quinolones.

D. Fungi and yeast

1. Most fungi and yeast are avirulent opportunistic pathogens that do not threaten healthy patients. However, such infections should also be unusual in the "typical" critically ill or injured patient. Unless occurring in a profoundly immunosuppressed patient (i.e., cancer chemotherapy with neutropenia, bone marrow transplant or nonrenal solid organ transplant) fungal infections are usually the result of antibiotic overuse. Prolonged broad-spectrum antibiotic therapy suppresses host flora, and creates the opportunity for overgrowth of commensal flora. The most common health care–acquired fungal infections are caused by *Candida* spp., which are part of gut flora in approximately one quarter of patients.

2. Some experts believe that high-risk patients (including those who require intensive antibiotic therapy) should be treated prophylactically with an azole antifungal agent (e.g., fluconazole) to prevent invasive infection, which can be lethal. Although colonization with *Candida* does precede invasive infection, the utility of antifungal prophylaxis requires confirmation. However, most surgical patients do not manifest fungemia.

3. Widespread prescribing of fluconazole has led to emergence of resistance among *Candida* sp. that are normally susceptible to fluconazole (e.g., *C. albicans, C. tropicalis*).

4. Empiric therapy of suspected invasive fungal infections is probably not necessary in most centers that have a low incidence of such infections, but must address the possibility of resistant *Candida* if administered. Therefore, fluconazole should not be used until an organism that is likely to be susceptible to fluconazole is identified (most centers do not perform fungal susceptibility testing). Empiric therapy choices include conventional amphotericin B, lipid formulations of amphotericin B, or the echinocandins, caspofungin or micafungin. Conventional amphotericin B is seldom used currently because of substantial toxicity (e.g., febrile reactions, hypokelemia, renal insufficiency). The lipid formulations mitigate the toxicity, but at high cost. Caspofungin is

broadly active against yeast and fungi including *Candida* spp. and *Aspergillus* sp., and a logical, if expensive, choice for empiric therapy, but data are scant, particularly in surgical patients. Comparative studies suggest that the triazole voriconazole may be more effective than amphotericin B for invasive aspergillosis.

VII. NOSOCOMIAL INFECTIONS. Among the nosocomial infections, pleuropulmonary infections (pneumonia, empyema) are more common than bacteremia, which in turn is more common than urinary tract infection. This section examines the factors that contribute to the increased risk of infection after trauma, considers what can be done to reduce the risk of infection, and determines how best to accomplish the risk reduction.

A. Pneumonia. The most common health care–associated infection following critical illness or injury is pneumonia (HAP). Trauma patients may be at specific risk for development of pneumonia (or empyema, which complicates 5% of cases of posttraumatic pneumonia) for several reasons.

1. Chest wall injury (e.g., rib fractures) decreases thoracic compliance and impair pulmonary toilet.
2. Direct (e.g., penetrating injury, pulmonary contusion) or indirect (e.g., acute respiratory distress syndrome, ARDS) pulmonary injury may depress local pulmonary host defenses directly.
3. Traumatic brain injury may produce obtundation or coma and impair airway reflexes, leading to an increased risk of aspiration of gastric contents.
4. Iatrogenic risk factors include prolonged bed rest, supine positioning, tracheal or nasogastric intubation, narcotic analgesics and sedatives, and prolonged mechanical ventilation. Even a single day of mechanical ventilation increases the risk of ventilator-associated pneumonia (VAP) demonstrably.
5. Pneumonia can be prevented by careful adherence to the principles of infection control.
   a. Positioning the head of the bed up 30 degrees at all times
   b. Daily sedation holidays and assessment for liberation from mechanical ventilation
   c. Prophylaxis of stress-related gastric mucosal hemorrhage and venous thromboembolic disease
6. Some authors describe HAP or VAP as **early-onset** or **late-onset**, with onset more than 5 days after admission or intubation, respectively, being the defining time. Whether this distinction is important is unclear.
   a. The microbiology of **early-onset HAP/VAP** differs, in that it is more likely to be caused by relatively antibiotic-susceptible bacteria such as *S. pneumoniae*, *H. influenzae*, or methicillin-sensitive *S. aureus* (MSSA).
   b. **Late-onset HAP** and especially VAP tend to be caused by methicillin-resistant *S. aureus* (MRSA), *P. aeruginosa*, *Acinetobacter* spp., and the *Enterobacteriaceae* (although *E. coli* pneumonia is relatively uncommon).
7. The diagnosis of VAP in particular is controversial. The pharynx becomes colonized soon after hospitalization with potential pathogens. Similarly, artificial airways (e.g., endotracheal or tracheostomy tubes) become coated with a glycocalyx biofilm that can sequester pathogens (especially *P. aeruginosa*) from the actions of antibiotics.
   a. Routine sputum collection for culture and susceptibility testing by standard endotracheal suctioning can contaminate the specimen with these upper airway "colonists," thereby leading to the overdiagnosis and consequent overtreatment of VAP.
   b. To reduce this risk, **quantitative microbiology testing of sputum** obtained by a technique that minimizes the possibility of contamination has been advocated. Fiberoptic bronchoscopy with bronchoalveolar lavage (BAL) or the use of a protected-specimen brush (PSB) catheter can reduce the risk of contamination of the specimen and increase the accuracy by increasing the specificity of the diagnosis, and make antibiotic administration more accurate. The

threshold for the diagnosis of VAP is 10^4 colony-forming units (cfu)/mL (some authors argue that the threshold should be 10^5 cfu/mL for trauma patients) of a single organism, and 10^3 cfu/mL for the PSB technique. Techniques for both BAL and PSB specimen collection without bronchoscopy have been developed, so quantitative microbiology may be more important than bronchoscopy.

8. The most common causative organisms for VAP are MRSA and *P. aeruginosa*; effective empiric antibiotic therapy must account for both. **Misdirected (against resistant pathogens) or delayed antibiotic therapy of VAP are major causes of therapeutic failure and death.** Recent data suggest that the duration of therapy for VAP should be as brief as eight days for most cases of VAP, with the possible exception of cases caused by non-fermenting gram-negative bacilli (e.g., *P. aeruginosa*, *Acinetobacter* spp., *Stenotrophomonas maltophilia*), which may require up to 2 weeks of therapy.

9. The mortality rate of pneumonia complicating trauma is approximately 20%, whereas it is approximately 35% for VAP in critically ill surgical patients. Whether this difference relates to the timing of onset, microbiology, or underlying host factors such as age or severity of illness/injury is conjectural. Management based on quantitative microbiology may be associated with lower mortality. It is clear, however, that reliance on quantitative microbiology can increase clinician confidence that pneumonia is not present when testing is non-revealing, allowing the withholding or truncation of antibiotic therapy, which is unquestionably beneficial for those who are not infected and who do not need antibiotics.

B. **Catheter-related bloodstream infection**

1. Trauma and hemodynamically unstable nontrauma ICU patients often require reliable large-bore intravenous access. Placed typically into central veins (e.g., femoral, internal jugular, or subclavian vein), these catheters are prone to local infection and bloodstream infection.

2. Prevention by strict adherence to infection control and proper insertion technique is crucial because trauma patients are at particularly high risk for infection of central venous catheters (Table 57-1). When placed under elective (controlled) circumstances, proper insertion technique mandates that the operator prepare the operative field with chlorhexidine (not povidone-iodine solution), drape the entire bed into a sterile field, and don a cap, mask, and sterile gown and gloves.

3. When sterile procedure or technique is breached, the risk of infection increases exponentially, and the catheter should be removed and replaced (if still needed) at a different site using strict sterile technique as soon as the patient's condition permits (ideally within 24 hours).

   a. Infection risk for femoral vein catheters is highest, and lowest for catheters placed via the subclavian route.

   b. Peripheral vein catheters, peripherally placed central catheters (PICC), and tunneled central venous catheters (e.g., Hickman, Broviac), pose less risk of infection than percutaneous central venous catheters.

   c. Information campaigns, educational initiatives, and strict adherence to insertion protocols are all effective to decrease the risk of CR-BSI.

   d. Antibiotic- and antiseptic-coated catheters are controversial, but may decrease the risk of infection.

4. Catheter infection is diagnosed by isolation of >15 cfu from a segment of catheter by the semi-quantitative roll-plate technique. The diagnosis of CR-BSI is confirmed when the isolates from blood and the cultured catheter are identical. The pathogens of CR-BSI are predominantly gram-positive cocci, most commonly MRSE, MRSA, and enterococci.

   a. Unfortunately MRSE is not only the most common cause of CR-BSI, but also the most common cause of false-positive blood cultures because of contamination during the collection process. Isolation of MRSE from a single blood culture is likely a contaminant (do not treat), especially if the patient has no indwelling hardware that might become infected secondarily (e.g., prosthetic joint or heart valve).

b. Gram-negative bacillary pathogens are less common, and fungal CR-BSI are unusual in trauma patients.

c. Treatment is by removal of the catheter (for peripheral or percutaneous central venous catheters) with parenteral antibiotics, at least initially. Catheter-related bloodstream infections caused by MRSA require at least 2 weeks of therapy; some authorities argue for a longer course because of the risk of metastatic infection. Vancomycin or linezolid may be chosen for MRSA CR-BSI (or MRSE when treatment is indicated), with daptomycin as an alternative. Therapy for enterococcal or gram-negative CR-BSI is dictated by bacterial susceptibility, without clear consensus as to duration of therapy. Beyond removal of the catheter, treatment of fungal CR-BSI is controversial. Some authorities recommend removal of the catheter as sole therapy; others recommend at least 2 weeks of systemic antifungal therapy.

C. Peritonitis

1. The peritonitis associated commonly with perforated viscus is referred to as **secondary peritonitis**. In the trauma setting, secondary peritonitis may occur after penetrating injury to the intestine that is not treated promptly (>12 hours delay). Other causes include dehiscence of a bowel anastomosis with leakage of succus entericus, or development of an intraabdominal abscess. **Secondary peritonitis is polymicrobial**, with anaerobic gram-negative bacilli (e.g., *B. fragilis*) predominating, and *E. coli* and *Klebsiella* spp. isolated commonly. Any of a number of antibiotic regimens of appropriate spectrum may be appropriate. Enterococci, *Pseudomonas*, and other bacteria may be isolated, but do not require specific therapy if the patient is otherwise healthy (e.g., not immunocompromised) and responding to therapy as prescribed.

2. When secondary peritonitis develops in a hospitalized patient as a complication of disease or therapy, the flora are likely to reflect those encountered in the hospital. For example, enterococci, *Enterobacter*, and *Pseudomonas* are more prevalent, whereas *E. coli* and *Klebsiella* are less common. Antibiotic therapy must be adjusted accordingly, and **surgical source control must be achieved**. Failure of two source control procedures with persistent intraabdominal collections is referred to as **tertiary peritonitis**.

a. Tertiary peritonitis represents complete failure of intraabdominal host defenses. Therefore, it is controversial whether tertiary peritonitis is a true invasive infection, or rather colonization of the peritoneal cavity with incompetent local host defenses. The latter view is supported by the observation that the commonly isolated bacteria in tertiary peritonitis are avirulent opportunists such as MRSE, enterococci, *Pseudomonas*, and *C. albicans*. Some authorities recommend that these patients be managed with an open-abdomen technique, so that manual peritoneal toilet can be provided under sedation or anesthesia, possibly at the bedside. At times, there is no alternative to open-abdomen management if the infection extends to involve the abdominal wall, and extensive debridement is required.

D. *Clostridium difficile*–associated disease

1. *Clostridium difficile*–associated disease (CDAD) (formerly pseudomembranous colitis) develops because antibiotic therapy disrupts the balance of colonic flora, allowing the selection and overgrowth of *C. difficile*, present in the fecal flora of 3% of normal hosts. Any antibiotic can induce this selection pressure, even when given appropriately as single-dose surgical prophylaxis, although clindamycin, third-generation cephalosporins, and fluoroquinolones have a predilection. Even antibiotics used to treat CDAD (e.g., metronizazole) have been associated with CDAD.

2. *Clostridium difficile*–associated disease is unquestionably a nosocomial infection. Spores can persist on inanimate surfaces for prolonged periods, and pathogens can be transmitted from patient-to-patient by contaminated equipment (e.g., bedpans, rectal thermometers) or on the hands of health care workers. **The alcohol gel that is used increasingly for hand disinfection is not active against spores of C. difficile. Therefore, handwashing with soap and water is necessary when caring for an infected patient or during outbreaks.**

3. The clinical spectrum of CDAD is wide, ranging from asymptomatic (8% of affected patients do not have diarrhea) to life-threatening transmural pan-colitis with perforation and severe sepsis or septic shock. The typical patient will have fever, abdominal distention, copious diarrhea, and leukocytosis. Bleeding from the colon is rare, and if observed should prompt strongly an alternative diagnosis.

4. Diagnosis by assay for the enterotoxins in a fresh stool specimen has largely supplanted colonoscopy. Up to 50% of patients do not have the "characteristic" colonic mucosal pseudomembranes (hence, the change in nomenclature as well).

5. Treatment of mild cases consists of withdrawal of the offending antibiotic; oral antibiotic therapy is often prescribed. More severe cases may require parenteral metronidazole or oral or enteral vancomycin (by lavage or enema, if ileus precludes oral therapy); parenteral vancomycin is ineffective. On occasion, patients with severe disease may require total abdominal colectomy. The prevalence of severe disease has increased markedly with the emergence of a new strain of *C. difficile*. The new strain has undergone a mutation of a gene that suppresses toxin production, such that far more toxin is elaborated, resulting in clinically severe, systemic disease.

E. Sinusitis

1. Nosocomial sinusitis is a dangerous, closed-space infection that is increasing in incidence, but difficult to diagnose and therefore controversial as to its incidence and importance.

2. Patients with transnasal tubes (particularly nasotracheal intubation, after 7 days of which the incidence is one third) and maxillofacial trauma are at particular risk. Purulent or foul-smelling nasal discharge is an obvious clue to the diagnosis, but not always present. So, sinusitis must be sought radiographically by CT of the facial bones to identify sinus mucosal thickening or opacification. Because the process is often occult, the more the diagnosis is sought, the more often it will be confirmed.

3. Sinusitis should be suspected in any patient with sepsis, particularly if initial cultures (e.g., blood, sputum, urine, indwelling vascular catheters) are unrevealing. If sinusitis is suspected, the diagnosis is confirmed by maxillary antral tap, lavage, and culture using aseptic technique. Gram-positive cocci, gram-negative bacilli (including *P. aeruginosa*), and fungi (incidence, 8%) are possible pathogens; initial therapy should be based on local susceptibility patterns. Most antibiotics that might be chosen achieve adequate tissue penetration. The duration of therapy should be based on the patient's clinical response. Refractory cases may require repetitive lavage of the sinus, or a formal drainage procedure.

4. Sinusitis is a predisposing factor for VAP, and may be a source of pathogens that gain access to the lower respiratory tract. The association may be temporal; both infections are associated with prolonged endotracheal intubation. However, there is 85% concordance between sinusitis pathogens and pneumonia pathogens in patients who develop VAP subsequently, lending credence to the hypothesis that purulent drainage from infected sinuses inoculates the lower airway.

F. Decubitus ulcer.

Infection from decubitus ulcer may be obvious or covert. Patients are at substantially increased risk with prolonged bed rest (>7 days), which may be mitigated by specialized bedding. Vasopressor therapy and poor nutrition may be additional risk factors, but any association is unsubstantiated. Morbid obesity is a clear risk factor, given that routine turning and positioning of such patients is a formidable undertaking. Most decubitus ulcers form in the presacral area, but can form anywhere unremitting pressure is placed upon tissue. For example, if the position of the endotracheal tube at the lips is not changed periodically, ulceration may occur at the corner of the mouth. Also, occipital decubitus ulceration results from ill-fitting cervical collars, when used for an obtunded patient or when "clearance" of the cervical spine is delayed. When evaluating a patient for occult infection, the skin must be inspected systematically for decubitus ulcers. **Deep ulcers** (Stage III, involving subcutaneous fat; Stage IV, involving fascia, muscle, or bone) may require debridement or systemic antibiotic therapy. In rare cases, a decubitus ulcer may transform into a life-threatening necrotizing soft-tissue infection.

VIII. MULTIPLE ORGAN DYSFUNCTION SYNDROME
A. Epidemiology
   1. The multiple organ dysfunction syndrome (MODS) is the leading cause of death following critical illness and injury (>24 hours postinjury). Patients who develop any component of organ dysfunction are 20-fold more likely to die. The development of MODS usually follows infection and sepsis (75%) but may follow massive tissue injury (25%; e.g., multiple, trauma, burns, severe pancreatitis). The degree (number of affected organs) and magnitude (severity of dysfunction) closely correlate with the initial severity of illness and the severity and persistence of the proinflammatory state (systemic inflammatory response syndrome, SIRS) in response to illness/injury.
   2. Several scoring systems have been described to quantify MODS (Table 57-8); descriptive utility is comparable. Quantification of MODS is useful for prognostication; the magnitude of MODS is related closely to the mortality rate, which is 70% or more when MODS is manifest fully.
B. Risk factors and pathogenesis
   1. The usual presentation of MODS is multifactorial and involves multiple organ systems. Only in occasional circumstances (e.g., transfusion-associated acute lung injury, TRALI) is the cause of MODS identifiable discretely or manifested by dysfunction of a single organ. Even though the inciting injury may be localized, the host response is usually systemic.
   2. **Severe sepsis** (by definition, sepsis with dysfunction of at least one organ) and tissue injury are the usual precipitants of MODS, but the pathogenesis is complex and usually multifactorial. Many hypotheses of the pathogenesis of MODS have complimentary or overlapping features with the pathophysiology still not elucidated.

TABLE 57-8 **Multiple Organ Dysfunction Score**

	0	1	2	3	4
Pulmonary (PaO_2:FiO_2 ratio)	>300	226–300	151–225	76–150	<76
Renal (serum creatinine, mg/dL)	≤1.1	1.2–2.3	2.4–4.0	4.1–5.7	>5.7
Cardiovascular (HR = HR × RAP/MAP)	≤10	10.1–15.0	15.1–20.0	20.1–30.0	>30.0
Hepatic (serum bilirubin, mg/dL)	≤1.2	1.3–3.5	3.6–7.0	7.1–14.0	>14.0
CNS (Glasgow Coma Scale score)	15	13–14	10–12	7–9	≤6
Hematologic (platelet count × 10^3/mm^3)	>120	81–120	51–80	21–50	<21

HR, heart rate; RAP, right atrial pressure; MAP, mean arterial pressure; CNS, central nervous system.
(From Marshall JC, Cook DJ, Christou NV, et al. Multiple organ dysfunction score: A reliable descriptor of a complex clinical syndrome. *Crit Care Med* 1995;23:1638–1652.)

C. Organ-specific manifestations

1. **Cardiovascular.** The cardiovascular manifestations of MODS relate to vasomotor instability and refractory shock, often culminating in a requirement for vasopressors. Vasodilation, decreased myocardial contractility, and low cardiac output contribute to hypoperfusion. In some cases, decreased heart rate variability (decreased sympathetic tone, increased parasympathetic tone, making the heart rate more regular) may be a manifestation of deranged cell-cell communication between the neurologic and cardiovascular systems.

2. **Central nervous system**
   a. The classical neurologic manifestation of MODS has been encephalopathy. Although there may be myriad potential causes of encephalopathy in sepsis (e.g., cerebral edema, septic microemboli, hypoperfusion, "metabolic" causes), it can be difficult to quantify because of the use of powerful sedatives and analgesics that have decreased sensorium as their desired therapeutic effect. Even correcting for an altered sensorium, central nervous system failure is a powerful predictor of death in MODS.
   b. Alternative neurologic manifestations of MODS may be ICU delirium, decreased heart rate variability, or critical illness polyneuropathy. **Critical illness polyneuropathy** may be the manifestation of failure of communication between motor neurons and skeletal myocytes, although toxicity (e.g., neuromuscular blockade, corticosteroids) has been hypothesized also, albeit unconvincingly. Critical illness encephalopathy represents an explanation for the profound muscle weakness and failure to wean from mechanical ventilation exhibited by some patients.

3. **Gastrointestinal.** Because overt upper gastrointestinal hemorrhage from gastric mucosal injury due to splanchnic ischemia-reperfusion injury has been largely eliminated by better (enteral) nutritional support and effective prophylaxis (e.g., H_2 antihistamines, proton pump inhibitors), many classifications of MODS now omit mention of gastrointestinal failure as part of the syndrome. In addition, gastrointestinal failure may be manifested by intolerance of enteral feedings, ileus, or acute acalculous cholecystitis (ischemia-reperfusion injury of the gallbladder).

4. **Hematologic.** Hematologic failure is defined by thrombocytopenia. Thrombocytopenia may be caused by sepsis, massive hemorrhage and transfusion, drug toxicity (e.g., heparin, β-lactam antibiotics), or myriad other causes, but bone marrow depression caused by sepsis is the paradigm. Coagulopathy from other causes, such as decreased clotting factor synthesis from hepatic failure, is accounted for by neither the definition of hematologic nor hepatic failure.

5. **Hepatic.** Hepatic failure is defined by hyperbilirubinemia characteristic of intrahepatic cholestasis. Proinflammatory cytokines (particularly interleukin-1) are profoundly cholestatic, disrupting active-transport processes that regulate bile secretion into the canaliculus. Another important cause of jaundice is metabolism of heme pigment from resorption of large hematomas (e.g., pelvic hematoma from blunt trauma), or from senescent red blood cells after large-volume transfusion. With metabolism of heme, hepatic metabolic pathways are saturated transiently. Hyperbilirubinema is usually conjugated (direct), but may be either.

   Hyperbilirubinemia is insensitive, presenting late and after substantial hepatic dysfunction has already occurred because normal hepatic metabolic capacity exceeds usual metabolic requirements by several-fold. As much as 80% of hepatic function may be lost before jaundice becomes apparent clinically. Investigators have shown that measurement of metabolites after administration of pharmaceuticals metabolized by the liver is more sensitive and may allow earlier detection of hepatic dysfunction.

6. **Pulmonary.** Although the consensus definition of acute respiratory distress syndrome (ARDS) includes not only hypoxemia (PaO_2:FiO_2 <200), but also a precipitant process, bilateral pulmonary infiltrates, and a pulmonary artery occlusion pressure <18 mmHg, the definition of pulmonary MODS is based on the degree

of hypoxemia only. Therefore, cases of respiratory failure other than ARDS may sometimes be considered a manifestation of ARDS. However, ARDS is the paradigm, and commonly caused by sepsis (the most common precipitant), aspiration of gastric contents, multiple long bone fractures with fat microembolism of the lungs, massive transfusion (TRALI), acute pancreatitis, and near-drowning.

Pulmonary dysfunction (TRALI excepted) rarely occurs in isolation, so ARDS is most often the pulmonary manifestation of systemic inflammation. There is no correlation between the degree of hypoxemia and the mortality of ARDS; mortality with ARDS is related to the magnitude of nonpulmonary MODS. Thus, although low tidal volume ventilation has decreased the mortality of ARDS, the benefit may be due as much or more to decreased pulmonary generation of proinflammatory mediators from overventilation than avoidance of exacerbation of local lung injury morphology.

7. **Renal.** Acute renal failure is usually caused by renal ischemia, sometimes with an added component of reperfusion injury either of the kidney itself or generation of oxygen free radicals from reperfusion of other ischemic tissues attendant to hemorrhage, hypovolemia, and the resuscitation of shock. Other common etiologies of acute renal failure include sepsis, crush injury, and drug toxicity. Proinflammatory mediators may play a role in renal ischemia as well, owing to the potent action of tumor necrosis factor as an activator of the renin-angiotensin-aldosterone axis and the regulation of renal blood flow by eicosanoids. The usual manifestation is acute tubular necrosis, which usually resolves. However, mortality of acute renal failure remains high, exceeding 50% despite new modes of renal replacement therapy. Some data suggest that aggressive hemofiltration regimens (as opposed to conventional, thrice-weekly hemodialysis) may improve outcomes.

Bibliography

Barie PS, Hydo LJ. Epidemiology of multiple organ dysfunction syndrome in critical surgical illness. *Surg Infect* 2000;1:173–186.

Bartlett JG, Perl TM. The new *Clostridium difficile*—What does it mean? *N Engl J Med* 2005;353:2503–2525.

Bercker S, Weber-Carstens S, Deja M, et al. Critical illness polyneuropathy and myopathy in patients with acute respiratory distress syndrome. *Crit Care Med* 2005;33:711–715.

Bozorgzadeh A, Pizzi WF, Barie PS, et al. The duration of antibiotic administration in penetrating abdominal trauma. *Am J Surg* 1999;177:125–131.

Buchman TG. Nonlinear dynamics, complex systems, and the pathobiology of critical illness. *Curr Opin Crit Care* 2004;10:378–382.

Buchman TG, Stein PK, Goldstein B. Heart rate variability in critical illness and critical care. *Curr Opin Crit Care* 2002;8:311–315.

Chastre J, Wolff M, Fagon JY, et al., and the PneumA Trial Group. Comparison of 8 vs 15 days of antibiotic therapy for ventilator-associated pneumonia in adults: A randomized trial. *JAMA* 2003;290:2588–2598.

Coopersmith CM, Rebmann TL, Zack JE, et al. Effect of an education program on decreasing catheter-related bloodstream infections in the surgical intensive care unit. *Crit Care Med* 2002;30:59–64.

Croce MA, Tolley EA, Claridge JA, Fabian TC. Transfusions result in pulmonary morbidity and death after a moderate degree of injury. *J Trauma* 2005;59:19–23.

Cummings P. Antibiotics to prevent infection in patients with dog bite wounds: A meta-analysis of randomized trials. *Ann Emerg Med* 1994;23:535–540.

Davidson RN, Wall RA. Prevention and management of infections in patients without a spleen. *Clin Microbiol Infect* 2001;7:657–660.

Dellinger EP. Increasing inspired oxygen to decrease surgical site infection: Time to shift the quality improvement research paradigm. *JAMA* 2005;294:2091–2092.

Dente CJ, Tyburski J, Wilson RF, et al. Ostomy as a risk factor for posttraumatic infection in penetrating colonic injuries: Univariate and multivariate analyses. *J Trauma* 2000;49:628–634.

Desborough JP. The stress response to trauma and surgery. *Br J Anaesth* 2000;85:109–117.

Diaz JJ Jr, Mauer A, May AK, et al. Bedside laparotomy for trauma: Are there risks? *Surg Infect* 2004;5:15–20.

Dunne JR, Malone DL, Tracy JK, Napolitano LM. Allogenic blood transfusion in the first 24 hours after trauma is associated with increased systemic inflammatory response syndrome (SIRS) and death. *Surg Infect* 2004;5:395–404.

Eachempati SR, Hydo LJ, Barie PS. Factors influencing the development of decubitus ulcers in critically ill surgical patients. *Crit Care Med* 2001;29:1678–1682.

Edwards PS, Lipp A, Holmes A. Preoperative skin antiseptics for preventing surgical wound infections after clean surgery. Cochrane Database Syst Rev 2004;3:CD003949.

Eggimann P, Calandra T, Fluckiger U, et al., and the Fungal Infection Network of Switzerland. Invasive candidiasis: Comparison of management choices by infectious disease and critical care specialists. *Intens Care Med* 2005;31:1514–1521.

Fagon JY, Chastre J, Wolff M, et al. Invasive and noninvasive strategies for management of suspected ventilator-associated pneumonia: A randomized trial. *Ann Intern Med* 2000;132:621–630.

Gannon CJ, Napolitano LM, Pasquale M, et al. A statewide population-based study of gender differences in trauma: Validation of a prior single-institution study. *J Am Coll Surg* 2002;195:11–18.

Gillespie WJ, Walenkamp G. Antibiotic prophylaxis for surgery for proximal femoral and other closed long bone fractures. Cochrane Database Syst Rev 2001;1: CD000244.

Gleason TG, May AK, Caparelli D, et al. Emerging evidence of selection of fluconazole-tolerant fungi in surgical intensive care units. *Arch Surg* 1997;132:1197–1201.

Gosselin RA, Roberts I, Gillespie WJ. Antibiotics for preventing infection in open limb fractures. Cochrane Database Syst Rev 2004;1:CD003764.

Grobmyer SR, Graham D, Brennan MF, Coit D. High-pressure gradients generated by closed-suction surgical drainage systems. *Surg Infect* 2002;3:245–249.

Hammerschmidt S, Kuhn H, Sack U, et al. Mechanical stretch alters alveolar type II cell mediator release toward a proinflammatory pattern. *Am J Respir Cell Mol Biol* 2005;33:203–210.

Hanna R, Raad II. Diagnosis of catheter-related bloodstream infection. *Curr Infect Dis Rep* 2005;7:413–419.

Hanna HA, Raad II, Hackett B, et al., and the Anderson Catheter Study Group. Antibiotic-impregnated catheters associated with significant decrease in nosocomial and multidrug-resistant bacteremias in critically ill patients. *Chest* 2003;124:1030–1038.

Hill GE, Frawley WH, Griffith KE. Allogeneic blood transfusion increases the risk of post-operative bacterial infection: A meta-analysis. *J Trauma* 2003;54:908–914.

Hollander JE, Singer AJ, Valentine SM, Shofer FS. Risk factors for infection in patients with traumatic lacerations. *Acad Emerg Med* 2001;8:716–720.

Kollef MH. Prevention of hospital-associated pneumonia and ventilator-associated pneumonia. *Crit Care Med* 2004;32:1396–1405.

Kurz A, Sessler DI, Lenhardt R. Perioperative normothermia to reduce the incidence of surgical-wound infection and shorten hospitalization. Study of Wound Infection and Temperature Group. *N Engl J Med* 1996;334:1209–1215.

Lambert PA. Bacterial resistance to antibiotics: Modified target sites. *Adv Drug Deliv Rev* 2005;57:1471–1485.

Leone M, Garnier F, Avidan M, Martin C. Catheter-associated urinary tract infections in intensive care units. *Microbes Infect* 2004;6:1026–1032.

Luchette FA, Barrie PS, Oswanski MF, et al. Practice management guidelines for prophy-lactic antibiotic use in tube thoracostomy for traumatic hemopneumothorax: The EAST Practice Management Guidelines Work Group. Eastern Association for Trauma. *J Trauma* 2000;48:753–757.

Malangoni MA. Evaluation and management of tertiary peritonitis. *Am Surg* 2000; 66:157–161.

Marik PE, Zaloga GP. Early enteral nutrition in acutely ill patients: A systematic review. *Crit Care Med* 2001;29:2264–2270.

Marshall JC, Cook DJ, Christou NV, et al. Multiple organ dysfunction score: A reliable descriptor of a complex clinical outcome. *Crit Care Med* 1995;23:1638–1652.

Maynard ND, Bihari DJ, Dalton RN, et al. Liver function and splanchnic ischemia in critically ill patients. *Chest* 1997;111:180–187.

McDonald LC, Killgore GE, Thompson A, et al. An epidemic, toxin gene-variant strain of Clostridium difficile. *N Engl J Med* 2005;353:2433–2441.

McGee DC, Gould MK. Preventing complications of central venous catheterization. *N Engl J Med* 2003;348:1123–1133.

McIntyre L, Hebert PC, Wells G, et al., and the Canadian Critical Care Trials Group. Is a restrictive transfusion strategy safe for resuscitated and critically ill trauma patients? *J Trauma* 2004;57:563–568.

Miller RS, Morris JA Jr, Diaz JJ Jr, et al. Complications after 344 damage-control open celiotomies. *J Trauma* 2005;59:1365–1371.

Montravers P, Chalfine A, Gauzit R, et al. Clinical and therapeutic features of nonpostoperative nosocomial intra-abdominal infections. *Ann Surg* 2004;239:409–416.

Mueller EW, Hanes SD, Croce MA, et al. Effect from multiple episodes of inadequate empiric antibiotic therapy for ventilator-associated pneumonia on morbidity and mortality among critically ill trauma patients. *J Trauma* 2005;58:94–101.

Napolitano LM, Faist E, Wichmann MW, Coimbra R. Immune dysfunction in trauma. *Surg Clin North Am* 1999;79:1385–1416.

National Nosocomial Infections Surveillance (NNIS) System report, data summary from January 1992 through June 2004, issued October 2004. *Am J Infect Control* 2004;232:470–485.

Neuhauser MM, Weinstein RA, Rydman R, et al. Antibiotic resistance among gram-negative bacilli in US intensive care units: Implications for fluoroquinolone use. *JAMA* 2003;289:885–888.

Nichols RL, Smith JW, Klein DB, et al. Risk of infection after penetrating abdominal trauma. *N Engl J Med* 1984;311:1065–1070.

Offner PJ, Moore EE, Biffl WL. Male gender is a risk factor for major infections after surgery. *Arch Surg* 1999;134:935–938.

O'Grady NP, Alexander M, Dellinger EP, et al., and the Healthcare Infection Control Practices Advisory Committee. Guidelines for the prevention of intravascular catheter-related infections. *Infect Control Hosp Epidemiol* 2002;23:759–769.

Papia G, McLellan BA, El-Helou P, et al. Infection in hospitalized trauma patients: Incidence, risk factors, and complications. *J Trauma* 1999;47:923–927.

Pelz RK, Hendrix CW, Swoboda SM, et al. Double-blind placebo-controlled trial of fluconazole to prevent candidal infections in critically ill surgical patients. *Ann Surg* 2001;233:542–548.

Phu NH, Hien TT, Mai NT, et al. Hemofiltration and peritoneal dialysis in infection-associated acute renal failure in Vietnam. *N Engl J Med* 2002;347:895–902.

Pittas AG, Siegel RD, Lau J. Insulin therapy for critically ill hospitalized patients: A meta-analysis of randomized controlled trials. *Arch Intern Med* 2004;164:2005–2011.

Powers JH, Ross DB, Lin D, Soreth J. Linezolid and vancomycin for methicillin-resistant *Staphylococcus aureus* nosocomial pneumonia: The subtleties of subgroup analyses. *Chest* 2004;126:314–315.

Resar R, Pronovost P, Haraden C, et al. Using a bundle approach to improve ventilator care processes and reduce ventilator-associated pneumonia. *Joint Comm J Qual Patient Saf* 2005;31:243–248.

Shah MR, Hasselblad V, Stevenson LW, et al. Impact of the pulmonary artery catheter in critically ill patients: Meta-analysis of randomized clinical trials. *JAMA* 2005; 294:1664–1670.

Shorr AF, Chung K, Jackson WL, et al. Fluconazole prophylaxis in critically ill surgical patients: A meta-analysis. *Crit Care Med* 2005;33:1928–1935.

Shorr AF, Sherner JH, Jackson WL, Kollef MH. Invasive approaches to the diagnosis of ventilator-associated pneumonia: A meta-analysis. *Crit Care Med* 2005;33:46–53.

Smith AW. Biofilms and antibiotic therapy: Is there a role for combating bacterial resistance by the use of novel drug delivery systems? *Adv Drug Deliv Rev* 2005; 57:1539–1550.

Stillwell M, Caplan ES. The septic multiple-trauma patient. *Infect Dis Clin North Am* 1989;3:155–183.

Talmor M, Hydo L, Barie PS. Relationship of systemic inflammatory response syndrome to organ dysfunction, length of stay, and mortality in critical surgical illness: Effect of intensive care unit resuscitation. *Arch Surg* 1999;134:81–87.

Talmor M, Li P, Barie PS. Acute paranasal sinusitis in critically ill patients: Guidelines for prevention, diagnosis, and treatment. *Clin Infect Dis* 1997;25:1441–1446.

van den Berghe G, Wouters P, Weekers F, et al. Intensive insulin therapy in the critically ill patients. *N Engl J Med* 2001;345:1359–1367.

Velmahos GC, Toutouzas KG, Sarkisyan G, et al. Severe trauma is not an excuse for prolonged antibiotic prophylaxis. *Arch Surg* 2002;137:537–541.

Wallace WC, Cinat M, Gornick WB, et al. Nosocomial infections in the surgical intensive care unit: A difference between trauma and surgical patients. *Am Surg* 1999; 65:987–990.

Weigelt J, Kaafarani HM, Itani KM, Swanson RN. Linezolid eradicates MRSA better than vancomycin from surgical-site infections. *Am J Surg* 2004;188:760–766.

Weigelt JA. Risk of wound infections in trauma patients. *Am J Surg* 1985;150:782–784.

Widmer AF. Replace hand washing with use of a waterless alcohol hand rub? *Clin Infect Dis* 2000;31:136–143.

Wright GD. Bacterial resistance to antibiotics: Enzymatic degradation and modification. *Adv Drug Deliv Rev* 2005;57:1451–1470.

Yendamuri S, Fulda GJ, Tinkoff GH. Admission hyperglycemia as a prognostic indicator in trauma. *J Trauma* 2003;55:33–38.

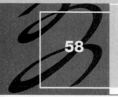

THE ACUTE ABDOMEN IN INTENSIVE CARE UNIT PATIENTS

58

ERIC L. MARDERSTEIN AND
MATTHEW ROSENGART

I. INTRODUCTION

A. It is estimated that intraabdominal pathology necessitating surgical intervention occurs in approximately 4% of patients admitted to the intensive care unit (ICU). The number of patients requiring surgical evaluation is several-fold higher. Differentiating those in need of surgical intervention from those who do not is difficult. Many characteristics of critical illness, such as mechanical ventilation, narcotics and sedatives, and distracting pathology, confound the ability to obtain an accurate historical and physical examination. Hence, diagnosis typically relies on ancillary laboratory and radiological studies (Table 58-1). However, even these can be difficult to obtain in the critically ill patient with tenuous physiology. Nevertheless, timely diagnosis is essential, as any delay, in either diagnosis or treatment, has been associated with a poor outcome.

B. The goals of this chapter are to provide a systematic approach, and the evidence in support of such recommendations, for the evaluation of the acute abdomen in critically ill patients. Particular difficulties in both diagnosis and treatment are emphasized, as are alternative strategies by which to facilitate achieving both endpoints.

II. EVALUATION

A. History. Many aspects of both the patient and the ICU environment make obtaining an accurate historical examination difficult. Preexisting comorbidities, such as underlying dementia or delirium consequent to the admission diagnosis (i.e., traumatic brain injury or sepsis), are common. Seventy percent or more of ICU patients experience delirium during their course. Many interventions (e.g., mechanical ventilation, surgery) and pathology (e.g., orthopedic trauma, elevated intracranial pressure) necessitate sedation, narcotic analgesics, or paralysis. Nevertheless, an exhaustive attempt to acquire any historical data is essential. If feasible, temporary discontinuation of any sedating agent may enable an objective examination. For the alert patient, a pen and pad may facilitate some degree of communication; though tedious, frustrating, and conveying small volumes of data, any information may prove decisive for either continued observation or surgical exploration. The lower nurse-to-patient ratio in the ICU makes the nurse an invaluable source of information. All available family members, prior caregivers, or other close associates should be interviewed for any salient information that might facilitate a diagnosis.

  1. Questions to be answered in the history are similar for any patient undergoing surgical evaluation of the acute abdomen.

  a. What aspects prompted a surgical evaluation?

  b. Is this the primary impetus for admission, or did it develop during the treatment of other pathology?

  2. Determining the duration of the signs or symptoms that have prompted the evaluation determines the acuity of the process, as it relates to rapidity with which a diagnosis needs to be made and definitive treatment instituted.

  3. The details of the abdominal pain are important including when it began and aspects of intensity, radiation, nature, and exacerbating and mitigating circumstances if available.

TABLE 58-1	Leading Causes for Abdominal Operative Exploration in ICU Patients and Characteristic Findings			
Diagnosis	**History and physical exam**	**Laboratory**	**Radiology**	**DPL/ laparoscopy**
Ulcer perforation (gastric/duodenal)	Hx of ulcer disease	Leukocytosis common	Free air on plain films/CT	Murky fluid in abdomen
Colon perforation	Hx diverticular disease	Leukocytosis common	Free air on plain films/CT	Murky fluid in abdomen
Bowel ischemia (small bowel)	AFIB or vascular disease; abdomen rigid with hemodynamic collapse	Leukocytosis common; lactate elevation and acidosis common	Finding subtle on plain films; CT may show thumbprinting or pneumatosis (air in bowel wall)	DPL should have elevated WBC; laparoscopy will demonstrate black or gray necrotic bowel
Cholecystitis	Presence of gallstones; pain more likely in upper right quadrant	LFT may be elevated	Thickened gallbladder wall with stones is classic by ultrasound	Inflammation in upper right quadrant by laparoscopy— adherence of structures to gallbladder
Bowel obstruction	Prior abdominal surgeries, vomiting, abdominal distension and absence of flatus or bowel movements	Leukocytosis may be present; acidosis may be present if associated with compromised bowel viability	Air fluid levels throughout abdomen on plain films/CT	DPL with elevated WBC when advanced; laparoscopy will show distended bowel; may be able to relieve obstruction laparoscopically
Sigmoid volvulus	Hx of constipation; abdominal distention on exam	Leukocytosis and acidosis may be present if advanced	"Omega loop" of colon seen on plain film; distended colon by CT	Should be able to make Dx with Hx/physical exam and radiology
Clostridium difficile colitis	Hx of prior antibiotic use	Profound leukocytosis often seen; stool assay for bacterial toxin or fecal leukocytes may be positive	Thickened colon by CT; free fluid in abdomen is a bad prognosis sign	Laparoscopy will show a diffusely inflamed colon

4. The gastrointestinal review of systems is also useful, for example knowing that the patient is not tolerating his or her tube feeds or has nausea, vomiting, hematemesis, melena, or hematochezia. Compromise of other subsystems, including the development of renal failure, acute lung injury, or hemodynamic instability, all suggest a significant insult.

5. Finally, if time permits, identification of the medical decision maker for this patient and any advanced directives can simplify the decision process and ensure that the process of care achieves the patient's wishes, which should

include aspects other than just survival, including quality and function of life. However, emergency intervention should never be delayed awaiting informed consent.

B. Physical examination. Many of the same conditions hindering a historical examination also make the abdominal examination unreliable. Patients often have an altered level of consciousness, either iatrogenic (e.g., narcotics) or because of concomitant pathology (e.g., stroke, trauma). Hence there is a lack of sensitivity for subtle findings, and even signs of abdominal catastrophe may be difficult to elicit. Medications such as steroids and immunosuppressants may mask the signs of peritoneal irritation. In this context, alternate endpoints and surrogate markers of tenderness, such as facial grimacing and localization, are utilized, which compromises specificity. Physiologic changes such as tachycardia or hypertension during the exam may also indicate tenderness. It is essential to judge the reliability of your examination in addition to the findings themselves.

1. The physical evaluation commences with a review of vital signs, including heart rate, blood pressure, and urine output. Because of the frequency with which both physiologic and biochemical data are recorded, trends may be tracked and can facilitate identifying the temporal sequence of events. For example, the detailed records can be reviewed to see when urinary output dropped off, when the ventilatory requirements increased, or when the dosage of pressors was raised. The combination of these data may lend insight into whether this process is acute, subacute, or has taken place over a period of hours or days.

2. A thorough abdominal exam follows. The presence and location of any prior abdominal operations should be noted and matched with the details of the past surgical history. The presence, character, and location of any tenderness should be elicited. Temporally related events (e.g., cardiac catheterization, ruptured abdominal aneurysms), including precipitating or alleviating factors (e.g., movement, meals, emesis) may assist in narrowing the differential. Peritonitis, in particular involuntary guarding, is particularly suggestive of surgical pathology. Distension and tympany, though nonspecific, usually suggests obstruction or ileus. A rectal exam should be performed to check for masses, distal passage of stool and presence of blood. Melena or hematochezia suggest significant mucosal injury (e.g., ischemia). The nature and volume of nasogastric aspirate (e.g., bloody vs. bilious) may provide insight. Hernias should be searched for and characterized as to reduced, incarcerated, or strangulated.

3. Extraabdominal findings may provide additional corroborating evidence of a particular diagnosis. Evidence of peripheral vascular disease supports a diagnosis of mesenteric ischemia/infarction. The lacelike livedo reticularis is an uncommon sign seen in cholesterol embolism. Similarly, atrial fibrillation may underlie distal embolization to the mesenteric circulation and bowel infarction.

C. Laboratory. Although tests should be specific to the differential diagnosis, the paucity of historical and physical data usually translates into the acquisition of a broad range of laboratory tests. Typically, a complete blood count with cell differential, electrolytes, liver function tests, amylase, lipase, urinalysis, and arterial blood gas with lactate should be obtained. Leukocytosis, a sign of inflammation, may be suggestive of an abdominal problem. However, its absence does not exclude surgical abdominal disease. In a cohort of patients older than 80 years, fever and leukocytosis were absent in 33% of cases of acute surgical disease. In the setting of a normal total white blood cell (WBC) count, which is not uncommon in the elderly or immunocompromised, a significant "left shift" (defined as a large proportion of neutrophils or immature band forms) may indicate that an acute problem is present. Electrolyte abnormalities such as a rising creatinine or low bicarbonate indicate poor perfusion and developing shock. Once again, these signs are sensitive to the presence of ischemia and shock, but lack any specificity in identifying a cause. Elevated bilirubin may indicate liver or gallbladder disease while an elevated amylase and lipase may result from acute pancreatitis. In a study of acute abdomens not caused by pancreatitis, 50% of patients had a normal amylase indicating that normal laboratory values do not exclude significant pathology. Serum lactate is produced through anaerobic tissue metabolism and is sensitive in abdominal disease. In one study it was elevated above the reference level in 100% of patients with mesenteric ischemia and 50% of patients with bowel obstruction. That same study points out that the specificity of lactate elevation was only 40%. Base deficit requires an arterial blood sample and a substantial base deficit provides similar information about tissue hypoperfusion as the lactate level. One study of outcome in critically ill surgical patients demonstrated that the persistent lactate elevation is more predictive of poor outcome than a persistent base deficit.

III. DIAGNOSTIC ADJUNCTS. The physiologic status of the patient may preclude transportation for diagnostic studies. Transportation typically involves a transition to more portable versions of complicated equipment such as ventilators and continuous infusions, as well as significant physical manipulation of the patient, which may not be tolerable. This tenuousity is more typical of patients requiring inotropic/vasopressor support or maximal ventilatory support. The location (e.g., CT scanner) to which the patient is transported creates a potentially hazardous environment to which it is difficult to summon qualified help immediately, to access the patient, and that lacks essential emergency equipment. In light of these dangers, the information to be gained from any diagnostic test and the extent to which this information may alter management must be interpreted in the context of the potential sacrifice to patient care.

  A. Plain radiographs. A supine and upright/decubitus abdominal radiograph is easy to obtain and may identify free air or evidence supporting the diagnosis of small- or large-bowel obstruction. More subtle signs include thumbprinting and pneumatosis that represent bowel ischemia. It is helpful to obtain three views of the abdomen. Compared to other tests, however, the sensitivity of plain radiographs is low. In known cases of bowel infarction, the abdominal films are normal in 25% and characteristic findings such as pneumatosis or thumbprinting are present in less than 40%.

  B. CT scan. While CT scan is a mainstay for diagnostic evaluation, and its use is widespread in the management of abdominal disease, it may not be as useful in the ICU patient population.

    1. The advantages of CT scan include its excellent resolution of most organs and identification of fluid collections and small amounts of free air if present. The CT scan has been used with variable success to identify features of mesenteric ischemia including bowel thickening, pneumatosis intestinalis (i.e., air in bowel wall), or atherosclerosis and vascular thrombus. Even with dynamic contrast the sensitivity for detection of features of ischemic intestine is 64%. As the technology and the resolution of the CT scan improves, the sensitivity may improve as well. CT findings (e.g., pancreatic and peripancreatic edema and stranding with pancreatitis) may also support a nonoperative diagnosis and continued observation. Liver and spleen hematomas and inflammatory diseases such as diverticulitis and appendicitis are well characterized by CT scan.

    2. The disadvantages include the need to transport the ill patient out of the ICU and to administer oral and intravenous contrast, which carry the risks of intolerance, emesis with aspiration, and renal toxicity. In one randomized controlled trial, orally administered N-acetylcysteine (600 mg orally twice daily) the day prior to and of CT imaging combined with hydration decreased the rise in creatinine in patients with chronic renal insufficiency receiving intravenous contrast. CT scans can be administered without oral and/or intravenous contrast, however, this may detract from image quality and utility. While fluid collections and free air can be seen, it may be difficult to characterize a collection as an abcess in the absence of the rim enhancement afforded by intravenous contrast. Likewise visualizing a contained perforation is facilitated by observing a pooling of extraluminal contrast.

  C. Abdominal ultrasound has the major advantages that it can be performed at the bedside and does not require an intravenous dye load; however, it is operator dependent. Ultrasound is good at imaging the gallbladder and biliary system, and can identify collections of intraabdominal fluid. It is limited in ability to provide information regarding hollow organs, and may be difficult to adequately perform in the obese or anasarcic patient.

D. Diagnostic peritoneal lavage (DPL). Borrowed from the trauma experience, the DPL attempts to determine the need for abdominal exploration. The procedure for performing a DPL and the criteria for a positive test is outlined in Chapter 26. In one study of general surgery patients, a WBC count greater than or equal to 200 cells/mm^3 was associated with a 99% probability of peritonitis. One retrospective study indicated that DPL is 100% sensitive and 88% specific in identifying abdominal pathology requiring operation in nontrauma patients. Their conclusion was that a negative DPL excludes intraabdominal pathology, but a positive DPL does not necessarily denote the presence of surgical disease; hence, it is sensitive, but lacks specificity. This in part is dependent on the laboratory threshold employed to identify pathology. Through the small entry site, some loops of small bowel can be examined for obvious ischemia. If justification for exploration is found the patient can be transported to the operating room (OR) for further management or, if the ICU is able to provide the support, the operation can be performed at the bedside.

E. Bedside laparoscopy is an extension of the DPL; the abdomen is insufflated and a camera introduced at the bedside.

  1. The advantage over DPL is that the viscera can be manipulated and directly visualized for pathology.

  2. The disadvantage involves the pneumoperitoneum that may decrease renal blood flow and venous return and induce unfavorable hemodynamic consequences in the critically ill patient. In addition, it requires general endotracheal anesthesia and mechanical ventilation, which are additional challenges for the spontaneously breathing patient. The procedure itself requires the availability and portability of appropriate sterile instrumentation, videoscopic monitors, and gas insufflation equipment. Depending on the individual institutional commitment, the ease and availability of these procedures will be variable.

  3. Multiple studies have demonstrated the feasibility and safety of performing diagnostic laparoscopy in critically ill patients. An exploration of the stomach, small bowel, colon, liver, and gallbladder can be performed with a camera port and two additional ports. Use of a 30- or 45-degree angled laparoscopic camera can facilitate inspection of the abdomen. Two atraumatic laparoscopic graspers can be used to manipulate and inspect the intestines. More recently, authors have described a technique for minilaparoscopy using a 3.3-mm laparoscope and 3-mm instruments with success. When compared to DPL, bedside laparoscopy may be more specific in that there were fewer negative laparotomies following laparoscopy than DPL.

IV. SURGICAL EXPLORATION. Refinements in diagnostic capabilities have allowed a more selective application of laparotomy, reducing the number of nontherapeutic laparotomies without increasing morbidity and mortality. In light of the compelling evidence that delay in surgical intervention is associated with worse outcome, preparation should occur concomitantly with diagnostic evaluation.

A. Preoperative preparation. Preoperative preparation includes a full laboratory analysis including electrolyes, complete blood count, and coagulation factors. Many patients will have either coagulopathy or electrolyte imbalances that will necessitate correction. Accomplishing this preoperatively may be difficult and cause undue, life-threatening delay. Thus, the patient should have a sample sent for type and screen and a type and cross if transfusion is anticipated. An EKG and CXR are helpful but should not delay emergency surgery. Active fluid resuscitation is critical prior to taking the patient to the operating room so that the induction of anesthesia is uneventful. A patient in profound shock who is intravascularly volume depleted may arrest when administered anesthestic agents. If possible, informed consent should be obtained from the patient or relative. This is not always possible or practical, depending on the clinical state of the patient and the urgency of surgical intervention; in such cases, the operation should proceed without life-threatening delays to obtain consent. In tenuous patients, it is our practice to have the resuscitation team accompany the patient to the operating room.

B. Preoperative OR. For urgent exploration, the patient should be positioned supine with both arms abducted and available for adequate access. Modifications in this positioning (e.g., lithotomy) should be tailored to the anticipated pathology. However, perineal and anorectal access can be achieved by "frogging" the legs under the sterile drapes. The disadvantage of stirrups includes the possibility of lower extremity nerve injury, especially if the legs are not padded properly and/or during prolonged cases.

After positioning, time should be permitted to enable the placement of necessary monitoring and resuscitation lines, including invasive arterial cannulas, central venous access, and Swan-Ganz catheterization. Sequential compression devices for DVT prophylaxis should be placed, preferably prior to the induction of general anesthesia. All patients require Foley catheterization and typically nasogastric intubation. Empiric broad-spectrum antibiotics should be administered. In the absence of known drug allergy, cefotetan or cefoxitin provide excellent coverage for both integument and enteric organisms. Ciprofloxacin and metronidazole are reasonable alternatives in the penicillin/cephalosporin-sensitive patient. Suspicion of nosocomial organisms should prompt broadening coverage to include nonlactose fermenting gram-negative rods (*Pseudomonas, Acinetobacter*), methicillin-resistant *Staphalococcus aureus* (MRSA), enterococcus, and yeast. A long duration of hospitalization and prior antibiotic usage during the stay increase the likelihood of these nosocomial organisms. The patient's skin should be prepped from the nipple line to the pubis. The prep may be modified to include the bilateral groins or chest if clinically indicated. Ensure that adequate help, light, and suction is available.

C. Operative. The goals of operation are the same regardless of the stability of the patient, but the techniques to achieve these goals modified depending on the clinical status of the patient. Much like a trauma celiotomy, the operative goal is to control hemorrhage if present, control contamination, and to identify and treat other pathology. Most patients can be explored through a midline laparotomy, and exposure must be optimal. The operation should not be compromised by inadequate exposure. An "indecisive" midline incision around the umbilicus is a reasonable initial approach to identify if the problem is in the upper or lower abdomen so as to avoid an unnecessarily lengthy incision. Alternatively, the incision may be tailored to a preoperative diagnosis (e.g., a right or left upper quadrant incision two fingerbreaths below the costal margin for work on the liver/gallbladder or spleen, respectively). The disadvantage of these incisions is that they provide exposure to only a portion of the abdomen, and if the pathology resides outside this area, a much larger incision will be necessary. Likewise, although the appendix is typically removed through an incision in the right lower quadrant, a vertical lower midline incision will also serve well for this purpose.

1. Once the abdomen is open, definitive care should be provided to any obvious pathology. Typically, the pathology threatening the patient is obvious. Any sources of contamination can be temporarily controlled with clamps or oversewing until all peritoneal viscera evaluated and all pathology identified. If bowel is nonviable, then it is resected. Doppler interrogation of the mesenteric vessels or fluorescein dye with Woods lamp illumination may objectively define the adequacy of perfusion to tenuous appearing bowel. The utilization of the GIA staplers has markedly facilitated the process of resection. The vascular endoGIA stapler can markedly reduce the time needed for mesenteric division.

2. Different approaches to reconstruction depend on the stability of the patient. If the patient is stable than definitive repair or anastomosis can be performed. Hypothermia, hypotension, and the need for blood transfusion are signs that reconstruction may best be performed another day, after resuscitation and restoration of homeostasis have been achieved. Borrowing from the trauma experience with damage control laparotomy, some of this logic has been extended to general surgery patients. The divided ends of bowel can be left in the abdomen with the plan to reexplore and restore intestinal continuity when homeostasis has been achieved. In addition, bowel of questionable viability can be reexamined at a later date so that the minimum length of bowel is resected.

3. A variety of temporary closure methods of the abdomen are available and covered elsewhere in this manual but include a sterile IV bag (Bogota bag), vacuum-assisted techniques, or a sticky drape over some towels. The advantage of these dressings is that the likelihood of developing an abdominal compartment syndrome is greatly decreased, though not eliminated. They also permit intraabdominal fluid to be drained continuously so that the patient does not retain quite so much fluid. The disadvantage of these dressings is that the patient generally must be sedated to prevent evisceration, the patient is committed to a second operation, and with time, the fascia will retract, thereby making primary closure more challenging and increasing the need for future incisional herniorrhaphy.

D. **Postoperative.** Once the operation has been completed and the responsible pathology addressed, efforts focus on resuscitation and subsystem support. Endpoints of resuscitation (i.e, markers of adequate tissue perfusion) include conventional parameters (e.g., heart rate, blood pressure, urine output), global parameters (e.g., lactate, base deficit, SvO_2), and regional measures (e.g., mucosal pH, capnometry, and near infrared spectroscopy). Normoglycemia should be maintained. For patients with severe sepsis, activated protein C may be utilized; we do not consider surgical intervention an absolute contraindication.

V. **OUTCOMES.** As ICU care continues to improve, the outcomes for emergency abdominal surgery in critically ill patients should improve. However, the frail state of the patient at the start of operation makes it difficult for them to handle and recover from the stress of surgery. The most common etiologies necessitating surgical intervention in ICU patients are bowel perforation, bowel ischemia, cholecystitis, bowel obstruction, and cecal/sigmoid volvulus. An emerging indication for operation in ICU patients is fulminant antibiotic associated colitis from *Clostridium difficile* infection. The overall mortality rate in the entire population remains high, approximately 38%, and it correlates with organ system failure index (OSFI) and Acute Physiology and Chronic Health Evaluation (APACHE) score. Not surprisingly, the greater degree of preoperative physiologic derangement the higher the mortality. In one observational study, a high OSFI and APACHE score was associated with a mortality of 89%, but if both scores were low, only 5% died. Diagnostic delay, if present, continues to be independently associated with a higher mortality.

VI. **SUMMARY.** The evaluation of the acute abdomen in the ICU patient can be challenging. Though the approach is similar to that of the noncritically ill patient, the source of the data is different. Often a history is not available and a physical exam is not reliable. These are compensated for by the wealth of physiologic and laboratory value available. Diagnostic studies are useful but their value must be weighed against the potential need to transport the patient off of the unit. At operation decisions need to be made regarding definitive reconstruction, creation of stomas, or leaving the abdomen open for planned reoperation. The outcome of ICU patients undergoing emergency surgery is poor and is dependent on the preoperative APACHE score. Diagnostic delay, a variable that the physician can control, results in increased mortality.

Bibliography

Alverdy JC, Saunders J, Chamberlin WH, Moss GS. Diagnostic peritoneal lavage in intra-abdominal sepsis. *Am Surg* 1988;54(7):456–459.

Dallal RM, Harbrecht EG, Boujoukas AJ, et al. Fulminant *Clostridium difficile*: An underappreciated and increasing cause of death and complications. *Ann Surg* 2002;235(3): 363–372.

Gagne DJ, Malay MB, Hogle NJ, Fowler DL. Bedside diagnostic minilaparoscopy in the intensive care patient. *Surgery* 2002;131:491–496.

Gajic O, Urrutia LE, Sewani H, et al. Acute abdomen in the medical intensive care unit. *Crit Care Med* 2002;30(6):1187–1190.

Husain FA, Martin MJ, Mullenix PS, et al. Serum lactate and base deficit as predictors of mortality and morbidity. *Am J Surg* 2003;185(5):485–491.

Kollef MH, Allen BT. Determinants of outcome for patients in the medical intensive care unit requiring abdominal surgery. *Chest* 1994;106(6):1822–1828.

Lange H, Jackel R. Usefulness of plasma lactate concentration in the diagnosis of acute abdominal disease. *Eur J Surg* 1994;160(6-7):381–384.

Larson FA, Haller CC, Delcore R, Thomas JH. Diagnostic peritoneal lavage in acute peritonitis. *Am J Surg* 1992;164(5):449–452.

McNicoll L, Pisani MA, Zhang Y, et al. Delirium in the intensive care unit: Occurrence and clinical course in older patients. *Am Geriatr Soc* 2003;51(5):591–598.

Oldenburg WA, Lau LL, Rodenberg TJ, et al. Acute mesenteric ischemia: A clinical review. *Arch Intern Med* 2004;164:1054–1062.

Pace BW, Bank S, Wise L, et al. Amylase isoenzymes in the acute abdomen: An adjunct in those patients with elevated total amylase. *Am J Gastroenterol* 1985;80(11):898–901.

Pitts FE, Vukov LF. Utility of fever and leukocytosis in acute surgical abdomens in octogenarians and beyond. *J Gerontol A Biol Sci Med Sci* 1999;54(2):M55–M58.

Taourel PG, Deneuville M, Pradel JA, et al. Acute mesenteric ischemia: Diagnosis with contrast-enhanced CT. *Radiology* 1996;199:632–636.

Tepel M, van der Giet M, Schwarzfeld C, et al. Prevention of radiographic-contrast-agent-induced reductions in renal function by acetylcysteine. *N Engl J Med* 2000; 343(3):180–184.

Walsh RM, Popovich MJ, Hoadley J. Bedside diagnostic laparoscopy and peritoneal lavage in the intensive care unit. *Surg Endosc* 1998;12:1405–1409.

59 VASCULAR EMERGENCIES
JOEL E. BARBATO AND EDITH TZENG

I. **INTRODUCTION.** The general surgeon is often called to evaluate patients in the emergency room or in consultation who are ultimately found to have a vascular etiology for their complaints. It is therefore incumbent on the acute care surgeon to include vascular surgical emergencies in the patient's differential diagnosis. Key in the determination of the morbidity and mortality associated with these vascular surgery conditions is the quick recognition and treatment of the vascular pathology.

II. **RUPTURED AORTIC ANEURYSMS**
   A. **Introduction.** An aneurysm is defined as a vascular structure whose diameter is enlarged to >1.5 times the normal caliber of that vessel. Abdominal aortic aneurysms (AAAs) are the most common form of true aneurysm. The most common form of aortic aneurysm is located below the renal arteries. Thoracoabdominal aortic aneurysms (TAAAs) are less common and present significant treatment challenges. Given the high mortality of a ruptured aortic aneurysm, attempts have been made to establish guidelines by which the asymptomatic aneurysm should be repaired. Controversy exists for "small aortic aneurysms" (4–5 cm). Most authorities agree that nonruptured aneurysms >5.5 cm should be repaired as there is a 5% annual rupture rate for aneurysms larger than 5 cm.
   B. **Diagnosis of ruptured AAA**
      1. Classification of thoracic and abdominal aneurysms (Fig. 59-1).
      2. History. Ninety-six percent of patients with ruptured AAA present with abdominal and/or back pain.
      3. Physical exam. The sensitivity of physical exam ranges from 29% to 76% depending on the size of the aneurysm. Obesity significantly affects the clinician's ability to palpate an aneurysm. Therefore, lack of pulsatile mass should not dissuade the examiner from considering a diagnosis of ruptured AAA. Abdominal pain and hypotension in a patient with a known AAA is assumed to be a ruptured aneurysm until proven otherwise.
      4. CT scan. The most commonly employed modality for the diagnosis of ruptured AAA. Only performed in hemodynamically stable patients. A noncontrast CT can be performed in stable patients who are suspected of having a leaking aneurysm. A fine-cut CT angiogram of the aorta may be helpful in determining if a stable patient with a leaking aneurysm may be a candidate for an endovascular aneurysm repair (EVAR).
      5. Ultrasound. Useful for emergent evaluation of patients in ED. Its accuracy is user-dependent and limits its widespread applicability. Examination is limited to the presence of an AAA and free fluid.
      6. There is no role for angiography or MRI/MRA in evaluation of ruptured AAA.
   C. **Treatment**
      1. Preoperative evaluation should be minimal in setting of presumed ruptured AAA. **Urgent operation is essential to minimize morbidity and mortality.** Elderly patients with abdominal pain, a pulsatile mass, and hypotension have a ruptured AAA until proven otherwise.
      2. Large-bore intravenous (IV) access—resuscitate to adequate perfusion pressures (systolic blood pressure [SBP] 60–80 mmHg to maintain mentation). Do

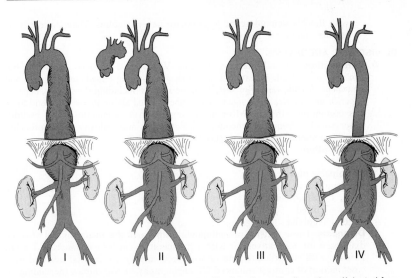

Figure 59-1. The Stanford and DeBakey classifications for aortic dissections. (Adapted from Brunicardi FC, Andersen DK, Billiar TR, et al. *Schwartz's Principles of Surgery*. 8th ed. New York, NY: McGraw-Hill; 2005:704, with permission.)

not attempt to overresuscitate as this may further exacerbate bleeding from the AAA.

3. Uncrossmatched blood should be available until type-specific blood is ready.

4. Control the airway if transfer of patient is necessary. In addition, a Foley catheter is inserted.

5. Prep chest, abdomen, and thighs. Make a long midline incision. Transabdominal exposure may be required for emergency operation.

6. Duodenum is mobilized to the right and proximal control is obtained either below renal vessels or supraceliac depending on the location of the hematoma, rupture site, and the stability of the patient. Distal control is obtained at the common iliac arteries.

7. The aneurysm is opened, lumbar vessels oversewn, and either a tube or bifurcated graft sewn into the aneurysm, depending on iliac artery involvement.

8. The aneurysm sac is closed over the graft and the abdomen closed.

9. Endovascular repair for ruptured aneurysm is gaining popularity in a select group of patients who are relatively stable hemodynamically and with favorable anatomy. It is performed in specialized centers that maintain an inventory of a wide selection of endografts.

D. Outcomes

1. Overall mortality of ruptured AAA is 80% to 90%.

2. Mortality of patients surviving to reach the operating room (in setting of rupture) is >50%.

3. EVAR appears to be associated with decreased morbidity and mortality compared with open repair of ruptured AAA but the number of patients undergoing EVAR for rupture is small. This difference in outcome may also be a reflection that patients undergoing EVAR are hemodynamically stable while those undergoing open repair are unstable.

4. No randomized controlled trials have been completed to compare ER versus open repair (OR).

5. Sixty percent of ruptured AAAs will develop bowel ischemia. Postoperative acidosis, bloody stools, or abdominal pain suggests this diagnosis. Proceed

with flexible sigmoidoscopy to assess for ischemic colitis. These patients may require urgent colectomy.

III. VISCERAL ANEURYSMS

A. Introduction. Visceral arterial aneurysms (VAAs) are a relatively rare entity but can present with life-threatening hemorrhage requiring expedient diagnosis and treatment. A wide variety of vessels can be affected including the splenic, hepatic, superior mesenteric, and celiac vessels. Other named abdominal vessels tend to be less commonly affected. Most aneurysms are true aneurysms, with pseudo-aneurysms less frequently encountered. Both open and endovascular approaches have been applied with varying success.

B. Presentation
1. Pain
2. Palpable mass
3. Hemorrhage
   a. Intraabdominal
   b. GI bleed
   c. Hemobilia

C. Diagnosis. Those patients presenting with rupture of the aneurysm will often be diagnosed intraoperatively or with a preoperative contrast enhanced CT scan. Patients with symptomatic, but nonruptured, aneurysms are best assessed by a combination of contrast enhanced CT, angiography, and/or duplex (depending on the expertise of the ultrasonographer).

D. Affected vessels
1. **Splenic.** The most commonly affected visceral vessel. These are associated with pregnancy and portal hypertension. Elective repair is recommended for aneurysms >2 cm in diameter.
2. **Hepatic.** The second most common VAA (roughly 20% of all VAA). One half are pseudoaneurysms as a result of invasive biliary procedures. May present with obstructive jaundice. The majority are single and extrahepatic.
3. **SMA.** Five percent of VAA. These are frequently mycotic/infectious in nature. Fifty percent of ruptures will present with hemodynamic instability and 25% will have evidence of bowel ischemia.
4. **Celiac.** Four percent of VAA. Risk of rupture estimated to be 13%. Most commonly felt to be atherosclerotic in nature.

E. Cause
1. Atherosclerosis
2. Vasculitis
3. Fibromuscular dysplasia
4. Trauma
5. Duodenal ulcer
6. Infection
7. Iatrogenic

F. Treatment
1. Percutaneous embolization successful in 70% to 90% of cases.
2. Aneurysm resection and interposition versus primary anastomosis. In patients with hemodynamic instability, selective ligation may be performed.
3. In select cases (e.g., contained rupture with hematoma formation), nonoperative management has been performed although newer endovascular technologies make this less appealing.

IV. AORTIC DISSECTION

A. Introduction. Aortic dissection may be similar to aortic aneurysms in their sometimes quite dramatic presentation and catastrophic consequence in the absence of prompt diagnosis. *Dissection* and *aneurysm* are frequently misused terms. Dissections may arise in the setting of an aneurysm. *Dissecting aneurysm* as a term should be confined to this particular setting.

B. Pathophysiology. Abnormal separation of walls of aorta (most commonly the intima and media) creating a "true lumen" and a "false lumen." Morbidity arises

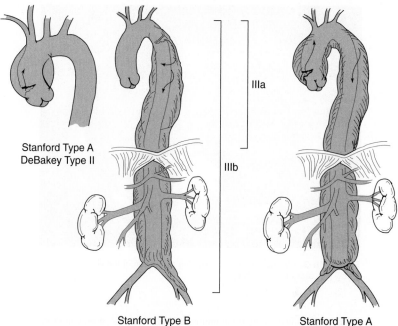

Stanford Type A
DeBakey Type II

IIIa

IIIb

Stanford Type B
DeBakey Type III

Stanford Type A
DeBakey Type I

Figure 59-2. Crawford's classification scheme of thoracic and thoracoabdominal aneurysms. (Adapted from Brunicardi FC, Andersen DK, Billiar TR, et al. *Schwartz's Principles of Surgery*. 8th ed. New York, NY: McGraw-Hill; 2005:700, with permission.)

from dissection into aortic branches with interruption of perfusion and from aneurysmal degeneration of the weakened aortic wall over time.

C. Classification

1. **Chronicity** of symptoms. "Acute" dissection refers to a dissection whose symptoms have occurred for <14 days. Longer than 14 days from the onset of symptoms, a dissection is classified as "chronic."

2. **DeBakey classification** (Fig. 59-2)
    a. **Type I:** ascending aorta and variable extent of descending
    b. **Type II:** limited to ascending aorta
    c. **Type III**
        i. IIIa: descending aorta without extension to abdomen
        ii. IIIb: descending aorta with extension to abdomen

3. **Stanford classification**
    a. **Type A:** proximal to takeoff of subclavian artery
    b. **Type B:** distal to takeoff of subclavian artery

D. Diagnosis

1. Severe pain. Eighty-five percent have abrupt onset of severe pain; anterior chest pain (Stanford type A) or back/abdominal pain (Type B)—most commonly sharp in nature; classically described as "tearing."

2. Discrepancy in pulse exam or BP in extremities. Right arm versus left arm for proximal dissection; upper extremities versus lower extremities for distal dissection.

3. Radiography
    a. CT angiogram (Fig. 59-3). Most commonly used modality and shows the intimal flap extending for multiple slices.

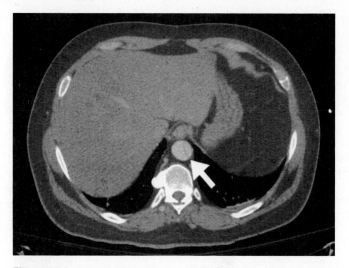

Figure 59-3. CT angiogram demonstrating dissection of the abdominal aorta (arrow indicates dissection flap).

  b. MRA. Availability often limited by urgent nature of presentation.
  c. Transesophageal echocardiogram. Good for emergent evaluation of proximal dissection.
  d. Arteriography. More difficult because it requires imaging both false and true lumens to demonstrate visceral perfusion.
  e. CXR. May show enlarged aortic knob, mediastinal widening, left effusion, deviation of NG tube, displacement of left mainstem bronchus in proximal dissection with aneurysmal changes.
E. Management
  1. Type A. Urgent operative intervention with replacement of ascending aorta is almost always warranted.
  2. Type B
    a. Medical management
      i. Initial management includes intensive monitoring with admission to ICU. Blood pressure (BP) should be measured frequently, preferably with an arterial catheter (extremity with highest BP should be used as dissection may decrease BP in extremity perfused by false lumen). Insertion of Foley catheter and central venous monitoring are also invaluable adjuncts.
      ii. BP and heart rate (HR) control to decrease wall stress. IV beta-blockers such as esmolol and labetalol (titrated to heart rate of 60–80 bpm with SBP of 100–110 mmHg) with direct vasodilators (e.g., nitroprusside), calcium channel blockers, and ACE inhibitors as necessary.
      iii. These patients should have follow-up CT scans during the acute phase (within first week) to assess for aortic expansion; followed by routine scans during chronic phase.
      iv. Long-term antihypertensives (preferably beta-blockers).
    b. Surgical management warranted in those patients with:
      i. Lower extremity ischemia
      ii. Impending rupture
      iii. Aneurysm degeneration
      iv. End-organ ischemia (e.g., renal failure, mesenteric ischemia)

    c. Surgical options

      i. Open repair

        a) Graft replacement

        b) Aortoplasty

        c) Open fenestration

      ii. Endovascular options

        a) Stent graft to obliterate the entry point and the false lumen

        b) Fenestration

      iii. Outcomes

        a) Ten percent to 30% mortality during acute phase

        b) Case series suggest high success (85%–100%) closure of false lumen in endovascular treatment, but complications may include aneurysmal degeneration, stroke, access site bleeding, and need for further open surgical interventions.

V. AORTOENTERIC FISTULA

A. Introduction. Patients with aortoenteric fistula may present with life-threatening hemorrhage. The vast majority of these cases result from prior aortic surgery, one half following AAA repair and one half from aortobifemoral bypass. Occurs in 0.9% of patients following open AAA repairs.

B. Etiology

  1. Primary: majority associated with AAA

  2. Secondary: occur in the presence of previous vascular surgery with prosthetic material; average time to formation after primary intervention is 5 years

    a. Graft enteric fistula—75%

    b. Graft enteric erosion—25%

C. Symptoms

  1. GI bleeding: with secondary and 94% with primary will present with bleeding.

  2. Graft infection: one half of patients will grow out an organism; most commonly mixed flora with *Strep, E. coli,* and *S. aureus.*

  3. Pain

  4. Palpable mass

  5. Fever

D. Treatment

  1. Extraanatomic bypass and excision of graft with debridement of aorta and surrounding tissues

  2. Reconstruction with autogenous graft

  3. In situ prosthetic reconstruction

E. Site of bowel involvement

  1. Duodenum—75%

  2. Small bowel—19%

  3. Colon—6%

F. Diagnosis

  1. Assume that a patient with history of aortic reconstruction presenting with GI bleed has an aortoenteric fistula from the onset; until proven definitely otherwise. The initial bleed may be a herald bleed, followed by exsanguination.

  2. CT scan (diagnostic sensitivity, 45%)

  3. UGI (29%)

  4. EGD (24%)

  5. Aortography (18%)

  6. Nuclear scan (16%)

  7. Colonoscopy (8%)

G. Incidence. Aortic graft infections occur in 1% to 2% of all patients who receive aortic reconstruction with prosthetic material. The percentage of those patients with reconstructions who will develop a fistula is approximately 0.4%.

H. Outcome

  1. Twenty percent to 50% mortality.

  2. Extraanatomic bypass in this setting results in amputation rates as high as 30%.

VI. MESENTERIC ISCHEMIA

A. Introduction. Despite improved technology, the mortality of acute mesenteric ischemia has remained unchanged. This results from the difficulty in diagnosis which often leads to bowel necrosis prior to appropriate recognition. The pathophysiology of acute mesenteric ischemia and its chronic form are different; only the acute version is discussed here. Characterized by subjective complaints of pain and a relative paucity of physical findings, **acute mesenteric ischemia can lead to mortality rates as high as 60% to 80%.**

B. Etiology
   1. **Arterial embolism**—40% to 50% of cases (most frequent cause). Most emboli originate from the heart, frequently following myocardial infarction or in the setting of atrial fibrillation. The SMA is more frequently involved because of the more gentle angle relative to the other visceral vessels (most arterial emboli lodge at first branch point of SMA).
   2. **Arterial thrombosis**—25% to 30%; generally in setting of advanced atherosclerosis and chronic mesenteric ischemia; most commonly at origin of SMA.
   3. **Nonocclusive**—20%; poorly understood; low cardiac output and vasoconstriction; most likely to effect watershed regions of bowel.
   4. **Venous thrombosis**—10%; may be secondary to underlying hypercoagulable state, malignancy, sepsis, or pancreatitis; usually segmental; most commonly involves SMV; slower onset than embolic or thrombotic.

C. Diagnosis
   1. History. The scenario relayed by the patient depends in part on the etiology of the occlusion. Patients with embolic events generally have an acute onset of diffuse pain which may be followed by diarrhea (perhaps bloody). Patients with thrombotic events may have a more insidious onset of symptoms, as they are more likely to have a well-developed collateral system due to chronic atherosclerosis. Rapid diagnosis and intervention are essential to optimize outcome; **the high mortality is related directly to delay in diagnosis and treatment.**
   2. Physical exam. "Pain out of proportion to exam"; may have evidence of dehydration, hemodynamic instability, tachypnea.
   3. Imaging. Plain films and CT are helpful to exclude other causes of abdominal pain; thrombus is infrequently seen on CT. Preoperative angiogram can be helpful but should not delay definitive intervention. Chronic occlusion may demonstrate well-formed collateral vessels.
   4. Laboratory tests. Metabolic acidosis; elevated lactate; increased base deficit; leukocytosis; may have evidence of dehydration (elevated BUN/creatinine ratio).

D. Treatment. The key to the treatment of mesenteric ischemia is early recognition and diagnosis with prompt restoration of mesenteric blood flow. This has been accomplished historically by surgical exploration. Newer endovascular techniques have been devised. Both are appropriate options in well-selected patients. **Initial management in all patients involves fluid resuscitation and anticoagulation.**
   1. **Operative.** Exploratory laparotomy with exposure of the superior mesenteric vessels. Transverse arteriotomy and thrombectomy is performed in the setting of an otherwise normal vessel. Mesenteric bypass should be performed if flow is unable to be reestablished or if severe underlying disease exists. Assessment of intestinal viability (e.g., Wood's lamp, Doppler of distal vessels) should be performed, in conjunction with resection of nonviable bowel. Second-look assessment of bowel can be performed in 24 to 48 hours if there is a question of bowel viability or if massive resection may be required.
   2. **Interventional.** Endovascular techniques have little application in this setting when bowel viability must be assessed. Thrombolytics are generally not indicated as mesenteric flow must be reestablished as the first priority.
   3. **Treatment of nonocclusive mesenteric ischemia** involves correction of low cardiac output state to improve mesenteric perfusion. Angiographic

delivery of vasodilators may be needed to relieve vasospasm in patients who do not respond to resuscitation alone.

4. **Treatment for mesenteric venous thrombosis** involves anticoagulation, bowel rest, and resuscitation. Questionable role for thrombolytic agents.

E. **Outcomes**
   1. Survival is 50% if diagnosis is made within 24 hours of onset of symptoms; mortality exceeds 70% if diagnosis is delayed.
   2. Thrombolytics have been used in select patients with anecdotal success.
   3. Prognosis for acute mesenteric ischemia is worse than for those patients with chronic ischemia.

VII. ACUTE LOWER EXTREMITY ISCHEMIA
A. **Clinical manifestations.** The **six P's:**
   1. **Pain** (the most common presenting symptom)
   2. **Pallor**
   3. **Paresthesias**
   4. **Paralysis**
   5. **Pulselessness**
   6. **Poikilothermia**

B. **Diagnosis.** Physical exam is key.
   1. The pulse exam may indicate the level of obstruction (i.e., absent femoral pulse indicates iliac or aortic occlusion; absent popliteal pulse with good femoral pulses indicates superficial femoral artery or popliteal occlusion).
   2. Motor and sensory exams indicate severity of ischemia and dictate the treatment.

C. **Etiology**
   1. **Thrombotic** (85%). Arises in setting of advanced underlying atherosclerotic disease; most commonly in superficial femoral artery in adductor canal. Overall, bypass graft thrombosis is the most common cause of acute limb ischemia.
   2. **Embolic** (15%). More likely in younger patients and those patients without prior cardiac or vascular history. After restoration of flow, investigation as to the etiology of the embolus should be undertaken; may include cardiac echocardiography (evaluate for valvular vegetation), abdominal CT (possible aortic aneurysm), or lower extremity duplex to assess for iliac, femoral, or popliteal aneurysms.

D. **Treatment**
   1. Underlying hemodynamic instability should be treated with aggressive hydration and institution of heparin to prevent propagation of clot or further embolus from the source.
   2. Urgent operative intervention is warranted in patients with significant motor function deficits. The level of exploration is dictated by level of vascular occlusion (i.e., absent femoral pulse, femoral exposure; absent popliteal pulse with good femoral pulse, popliteal exploration). The thrombus is removed with the embolectomy catheter passed proximally and distally. Additional procedures may be required to restore adequate blood flow to foot, such as endarterectomy or bypass.
   3. Lytics. Appropriate for those patients presenting <14 days from occurrence, thromboemboli not accessible to embolectomy catheters, and thrombosed popliteal artery aneurysms with little or no runoff. Lysis should be followed by endovascular or open surgical repair of any underlying lesions.
   4. Prophylactic fasciotomies are warranted with prolonged ischemia prior to revascularization. Release of all four compartments must be performed (this can be done either through a single lateral incision or by medial and lateral incisions) (Fig. 59-4).
   5. Prophylaxis for rhabdomyolysis following reperfusion in profound ischemia. Begin aggressive hydration prior to reperfusion, mannitol, and possible alkalinization of urine to prevent precipitation of myoglobin and renal failure (Chapter 34).

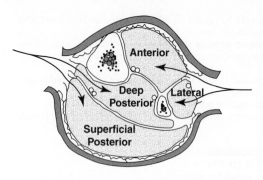

Figure 59-4. Surgical approach for four-compartment fasciotomy in the lower leg. (Reprinted from Rutherford RB, ed. *Rutherford's Vascular Surgery.* 5th ed. Philadelphia, Pa: Elsevier Science; 2000:905.)

E. Outcome

1. Reperfusion of the extremity may result in the release of toxic oxygen metabolites which can result in local edema leading to compartment syndrome and systemic metabolic derangements.
2. Amputation rates of 10% to 30% and mortality as high as 15% at 30 days.
3. Extremities should be monitored frequently postoperatively for changes in sensation or compartment pressures as these patients are at risk for compartment syndrome.

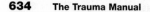

AXIOMS

- A patient with a pulsatile mass and abdominal pain has a ruptured AAA until proven otherwise.
- Aortic dissection of the ascending aorta is a surgical emergency. Dissection of the descending aorta is generally managed medically with antihypertensive medications.
- GI bleeding in a patient with prior aortic surgery should be presumed to be from an aortoenteric fistula until proven otherwise.
- Pain out of proportion to exam should suggest the diagnosis of mesenteric ischemia, the majority of which are the result of embolic or thrombotic events requiring operative intervention.
- Acute lower extremity ischemia most often arises in setting of prior lower extremity bypass. The development of compartment syndrome must be monitored with vigilance after reperfusion.

Bibliography

Boley SJ, Feinstein FR, Sammartano R. New concepts in the management of emboli of the superior mesenteric artery. *Surg Gynecol Obstet* 1981;153(4):561–569.

Crawford ES, Saleh SA, Babb JW III, et al. Infrarenal abdominal aortic aneurysm: Factors influencing survival after operation performed over a 25-year period. *Ann Surg* 1981;193(6):699–709

Donaldson MC, Rosenberg JM, Bucknam CA. Factors affecting survival after ruptured abdominal aortic aneurysms. *J Vasc Surg* 1985;2(4):564–570.

Dormandy J, Heeck L, Vig S. Acute limb ischemia. *Semin Vasc Surg* 1999;12(2):148–153.

Gabelmann A, Gorich J, Merkle EM. Endovascular treatment of visceral artery aneurysms. *J Endovasc Ther* 2002;9(1):38–47.

Hagan PG, Nienaber CA, Isselbacher EM, et al. The International Registry of Acute Aortic Dissection (IRAD): New insights into an old disease. *JAMA* 2000;283(7):897–903.

Lederle FA, Simel DL. The rational clinical examination: Does this patient have abdominal aortic aneurysm? *JAMA* 1999;281(1):77–82.

O'Hara PJ, Hertzer NR, Beven EG, Krajewski LP. Surgical management of infected abdominal aortic grafts: Review of a 25-year experience. *J Vasc Surg* 1986;3(5):725–731.

Oldenburg WA, Lau LL, Rodenberg TJ, et al. Acute mesenteric ischemia: A clinical review. *Arch Intern Med* 2004;164(10):1054–1062.

Pipinos II, Carr JA, Haithcock BE. Secondary aortoenteric fistula. *Ann Vasc Surg* 2000;14(6):688–696.

Zelenock GB, Strodel WE, Knol JA, et al. A prospective study of clinically and endoscopically documented colonic ischemia in 100 patients undergoing aortic reconstructive surgery with aggressive colonic and direct pelvic revascularization, compared with historic controls. *Surgery* 1989;106(4):771–779.

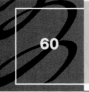

60 GASTROINTESTINAL BLEEDING
ANDREW WATSON AND JAMES MOSER

I. GASTROINTESTINAL BLEEDING

A. Overview. A patient bleeding into the gastrointestinal tract encompasses a diverse array of pathology that leads to either an upper or lower gastrointestinal bleed (GIB). Bleeding is typically caused by vascular disease, neoplasms, inflammation, or anatomic lesions such as an arteriovenous malformation (AVM). Other sources include postsurgical, traumatic, and medication-induced bleeding. A GIB can be either acute, chronic, or occult. We will focus on the acute sources and their management.

B. Statistics. A GIB leads to approximately 300,000 hospitalizations each year and is more commonly found in men and the elderly with increasing incidence in the latter. Of those being hospitalized, 75% are for upper sources and 25% for lower sources. The morbidity is significant as the patient population is typically older with multiple medical comorbidities. Mortality of an upper GIB approaches 10%.

C. Initial patient evaluation, history, and physical examination.

1. There are many diverse causes of a GIB and one must have a basic understanding of the patient's underlying diseases, as well as likely sources of bleeding and his or her age.

2. A bleed may range from a positive fecal occult blood test to hypovolemic shock with cardiovascular collapse. Vomiting ranges from frank blood (hematemesis) to coffee grounds emesis (old blood broken down by gastric acid). A bowel movement may be maroon, tarry, or frank blood with clots (hematochezia).

3. It is important to ask a patient about abdominal pain, weight loss, change in bowel habits, vomiting blood, blood per rectum, color of their vomit or feces, and presence or absence of clots in their vomitus or feces.

4. Look for medications that interfere with hemostasis: Lovenox, heparin, Coumadin, NSAIDs (excessive or routine), Plavix.

5. Past medical history:

   a. Bleeding-specific diseases. Prior GIB, cancer, liver disease, alcohol abuse, *Helicobacter pylori* infection or treatment for known peptic ulcer disease (PUD), esophageal varicies.

   b. General diseases that may cause bleeding. Prior operations (intestinal, liver, pancreatic, vascular), colon cancer screening or a history of colon polyps, inflammatory bowel disease, radiation, pancreatitis (pseudocysts, splenic vein thrombosis), recent trauma.

   c. Check for significant comorbidities that may impair resuscitation or be exacerbated by resuscitation. Renal failure, congestive heart failure, myocardial infarctions, underlying coagulopathy, transfusion reactions.

6. Family history. Cancer (colon, pancreatic, gastric), AVMs, GIB, diverticular disease, aneurysms.

7. Physical examination. A complete examination should be performed with particular attention to the following:

   a. Vital signs and orthostatic hypotension. The goal is to determine the degree of shock (Chapter 5).

   b. HEENT (head, ears, eyes, nose, throat). Scleral icterus or pale sclerae.

    c. Cardiac examination looking for signs of failure or murmurs from an underlying cardiomyopathy or previous infarction, rhythm.

    d. Abdomen. Signs of liver disease: jaundice, liver masses (primary or metastatic disease). Splenomegaly: coagulopathy or portal hypertension. Scars indicating previous operations. Focal tenderness or masses: perforation, strictures, or cancer.

    e. Neurologic. Asterixis.

    f. Rectal. Mass, tenderness, hemorrhoids, presence of stool or blood, guaiac if necessary, masses, hemorrhoids, or fissures.

  8. You must understand the patient's **cardiovascular reserve** and his or her ability to tolerate anemia and hypotension.

D. Causes of gastrointestinal bleeding

  1. The most common cause of a lower GIB is an upper GI source (five times more common).

  2. There are population specific causes of a GIB that may help differentiate the source.

    a. Young patients. Inflammatory bowel disease (IBD), Meckel's diverticulum, HIV/CMV infection.

    b. Middle-aged patients. IBD, polyps, cancer, hemorrhoids, ulcers, varicies, diverticulosis.

    c. Older patients. Same as the middle-aged patient but also including AVM and ischemia.

  3. Use the history to pinpoint the cause (i.e., history of surgery and anticoagulation with staple line bleeding; an alcoholic with esophageal variceal bleeding; excessive NSAID use leading to an ulcer; or recent weight loss, pain, and thin stools that may indicate the presence of a bleeding colon cancer.

  4. Use the output to judge the location of the bleeding.

    a. Hematemesis or coffee ground emesis imply an upper source or one that is proximal to the Ligament of Treitz.

    b. Hematochezia and clots per rectum imply a lower source or a very brisk upper source.

    c. Melena is black, tarry stool that is usually from an upper source. Fifty cubic centimeters of blood can produce this color and it is foul smelling (unlike the stool from a patient taking bismuth compounds). Melena represents blood that has been in the GI tract for some period of time.

    d. Note that left colon bleeding is usually red; right colon bleeding typically produces melena.

  5. To determine the cause of a bleed, consider site specific pathology in combination with the four main categories of pathology: vascular lesions, inflammation, cancer, and specific anatomic lesions.

  a. Upper sources of GIB

    i. These are proximal to the Ligament of Treitz and 80% will stop spontaneously with supportive care only.

    ii. Esophagus. Varicies, Mallory Weiss tear at the gastroesophageal junction (most will stop spontaneously), esophagitis, cancer, Boerhaave's syndrome.

    iii. Stomach. A highly vascular organ with many collaterals.

      a) Ulcers. Check for NSAID use or abuse; the location indicates the type of ulcer and whether associated with high acid secretion. *Helicobacter pylori* infection leads to ulcers and GI bleeding.

      b) Other causes. Bleeding pancreatic pseudocyst, lymphoma, cancer, polyp, gastrointestinal stromal tumor, hiatal hernia, Dieulafoy's lesion, varicies secondary to splenic vein thrombosis or portal hypertension.

    iv. Duodenum

      a) Ulcers in this location cause 50% of upper GIB; most are in the duodenal bulb and if posterior involve the gastroduodenal artery. Rarely, they are caused by Zollinger-Ellison syndrome.

b) Other causes. Cancer, diverticulum, hemobilia, aortoenteric fistula (after an abdominal aortic aneurysm repair).

c) Lower sources of GIB. These are distal to the Ligament of Treitz.

  1) These usually will stop with supportive care only. Most present at an older age (65–70 years), hence these patients are sicker and less able to tolerate the consequences of a major bleed. Bleeding from a lower source is more likely to be bright red.

v. Small bowel

  a) Meckel's diverticulum. Typically found in 2% of the population, within 2 feet of the ileocecal valve in the terminal ileum.

  b) Other causes. Intussusception, sprue, IBD, radiation, cancer, fistula, melanoma, lymphoma, infection, ischemia, diverticulum, Zollinger-Ellison syndrome causing an ulcer.

vi. Large bowel

  a) Diverticulosis. Most will stop spontaneously and not recur. Thirty percent to 50% of diverticular bleeding will be massive; 25% will rebleed after the initial bleed stops spontaneously.

  b) AVM. Cause 20% to 30% of massive lower GIB. These are acquired later in life (age >60 years) when ectatic and dilated vessels become thin walled. The right colon is more often affected and they are usually multiple.

  c) IBD. The majority of ulcerative colitis and one third of Crohn's patients will present with a GIB.

  d) Cancer. Can be from precancerous polyps or cancer itself. It is important to check for colorectal cancer screening when taking a history and specifically ask when the patient last had a flexible sigmoidoscopy or colonoscopy. Also, note the history of fecal occult blood testing and if there was a positive test.

vii. Rectum/perianal disease. Fistulas, fissures, hemorrhoids, rectal prolapse. Usually patients will know if they have a history of pathology in this region and an external examination and anoscopy may be helpful.

viii. Other causes. Ischemia, radiation, volvulus, endometriosis.

II. INITIAL RESUSCITATION AND DEVELOPMENT OF A TREATMENT PLAN

A. Initial resuscitation. Resuscitate the patient according to ATLS protocol (Chapter 10).

  1. Check the ABCs, start two large-bore IVs, and resuscitate initially with colloid.

  a. Attempt to resuscitate to normal vital signs. Recognize that if vital signs are unstable and certainly if they remain so a patient is likely to need transfusion. Failure to respond to resuscitation also categorizes the patient as one likely to need operative intervention. Focus on the history to determine the cause/location of the bleed while resuscitating the patient.

  b. Try to determine the degree of shock to anticipate making a plan (i.e., class III shock in an 80-year-old woman will need a far more aggressive plan than a 20-year-old with blood on his toilet paper from hemorrhoidal bleeding).

  c. In the setting of the initial resuscitation, protect the airway.

  d. Access is critical for both resuscitation and lab draws so an introducer is typically used for the unstable patient.

B. Development of a treatment plan

  1. A plan must be quickly thought through and clearly delineated in the chart so that other consulting teams or on-call physicians can effectively and efficiently care for a bleeding patient.

  2. Risk stratify the patient: Try to determine what degree of anemia can be tolerated and what is the best setting in which to resuscitate the patient and diagnose the source of bleeding. Focus on the ability of a patient to tolerate bleeding.

3. Location. Unstable patients, elderly patients, or patients with the signs of a massive hemorrhage should be quickly transferred to the ICU. Other relatively more stable patients may be best managed in a monitored floor setting.

4. Transfusions. The decision to transfuse may be complicated. The two important factors are: the cardiovascular reserve and the cause of the bleed (severity of the initial bleed with unstable vital signs coupled with the chance of a rebleed).

5. For larger bleeds or massive bleeds review the chapter in this book on massive transfusion syndrome. Call the blood bank to ensure they have a specimen for a type and cross. Stay four units ahead and get platelets and fresh frozen plasma (FFP) ready.

6. Transfuse the patient with unstable vital signs (persistent tachycardia or hypotension). If a patient has stable vital signs but continues to pass a significant amount of blood, be aware that the GI tract can hold and then later evacuate blood long after the bleed source itself has stopped.

7. How much to transfuse depends on the source, the patient's reserve, and the initial hematocrit (HCT). Remember that the patient is actively bleeding and some margin for this must be allowed when transfusing to an HCT. Be sure to check for medications that may interfere with clotting and be wary of transfusion reactions.

8. For cardiac patients with active disease attempt to keep an HCT >30; most other patients can tolerate an HCT drop to approximately 22. If a patient is rapidly bleeding do not wait for the HCT to reach a specific number, especially if he or she has significant comorbidity. Also, know that a patient can experience isovolemic blood loss and that the HCT may be falsely elevated with intravascular volume depletion.

9. Correct all coagulation defects.

10. Massive transfusion may lead to hypothermia which must be avoided as this further impairs coagulation. Warming blankets and warmed intravenous (IV) fluids may be of assistance.

11. Each day, chart the amount of blood products transfused to keep track of the overall scale of the resuscitation and to watch for massive transfusion syndrome or dilutional coagulopathy.

12. Interaction with other teams.
    a. Bleeding patients will likely need to be transferred to an intensive care unit (ICU) with a critical care team following them.
    b. A gastroenterologist will almost certainly be needed for either an upper or lower endoscopy (or both) and they should be notified immediately.
    c. Surgery. In all cases of massive blood loss and for unstable patients, a surgeon must be consulted immediately. A small proportion of patients may be too unstable for diagnostic testing; these patients should be resuscitated and taken promptly to the operating room (OR). For such a patient the OR and anesthesia must be notified immediately.
    d. Frequently cardiology or hematology may be consulted.
    e. Due to the severity of the disease and the complexity of the patient, frequent communication will be necessary, especially with the GI team.

13. Labs. There are not exact values that one should adhere to, but in general the following are reasonable goals:
    a. HCT >30 in a cardiac patient who is symptomatic; HCT >21 in other patients. If the patient is actively bleeding, a higher HCT is maintained. Platelets >100, INR ≤1.3, PTT ≤35.
    b. Frequent blood draws should include serial HCT every 4 to 6 hours as needed, platelets, coagulation profile, and (if needed) a thromboelastogram or fibrinogen level.
    c. If bleeding continues despite resuscitation and therapeutic interventions, consider an underlying coagulopathy that may require a hematology consult and specific labs to be drawn. Realize that the likely cause for coagulopathy is ongoing hemorrhage.

d. Remember that the initial HCT value may represent isovolemic blood loss.

e. Look for an elevated BUN as seen with blood loss into the GI tract, a low MCV consistent with chronic blood loss as in a cancer, and an elevated creatinine or cardiac enzymes that will complicate resuscitation.

14. Family. Due to the potential mortality and morbidity, the physician in charge should contact the family. Pertinent details of a history should be obtained, especially if the patient is unresponsive or intubated at the time of admission. The potential need for an invasive procedure (EGD, colonoscopy, surgery) should be explained and a contact number should be obtained in order to facilitate informed consent.

15. The last aspect of a plan is repeated examinations and close monitoring of vital signs and lab values. Anticipating problems is far better than reacting to a crashing patient.

III. DIAGNOSTIC TESTS

A. These should be used after an attempt has been made to determine the site of the bleeding. Such tests may involve the patient leaving the safe environment of an ICU.

B. Primary modalities to determine the location of bleeding

1. Nasogastric tube (NGT). A nasogastric lavage with 250 cc of normal sterile saline may return clots, red blood, or coffee grounds indicating an upper GIB. If it is bilious, then the pylorus is open. The false negative rate is 25% for an upper source.

2. Esophagogastroduodenoscopy (EGD): Performed by a GI consultant.

a. This may be both a diagnostic and therapeutic procedure. Bleeding varicies may be banded or bleeding ulcers can be clipped, injected with epinephrine or coagulated with a heater probe. Based on the appearance of the ulcer or vessel, prognostic information about the rate of rebleeding can be provided.

b. For unstable patients or those with massive blood loss it is important for a surgeon to watch the EGD to understand the anatomy prior to operation.

3. Bleeding scan. Detects bleeding to a rate >0.5 cc/minute. This test will find a source 45% of the time. The advantages are the low rate of bleeding needed to get a positive scan and that it requires no contrast. The disadvantages are that it is not therapeutic and that the patient has to leave the ICU setting for an extended period. It also poorly localizes the lesion to a specific source (due to peristalsis) which in the face of pending surgery may limit its usefulness. It is not suitable for unstable patients.

4. Angiogram. Detects bleeding to a rate of 1 cc/minute. Similar to a bleeding scan, the patient must leave the ICU, but this test may be both diagnostic and therapeutic. It can provide good localization and a bleeding vessel may be coiled or vasopressin may be injected. Disadvantages include the administration of contrast, especially with an elderly patient with abnormal renal function, the risk of bowel infarction with coiling or vasopressin, and the patient having to leave the ICU. If a bleeding scan is positive there is a high rate of operative intervention.

5. Colonoscopy. Depending on the hospital and consulting GI team, a colonoscopy may be a diagnostic and therapeutic test for a lower GIB. As blood may function as a cathartic, a bowel preparation may not be necessary. Its use as a first-line diagnostic or therapeutic modality is not clearly established. In the face of a massive lower GI bleed its utility may be limited due to poor visibility.

6. Anoscopy or proctoscopy. For patients with suspected perianal or rectal disease hemorrhoids, fistulas or low cancers may be seen.

7. Other diagnostic tests

a. Endoscopic retrograde cholangiopancreaticography looking for hemobilia or other biliary or pancreatic lesions.

b. Enteroclysis looking for small-bowel polyps or signs of Crohn's such as a stricture or fistula.

    c. Capsule endoscopy. Its role in GI bleeding has not be established, but for occult or sources that are difficult to access with other modalities (small-bowel polyp or AVM) it may be useful.

    d. Meckel's scan.

IV. TREATMENT OF THE SOURCE OF BLEEDING

    A. Most GIBs will stop spontaneously. When developing a plan, localize the site of bleeding and determine the risk of rebleeding. The algorithm for an upper GIB (Fig. 60-1) is different than that for a lower GIB (Fig. 60-2).

    B. Note which procedures can be done in the ICU—EGD, colonoscopy, anoscopy, or proctoscopy.

    C. Protect the airway at all times; if a patient is unstable or likely to go to the OR, intubate the patient.

       1. EGD is always performed for an upper GIB. Protecting the airway during this procedure is critical.

       2. Variceal bleeding. Band ligation and sclerotherapy are effective. Mortality is 30% during the first hospitalization.

       3. Bleeding ulcers. Clips, heater probe, and epinephrine injection can all be used to stop bleeding. Even after stopping bleeding with an EGD, the ulcer may rebleed. The risk of rebleeding is as follows: active bleeding (20%), visible vessel (15%), adherent clot (5%). There are a number of features of an ulcer as seen on an EGD that may predict rebleeding, especially size >2 cm.

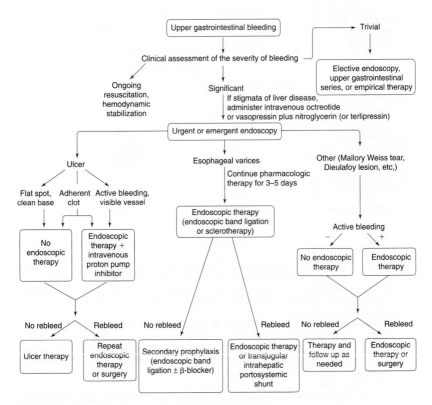

Figure 60-1. Algorithm for an upper gastrointestinal bleed.

MANAGEMENT OF LOWER GASTROINTESTINAL BLEEDING

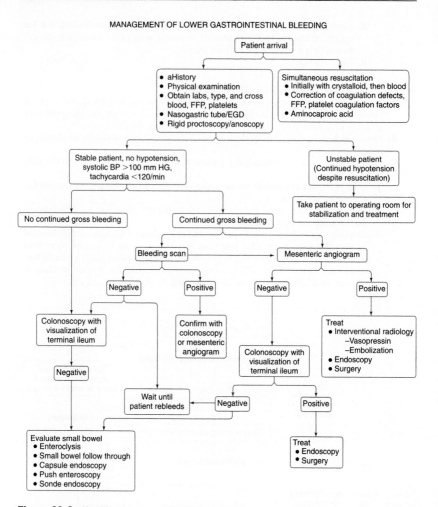

Figure 60-2. Algorithm for a lower gastrointestinal bleed.

    4. Again, a surgeon should watch the endoscopy for a massive bleed or with an unstable patient to help determine the best approach to take in the OR.

D. Transjugular insertion of a portocaval shunt (TIPS). In cases of bleeding esophageal varices that cannot be controlled with an EGD or medications, a TIPS procedure is indicated.

E. Operation. If a patient is at a high risk of rebleeding, has failed nonsurgical therapy, or may not tolerate rebleeding, operative intervention is the best option. In these circumstances a definitive surgical procedure is preferable to a diagnostic test with a low probability of localizing the lesion (Chapter 62). Some commonly performed procedures are as follows.

    1. Upper GIB

        a. Vagotomy and antrectomy. The antrectomy removes the gastrin secreting cells of the stomach. Depending on the condition of the patient, the vagotomy can be aborted and postoperative pharmacologic antisecretory therapy be utilized.

  b. Oversew of a bleeding duodenal ulcer. Relative indications for surgery are a patient that bleeds more than 4 units in 24 hours or a total of 10 units. The gastroduodenal artery is the artery most likely to bleed with a posterior duodenal bulb ulcer and it is oversewn with three stitches (superior, inferior, medial).

  c. For stabilized patients with varicies, decompressive shunting procedure (including a TIPS) may prevent rebleeding by decompressing the portal system.

2. Lower GIB

  a. Bleeding cancer. As long as this is clearly the source of bleeding, a segmental cancer resection is appropriate. Be wary of a synchronous lesion that is the cause of bleeding—carefully examine the entire colon at the time of surgery.

  b. Total abdominal colectomy. For patients who have bleeding localized to the colon (but it cannot be determined whether it is left or right). The source of major lower GIB is more commonly right colon. For a blind hemicolectomy there is at least a 20% chance of a rebleed. A total colectomy is currently the procedure of choice; this prevents the chance of a rebleed from the remaining colon and a second operation.

3. Medications. Consider starting medications that may stop bleeding or prevent rebleeding.

  a. Discontinue all anticoagulation.

  b. Varicies. ADH analogue (vasopressin, terlipressin), beta-blockers, octreotide.

  c. Ulcers. Acid secretion may block clot formation. Antisecretory therapy with IV Protonix (a proton-pump inhibitor), 80-mg bolus once and then start a drip at 8 mg/hour. Histamine-2 blockers.

  d. Aminocaproic acid. Plasminogen inhibitor, antifibrinolytic agent used primarily after cardiac surgery.

V. PITFALLS

A. Lack of planning

  1. Failure to notify the blood bank

  2. Failure to notify surgeon in advance

  3. Not recognizing a patient with limited cardiovascular reserve

  4. Inadequate IV access

  5. Loss of airway while performing a test or procedure

  6. Dilutional coagulopathy during resuscitation and massive transfusion syndrome

Bibliography

Chung IK, Kim EJ, Lee MS, et al. Endoscopic factors predisposing to rebleeding following endoscopic hemostasis in bleeding peptic ulcers. *Endoscopy* 2001;33:969–975.

Elta GH. Urgent colonoscopy for acute lower-GI bleeding. *Gastrointest Endosc* 2004;59:402–408.

Farner R, Lichliter W, Juhn J, et al. Total colectomy versus limited colonic resection for acute lower gastrointestinal bleeding. *Am J Surg* 1999;178:587–591.

Fireman Z, Friedman S. Diagnostic yield of capsule endoscopy in obscure gastrointestinal bleeding. *Digestion* 2004;70:201–206.

Hebert PC, Yetisir E, Martin C, et al. Is a low transfusion safe in critically ill patients with cardiovascular disease? *Crit Care Med* 2001;29:227–234.

ESOPHAGEAL EMERGENCIES
PERCIVAL BUENAVENTURA AND
JAMES D. LUKETICH

$\mathcal{E}$sophageal emergencies can be classified into perforation and obstruction. These emergencies require a high index of suspicion to diagnose quickly and treat appropriately. Delayed treatment carries a high rate of morbidity and mortality. The aim of this chapter is to provide practical guidelines for the diagnosis and management of esophageal emergencies.

I. PERFORATION: CLINICAL PRESENTATION

  A. Perforation of the esophagus is seen in many clinical scenarios. **Boerhaave's syndrome** is a frequently encountered syndrome of postemetic esophageal perforation. This may occur in previously normal patients. The pathophysiology involves a violent episode of vomiting or retching that results in a rapid increase in intraluminal pressure within the esophagus. Most commonly, the perforation is seen in the distal or lower third of the esophagus.

  B. Perforation of the esophagus is seen not infrequently in the setting of upper endoscopy. This can be seen in both normal patients and in patients with esophageal pathology.

  1. Typically, when encountered in the normal patient, perforation occurs in the cervical esophagus. This is a result of failure to navigate the cricopharyngeus muscle that guards the upper portion of the esophagus. Aggressive blind passage through this region of the esophagus can result in passage of the endoscope to the pyriform sinus. If the endoscope is forcibly advanced in the pyriform sinus, perforation of the pyriform sinus will ensue.

  2. Perforation can occur in patients with esophageal pathology during upper endoscopy.

  a. In patients with **Zenker's diverticulum**, failure to negotiate past the hypertensive cricopharyngeus can lead to perforation of the pyriform sinus, as described previously. Additionally, inadvertent forcible passage of the scope within the Zenker's diverticulum can lead to perforation of the diverticulum itself.

  b. Perforation can be seen during endoscopy for **obstructing malignancy**. Perforation can occur proximal to the obstruction or within the obstructing lesion itself.

  3. Rarely, perforation can occur with **endoscopic interventional procedures**. Patients with achalasia who are being treated with distal esophageal dilation or botulinum injection can suffer from distal esophageal perforation. Perforation can be seen in the setting of laser therapy, sclerotherapy, and photodynamic therapy. Attempts at retrieval of foreign objects within the esophagus can lead to perforation of the esophagus, particularly with the aggressive use of a rigid esophagoscope. In addition, the foreign object itself may perforate the esophagus.

  C. Perforation of the esophagus can be seen **perioperatively**. Manipulation and instrumentation of the esophagus, particularly in procedures such as fundoplication and Heller myotomy, may result in delayed presentation of esophageal perforation.

  D. Perforation can occur with **ingestion of caustic materials**. The esophagus is particularly susceptible to ingestion of alkali but relatively immune to ingestion of acidic material. Lye ingestion is commonly seen in clinical practice. Ingestion of lye can lead to both acute and subacute full-thickness necrosis and subsequent perforation of the entire length of the esophagus. Those who survive the acute event are at risk for recalcitrant stricture. In addition, there is increased risk of malignancy in the future.

E. Infrequently, perforation of the esophagus can occur in the setting of **esophageal malignancy**. Tumor necrosis can extend to the full thickness of the esophageal wall. This can be seen spontaneously or after treatment of the esophageal malignancy. This is a particular concern after photodynamic therapy ablation of obstructing esophageal malignancy.

F. Perforation of the esophagus can occur in the setting of both **penetrating and blunt trauma**. The entire length of the esophagus can be injured depending on the path of the offending agent. The cervical esophagus is particularly prone to injuries sustained either from knife or gunshot wounds in the neck because of its readily accessible and unprotected location. Esophageal perforation secondary to blunt trauma associated with motor vehicle accidents is less common.

II. PERFORATION: MANAGEMENT

A. The diagnosis of esophageal perforation begins with a **history and physical exam**. The patient's history may suggest perforation as described. Clinically, the patients may present with neck, chest, or abdominal pain. They may present with an acute abdomen. They may be moribund. The physical exam may reveal neck or upper body crepitus secondary to subcutaneous emphysema. The patients may be hemodynamically unstable secondary to associated mediastinitis or frank peritonitis.

B. A **baseline electrocardiogram, complete blood count with differential, coagulation profile, and electrolyte assay** should be obtained. In addition, a type and screen may be obtained if time permits in preparation for surgery.

C. A **chest radiograph** is the first radiographic exam to be performed. This may reveal an associated pleural effusion, hydropneumothorax, or pneumoperitoneum.

  1. **CT scan** of the chest and abdomen should be obtained with oral contrast when possible. This may reveal pneumomediastinum, pneumoperitoneum, and extraluminal contrast.

  2. This should be followed by an **esophagogram** with water-soluble contrast followed by thin dilute barium to identify the location of the perforation. In addition, the contrast esophagogram may demonstrate whether the leak is contained or drains spontaneously from the lumen of the esophagus. Special care should be taken when an associated obstruction is suspected to prevent aspiration of the water-soluble contrast. Aspiration of water-soluble contrast may lead to severe chemical pneumonitis and can further complicate the care of the patient.

  3. **Endoscopy** should be performed to identify the extent of the injury as well as assess viability of the esophagus. This can be done on the table at the time of planned surgery. However, in patients with contained leaks who are stable and are to be managed nonoperatively, endoscopy should be avoided for fear of worsening the perforation. Insufflation during endoscopy may blow out a contained leak and necessitate surgery.

D. **Surgical management** begins with resuscitative measures. Broad-spectrum antibiotics should be started with the aim of covering for enteric organisms and anaerobes. Fluid resuscitation with wide-bore intravenous (IV) lines is mandatory. Foley insertion should be performed to assess the adequacy of resuscitation.

  1. In a patient who is hemodynamically stable, the radiographic studies outlined previously should be performed (CXR, CT scan, contrast esophagogram).

  2. If the leak is contained, drains spontaneously in the esophagus, and is associated with a mildly elevated white blood cell count, nonoperative management consisting of IV fluids and antibiotics may be sufficient. These patients should be NPO (nothing by mouth). A repeat contrast esophagogram should be

considered in a week if the patient remains stable. If the esophagogram shows improvement, then liquids by mouth may be started. If the patient deteriorates during nonoperative management, surgery is warranted.

3. Surgery for esophageal perforation can be classified into **four broad categories: repair, resection, diversion, and wide drainage**. Regardless of the type of surgical intervention, upper endoscopy is done at the time of surgery to assess mucosal viability and to assess the integrity of the repair.

  a. If the patient is hemodynamically stable, attempt at primary repair should be performed regardless of time of presentation. Nonviable and necrotic tissue should be debrided. A two-layer repair (mucosa to mucosa and muscle to muscle) over a 42 F bougie or a gastroscope is recommended. It is potentially helpful to buttress the repair with soft tissue such as intercostal muscle or pericardium. Drains should be placed in the proximity of the repair. If the esophageal tissue is marginal, repair over a T-tube (size 14 F) can be done in addition to placement of periesophageal drains.

    i. Perforation in the setting of dilation or botulinum injection for achalasia may be repaired primarily. Typically, the perforation occurs at the site of or just above the hypertensive lower esophageal sphincter. A Heller myotomy needs to be performed 180 degrees away from the site of perforation. The myotomy needs to be at least 6 cm in length and extend to the very proximal gastric cardia. Additionally, a partial fundoplication (Toupet or Dor fundoplication) should be performed in conjunction with the repair and myotomy.

  b. In patients with esophageal malignancy, end-stage achalasia, or caustic injury with esophageal necrosis, esophagectomy should be done as long as the patient is hemodynamically stable. Drainage of the mediastinum with large-bore chest tubes or soft drains (e.g., Jackson-Pratt drain) is needed if there is extensive soilage.

  c. Diversion can be considered in a few patients in whom repair or resection is not possible either because of anatomic considerations (e.g., locally unresectable esophageal cancer) or in patients who are potentially resectable but have become unstable. In addition, as with caustic injuries, the final proximal and distal extent of the necrotic injury may not be readily apparent. In particular, this is an issue when there is necrosis of the stomach that may need to utilized as the conduit for reconstruction. Diversion can be accomplished with a lateral cervical esophagostomy. However, it is preferable to dissect the proximal esophagus and bring an end stoma of esophagus out below the clavicle. This allows for easier management of the stoma appliance. In addition, it allows for a longer length of proximal esophagus for potential future reconstruction. A gastrostomy should be placed. Wide drainage with large-bore tubes should be placed at the site of perforation.

  d. In a patient who is in extremis, emergent operation is required. However, this patient may not tolerate a prolonged procedure. In this patient, wide debridement and drainage may be the only option. This maneuver may allow for the patient to become stable enough to undergo repair or resection at a later date. A nasogastric tube should be placed with the tip in the distal esophagus to allow for drainage of saliva within the esophagus. A gastrostomy tube should be placed to prevent reflux of gastric contents.

    i. Debridement and drainage is appropriate and sufficient for perforations of the cervical esophagus. In these patients, one should be concerned about extension of soilage from the cervical area into the mediastinum. Drainage of the mediastinum in these cases can be accomplished through the cervical incision. Rarely, video-assisted thoracoscopy or even thoracotomy may be necessary to fully drain the superior mediastinum. Figure 61-1 describes an algorithm for the management of esophageal perforation.

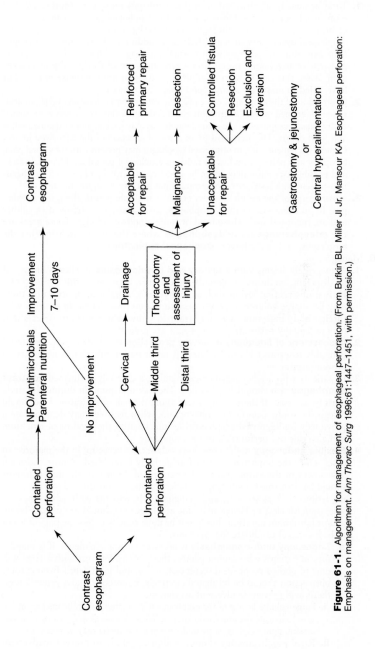

Figure 61-1. Algorithm for management of esophageal perforation. (From Bufkin BL, Miller JI Jr, Mansour KA. Esophageal perforation: Emphasis on management. *Ann Thorac Surg* 1996;61:1447–1451, with permission.)

III. OBSTRUCTION

A. Presentation

  1. Total or near total obstruction of the esophagus represents another class of esophageal emergencies. Obstruction of the esophagus can occur in the setting of primary esophageal pathology such as malignancy, benign strictures, and esophageal dysmotility such as achalasia. In addition, obstruction of the esophagus can occur in patients with normal esophagus. This can be seen in the pediatric or psychiatric population where ingestion of foreign objects is common. Also, this can be seen in adult patients who are otherwise normal but have failed to masticate a large food bolus (e.g., meat).

  2. Obstruction of the esophagus can cause respiratory compromise secondary to aspiration of retained saliva. Obstruction associated with a chronic process is associated with a dilated esophagus. The dilated esophagus may have a pool of retained saliva and food debris. This may lead to an acute obstruction of the narrowed lumen. Clinically, a patient with an obstructed esophagus may present with substernal pain, especially in a patient who has no previous esophageal pathology. Hypersalivation and possible aspiration may occur. In severe cases, a totally obstructed esophagus may present with respiratory compromise and inability to protect the airway.

  3. Obstruction of the esophagus can occur at multiple points along the esophagus. In an otherwise normal esophagus, three areas are narrowed in caliber and are the usual sites where food or foreign body can lodge. These areas are the **cricopharyngeus, midesophagus** where the aortic arch indents the esophagus, and at the **lower esophageal sphincter**.

B. Management

  1. Management begins with a **history and physical exam** to elicit a history of predisposing conditions as described previously. In patients with a history of a known obstructing lesion such as malignancy, achalasia, or stricture, there may be a large volume of pooled secretions and food debris. In patients with foreign body ingestion, it is important to know whether sharp objects that may potentially perforate the esophagus are present.

  2. **Assessment of adequacy of airway protection** is mandatory. If the patient is unable to protect his or her airway, immediate intubation is necessary to prevent aspiration.

  3. In patients who are hemodynamically stable, a carefully performed **contrast esophagogram** should be obtained. The risk of aspiration during the study must be assessed. If there is any doubt about the risk of aspiration, one should forego the study. Contrast esophagogram, when feasible, may demonstrate a previously undiagnosed esophageal lesion, identify the level of obstruction, and also rule out perforation of the esophagus.

  4. **Flexible endoscopy** under conscious sedation is successful in the majority of cases. Once the impacted food or foreign body is retrieved, a more thorough assessment of the esophagus can be performed. Biopsy of suspicious lesions should be performed. Endoscopic dilation can be performed to dilate obstructing lesions such as stricture and malignancy. In patients with achalasia, consideration for elective Heller myotomy at a later time should be made. Dilation and/or botulinum injection should not be done acutely unless the patient is not to be a surgical candidate for myotomy.

  a. **Endoscopy under anesthesia** is necessary in some patients. It is mandatory in patients who cannot protect their airway. Patients with a large volume of pooled esophageal secretions, saliva, and food debris from chronic obstruction should be intubated electively. Endoscopy under general anesthesia will prevent inadvertent aspiration.

  i. Large-volume lavage of the esophagus with a large-bore tube may be necessary to irrigate the impacted material. When flexible esophagocopy is unsuccessful, rigid esophagocopy under general anesthesia may be necessary.

  ii. Rigid esophagoscopy should be done carefully to prevent inadvertent perforation.

STOMACH, DUODENUM, SMALL INTESTINE, APPENDIX, AND COLON

RAGHUVEER VALLABHANENI, MICHAEL STANG, AND JOSE PRINCE

62

*T*his chapter reviews diseases of the stomach, duodenum, small bowel, appendix, and colon. The focus of the chapter is on diseases that cause inflammation or perforation of the gastrointestinal tract, often requiring operative intervention. A key principle is that **one must promptly recognize the patient who requires laparotomy**, rather than expending time and effort on diagnosis of the specific pathology in this patient.

I. PEPTIC ULCER DISEASE (PUD)

- **A. General.** Peptic ulcers represent either acute or chronic pathologic focal defects in the gastric and/or duodenal mucosa. Complications from this disease process result from the erosion into the surrounding deeper layers of the submucosa and muscularis propia with violation of surrounding vascular structures (hemorrhage) or full-thickness intestinal wall damage (viscus perforation). The concurrent inflammatory process leads to significant scarring and potential compromise of the intestinal lumen (obstruction).

- **B. Incidence.**
  1. Peptic ulcers continue to be a common outpatient diagnosis; however, over the past two decades the treatment has changed dramatically and the need for elective surgical management has decreased steadily.
  2. The estimated incidence of PUD is between 1,500 and 3,000 cases per 100,000 people per year. The overall prevalence of PUD in the United States is about 2%, with a current lifetime risk of 10%.
  3. Despite the advances in medical therapy and increased understanding of the pathogenesis of PUD, emergent surgery for complications of PUD has remained steady.
  4. During the natural course of their disease, peptic ulcer patients carry a lifetime risk of hemorrhage (15%–20%), perforation (5%), and obstruction (2%) if left untreated.

- **C. Risk factors.**
  1. *Helicobacter pylori* **infection in the upper gastrointestinal tract.** *H. Pylori* infection is associated with more than 90% of duodenal ulcers and 75% of gastric ulcers. As much as 50% of the adult population in the United States has *H. pylori*. However, only 15% to 20% of those patients colonized will develop PUD in their lifetime.
  2. **Nonsteroidal antiinflammatory drugs (NSAIDs).** The intake of nonsteroidal antiinflammatory medications is associated with approximately 15% to 20% of peptic ulcers. Complications of PUD are more common in patients taking NSAIDs.
  3. Physiologic stressors including trauma, shock, severe head injuries, sepsis, and surgery.
  4. Uremia.
  5. Cigarette smoking. People who smoke are twice as likely to develop PUD compared with nonsmokers.
  6. Zollinger-Ellison syndrome.

649

D. Pathogenesis/Etiology

1. Peptic ulcers are caused by an imbalance in either the action of peptic acid or a compromise of the mucosal defense mechanisms or both.
2. *H. Pylori* infection plays a major role in the weakening of mucosal defenses and subsequent ulcer development. Further, the inflammation and local alkalinization that accompanies *H. Pylori* infection decreases antral somatostatin secretion (antral D-cells) and disrupts the inhibitory control of gastrin release (antral G-cells). The result is a hypergastrinemic state promoting parietal cell hypertrophy and hypersecretion of gastric acid.
3. NSAID use is believed to compromise normal mucosal defense mechanisms.
4. Duodenal ulcerations are most commonly found in the first portion of the duodenum and are associated with acid hypersecretion.
5. Gastric ulcerations may or may not be associated with peptic acid hypersecretion and are classified further based on their anatomical features.
   a. Type 1 gastric ulcer (most common) is typically located near the incisura on the lesser curvature and is associated with normal or decreased acid secretion.
   b. Type 2 gastric ulcer is stomach body ulceration in combination with a duodenal ulcer and is associated with acid hypersecretion.
   c. Type 3 gastric ulcer is prepyloric and associated with increased acid secretion.
   d. Type 4 gastric ulcer occurs at the gastroesophageal junction and acid secretion is normal or below normal.

E. Clinical manifestations

1. Epigastric pain is a cardinal feature of PUD for >90% of patients and is typically described as a burning, stabbing, or gnawing discomfort. Ingestion of food or antacids may temporarily alleviate symptoms for those with duodenal ulcers and may exacerbate symptoms for those with gastric ulceration.
2. Other clinical history findings may include nausea, vomiting, and anorexia.
3. Significant upper GI bleeding from peptic ulcer can present with hematemesis (coffee ground emesis), melena, guaiac positive stools, or symptoms of hypotension secondary to hemorrhage (syncope).
4. Perforated peptic ulcers typically present with a sudden onset of severe abdominal pain and findings of generalized peritonitis on exam. Patients may also exhibit fever, tachycardia, and leukocytosis.

F. Diagnostic modalities

1. Early endoscopic evaluation with diagnostic and therapeutic intent is necessary in acute upper gastrointestinal bleeding.
2. In suspected perforation with obvious clinical signs of peritonitis, upright or left lateral decubitus abdominal plain films can be obtained to assess for the presence of free air in the abdomen (about 80%–85% of cases). In those patients with less dramatic presentations, abdominal CT may be warranted.
3. In nonemergent presentations of PUD, esophagogastroduodenoscopy (EGD) is the preferred diagnostic method allowing for both visualization of the ulcer disease and biopsy (*H. Pylori* can be confirmed on biopsy). Alternatively (with less sensitivity), upper gastrointestinal contrast radiograph may demonstrate retention of contrast in the ulcer.

G. Operative indications

1. Surgery for PUD is largely restricted to the treatment of life-threatening complications.
2. Evidence of perforation with signs of peritonitis on exam and free air on plain abdominal x-ray necessitate emergent surgical exploration.
3. About 80% of patients who present with bleeding from peptic ulceration stop bleeding without surgical or medical intervention. Endoscopic hemostasis can control the bleeding in 85% to 95% of patients who do not resolve spontaneously.
   a. About 1% to 2% of patients continue to bleed despite endoscopic hemostatic attempts and require early, emergent surgery (primary emergent surgery).

    b. Between 15% and 20% of ulcers rebleed after successful endoscopic treatment and also warrant surgical intervention (secondary emergent surgery). Patients with repeated episodes of bleeding and ongoing transfusion requirement of more than 4 to 6 units over 24 hours require surgery.

  4. Early elective surgery following initial endoscopic hemostasis within 48 hours should be performed for those patients with significant risk factors for rebleeding:

    a. Patients who present with shock and acute anemia

    b. Coagulopathy

    c. Patients hospitalized for other significant comorbidities

    d. Active bleeding at endoscopy or a visible vessel in base of ulcer

  5. Obstruction (Section II)

H. Treatment

  1. The goal of surgical treatment of PUD is to decrease acid production; this is accomplished through disruption of the nerve supply to the parietal cell mass of the stomach. In the case of complete truncal vagotomy, antropyloric dysfunction restricts gastric emptying and necessitates a concomitant drainage procedure (pyloromyotomy or pyloroplasty) or gastrectomy. The majority of peptic ulcers are adequately treated by one of three operations: highly selective vagotomy (HSV), truncal vagotomy and drainage procedure (V + D), or vagotomy and antrectomy/distal gastrectomy (V + A).

  2. Following antrectomy or distal gastrectomy, intestinal continuity can be reestablished with either a Billroth I gastroduodenostomy or a Billroth II loop gastrojejunostomy.

  3. Perforation

    a. Duodenal perforations are surgically managed with debridement and simple closure +/− omental patch oversewing (Graham patch). Omental patching alone may be necessary if significant duodenal fibrosis prohibits a tension free closure. Surgery should be followed by *H. pylori* eradication. A definitive ulcer operation (HSV or V + D) should be performed in stable patients that are known to be *H. pylori* negative or have failed previous medical therapy.

    b. Gastric perforation is treated with wedge resection/ulcer excision followed by acid-reducing surgery (HSV or V + D) for Type 2 and 3 gastric ulcers. Histologic investigation of the ulcer site is essential because gastric cancer may present as perforated gastric ulcer.

  4. Hemorrhage (Chapter 60)

    a. Initial management for hemorrhage secondary to peptic ulcer should include aggressive resuscitation, transfusion, and correction of any underlying coagulopathy.

    b. Duodenal peptic ulcer bleeding is approached through a duodenotomy followed by direct vessel suture ligation. In the case of large posterior ulcers, extraduodenal ligation of the gastroduodenal artery is obligatory. Proximity of the ulcer to the pylorus or the size of the ulcer (>2 cm) may necessitate a pyloroplasty or gastric resection (antrectomy). Addition of an acid-reducing procedure (preferably V + D) can be considered in those patients who are stable and have failed previous medical therapy. However, with the current availability of potent anti-secretory medications most patients will not require this.

    c. Gastric peptic ulcer bleeding is treated if possible with wedge resection/ulcer excision (for histologic exclusion of cancer) followed by V + D for Type 2 and 3 gastric ulcers. Distal gastrectomy in stable patients. If a large penetrating ulcer is found

      i. Same options as duodenal except all gastric ulcers should be sufficiently biopsied

      ii. If possible, should consider wedge resection +/− vagotomy + drainage

      iii. Distal gastrectomy

I. Obstruction (Section II)

J. *H. pylori* **eradication** is best attempted with a triple combination of a proton pump inhibitor (PPI) plus clarithromycin and amoxicillin/metronidazole or a quadruple regimen of PPI, bismuth, metronidazole, and tetracycline.

K. **Discontinuation** of NSAIDs (or addition of antisecretory medications including H_2 blockers or PPI if antacid surgery is not performed).

L. **Outcomes**
   1. Emergency operations for bleeding peptic ulcers carry a mortality risk as high as 25% to 30% with age >70 years, significant medical comorbidities, and evidence of shock on presentation being the most significant predictors.
   2. Emergent operations for peptic ulcer perforation carry a mortality risk of 6% to 30%. Risk factors for increased mortality include evidence of shock on admission, renal failure, delayed laparotomy >12 hours, concurrent medical illness, age, liver cirrhosis, and an immunocompromised state.
   3. Overall, complications from gastric ulceration carry a higher mortality rate when compared to duodenal ulcers because of the increased prevalence of gastric ulcers in the elderly population and the ubiquitous use of NSAIDs in this population.
   4. Successful eradication of *H. pylori* infection fundamentally changes the natural history of ulcer disease and nearly eliminates recurrence.
   5. Ulcer recurrence rate after antisecretory surgery is comparable between HSV and V + D (5%–15%) and superior with V + A (<2%). However, V + A does carry a higher risk of mortality if attempted in moribund patients.

M. **Complications**
   1. After gastric operations are performed for PUD, a variety of abnormalities may affect some patients due to the disturbance of normal physiologic mechanisms that control gastric function. Dumping syndrome occurs in 5% to 10% of patients after pyloroplasty or distal gastrectomy. Clinically significant diarrhea occurs in 5% to 10% of patients after truncal vagotomy. Other complications include gastric stasis, bile reflux gastritis, marginal ulceration, cholelithiasis, weight loss, anemia, and osteopenia.
   2. Performing a complete truncal vagotomy carries a risk of esophageal perforation.

II. GASTRIC OUTLET OBSTRUCTION

A. **General.** Gastric obstruction results from the fibrotic narrowing of the pyloric channel, mechanical twisting of the stomach, or impaction of undigestible matter or objects. However, a malignant process should always be considered and excluded as a potential cause, especially in older patients.

B. **Incidence**
   1. Gastric outlet obstruction secondary to PUD represents about 5% of ulcer-related complications with operations for obstruction totaling about 2,000 per year in the United States.
   2. The incidence of malignancy in patients presenting with gastric outlet obstruction is >50%.
   3. Obstruction from gastric volvulus, bezoars, and foreign objects is uncommon.

C. **Risk factors**
   1. Chronic PUD or other inflammatory processes of the upper GI tract. The risk of gastric cancer is increased in those patients that have a family history, a diet high in nitrates, history of gastric adenomas, hereditary nonpolyposis colorectal cancer (HNPCC), *H. pylori*, tobacco use, and a >10 year history of gastrectomy or gastrojejunosotomy.
   2. Large paraesophageal hiatal hernia or diaphragmatic defect from other cause (congenital or traumatic) may lead to gastric volvulus. The majority (80%) of cases of gastric volvulus occur in adults with peak incidence in the fifth decade of life. The remaining 20% occur in infants under 1 year of age.
   3. Bezoars are typically associated with gastroparesis, a history of previous gastric surgery, or patients with a propensity for ingesting hair (trichophagia).

D. **Etiology**
   1. The chronic inflammation associated with PUD may lead to pyloric channel stenosis. This promotes gastric stasis and increased gastric pH resulting in

pronounced gastrin release and excess acid production. The resulting acute inflammation compounds preexisting chronic fibrosis and leads to outlet obstruction. Other less common inflammatory causes of outlet obstruction include Crohn's disease, pancreatitis, cholecystitis, corrosive stricture, sarcoidosis, tuberculosis, and amyloidosis.

2. Malignant processes that may result in gastric obstruction include gastric adenocarcinoma, pancreatic adenocarcinoma, and lymphoma.

3. Mechanical obstruction from gastric volvulus. Twisting of the stomach usually occurs in association with a large hiatal or paraesophageal hernia. Organoaxial volvulus is an anterior and superior rotation of the greater curvature over the long axis of the stomach. Mesenteroaxial volvulus is the rotation of a very lax and floppy distal stomach and duodenum over the shorter transverse axis of the stomach and occurs in one third of all cases of gastric volvulus. This is more common secondary to ligamentous laxity around the crura.

4. Bezoars are concretions of undigestible materials that accumulate in the stomach. Phytobezoars are composed of vegetable matter (classically citrus fruits and persimmons) and are associated with altered gastric emptying. Trichobezoars consist of a mass of ingested hair and other fibers. Other less common causes include medications (pharmacobezoar) and chemical ingestion (shellac).

E. Clinical manifestations

1. Patients typically present with nonbilious vomiting or regurgitation of nondigested food and have significant pain or discomfort.

2. Hypochloremic alkalosis.

3. If the condition is long-standing, the patient may have experienced significant weight loss.

4. Volvulus may present with sudden, severe pain in the upper abdomen or lower chest with radiation to the back and shoulders, and is accompanied by nonproductive retching. Pressure on the adjacent thoracic organs may result in dyspnea, palpitations, or dysphagia. Chest film reveals a gas-filled viscus in the lower chest and a nasogatric tube may be difficult or impossible to pass. Gastric infarction results in a moribund state.

5. Large bezoars may elicit sensations of epigastric fullness and early satiety.

F. Diagnostic modalities

1. The etiology of the gastric outlet obstruction is best confirmed by endoscopy. Generous biopsies should be performed to exclude malignancy. The sensitivity of endoscopic biopsies in the setting of gastric obstruction is poor (<40%). Thus, a benign pathologic report does not eliminate the possibility of cancer.

2. The diagnosis of volvulus is made on clinical findings and confirmed by plain chest x-ray; however, if the diagnosis is unclear an upper GI contrast study is diagnostic.

G. Operative indications

1. Obstruction due to complicated PUD may respond to conservative management (nasogastric suction, NPO, gastric acid suppression, and IV resuscitation) for 3 to 5 days. However, most patients will ultimately require a definitive surgical procedure.

2. Gastric obstruction from malignant tumors requires operative resection or gastric bypass for palliation.

3. Obstruction from volvulus carries a risk of strangulation; thus, prompt surgical intervention is invariably necessary. Trichobezoars should be managed surgically. Phytobezoars are usually amenable to endoscopic fragmentation and removal.

H. Treatment

1. Initial management includes aggressive correction of volume and electrolyte abnormalities.

2. Nonoperative management of obstructing PUD with endoscopic pneumatic dilation may be utilized to temporarily alleviate symptoms and allow for an elective surgical procedure in poor surgical candidates.

3. Obstruction secondary to peptic ulcer is treated with HSV + gastrojejunostomy, V + A, or distal gastrectomy and gastrojejunostomy reconstruction after at least 72 hours of nasogastric decompression (to minimize gastric atony). In cases of significantly dilated, atonic gastrum, subtotal gastrectomy with Roux-en-Y reconstruction is necessary.
4. Surgical resection (preferably 5-cm margin) and lymphadenectomy is optimal for palliation and potential cure for gastric adenocarcinoma. Reconstruction is determined by the location of the lesion and degree of gastric resection that is needed. Obstructing pancreatic cancer may be palliated with loop gastrojejunostomy.
5. Gastric volvulus is a surgical emergency. Initial decompression with a nasogastric tube should be attempted along with aggressive resuscitation. The volvulized organ is reduced via an open or laparoscopic approach and appropriate gastric resection (partial or subtotal) performed if necrosis is present. Closure and repair of diaphragmatic defects with or without gastropexy should be attempted to prevent recurrence.
6. Uncomplicated phytobezoar can usually be managed medically with repeated doses of cellulase (or less commonly papain and acetylcysteine). Persistent phytobezoar can be managed with endoscopic fragmentation and removal. Trichobezoars and obstructing phytobezoars are surgically removed through a gastrotomy.

I. Outcomes
1. Long-term results of endoscopic dilation for obstructing PUD are poor. Short-term alleviation of symptoms is attained in 83% to 100% of patients. However, only a third of patients have lasting improvement (>3 months). Surgery for gastric outlet obstruction secondary to peptic ulcer is associated with a mortality of 5%.
2. Mortality for gastric volvulus may be as high as 30% to 50%. Thus, early recognition and prompt surgical correction of gastric volvulus is essential.

J. Complications
1. Sequelae of gastric resection. (Section I.M)
2. Gastric volvulus may result in ulceration, perforation, hemorrhage, pancreatic necrosis, and omental avulsion. Rarely, the rotation of the stomach may also disrupt the splenic vasculature and result in hemorrhage or splenic rupture.

III. DIVERTICULAR DISEASE
A. General. Diverticula may occur anywhere in the gastrointestinal tract. It is either described as being acquired as in the small bowel or colon or congenital as in Meckel's diverticulum. Congenital diverticula tend to be true diverticula in that they incorporate all layers of the intestine, whereas acquired diverticula tend to be considered "false" diverticula in that they only contain mucosa and submucosa.
B. Duodenal diverticula.
1. Incidence
   a. Duodenal diverticula are a relatively common entity with a prevalence measured by autopsy reports of about 9% of the population.
   b. They are most commonly found between the sixth and eighth decades of life.
   c. Approximately 75% of duodenal diverticula are periampullary and located within 2 cm of the ampulla. This concentration may be secondary to there being less dense muscle layers in that area.
2. Etiology. The exact pathophysiology of duodenal diverticula remains unclear; however, it appears that they occur secondary to a combination of:
   a. Disordered duodenal motility.
   b. Advancing age.
   c. Weakness of duodenal musculature.
   d. Congenital defects all contribute to their origin.
   e. Traction diverticula may occur near the first part of the duodenum secondary to scarring from PUD.

3. Clinical manifestations

    a. Duodenal diverticula are usually asymptomatic and not treated. The symptoms that can occur may be secondary to compression of the pancreaticobiliary tree such as jaundice or pancreatitis.

    b. There has been a slight association made between periampullary duodenal diverticula, bacterobilia, as well as primary and recurrent common bile duct stones.

    c. Patients may also present with upper or lower GI bleeding from the diverticula, anemia, signs of diverticulitis, perforation, or ulceration.

4. Diagnostic modalities

    a. Upper endoscopy may be used to evaluate the cause of bleeding in upper GI tract and may help treat bleeding as well.

    b. Endoscopic retrograde cholangiopancreatography (ERCP) can evaluate the biliopancreatic tree as well as help relieve jaundice.

    c. Upper GI barium meal examination.

    d. Incidental findings on CT scan may also be present.

5. Operative indications

    a. Asymptomatic patients should not be treated.

    b. Massive hemorrhage unable to be controlled by endoscopy.

    c. Perforation.

6. Treatment

    a. Patients with evidence of upper or brisk lower GI bleeding should have an upper endoscopy. Endoscopic management should be attempted whenever possible because of the difficulty in gaining intraoperative access to the region as well as the high morbidity rates associated with the procedure.

    b. Operative intervention should be utilized when unable to stop bleeding with endoscopy or if perforation is present. A wide Kocher maneuver is utilized to gain access to the second part of the duodenum and a diverticulectomy can be performed with a transverse two layer closure.

    c. Hemorrhage may also be controlled by performing a lateral duodenotomy and oversewing the vessel.

    d. Diverticulectomy is generally not recommended in patients presenting with pancreaticobiliary symptoms.

C. Jejunoileal diverticula.

    1. Incidence. These small-bowel diverticula (excluding Meckel's diverticulum) are acquired diverticula and have a prevalence of 1% to 5%.

    2. Epidemiology and etiology

        a. Diverticula may occur anywhere in the small bowel and occur with decreasing frequency from the ligament of Treitz to the ileocecal valve

        b. They tend to occur on the mesenteric side of the bowel at areas of weakness in the muscular layer.

    3. Clinical manifestations

        a. Five percent to 10% of patients with diverticula will experience symptoms.

        b. Nonspecific symptoms include intermittent crampy abdominal pain, flatulence, diarrhea, and constipation. However, no clear link between these symptoms and associated diverticula have been established. These symptoms may occur because of obstruction, diverticulitis, hemorrhage, perforation, or malabsorption.

    4. Diagnosis

        a. Jejunoileal diverticula are diagnosed most often as an incidental finding on ultrasound, GI series, or computerized tomography (CT).

        b. The most sensitive test for detection is enteroclysis.

        c. Endoscopy is technically limited past the ligament of Treitz. It is difficult to diagnose distal lesions.

        d. Wireless endoscopy may be utilized to visualize diverticula or when dealing with obscure sources of bleeding.

    5. Operative indications

        a. In asymptomatic patients, treatment is not indicated.

  b. Perforation.
  c. Uncontrolled hemorrhage if localized.
  d. Diverticulitis.
  6. Treatment. In cases of hemorrhage, diverticulitis, or perforation, segmental intestinal resection with primary anastomosis is performed.

D. Meckel's diverticulum.

  1. Incidence
  a. Meckel's diverticulum is the most prevalent congenital anomaly of the gastrointestinal tract affecting approximately 2% of the population.
  b. They are typically located within 100 cm proximal to the ileocecal valve.

  2. Pathogenesis/etiology
  a. Meckel's diverticulum occurs secondary to failure of the omphalomesenteric (vitelline) duct to obliterate during development.
  b. This duct is present during embryological development to connect the midgut of the embryo and the yolk sac. The duct has its own mesentery as well as blood supply.
  c. Most Meckel's diverticula have heterotopic mucosa, most often gastric followed by pancreatic.
  d. The "rule of two" is said to govern Meckel's diverticulum
    i. Affects 2% of the population.
    ii. Occurs approximately 2 feet proximal to the ileocecal valve.
    iii. Affects males twice as often as females.
    iv. The diverticulum is usually 2 inches long.
    v. Approximately 2% of patients develop symptoms.

  3. Clinical manifestations. Patients may present with symptoms of:
  a. Bleeding may occur from ileal ulceration because of excess acid secretion from heterotopic gastric mucosa in the diverticulum.
  b. Obstruction may occur from many reasons including intussusception with the diverticulum acting as a lead point, volvulus around the fibrous band attaching the diverticulum to the umbilicus, stricture secondary to chronic diverticulitis, or entrapment of intestine by mesodiverticular band.
  c. Diverticultis may also occur and may be difficult to distinguish from appendicitis.

  4. Diagnostic modalities
  a. Preoperative diagnosis may be made in patient's that are bleeding by utilizing a ^{99}technetium-pertechnate scan. This will identify heterotopic gastric mucosa.
  b. Patients presenting with obstruction or diverticulitis are typically diagnosed with Meckel's diverticulum intraoperatively.
  c. CT scan may also be used to denote mesenteric inflammation, volvulus, or evidence of obstruction

  5. Operative indications
  a. Incidental Meckel's diverticulum should be resected in children <18 years old or evidence of presence of heterotopic mucosa, narrow base of diverticulum, or presence of a mesodiverticular band.
  b. Bleeding.
  c. Perforation.

  6. Treatment
  a. Intraoperative treatment options include wedge resection of diverticulum or, if there is significant induration and inflammation, segmental intestinal resection with primary anastomosis.
  b. Appendectomy should also be performed at time of operation.

E. Colonic diverticular disease.

  1. Incidence
  a. Colonic diverticula occur predominantly in the sigmoid areas in residents of Western countries.
  b. They tend to occur as people get older and two thirds of adults over 85 have diverticulosis.

    c. Approximately 10% to 25% of patients with diverticulitis will have symptoms or complications of their diverticular disease.

2. Pathogenesis/Etiology

    a. Colonic diverticula are acquired false diverticula that tend to occur at areas of weakness where the vasa recta enter the muscularis.

    b. In Asian countries there is a congenital diverticular disease that tends to be right sided.

3. Risk factors. It is theorized that lack of fiber intake in the Western diet is associated with increasing incidence of acquired diverticular disease.

4. Clinical manifestations

    a. Diverticulosis may be **asymptomatic** and found incidentally.

    b. In patients who have **acute uncomplicated diverticulitis**, they typically present with a triad of left lower quadrant pain, fever, and leukocytosis. They may also have symptoms of nausea, vomiting, dysuria, diarrhea, and constipation.

    c. **Complicated diverticulitis** may present with the previously mentioned triad as well as diffuse abdominal tenderness and rebound tenderness. They may also present in septic shock secondary to gross contamination of the abdomen.

5. Diagnostic modalities. Colonic diverticulitis is a clinical diagnosis and does not require further studies if the patient's symptoms are relatively mild.

    a. If there is any question of the diagnosis or suspicion of complications of diverticulitis, a CT scan with IV contrast is the diagnostic test of choice. This may help determine if there is localized abscess formation in a patient not improving on antibiotics, determine the degree of inflammation, or help in an unclear diagnosis.

    b. **Barium enema or lower endoscopy should not be performed in patients with acute diverticulitis for risk of perforation and extravasation of barium.** These tests may be performed several weeks later prior to operative intervention if indicated to rule out distal obstruction and evaluate the rest of the colon prior to resection, especially in patients over the age of 40 years.

6. Operative indications

    a. Diffuse peritoneal signs on initial examination, due to nonlocalized perforation.

    b. Clinical deterioration 48 to 72 hours after medical management is instituted.

    c. Obstruction with failure of conservative management.

    d. Perforation.

    e. Complex abscess unable to be drained percutaneously.

    f. Fistula formation. Antibiotics should be implemented to help resolve inflammation prior to operating.

7. Treatment

    a. **Asymptomatic diverticulosis.** These patients do not need any operative intervention. They should be recommended to begin a high fiber diet with ingestion of >35 grams of fiber per day.

    b. **Acute uncomplicated diverticulitis.** The initial treatment in mild presentations where the patient can tolerate oral intake is broad-spectrum oral antibiotics and a liquid diet.

        i. If symptoms do not resolve after 48 hours, CT scan should be performed and patient should be admitted with IV antibiotics and bowel rest. Antibiotic treatment should be continued for 7 to 10 days with a broad-spectrum antibiotic as long as the patient continues to improve. If patients improve and are able to tolerate oral intake, they may finish a 7- to 10-day course of oral antibiotics as an outpatient.

        ii. Although most patients respond to conservative therapy with diverticulitis, approximately 15% to 30% of patients with acute diverticulitis will need surgery for failure to improve or associated complications. Free perforation with generalized peritonitis causes a high mortality (up to 35%) and should be treated emergently in the OR.

iii. Elective resection is indicated after two attacks of diverticulitis after the age of 50 years or if there is one before the age of 40 years. This is because there is a higher incidence of complications with every ensuing attack and younger patients tend to have more morbid episodes. This point remains **controversial** since recent epidemiological data suggest that several episodes of **uncomplicated** diverticulitis may be treated nonoperatively with no change in complication rates.

c. Complicated diverticulitis. Diverticulitis of the colon may be complicated by presence of abscess, fistula, obstruction, or free perforation.

  i. Abscess. Abscess may be localized secondary to a microperforation and formation of small well contained abscesses with pericolic inflammation. These patients may be treated conservatively with oral or IV antibiotics. Larger abscesses that are contained may be treated by percutaneous drainage to control sepsis and let the patient recover to undergo elective colonic resection 8 to 12 weeks following resolution of symptoms. Patients who fail conservative therapy or are unable to be drained percutaneously require operation.

  ii. Fistula. Formation of fistulas with diverticular disease most commonly involve the bladder. These fistulas occur twice as commonly in men compared to women because of the protective effect of the uterus. Colovesicular fistulas account for 50% of all diverticular-related fistula. They may present with pneumaturia, fecaluria, and recurrent urinary tract infections. Colovaginal fistulas comprise 25% of diverticular-related fistulas. These fistulas are treated by colonic segmental resection and repair of the bladder or vaginal wall, generally as delayed procedure after the acute episode has resolved.

  iii. Obstruction. Patients may present with obstruction from either narrowing of the colonic lumen during an attack or by a loop of small bowel incorporated into the inflammatory phlegmon causing obstruction. This may resolve with conservative management but should be closely monitored for potential need for operation.

  iv. Free perforation. Free perforation of colonic diverticula is a morbid complication associated with up to a 35% mortality rate. Intravenous broad-spectrum antibiotics and aggressive fluid resuscitation should be instituted immediately. The patient should then be taken directly to OR.

d. Operative management of complicated diverticulitis. The goal of the operation should be resection of the diseased bowel under most circumstances.

  i. If there is little pericolonic inflammation and minimal contamination of the peritoneal cavity without peritonitis, it may be safe in some situations to do an intraoperative colonic lavage and perform a primary anastomosis with proximal diversion.

  ii. If the patient is unstable, has peritonitis, or has significant pericolonic inflammation or large amounts of gross contamination, a Hartmann pouch should be performed with diverting colostomy and stapled blind rectal pouch.

  iii. The three-stage approach to complicated diverticulitis with proximal diversion followed by resection and primary anastomosis in three operations is no longer recommended.

IV. APPENDICITIS

A. General. Appendicitis is the most common surgical emergency in the United States. It is essential that physicians evaluating abdominal pain have a clear understanding of its presentation and differential diagnosis, and move toward early treatment to help prevent complications.

B. Incidence.

1. Approximately 250,000 people a year in the United States develop appendicitis.

2. It occurs more frequently in males (1.4:1).

TABLE 62-1	Differential Diagnosis of Acute Appendicitis

Inflammatory conditions	Gynecological conditions
Acute mesenteric adenitis	Pelvic inflammatory disease
Acute gastroenteritis	Ruptured ovarian follicle
Acute epididymitis	Ruptured ectopic pregnancy
Meckel's diverticulitis	
Crohn's disease	**Mechanical problems**
Peptic ulcer disease	Testicular torsion
Urinary tract infection	Intussusception
Yersinia infection	Ovarian torsion

3. It presents most commonly in the second and third decades of life, although it can occur at any age.

4. Appendicitis has a lifetime incidence of 7% in the United States.

C. **Etiology.** The cause of acute appendicitis is occlusion of the appendiceal lumen—90% of cases. This may be secondary to:

1. Fecalith
2. Lymphoid tissue
3. Malignancy
4. Parasites
5. Etiology unknown 90% of time

D. **Clinical manifestations.**

1. The classical presentation of appendicitis is present in approximately 50% of cases. It includes anorexia, pain originating around the umbilicus and moving to the right lower quadrant, pain followed by nausea and vomiting and peritoneal signs localizing to McBurney's point (two thirds the distance from the umbilicus to the right anterior superior iliac spine).

2. It is important to make the diagnosis of appendicitis as quickly as possible, for the rate of rupture increases significantly after the first 24 hours of symptoms.

3. However, there are many other entities that may give similar symptoms to appendicitis that must be considered in the differential (Table 62-1).

E. **Evaluation.** The history and physical exam are critical in differentiation of appendicitis from other ailments.

1. Key points from the history include:

a. **Onset of pain.** The time to presentation from initial onset of pain is important to note, for it may alter management decisions. If the symptoms have been present for more than 3 days, a CT scan is warranted to rule out possible perforation and abscess formation. Patients presenting earlier may either be admitted and followed by serial exams or taken to the OR for diagnostic laparoscopy and appendectomy or open appendectomy.

b. **Localization.** The initial pain is usually of sudden onset and is a visceral pain (vague, constant, poorly localized, not very severe) and periumbilical in location. This pain tends to progress to a pain localized in the right lower quadrant over the next several hours as the appendiceal lumen becomes increasingly distended and irritates the parietal peritoneum.

c. **Children and elderly patients.** It may be more difficult to elicit a complete history and physical exam in young children. The elderly may have a vague abdominal pain or no pain at all.

d. **Relief of pain.** This may be a worrisome sign in someone with continued abdominal pain for over 24 hours; may indicate rupture with relief of the pressure of the distended appendix on the peritoneum.

e. **Anorexia.** This is a very common symptom of acute onset appendicitis. If the patient desires to eat a large meal, the diagnosis of acute appendicitis should be reconsidered.

2. **Physical examination.** There are many factors of the physical examination that may help clarify the diagnosis of acute appendicitis.
   a. **Fever.** This is usually a low-grade fever, <38.5°C (101°F). If the fever is >39.4°C (103°F), the diagnosis of ruptured appendix should be considered.
   b. **Tenderness at McBurney's point.** May be minimal in the patient with a retrocecal appendix.
   c. **Rectal exam.** Helps identify if the appendix is inflamed and lies in the pelvis.
   d. **Psoas sign.** Performed with patient laying on left side while the examiner slowly extends the right thigh. If extension produces pain, this may suggest a retrocecal appendix.
   e. **Rovsing's sign.** Pain in the right lower quadrant when left lower quadrant is palpated. Suggests localized peritoneal process in right lower quadrant.
   f. **Obturator sign.** Performed with patient laying supine while the examiner internally rotates the patient's flexed thigh. Pain in hypogastric region suggests irritation of the obturator muscle by a low-lying pelvic appendix.

3. **Laboratory evaluation.** Because of the acute onset of appendicitis, laboratory abnormalities in patients with acute appendicitis are few.
   a. There is typically a mild leukocytosis ranging from 10,000 to 15,000/mm^3. This mild leukocytosis is usually associated with a left shift in the differential. Leukocytosis much greater than these values may be suggestive of a perforated appendix or another disease process, such as pelvic inflammatory disease.
   b. Urinalysis is also important to obtain to rule out a urinary tract infection as the cause of the symptoms. Although it is not uncommon for there to be pyuria or microscopic hematuria with inflammation from appendicitis, there typically is no bacteriuria.

F. **Imaging studies.** Should only be utilized if the history and physical do not clearly fit the picture of acute appendicitis.
   1. **Plain-film radiography.** Rarely shows a fecalith, but if it does it is suggestive of appendicitis. May be useful in evaluation of other pathology.
   2. **Sonography.** Reported sensitivity of 55% to 96% and specificity of 85% to 98%. Improved detection if ultrasonagrapher utilizes posterior flank manual compression while performing exam and in children. Disadvantages include operator dependence and difficulty in transabdominal ultrasound in obese patients. Transvaginal ultrasonagraphy may help rule out pelvic pathology in female patients with nonclassical presentation or pregnant women.
   3. **Helical computed tomagraphy (CT).** A helical CT is sensitive and specific for diagnosis of CT scan. Oral and IV contrast should be given if no contraindication, however rectal contrast has been shown to not be necessary. Should not delay treatment in someone whose history and physical clearly suggests appendicitis.
   4. **Diagnostic laparoscopy.** In times of uncertainty of the diagnosis of appendicitis, diagnostic laparoscopy may be performed. This is especially useful in women, where there may be a gynecological problem causing the symptoms. Incidental appendectomy should be performed in these patients even when it appears normal so that a recurrence of symptoms does not raise the question of appendicitis again.

G. **Operative indications.**
   1. Because of the complications and prolonged morbidity of ruptured appendicitis, prompt operative intervention when clinical judgment or diagnostic modalities suggest appendicitis should occur. Up to a 20% negative appendicitis rate may result in females. The long-term consequences of ruptured appendicitis in females includes an infertility rate as high as 40%.

2. Perforation with diffuse peritonitis and free air should also be operated on urgently.

H. Treatment. Once diagnosis of acute appendicitis is made, early operative intervention is important to prevent complications of rupture and sepsis if left untreated. Antibiotic therapy should be instituted immediately. Single-agent therapy with cefotetan, cefoxitin, or ticarcillin-clavulanic acid has been recommended by the Surgical Infection Society.

1. **Uncomplicated appendicitis.** Acute appendicitis that is uncomplicated may be approached either by laparoscopy or open technique. Technique used should be surgeon's preference and comfort level.

   a. Laparoscopy has been shown in many studies to have a slightly lower length of stay (LOS) and as well as a decreased length of return to activity; however, the cost and the length of operation may be greater. Laparoscopy may be useful as both a diagnostic and therapeutic technique in women and patients with unclear diagnoses.

   b. For an open technique, an incision is made transversely (Rockey-Davis) or obliquely (McBurney's) in the right lower quadrant at McBurney's point.

   c. In either operative approach, if appendicitis is not found, a thorough search to find missed pathology should be performed. This should extend at least 2 feet proximal from the ileocecal valve as well as examine the ovaries in women. An appendectomy is still performed to avoid later confusion.

2. **Complicated appendicitis.** Ruptured appendicitis has an incidence of 25% of the time in acute appendicitis. Patients may present with a right lower quadrant mass if they have had appendicitis for at least 5 days.

   a. If small abscesses or a phlegmon are present, conservative management with IV antibiotics and hydration may be used initially.

   b. When there is a well-localized abscess, this can typically be treated with antibiotics and percutaneous CT or ultrasound-guided drainage of the abscess. This should be followed by interval appendectomy in 6 weeks.

   c. A complex abscess may need operative drainage, and this is best approached extraperitoneally. Operative drainage of a complex abscess should involve appendectomy at time of drainage only if easily accessible.

3. **Incidental appendectomy.** Appendectomy should typically not be performed at the time of another abdominal operation. It should be performed prophylactically only if:

   a. The patient is a child about to receive chemotherapy.

   b. The patient is about to travel to a location where there is no access to medical care.

   c. The individual is unable to respond appropriately to abdominal pain

   d. The patient has Crohn's disease and has a cecum that is grossly free of disease.

V. MIDGUT VOLVULUS. Midgut volvulus, and its predisposing condition of malrotation, is seen mainly in the pediatric population, but may also be seen in adults. It can lead to abdominal catastrophe and should be dealt with in an urgent manner when present.

A. Incidence. Ninety percent of malrotation is diagnosed in children, but 10% may present in adulthood.

B. Etiology. The predisposing condition to midgut volvulus is malrotation of the abdominal contents.

1. Malrotation occurs secondary to the intestines not completing a 270-degree rotation once they return to the abdomen during Week 11 of embryological development.

2. Although 90% of cases of malrotation present in infancy, patients may remain asymptomatic into adulthood.

3. The midgut is supplied by the superior mesenteric artery (SMA). Malrotation predisposes the nonfixed small-bowel mesentery to twist around the SMA leading to compromised blood supply of the bowel.

C. Clinical presentation

1. Patients may present with vague abdominal pain, diarrhea, nausea, and vomiting since they were children or may be asymptomatic until the current episode.

2. They may have been labeled as having irritable bowel syndrome or another nonsurgical condition.

3. In the acute setting they may present with nausea, bilious vomiting, leukocytosis, and heme positive stools.

4. Diffuse tenderness of the abdomen with or without peritoneal signs may be present.

D. Diagnostic modalities

1. Abdominal radiographs may show evidence of intestinal obstruction with air fluid levels and dilated bowel.

2. If there is not a clear need for operation, a CT scan may be warranted to help with the diagnosis. A classic "whirlpool sign" is typically present with the mesentery wrapped around the SMA.

3. Upper GI series may be useful in patients with suspected malrotation, but in adults CT scan is usually initially obtained for unclear causes of abdominal pain.

4. Base deficit and lactate levels may show evidence of severe ischemia.

E. Operative indications

1. Any patient presenting with midgut volvulus is a surgical emergency and should be taken promptly to the OR.

2. Patients with malrotation who are symptomatic.

F. Treatment. The treatment of a midgut volvulus is surgical. This may be approached either laparoscopically or by laparotomy, based on the surgeon's comfort level. The bowel should be visualized to assess it for viability.

1. Untwisting of the mesentery should be performed in a counterclockwise manner.

2. Resecting necrotic bowel if present prior to untwisting the mesentery may decrease the systemic inflammatory response by limiting circulation of inflammatory mediators.

3. If no necrosis is visible, the bowel should be reduced. Untwisting of the mesentery should be performed in a counterclockwise manner. If there is a question of viability, a second-look operation should be performed.

4. Ladd's procedure should be performed with lysis of all abdominal bands, straightening of the duodenum so it enters the right lower quadrant, and widening of the small bowel mesentery and appendectomy.

5. There is no evidence that performing a cecopexy improves outcome.

VI. FOREIGN BODY INGESTION AND RETENTION

A. Ingestion of foreign bodies

1. Incidence

a. The majority of foreign body ingestions occur in children with a peak incidence between the ages of 6 and 36 months.

b. In adults, the majority of foreign body ingestions occur in those who are mentally retarded, have psychiatric disorders, are illegally smuggling drugs in ingested condoms, or are in the prison population seeking secondary gain.

c. Food bolus impaction is also a problem, especially if underlying esophageal pathology is present.

2. Clinical manifestations

a. **History**

i. In an alert older child or adult, the patient may be able to report the item that was ingested as well as the amount of time passed since ingestion.

ii. The size, shape, and sharpness of the object should be elicited if possible.

iii. Prior history of dysphagia is important, for many esophageal impactions occur at sites of underlying esophageal pathology.

   b. Physical exam
      i. Drooling, respiratory distress, substernal chest pain, or choking may be signs of esophageal impaction or compression of the tracheobronchial tree.
      ii. Subcutaneous emphysema, new-onset pleural effusion, abdominal distension, evidence of gross blood per rectum, and peritonitis are important aspects of the physical exam that may signify complications of ingestion.
3. Diagnostic modalities
   a. Radiographs give pertinent information as to the location of the object, and presence of mediastinal or intraperitoneal free air. Anteroposterior and lateral radiographs of the neck, chest, and abdomen should be performed to help identify radiopaque objects; however, they are unable to diagnose radiolucent objects such as fish bones, wood, plastic, and most glass.
   b. Contrast examinations should not be performed routinely secondary to increased risk of aspiration if foreign body impaction and obstruction are present.
   c. In a patient who has no visible object on radiography and is asymptomatic, no further treatment is necessary.
4. Operative indications
   a. Any object in oropharynx or esophagus that is not able to be removed endoscopically
   b. Any evidence of perforation or obstruction
   c. Narcotic packets that have not passed and have shown signs of rupture or obstruction
5. Treatment. The management of foreign body ingestion varies depending on the location of the foreign body at time of diagnosis as well as its type and size.
   a. Oropharynx. Objects stuck in the oropharynx should be removed expeditiously upon diagnosis using direct laryngoscopy and a McGill forceps, or upper rigid or flexible endoscopy. Bones have a tendency to get caught in the valleculae or piriform sinuses and may cause retropharyngeal abscesses or erode into the trachea or neighboring blood vessels if not treated.
   b. Esophagus
      i. Objects identified in the esophagus that have not progressed within 24 hours should be attempted to be removed endoscopically to limit risk of perforation.
      ii. Sharp objects should be retrieved upon diagnosis as well.
      iii. Food bolus impactions can be removed piecemeal using an endoscope. However, it is not encouraged to blindly push an impaction into the stomach secondary to possible pathology distal to impaction and risk of perforation.
      iv. Glucagon (1-mg IV) may also be administered to relax the esophageal sphincter and allow the bolus to pass.
      v. Foley balloons have also been utilized to retrieve objects in the esophagus safely, but care must be taken to protect the airway when bringing the foreign body through the oropharynx to prevent aspiration.
   c. Stomach. The majority of objects entering the stomach will pass through the rest of the gastrointestinal tract without problems.
      i. For objects >10 cm, such as toothbrushes, that are unlikely to pass the duodenal sweep, endoscopic removal is indicated.
      ii. Sharp objects should be attempted to be retrieved endoscopically if it can be accomplished safely. Otherwise, the patient should be followed with serial radiographs and physical examination to make sure the object progresses. Any nausea, vomiting, fever, abdominal pain, or GI bleeding should warrant consideration for operative intervention.
      iii. Blunt objects that do not pass the stomach and pylorus in 3 to 4 weeks should be removed endoscopically.
      iv. Batteries should be retrieved if they have not passed the pylorus within 72 hours.

v. If endoscopic retrieval fails, patients can be managed conservatively for symptoms to develop prior to operative intervention, for the majority of all objects, including sharp ones, will pass without complications.

d. Narcotic packets. Narcotics such as heroin and cocaine are occasionally smuggled by people ingesting latex condoms or plastic bags filled with the drugs. Care should be taken not to rupture these bags, for it can cause lethal overdose. Thus, **endoscopic retrieval is contraindicated**. Observation should be the rule, and surgery considered if there is evidence of obstruction or a signs of rupture.

B. Retained foreign body. Retained foreign bodies in the rectum are an underreported problem that typically has a delay in presentation secondary to embarrassment of the patient. It is important to have a clear understanding of the proper approach to this problem in order to prevent serious complications.

  1. History and physical examination. Important information may be gleaned from a thorough history and physical when approaching a patient with a retained foreign body.

  a. Important questions to ask include the timing of the placement of foreign object, the shape and size of the object, as well as descriptions of removal attempts.

  b. A review of systems including history of fever, nausea, vomiting, abdominal pain, obstipation, and last bowel movement is also important to ascertain.

  c. Physical exam should focus on the abdomen evaluating for peritonitis, distension, and masses. Digital rectal examination and anoscopic evaluation should also be performed to help locate the object if possible.

  2. Diagnostic modalities

  a. Abdominal radiographs in the emergency department (ED) are important to help further guide management for removal of the foreign body. These may demonstrate evidence of free air and also help determine the location of the object in the rectum versus the sigmoid colon if it is radiopaque.

  b. CT scan may be useful in determining the extent of inflammation of the rectum and any fluid collections or pockets of free air suggestive of occult perforation.

  3. Operative indications

  a. Inability to remove object in the ED

  b. Evidence of peritonitis or perforation

  4. Treatment

  a. Bedside removal in the ED. Sixty % to 75% of retained foreign bodies in the rectum can be removed in the ED at the bedside. In the awake patient, a valsalva maneuver is typically attempted first. If this is unsuccessful, a variety of other techniques may be employed to facilitate removal.

  i. IV sedation and local anesthesia. Sedation with benzodiazepine such as midazolam combined with local anesthesia of the sphincter is an effective way to relax the anal sphincter to allow further procedures.

  ii. Digital extraction

  iii. Rigid proctoscopy. Using forceps or clamps in conjunction with proctoscopy may help extract the object. It is important to be careful not to advance the object more proximally while performing proctoscopy.

  iv. Foley catheter. There is usually a vacuum of the rectum around the object. Using a Foley catheter balloon to pass the object and inflating the balloon may disrupt the vacuum and traction on the Foley proximal to the object may allow for easier removal.

  b. Operative interventions

  i. Exam under anesthesia (EUA). If bedside removal of object is not successful, EUA is necessary to help extract the foreign body. Spinal or general anesthesia are both effective in further relaxing the sphincter. Serial anal dilations and lateral internal sphincterotomy may also be necessary to deliver the object.

    ii. Laparotomy. Should be performed on anybody who has evidence of peritonitis or free air on initial presentation. Transabdominal manipulation to help advance the object through the anus should be the goal. Colotomy should be performed if unable to remove the object transanally. Diverting colostomy may be necessary if gross contamination is present.

    5. Postextraction sigmoidoscopy. Postextraction sigmoidoscopy should be performed following removal of a foreign object from the rectum to evaluate for perforating injuries or injuries that enter the muscularis and need repair. Water-soluble enema may also be utilized to exclude rectal injury.

VII. COLITIS

    A. General. Colonic inflammation or colitis may be of very different etiologies ranging from inflammatory bowel disease (IBD), to infectious, neutropenic, and ischemic colitis. Ulcerative colitis is discussed in Section VIII. Ischemic colitis is discussed in the next section. Management and definitive treatment varies among the different etiologies and is discussed in this section.

    B. Infectious colitis. Infectious colitis may be secondary to overgrowth of a pathogenic bacteria, virus, fungi, or parasite. These tend to occur more commonly in immunocompromised individuals who cannot defend against these pathogens. Transplant patients are at very high risk.

    1. *Clostridium difficile* colitis (*Pseudomembranous colitis*). Pseudomembranous colitis is the most common infectious colitis that may require operative intervention. This is most commonly associated with recent antibiotic use and presents as watery diarrhea. Most patients may be able to be treated with oral metronidazole or vancomycin with resolution of symptoms. However, there is also an extremely fulminant colitis that may develop which may lead to a severe inflammatory response syndrome (SIRS) or even death if appropriate medical therapy or emergent colectomy is not performed.

    a. Etiology

      i. *C. difficile* colitis is the leading cause of nosocomially acquired diarrhea. Antibiotic use causes an alteration of the normal colonic flora leading to an overgrowth of *C. difficile* bacteria. Toxins are released that may cause symptoms ranging from simple diarrhea to toxicity including hypotension, mental status changes, multiple organ failure, and death.

      ii. Patients may present without diarrhea in the setting of severe colonic dysmotility.

    b. Risk factors

      i. A single dose of preoperative antibiotics is sufficient to cause this nosocomial infection.

      ii. Immunosuppression, medical comorbidities, and a recent surgical procedure increase the risk of complications.

    c. Clinical manifestations. Patients have varying presentations with pseudomembranous colitis.

      i. Clinical suspicion is usually raised from loose, watery diarrhea. There may be mucoid material in the diarrhea as well. Diarrhea does not necessarily have to be present.

      ii. Abdominal distension secondary to obstruction or ascites may be present.

      iii. In the severe form of colitis, the patient may present with evidence of obstipation or obstruction. Patients may also have abdominal pain in the more severe form.

      iv. There is a significant leuckocytosis, with peripheral white blood cell (WBC) counts possibly reaching levels of 30,000 to 50,000 with a bandemia in immunocompetent patients.

    d. Diagnostic modalities

      i. History should be obtained to establish recent antibiotic use, recent hospitalization, domicile in a nursing facility, and medical comorbidities.

ii. Patients who present with diarrhea should have a cytotoxin assay or immunoassay sent to determine the presence of toxin A in the stool. A negative stool assay should be repeated up to three times if there is sufficient clinical concern for *C. difficile* infection.

iii. A WBC count with differential should be sent as well, for there is typically a severe leukomoid reaction in patients with impending fulminant colitis. Peripheral WBC counts reaching levels of 30,000 to 50,000 with bandemia are common in immunocompetent patients.

iv. The diagnosis may also be made with endoscopy to search for pseudomembranes in the colon.

v. If there is significant abdominal distension and the patient does not appear to be improving on medical therapy, a CT scan may be obtained. Patients with thickening of the colonic wall, dilation of the colon, and ascites who have systemic symptoms require a total abdominal colectomy.

e. Operative indications

i. If there is failure of medical management with patients developing hypotension, elevated WBC, or signs of end-organ failure (such as worsening pulmonary status, oliguria or increasing creatinine, or mental status changes) with abdominal pain or evidence of colonic wall thickening with ascites on CT scan, emergent laparotomy and total abdominal colectomy with end ileostomy should be performed.

ii. Immunosuppressed patients may not develop elevation of WBC or abdominal pain, so evidence on CT scan of fulminant colitis with hypotension or organ failure should prompt operation.

f. Treatment

i. Initial prophylactic therapy with oral metronidazole should be instituted as soon as suspicion of *C. difficile* is entertained. **Do not delay treatment awaiting confirmatory test results.** Mild cases may be treated as an outpatient for 10 days. Recurrence rate may be 30% even after treatment.

ii. Unnecessary antibiotics should be stopped immediately.

iii. In patients who are allergic to metronidazole or are refractory, oral vancomycin may be used.

iv. In severely dehydrated patients with fever and abdominal pain, IV hydration, bowel rest, and continuation of metronidazole and/or vancomycin is indicated.

v. In recurrent cases, prolonged therapy is indicated.

vi. If operation is indicated, total abdominal colectomy should be performed because there is a very high incidence of recurrence and need for reoperation in patients who have colon left behind. The typical findings are a boggy, edematous colon. The serosa of the colon is generally not impressively abnormal. Do not be misled by this. The patient still requires a total abdominal colectomy. Take the colon distally as far as can be easily accomplished, staying above peritoneal reflection. If too much colon is left behind, the patient will not improve.

g. Outcomes. Colectomy from *C. difficile* colitis is associated with a mortality as high as 57%.

2. Neutropenic enterocolitis. Neutropenic enterocolitis has been referred to as typhlitis, ileocecal syndrome, or necrotizing enterocolitis.

a. Incidence. Neutropenic enterocolitis is a rare entity in adults with fewer than 150 cases reported in the literature. It is more common among the pediatric population. The incidence ranges from up to 40% of patients with childhood leukemia to 1% to 5% of adult leukemic patients treated with chemotherapy.

b. Pathogenesis/Etiology. Typically, the cause of the colitis is secondary to the toxic effects of chemotherapeutic agents on the mucosa of the colon secondary to its rapidly dividing nature. Enterocolitis is believed to occur when the injured bowel mucosa develops microbial invasion in the face of immunosuppression.

c. Risk factors
  i. Chemotherapy
  ii. Malignancy
  iii. Systemic antibiotics changing the bowel flora
d. Diagnosis. Diagnostic studies should include CBC with differential. Anemia, neutropenia, and thrombocytopenia may all be present. Radiographic studies should be obtained as with other forms of colitis.
e. Operative indications
  i. Perforation
  ii. Pneumoperitoneum
  iii. Peritonitis
f. Treatment
  i. Aggressive fluid resuscitation.
  ii. Systemic antibiotics.
  iii. Operation should remove all areas of transmural necrosis. Second-look operation may be necessary in questionable areas of bowel.
g. Outcomes. Patients have a very poor prognosis if necrosis is present and no operative intervention is performed. Medical management with antibiotics and fluid resuscitation and halting chemotherapy may be successful if no necrosis is present.

3. Cytomegalovirus (CMV) colitis
  a. CMV colitis is rare in immunocompetent hosts. However, CMV is common in immunocompromised patients. CMV may target multiple organs, with the esophagus and colon being the most common sites of infection. Patients typically present with ulcerations, mucosal hemorrhage, or erosions of the colon.
  b. In immunocompetent hosts, IBD may be the underlying diagnosis with CMV superinfection. Spontaneous resolution occurs in around 30% of patients.
  c. Immunoassays can help determine the diagnosis.
  d. Aggressive fluid resuscitation and antiviral therapy should be instituted immediately.
  e. Colectomy is indicated in patients presenting with toxic colitis.
  f. In patients undergoing colectomy, the mortality is over 30%.

VIII. MESENTERIC ISCHEMIA AND ISCHEMIC COLITIS (Chapter 59). There are many causes of ischemia to the small bowel and colon and it may appear in various degrees of injury. It is important to have a high level of clinical suspicion to treat these patients rapidly and minimize complications.
  A. Incidence. Occurs most commonly in elderly critically ill patients; however, 10% to 20% of cases may occur in patients younger than 40 years old.
  B. Etiology. The end-cause of ischemic colitis or mesenteric ischemia is hypoperfusion of the bowel or colon. This may be broken down into occlusive and nonocclusive disease.
    1. Occlusive disease
      a. Arterial occlusive disease may be secondary to atherosclerotic plaque, emboli, dissection of the artery, diabetic small vessel disease, autoimmune arteritis, or volvulus.
      b. Venous occlusion may be secondary to thrombus from hypercoaguable states, portal hypertension, CHF, or pancreatitis.
      c. In mesenteric ischemia embolic occlusion of the superior mesenteric artery (SMA) occurs in about 50% of cases.
      d. Twenty-five percent of cases of mesenteric ischemia occur secondary to thrombosis of preexisting atherosclerotic lesions.
    2. Nonocclusive disease. The most common cause of nonocclusive disease is a low flow state. The low flow state typically causes acute mesenteric vasoconstriction, especially watershed areas of the colon. Drugs may cause this

mesenteric vasoconstriction as well, including cocaine, nasal decongestants, digitalis, and NSAIDs.

3. **Anatomy.** Although there is an abundant collateral circulation to the intestine, this may, especially in the elderly, be compromised secondary to calcifications, plaque, or iatrogenically because of AAA surgery or prior surgical bowel resections. The superior mesenteric artery supplies the small bowel as well as the right side of the colon and two thirds of the transverse colon. The watershed areas of the colon, the splenic flexure and the descending and sigmoid colon, are most susceptible to the low flow state in nonocclusive ischemia. Occlusive disease typically causes ischemia in a more segmental fashion.

C. **Clinical manifestations.** The clinical presentation of patients with mesenteric ischemia or ischemic colitis varies according to the severity of ischemia.

1. **Acute mesenteric ischemia.** These patients classically present with nonspecific symptoms of abdominal pain that is disproportional to relatively unremarkable physical findings. If presentation is delayed, patients may present with a rigid abdomen, hypotension, and obtunded mental status. Nausea, vomiting, fever, diarrhea, heme positive stools, and hematochezia are also common symptoms.

2. **Ischemic colitis**

   a. In patients with partial-thickness mucosal injuries, they may present with a fever, tachycardia, and sudden-onset left-sided abdominal tenderness. The patients may have heme positive stools as well.

   b. In patients with injury extending to the submucosa, they have the same presentation as someone with a mucosal injury, but may also present with hypotension and gross blood.

   c. In a patient with full-thickness ischemia, which affects 10% to 20% of patients, septic shock with peritonitis is the typical presentation.

3. A thorough history should be obtained focusing on prior operations, acuity of onset of pain, fevers, chills, nausea, vomiting, change in bowel habits, blood in stool, history of arrhythmias, hypercoaguable state, and peripheral vascular disease.

4. Physical exam should focus on cardiac exam, evidence of peritonitis, distension, abdominal exam, and rectal exam with stool sample for occult blood.

D. **Diagnostic modalities**

1. **Acute mesenteric ischemia**

   a. Radiographs of the abdomen may show a nonspecific ileus in early ischemia. Thumbprinting, intramural pneumatosis, and portal venous gas may be present in late ischemia or transmural infarction.

   b. Angiography has traditionally been the gold standard imaging method for both diagnosing intestinal ischemia and being a modality for possible therapeutic intervention.

   c. Magnetic resonance angiography (MRA) has been increasingly helpful in diagnosing ischemia, especially with gadolinium. Benefits include prevention of contrast nephropathy and excellent vascular visualization in mesenteric venous disease. Disadvantages include inability to perform therapeutic procedures and insufficient resolution to diagnose distal embolic events.

   d. Helical CT may show mesenteric ischemia with a sensitivity >90% and is the diagnostic test of choice in excluding other abdominal pathologies. Signs of segmental edema or bowel wall thickening, portal venous gas, or pneumatosis may be seen.

   e. Elevated lactate level and leuckocytosis with a left shift and bandemia are common lab abnormalities.

2. The diagnosis of ischemic colitis is made based on a combination of clinical, endoscopic, and pathological findings. Both laboratory tests and radiological studies may be used as adjuncts but are relatively nonspecific.

   a. Initial diagnosis commonly includes an endoscopy which can be used to grade the severity of disease. It is important that the endoscopist does not attempt to advance past areas of necrosis. Biopsy may be helpful to differentiate ischemic colitis from infectious, inflammatory, or other forms of colitis.

   b. Plain films of the abdomen may show evidence of free air, pneumatosis, or portal venous gas in full-thickness ischemia.

   c. CT scan, which is frequently done in the evaluation of abdominal pain, typically demonstrates nonspecific colonic wall thickening in mild cases, but can also show pneumatosis, portal venous gas, or another source of abdominal pain.

   d. Angiography is more helpful in diagnosing ischemia of the small bowel than in the colon, for occlusive disease in the colon typically takes place at the level of the arteriole.

   e. Peripheral WBC count is typically elevated, with a left shift and bandemia being present in severe ischemic colitis.

   f. Other laboratory value abnormalities may be a base deficit, acidosis, or elevated lactate levels.

E. Operative indications. Most cases of ischemic colitis may be treated nonoperatively and respond to fluid resuscitation. Patients should be taken to operation who have:

   1. Free air or pneumatosis intestinalis on CT scan or plain films

   2. Deterioration or failure to improve with fluid resuscitation and antibiotics

   3. Clear signs of peritonitis, indicative of infarcted intestine

F. Treatment.

   1. Initial treatment with bowel ischemia with is aggressive fluid resuscitation for the large degree of third spacing. Nasogastric tube should be placed.

   2. Broad-spectrum antibiotics if ischemic colitis is suspected and *C. difficile* colitis is unlikely to be the disease process.

   3. If mesenteric venous thrombosis is diagnosed based on CT scan or angiographic findings, systemic anticoagulation with heparin is instituted, followed by chronic anticoagulation with warfarin. Search for underlying thrombotic disorders.

   4. If arterial insufficiency is suspected on CT scan and there is no evidence of full-thickness infarction on CT scan, angiography may play a role for preoperative planning and possible infusion of papaverine into the SMA.

   5. Angioplasty and stents have recently been used in place of surgical bypass in patients with chronic mesenteric ischemia. This technique has been advocated in very high-risk patients.

   6. Intrarterial thrombolytics, such as urokinase, streptokinase, or recombinant tissue plasminogen activator, may also be useful in patients with high operative risk.

   7. There is no role of angiography in suspected ischemic colitis following aortic surgery because the etiology is known to be from ligation of the inferior mesenteric artery and there are no effective radiologic or pharmacologic interventions that are feasible.

   8. Surgical exploration.

      a. Laparoscopy may be performed if the diagnosis is unclear and the abdomen is not distended.

      b. The degree of ischemia should be determined as well as examination of all pulses and venous congestion.

      c. If the superior mesenteric artery (SMA) is occluded at the origin from an embolic event, an embolectomy can be attempted with a patch or transverse closure.

      d. If the SMA is occluded secondary to atherosclerotic disease there are two approaches.

         i. Bypass of atherosclerotic SMA from aorta prior to resection can help salvage some ischemic bowel, although there is high failure rate, reperfusion injury, and prolonged operative time.

         ii. Resection of all infarcted bowel. Marginally perfused bowel should be preserved if resection will result in short gut syndrome.

    e. Viability may be assessed intraoperatively by palpation of mesenteric pulses, Doppler of the mesenteric vessels, or IV fluorescein dye and use of the Wood's lamp.

    f. Second-look operation should be decided on before closing the abdomen, especially if there is a question of viability for long segments of intestine.

    g. Anastomosis is generally not recommended when there are large areas of ischemia and resected ends should be either left in the abdomen for a second-look operation or brought out as stomas.

G. Outcomes.

  1. Mortality is directly related to delay in diagnosis and treatment.

  2. Mortality rates for acute arterial mesenteric ischemia range from 60% to 80%.

  3. Mortality rates for acute mesenteric venous thrombosis ranges from 20% to 50%.

  4. Recurrent mesenteric ischemia from angioplasty is higher than surgical revascularization, ranging from 10% to 67%.

  5. Mortality from ischemic colitis may be as high as 50%, and is higher for patients who require surgical intervention.

H. Complications

  1. Short-bowel syndrome may develop if >50% to 80% of small intestine has been resected. Lifelong parenteral nutrition may ensue.

  2. Long-term stricture may occur in 10% to 15% of patients with ischemic colitis.

IX. COMPLICATIONS OF INFLAMMATORY BOWEL DISEASE

A. General. Inflammatory bowel disease (IBD) can be broadly classified as three types: Crohn's disease, ulcerative colitis, and indeterminate colitis. Although the etiology for these conditions remains generally unknown, all are characterized by intestinal inflammation. The first line of therapy consists of medical therapy aimed at reducing the inflammation. Many of these patients will first come to the attention of a surgeon in the setting of an ED with an acute complication of their disease. We review some of the more common acute presentations of these conditions and their management.

B. Crohn's disease

  1. Incidence. Approximately 1 to 5 people per 100,000 in the United States and Europe, with a greater proportion noted in the White populations. Crohn's presents in a bimodal distribution around the ages of 15 to 30 years and again at 55 to 60 years. Up to 80% of Crohn's patients will require some form of bowel resection within 10 years of diagnosis.

  2. Risk factors

    a. Genetic conditions: NOD2/CARD15 mutations, chronic granulomatous disease, glycogen storage disease type 1B.

    b. Smoking

    c. Family history of IBD

  3. Pathogenesis/Etiology. A transmural inflammatory process that may affect **any part of the gastrointestinal tract** from mouth to anus. Pathologic hallmarks of the disease include mucosal ulcerations, inflammatory cell infiltrates, and noncaseating granulomas. Chronic inflammation may result in fibrosis, strictures, and fistulas.

  4. Clinical manifestations. Depending on the site of disease, Crohn's disease may present with almost any gastrointestinal symptom as well as systemic symptoms. Most common location is ileocolic disease (40%), followed by ileal disease (30%), and colonic only (25%).

    a. Colitis

      i. Fever

      ii. Chronic colicky abdominal pain, which may mimic acute appendicitis

      iii. Obstruction, often from the presence of strictures

      iv. Weight loss from protein loss and obstruction

      v. Night sweats

      vi. Right lower quadrant mass may be palpable

    b. Toxic colitis or "fulminant" colitis presents with fever, sudden onset of bloody diarrhea, abdominal tenderness, colicky pain, and anorexia. As a result, patients may have dehydration, altered mental status, electrolyte disturbances, and hypotension. Toxic colitis may be the initial presentation of Crohn's in up to 30% of cases.

        i. Toxic colitis is defined by the presence of severe colitis with at least two of the following:

            a) Fever (T $>38.5°C$)

            b) Tachycardia (HR >100 bpm)

            c) Leukocytosis (WBC $>10.5/mm^3$)

            d) Hypoalbuminemia (<3.0 g/dL)

        ii. Gross pathology shows transmural vascular congestion and muscle disintegration. Histology shows acute inflammation in all layers of the colon with myocyte degeneration, necrosis, and inflammatory cell infiltrates.

        iii. Precipitating factors. Hypokalemia, antiinflammatory medications, narcotics, anticholinergics, abrupt steroid therapy discontinuation, recent barium enema, and colonscopy.

    c. Toxic megacolon. Toxic colitis with either total or segmental nonobstructive dilation of the colon (>6 cm transverse diameter). Usually the transverse or right colon are the most dilated. Occurs in 4% to 6% of cases of toxic colitis.

5. Diagnostic evaluation

    a. In the emergent setting, complete evaluation with colonoscopy or barium enema is contraindicated in a patient with toxic megacolon or toxic colitis because of the risk of perforation. Radiographic evaluation usually consists of:

        i. Plain abdominal radiograph helps exclude toxic megacolon and identify pneumoperitoneum. Only 20% of cases of perforated Crohn's disease may show pneumoperitoneum.

        ii. CT of abdomen/pelvis is recommended to identify pericolic abscesses amenable to percutaneous drainage, colonic thickening, and the presence of fistulas.

    b. In the nonacute setting, endoscopic evaluation may demonstrate normal mucosa with areas of ulcerated mucosa, a "cobblestone" appearance with skip lesions, or rectal sparing. Air-contrast barium enema will also provide full evaluation of the colon. A small-bowel series may be performed to evaluate small bowel Crohn's disease.

    c. Stool culture for ova and parasites to exclude infectious colitis.

6. Emergency operative indications

    a. Failure of medical therapy is the most common overall indication for surgery due to chronic unremitting symptoms or an acute exacerbation that fails to respond to optimal medical therapy. A bout of acute colitis that fails to improve after 2 weeks of medical therapy should be managed as toxic colitis.

    b. Toxic colitis requires aggressive resuscitation and stabilization upon admission to the hospital. Failure to respond to maximal medical therapy within 7 to 10 days of starting intravenous corticosteroids is an indication for colectomy. Further delay carries a significant risk of perforation that carries a mortality rate of more than 40% in this setting.

    c. Toxic megacolon requires operative intervention within 48 to 72 hours if there is no response to medical therapy.

    d. Perforation occurs in 1% to 3% of Crohn's patients. Mandates emergent surgical exploration. May occur in any segment of the gastrointestinal tract.

        i. Gastroduodenal debridement and primary repair.

        ii. Jejunum and ileum resection with primary anastomosis or diversion.

        iii. Colon usually occurs in the setting of toxic colitis, total abdominal colectomy, and end ileostomy. Postcolonoscopic perforation in a diseased segment—the diseased segment and the perforation should be resected.

e. Obstruction affects up to 50% of Crohn's patients.

  i. Etiology

    a) Fibrosis and scarring with stricture formation

    b) Acute active inflammation involving a stenotic bowel segment

    c) Mass effect from a phlegmon/abscess

    d) Malignancy

  ii. Management. With initial course of medical therapy, most obstructions will resolve. Should operative therapy be required:

    a) Benign stricture—segmental resection of stricture is preferred therapy, though strictureplasty may rarely be an option.

    b) Malignant stricture—formal cancer resection required.

f. Abscess. May be perianal, intraperitoneal, retroperitoneal, or intramesenteric.

  i. Within the abdomen, most commonly found in the right lower quadrant. Abscesses require drainage, which may often be accomplished with a radiographic percutaneous procedure. When required, operative goals should include drainage of the abscess, resection of diseased intestine, and fecal diversion.

  ii. For perianal collections, goals of drainage should include minimizing tissue trauma, placing the incision as close to the anal verge as possible, and ensuring adequate drainage with setons and mushroom catheters.

g. Bleeding. Two percent to 3% incidence. Usually from a localized source, most commonly in small bowel (65%) Crohn's involvement. A complete evaluation for gastrointestinal hemorrhage should be performed as nearly 30% of GI bleeds in Crohn's patients are due to a bleeding duodenal ulcer. Continued bleeding after a 4- to 6-unit transfusion requirement or recurrent bleeding may require surgical exploration to stop life-threatening bleeding if angiographic treatment is not successful. If localized to a segment of small bowel, then a small-bowel resection and anastomosis should be performed. In Crohn's colitis, a total abdominal colectomy may be needed with patient condition dictating whether an ileorectal anastomosis should be performed.

7. Treatment

  a. Medical management. Initial therapy should consist of aggressive resuscitation, broad-spectrum antibiotics, bowel rest, and parenteral corticosteroids. Antidiarrheal agents should be avoided.

  b. Emergent operative management. Focuses on removal of grossly diseased intestine with maximal preservation of intestinal length. Midline abdominal incision or laparoscopy are the preferred approaches for exploration. Unlike in bowel resections for malignancy, high ligation of the mesenteric vessels is unnecessary.

    i. Segmental resection may be an option in disease limited to a discrete region.

    ii. Subtotal colectomy with or without ileostomy should be considered for colonic disease in which rectal sparing is noted. In the setting of **toxic colitis, subtotal colectomy with end ileostomy** is the procedure of choice. The distal rectal stump may be implanted subcutaneously in the wound, left at the pelvic brim, or matured as a mucous fistula. With toxic megacolon, colonic decompression intraoperatively may facilitate surgery.

    iii. Proctocolectomy with end ileostomy may be required for pancolonic disease; however, it carries a higher morbidity and mortality than subtotal colectomy. It is important to preserve the anal musculature for future surgical procedures. A restorative proctocolectomy is not advised when treating toxic colitis.

8. Outcomes. In Crohn's disease, it is impossible to cure the patient with operative therapy. Mortality rates in the setting of toxic megacolon without perforation are 2% to 8%.

C. Ulcerative colitis (UC)

1. **Incidence.** About 10 in 100,000 people in the American and European populace. The incidence tends to be lower in the non-White population in the United States. There is a bimodal distribution for the onset of symptoms in the third and seventh decades of life.

2. **Risk factors**
   a. Autoantibodies such as pANCA, antiepithelial antibodies
   b. HLA class II DRB1*0103
   c. Family history of IBD

3. **Pathogenesis/Etiology.** A **mucosal process** limited to the colon in which colonic mucosa and submucosa are infiltrated by inflammatory cells. Pathologic evaluation shows atrophic mucosa with crypt abscesses with **continuous involvement** of the rectum and colon. Unlike in Crohn's disease, the rectum is always involved in UC attacks.

4. **Clinical manifestation.** UC typically presents with **bloody diarrhea** or rectal bleeding, but may also include:
   a. Tenesmus as a result of proctitis
   b. Anemia
   c. Backwash ileitis—inflammatory changes may be seen in the terminal ileum
   d. Toxic colitis (overall incidence of 10%) and toxic megacolon (as mentioned previously regarding Crohn's disease)

5. **Diagnostic evaluation.** Refer to the previous discussion about Crohn's disease.

6. **Emergency operative indications.** Essentially the same indications as for Crohn's disease.
   a. Life-threatening hemorrhage.
   b. Toxic colitis failing to respond to medical therapy.
   c. Toxic megacolon.
   d. Obstruction—stricture formation is less common in UC than Crohn's, therefore the presence of obstruction or stricture should be concerning for a malignancy.

7. **Treatment**
   a. Medical management. Essentially the same initial therapy as in Crohn's disease.
   b. Emergent operative management:
      i. **Total abdominal colectomy with end ileostomy**—procedure of choice for perforation, toxic megacolon, toxic colitis, or life-threatening hemorrhage from UC.
      ii. Total proctocolectomy with end ileostomy—increases morbidity and may compromise future sphincter preserving procedures.
      iii. Loop ileostomy and decompressing colostomy may be required in critically ill and unstable patient.

8. **Outcomes.** Unlike in Crohn's disease, complete surgical resection of the colon and rectum removes the cause of ulcerative colitis. Mortality rates are <1%. Patients undergoing emergency operation may require a second operation for definitive treatment and to establish intestinal continuity. In cases where the rectum is not resected, patients will require continued proctoscopic screening for malignancy and remain at risk for continued complications from UC.

9. **Complications**
   a. Bleeding. In unusual cases undertaken for bleeding, a total abdominal resection will fail to treat bleeding from the rectal stump (<12%). Epinephrine enemas may be utilized to help control this bleeding. In rare cases, a proctectomy will be required.
   b. Autonomic nerve injury during proctectomy resulting in impotence, ejaculatory dysfunction, or bladder dysfunction.
   c. Common postoperative complications: small bowel obstructions, wound infections, and thromboembolic events.

D. **Indeterminate colitis.** In up to 15% of patients, the distinction between Crohn's colitis and ulcerative colitis cannot be made even after a complete diagnostic evaluation. In the acute setting, these patients should be evaluated and managed in a manner similar to the patient with ulcerative colitis.

Bibliography

Behrman SW. Management of complicated PUD. *Arch Surg* 2005;140:201–208.

Berg DF, Bahadursingh AM, Kaminski DL, Longo WE. Acute surgical emergencies in inflammatory bowel disease. *Am J Surg* 2002;184:45–51.

Blaho KE, Merigian KS, Winbery SL, et al. Foreign body ingestions in the emergency department: Case reports and review of treatment. *J Emerg Med* 1998;16:21–26.

Brunicardi FC, Andersen DK, Billiar TR, et al. *Schwartz's Principles of Surgery.* 8th ed. New York, NY: McGraw-Hill; 2005.

Cameron JL, ed. *Current Surgical Therapy.* 8th ed. Philadelphia, Pa: Mosby; 2004.

Cohen H. Peptic ulcer and Helicobacter pylori. *Gastroenterol Clin North Am* 2000;29:775–789.

Cunningham SC, Fakhry K, Bass BL, Napolitano LM. Neutropenic enterocolitis in adults: Case series and review of the literature. *Dig Dis Sci* 2005;50:215–220.

Dallal RM, Harbrecht BG, Boujoukas AJ, et al. Fulminant Clostridium difficile: An underappreciated and increasing cause of death and complications. *Ann Surg* 2002;235:363–372.

Donahue PE. Ulcer surgery and highly selective vagotomy—Y2K. *Arch Surg* 1999;134:1373–1377.

Eisen GM, Baron TH, Dominitz JA, et al. Guideline for the management of ingested foreign bodies. *Gastrointest Endosc* 2002;55:802–806.

Galiatsatos P, Shrier I, Lamoureux E, Szilagyi A. Meta-analysis of outcome of cytomegalovirus colitis in immunocompetent hosts. *Dig Dis Sci* 2005;50:609–616.

Hellinger MD. Anal trauma and foreign bodies. *Surg Clin North Am* 2002;82:1253–1260.

Khullar SK, DiSario JA. Gastric outlet obstruction. *Gastrointest Endosc Clin North Am* 1996;6:585–603.

Lai AT, Chow TL, Lee DT, Kwok SP. Risk factors predicting the development of complications after foreign body ingestion. *Br J Surg* 2003;90:1531–1535.

Lake JP, Essani R, Petrone P, et al. Management of retained colorectal foreign bodies: Predictors of operative intervention. *Dis Colon Rectum* 2004;47:1694–1698.

Lee J. Bezoars and foreign bodies of the stomach. *Gastrointest Endosc Clin N Am* 1996;6:605–619.

Millat B, Fingerhut A, Borie F. Surgical treatment of complicated duodenal ulcers: Controlled trials. *World J Surg* 2000;24:299–306.

Modigliani R. Medical management of fulminant colitis. *Inflamm Bowel Dis* 2002;8:129–134.

Nayar M, Rhodes JM. Management of inflammatory bowel disease. *Postgrad Med J* 2004;80:206–213.

Ohmann C, Imhof M, Roher HD. Trends in peptic ulcer bleeding and surgical treatment. *World J Surg* 2000;24:284–293.

Shelton T, McKinlay R, Schwartz RW. Acute appendicitis: Current diagnosis and treatment. *Curr Surg* 2003;60:502–505.

Sheth SG, LaMont JT. Toxic megacolon. *Lancet* 1998;351:509–513.

Sreenarasimhaiah J. Diagnosis and management of intestinal ischaemic disorders. *BMJ* 2003;326:1372–1376.

Svanes C. Trends in perforated peptic ulcer: Incidence, etiology, treatment, and prognosis. *World J Surg* 2000;24:277–283.

Toursarkissian B, Thompson RW. Ischemic colitis. *Surg Clin North Am* 1997;77:461–470.

Wasselle JA, Norman J. Acute gastric volvulus: Pathogenesis, diagnosis, and treatment. *Am J Gastroenterol* 1993;88:1780–1784.

Weiland ST, Schurr MJ. Conservative management of ingested foreign bodies. *J Gastrointest Surg* 2002;6:496–500.

Zittel TT, Jehle EC, Becker HD. Surgical management of PUD today—Indication, technique and outcome. *Langenbecks Arch Surg* 2000;385:84–96.

BOWEL OBSTRUCTION
PAUL R. KLEPCHICK AND
STEVEN J. HUGHES

63

I. OVERVIEW. Small- and large-bowel obstruction represent two distinct clinical entities that require different evaluation and treatment. Understanding potential etiologies of obstruction, clinically differentiating these types of bowel obstruction, and recognizing adynamic ileus when present are essential for optimal management. This chapter provides a systematic approach to evaluation of a patient with suspected bowel obstruction.

II. DEFINITIONS
   A. Partial bowel obstruction. Bowel lumen is narrowed but permits passage of some air and fluid as evidenced by flatus or distal gas radiographically.
   B. Complete bowel obstruction. Lumen is totally occluded and does not allow passage of air or fluid as evidenced by a **lack** of flatus or distal gas radiographically.
   C. Simple bowel obstruction. Lumen is partially or completely obstructed without compromise of intestinal blood flow.
   D. Complicated bowel obstruction. Blood flow to a portion of bowel is compromised, either from increased intraluminal pressure interrupting venous outflow, or interruption of mesenteric flow by twisting or entrapment.
   E. Closed-loop obstruction. Outflow of bowel contents obstructed at both ends of bowel preventing prograde **and** retrograde decompression which leads to more rapid distention and increased likelihood of bowel ischemia.
   F. Volvulus. A segment of intestine twists around its mesentery.

III. INITIAL EVALUATION (See Fig. 63-1 for management algorithm)
   A. Patients presenting with bowel obstruction typically require attention to intravascular volume status. Depending on the duration of symptoms and level of obstruction, patients will present with volume depletion that may be severe. While diagnostic evaluation is being completed, early fluid resuscitation should be instituted.
      1. Initial resuscitation should begin with isotonic fluids.
      2. The frequently present potassium deficiency should be corrected with potassium chloride after restoration of intravascular volume, usually noted by the return of adequate urine output.
      3. Treatment with sodium bicarbonate is only a temporizing measure and generally should be avoided.
   B. Adjuncts to resuscitation, including nasogastric decompression and bladder catheter placement, are beneficial in all but the mildest cases of partial bowel obstruction. Invasive monitoring may be indicated in patients with cardiac, pulmonary, or renal insufficiency.
   C. Evaluation for the possibility of a complicated obstruction should take first priority. These patients require few if any imaging studies and treatment centers on rapid resuscitation and emergent exploratory laparotomy. Although there are no specific findings or diagnostic tests that confirm or exclude strangulating obstruction, the following findings are worrisome for this diagnosis and should prompt consideration for urgent intervention.
      1. Physical findings—fever, severe continuous abdominal pain, tachycardia, rebound tenderness, and abdominal rigidity.

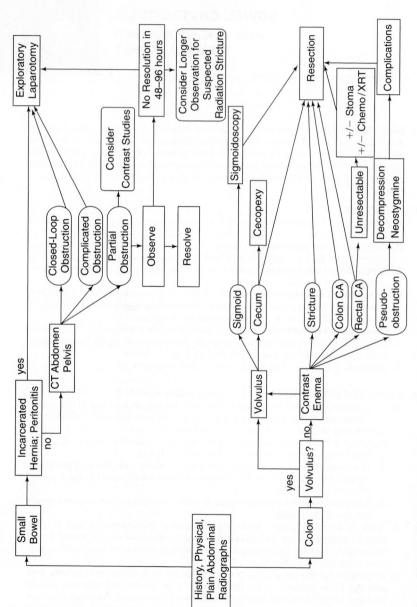

Figure 63-1. Algorithm for evaluation and management of bowel obstruction.

2. Laboratory findings—acidosis, leukocytosis.
3. Radiologic findings of complicated obstruction.
   a. Plain films—pneumatosis intestinalis, portal venous gas, or pneumoperitoneum are findings indicating that necrosis has already occurred. Thumbprinting, loss of mucosal pattern, and bowel wall gas are also ominous findings that usually warrant surgical exploration.
   b. Computerized tomography (CT)—pneumoperitoneum, pneumatosis intestinalis, and portal venous gas all indicate that necrosis is present. CT is also a good modality for identifying volvulus, intussusception, or complete obstruction. These findings generally culminate in surgical intervention.
   D. The history and physical examination provide important diagnostic information.
   1. **The presence of peritonitis suggests the need for emergent surgical intervention.** Any additional evaluation should focus on preoperative optimization of the patient.
   2. Patients with **small-bowel obstruction (SBO)** typically present with nausea, vomiting, and colicky abdominal pain. A lack of abdominal distention on physical exam may be observed in proximal obstruction. Presentation is usually within 24 to 48 hours of onset of symptoms.
   3. Patients with large-bowel obstruction (LBO) typically complain of distention, fullness, and obstipation. Nausea and abdominal pain are also common. The onset of symptoms is typically more gradual that in SBO, and patients often present more than 48 hours after first experiencing symptoms.
   4. A previous history of abdominal surgery or the presence of surgical incisions provides information regarding possible etiology of obstruction. SBO is caused by adhesive bands in up to 75% of cases. Incisional, inguinal, and umbilical hernia are also common etiologies of SBO and the physical exam must specifically search for their presence.
   5. LBO is most commonly due to colon cancer. Other common etiologies include diverticulitis, ischemic stricture, volvulus, and fecal impaction.

IV. LABORATORY EVALUATION. In the absence of peritonitis, further workup is necessary to determine both the location of obstruction and likely etiology that are necessary for appropriate management.
   A. A complete blood count and electrolyte panel are routinely obtained; however, these findings are nonspecific. No abnormalities may be present in patients with a complicated obstruction, and significant abnormalities may be present in a patient that is a candidate for conservative management. Additional laboratory studies should be obtained as indicated for coexisting medical conditions or preoperative screening.
   B. **Radiographic evaluation**
   1. An acute abdominal series, including supine and upright images of the abdomen and an upright chest film, is indicated for all patients presenting with symptoms consistent with small-bowel or colonic obstruction.
      a. Presence of dilated small-bowel loops on supine exam and air-fluid levels on upright exam is consistent with SBO. The absence of gas in the colon and rectum suggests complete obstruction.
      b. Plain films in colonic obstruction typically demonstrate dilated large-bowel loops with a point of decompression in the colon defining the site of obstruction. An incompetent ileocecal valve will also permit gas to distend the distal small bowel. Specific patterns on plain film can suggest certain etiologies.
         i. Sigmoid volvulus appears as a "bent inner-tube" with convexity of the loop in right upper quadrant (away from point of fixation).
         ii. Cecal volvulus demonstrates classic kidney-shaped air-filled structure with convexity of loop in left upper quadrant. Dilated loops of small bowel with air-fluid levels are often present with cecal volvulus.
   2. CT scan may be evolving as the initial imaging study of choice. Dilated bowel that is fluid filled and devoid of gas will be apparent on CT, but not noted on

plain films. Intravenous contrast improves diagnostic accuracy because it highlights the bowel wall, the mesenteric vasculature, and may demonstrate pathologic process responsible for SBO. Enteric contrast is rarely necessary as intraluminal air and fluid provide sufficient contrast. Rectal contrast is indicated for studies obtained to evaluate suspected LBO. Key findings may include:

   a. Dilated, fluid-filled bowel loops with thin walls.
   b. Transition zone—a dilated and/or air-filled small bowel proximal with collapsed distal bowel is the most reliable CT criterion to differentiate SBO from adynamic ileus.
   c. Closed-loop obstruction is suggested by U-shaped or C-shaped dilated bowel loop associated with radial distribution of mesenteric vessels.
   d. CT indications of strangulation
      i. Poor contrast enhancement of the bowel wall
      ii. Engorgement of mesenteric vasculature
      iii. Mesenteric haziness (congestion)
      iv. "Target" sign—slight circumferential thickening of bowel walls
      v. Intestinal pneumatosis
      vi. Portal venous gas
   3. After initial radiologic evaluation, contrast studies may be helpful in several scenarios.
      a. CT scan has limited sensitivity for low-grade or partial SBO. Under these circumstances, small-bowel contrast studies, either small-bowel follow-through or enteroclysis, can be helpful and at times therapeutic.
      b. Contrast enema can help identify the site of a colonic obstruction. Water-soluble contrast should be used if the possibility of perforation exists. A water-soluble-contrast enema is also therapeutic in cases of fecal impaction.
   C. Flexible sigmoidoscopy or rigid proctoscopy may be used in place of colonic contrast studies when sigmoid volvulus or an obstructing sigmoid or rectal cancer is suspected. Passage of the endoscope typically detorses the volvulus, and visualization allows evaluation of mucosa for viability and allows biopsy of luminal irregularities.

V. TREATMENT is based on location of obstruction and suspicion for strangulation.
   A. Strangulating obstruction requires emergent surgical intervention to prevent progression to frank bowel necrosis. Patients should be rapidly evaluated and resuscitated, and undergo exploration without delay.
   B. Small-bowel obstruction. Management of SBO differs depending on the etiology and degree of obstruction.
      1. Obstruction in a patient without history of abdominal surgery is unlikely to be caused by adhesions and typically does not resolve without operation. Hernia and neoplasm are the most common causes of bowel obstruction under these circumstances. Hernias that are not reducible frequently progress to strangulating obstruction and should be repaired as soon as fluid resuscitation is complete. Neoplastic obstruction, due to intrinsic or extrinsic obstruction, requires resection or bypass for relief. **Intussusception** may be responsible for obstruction in this group of patients. When this condition occurs in adults, preexisting small-bowel pathology serves as a lead point for intussusception. Therefore, treatment involves resection of the intussuscepted mass en bloc without attempting nonsurgical reduction.
      2. When adhesive obstruction is suspected, **differentiation of complete versus partial SBO is important**. Patients who have not passed flatus or stool in the previous 12 hours and have no colonic gas on abdominal plain film are likely to have complete small SBO. In such circumstances, the frequency of ischemic bowel is higher than in patients with incomplete obstruction. Ischemic bowel may be present in the absence of peritonitis or laboratory abnormalities, and up to 80% do not resolve with nasogastric suction alone. Thus, **early operative intervention is indicated for complete SBO once fluid resuscitation is complete.**

3. Patients with incomplete SBO and without evidence of ischemic bowel may be managed expectantly with nasogastric suction and frequent, serial abdominal exam. Resolution can be expected in up to 80% of patients. Greater than 90% of patients successfully treated nonoperatively show substantial improvement within 48 hours of initiation of resuscitation and enteric decompression. Thus, there is little sense to continue nonoperative management for more than 3 to 4 days.

4. Early operation is indicated after adequate resuscitation if the following are present or develop in a patient under observation: rapidly progressive abdominal pain or distention, development of peritoneal findings, fever, leukocytosis, metabolic acidosis, or diminished urine output unresponsive to fluid challenge.

5. Other, less common causes of SBO should always be considered (Table 63-1).

C. **Large-bowel obstruction** generally requires operative intervention.

1. **Complete colonic obstruction is an indication for urgent surgery.** The condition of the patient typically allows for the necessary planning and resuscitation to be completed prior to surgical intervention. Diameter of the proximally dilated cecum is a determinant in urgency for operation. Due to the law of LaPlace (thinner wall and larger lumen than the distal colon), the cecum becomes distended with distal obstruction in the colon. With the cecal diameter >10 or 12 cm, the need for operation becomes urgent.

2. Modified bowel preparation should be considered. In cases of partial bowel obstruction, an attempt at careful mechanical preparation with oral antibiotics is reasonable if immediate anastomosis is desired.

3. **Sigmoid volvulus** can often be detorsed preoperatively using rigid or flexible sigmoidoscopy to facilitate preoperative bowel preparation when primary anastomosis is desired, and to complete preoperative risk assessment and planning. Without sigmoid resection, up to 90% of patients suffer recurrence.

   a. If the patient with sigmoid volvulus presents with peritonitis, systemic signs of compromised bowel, or nonviable bowel with initial insertion of the sigmoidoscope, do not attempt reduction of the volvulus; these patients require immediate operation.

4. **Cecal volvulus** requires urgent operative intervention as visualization of the bowel is the best method of evaluation of vascular integrity. Optimal treatment is resection with primary anastomosis; however, cecopexy may *rarely* be indicated when the patient's condition precludes extensive operation.

5. **Malignant obstruction** typically occurs in the left colon, hepatic flexure, or proximal transverse colon—areas in which narrow lumen diameter predisposes to obstruction. Malignant obstruction of the cecum and ascending colon is unusual.

   a. Temporary formation of end colostomy and blind distal pouch is the most conservative option for managing obstructing colorectal cancers and is appropriate when a bowel preparation is not possible. Some surgeons advocate on-table lavage and primary anastomosis when preoperative preparation of the bowel is not technically feasible, as future reversal of colostomy is associated with a significant rate of major morbidity.

   b. Hepatic flexure tumors are managed by extended right hemicolectomy and primary anastomosis, even without bowel preparation.

   c. Obstructing rectal tumors are often caused by large tumors that may be fixed to surrounding tissues precluding primary resection. In settings of complete obstruction, proximal diverting colostomy and mucus fistula are appropriate followed by chemoradiation in appropriate patients. With partial obstruction, neoadjuvant chemoradiation is the ideal approach prior to resection and primary anastomosis. If the neoplasm is resectable but causing obstruction requiring palliation, the subtle benefits of the neoadjuvant approach should probably not preclude proceeding with definitive resection prior to adjuvant therapy.

6. **Diverticular stricture** may occur in setting of acute diverticulitis or at any time thereafter. In acute diverticulitis, contamination precludes formation of

TABLE 63-1 Small-Bowel Obstruction

Condition	Suggestive factors	Identifying features	Treatment	Other
Adhesion	Attempt to identify degree of obstruction.	History of laparotomy.	Up to 80% of simple SBO associated with adhesions resolve without surgery.	Most common cause of SBO.
Hernia	History and exam.	Physical exam. Internal hernia may be demonstrated on CT scan.	Resuscitate, reduce, and repair. Resect nonviable bowel.	Second most common cause of SBO, most common cause in patients without prior operation.
Neoplasm	History may be suggestive.	Typically requires enteroclysis for identification.	Resection vs. bypass.	May be primary or secondary (metastasis, extrinsic compression).
Crohn's disease	History.	Diagnosis based on clinical assessment with confirmatory findings based on radiologic, endoscopic, and pathologic tests.	Acute flare may respond to conservative treatment. Chronic strictures require operative treatment.	A third of patients with Crohn's disease will eventually require surgery for intestinal obstruction.
Intussusception	5% of intussusception cases occur in adults.	Occasionally sausage-shaped soft-tissue density identified on exam. Most diagnosed by contrast studies.	En block resection—lead point is commonly neoplasm in adult patients.	May occur in postoperative setting for other abdominal conditions.
Radiation stricture	History of abdomino-pelvic irradiation. May have recurring low-grade obstruction.	Enteroclysis is most accurate diagnostic test.	Most cases self-limiting. Surgery for incapacitating symptoms.	Surgery associated with increased risk of abscess and fistula formation.
Meckel's diverticulum	SBO most common presentation in adults.	Typically identified at time of surgery.	Diverticulectomy with removal of associated bands.	May act as lead point for intussusception.
Foreign body	History of ingestion.	May be evident on radiographic studies.	Enterotomy and removal vs. enterectomy.	
Gallstone ileus	Typically older patients.	Biliary air, gallstone in right lower quadrant.	Enterotomy for stone removal. Resect necrotic bowel.	Most stones impacted just proximal to ileocecal valve.

TABLE 63-2   Large-Bowel Obstruction

Condition	Suggestive factors	Identifying features	Treatment	Other
Neoplasm	Typically gradual progression.	Contrast enema—irregular luminal narrowing. Colonoscopy and biopsy.	Resection vs. stoma.	Neoadjuvent chemoradiaton for rectal cancers. Recurrence up to 90% without resection.
Sigmoid volvulus	Chronic constipation may be predisposing factor.	"Bent inner-tube" with convexity in right upper quadrant. Rare small-bowel dilatation.	Endoscopic detorsion. Resection.	
Cecal volvulus	Occurs from nonfixation of right colon.	Kidney-shaped air-filled obstruction in left upper quadrant. Small-bowel dilatation is common.	Resection. Cecopexy should be avoided.	Vascular impairment occurs early.
Colonic pseudoobstruction	No identifiable mechanical obstruction.	Contrast enema shows no obstructing lesion.	Colonoscopic decompression; neostygmine 2.5-mg IV. (Requires telemetry; contraindicated with heart block.)	Perforation and necrosis may occur if untreated.
Diverticulitis	Obstruction can occur as part of acute diverticulitis or as late sequelae.	Malignant involvement may be difficult to assess in acute setting, but should be evaluated with colonoscopy or contrast studies after resolution.	Resection with primary anastomosis if bowel preparation can be completed. Resection and colostomy if excessive peritoneal contamination.	
Inflammatory bowel disease	Typically identified by history.	Identification by clinical assessment and biopsy for confirmation.	Conservative management for inflammatory strictures. Resection if unable to exclude malignancy.	Malignant until proven otherwise.
Ischemic stricture	History of ischemic colitis or prior abdominal aortic surgery.	Contrast enema—concentric luminal narrowing with minimal irregularity.	Resection.	
Anastomotic stricture	Prior colon resection.	Contrast enema—short segment luminal narrowing.	Resection.	
Inspissated feces	May have underlying medical etiology.	Feces may be evident on plain abdominal radiograph, CT scan, or contrast enema.	Gastrograffin enema may be therapeutic. Disempaction.	Correct underlying medical causes.

anastomosis and temporary formation of end colostomy and blind rectal pouch is recommended. Unless it is technically impossible, the inflamed segment of large bowel should be resected in almost all cases, as simple proximal diversion results in considerably worse outcome. Treatment of late fibrotic strictures should be treated as described for obstructing malignancy with resection and primary anastomosis.

7. Less common etiologies of LBO should also be considered (Table 63-2).

　　a. Colonic pseudoobstruction (Ogilvie's syndrome) is relatively common in hospitalized patients. This must be differentiated from mechanical large-bowel obstruction, at times requiring contrast studies. Decompression with colonoscopy may be required to avoid ischemia or perforation in more severe cases.

Bibliography

Baradi H, Ponsky F. Large bowel obstruction. In: Cameron JL, ed. *Current Surgical Therapy.* Philadelphia, Pa: Mosby; 2004.

Bullard KM, Rothenberger DA. Colon, rectum, and anus. In: Brunicardi FC, Andersen DK, Billiar TR, et al. *Schwartz's Principles of Surgery.* 8th ed. New York, NY: McGraw-Hill; 2005.

Dayton MT. Small bowel obstruction. In: Cameron JL, ed. *Current Surgical Therapy.* Philadelphia, Pa: Mosby; 2004.

Drelichman ER, Nelson H. Colonic volvulus. In: Cameron JL, ed. *Current Surgical Therapy.* Philadelphia, Pa: Mosby; 2004.

Frager DH, Baer JW. Role of CT in evaluating patients with small-bowel obstruction. *Semin Ultrasound CT MR* 1995;16(2):127–140.

Girvent M, Carlson GL, Anderson I, et al. Intestinal failure after surgery for complicated radiation enteritis. *Ann R Coll Surg Engl* 2000;82(3):198–201.

Hughes SJ. Large bowel obstruction. In: Bland K, ed. *The Practice of General Surgery.* New York, NY: WB Saunders; 2001.

Keck JO, Collopy BT, Ryan PJ, et al. Reversal of Hartmann's procedure: Effect of timing and technique on ease and safety. *Dis Colon Rectum* 1994;37(3):243–248.

Korman MU. Radiologic evaluation and staging of small intestinal neoplasms. *Eur J Radiol* 2002;42(3):193–205.

Lee EC, Murray JJ, Coller JA, et al. Intraoperative colonic lavage and primary anastomosis in nonelective surgery for diverticular disease. *Dis Colon Rectum* 1997; 40(6):669–674.

Maggard MA, Zingmond D, O'Connell, Ko CY. What proportion of patients with an ostomy (for diverticulitis) get reversed? *Am Surg* 2004;70(10):928–931.

Mallo RD, Salem L, Lalani T, et al. Computed tomography diagnosis of ischemia and complete obstruction in small bowel obstruction: A systematic review. *J Gastrointest Surg* 2005;9(5):690–694.

Murray JJ, Schoetz DJ Jr, Coller JA, et al. Intraoperative colonic lavage and primary anastomosis in nonelective colon resection. *Dis Colon Rectum* 1991;34(7):527–531.

Runkel NS, Schlag P, Schwarz V, Herfarth C. Outcome after emergency surgery for cancer of the large intestine. *Br J Surg* 1991;78(2):183–188.

Sarr MG, Blukley GB, Zuidema GD. Preoperative recognition of intestinal strangulation obstruction: Prospective evaluation of diagnostic capability. *Am J Surg* 1983; 145(1):176–182.

Toaurel P, Kessler N, Lesnik A, et al. Helical CT of large bowel obstruction. *Abdominal Imaging* 2003;28(2):267–275.

Varana AM III, DeBaros J. Ogilve's syndrome (colonic pseudo-obstruction). In: Cameron JL, ed. *Current Surgical Therapy.* Philadelphia, Pa: Mosby; 2004.

Whang EE, Ashley SW, Zinner MJ. Small intestine. In: Brunicardi FC, Andersen DK, Billiar TR, et al. *Schwartz's Principles of Surgery.* 8th ed. New York, NY: McGraw-Hill; 2005.

ACUTE ANORECTAL PAIN

LINDA M. FARKAS AND
FREDERICK J. DENSTMAN

64

I. INTRODUCTION

A. The most common causes of anal pain are fissure, hemorrhoidal thrombosis, and infection. Most patients afflicted by one of these lesions presents with a chief complaint of "rectal pain." The key first step in the history-taking process is garnering a more precise description of the pain location.

B. Most etiologies of anal pain can be diagnosed on the history coupled with a simple exam, which generally consists of inspection and palpation.

C. Only a few simple instruments are required for the diagnosis and treatment of most acute cases of anorectal pain. Many colon and rectal surgeons employ a proctology table which allows examination in the prone jackknife position. Although ideal, these tables are seldom available in most emergency departments (EDs), and a standard exam table with a decibitus positioned patient is adequate. A good exam light is imperative and this need be little more than the light provided by a 60-watt light bulb. Although anoscopes and rigid sigmoidoscopes should be available in the ED and acute care clinic, it should be stressed that in most patients with severe anal or rectal pain, endoscopy is usually unnecessary for arrival at the correct diagnosis and is often inhumane.

D. Lidocaine 0.5% with epinephrine is an excellent choice for local anesthesia. Some practitioners will mix this with bicarbonate solution to decrease the acidity of the lidocaine and therefore the pain of injection. Bupivicaine 0.25% can also be mixed with the lidocaine or used alone or after initial anesthesia to extend the duration of relief.

E. To deliver the local anesthesia, a 1.5-cc or 3-cc syringe with a 21- or 22-gauge needle with which to draw up local anesthesia is adequate. A 27- or 30-gauge needle is sufficient to inject the local anesthesia; larger needles are unnecessarily more uncomfortable. A larger gauge needle, such as a 16 gauge, is excellent for aspirating a suspected site of abscess.

II. ANATOMY

A. The rectum and anus are specialized segments of the gastrointestinal tract. The rectum functions primarily as a reservoir for stool. The rectosigmoid junction is marked by the merging of the taenia coli into the complete layer of longitudinal muscularis propria of the rectum. This junction is easily defined during laparotomy but can only be estimated during endoscopy. The distance between anal verge and rectosigmoid junction varies over a fairly wide range from patient to patient, from approximately 12 to 16 cm.

B. The surgical rectum ends at the level of the puborectalis muscle, which marks the hiatus through the levator ani muscles. This hiatus is palpable during digital rectal exam as the **anorectal ring**. The anal canal begins at the anorectal ring and extends to the anal verge. It is embraced by the anal sphincter muscles. The **dentate line** is the line between mucosa and skin and is located several centimeters proximally within the canal. The skin immediately distal to this line is the anoderm. The anoderm is a modified squamous epithelium, containing no accessory glands. The anoderm is very sensitive. The **anal** verge marks the junction between the anoderm and normal skin. This is easily identified by the appearance of hair-bearing skin.

C. Hemorrhoids are normal anatomic structures surrounding the anus. This collection of arteries and veins form an anal cushion and are thought to participate in the mechanism of fecal continence. The vessels proximal to the dentate line or mucocutaneous border and covered by mucosa are called **internal hemorrhoids**. Those vessels distal to the dentate line and covered by skin are called **external hemorrhoids**. These vessels are supported by surrounding connective tissue. Degeneration of this supporting connective tissue seems to be a common pathway to the development of hemorrhoidal disease.

III. FISSURE-IN-ANO

A. **Anal fissure** is the most common cause of acute anal pain. When asked to describe the pain from a fissure, most patients will use terms such as "sharp," "cutting," or "it feels like something tore." The pain usually is brought on by a bowel movement, but often the pain becomes most severe immediately following the movement and persists for 5 to 10 minutes. Occasionally, it is constant or increased by sitting.

B. When asked, most patients will describe minor anal bleeding, usually on the toilet tissue, streaking the outside of the stool or occasionally, dripping into the bowl. Patients will occasionally ascribe the pain to a swelling, but unlike the swelling described for hemorrhoids or abscesses, this swelling is usually chronic and small. The swelling is in fact not the exact site of the pain but is the sentinel skin tag that is adjacent but distal to the actual fissure.

C. Fissures are typically classified as either acute or chronic, although many patients will have features of both. The typical **acute fissure** occurs following some excessive wear and tear on the anoderm, which is the very sensitive ring of skin that extends from the dentate line to the anal verge. This is usually a hard, forceful bowel movement, although multiple loose stools over a short period of time (e.g., following colonoscopy bowel prep) can have an equally harmful effect. Patients with irritable bowel syndrome are prone to multiple, acute anal fissures. In an otherwise normal anal canal, an acute fissure will heal in a day or two.

D. In patients with **chronic fissure**, the fissure fails to heal. Excessively high tone in the internal anal sphincter muscle is the accepted etiology of the chronic fissure, and this is thought to act by decreasing blood flow to the anoderm. As the fissure matures, it becomes deeper and wider, eventually exposing the fibers of the internal sphincter muscle.

E. Many patients seem to have a subacute syndrome, with overlapping features of both acute and chronic fissure. Their pain is characterized by good weeks and bad weeks. The fissure becomes relatively asymptomatic as is covered by a thin layer of immature scar, only to be split open again by a difficult bowel movement. This pattern of alternating severe pain and relief persists over a course of months. Even though these patients may present with acute pain, these fissures are best treated as chronic fissures.

F. Occasionally the fissures become infected. This usually occurs as a result of incomplete healing of the fissure, such that a hood of skin forms over the fissure and traps stool particles beneath. These lesions are more practically treated as infections than fissures in the acute setting (*vide infra*).

G. **Diagnosis.** In most cases, a careful history clarifies the diagnosis, which can be verified on physical exam. Typical anal fissures are located in either the posterior or anterior midline. Since fissures reside in the anoderm, the most superficial aspect of the anal canal, an anoscope is usually not required to make this diagnosis. The anoderm can usually be well visualized by simply spreading apart the buttocks.

1. The acute fissure is usually superficial and linear. The classic chronic fissure is a teardrop-shaped ulceration of the anoderm, with an associated "sentinel tag" on its distal end and a hypertrophied papilla on its proximal end. The transversely oriented fibers of the internal sphincter are visible within the bed of the chronic fissure. The sphincter will not be visible in an acute fissure. As stated, patients can sometimes manifest features of both acute and chronic fissure.

2. Once a typical midline fissure is visualized, no further immediate diagnostic maneuvers are required. If no fissure is visualized, proceed with a gentle digital exam. If the exam fails to evoke tenderness, anoscopy can be performed. If anoscopy is negative, assume the patient had an acute fissure that has healed. If digital exam is tender in the absence of a fissure, move down the list of differential diagnoses.

3. If the fissure is located well off the midline, this is referred to as an **atypical fissure**, and this must be noted as such because it may have special diagnostic and therapeutic significance.

H. **Treatment.** By definition, an acute fissure should heal after the precipitating problems with bowel habit are corrected. This is usually a matter of prescribing a better diet for the patient, including more fiber, water, or a bulk laxative. Constipating medications, such as narcotics, should be avoided when possible. An antidiarrheal medication may be helpful in patients with chronic loose stools

1. To treat the acute pain, topical anesthetic in the form of 5% lidocaine ointment is helpful. The patient places 0.5 to 1.0 inch of the ointment into the anal canal by fingertip about 5 minutes before a bowel movement. This will usually provide the patient with good pain relief while waiting for the fissure to heal.

2. With proper diet most acute fissures, and even some chronic fissures, will heal. However, if healing does not occur within 3 to 4 weeks of good conservative management, additional treatment is required. The gold standard for treatment of chronic fissure is a partial, lateral internal sphincterotomy. This surgical treatment has the advantage of a rapid and lasting relief of symptoms in 95% of patients.

3. Several topical medications are potential alternatives to sphincterotomy. These include injectable botulinim toxin and ointment formulations of 0.2% nitroglycerin, 2% diltiazem, or 0.3% nifedipine applied twice daily. Unlike an operation, they tend to work slowly and their effectiveness is usually measured over a period of months rather than days or weeks.

I. **Atypical fissures.** Fissures located well off the midline are called **atypical fissures**. Occasionally patients with diarrhea will develop multiple, very superficial fissures related to excessive bowel movements and wiping. This type of atypical fissure usually will heal spontaneously.

1. **Solitary atypical fissures that do not heal quickly are a reason for concern.** The differential diagnosis includes squamous cell carcinoma of the anus, Crohn's disease, and syphilis. Many patients with Crohn's will already carry a diagnosis. Even for the undiagnosed Crohn's patient, there will usually be other signs or symptoms of the disease. However, there are rare patients whose initial presentation consists only of a painful, persistent atypical fissure. Squamous cell carcinoma of the anus can present as a small fissure. These early cancers tend to be extremely painful. As the disease progresses, the lesion takes on the more typical appearance of an ulcerated, hard mass. Diagnosis requires biopsy.

IV. THROMBOSED AND PROLAPSED HEMORRHOIDS

A. Generally, the patient will describe the sudden appearance of a hard, painful external swelling around the anus. This often follows a difficult bowel movement, but may present without obvious precipitating cause.

1. Frequently, the patient will have a long history of hemorrhoidal problems. Typically, the pain progresses for 1 to 2 days, plateaus, and then begins to improve. The pain is steady and is not increased by a bowel movement; these features distinguish it from fissure pain. It tends to be aggravated mainly by direct pressure. Patients will compare the swelling to a hard pea beneath the skin or a cluster of grapes. Many patients (and even some physicians) attempt to push thrombosed external hemorrhoids back up into the anal canal. This obviously does not work, but it is commonly related during the history. Prolapsing internal hemorrhoids may be successfully reduced.

B. Etiology. When the external hemorrhoids lose their connective tissue support, they tend to dilate and blood flow through the veins tends to slow, leading to clot formation or thrombosis. As the skin becomes ischemic, pain can become intense. Small areas of gangrene may develop, and if the skin sloughs, clot will extrude from the external hemorrhoid leading to some relief in pain.

C. Internal hemorrhoids are much less prone to thrombosis than external hemorrhoids. As internal hemorrhoids lose support, they tend to **prolapse** into the anal canal. Although severe prolapse can lead to pain, the common symptom of prolapsing internal hemorrhoids is painless anal bleeding.

1. Although pregnancy seems to be a common cause of hemorrhoidal disease, for many patients there is no obvious etiology.

2. Patients often describe the onset of problems after a particularly painful bowel movement or a day of diarrhea. Very rarely a low rectal carcinoma can lead to thrombosed hemorrhoids.

D. Diagnosis. A thrombosed external hemorrhoid should be apparent on physical exam. Most commonly, it is a distinct lateral swelling of the hair-bearing skin, often with a blue tint. Midline swelling should suggest either a sentinel tag from a fissure or an infection. The swelling is usually firm and tender. Beyond 2 days' duration, the thrombosis tends to be softer and less tender. Internal exam may be painful and can be deferred in patients with severely painful hemorrhoids. Internal exam should be completed at a later date.

E. Treatment. In the acute setting of the first 24 to 48 hours, the best treatment for a simple thrombosed hemorrhoid is surgical excision.

1. This is best done in prone jackknife position, although it can be done in lateral position as well. The skin overlying the hemorrhoid is infiltrated with **0.5% lidocaine with 1:200,000 epinephrine.** An unhurried injection through a 30-gauge needle will decrease the discomfort from this injection. Both the overlying skin and underlying subcutaneous tissue should be infiltrated.

2. Using a fine, sharp scissors (Metzenbaum or iris scissors) an ellipse of overlying skin will expose the underlying thrombus, which can then be excised as well. Since multiple small clots are generally encountered, simple "lancing" or incision of the hemorrhoid is usually inadequate and should be avoided.

3. Excision may also avoid a recurrence of future thrombosis in the hemorrhoid. **Do not excise the anoderm**; keep the excision well lateral in the hair-bearing region only. Involving the anoderm will lead to more postoperative pain and perhaps the development of a chronic fissure.

4. Since the hemorrhoid is thrombosed, little bleeding is encountered, especially if local anesthesia contains epinephrine. Silver nitrate can be applied for nuisance bleeding. Traditionally, this small wound is left open and heals very nicely, although suturing the wound closed with chromic catgut or some other absorbable material is an option.

5. **Bupivicaine** can be injected to prolong duration of anesthesia. The patient is advised to take two to three sitz baths or tub baths a day, for 2 to 3 days, or until minor bleeding on a clean pad or gauze stops. Provide a prescription for an opioid for 24 to 48 hours.

6. If the hemorrhoid has been present for longer than 48 to 72 hours, and is beginning to soften or hurt less, excision will generally not be necessary. If the hemorrhoid has already necrosed and begun to drain, no operation is required, although occasionally there is a role for minor debridement of the gangrenous tissue or assistance with complete evacuation of the clot. This requires local anesthesia.

F. Complicated hemorrhoid disease. Patients may present with multiple discrete areas of external thrombosis. They may develop a more involved process with nearly circumferential or confluent areas of thrombosis and extensive edema. These patients may also have irreducible, circumferential prolapse of the internal hemorrhoids (grade 4 prolapse). The internal hemorrhoids can then begin to thrombose. This can further progress to the development of gangrenous changes in the skin and anal mucosa.

1. These more severe expressions of hemorrhoidal disease cannot be treated by the acute care physician in a simple outpatient setting. These patients are probably best served by referral to a surgeon who is experienced in the treatment of severe anorectal disease. The surgeon may elect to attempt a bedside reduction after injection with local anesthesia (and hyaluronidase if available). Alternatively this patient may require more formal operative intervention.

V. PERIANAL INFECTIONS

A. Perianal and ischiorectal abscesses are common causes of perianal pain. The pain is usually severe, constant, and tends to increase with time. Most abscesses develop over the course of a day or two; occasionally, with a more chronic presentation.

B. Patients will usually describe a tender swelling. Unlike fissures, the pain is usually not strongly associated with bowel movements. When present, the symptoms of fever and malaise can suggest abscess, but fever is often absent.

C. Etiology. Most perianal suppurative disease begins in the cryptoglandular space. The infection migrates along the course of the anal gland's ducts. These ducts travel to various anatomic spaces around the anus, and the abscess evolves where these ducts terminate.

　　1. Anal fissures probably are responsible for many perianal infections. In this case, the fissure is a direct portal for bacterial invasion into the underlying subcutaneous or intersphincteric space. These patients will usually describe a typical fissure type history which precedes the development of the constantly tender swelling.

　　2. Although only a small percentage of abscesses are caused by Crohn's disease, it is important to consider this in patients with an abscess. All patients with abscesses should be questioned about chronic diarrhea and abdominal pain, the presence of which should at least raise the suspicion of inflammatory bowel disease.

D. Diagnosis. Most perianal infection is apparent on simple inspection as a raised, erythematous swelling near the anal verge. The swelling is usually quite tender and often fluctuant.

　　1. Abscesses deep in the ischiorectal or posterior anal spaces may be less obvious on inspection, lacking the erythematous skin changes, but can be identified by a tender area of induration and swelling. The swelling is sometimes subtle when palpated through the skin, but generally obvious on palpation through the anal mucosa during digital exam.

　　2. Abscesses confined to the intersphincteric space are less common and more difficult to identify. These tend to be small with only subtle amounts of swelling palpable on digital exam. These patients will give a history more suggestive of fissure, with pain strongly associated with bowel movements, but on physical exam no fissure is seen. There may be a complete absence of physical findings, other than tenderness.

E. Treatment. The treatment for an abscess is operative drainage. There is no indication for allowing an abscess to "mature" or "ripen." Furthermore, antibiotics are not a substitute for drainage.

　　1. Most abscesses are superficial and easily drained with simple instruments and techniques. The deeper infections may require consultation with a surgeon and exam under anesthesia and drainage in the operating room.

　　2. For the majority of patients, the overlying skin is anesthetized with 0.5% lidocaine and epinephrine. The skin is then incised with the no. 11 scalpel blade, allowing drainage of the pus. A generous disk of skin, at least 5 mm in diameter, should be excised to allow ongoing drainage of the pus, and to prevent premature closure of the skin, which leads to rapid recurrence of the infection.

　　3. If the abscess is deep and not easily demonstrated by simple inspection or palpation, a trial aspiration with the larger 16-gauge needle may be employed as a localizing maneuver.

　　4. Many physicians incise then insert packing into the abscess cavity. This painful practice of packing and repacking serves no useful purpose, except in the rare case of controlling bleeding from deep in the wound. If an adequately large drainage incision is created, the abscess will drain very well without packing and, in fact, packing the wound inhibits adequate drainage. An indwelling drain may be left in place for several days, but this is not our practice.

5. Probing into the abscess cavity should be avoided. This can lead to creation of false openings into the anal canal as well as unnecessary bleeding from the depth of the wound.

6. In some cases, drainage of an abscess is a definitive therapy leading to a complete resolution of the suppurative process. Unfortunately, more than 50% of patients will develop a recurrent abscess or form an anal fistula, indicating the presence of a persistent internal opening within the anal canal. Follow-up is required and is most appropriately performed by a surgeon experienced in the treatment of anal fistulae.

7. Although antibiotics are not appropriate as primary treatment of an abscess, they may be added as an adjunct to drainage in patients who are immunocompromised or those with cellulitis surrounding a well-drained abscess cavity. The resolution of erythema within a few minutes of the incision and drainage procedure is a good sign that antibiotics will not be required. If needed, antibiotic therapy should be directed toward gram negative and anaerobic organisms.

VI. PILONIDAL DISEASE

A. Pilonidal disease typically presents during puberty or young adulthood. It is more common among young men and presents similar to most abscess processes. The patient is more likely to describe this in relation to the tailbone as opposed to the anus.

B. Etiology. Pilonidal disease is believed to be initiated by the ingrowth of hair follicles. It is most common in hirsute males, although occasionally seen in women with little hair. The process is encouraged by the presence of a deep gluteal cleft. It is believed to begin as one or a series of several midline sinuses. Skin flora migrate down the sinus tracts and cause midline abscess formation, which frequently extends bilaterally. Hair shafts frequently migrate down the sinus tracts and on occasion rather large hair plugs are trapped within the abscess cavity.

C. Diagnosis. Pilonidal abscess is easily diagnosed as a tender, erythematous midline swelling. The lesions generally originate superior to the coccyx, although extension of the primary process toward the coccyx is not unusual. Careful scrutiny will usually reveal one or more sinuses with protruding hair shafts.

D. Treatment for pilonidal abscess is drainage, often performed in the emergency department or clinic setting.

1. With the patient placed in either prone jackknife or Sims position, the skin overlying the abscess is infiltrated with local anesthesia. The abscess is then incised with a no. 11 scalpel blade. Following this a disk of skin should be excised to enhance adequate drainage. Hair plugs should be removed if present.

2. Packing is not indicated except to control bleeding. The overlying skin may be several millimeters thick and require a fairly deep incision to initiate the drainage. An exploratory needle aspiration may be helpful.

3. Antibiotics may be used as an adjunct in immunocompromised patients or in cases with extensive cellulitis.

4. With pilonidal disease, abscess recurrence is the rule rather than the exception. Referral to a surgeon for follow-up is required. Definitive treatment of pilonidal disease is controversial.

VII. FOURNIER'S (PERINEAL) GANGRENE

A. Fournier's gangrene is a true surgical emergency, albeit rare. These patients generally present with systemic signs of infection. This is a disease that tends to afflict diabetics and immunocompromised adults.

B. These patients will complain of severe, diffuse perineal and perianal pain. Although urinary retention is associated with any form of perianal pain, it is very common with Fournier's gangrene. There may be an antecedent history of trauma. These patients are often brought in by ambulance because the pain prohibits them from walking. They are often febrile and have a significant leukocytosis.

C. Fournier's gangrene is a necrotizing infection of the deep perianal or perineal fascia. The portal of entry can be any form of perianal infection, but breaks in the perineal, vaginal, or scrotal skin are often the source of infection. Blunt trauma can be the initiator. In many cases the first site of bacterial entry is never identified.

D. Diagnosis. The classic finding is crepitance on palpation of the exquisitely tender perineal skin or a blackened area of ischemic skin in the perineum, perianum, scrotum, or vaginal labia. A worrisome clue to the diagnosis of Fournier's gangrene is a gray, watery discharge from an abscess cavity, or the presence of gray subcutaneous tissue at the base of the abscess. Although imaging studies are usually not necessary to make this diagnosis, the presence of gas in the soft tissues can be seen on plain x-ray or CT films. Systemic signs—fever, tachycardia, tachypnea, and chills—are seen often.

E. Fournier's gangrene is a life-threatening disease and requires prompt attention, with both immediate broad-spectrum antibiotics and surgical evaluation.

  1. Once resuscitated, these patients must be treated in the operating room with very aggressive, wide surgical debridement.

  2. Although not necessary in all cases, many patients will require fecal diversion at some point in the course of their disease.

VIII. RECTAL PAIN FOLLOWING THE TREATMENT OF HEMORRHOIDS

A. Barron ligation is a common and time-proven treatment for prolapsing hemorrhoids. With this technique a small rubber band is applied to a small section of mucosa at the apex of a prolapsing internal hemorrhoid. The band strangulates this small disk of mucosa which then sloughs in 2 to 3 days, leading to the formation of a small ulcer and ultimately a small scar. The scar leads to fixation of the hemorrhoid so it no longer prolapses into the anal canal during bowel movements, and is therefore less likely to bleed.

  1. The properly applied rubber band should be placed at least 2 cm above the dentate line where there are no somatic pain receptors; ideally, the patient should have no pain following proper application of the band. However, three different types of discomfort may be experienced and need to be differentiated.

  a. The most common discomfort is a vague pressure or sense of tenesmus that is noted soon after band application. This is due to the physical presence of a small mass in the anal canal which visceral receptors interpret as a stool bolus. This is usually a mild discomfort and generally passes within 24 hours, requiring no treatment beyond reassurance of the patient.

  b. The second most common discomfort is a severe, sharp pain which the patient feels very soon or immediately with application of the band. This occurs when the band is applied too far distally (i.e., at the level of somatic skin sensation). This should hopefully be recognized by the doctor applying the band and remedied by either removing or repositioning the band more proximally.

  c. The third type of discomfort is very rare but must be recognized and treated aggressively. This presents in a delayed fashion as severe rectal pain, perhaps a day or two after the procedure. It is frequently accompanied by urinary retention, fever, and other signs of sepsis. This pain results from infection and possibly necrosis, extending from the anal mucosa to deeper layers of the rectum and ultimately into the pelvis. Recognition of this entity requires institution of broad-spectrum parenteral antibiotics and possible debridement of the rectal wall. Left untreated, this rectal sepsis can lead to death.

B. Procedure for prolapsing hemorrhoids (PPH). PPH is a relatively new method of treating prolapsing internal hemorrhoids. The PPH device is a modified form of the intraluminal circular stapling device employed for creating low anterior anastomoses. The PPH device excises a ring of anal mucosa and then reanatomoses it, causing fixation of the mucosa. This then prevents prolapse of the internal hemorrhoids. It is analogous to Barron ligation, but creates a circumferential fixation as opposed to scarring down one hemorrhoid at a time.

1. Similar to the rubber banding technique, this device ideally should cause no sensation. However, this is not always the case and discomfort is common. The acute care physician should be aware of two different types of discomfort following the PPH procedure.

  a. The most common discomfort is best described as severe tenesmus, or a very strong and false urge to defecate. This can be distressing enough for the patient to request narcotic pain relief. It can persist for days or weeks after surgery.

  b. A rare but much more serious pain can occur as a symptom of pelvic sepsis, similar to the situation of infection developing after Barron ligation. These patients present with various other symptoms and signs of systemic sepsis, and again must be treated aggressively with parenteral antibiotics and require surgical consultation.

IX. PELVIC FLOOR PAIN

A. Levator pain. The floor of the pelvis is formed primarily by the levator and puborectalis muscles. A hiatus exists for the ostia of the gastrointestinal and genitourinary systems. Pains in the levator muscle or any organ traveling through its hiatus is frequently perceived as a rectal pain.

  1. Levator spasm can present with a constant feeling of fullness or pain. This is frequently compared by the patient as the sense of sitting on a ball. This pain tends to be chronic and is unlikely to be a presenting symptom in the ED.

  2. Proctalgia fugax is a severe, acute pain that frequently will awaken a patient from sleep. It is typically self-limited, lasting only minutes, but can be quite alarming to the patient with its first presentation and may trigger a visit to the ED. This is a poorly understood entity and is thought to be an acute spasm of some portion of the levator muscle. These patients are almost always pain free by the time they present to the physician and the sudden onset and brief duration of this rectal pain is pathognomonic of this disorder. There is a complete absence of visible physical findings. The main treatment of proctalgia fugax is to make the diagnosis and then reassure the patient that the pain, no matter how distressing, is a form of muscle cramp, is not a serious health problem, but may be prone to recurrence.

B. Uterine pain. Lesions arising from the uterus or uterine adnexae can present with pain radiating to the rectum. The gynecologic origin of this pain may at least be suspected by the history. A gentle but thorough digital exam that includes manipulation of the uterine cervix should also suggest the extrarectal origin of this pain. This should then be followed by a bimanual pelvic exam.

C. Prostatic pain. Men frequently describe pain arising in the prostate gland as rectal pain. This will most likely be prostatitis, with the finding of a tender, soft prostate gland on digital rectal exam. This pain usually responds to antibiotic therapy directed against the usual urinary pathogens. A more problematic entity is prostadynia, a pain in the prostate not necessarily caused by acute infection. This is a chronic disorder, more appropriately treated by an urologist on a nonurgent basis.

AXIOMS

- Careful history and simple examination will diagnose most causes of anal pain.
- An anal fissure that is off the midline, an atypical fissure, may be a squamous cell carcinoma.
- The treatment for a perianal abscess is operative drainage. A 5-mm disc of skin should be excised to ensure adequate drainage.

65

MICHAEL C. COELLO AND
VAISHALI DIXIT SCHUCHERT

I. INTRODUCTION. Hernias are problems frequently encountered faced by surgeons in both the elective and emergency setting. The estimated lifetime risk of developing a spontaneous hernia worldwide is 5%, while the incidence of secondary hernias arising from abdominal incisions is 10% to 15%. Inguinal hernias display a 7:1 male-to-female predominance, with the prevalence correlating with advancing age.

II. ANATOMY. An intimate knowledge of the anatomy and understanding of the physical concepts is essential to approaching the diagnosis and treatment of hernias. The abdominal wall consists of layers of musculature with crossing fibers inserting into aponeuroses of relatively dense connective tissue. Defects in these aponeurotic areas, along with penetrating structures (nerves, vessels, gonadal structures) can lead to herniation of abdominal contents, most often small bowel. There are a number of abdominal wall hernias defined by the hernia contents and by the anatomical relationship of the sac to the abdominal wall and structures. A particularly susceptible area is the groin, where indirect and direct inguinal hernias as well as femoral hernias arise, as distinguished by their relationship to the inferior epigastric vessels and the inguinal ligament (Fig. 65-1).

III. COMPLICATIONS OF HERNIAS. Existing literature indicates that 5% to 15% of patients with groin hernias undergo emergency surgery secondary to incarceration or strangulation. However, in any type of hernia, the general practice of repairing even asymptomatic hernias at the time of diagnosis has made it difficult to accurately determine the actual risk of developing complications (i.e., incarceration, obstruction, strangulation). A recent prospective study suggested that asymptomatic inguinal hernias can be followed safely.

  A. Incarceration. Abdominal contents are contained within the hernia sac and cannot be reduced.
  B. Obstruction. Hernias are the leading cause of intestinal obstruction worldwide and the third most common cause in the United States and other Western countries. Obstruction may be acute or intermittent and chronic.
  C. Strangulation involves compromise of the blood supply leading to ischemia, necrosis, and eventual perforation of the bowel wall. The pathophysiology of strangulation generally involves obstruction—with subsequent edema of the bowel wall, venous engorgement, and ultimately arteriolar compression—leading to both venous and arterial ischemia. Up to 15% of incarcerated hernias are associated with bowel necrosis. An exception to this is a **Richter's hernia** where a segment of the intestinal wall can become strangulated without obstruction of the viscus. Strangulation is a true surgical emergency associated with a 30% to 40% morbidity and 10% mortality rate.

IV. PRESENTATION. Uncomplicated hernias may be asymptomatic but may often present as a bulge associated with vague discomfort or neuralgia. An incarcerated hernia may also be asymptomatic except for the presence of a persistent bulge. Patients with an incarcerated hernia may present with a history and physical findings consistent with obstruction including nausea, vomiting, abdominal distension, obstipation, or diarrhea. Certainly, any patient presenting with suspected bowel obstruction should be

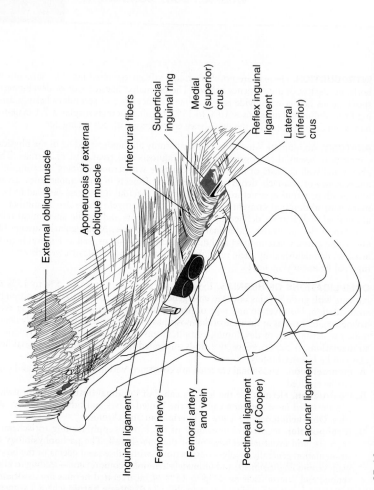

External oblique muscle

Aponeurosis of external oblique muscle

Intercrural fibers

Superficial inguinal ring

Medial (superior) crus

Reflex inguinal ligament

Lateral (inferior) crus

Inguinal ligament

Femoral nerve

Femoral artery and vein

Pectineal ligament (of Cooper)

Lacunar ligament

Figure 65-1A. The inguinal, lacunar, and pectineal ligaments, and the superficial inguinal ring. (From Clemente CD. *Clemente's Anatomy Dissector.* 2nd ed. Baltimore, Md: Lippincott Williams & Wilkins; 2007:127, with permission.)

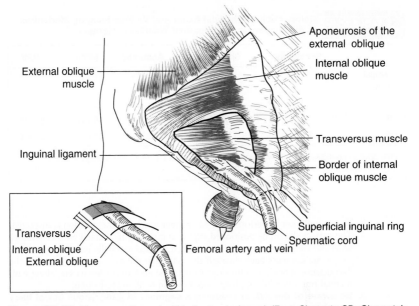

Figure 65-1B. The spermatic cord within the inguinal canal. (From Clemente CD. *Clemente's Anatomy Dissector.* 2nd ed. Baltimore, Md: Lippincott Williams & Wilkins; 2007:127, with permission.)

evaluated for the presence of a hernia. Signs and symptoms of strangulation include a tender, tense, irreducible bulge, with erythema or bluish discoloration of the overlying skin. The patient may be ill-appearing, febrile, have a leukocytosis with left shift, acidosis, or have signs of local or diffuse peritonitis.

V. DIAGNOSIS. Diagnosis is most often based solely on a thorough history and physical examination. The patient should be examined in both the recumbent and standing positions, if feasible, to look for intermittent or persistent bulging in the abdominal wall or groin. Diligent clinical examination is paramount, as a patient with even life-threatening strangulation may not exhibit classical signs and symptoms. In the setting of diagnostic uncertainty, radiologic adjuncts may play a role:

A. Plain roentgenogram may demonstrate evidence of obstruction (air-fluid levels, bowel distention).

B. Ultrasound may be useful to evaluate contents of an abdominal mass, but is highly operator dependent.

C. Computed tomography (CT) and magnetic resonance imaging (MRI) identify abdominal and pelvic anatomical structures in relation to the abdominal wall and may display evidence of necrosis/ischemia (bowel wall thickening, lack of bowel wall enhancement, free air, etc.). These modalities have the added benefit of identifying other potential etiologies of abdominal or groin pain. Given the high specificity of physical exam findings, the utility of these imaging modalities should be limited to cases in which the diagnosis is in doubt (Table 65-1).

VI. MANAGEMENT (Fig. 65-2)

A. Nonoperative management

1. Incarceration in itself is not a surgical emergency. Chronically incarcerated hernias, without sign of obstruction or strangulation, should undergo repair, but this can be done on an elective basis. Reduction of an incarcerated hernia by gentle manual pressure (taxis) may be attempted.

TABLE 65-1	Comparison of Physical Exam and Various Imaging Modalities in the Diagnosis of Abdominal Wall/Groin Hernias				
	Sensitivity	**Specificity**	**Accuracy**	**PPV**	**NPV**
Physical exam	74.5%	96.3%	81.7%	97.6%	65%
CT	83%	67%–83%			
MRI	94.5%	96.3%	95.1%	98.1%	89.7%
US	92.7%	81.5%	89.0%	91.0%	84.6%

PPV, positive predictive value; NPV, negative predictive value; CT, computed tomography; MRI, magnetic resonance imaging; US, ultrasound.

2. Taxis should not be performed in any patient in whom strangulation is suspected. The patient should be positioned supine and should be relaxed with or without sedation. Gentle kneading pressure is then applied manually to coax and reduce the hernia contents back through the defect. In the case of a groin hernia, the Trendelenberg position with elongation of the neck of the hernia sac, along with manual traction while applying pressure, can facilitate reduction.

3. **Be aware of the risk of reducing a segment of gangrenous bowel back into the peritoneal cavity.**

   a. Overly forceful manual pressure may also result in the rare occurrence of **reductio en masse**, whereby the entire sac is rapidly reduced with the visceral contents remaining entrapped and compromised within the hernia sac itself. The potential for these complications demands continued monitoring and assessment of the patient to look for signs of worsening clinical condition suggestive of ongoing pathology. Once an incarcerated hernia is manually reduced, early definitive surgical repair during the same hospitalization is recommended, unless medical contraindications exist.

B. **Operative repair**

   1. In the case of a patient with signs of obstruction or strangulation, timely diagnosis and intervention is paramount. The duration of symptoms (>6 hours) has been shown to be a significant factor in the need for bowel resection. Such patients require rapid fluid and electrolyte resuscitation, nasogastric decompression, and antibiotics, coupled with timely surgical intervention. The basic principles of surgical repair of an incarcerated hernia are the same regardless of type of hernia: **Explore the hernia sac for compromised viscera, reduce the hernia, and repair the defect.**

   2. The use of synthetic mesh is generally contraindicated in the setting of strangulated bowel or contamination. If primary repair is not feasible and mesh is necessary to close the defect, absorbable synthetic polyglactin (Vicryl) or porcine extracellular matrix (Surgisis) may be used. These materials serve a role in contaminated scenarios, but are not suitable for permanent repair as they leave a fascial defect behind when they are absorbed. Once the infection has cleared and the patient has recovered, one can consider reoperation, either open or laparoscopically, with placement of synthetic mesh for definitive repair.

   3. There have been several recent small studies and case reports describing laparoscopic repair of incarcerated hernias. Proponents of this approach cite the ability to evaluate the viability of the hernia contents using the laparoscope and suggest such an approach would decrease the morbidity and mortality associated with emergency laparotomy. To date, however, there are no adequate trials to compare open versus laparoscopic repair of incarcerated hernias.

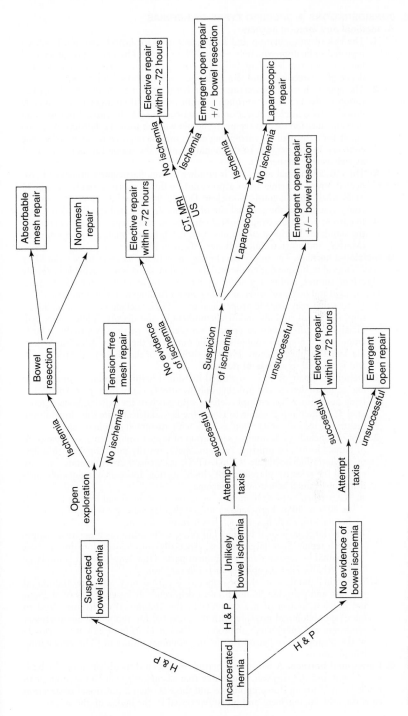

Figure 65-2. Incarcerated hernia decision tree.

VII. CONSIDERATIONS IN SPECIFIC TYPES OF HERNIAS

A. Inguinal and femoral hernias

1. The risk of strangulation and subsequent need for bowel resection has been reported to be approximately 4% to 8% in inguinal hernias. Though femoral hernias comprise less than 10% of hernias, these femoral hernias carry a 40% incidence of incarceration and strangulation requiring bowel resection.

2. The approach to an incarcerated groin hernia is best taken directly, by exploration of the hernia sac through a groin incision. If strangulated, nonviable bowel is encountered, resection and anastomosis can be carried out through the same incision used to repair the hernia without formal celiotomy. A releasing incision through the entrapping defect may be required to safely reduce the contents. It is imperative to thoroughly explore the region for indirect, direct, as well as femoral hernias.

3. The intraabdominal approach is another option, particularly in cases of suspected bowel ischemia from a previously reduced incarcerated hernia, or in cases where the diagnosis is unclear. During the intraabdominal approach, a counterincision at the external site of the hernia may facilitate reduction.

4. In current practice, extraperitoneal tension-free mesh repair of groin hernias is the standard. The most commonly used synthetic materials are polypropylene (Marlex) and polytetrafluoroethylene (GORE-TEX).

B. Incisional hernias.
The risk of developing an incisional hernia can be reduced by good surgical technique during the initial operation, using nonabsorbable or slowly absorbing sutures, and taking adequate bites, approximately 2 cm back from the fascial edge and one centimeter apart in either a running or interrupted fashion.

1. Factors that may impede proper healing of fascia include infection, malnutrition, the use of steroids and/or chemotherapy, and obesity. If left unrepaired, incisional hernias tend to enlarge progressively so that eventually a large amount of abdominal contents will lie outside of the fascial defect in the hernia sac. This phenomenon results in shrinkage of the abdominal cavity itself, and is referred to as **loss of domain**.

2. Definitive repair of an incarcerated incisional hernia mandates removing or excluding all defects and utilizing only healthy fascia in the repair. The underlying fascia often has multiple defects with much of the existing fascia attenuated. It is often not possible to repair the fascial defect primarily. In addition, recurrence may occur as often as 50% with attempted simple repair.

3. Options include performing a separation of fascial components, or separation of parts, closure, or utilizing synthetic mesh, usually polypropylene (Marlex) or polytetrafluoroethylene (GORE-TEX). If extensive subcutaneous flaps are created the selective placement of closed suction drains may reduce the incidence of retained hematoma or seroma.

   a. Recurrence rates with anterior mesh repair of incisional hernias is as high as 30% to 40%. Early reports suggest that laparoscopic repair of incisional hernia with mesh has a much lower recurrence rate.

   b. Very large incisional hernias fail often with either open or laparoscopic mesh repair. Such large hernias, especially with loss of domain, are best repaired by separation of component parts. How large a defect is too large for reliable laparoscopic repair is not yet clear.

4. Abdominal binders in the postoperative period may alleviate abdominal pressure and pain, but do not prevent dehiscence. In cases of loss of abdominal domain, return of the contents to the abdominal cavity may lead to increased abdominal pressure with the potential for abdominal compartment syndrome and pulmonary compromise. These patients must be watched closely in the postoperative period for the development of any of these devastating complications.

C. Peristomal hernias.
A peristomal hernia presents a difficult situation for both the patient and the surgeon. The bulge that occurs adjacent to the stoma can result in an ill-fitting stoma appliance and there is often a functional obstruction caused by the impingement and pressure exerted by the hernia on the stoma.

1. The presentation of an incarcerated peristomal hernia is similar to that of any external abdominal hernia, typically featuring a painful, tender bulge that is not reducible, with possible bowel obstruction with or without strangulation.

2. The simplest way to address a peristomal hernia is with relocation of the stoma and closure of the abdominal wall defect. This generally requires formal celiotomy. If the stoma cannot be moved, either a primary repair (if the defect involves less than one third of the stoma circumference) or in situ repair with mesh can be performed. Examination of the hernia sac prior to reduction of the hernia should be performed regardless of the surgical approach undertaken.

D. Traumatic diaphragmatic hernias

1. Both blunt and penetrating trauma can cause diaphragmatic injury. Blunt forces cause an abrupt increase in intraabdominal pressure, leading to rupture and extensive tears across the dome of the diaphragm. In penetrating trauma, the appropriate level of suspicion comes from an understanding of the anatomy of the diaphragm. The diaphragm is a dome that is projected on the external surface area of the torso from the 4th intercostal space to the 12th thoracic vertebra. Diagnosis of diaphragmatic injury requires a high index of suspicion. Approximately 25% to 40% of such injuries are readily apparent on chest roentgenograms. In the other 60% the findings are equivocal or negative. Diaphragmatic injures are easily missed by CT scan.

2. Early repair of diaphragmatic injury is best approached transabdominally as there is a high incidence (60%–80%) of concomitant intraabdominal injury. Late repair of diaphragmatic hernias after delayed diagnosis is usually best approached via thoracotomy, which facilitates lysis of adhesions between the lung parenchyma and abdominal viscera.

E. Spigelian hernias

1. The semilunar line (Spigelian line) marks the transition from muscular fibers to aponeurotic fibers of the transversus abdominis. A Spigelian hernia is one in which the sac passes through a defect in the Spigelian aponeurosis usually just lateral to the rectus abdominis sheath. Ninety percent occur within 6 cm above the level of the anterior superior iliac spines (Fig. 65-3).

2. The hernia sac is intraparietal, lying between the various muscle layers of the abdominal wall, and is therefore difficult to diagnose. These hernias usually present with vague abdominal pain, less commonly with signs of incarceration or obstruction, and are often not associated with a definable mass. Most commonly,

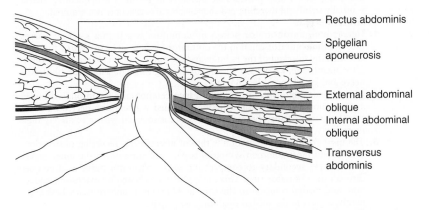

Figure 65-3A. Site of Spigelian hernia. Cross-sectional view of bowel protruding through defect in Spigelian aponeurosis. (From Richard AT, Quinn TH, Fitzgibbons RJ Jr. Abdominal wall hernias. In: Mullholland MW, Lillemoe KD, Doherty GM, et al., eds. *Greenfield's Surgery: Scientific Principles and Practice.* 4th ed. Philadelphia, Pa: Lippincott Williams & Wilkins; 2006:1187.)

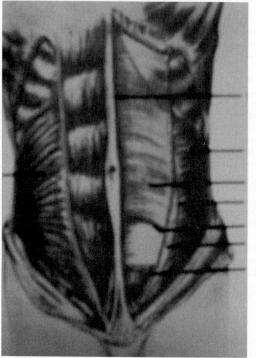

Linea alba

Tranversus abdominis

Rectus sheath
Spigelian line
Semicircular line
Spigelian aponeurosis
Rectus abdominis

Figure 65-3B. Ventral view of abdominal wall demonstrating Spigelian aponeurosis. (From Bennett D. Incidence and management of primary abdominal wall hernias: Spigelian hernia. In: Fitzgibbons RJ, Greenburg AG, eds. *Nyhus & Condon's Hernia.* 5th ed. Philadelphia, Pa: Lippincott Williams & Wilkins; 2002:406.)

ultrasound or CT scan provides the definitive diagnosis. The aponeurotic defect is usually small and therefore prosthetic material is generally not required.

F. Obturator hernias

1. Uncommon, an obturator hernia by definition is a hernia sac that passes through the obturator canal in the obturator foramen. The obturator foramen is formed by the rami of the ischium and the pubis, and is covered by the obturator membrane, except for the small opening through which the obturator nerve and vessels pass (Fig. 65-1).

2. These hernias frequently present with incarceration and compromised bowel and are most often found in elderly, emaciated women with decreased functional capacity. Thus obturator hernias are associated with a relatively high mortality.

3. The most common presentation is that of intermittent, recurring obstruction. The second most common symptom is pain radiating down the inner aspect of the thigh, secondary to compression of the obturator nerve as it courses through the obturator ring. This finding may be elicited by extension, adduction, and medial rotation of the leg (the Howship-Romberg sign). Less commonly, a mass in the medial thigh may be palpated.

4. The generally accepted approach to the obturator hernia is transabdominal. This approach allows the surgeon to establish the cause of obstruction when the diagnosis is in doubt, provides the best exposure to the obturator ring, and allows for intestinal resection which is frequently necessary.

G. Umbilical hernias. Umbilical hernias account for approximately 14% of all hernias. They are divided into congenital infantile hernias and adult acquired hernias.

1. The majority of infantile hernias will spontaneously close and rarely result in incarceration. Larger hernias and those that persist past 4 to 5 years of age are less likely to resolve. For these reasons, surgical repair is generally deferred until around 5 years of age, though at this point most families will seek surgical intervention for cosmetic and psychological considerations of the children.

2. Acquired umbilical hernias are often a result of chronically increased intraabdominal pressure secondary to pathologic conditions such as cirrhosis, congestive heart failure, chronic obstructive pulmonary disease (COPD), obesity, and renal failure.

3. The incidence of incarceration of umbilical hernias is 14 times higher in adults than in children, and such hernias are more likely to cause obstruction and strangulation. Therefore, for those whose medical comorbidities do not preclude surgery, surgical repair should be undertaken to avoid the increased morbidity of complications in this population of patients.

   a. A particularly difficult situation involves the patient with severe ascites, usually secondary to cirrhosis, and an umbilical hernia. Any operation in this type of patient is associated with an exceedingly high morbidity and mortality. Continued pressure exerted from within the peritoneal cavity leads to chronic incarceration and skin necrosis leading to leakage of ascites and peritonitis.

   b. The ideal management is through prevention (i.e., control of ascites with meticulous medical management and paracentesis if necessary). It is wise to counsel the patient and family regarding the high risk of an operation should surgical intervention become absolutely necessary.

H. Internal hernias

1. Internal hernias are defects in the peritoneum through which bowel and other abdominal viscera may pass. Internal hernias can be spontaneous, but are more frequently the iatrogenic result of a previous operation, whereby a defect created in the peritoneum, mesentery, or omentum has not been closed or has reopened.

2. Often the primary presentation is that of bowel obstruction, strangulation, or frank peritonitis. Though rare, malrotation may present in adults as an acute abdomen secondary to obstruction related to an internal hernia. An incarcerated internal hernia should be considered in the differential diagnosis of any patient who presents with a bowel obstruction or acute abdomen with no clearly identifiable etiology. Prompt celiotomy with repair of the anatomic defect or correction of the malrotation is the definitive treatment.

AXIOMS

- An incarcerated hernia is an irreducible hernia.
- An incarcerated hernia with signs of bowel obstruction and/or strangulation is a surgical emergency.
- History and physical exam is the most important diagnostic tool, with the use of adjunctive radiologic tests in the setting of diagnostic uncertainty.
- Patients with evidence of strangulated hernias require rapid fluid and electrolyte resuscitation, nasogastric suction, and antibiotics, followed by timely surgical intervention.
- Repair of the abdominal wall defect is the sine qua non of herniorrhaphy.
- Use of mesh is contraindicated in the setting of contamination and compromised bowel due to strangulation or bowel injury.

Bibliography

Abramson JH, Gofin J, Hopp C, et al. The epidemiology of inguinal hernia, a survey in western Jerusalem. *J Epidemiol Comm Health* 1978;32:59.

Bekoe S. Prospective analysis of the management of incarcerated and strangulated inguinal hernias. *Am J Surg* 1973;126:665–668.

Brasso K, Nielsen KL, Christiansen J. Long term results of surgery for incarcerated groin hernia. *Acta Chir Scand* 1989;155:583–585.

Brunicardi FC, Andersen DK, Billiar TR, et al. *Schwartz's Principles of Surgery*. 8th ed. New York, NY: McGraw-Hill; 2005.

Cameron JL, ed. *Current Surgical Therapy*. 6th ed. St. Louis, Mo: Mosby; 1998.

Ferzli G, Shapiro K, Chaudry G, Patel S. Laparoscopic extraperitoneal approach to acutely incarcerated inguinal hernia. *Surg Endosc* 2004;18:228–231.

Ishihara T, Kubota K, Eda N, et al. Laparoscopic approach to incarcerated inguinal hernia. *Surg Endosc* 1996;10:1111–1113.

Kulah B, Kulacoglu IH, Oruc MT, et al. Presentation and outcome of incarcerated external hernias in adults. *Am J Surg* 2001;181:101–104.

Kurt N, Oncel M, Ozkan Z, Bingul S. Risk and outcome of bowel resection in patients with incarcerated groin hernias: Retrospective study. *World J Surg* 2003;27:741–743.

Leibl BJ, Daubler P, Schmedt G, et al. Laparoscopic transperitoneal hernia repair of incarcerated hernias: Is it feasible? Results of a prospective study. *Surg Endosc* 2000;15:1179–1183.

Liao K, Ramirez J, Carryl S, Shaftan GW. A new approach in the management of incarcerated hernia: Emergency laparoscopic hernia repair. *Surg Endosc* 1997;11:944–945.

Mulholland MW, Lillemoe KD, Doherty GM, et al., eds. *Greenfield's Surgery: Scientific Principles and Practice*. 4th ed. Philadelphia, Pa: Lippincott Williams & Wilkins; 2006.

Nesterenko IA, Shovskii OL. Outcome of treatment of incarcerated hernia. *Khirurgia Mosk* 1993;9:26–30.

Nyhus LM, Condon RE, eds. *Hernia*. 4th ed. Philadelphia, Pa: JB Lippincott Co; 1995.

Shackleford RT. *Surgery of the Alimentary Tract*. Philadelphia, Pa: WB Saunders; 1995:2369.

Toms AP, Dixon AK, Murphy JMP, Jamieson NV. Illustrated review of new imaging techniques in the diagnosis of abdominal wall hernias. *Brit J Surg* 1999;86:1243–1249.

van den Berg JC, de Valois JC, Go PM, Rosenbusch G. Detection of groin hernia with physical examination, ultrasound, and MRI compared with laparoscopic findings. *Invest Radiol* 1999;34(12):739–743.

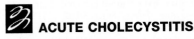

ACUTE CHOLECYSTITIS

I. INTRODUCTION

A. Laparoscopic cholecystectomy for symptomatic cholelithiasis is one of the most common *elective* operations performed in the United States. Acute cholecystitis, in contrast, requires *urgent* treatment. The incidence of gallstones and development of acute cholecystitis may differ according to various risk factors such as gender, age, obesity, pregnancy, cirrhosis, and concomitant critical illness. In large demographic studies, only a small percentage of patients with gallstones have been found to develop symptoms during a 10-year period of follow-up. Among patients who are symptomatic, a significant portion develop recurrent symptoms with a smaller subset developing complications such as acute cholecystitis or pancreatitis. The following discussion will focus on the typical presentation of acute cholecystitis in the general population and will address some of the unique issues pertaining to patients who are pregnant, critically ill, or cirrhotic.

B. Common clinical scenarios in which the general surgery consultant may be involved include the following: assessing the patient with right upper quadrant abdominal pain or with less specific complaints such as fevers in association with nausea, vomiting, and abdominal pain. These patients may present to the emergency department (ED) or may already be hospitalized. The intensive care unit (ICU) patient with an unknown source of abdominal sepsis is another frequent circumstance in which the general surgery team may be involved in the diagnostic process. It is important to exclude other "extraabdominal" diagnoses that mimic gallbladder pathology, such as diaphragmatic, cardiac, and pulmonary processes. Atypical chest pain, myocardial infarction, pneumonia, pulmonary embolism, and costochondritis should all be considered. Epidemiology and natural history studies suggest that patients with biliary symptoms or prior complications related to gallstones (such as pancreatitis, common duct stones, cholecystitis, or cholangitis) have a very high likelihood of developing recurrent symptoms over a period of approximately 2 years: when questioned, many of the patients presenting to the ED with these symptoms are found to have had prior episodes of biliary colic.

II. PATHOGENESIS

A. Acute cholecystitis is an inflammatory process involving the gallbladder that is most often related to gallstone disease causing obstruction of the cystic duct. A subset of patients develop biliary tract infection during the course of acute cholecystitis, with the most common isolates being *Escherichia coli, Klebsiella, Enterobacter,* and *Enterococcus.* The most common type of gallstone is "mixed," consisting of cholesterol and pigmented components. Pure cholesterol and pure pigment gallstones (composed of unconjugated bilirubin, calcium, and other organic material) are found more commonly in certain populations (e.g., Pima Indians and patients with certain hemolytic anemias).

B. Ischemia of the gallbladder wall can result in emphysematous or gangrenous cholecystitis. Potential complications of unrecognized or untreated acute cholecystitis include abscess formation, gallstone ileus, enteric fistulae, perforation leading to bile peritonitis, sepsis, cholangitis, and hydrops of the gallbladder.

III. CLINICAL PRESENTATION AND DIAGNOSIS

A. Clinical presentation. Acute cholecystitis commonly presents as acute onset of right upper quadrant or epigastric pain, fever, and increased white blood cell (WBC) count. Radiation of the pain to the back, right shoulder or scapula, is not uncommon. Murphy's sign, which is right upper quadrant tenderness to palpation elicited when the patient inspires deeply, may be present. Some patients have had prior symptoms of biliary colic and may have radiologic confirmation of cholelithiasis on prior workup.

B. History

1. Important historical data to gather are duration of symptoms, location, quality, and radiation of pain, and associated symptoms (fevers/chills, nausea/vomiting, acholic or clay-colored stool, jaundice, pruritis, fatty food intolerance). A thorough review of systems (constitutional symptoms such as recent unexplained weight loss) should be documented.

2. A detailed past medical and past surgical history should be obtained with special attention paid to certain risk factors including age, gender, oral contraceptive or estrogen replacement therapy, recent rapid weight loss (as may occur after obesity surgery), obesity, hypercholesterolemia/hyperlipidemia, prior history of biliary colic, pancreatitis, cirrhosis, diabetes mellitus, Crohn's disease, hemolytic anemias, and recent prolonged use of total parenteral nutrition (TPN). Prior endoscopies and abdominal operations should also be noted.

3. Medications associated with gallstone formation include estrogens, octreotide, clofibrate, and certain antibiotics and should be detailed in the history.

4. Allergy history, social history, and family history should also be obtained.

5. The differential diagnosis with these typical presenting symptoms includes biliary colic, choledocholithiasis, cholangitis, acid reflux, ulcer disease, pancreatitis, bowel obstruction, appendicitis (especially in the pregnant patient), acute hepatitis, pyelonephritis, renal calculi, diaphragmatic process, pneumonia, atypical chest pain/myocardial infarction, and aortic dissection. The pain of biliary colic resolves after several hours and is not accompanied by signs of inflammation such as fever, leukocytosis, or tenderness.

C. Physical exam. Vital signs may demonstrate fever, tachycardia, or hypotension depending on how advanced the inflammatory process has become. Immunosuppressed, elderly, or diabetic patients may not exhibit the typical signs and symptoms seen in healthier individuals.

1. The physical exam should focus on the abdominal exam without excluding other essential parts of a general physical exam. Sclerae should be examined for jaundice and a heart and lung exam should be completed.

2. A complete abdominal exam includes inspection (distension, stigmata of cirrhosis), auscultation (absent bowel sounds), percussion, and palpation (Murphy's sign). Distension may be due to ileus secondary to gallbladder inflammation. Local signs of peritoneal irritation in the region of the gallbladder may be present. Tenderness to palpation in the subhepatic region during inspiration is a positive **Murphy's sign** and indicates local peritoneal irritation from an inflamed gallbladder or other underlying inflammatory process. Diffuse peritoneal signs include tenderness to palpation, involuntary guarding, and rebound and can signal a complication of cholecystitis such as gangrene or perforation, or possibly another diagnosis.

D. Laboratory data. The following are important to aid in the diagnosis of acute cholecystitis: WBC count with differential, liver function tests (LFTs; including coagulation parameters), total bilirubin and direct/indirect bilirubin, alkaline phosphatase, amylase, and lipase. A leukocytosis may suggest either inflammation of the gallbladder from an obstructed cystic duct or may represent more significant complications, such as cholangitis. Elevation of total bilirubin, alkaline phosphatase, and LFTs may arise from passage of a gallstone into the bile duct (common bile duct [CBD] stones) or **Mirizzi's syndrome** (local compression of the CBD by a large, impacted cystic duct stone). Elevated pancreatic enzymes suggest a diagnosis of gallstone pancreatitis.

E. Imaging

1. **Plain films of the abdomen or an upright chest film** are generally useful if there is a concern for alternate diagnoses and to evaluate for free air. In a small percentage of patients, gallstones will be radiopaque and detectable on plain x-rays ($\sim$15%).

2. **Ultrasonography and HIDA** (technetium-labeled hepatobiliary iminodiacetic acid) scan remain the mainstays of imaging in the diagnosis of acute cholecystitis. If the clinical presentation, history, and physical exam strongly suggest acute cholecystitis, ultrasonography can provide evidence to support the diagnosis. Ultrasound may also confirm the presence of gallstones or biliary sludge. Ultrasound findings suggestive of acute cholecystitis include **gallbladder wall thickening greater than 3 mm, pericholecystic fluid, a sonographic Murphy's sign, and gallbladder distension**. Biliary ductal dilatation (CBD >8 mm in a patient without prior papillotomy or cholecystectomy) suggests CBD obstruction. The sensitivity and specificity of ultrasound in diagnosing acute cholecystitis have been reported to be 88% and 80%, respectively.

3. When ultrasonography is equivocal and the clinical scenario is still suspicious for acute cholecystitis, a HIDA scan is a useful adjunct. The HIDA scan has a sensitivity and specificity of 97% and 90%, respectively. A technetium-labeled acid is taken up preferentially by hepatocytes and excreted into the biliary system. In acute cholecystitis, the obstructed cystic duct does not allow passage of tracer into the gallbladder.

   a. Filling of the gallbladder with tracer within 30 to 60 minutes of the intravenous (IV) injection indicates patency of the cystic duct and excludes the diagnosis of acute cholecystitis.

   b. Nonvisualization of the gallbladder (a "positive" HIDA scan) is consistent with but not diagnostic of acute cholecystitis. False positive HIDA scans can occur with such conditions as prolonged fasting, prior sphincterotomy, hyperbilirubinemia, and liver disease/dysfunction. In ICU patients or TPN-dependent patients in whom the gallbladder is already distended from lack of stimulation, a morphine-assisted HIDA scan may be helpful. IV morphine increases sphincter of Oddi pressure and can assist in filling of a nonobstructed cystic duct and gallbladder.

4. Abdominal computed tomography (CT) can demonstrate complications related to acute cholecystitis such as perforation, gangrene, emphysema in the gallbladder wall, cholecystoenteric fistula, and abscess. Pericholecystic fluid, fat stranding, and gallbladder wall edema can be visualized on CT.

IV. TREATMENT/MANAGEMENT STRATEGIES

A. **Initial management.** As with other acute surgical disease processes, the initial assessment of the patient presenting with symptoms of acute cholecystitis should include monitoring of the ABCs (airway, breathing, circulation). Hemodynamic instability with associated airway compromise may be present in septic patients who have not yet been resuscitated. The patient should be admitted to a surgical service and kept NPO (nothing by mouth). Nasogastric decompression and Foley catheter placement should be decided on an individual basis, depending on the patient's hydration status and symptoms. IV fluid resuscitation and broad-spectrum antibiotic therapy should be instituted.

   1. As many patients will have positive biliary cultures, antibiotics should be given that provide coverage for enteric pathogens including *Enterococcus*. Interestingly, antibiotic use does not seem to alter the development of abscesses related to cholecystitis but may decrease rates of wound infection and bacteremia. Typically, a fourth-generation cephalosporin or a penicillin

in combination with an aminoglycoside is adequate. Certain fluoroquinolones and carbapenems may also be employed if the patient is allergic to penicillins. Duration of antibiotic therapy in the postoperative period is dependent on how systemically ill the patient is or the presence of a subhepatic abscess or other complication of the cholecystitis. The initial choice of antibiotics may need to be modified based upon subsequent culture results.

B. Operative treatment. The timing and manner of intervention and type of biliary drainage depend on the patient's overall health status, ability to tolerate an operation under general anesthesia, and duration of the acute inflammatory process. Minimally invasive methods of biliary drainage in the critically ill patient are discussed later in this chapter.

   1. If common duct stones are suspected based on imaging and laboratory data (persistently high or increasing LFTs, total bilirubin, pancreatic enzymes), then preoperative endoscopic retrograde cholangiopancreatography (ERCP) with stone extraction and/or sphincterotomy should be considered. Magnetic resonance imaging of the bile duct to confirm the presence of common duct stones may increase the yield of ERCP (preoperative versus postoperative) may depend upon the degree to which cholangitis is suspected and the availability of endoscopic expertise. Biliary pancreatitis infrequently occurs concurrently with acute cholecystitis, but if present needs to be treated appropriately prior to proceeding with cholecystectomy. If pancreatitis is severe and acute cholecystitis is not responsive to antibiotic therapy, treatment of the acute cholecystitis by means of percutaneous drainage should be considered.

   2. The surgical management of uncomplicated acute cholecystitis is focused on here. After a period of approximately 24 to 48 hours of resuscitation and empiric IV antibiotics, a laparoscopic cholecystectomy during the same hospital admission is performed. Generally, we perform a cholecystectomy on these patients as soon as possible during daylight hours—ideally within 24 hours of admission. This approach is advisable in patients of low surgical risk.

   a. As the interval from onset of acute cholecystitis to surgical treatment increases, the frequency of conversion to open cholecystectomy and likelihood of common duct injury increase because of progressive inflammation in the right upper quadrant.

   b. Patients who are poor operative risks may require treatment with IV antibiotics and placement of a percutaneous cholecystostomy tube.

   3. Earlier operative intervention is warranted in patients who develop systemic signs of sepsis, generalized peritonitis, gangrene, or perforation of the gallbladder.

   4. In summary, antibiotics should be administered, fluid resuscitation should be provided if needed, and with uncomplicated acute cholecystitis, a cholecystectomy should be performed. ERCP with drainage of the bile duct and extraction of common bile duct (CBD) stones prior to cholecystectomy should be considered in patients with cholangitis or evidence of CBD stones on preoperative imaging.

C. Operative strategy. Acute inflammation found with acute cholecystitis may make safe laparoscopic removal of the gallbladder difficult, but does not preclude an initial laparoscopic attempt. Relative contraindications include severe chronic obstructive pulmonary disease with significant hypercarbia, hostile abdominal anatomy from prior operations or injury, and advanced stages of pregnancy. Surgeon inexperience in combination with some of the aforementioned conditions may lead to an open approach. Preoperative coagulation studies, informed consent (should include "laparoscopic, possible open, cholecystectomy with possible intraoperative cholangiogram"), 12-lead EKG, and chest x-ray should be obtained. The patient is placed supine on an OR table that is capable of fluoroscopy.

   1. Whether performed as a laparoscopic or open procedure, the critical steps in the cholecystectomy are accurate identification, ligation, and division of the cystic duct and artery and mobilization of the gallbladder from its attachments to the gallbladder fossa. An operative cholangiogram may be performed via the gallbladder or cystic duct and should be performed to define bile duct anatomy or if CBD stones are suspected. If the cholangiogram demonstrates the presence of CBD stones, a CBD exploration or postoperative ERCP with duct clearance should be performed.

2. Factors influencing the choice include the surgeon's expertise with laparoscopic CBD exploration, the available expertise with ERCP, and whether the surgical procedure is open or laparoscopic. Recent data also suggest that routine cholangiography may decrease the incidence of bile duct injury during laparoscopic cholecystectomy. Conversion from a laparoscopic to open procedure may be necessary if anatomy is unclear in order to avoid injury to the bile ducts, blood vessels, liver, and other structures, or if a neoplastic process or fistula is identified.

D. **Complications.** A detailed review of potential complications of laparoscopic cholecystectomy and their management is beyond the scope of this chapter. However, certain specific complications should be recognized. Intraoperative complications can include cardiopulmonary instability related to general anesthesia, intolerance of the pneumoperitoneum necessary for laparoscopy, gas embolism, CBD injury, bowel injury related to trocar placement or cautery injury, and hemorrhage. Postoperative complications can present in an immediate or delayed fashion and include the following: **cystic duct leak, bile duct injury that may present acutely or as a subsequent stricture, wound infection, cautery injury to the intestine with delayed perforation, hemorrhage, biloma, and abscess.** Complications need to be recognized and treated in a prompt manner.

E. **Postoperative management.** Duration of antibiotic therapy depends on how systemically ill the patient is and whether complications of acute cholecystitis were present at the time of the operation (e.g., abscess, perforation). After an uncomplicated laparoscopic cholecystectomy most patients are started on a clear liquid diet and advanced as tolerated to a regular diet. In the majority of cases, patients can be discharged safely to home on oral narcotics and wound care instructions on postoperative day one. Length of hospital stay is longer and postoperative pain is greater with the open technique.

V. SPECIAL POPULATIONS

A. **Pregnant patients.** Possibly due to the high estrogen state of pregnancy, symptomatic cholelithiasis is common. Special considerations for the care of the pregnant patient with acute cholecystitis include the following: gestational age (and risk of premature labor or fetal loss); close fetal monitoring (depending on gestational age); appropriate antibiotic therapy; altered port placement for laparoscopy to avoid injuring the gravid uterus; proper OR positioning of the patient to ensure adequate venous return to the heart (left side down with reverse Trendelenberg); and judicious use of cholangiography. Multidisciplinary care of the pregnant patient with close involvement of maternal–fetal medicine specialists and gastroenterologists is imperative. Tocolytics are used on an individual case basis. In evaluation of patients in later stages of pregnancy, it is important to note that the appendix is displaced to the right upper quadrant by the gravid uterus and may mimic acute cholecystitis.

B. **Critically ill patients.** The clinical presentation of acute cholecystitis in the critically ill patient may be significantly altered by concomitant multiorgan dysfunction. Gram-negative bacteremia along with systemic signs of sepsis (fever, elevated WBC count, and acidosis) may be the only indication of an abdominal source of sepsis.

1. Bedside imaging with ultrasound may identify evidence of acute cholecystitis and is potentially valuable if the patient is too unstable to transport for a CT scan.

2. Critically ill patients, immunocompromised and transplant patients, patients with recent trauma, burns, or following major surgery such as coronary artery bypass grafting are at risk for developing acute cholecystitis in the absence of gallstones—**acute acalculous cholecystitis.** Ultrasonographic signs will be similar to those of acute cholecystitis except for the absence of visible stones. Mortality rates for acute acalculous cholecystitis are high due to the patient population in which it occurs.

3. Any patient with acute cholecystitis who is unable to tolerate an operative intervention (laparoscopic or open cholecystectomy) due to his or her medical comorbidities may be a candidate for a percutaneous cholecystostomy. **Percutaneous cholecystostomy** tube placement can be performed at the bedside under local anesthesia using ultrasound guidance and, in the properly selected patient, may be less risky than general anesthesia and formal cholecystectomy. Percutaneous gallbladder drainage temporarily relieves the cystic duct obstruction and drains the functional equivalent of an abscess. Bile cultures are obtained and monitored for growth and appropriate antibiotics are given. A tube study can be performed a few weeks following placement and plans for an interval cholecystectomy can be determined based on the patient's overall condition.

C. **Cirrhotic patients.** Patients with cirrhosis must be evaluated carefully when assessing surgical risk for cholecystectomy. Careful attention should be paid to the patient's Child-Pugh class (assessment of liver function) since this may be the most important prognostic indicator of overall morbidity and mortality. It is important to note that hypoalbuminemia (often seen in liver and heart failure patients) can cause gallbladder wall thickening that is not necessarily pathologic.

ACUTE CHOLANGITIS

I. INTRODUCTION

A. Acute cholangitis results from a variety of biliary pathology but ultimately refers to the systemic consequences of biliary infection resulting from biliary obstruction and stasis. Gallstones causing CBD obstruction are a frequent cause of cholangitis, followed by instrumentation of the biliary tract, indwelling biliary stents, malignant obstruction, benign strictures of the biliary tract, primary sclerosing cholangitis, anatomic abnormalities such as choledochal cysts, papillary stenosis, and postoperative strictures (e.g., stricture of bilioenteric anastamoses). The transplant population is a special group in which cholangitis can be caused by ductal anastomotic strictures and hepatic artery strictures.

B. **Common clinical scenarios** in which the general surgery team will be involved are similar to those discussed in the section on acute cholecystitis. However, it is important to gather information about recent surgical or endoscopic manipulation of the biliary tract early in the assessment. It is also essential to decide whether the patient needs a higher level of care such as the ICU for adequate resuscitation and monitoring.

II. PATHOGENESIS

A. Biliary tract obstruction is the predisposing factor for bacterial seeding of the biliary tract. Increased biliary pressure can lead to alteration of normal bile flow, hepatic tight junctions, and the normal immunologic microenvironment of the liver. Bacteria can then ascend from the gastrointestinal tract and subsequently enter the systemic circulation causing systemic manifestations of biliary sepsis. Common organisms include *E. coli*, *Klebsiella*, and *Enterococcus* species. It is important to tailor antibiotic coverage to the hospital antibiotic sensitivity profile. Since *Enterococcus* is the most common gram-positive isolate from biliary cultures, determining whether vancomycin-resistant *Enterococcus* is present is important for antibiotic choice.

III. CLINICAL PRESENTATION AND DIAGNOSIS

A. **History.** The patient should be simultaneously assessed resuscitated while obtaining relevant historical and physical exam information. **Charcot's triad**, which consists of fever, jaundice, and right upper quadrant pain, may be present in up to half of patients with cholangitis. Associated systemic signs of sepsis include hypotension and mental status changes and complete the symptom complex known as **Reynold's pentad**. In addition to inquiring about recent procedures or remote operations involving the hepatobiliary system, it is important to characterize the duration and onset of abdominal pain and jaundice. Prior history of gallstone disease should be noted. Recent antibiotic usage should be documented. Most patients having undergone ERCP will have received prophylactic antibiotic coverage prior to and after the procedure. Information regarding type (metal or plastic) of and duration of indwelling biliary stents from the medical record or patient is also important in formulating a differential diagnosis and guiding therapy. In addition to all of the differential diagnoses listed for acute cholecystitis, other diagnostic considerations include choledocholithiasis, benign or malignant biliary strictures, obstructed endobiliary stents, bile leak from recent operative intervention (e.g., common duct or cystic duct injury status postcholecystectomy), infected or obstructed choledochal cysts, liver abscess, or post procedure cholangitis (post-ERCP or post-PTC tube placement).

B. Physical exam. Fever, tachycardia, and hypotension should be noted in the initial assessment of the patient and IV fluid resuscitation should be initiated promptly. Scleral icterus should be noted. Physical exam should focus primarily on the abdominal exam. External biliary drains, if present, should be examined for patency and be left open for drainage. Gram stain and cultures of bile should be obtained. Inspection, auscultation, percussion, and palpation should be included in a thorough abdominal exam. Nonbiliary sources of sepsis (intraabdominal or otherwise) should be considered, as jaundice can be a nonspecific finding in sepsis. Therefore, a cardiopulmonary exam should not be omitted and an ICU patient should be examined thoroughly for signs of decubitus ulcers, line sepsis, and nosocomial pneumonia. If suspicion is high for cholangitis, broad-spectrum antibiotic therapy should be initiated after blood and bile cultures are taken. Surgical scars that suggest prior biliary tract surgery should be noted (i.e., right upper quadrant incisions or laparoscopy incisions).

C. Laboratory data. A WBC count with differential, LFTs (including coagulation parameters and serum albumin), total bilirubin and direct/indirect bilirubin, alkaline phosphatase, amylase, and lipase are useful in determining the etiology and severity of the cholangitis. Significantly elevated bilirubin, alkaline phosphatase, and LFTs strongly suggest CBD obstruction secondary to gallstones, stricture, or a clogged stent. Tumor markers such as CA 19-9 and alpha-feto protein should be measured if malignancy is suspected. Blood and bile cultures should be taken and prior biliary cultures with sensitivity profiles should be examined to guide antibiotic therapy.

D. Imaging. As with most biliary pathology, it is useful to start with noninvasive ultrasonography looking for evidence of ductal obstruction (either from gallstones, clogged stent, or stricture) or signs of a right upper quadrant inflammatory process. Early ductal dilatation, however, may not be visualized on ultrasound. In the transplant population who may have a more complicated problem such as hepatic artery thrombosis or ductal anastamotic strictures, ultrasound can be obtained with Doppler flow studies to evaluate direction of blood flow and resistive indices. CT scanning can be helpful in identifying potential causes of ductal obstruction ranging from malignancy with mass effect to inflammatory processes involving the gallbladder. Magnetic resonance cholangiopancreatography (MRCP) is less invasive than ERCP and allows for evaluation of intra- and extrahepatic ductal anatomy. The availability of MRCP varies considerably between institutions and may not be a practical option for a critically ill patient. Risks of ERCP include pancreatitis, bleeding from sphincterotomy, perforation, worsening cholangitis, and risks associated with general anesthesia if necessary for the procedure. However, ERCP provides both a diagnostic and therapeutic option. Choledocholithiasis can be identified and treated with sphincterotomy and stone extraction with ERCP. Drainage of an obstructed bile duct can be accomplished by placement of a stent. An occluded stent can also be removed and exchanged with this technique. Percutaneous transhepatic cholangiography (PTC) can identify the cause of biliary obstruction and provide external biliary drainage and stent placement. Risks with PTC include hemobilia and electrolyte abnormalities associated with external biliary drainage. Which method is employed depends on the overall status of the patient and the etiology of the cholangitis, and is discussed more extensively in the next section.

IV. TREATMENT/MANAGEMENT STRATEGIES

A. Initial management. Because these patients may be systemically ill, it is important to transfer them to an **intensive care setting** for close hemodynamic monitoring. Intubation for definitive airway management may be necessary if the patient is obtunded secondary to septic or hypovolemic shock. Large-bore **IV access** should be obtained and isotonic crystalloid and/or colloid resuscitation should be initiated early. **Broad-spectrum IV antibiotics** can also be administered after drawing appropriate blood and biliary cultures. Prior cultures should be examined for specific organisms and sensitivity profiles. Empiric antibiotic therapy should be initiated for gram-negative organisms and *Enterococcus*. A penicillin in combination with an aminoglycoside (e.g., ampicillin and gentamicin) is effective in patients without significant renal or hepatic dysfunction. Extended-spectrum penicillins with beta-lactamase inhibitors (e.g., piperacillin-tazobactam) can be effective as a single agent. Addition of anaerobic coverage with metronidazole can be useful in patients who are at risk for *Clostridium difficile* colitis (e.g., transplant patients), are particularly ill, or are suspected of having an anaerobic infection. Carbapenems or fluoroquinolones are effective and can be used in patients who are allergic to penicillins. Antifungal therapy may be appropriate as *Candida* species are becoming more common. Externally dwelling catheters, such as PTC catheters, should be irrigated and placed to a gravity bag for adequate drainage. Nasogastric tube placement may be necessary for associated ileus. Foley catheter placement will help guide volume resuscitation. Tight glycemic control and insulin therapy play an important role in the care of the septic patient. Consideration of administration of recombinant human-activated protein C may be appropriate, depending on how critically ill the patient is and whether he or she responds to initial resuscitation efforts.

B. Interventions. Determining the etiology of cholangitis during the initial resuscitation will expedite implementation of treatment. As discussed, several etiologies of biliary obstruction can contribute to acute cholangitis.

   1. Regardless of etiology, establishing **biliary decompression** quickly and effectively is imperative if obstruction is present and there is ongoing sepsis. Irrigating an obstructed PTC catheter and treating supportively with fluid resuscitation and antibiotics may be enough to successfully treat an episode of cholangitis.

   2. Whether the patient can be treated with a less invasive procedure such as endoscopic decompression or percutaneous measures depends on whether there exist specific contraindications to the various procedures. Patients with altered anatomy from prior biliary or gastrointestinal tract operations may be technically difficult to instrument endoscopically. Percutaneous approaches usually involve instrumentation of the liver and will not be safe in coagulopathic patients. Sphincterotomy may also be contraindicated in coagulopathic patients and may limit approaches with ERCP to just balloon dilation and/or stent placement. In patients who have malignant obstruction, ERCP with stent placement may be a temporizing measure prior to a complete staging workup and a definitive operation.

   3. For gallstone disease, an ERCP with stone extraction is effective in the vast majority of cases. Surgical CBD exploration and cholecystectomy may be necessary if ERCP is unable to remove the stones and cholangitis is still present. PTC may be an initial temporizing measure to decompress the biliary tree prior to operative intervention. Cholangitis from benign biliary strictures from prior operations or instrumentation can be both diagnosed and treated acutely with ERCP and decompression (often with balloon dilation alone). Poor prognostic factors include systemic signs of infection and mandate earlier interventions and more aggressive resuscitation. Duration of antibiotic therapy after decompression depends on the clinical status of the patient and whether they are immunocompromised. The majority of patients respond to resuscitation and antibiotics and can undergo semielective biliary decompression either through percutaneous or endoscopic approaches. While only a minority of patients with cholangitis will not respond in the initial period to antibiotics and fluid resuscitation, they must be recognized as they require urgent decompression within the first 24 hours of presentation.

ACUTE PANCREATITIS

I. INTRODUCTION. Although most cases of acute pancreatitis resolve without serious sequelae, severe morbidity and possibly death may result in patients with severe acute pancreatitis. Among these patients, mortality rates may exceed 10%, and in contrast to patients with mild acute pancreatitis, lengthy ICU stays and hospitalizations, operative interventions, nutritional support, and other supportive measures are commonly necessary. While the etiology of pancreatitis may vary, common principles of management apply to patients with acute pancreatitis.

II. ETIOLOGY AND PATHOGENESIS
   A. Passage of **gallstones** into the bile duct is one of the most common causes of acute pancreatitis, although only a small subset of patients with cholelithiasis develops this complication.
   B. Alcohol consumption, particularly binge drinking, is another common cause of acute pancreatitis.
   C. Familial hereditary pancreatitis is an uncommon cause of recurrent pancreatitis, but is associated with a high incidence of pancreatic cancer. Mutations of the genes for cystic fibrosis transmembrane conductance regulator (CFTR) and cationic trypsinogen may also predispose to the development of acute pancreatitis.
   D. Metabolic abnormalities such as **hypertriglyceridemia and hypercalcemia** are less common causes of acute pancreatitis.
   E. Medications (e.g., steroids, exogenous estrogens, certain antibiotics such as sulfa drugs, antiviral therapies, diuretics, azathioprine, valproic acid, and tamoxifen), viral infections, ERCP, blunt or penetrating trauma, anatomic variations such as pancreas divisum, pancreatic or ampullary tumors, and sphincter of Oddi dysfunction constitute other causes of acute pancreatitis. Finally, in a significant subset of patients the cause of acute pancreatitis remains undetermined (idiopathic).
   F. The precise cascade of events leading to acute pancreatitis is not completely understood. Premature activation of zymogens and intraacinar activation of proteolytic enzymes may lead to autodigestion of pancreatic tissue. Subsequently, the inflammatory cascade is perpetuated both locally and systemically with release of cytokines and migration of inflammatory cells to the area of damage. This can lead to further activation of inflammatory mediators, in addition to changes in the pancreatic microcirculation.
   G. In severe cases of acute pancreatitis, systemic manifestations include acute respiratory distress syndrome, metabolic derangements of calcium, glucose, acid-base regulation, and acute renal failure. Hypovolemic shock may also ensue.

III. CLINICAL PRESENTATION AND DIAGNOSIS
   A. History. The general surgery consultant is most often asked to evaluate a patient who complains of abdominal pain radiating to the back. Other nonspecific symptoms may include nausea, vomiting, or fever. Eliciting the following historical information can aid in diagnosis: prior episodes of pancreatitis or history of chronic pancreatitis, symptoms of biliary colic or known gallstone disease, history of significant alcohol use, new medication use, recent infections, history of high triglycerides, hypercalcemia, recent abdominal trauma, or procedures such as ERCP. Information regarding duration of symptoms, characterization of pain (e.g., colicky vs. constant, radiation to the back), and associated symptoms (change in bowel movements, nausea, or vomiting) should be gathered. Constitutional symptoms such as fevers, anorexia, or weight loss should also be documented. Systemic signs and symptoms of sepsis, cholangitis, or infected pancreatic necrosis such as fever or mental status changes are

important to note early in the assessment. In a patient unable to provide satisfactory history, acute pancreatitis should be considered in patients with unexplained sepsis, hemodynamic instability, ileus, or jaundice. The differential diagnosis for symptoms consistent with acute pancreatitis is similar to that for acute cholecystitis and includes biliary colic, cholangitis, choledocholithiasis without pancreatitis, peptic ulcer disease, abdominal aortic dissection or aneurysm, reflux disease, bowel obstruction, atypical chest pain/myocardial infarction, and acute hepatitis.

B. **Physical exam.** Airway management should precede any further assessment if mental status changes are present or airway protection is an issue. Additionally, hypovolemia is common with severe acute pancreatitis. If tachycardia or hypotension is present, fluid resuscitation with IV fluids should begin promptly. Vital signs should be monitored and urine output should be measured. Particular attention should be paid to the abdominal examination. Distention resulting from ileus may be present and require nasogastric decompression. Retroperitoneal bleeding may result in discoloration of the flanks (Grey-Turner's sign) or periumbilical region (Cullen's sign). Palpation may reveal evidence of either localized or generalized peritoneal irritation. A peripancreatic inflammatory mass, often referred to as a phlegmon, or an evolving acute peripancreatic fluid collection may be palpable. Stigmata of chronic liver disease or hyperlipidemia may be evident on physical examination and may provide clues as to the etiology of the episode of acute pancreatitis.

C. **Laboratory data.** A complete blood count with differential, arterial blood gas with base deficit, complete electrolyte panel including serum calcium, BUN, creatinine, liver functions including total bilirubin and alkaline phosphatase, serum amylase and lipase, and triglycerides should be measured. The degree of pancreatic enzyme elevation is not by itself an indication of the severity of pancreatitis. However, the various laboratory tests already discussed may help establish the diagnosis and possibly the cause of acute pancreatitis, as well as stratify the patient's risk for significant morbidity or mortality resulting from the episode of acute pancreatitis. Several clinical stratification scales have been devised that are based on such laboratory measures. Table 66-1 shows Ranson's criteria, consisting of 11 measurements made at the time of presentation or after 48 hours that predict mortality. The Glasgow criteria consist of similar measurements made at the time of presentation. Serum C-reactive protein level is also a useful indicator of disease severity.

TABLE 66-1	Ranson's Criteria—Prognostic Signs in Acute Pancreatitis
Admission	**48 hours postadmission**
Age >55 y	Hematocrit decrease >10%
WBC >16,000 cells/mm^3	BUN increase >5 mg/dL
Glucose >200 mg/dL	Serum calcium <8 mg/dL
LDH >350 IU/L	Arterial PaO$_2$ <60 mmHg
SGOT >250 IU/L	Base deficit >4 mEq/L
	Fluid sequestration >6 L
Mortality	
<3 signs = 1%	
3–4 signs = 15%	
5–6 signs = 50%	
>6 signs = approximately 100%	

WBC, white blood cell; BUN, blood urea nitrogen; LDH, lactate dehydrogenase; IU/L, international units per liter; SGOT, serum glutamic-oxaloacetic transaminase.

D. Imaging

1. As acute pancreatitis may present with the clinical picture of an acute abdomen, **plain abdominal and chest radiographs** should be obtained to evaluate for free air, evidence of intestinal obstruction, or a cardiopulmonary process. A localized ileus caused by acute pancreatitis may be visible as a "sentinel loop" on plain radiographs.

2. **Abdominal CT scan** performed with rapid bolus infusion of IV contrast (dynamic CT scan) is particularly useful in the evaluation of acute pancreatitis. When the abdominal CT is performed in this manner, acute necrotizing pancreatitis can be distinguished from acute edematous interstitial pancreatitis by the failure of areas of pancreatic necrosis to enhance with IV contrast. The presence of pancreatic necrosis is associated with a greater risk of pancreatic infection and of severe morbidity and mortality and can be used to stratify treatment of these patients. Pancreatic or peripancreatic infections are unusual in the absence of necrosis, and the need for surgical intervention is very uncommon in the absence of necrosis. CT can also help identify other causes for the patient's acute presentation or other complications of acute pancreatitis such as intestinal ischemia or biliary obstruction. However, to avoid the potentially harmful effects of IV contrast on the patient's renal function, a CT with IV contrast should be delayed until the patient has been satisfactorily volume resuscitated unless the study is needed to exclude other intraabdominal emergencies for which immediate surgical intervention is necessary.

3. **Ultrasonography** is useful to identify gallstones or common duct stones in suspected cases of biliary pancreatitis. Ultrasonography may also aid in determining if abnormal liver function studies are due to biliary obstruction.

4. **ERCP** (Section IV.B) should not be performed routinely in patients with acute pancreatitis, but should be considered when cholangitis or choledocholithiasis are suspected. Endoscopic placement of pancreatic duct stents may occasionally be useful for treatment of pancreatic duct disruptions. However, instrumentation of the pancreatic duct in this setting may risk worsening of the pancreatitis or infection of areas of necrosis.

IV. TREATMENT/MANAGEMENT STRATEGIES

A. General management

1. Mild pancreatitis. In approximately 85% of patients with acute pancreatitis, the disease follows a mild course and typically resolves without significant sequelae within several days. Pancreatic necrosis is uncommon among these patients and clinical and CT severity scores are usually low. These patients should initially be kept NPO and may require nasogastric decompression if an ileus is present. IV fluids should be administered, and frequently large volumes are needed to correct substantial intravascular volume deficits. Foley catheter placement is useful in even mild pancreatitis in order to monitor the adequacy of intravascular volume replacement. Adequate analgesia in the form of a patient-controlled analgesic (PCA) pump can be used in the awake patient. As symptoms and physical findings improve, oral intake can resume. Supplemental nutritional support is generally not necessary. While providing supportive care, the underlying cause of acute pancreatitis should be investigated and treated as necessary. Improvement should be progressive, and if not, investigations should be undertaken for the development of complications such as formation of a pseudocyst or development of infection.

2. Severe pancreatitis. In approximately 15% of patients with acute pancreatitis, the disease follows a severe course with a greater likelihood of local and systemic complications, need for ICU care and surgical or other invasive interventions, and risk of mortality. Among these patients, early mortality (within the first week) most often results from cardiopulmonary complications. Early transfer to the ICU should be considered to facilitate aggressive fluid resuscitation and close hemodynamic monitoring. Additionally, respiratory support including endotracheal intubation is frequently necessary among these patients. Once stabilized,

subsequent acute clinical deterioration should prompt investigation into the possibility of intraabdominal infection (infected necrosis, ascites, or abscess formation), hemorrhage, or perforated viscus.

a. Nutritional support. In contrast to mild acute pancreatitis, in severe pancreatitis a highly catabolic state arises and supplemental nutritional support is frequently required. In acute pancreatitis, pancreatic stimulation is generally held to be potentially detrimental. Parenteral nutrition avoids pancreatic stimulation but is associated with catheter-related complications (line sepsis, pneumothorax, etc.) in addition to hepatic and intestinal dysfunction. Enteral nutrition has been shown to be safe in patients with acute pancreatitis. Several small controlled clinical trials as well as a meta-analysis have shown benefit of enteral over parenteral feeding in patients with acute pancreatitis. Reduction in hospital stay, infections, and surgical interventions was seen in most of these studies without a significant difference in mortality. To minimize stimulation of the pancreas, feeding through a nasojejunal tube is advocated and should be started early in the hospitalization for patients with moderate to severe pancreatitis.

b. Antibiotic treatment and infectious complications. Infectious complications are a cause of significant morbidity and are the most frequent cause of mortality after the first week. Areas of peripancreatic or pancreatic necrosis are prone to become infected. Such infections should be suspected when fevers, leukocytosis, positive blood cultures, or other signs of sepsis develop in patients with known peripancreatic or pancreatic necrosis. CT- or ultrasound-guided fine-needle aspiration of such areas of necrosis can provide specimens for gram stain and culture and sensitivity testing. If fluid cannot be readily aspirated, a small amount of sterile fluid can be injected and then aspirated. If infection is confirmed, mortality is high, unless adequate debridement and drainage of infected tissues is performed. Open surgical debridement and drainage procedures (necrosectomy) remain the standard treatment for infected pancreatic or peripancreatic necrosis, although recently percutaneous drainage or laparoscopic debridement have been reported with encouraging results even in the presence of extensive necrosis. Discrete infected fluid collections that do not contain necrotic tissue may be especially suitable for percutaneous drainage.

  i. The use of prophylactic antibiotics to prevent infection of pancreatic or peripancreatic necrosis remains controversial, as prospective randomized trials have yielded conflicting results. Additionally, the use of prophylactic antibiotics may predispose to development of resistant organism infections or fungal infections. If prophylactic antibiotics are to be used, their use should be limited to patients with areas of necrosis, as the risk of local infection is very low in the absence of necrosis.

  ii. Common isolates from infected pancreatic necrosis include *Klebsiella, E. coli, Pseudomonas, Enterobacter,* and *Enterococcus,* as well as *Streptococcus* and *Staphylococcus.* Thus, prophylactic treatment should be effective against a broad range of organisms and have good penetrance into pancreatic tissue. Such antibiotics include imipenem, fluoroquinolones, piperacillin, third-generation cephalosporins, and metronidazole. As fungal isolates are increasingly common, antifungal agents should be considered also, especially in patients who have already been receiving antibiotic therapy. Finally, secondary sources of sepsis in acute pancreatitis such as line sepsis and ventilator-associated pneumonia can be treated with appropriate antibiotics and ICU management.

c. Protease inhibitors and octreotide. Neither protease inhibitors nor octreotide have been shown to be of benefit in the treatment of acute pancreatitis, although octreotide may be useful for the treatment of such complications of pancreatitis as a pancreatic fistula.

d. Operative intervention. Except as noted previously, infected pancreatic and peripancreatic necrosis should be treated by means of surgical debridement and drainage. The role of percutaneous drainage or surgical debridement or necrosectomy in the setting of sterile necrosis is less clear. If the patient has not responded to aggressive ICU care and is experiencing progressive multiorgan failure, then such interventions may be considered. Surgical intervention may also be indicated for complications of acute pancreatitis such as intestinal perforation that may arise from direct injury to the wall or the intestine or thrombosis of mesenteric vessels, or intestinal obstruction. Vascular complications such as splenic artery pseudoaneurysms or hemorrhage can occur from direct contact with proteolytic enzymes. Angiography with embolization of actively bleeding vessels is the preferred treatment of bleeding pseudoaneurysms. Packing may be necessary to control bleeding from the pancreatic bed. Pancreatic ductal disruption from necrosis can lead to accumulation of **pancreatic ascites** or development of either a pancreatic fistula or pseudocyst formation. Pseudocyst themselves can cause obstruction or can become secondarily infected. Various criteria and procedures exist for decompression of these pseudocysts depending on size, symptoms, infection, and obstruction.

B. **Management of biliary (gallstone) pancreatitis.** When acute pancreatitis is believed to be caused by gallstones, a cholecystectomy should be performed once the acute pancreatitis has resolved clinically (indicated by resolution of symptoms and decreasing biochemical markers). Preferably, this is performed during the same hospitalization, as the risk of recurrent pancreatitis is significant if instead an interval cholecystectomy is performed. If a pseudocyst or other pancreatic changes are still evolving, however, consideration may be given to delaying the cholecystectomy until the outcome of these changes and the need for any additional interventions has been determined. In the case of pancreatic complications, the cholecystectomy can be performed in conjunction with treatment of the pseudocyst. If a lengthy delay is expected before the cholecystectomy is performed, an ERCP with endoscopic sphincterotomy may reduce the risk of recurrent biliary pancreatitis. At the time of the cholecystectomy, an operative cholangiogram should be performed to evaluate for the presence of common duct stones. If these are found, either a concurrent common duct exploration or postoperative ERCP should be performed.

Pancreatic inflammation often results in LFT abnormalities and mild hyperbilirubinemia. Such changes can be evaluated noninvasively with either ultrasonography or MRCP. If the patient does not improve with initial supportive care and has persistent jaundice, urgent ERCP should be considered for drainage of the bile duct and treatment of possible cholangitis. In experienced hands, urgent ERCP can be performed safely in this setting and may improve outcome among patients with severe acute pancreatitis. Again, ERCP can be both diagnostic and therapeutic but does carry a risk of procedure-related pancreatitis (up to 5%). If ERCP is unavailable or technically difficult, then emergent surgical exploration with laparoscopic or open cholecystectomy with common duct exploration may be required in a patient with ongoing ductal obstruction and cholangitis.

C. **Management of other causes of acute pancreatitis**

1. In the case of **alcohol-related pancreatitis**, careful attention should be paid to signs of alcohol withdrawal. Appropriate prophylaxis against delirium tremens should be administered and alcohol cessation counseling should be provided to prevent further episodes of acute pancreatitis.

2. If acute pancreatitis has been caused by **hypertriglyceridemia, hypercalcemia,** or other metabolic abnormalities, the cause of the metabolic abnormality should be determined and appropriate therapy should be instituted. In the case of high serum triglycerides, pharmacologic therapy should be instituted (e.g., nicotinic acid, fibrates, and/or statins). **Drugs** implicated in the episode of acute pancreatitis should be withdrawn.

3. General management principles for acute pancreatitis apply to post-ERCP pancreatitis. As elevation of serum amylase and lipase levels is common following ERCP, the diagnosis of acute pancreatitis in this setting is additionally

based upon symptoms and radiographic studies. If a sphincterotomy has been performed at the time of ERCP, perforation of the duodenum should be excluded by means of a CT scan or upper GI series.

Bibliography

Abuabara SF, Gross GW, Sirinek KR. Laparoscopic cholecystectomy during pregnancy is safe for both mother and fetus. *J Gastrointest Surg* 1997;1:48.

Al-Omran M, Groof A, Wilke D. Enteral versus parenteral nutrition for acute pancreatitis. *Cochrane Database Syst Rev* 2003;(1):CD002827.

Andruilli A, Leandro G, Clemente R, et al. Meta-analysis of somatostatin, octreotide, and gabexate mesilate in the therapy of acute pancreatitis. *Aliment Pharmacol Ther* 1998;12:237.

Arvanitakis M, Delhate M, DeMaertellaere V, et al. Computed tomography and magnetic resonance imaging in the assessment of acute pancreatitis. *Gastroenterology* 2004;126:715.

Attili AF, De Santis A, Capri R, et al. The natural history of gallstones: The GREPCO experience. *Hepatology* 1995;21:655.

Barbara L, Sama C, Morselli Labate AM, et al. A population study on the prevalence of gallstone disease: The Sirmione study. *Hepatology* 1987;7:913.

Bassi C, Falconi M, Talamini G, et al. Controlled clinical trial of pefloxacin versus imipenem in severe acute pancreatitis. *Gastroenterology* 1998;115:1513.

Bassi C, Larvin M, Villatoro E. Antibiotic therapy for prophylaxis against infection of pancreatic necrosis in acute pancreatitis. *Cochrane Database Syst Rev* 2003;(4):CD002941.

Beger HG, Bittner R, Block S, et al. Bacterial contamination of pancreatic necrosis: A prospective clinical study. *Gastroenterology* 1986;91:433.

Bennett GL, Balthazar EJ. Ultrasound and CT evaluation of emergent gallbladder pathology. *Radiol Clin North Am* 2003;41:1203.

Bisharah M, Tulandi T. Laparoscopic surgery in pregnancy. *Clin Obstet Gynecol* 2003;46:92.

Byrne MF, Suhocki P, Mitchell RM, et al. Percutaneous cholecystostomy in patients with acute cholecystitis: Experience of 45 patients at a US referral center. *J Am Coll Surg* 2003;197:206.

Chan Y, Chan AC, Lam WW, et al. Choledocholithiasis: Comparison of MR cholangiography and endoscopic retrograde cholangiography. *Radiology* 1996;200:85.

Cirillo DJ, Wallace RB, Rodabough RJ, et al. Effect of estrogen therapy on gallbladder disease. *JAMA* 2005;293:330.

Cohen S, Bacon BR, Berlin JA, et al. National Institutes of Health State-of-the-Science Conference Statement: ERCP for diagnosis and therapy. *Gastrointest Endosc* 2002;56:803.

Cohn JA, Friedman KJ, Noone PG, et al. Relation between mutations of the cystic fibrosis gene and idiopathic pancreatitis. *N Engl J Med* 1998;339:645.

Corfield AP, Cooper MJ, Williamson RC, et al. Prediction of severity in acute pancreatitis: Prospective comparison of three prognostic indices. *Lancet* 1985;2:403.

Csendes A, Burdiles P, Maluenda F, et al. Simultaneous bacteriologic assessment of bile from gallbladder and CBD in control subjects and patients with gallstones and common duct stones. *Arch Surg* 1996;131:389.

Curro G, Iapichino G, Melita G, et al. Laparoscopic cholecystectomy in Child-Pugh class C cirrhotic patients. *JSLS* 2005;9:311.

Davis CA, Landercasper J, Gundersen LH, et al. Effective use of percutaneous cholecystostomy in high-risk surgical patients: Techniques, tube management, and results. *Arch Surg* 1999;134:727.

Eland IA, Sturkenboom MJ, Wilson JH, et al. Incidence and mortality of acute pancreatitis between 1985 and 1995. *Scand J Gastroenterol* 2000;17:S1.

Everhart JE, Yeh F, Lee ET, et al. Prevalence of gallbladder disease in American Indian populations: Findings from the Strong Heart Study. *Hepatology* 2002;35:1507.

Fan ST, Lai EC, Mok FP, et al. Early treatment of acute biliary pancreatitis by endoscopic papillotomy. *N Engl J Med* 1993;328:228.

Fidler J, Paulson EK, Layfield L. CT evaluation of acute cholecystitis: Findings and usefulness in diagnosis. *Am J Roentgenol* 1996;166:1085.

Fink-Bennett D, Freitas JE, Ripley SD, et al. The sensitivity of hepatobiliary imaging and real time ultrasonography in the detection of acute cholecystitis. *Arch Surg* 1985;120:904.

Flancbaum L, Choban PS, Sinha R, et al. Morphine cholescintigraphy in the evaluation of hospitalized patients with suspected acute cholecystitis. *Ann Surg* 1994;220:25.

Flum DR, Dellinger EP, Cheadle A, et al. Intraoperative cholangiography and risk of common bile duct injury during cholecystectomy. *JAMA* 2003;289:1639.

Fortson MR, Freedman SN, Webster PD. Clinical assessment of hyperlipidemic pancreatitis. *Am J Gastroenterol* 1995;90:2134.

Freeman ML, Nelson DB, Sherman S, et al. Complications of endoscopic biliary sphincterotomy. *N Engl J Med* 1996;335:909.

Freeny PC, Hauptmann E, Althaus AJ, et al. Percutaneous CT-guided catheter drainage of infected acute necrotizing pancreatitis: Techniques and results. *Am J Roentenol* 1998;170:969.

Friedman GD, Raviola CA, Fireman B. Prognosis of gallstone with mild or no symptoms: 25 year follow up in a health maintenance organization. *J Clin Epidemiol* 1989;42:127.

Gallstones and laparoscopic cholecystectomy. NIH Consens Statement 1992;10:1.

Gerzof SG, Banks PA, Robbins AH, et al. Early diagnosis of pancreatic infection by computer tomography guided aspiration. *Gastroenterology* 1987;93:1315.

Gloor B, Muller CA, Worni M, et al. Late mortality in patients with severe acute pancreatitis. *Br J Surg* 2001;88:975.

Gloor B, Muller CA, Worni M, et al. Pancreatic infection in severe pancreatitis: The role of fungus and multiresistant organisms. *Arch Surg* 2001;136:592.

Golub R, Siddiqi F, Pohl D. Role of antibiotics in acute pancreatitis: A meta-analysis. *J Gastrointest Surg* 1998;2:496.

Halangk W, Lerch MM, Brandt-Nedelev B, et al. Role of cathepsin B in intracellular trypsinogen activation and onset of acute pancreatitis. *J Clin Invest* 2000;106:773.

Hanck C, Singer MV. Does acute alcoholic pancreatitis exist without preexisting chronic pancreatitis? *Scand J Gastroenterol* 1997;32:625.

Hernandez V, Pascual I, Almela P, et al. Recurrence of acute gallstone pancreatitis and relationship with cholecystectomy or endoscopic sphincterotomy. *Am J Gastroenterol* 2004;99:2417.

Hussaini SH, Murphy GM, Kennedy C, et al. The role of bile composition and physical chemistry in the pathogenesis of octreotide-associated gallbladder stones. *Gastroenterology* 1994;107:1503.

Isenmann R, Ran B, Berger HG. Early severe acute pancreatitis: Characteristics of a new subgroup. *Pancreas* 2001;22:274.

Isenmann R, Runzi M, Kron M, et al. Prophylactic antibiotic treatment in patients with predicted severe acute pancreatitis: A placebo-controlled, double-blind trial. *Gastroenterology* 2004;126:997.

Johansson M, Thune A, Nelvin L, et al. Randomized clinical trial of open versus laparoscopic cholecystectomy in the treatment of acute cholecystitis. *Br J Surg* 2005;92:44.

Kaminski DL. Arachidonic acid metabolites in hepatobiliary physiology and disease. *Gastroenterology* 1989;97:781.

Kasholm-Tengve B. Selective antibiotic prophylaxis in biliary tract operations. *Surg Gynecol Obstet* 1991;173:25.

Kim EE, Moon T, Delpassand ES, et al. Nuclear hepatobiliary imaging. *Radiol Clin North Am* 1993;31:923.

Kingsnorth A. Role of cytokines and their inhibitors in acute pancreatitis. *Gut* 1997;40:1.

Kiviluoto T, Siren J, Luukkonen P, et al. Randomised trial of laparoscopic versus open cholecystectomy for acute and gangrenous cholecystitis. *Lancet* 1998;351:321.

Lahtinen J, Alhava EM, Aukee S. Acute cholecystitis treated by early and delayed surgery: A controlled clinical trial. *Scand J Gastroenterol* 1978;13:673.

Lai EC, Tam PC, Paterson IA. Emergency surgery for acute cholangitis. *Ann Surg* 1990; 211:55.

Landau I, Kott AA, Deutsch E, et al. Multifactorial analysis of septic bile and septic complications in biliary surgery. *World J Surg* 1992;16:962.

Leung JW, Ling TK, Chan RC, et al. Antibiotics, biliary sepsis, and bile duct stones. *Gastrointest Endosc* 1994;40:716.

Lo CM, Liu CL, Fan ST, et al. Prospective randomized study of early versus delayed laparoscopic cholecystectomy for acute cholecystitis. *Ann Surg* 1998;227:461.

Lu EJ, Curet MJ, El-Sayed YY, et al. Medical versus surgical management of biliary tract disease in pregnancy. *Am J Surg* 2004;188:755.

Ludwig K, Bernhardt J, Steffen H, et al. Contribution of intraoperative cholangiography to incidence and outcome of common bile duct injuries during laparoscopic cholecystectomy. *Surg Endosc* 2002;16:1098.

Lujan JA, Parrilla P, Robles R, et al. Laparoscopic cholecystectomy versus open cholecystectomy in the treatment of acute cholecystitis: A prospective study. *Arch Surg* 1998; 133:173.

Marik PE, Zaloga GP. Meta-analysis of parenteral nutrition versus enteral nutrition in patients with acute pancreatitis. *BMJ* 2004;328:1407.

McArthur P, Cuschieri A, Sells RA, et al. Controlled clinical trial comparing early versus interval cholecystectomy for acute cholecystitis. *Br J Surg* 1975;62:850.

McClave SA, Greene LM, Snider HL, et al. Comparison of the safety of early enteral vs. parenteral nutrition in mild acute pancreatitis. *J Parenter Enteral Nutr* 1997;21:14.

Mier J, Leon EL, Castillo A, et al. Early versus late necrosectomy in severe necrotizing pancreatitis. *Am J Surg* 1997;173:71.

Myers SI, Bartula L. Human cholecystitis is associated with increased prostaglandin I2 and prostaglandin E2 synthesis. *Hepatology* 1992;16:1176.

Nieewenhuijs VB, Besselink MGH, van Minnen LP, et al. Surgical management of acute necrotizing pancreatitis: A 13-year experience and systematic review. *Scand J Gastroenterol* 2003;38:111.

Nielsen ML, Moesgaard F, Justesen T, et al. Wound sepsis after elective cholecystectomy. Restriction of prophylactic antibiotics to risk groups. *Scand J Gastroenterol* 1981; 16:937.

Norrby S, Herlin P, Holmin T, et al. Early or delayed cholecystectomy for acute cholecystectomy? A clinical trial. *Br J Surg* 1983;70:163.

Papi C, D'Ambrosio L, Capurso L. Timing of cholecystectomy for acute calculous cholecystitis: A meta-analysis. *Am J Gastroenterol* 2004;99:147.

Puggioni A, Wong L. A metaanalysis of laparoscopic cholecystectomy in patients with cirrhosis. *J Am Coll Surg* 2003;197:921.

Quigley EM, Marsh MN, Shaffer JL, et al. Hepatobiliary complications of total parenteral nutrition. *Gastroenterology* 1993;104:286.

Ranson JH, Rifkind KM, Roses DF, et al. Prognostic signs and the role of operative management in acute pancreatitis. *Surg Gynecol Obstet* 1974;139:69.

Roslyn JJ, Den Besten L, Thompson JE, et al. Roles of lithogenic bile and cystic duct occlusion in the pathogenesis of acute cholecystitis. *Am J Surg* 1980;140:126.

Saino V, Kemppainen E, Puolakkainen P, et al. Early antibiotic treatment in acute necrotizing pancreatitis. *Lancet* 1995;346:663.

Sampliner RE, Bennet PH, Comess LJ, et al. Gallbladder disease in Pima Indians. Demonstration of high prevalence and early onset by cholecystography. *N Engl J Med* 1970;283:1358.

Sawyer RG, Scott Jones R. Acute cholangitis. In: Cameron JL, ed. *Current Surgical Therapy.* 8th ed. Philadelphia, Pa: Mosby; 2004:407–410.

Shea JA, Berlin JA, Escarce JJ, et al. Revised estimates of diagnostic test sensitivity and specificity in suspected biliary tract disease. *Arch Intern Med* 1994;154:2573.

Shiffman ML, Keith FM, Moore EW. Pathogenesis of ceftriaxone-associated biliary sludge: In vitro studies of calcium-ceftriaxone binding and solubility. *Gastroenterology* 1990;99:1772.

Simchuk EJ, Traverso LW, Nukui Y, et al. Computed tomography severity index is a predictor of outcomes for severe pancreatitis. *Am J Surg* 2000;179:352.

Simopoulos C, Botaitis S, Polychronidis A, et al. Risk factors for conversion of laparoscopic cholecystectomy to open cholecystectomy. *Surg Endosc* 2005;19:905.

Singh AK, Sagar P. Gangrenous cholecystitis: Prediction with CT imaging. *Abdom Imaging* 2005;30:218.

Sirinek KR, Schauer PR, Yellin AE, et al. Single-dose cefuroxime versus multiple-dose cefazolin as prophylactic therapy for high-risk cholecystectomy. *J Am Coll Surg* 1994;178:321.

Soto JA, Yucel EK, Barish MA, et al. MR cholangiopancreatography after unsuccessful or incomplete ERCP. *Radiology* 1996;199:91.

Stahlberg D, Reihner E, Rudling M, et al. Influence of bezafibrate on hepatic cholesterol metabolism in gallstone patients: Reduced activity of cholesterol 7-alpha-hydroxylase. *Hepatology* 1995;21:1025.

Stone K. Acute abdominal emergencies associated with pregnancy. *Clin Obstet Gynecol* 2002;45:553.

Sung JY, Costeron JW, Shaffer EA. Defense system in the biliary tract against bacterial infection. *Dig Dis Sci* 1992;37:689.

Sung JY, Lyon DJ, Seun R, et al. Intravenous ciprofloxacin as treatment for patients with acute suppurative cholangitis: A randomized, controlled clinical trial. *J Antimicrob Chemother* 1995;35:855.

Swaroop VS, Chari ST, Clain JE. Severe acute pancreatitis. *JAMA* 2004;291:2865.

Thistle JL, Cleary PA, Lachin JM, et al., and the Steering Committee, National Cooperative Gallstone Study Group. The natural history of cholelithiasis: The National Cooperative Gallstone Study. *Ann Intern Med* 1984;101:171.

Triester SL, Kowdley KV. Prognostic factors in acute pancreatitis. *J Clin Gastroenterol* 2002;34:167.

Uhl W, Buchler MW, Malfertheiner P, et al. A randomized, double blind, multicentre trial of octreotide in moderate to severe acute pancreatitis. *Gut* 1999;45:97.

Uhl W, Muller CA, Krahenbuhl L, et al. Acute gallstone pancreatitis: Timing of laparoscopic cholecystectomy in mild and severe disease. *Surg Endosc* 1999;13:1070.

Van den Hazel SJ, Speelman P, Tygat GN, et al. Role of antibiotics in the treatment and prevention of acute and recurrent cholangitis. *Clin Infect Dis* 1994;19:279.

Welschbillig-Meunier K, Pessaux P, Lebigot J, et al. Percuataneous cholecystostomy for high-risk patients with acute cholecystitis. *Surg Endosc* 2005;19:1256.

Werner J, Uhl W, Buchler M. Acute pancreatitis. In: Cameron JL, ed. *Current Surgical Therapy.* 8th ed. Philadelphia, Pa: Mosby; 2004:407–410.

Whitcomb C, Preston RA, Aston CE, et al. Hereditary pancreatitis is caused by a mutation in the cationic trypsinogen gene. *Nat Genet* 1996;14:141.

Williams M, Simms HH. Prognostic usefulness of scoring systems in critically ill patients with severe acute pancreatitis. *Crit Care Med* 1999;27:901.

Windsor AC, Kanwar S, Li AG, et al. Compared with parenteral nutrition, enteral feeding attenuates the acute phase response and improves disease severity in acute pancreatitis. *Gut* 1998;42:431.

Yellin AE, Berne TV, Appleman MD, et al. A randomized study of cefepime versus the combination of gentamicin and mezlocillin as an adjunct to surgical treatment in patients with acute cholecystitis. *Surg Gynecol Obstet* 1993;177:S23.

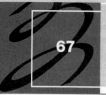

67 OBSTETRIC AND GYNECOLOGIC EMERGENCIES
GLENN UPDIKE

I. INTRODUCTION. A wide variety of emergent obstetric and gynecologic issues bring women to seek care. This chapter outlines the pathophysiology, diagnosis, and management of the common obstetric and gynecologic conditions encountered by surgeons and emergency physicians.

II. ECTOPIC PREGNANCY
- **A. Introduction.** Ectopic pregnancy refers to those pregnancies that occur outside the fundus of the uterus. While most ectopic pregnancies occur in the fallopian tube, they may also occur in the abdomen, cervix, and cornua of the uterus. Ectopic pregnancy is a significant cause of maternal morbidity. Prompt diagnosis and appropriate management, whether medical or surgical, are critical to prevent intraperitoneal hemorrhage and its complications.
- **B. Incidence and epidemiology**
    1. Approximately 19 per 10,000 pregnancies
    2. Most commonly occurs in the fallopian tube (96%)
    3. Risk factors include:
        - **a.** Previous ectopic pregnancy. In a patient with a prior ectopic pregnancy, the chance of having a subsequent ectopic pregnancy is between 8% and 15%.
        - **b.** Previous pelvic inflammatory disease
        - **c.** A history of tubal surgery including tubal ligation. Nearly 50% of pregnancies are ectopic after having tubal ligation.
        - **d.** Having an intrauterine device in place
        - **e.** Cigarette smoking
- **C. Diagnosis**
    1. The **triad of a missed menstrual cycle, vaginal bleeding, and abdominal pain** should raise the suspicion for ectopic pregnancy.
    2. The most common symptom is abdominal pain (94% of patients).
    3. Physical examination may reveal unilateral tenderness and/or an adnexal mass.
    4. May screen with a urine pregnancy test, but diagnosis will require a quantitative serum human chorionic gonadotropin (hCG).
    5. When ectopic pregnancy is suspected, the patient should have a pelvic ultrasound by a sonographer experienced in gynecologic ultrasound.
    6. If the serum hCG is >1,500 milli-international units per milliliter (mIU/mL), an intrauterine gestational sac should be visualized by transvaginal pelvic ultrasound.
    7. An adnexal mass may or may not be visualized by ultrasound with ectopic pregnancy. An adnexal gestational sac, yolk sac, and embryo may be visualized.
    8. If extrauterine or intrauterine pregnancy are not visualized and the serum quantitative hCG is <1,500 mIU/mL, the serum quantitative hCG should be repeated in 48 hours.
    9. In a normal pregnancy, the serum quantitative hCG should approximately double every 48 hours. The median increase of the hCG in 48 hours in normal pregnancies is 124%, with a minimum of 52%.
    10. If the serum quantitative hCG is rising abnormally but it is unclear by ultrasound whether the pregnancy is extra- or intrauterine, a diagnostic dilation

and curettage may be performed to assess for the presence of villi. The absence of villi and intermediate trophoblast cells on pathologic examination suggests the presence of an ectopic pregnancy.

D. Management

1. **Surgical management**
   a. Gold standard for the management of ectopic pregnancy.
   b. Laparoscopic approach is favored in most cases except in the setting of hemodynamic instability.
   c. If possible, the ectopic pregnancy should be removed through an incision in the fallopian tube (salpingostomy). The quantitative serum hCG should be followed after salpingostomy to ensure complete removal of the pregnancy.
   d. If salpingostomy is not possible, the entire affected fallopian tube should be removed (salpingectomy).
   e. Limited data suggest that there may be a higher rate of successful pregnancies following salpingostomy when compared to salpingectomy.

2. **Expectant management**
   a. Reserved only for highly specialized circumstances.
   b. Patients should be highly compliant with a documented falling quantitative serum hCG that is <1,000 mIU/mL.

3. **Medical management**
   a. Also reserved for highly specialized circumstances in the compliant patient.
   b. Contraindications to medical management include:
      i. Poor compliance
      ii. Hemodynamic instability
      iii. Adnexal mass >3 cm
      iv. Presence of embryonic cardiac activity
      v. Quantitative serum hCG >10,000 mIU/mL
   c. Therapy consists of the administration of methotrexate delivered as a single dose of 50 mg/m^2.
   d. The serum hCG is assessed on day 4 and day 7 after administration.
   e. If the serum hCG has not fallen by 15% between days 4 and 7, the patient may be given a second dose of methotrexate or offered surgical management.
   f. If the serum hCG decreases by 15% between days 4 and 7, the serum quantitative hCG should be assessed at weekly intervals until it is less than 20 mIU/mL.

III. MISCARRIAGE

A. Introduction.
Spontaneous abortion, defined as loss of the pregnancy prior to 20 weeks of gestation, is a common occurrence. When women experience bleeding during pregnancy, they often present to the ED for initial care.

1. The term **threatened abortion** is used when there is vaginal bleeding in the first half of pregnancy and the cervical os is closed.
2. A **missed abortion** is a pregnancy in which there is embryonic demise or lack of progression of the pregnancy in the setting of a closed cervical os.
3. **Inevitable abortion** is used to describe pregnancies in the first 20 weeks in which the cervix has begun to dilate or there is gross rupture of fetal membranes, but the pregnancy has not yet been expelled.
4. **Incomplete abortion** refers to pregnancies in which the cervix has dilated and delivery of the fetus or placenta has begun, but products of conception remain in the uterus. This may be accompanied by heavy bleeding.
5. **Complete abortion** refers to the passage of all products of conception and subsequent closure of the cervix.

B. Epidemiology and Pathophysiology
1. Fifteen percent of pregnancies end in spontaneous abortion.
2. Risk factors include advanced maternal age and short interpregnancy interval.
3. Sixty percent of spontaneous abortions are because of chromosomal anomalies.

C. Diagnosis
1. Patients may present to the ED with vaginal bleeding or cramping.

2. Physical examination may reveal blood in the vaginal vault. The cervix may appear dilated and the uterus is enlarged.
3. Gestational age by ultrasound may be inconsistent with the last menstrual period and may reveal an empty gestational sac or an embryo without a heartbeat. Cardiac activity should be noted in the embryo when the crown rump length is 5 mm, or by 5 to 6 weeks' gestation
4. It is essential to rule out the presence of ectopic pregnancy with ultrasound.

D. Management

1. No therapies are effective in the prevention of miscarriage in the case of threatened abortion. Pelvic rest and limited activity does not decrease the chance of spontaneous abortion.
2. Patients who are not bleeding heavily, are hemodynamically stable, and are not in excessive pain can be managed expectantly.
3. Medical management with drugs such as misoprostil and mifepristone are currently being studied.
4. Dilation and curettage is the treatment for patients who are bleeding heavily, are hemodynamically unstable, or unwilling to undergo expectant or medical management.
5. All patients who have bleeding during pregnancy should have a blood type and antibody screen. In patients who are Rh negative and bleeding during the first trimester, MICRhoGAM 50 mg intramuscularly (IM) should be administered.

IV. THIRD TRIMESTER BLEEDING

A. Introduction. During the third trimester, uterine blood flow increases by 500 cc per minute. As such, a variety of pathologic states involving the placenta and uterus can result in massive blood loss in a short period of time. Prompt recognition and appropriate resuscitation are critical in preventing serious morbidity and mortality from obstetric hemorrhage in the third trimester.

B. Placental abruption

1. Refers to the state in which all (**total abruption**) or part (**partial abruption**) of the placenta separates from the uterus after 20 weeks' gestation but prior to delivery.
2. Incidence is 0.4% to 1.3% of pregnancies, with 80% occurring prior to the onset of labor.
3. Fetal demise from placental abruption occurs in 0.12% of pregnancies.
4. Risk factors include trauma, hypertension, cocaine use, thrombophilias, and rapid decompression of the amniotic fluid.
5. Placental abruption results from a disruption of maternal vessels in the decidua basalis where they interface with the villi of the placental cytotrophoblast. May result from trauma or a chronic pathological vascular process.
6. Most common presentation is vaginal bleeding, although 20% of patients will not exhibit bleeding. Fifty percent of patients will have abdominal pain and uterine contractions.
7. Physical examination may reveal a rigid, firm uterine fundus.
8. The fetal heart rate may show signs of fetal distress.
9. Ultrasound may show a retroplacental hematoma, but the sensitivity of ultrasound for detecting placental abruption is poor.
10. If massive bleeding is present, there may be clinical and laboratory evidence of disseminated intravascular coagulation.

C. Placenta previa

1. Placenta previa refers to the implantation of the placenta over the cervical os. This may be **complete** (entirely covering the cervical os), **partial** (only a portion of the placental covers the cervical os), or **marginal** (the placenta approaches but does not cover the cervical os).
2. Placenta previa complicates approximately 0.5% of pregnancies.
3. Risk factors include advanced maternal age, ethnicity (with an increased incidence in African Americans), and previous cesarean section. Previous cesarean section remains the most important risk factor for development of placenta previa, with the risk increasing with the number of previous cesarean sections.

4. The **classic presentation of placenta previa is painless vaginal bleeding**. All patients presenting with vaginal bleeding should be imaged with ultrasound to determine the location of the placenta.

5. **Do not perform digital examination of the cervix** in patients with placenta previa—this manipulation may precipitate hemorrhage.

D. Management of third trimester bleeding

1. The maternal hemodynamic status should be monitored closely and fetal status should be assessed with continuous fetal heart rate monitoring.

2. Two large-bore intravenous lines should be placed with prompt administration of crystalloid to replace lost intravascular volume.

3. If blood loss is large, ongoing, or associated with hypotension, transfuse with packed red blood cells.

4. In addition to measurement of a hemoglobin, platelet count, and blood type, assess coagulation with measurements of prothrombin time, activated partial thromboplastin time, and fibrinogen. Coagulopathy should be corrected with fresh frozen plasma or cryoprecipitate as necessary.

5. When severe bleeding is present, marked by evidence of maternal hypovolemia, coagulopathy, or nonreassuring fetal heart rate status, delivery must be expedited to prevent maternal and fetal morbidity.

6. In patients with placenta previa, delivery will always be by cesarean section.

7. Patients with placental abruption and hypovolemia, coagulopathy, or nonreassuring fetal heart rate status should likewise be delivered by cesarean section.

8. In general, cesarean section should be delayed only as long as it takes to correct maternal hypovolemia and coagulopathy.

V. LABOR AND DELIVERY

A. Introduction. Occasionally women present to locations other than a delivery suite in the advanced stages of labor, and movement to the labor and delivery suite to deliver may not be possible. Some basic aspects of labor and delivery are reviewed here.

B. Normal labor

1. Normal labor is divided into three stages:

   a. The first stage of labor starts with the onset of contractions until the cervix is completely dilated. The first stage of labor is divided into a latent phase (from closed to 4-cm dilation) and active phase (from 4-cm dilation to complete dilation). The active phase progresses at a minimum of 1.2 cm per hour.

   b. The second stage of labor is time from complete cervical dilation until delivery of the fetus.

   c. The third stage of labor is the time from delivery of the fetus until delivery of the placenta. This should last less than 30 minutes.

2. Labor progresses in an orderly fashion.

   a. The head becomes engaged in the maternal pelvis.

   b. The head of the fetus flexes, minimizing the diameter passing through the pelvic inlet.

   c. The head descends through the pelvis.

   d. The fetal head rotates internally.

   e. The fetal head extends and passes through the budging introitus.

   f. The fetal head rotates externally.

   g. The shoulders pass below the pubic symphysis and the remainder of the fetus is delivered.

3. The role of the delivering clinician is as follows:

   a. As the fetal head extends and delivers through the introitus, the delivering clinician should place his or her hands on the fetus and support the perineum to ensure that the head delivers in a controlled fashion. Rapid extension and delivery can result in increased perineal trauma and increased damage to the anal sphincter.

   b. After delivery of the head, a bulb suction device is used to clear amniotic fluid and blood from the mouth and nares of the infant.

    c. The finger should be swept over the neck to assess for the presence of a nuchal umbilical cord. The cord usually sweeps easily over the fetal head. If the cord is too tight to move over the fetal head easily, it may be doubly clamped and ligated to facilitate delivery.

    d. After delivery of the head and restitution (external rotation), the fetal shoulders should be gently guided below the pubic symphysis. It is important to not apply excessive traction at this point as doing so may result in brachial plexus injury. The posterior shoulder is then delivered.

    e. Perineal lacerations are common following delivery. Consultation with an obstetrician should be made in the ED setting for repair of perineal lacerations.

  4. Shoulder dystocia refers to a delay in delivery of the fetal shoulder after delivery of the fetal head. It is an obstetric emergency and should be managed in an orderly fashion.

    a. Call for assistance and immediate backup by an obstetrician.

    b. The maternal legs should be hyperflexed toward the maternal abdomen, thus widening the pelvic outlet (McRobert's maneuver).

    c. Suprapubic pressure should be applied on the maternal abdomen to attempt to displace the fetal shoulder below the pubic symphysis.

    d. If these maneuvers are not successful, two fingers are placed against the posterior shoulder and pressure is applied towards the fetal back. This should rotate the shoulders into the wider diameter of the pelvis (Wood's screw maneuver).

    e. The posterior arm is delivered.

    f. With failure of these maneuvers, deliberate fracture of the fetal clavicle may facilitate delivery.

VI. ACUTE PELVIC INFLAMMATORY DISEASE

  A. Introduction. Pelvic inflammatory disease (PID) is an inflammatory condition of the upper genital tract thought to be caused by upward ascension of microorganisms from the lower genital tract. This disease may include infection of the endometrium (**endometritis**), fallopian tubes (**salpingitis**), or peritoneal cavity. The disease may also include the development of tuboovarian abscess. Prompt diagnosis and treatment of PID is important to prevent both short- and long-term morbidity in women with the diagnosis. The consequences of PID include infertility, increased risk of ectopic pregnancy, and chronic pelvic pain.

  B. Epidemiology and pathophysiology

    1. The Centers for Disease Control and Prevention (CDC) estimates that there are approximately 780,000 new cases of PID diagnosed annually in the United States.

    2. Many cases of PID are unrecognized and undiagnosed (**silent PID**).

    3. Risk factors for development of PID include:

      a. Young age

      b. Multiple sex partners

      c. Young age of sexual debut

      d. Lack of use of barrier contraception

    4. Occurs as a result of the ascension of microorganisms from the vagina and endocervix into the endometrium, fallopian tubes, and pelvic peritoneum.

    5. Most cases are caused by *Neisseria gonorrhea* (43%), 10% caused by *Chlamydia trachomatis* alone, and 12% caused by coinfection with both organisms.

    6. The remaining 30% of PID is caused by infection with anaerobic bacteria, *Mycoplasma,* and *Ureaplasma.*

  C. Diagnosis

    1. Often a difficult diagnosis and is quite inaccurate secondary to wide variation in severity of symptoms.

    2. Gold standard for diagnosis remains laparoscopy with directed biopsy and culture, although this is not practical or necessary for most patients.

3. The CDC provides criteria for the diagnosis of PID. These criteria require the presence of uterine or adnexal tenderness **and** cervical motion tenderness. The patient may also have one or more of the following: temperature of greater than 101°F, a mucopurulent cervical discharge, white blood cells on wet mount, an elevated sedimentation rate, an elevated C-reactive protein, or positive testing for *Neisseria gonorrhea* and/or *Chlamydia trachomatis.*

D. Management
1. The goal of management is not only to treat the immediate symptoms of abdominal pain and pelvic pain, but also to prevent later consequences such as infertility, ectopic pregnancy, and chronic pelvic pain.
2. Table 67-1 shows the CDC criteria for hospitalization of patients with PID.
3. Table 67-2 shows the CDC parenteral treatment regimens for acute PID.
4. Table 67-3 shows the CDC oral treatment regimens for acute PID.

E. Tuboovarian abscess
1. Common complication of PID (up to one third of hospitalized patients).
2. Suspected when abdominal pain is lateralized. On physical examination there is usually a tender palpable adnexal mass. Ultrasound confirms the diagnosis.
3. Patients with tuboovarian abscess should initially have a trial of medical therapy with a CDC-recommended treatment regimen. All patients should be admitted.

TABLE 67-1   Criteria for Hospitalization of Patients with Acute PID

Surgical emergencies such as appendicitis cannot be excluded.
The patient is pregnant.
The patient does not respond clinically to oral antibiotic therapy.
The patient is unable to tolerate or follow an outpatient treatment regimen.
The patient has severe illness with nausea, vomiting, or high fever.
The patient has a tuboovarian abscess.
The patient is immunodeficient.

TABLE 67-2   CDC-Recommended Treatment Schedules for Parenteral Treatment of Acute PID

Regimen A
Cefotetan 2-g IV every 12 h
  or
Cefoxitin 2-g IV every 6 h
  plus
Doxycycline 100-mg IV or orally every 12 h

The regimen is given for at least 24 hours after patient clinically improves. After discharge from the hospital, continue doxycycline 100 mg orally twice daily for 14 days.

Regimen B
Clindamycin 900-mg IV every 8 h
  plus
Gentamicin loading dose IV or IM (2 mg/kg) followed by a maintenance dose (1.5 mg/kg) every 8 h

The regimen is given for at least 24 hours after patient clinically improves. After discharge from the hospital, continue doxycycline 100 mg orally twice daily for 14 days, or clindamycin 450 mg orally four times daily to complete 14 days of therapy.

TABLE 67-3	CDC Treatment Schedule for Oral Treatment of Acute PID

Regimen A

Ofloxacin 400 mg orally every 12 h for 14 d or levofloxacin 500 mg orally once daily
  with or without

Metronidazole 500 mg orally every 12 h for 14 d

Regimen B

Ceftriaxone 250 mg IM once
  or
Cefoxitin 2 g IM plus probenecid 1 g orally in a single dose
  or
Other parenteral third-generation cephalosporin
  plus
Doxycycline 100 mg orally every 12 h for 14 d with or without metronidazole 500 mg orally
every 12 h for 14 d

4. If patients do not have an objective clinical response in 2 to 4 days, the abscess should be surgically managed. Consideration may be given to ultrasound-guided drainage, although recurrences are common.

VII. ABNORMAL UTERINE BLEEDING

A. Introduction. Abnormal uterine bleeding can be caused by both anatomic abnormalities and by abnormalities of the menstrual cycle. The term **dysfunctional uterine bleeding** is used to describe bleeding that is unrelated to anatomic abnormalities. **Menorrhagia** refers to heavy uterine bleeding at the expected time of menses. The normal menses usually results in approximately 80 mL of blood loss and lasts for <7 days. Bleeding in excess of this amount, or bleeding that lasts >7 days, constitutes menorrhagia. As a practical matter, it is difficult to quantify the volume of blood loss with each menses. The number of pads or tampons used during menses serves as a surrogate measure of blood loss, although even pad counts may not accurately estimate blood loss. **Metrorrhagia** is the term used to describe bleeding that occurs between menses. **Menometrorrhagia** refers to heavy menses in addition to bleeding between menses.

B. Pathophysiology

1. Anatomic causes of abnormal uterine bleeding include:

  a. Leiomyomas (fibroids) are especially related to abnormal bleeding when located in an intracavitary or submucosal location, but intramural leiomyomas may also be related to abnormal uterine bleeding.

  b. Endometrial polyps

  c. Endometritis

  d. Endometrial hyperplasia

  e. Endometrial cancer

2. Dysfunctional uterine bleeding is bleeding that occurs in the absence of an anatomic cause. The most common cause of dysfunctional uterine bleeding is anovulation. Risk factors for dysfunctional uterine bleeding include obesity, thyroid dysfunction, endometrial atrophy, and bleeding dyscrasias.

C. Evaluation

1. Patients with abnormal uterine bleeding should have a thorough history and physical examination performed. Measure vital signs, including orthostatic testing, to assess physiologic responses. A pelvic examination including a speculum examination is mandatory. Look for lower genital tract causes of vaginal bleeding. In addition, assess the size, texture, and mobility of the uterus.

2. Laboratory testing should begin with a urine hCG to assess potential pregnancy. Also, a hematocrit should be obtained to assess for anemia. In select cases of very heavy, recurrent of bleeding in more than one site, assess coagulation with a prothrombin time, activated partial thromboplastin time, and fibrinogen level.

3. Pelvic imaging with ultrasound should be considered, but often is not needed initially.

D. Management

1. Patients presenting with profuse vaginal hemorrhage should receive the same care as any patient presenting with life-threatening bleeding. Intravenous volume replacement initiated with crystalloids or packed red blood cells if necessary. Consult a gynecologist while resuscitating, since the quickest and most effective way to relieve profuse hemorrhage often is dilation and curettage.

2. Medical therapy for heavy bleeding in the absence of life-threatening hemorrhage includes:

   a. Intravenous estrogen administered as conjugated equine estrogens, 25 mg every 6 hours.

   b. Oral estrogen administered as conjugated equine estrogens, 2.5 mg every 6 hours.

   c. Oral contraceptives.

   d. Medroxyprogesterone acetate.

   e. Patients should receive iron supplementation.

E. Gynecologic causes of abdominal pain

1. Ovarian cysts

   a. Commonly cause pelvic pain, and are classified as either functional (arise as a result of the normal menstrual cycle) or neoplastic (a true cyst that arises from the epithelium).

   b. The pain is from rupture, hemorrhage, or torsion.

   c. Diagnosis is made by history and physical examination. Pelvic exam will confirm the diagnosis and define the type of cyst.

   d. Management is supportive, including appropriate pain therapy. Nonsteriodal agents are first line choices, with opioids using for more severe discomfort (though more pain should prompt a search for ovarian torsion).

   e. Hemorrhagic cysts may require surgical management if there is severe or evolving anemia. Oral contraceptives do not cause regression of existing ovarian cysts.

2. Ovarian torsion

   a. Ovarian torsion occurs when the ovary (and most often the fallopian tube) twists and compromise blood flow to the adnexa. As the ovarian veins and lymphatic system are obstructed, the adnexa becomes increasingly edematous.

   b. Patients present with unilateral exquisite abdominal pain that is sudden and severe.

   c. Pain may be accompanied by nausea and vomiting, mimicking appendicitis.

   d. An adnexal mass is found, and exam should also reveal severe lower abdominal tenderness that is often lateralized.

   e. Pelvic ultrasound may aid in diagnosis by demonstrating an adnexal mass. Color Doppler to detect obstructed flow may further aid in the diagnosis of ovarian torsion, but should not be relied upon to make or exclude the diagnosis.

   f. Gynecologic consultation is necessary to provide relief of pain and possible preservation of ovarian function using a surgical intervention. The adnexa may be "untwisted" with removal of the causative mass. If there is evidence of tissue necrosis (failure of return of pink color 30 minutes after untwisting) the adnexa should be removed.

3. Endomyometritis

   a. Infection of the endometrium with extension to the myometrium.

   b. Commonly diagnosed following a therapeutic termination of pregnancy, with an incidence of 1 per 100 procedures.

    c. Pathogens include group B beta streptococcus, *Staphylococcus aureus*, *Bacteroides* species, *Neisseria gonorrhea,* and *Chlamydia trachomatis.* New reports also note *Clostridium sordelli* as an uncommon but lethal (toxic shock producing trigger) pathogen.

    d. Commonly presents within 5 days after procedure or delivery.

    e. Symptoms include abdominopelvic pain, fever, and a foul-smelling discharge.

    f. Physical examination reveals uterine tenderness.

    g. Requires admission to the hospital and broad-spectrum parenteral antibiotics.

    h. Ultrasound to search for retained products of conception is helpful in patients not responding to antibiotic therapy. Dilation and curettage is necessary in patients with endometritis and retained products of conception.

4. Endometriosis

    a. Condition in which hormonally responsive implants of endometrial tissue are present in the abdominopelvic cavity on areas such as the peritoneum, bladder, and bowel.

    b. Present in up to 15% of premenopausal women.

    c. The etiology of endometriosis is uncertain but may be related to retrograde menstruation through the fallopian tube.

    d. The most common complaint is cyclic abdominal pain and painful menses (**dysmenorrhea**).

    e. Physical examination reveals abdominal and pelvic tenderness. An ovarian mass may be palpated and may represent an endometrioma, or the so-called chocolate cyst. Rectovaginal examination may reveal nodularity in the rectovaginal septum or uterosacral ligaments.

    f. Like simple ovarian cysts, acute management centers on pain control. Patients with endometriosis will need outpatient gynecologic management to determine what medical or surgical treatment plan is most appropriate.

5. Adenomyosis

    a. Adenomyosis is the proliferation of endometrial glands within the myometrial walls.

    b. Patients present with abnormal uterine bleeding and dysmenorrheal/dysmenorrhea.

    c. Physical examination reveals an enlarged, globular, tender uterus.

    d. The diagnosis of adenomyosis is clinical, with pelvic ultrasound adding little to the diagnosis. MRI may confirm the diagnosis.

    e. Acute management of adenomyosis includes pain control.

6. Intraabdominal adhesions

    a. May be a cause of abdominal pain and may be associated with bowel obstruction.

    b. Risk factors include prior pelvic surgery, endometriosis, a history of pelvic inflammatory disease, and radiation therapy.

    c. Initial management of patients suspected of pain secondary to adhesions is supportive, with parenteral fluids and suctioning as needed, and analgesics used as necessary. Surgical lysis is reserved for refractory or severe cases of adhesion with obstruction.

VIII. BARTHOLIN'S ABSCESSES

  A. Introduction. Bartholin's glands are located at four and eight o'clock in the posterior introitus and drain through duct openings in the vulvar vestibule. The glands can become obstructed resulting in a cyst or, if infected, an abscess.

  B. Epidemiology and pathophysiology

    1. Most commonly affects women in their third decade, and 2% of women develop a Bartholin's cyst or abscess during their lifetime.

    2. Infections are generally polymicrobial and caused by a wide variety of organisms. Anaerobes are the most commonly isolates, and *N. gonorrhea* is the most common aerobic species isolated.

C. Diagnosis

1. Patients with Bartholin's gland abscess usually present with the complaint of a painful mass in the posterior vulva.

2. Physical examination reveals a tender, indurated, erythematous mass at the posterior vulvar vestibule. Occasionally, spontaneous drainage of purulent material occurs.

3. Induration and swelling that is more anterior is likely not a Bartholin's abscess but rather a labial abscess.

D. Management

1. Simple incision and drainage of Bartholin's abscesses **should not be performed** as the recurrence of abscesses is common (13%).

2. A preferred option is use of a **Word catheter**.

   a. The vulva is prepared with betadine.

   b. A 5-mm incision is made distal to the hymeneal ring, but proximal to the labia minora in the vulvar vestibule.

   c. The abscess is drained completely and an instrument is used to break up loculations. Cultures can be sent at this time. The abscess is then irrigated copiously with normal saline.

   d. The Word catheter is placed and filled with 3 mm of saline.

   e. The catheter should be left in place for at least 4 weeks to allow epithelialization.

   f. Unless there is surrounding cellulitis or the patient is diabetic, antibiotics are not necessary.

3. Another option is marsupialization of a Bartholin's cyst.

   a. The vulva is prepared with betadine.

   b. A 3-cm incision is made distal to the hymeneal ring, but proximal to the labia minora in the vulvar vestibule.

   c. The abscess is drained completely and an instrument is used to break up loculations. Cultures can be sent at this time. The abscess is then irrigated copiously with normal saline.

   d. The cyst wall is then everted and sutured to the mucosa of the vestibule with interrupted suture.

4. Excision of Bartholin's gland is performed for recurrent abscesses. This procedure should only be performed in the operating room setting by an experienced gynecologist.

IX. MASTITIS

A. Introduction. Mastitis is infection of the breast tissue.

B. Epidemiology and athophysiology

1. Occurs in 2% to 3% of lactating women.

2. Most common during the first 3 weeks after delivery.

3. Cracks in the skin of the nipple or breast allows the entry of bacteria. The most common pathogens are *Staphylococcus* species, *E. Coli*, and *Streptococcus*.

C. Diagnosis

1. Patients present with the complaint of breast pain, usually unilateral. In addition, they may complain of fever, chills, malaise, and body aches.

2. Physical examination reveals erythema, tenderness, and warmth to the touch. Careful palpation should be performed to rule out the presence of a breast abscess.

D. Management

1. Treatment consists of antibiotic therapy, usually with an extended penicillin (such as dicloxacillin or nafcillin) or first-generation cephalosporin for 10 to 14 days.

2. Lactating mothers should continue to breast feed or pump on the affected breast, although this may be somewhat painful.

3. Warm or cold compresses should be encouraged.

4. Patients should wear a well-supporting bra and wear a bra while sleeping.

5. Follow-up should be arranged within several days to ensure that the mastitis is resolving.

6. Breast abscess develops in 10% of women with mastitis. Findings include a tender, fluctuant mass in the breast and can be confirmed by ultrasound. The breast abscess should be surgically treated with incision and drainage. Cultures and antibiotic sensitivities should be obtained from abscess material.

X. SEXUAL ASSAULT

A. Introduction. Sexual assault is a common problem in the United States and with increasing prevalence. Although most sexual assaults go unreported, many victims present for care following an assault.

B. Incidence and epidemiology

  1. The true population incidence is unknown, although some studies suggest that up to 24% of women have been the victim of a completed rape, with another 20% reporting that they have been the victim of an attempted rape.

  2. Women between the ages of 17 and 25 years are the most common victims of rape, and nearly three quarters of women know the assailant.

  3. One third of rapes involve oral and/or anal penetration.

C. Management

  1. Victims should be immediately taken to a private room in the ED or care site. With the permission of the victim, and not to impede evaluation and treatment of medical/traumatic needs, law enforcement personnel should be contacted early to aid with the combined medical–legal needs. Also, a sexual assault team, or an experienced clinician, is preferred to provide the best possible evaluation and care.

  2. A thorough history should be taken detailing all of the specifics of the assault that the patient can remember.

  3. Clothes should be gathered and labeled with the patient's name, date, and time of collection. Evidence should never be left unattended to maintain the chain of evidence from clinician to law enforcement.

  4. Physical examination should include a complete body examination. Any moist or dried secretions, stains, hair, or foreign material should be collected. A Wood's lamp might make collection easier. A complete pelvic examination should be performed, again with attention to the presence of any secretions, stains, hair, or foreign material. The pubic hair must be combed and the material collected sent with the comb to the laboratory. A speculum examination should be performed, with careful attention to find any trauma to the vaginal walls. Also, collect vaginal fluid, to be examined for the presence of sperm. If intercourse was >72 hours prior to presentation, swabs of the cervix may yield the presence of sperm. Obtain swabs to examine for gonorrhea, chlamydia, and trichomonas. Perform a bimanual examination to assess for pelvic trauma. Rectal examination should be included as necessary with the collection of appropriate specimens. Finally, obtain blood to test for HIV, hepatitis B, and syphilis. In select cases, directed toxicology screening may be needed.

  5. Emergency contraception should be offered to all victims of sexual assault as indicated. Immediate counseling should be available, along with structured follow-up for medical and psychologic assessment after the initial evaluation.

  6. Depending on state and local regulations, other specimens may be collected such as blood, saliva, and fingernail debris. It is important to be familiar with local regulations and hospital policy when gathering evidence and caring for the victim of sexual assault—this is another reason for creating trained sexual assault teams or clinicians.

XI. LOWER GENITAL TRACT TRAUMA

A. Introduction. Vulvar and vaginal trauma may occur in both the obstetric and nonobstetric setting, and may be penetrating or nonpenetrating.

B. Vulvar and vaginal hematoma

  1. Most commonly encountered trauma in the vulva is the straddle injury.

  2. Because of the dense vascularity of the vulva and vagina, bleeding is often profuse. Contained bleeding may result in a vulvar or vaginal hematoma.

3. Nonexpanding hematomas should be observed. The pressure of the hematoma may be sufficient to tamponade bleeding. Insert a urinary catheter if outflow is obstructed.
4. If the hematoma is expanding or the patient's vital signs suggest decompensation or ongoing physiologic losses, surgical exploration is required to identify and stop the bleeding site.

C. Vulvar and vaginal lacerations
1. If the laceration is superficial and hemostatic, it is not necessary to suture the injury. If bleeding is light, use a hemostatic agent (such as silver nitrate and Monsel's solution).
2. Deep lacerations are best repaired in the OR.
3. Deep lacerations should be repaired in layers with absorbable suture after copious irrigation. Avoid placement of sutures in the bladder anteriorly and the rectum posteriorly.
4. If there is evidence of infection, leave the wound open and repair later or by allowing healing by secondary intention.

Bibliography
Barnhart KT, Sammel MD, Rinaudo PF, et al. Symptomatic patients with an early viable intrauterine pregnancy: HCG curves redefined. *Obstet Gynecol* 2004;105(1):50–55.
Bangsgaard N, Lund CO, Ottesen B, Nilas L. Improved fertility following conservative surgical treatment of ectopic pregnancy. *BJOG* 2003;110(8):765–770.
Centers for Disease Control and Prevention. Sexually transmitted disease treatment guidelines 2002. *MMWR Morb Mortal Wkly Rep* 2002;51(RR-6).
Nelson AL, Sinow RM, Renslo R, et al. Endovaginal ultrasonographically guided transvaginal drainage for treatment of pelvic abscesses. *Am J Obstet Gynecol* 1995;172(6): 1926–1932; discussion 1932–1935.
Zweizig S, Perron J, Grubb F, Mishell DR. Conservative management of adnexal torsion. *Am J Obstet Gynecol* 1993;168(6 pt 1):1791–1795.

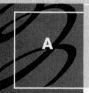

INJURY SCALES

Cervical vascular organ injury scale

Grade*	Description of injury	AIS-90
I	Thyroid vein	1–3
	Common facial vein	1–3
	External jugular vein	1–3
	Unnamed arterial or venous branches	1–3
II	External carotid arterial branches (ascending pharyngeal, superior thyroid, lingual, facial, maxillary, occipital, posterior auricular)	1–3
	Thyrocervical trunk or primary branches	1–3
	Internal jugular vein	1–3
III	External carotid artery	2–3
	Subclavian vein	3–4
	Vertebral artery	2–4
IV	Common carotid artery	3–5
	Subclavian artery	3–4
V	Internal carotid artery (extracranial)	3–5

*Increase one grade for multiple grade III or IV injuries involving >50% vessel circumference.
Decrease one grade for <25% vessel circumference disruption for grade IV or V.
AIS, Abbreviated Injury Score.

Chest wall injury scale

Grade*	Injury type	Description of injury	AIS-90
I	Contusion	Any size	1
	Laceration	Skin and subcutaneous tissue	1
	Fracture	Fewer than three ribs, closed; nondisplaced clavicle, closed	1–2
II	Laceration	Skin, subcutaneous tissue, and muscle	1
	Fracture	Three or more adjacent ribs, closed	2–3
		Open or displaced clavicle	2
		Nondisplaced sternum, closed	2
		Scapular body, open or closed	2
III	Laceration	Full thickness, including pleural penetration	2
	Fracture	Open or displaced sternum, flail sternum	2
		Unilateral flail segment (<3 ribs)	3–4

(continued)

IV	Laceration	Avulsion of chest wall tissues with underlying rib fractures	4
	Fracture	Unilateral flail chest (≥3 ribs)	3–4
V	Fracture	Bilateral flail chest (≥3 ribs on both sides)	5

*This scale is confined to the chest wall alone and does not reflect associated internal thoracic or abdominal injuries. Therefore, further delineation of upper versus lower or anterior versus posterior chest wall was not considered, and a grade VI was not warranted. Specifically, thoracic crush was not used as a descriptive term; instead, the geography and extent of fractures and soft-tissue injury were used to define the grade. Advance by one grade for bilateral injuries up to grade III.
AIS, Abbreviated Injury Score.

Heart injury scale

Grade*	Description of injury	AIS-90
I	Blunt cardiac injury with minor electrocardiographic abnormality (nonspecific ST- or T-wave changes, premature atrial or ventricular contraction, or persistent sinus tachycardia)	3
	Blunt or penetrating pericardial wound without cardiac injury, cardiac tamponade, or cardiac herniation	
II	Blunt cardiac injury with heart block (right or left bundle branch, left anterior fascicular, or atrioventricular) or ischemic changes (ST-depression or T-wave inversion) without cardiac failure	3
	Penetrating tangential myocardial wound up to, but not extending through, endocardium, without tamponade	3
III	Blunt cardiac injury with sustained (≥6 bpm) or multifocal ventricular contractions	3–4
	Blunt or penetrating cardiac injury with septal rupture, pulmonary or tricuspid valvular incompetence, papillary muscle dysfunction, or distal coronary arterial occlusion without cardiac failure	3–4
	Blunt pericardial laceration with cardiac herniation	
	Blunt cardiac injury with cardiac failure	3–4
	Penetrating tangential myocardial wound up to, but extending through, endocardium, with tamponade	3
IV	Blunt or penetrating cardiac injury with septal rupture, pulmonary or tricuspid valvular incompetence, papillary muscle dysfunction, or distal coronary arterial occlusion producing cardiac failure	3
	Blunt or penetrating cardiac injury with aortic mitral valve incompetence	
	Blunt or penetrating cardiac injury of the right ventricle, right atrium, or left atrium	5

(*continued*)

V	Blunt or penetrating cardiac injury with proximal coronary arterial occlusion	5
	Blunt or penetrating left ventricular perforation	5
	Stellate wound with <50% tissue loss of the right ventricle, right atrium, or left atrium	5
VI	Blunt avulsion of the heart; penetrating wound producing >50% tissue loss of a chamber	6

*Advance one grade for multiple wounds to a single chamber or multiple chamber involvement.
AIS, Abbreviated Injury Score.

Lung injury scale

Grade*	Injury type	Description of injury	AIS-90
I	Contusion	Unilateral, less than one lobe	3
II	Contusion	Unilateral, single lobe	3
	Laceration	Simple pneumothorax	3
III	Contusion	Unilateral, more than one lobe	3
	Laceration	Persistent (>72 hours) air leak from distal airway	3–4
	Hematoma	Nonexpanding intraparenchymal	
IV	Laceration	Major (segmental or lobar) air leak	4–5
	Hematoma	Expanding intraparenchymal	
	Vascular	Primary branch intrapulmonary vessel disruption	3–5
V	Vascular	Hilar vessel disruption	4
VI	Vascular	Total uncontained transection of pulmonary hilum	4

*Advance one grade for bilateral injuries up to grade III. Hemothorax is scored under thoracic vascular injury scale.
AIS, Abbreviated Injury Score.

Thoracic vascular injury scale

Grade*	Description of injury	AIS-90
I	Intercostal artery or vein	2–3
	Internal mammary artery or vein	2–3
	Bronchial artery or vein	2–3
	Esophageal artery or vein	2–3
	Hemiazygous vein	2–3
	Unnamed artery or vein	2–3
II	Azygos vein	2–3
	Internal jugular vein	2–3
	Subclavian vein	3–4
	Innominate vein	3–4
III	Carotid artery	3–5
	Innominate artery	3–4
	Subclavian artery	3–4

(continued)

IV	Thoracic aorta, descending	4–5
	Inferior vena cava (intrathoracic)	3–4
	Pulmonary artery, primary intraparenchymal branch	3
	Pulmonary vein, primary intraparenchymal branch	3
V	Thoracic aorta, ascending and arch	5
	Superior vena cava	3–4
	Pulmonary artery, main trunk	4
	Pulmonary vein, main trunk	4
VI	Uncontained total transection of thoracic aorta or pulmonary hilum	5

*Increase one grade for multiple grade III or IV injuries if >50% circumference; decrease one grade for grade IV or V injuries if <25% circumference.
AIS, Abbreviated Injury Score.

Diaphragm injury scale

Grade*	Description of injury	AIS-90
I	Contusion	2
II	Laceration <2 cm	3
III	Laceration 2–10 cm	3
IV	Laceration >10 cm with tissue loss ≤ 25 cm^2	3
V	Laceration with tissue loss >25 cm^2	3

*Advance one grade for bilateral injuries up to grade III.
AIS, Abbreviated Injury Score.

Spleen injury scale (1994 revision)

Grade*	Injury type	Description of injury	AIS-90
I	Hematoma	Subcapsular, <10% surface area	2
	Laceration	Capsular tear, <1 cm parenchymal depth	2
II	Hematoma	Subcapsular, 10% to 50% surface area; intraparenchymal, <5 cm in diameter	2
	Laceration	Capsular tear, 1–3 cm parenchymal depth that does not involve a trabecular vessel	2
III	Hematoma	Subcapsular, >50% surface area or expanding; ruptured subcapsular or parenchymal hematoma; intraparenchymal hematoma ≥ 5 cm or expanding	3
	Laceration	Parenchymal depth >3 cm or involving trabecular vessels	3
IV	Laceration	Laceration involving segmental or hilar vessels producing major devascularization (>25% of spleen)	4

(continued)

| V | Laceration | Completely shattered spleen | 5 |
| | Vascular | Hilar vascular injury that devascularizes spleen | 5 |

*Advance one grade for multiple injuries up to grade III.
AIS, Abbreviated Injury Score.

Liver injury scale (1994 revision)

Grade*	Type of injury	Description of injury	AIS-90
I	Hematoma	Subcapsular, <10% surface area	2
	Laceration	Capsular tear, <1 cm parenchymal depth	2
II	Hematoma	Subcapsular, 10% to 50% surface area; intraparenchymal <10 cm in diameter	2
	Laceration	Capsular tear 1–3 cm parenchymal depth, <10 cm in length	2
III	Hematoma	Subcapsular, >50% surface area or expanding; ruptured subcapsular or parenchymal hematoma; intraparenchymal hematoma >10 cm or expanding	3
	Laceration	Parenchymal depth >3 cm	3
IV	Laceration	Parenchymal disruption involving 25% to 75% hepatic lobe or 1–3 Couinaud's segments	4
V	Laceration	Parenchymal disruption involving >75% of hepatic lobe or >3 Couinaud's segments within a single lobe	5
	Vascular	Juxtahepatic venous injuries (i.e., retrohepatic vena cava/central major hepatic veins)	5
VI	Vascular	Hepatic avulsion	6

*Advance one grade for multiple injuries up to grade III.
AIS, Abbreviated Injury Score.

Extrahepatic biliary tree injury scale (1995 revision)

Grade*	Description of injury	AIS-90
I	Gallbladder contusion/hematoma	2
	Portal triad contusion	2
II	Partial gallbladder avulsion from liver bed; cystic duct intact	2
	Laceration or perforation of the gallbladder	2
III	Complete gallbladder avulsion from liver bed	3
	Cystic duct laceration	3
IV	Partial or complete right hepatic duct laceration	3
	Partial or complete left hepatic duct laceration	3
	Partial common hepatic duct laceration (<50%)	3
	Partial common bile duct laceration (<50%)	3
V	Transection of common hepatic duct (≥50%)	3–4
	Transection of common bile duct (≥50%)	3–4
	Combined right and left hepatic duct injuries	3–4
	Intraduodenal or intrapancreatic bile duct injuries	3–4

*Advance one grade for multiple injuries up to grade III.
AIS, Abbreviated Injury Score.

Pancreas injury scale

Grade*	Type of injury	Description of injury	AIS-90
I	Hematoma	Minor contusion without duct injury	2
	Laceration	Superficial laceration without duct injury	2
II	Hematoma	Major contusion without duct injury or tissue loss	2
	Laceration	Major laceration without duct injury or tissue loss	3
III	Laceration	Distal transection or parenchymal injury with duct injury	3
IV	Laceration	Proximal transection or parenchymal injury involving ampulla†	4
V	Laceration	Massive disruption of pancreatic head	5

*Advance one grade for multiple injuries up to grade III.
† Proximal pancreas is to the patient's right of the superior mesenteric vein.
AIS, Abbreviated Injury Score.

Esophagus injury scale

Grade*	Description of injury	AIS-90
I	Contusion or hematoma	2
	Partial thickness laceration	3
II	Laceration circumference <50%	4
III	Laceration circumference ≥50%	4
IV	Segmental loss or devascularization <2 cm	5
V	Segmental loss or devascularization ≥2 cm	5

*Advance one grade for multiple injuries up to grade III.
AIS, Abbreviated Injury Score.

Stomach injury scale

Grade*	Description of injury	AIS-90
I	Contusion or hematoma	2
	Partial thickness laceration	2
II	Laceration in GE junction or pylorus <2 cm	3
	In proximal one third of stomach <5 cm	3
	In distal two thirds of stomach <10 cm	3
III	Laceration >2 cm in GE junction or pylorus	3
	In proximal one third of stomach ≥5 cm	3
	In distal two thirds of stomach ≥10 cm	3
IV	Tissue loss or devascularization <two thirds of stomach	4
V	Tissue loss or devascularization >two thirds of stomach	4

*Advance one grade for multiple injuries up to grade III.
GE, gastroesophageal.

Duodenum injury scale

Grade*	Type of injury	Description of injury	AIS-90
I	Hematoma	Involving single portion of duodenum	2
	Laceration	Partial thickness, no perforation	3
II	Hematoma	Involving more than one portion	2
	Laceration	Disruption <50% of circumference	4
III	Laceration	Disruption 50% to 75% of circumference of D2	4
		Disruption 50% to 100% of circumference of D1, D3, D4	4
IV	Laceration	Disruption >75% of circumference of D2	5
		Involving ampulla or distal common bile duct	5
V	Laceration	Massive disruption of duodenopancreatic complex	5
	Vascular	Devascularization of duodenum	5

*Advance one grade for multiple injuries up to grade III.
D1, first position of duodenum; D2, second portion of duodenum; D3, third portion of duodenum; D4, fourth portion of duodenum.
AIS, Abbreviated Injury Score.

Small bowel injury scale

Grade*	Type of injury	Description of injury	AIS-90
I	Hematoma	Contusion or hematoma without devascularization	2
	Laceration	Partial thickness, no perforation	2
II	Laceration	Laceration <50% of circumference	3
III	Laceration	Laceration ≥50% of circumference without transection	3
IV	Laceration	Transection of the small bowel	4
V	Laceration	Transection of the small bowel with segmental tissue loss	4
	Vascular	Devascularized segment	4

*Advance one grade for multiple injuries up to grade III.
AIS, Abbreviated Injury Score.

Colon injury scale

Grade*	Type of injury	Description of injury	AIS-90
I	Hematoma	Contusion or hematoma without devascularization	2
	Laceration	Partial thickness, no perforation	2
II	Laceration	Laceration <50% of circumference	3
III	Laceration	Laceration ≥50% of circumference without transection	3
IV	Laceration	Transection of the colon	4
V	Laceration	Transection of the colon with segmental tissue loss	4

*Advance one grade for multiple injuries up to grade III.
AIS, Abbreviated Injury Score.

Rectum injury scale

Grade*	Type of injury	Description of injury	AIS-90
I	Hematoma	Contusion or hematoma without devascularization	2
	Laceration	Partial-thickness laceration	2
II	Laceration	Laceration <50% of circumference	3
III	Laceration	Laceration ≥50% of circumference	4
IV	Laceration	Full-thickness laceration with extension into the perineum	5
V	Vascular	Devascularized segment	5

*Advance one grade for multiple injuries up to grade III.
AIS, Abbreviated Injury Score.

Abdominal vascular injury scale

Grade*	Description of injury	AIS-90
I	Non-named superior mesenteric artery or superior mesenteric vein branches	NS
	Non-named inferior mesenteric artery or inferior mesenteric vein branches	NS
	Phrenic artery or vein	NS
	Lumbar artery or vein	NS
	Gonadal artery or vein	NS
	Ovarian artery or vein	NS
	Other non-named, small arterial or venous structures requiring ligation	NS
II	Right, left, or common hepatic artery	3
	Splenic artery or vein	3
	Right or left gastric arteries	3
	Gastroduodenal artery	3
	Inferior mesenteric artery, or inferior mesenteric vein, trunk	3
	Primary named branches of mesenteric artery (e.g., ileocolic artery) or mesenteric vein	3
	Other named abdominal vessels requiring ligation or repair	3
III	Superior mesenteric vein, trunk	3
	Renal artery or vein	3
	Iliac artery or vein	3
	Hypogastric artery or vein	3
	Vena cava, infrarenal	3
IV	Superior mesenteric artery, trunk	3
	Celiac axis proper	3
	Vena cava, suprarenal and infrahepatic	3
	Aorta, infrarenal	4
V	Portal vein	3
	Extraparenchymal hepatic vein	3–5
	Vena cava, retrohepatic or suprahepatic	5
	Aorta suprarenal, subdiaphragmatic	4

*This classification system is applicable to extraparenchymal vascular injuries. If the vessel injury is within 2 cm of the organ parenchyma, refer to specific organ injury scale. Increase one grade for multiple grade III or IV injuries involving >50% vessel circumference. Downgrade one grade if <25% vessel circumference laceration for grade IV or V.
NS, not scored.
AIS, Abbreviated Injury Score.

Adrenal organ injury scale

Grade*	Description of injury	AIS-90
I	Contusion	1
II	Laceration involving only cortex (<2 cm)	1
III	Laceration extending into medulla (≥2 cm)	2
IV	Parenchymal destruction (>50%)	2
V	Total parenchymal destruction (including massive intraparenchymal hemorrhage)	3
	Avulsion from blood supply	3

*Advance one grade for bilateral lesion up to grade V.
AIS, Abbreviated Injury Score.

Kidney injury scale

Grade*	Type of injury	Description of injury	AIS-90
I	Contusion	Microscopic or gross hematuria, urologic studies normal	2
	Hematoma	Subcapsular, nonexpanding without parenchymal laceration	2
II	Hematoma	Nonexpanding perirenal hematoma confined to renal retroperitoneum	2
	Laceration	Parenchymal depth of renal cortex (<1.0 cm) without urinary extravasation	2
III	Laceration	Parenchymal depth of renal cortex (>1.0 cm) without collecting system rupture or urinary extravasation	3
IV	Laceration	Parenchymal laceration extending through the renal cortex, medulla, and collecting system	4
	Vascular	Main renal artery or vein injury with contained hemorrhage	4
V	Laceration	Completely shattered kidney	5
	Vascular	Avulsion of renal hilum which devascularizes kidney	5

*Advance one grade for bilateral injuries up to grade III.
AIS, Abbreviated Injury Score.

Ureter injury scale

Grade*	Type of injury	Description of injury	AIS-90
I	Hematoma	Contusion or hematoma without devascularization	2
II	Laceration	Transecection <50%	2
III	Laceration	Transection ≥50%	3
IV	Laceration	Complete transection with <2 cm devascularization	3
V	Laceration	Avulsion with >2 cm of devascularization	3

*Advance one grade for bilateral lesions up to grade III.
AIS, Abbreviated Injury Score.

Bladder injury scale

Grade*	Injury type	Description of injury	AIS-90
I	Hematoma	Contusion, intramural hematoma	2
	Laceration	Partial thickness	3
II	Laceration	Extraperitoneal bladder wall laceration <2 cm	4
III	Laceration	Extraperitoneal (≥2 cm) or intraperitoneal (<2 cm) bladder wall laceration	4
IV	Laceration	Intraperitoneal bladder wall laceration ≥2 cm	4
V	Laceration	Intraperitoneal or extraperitoneal bladder wall laceration extending into the bladder neck or ureteral orifice (trigone)	4

*Advance one grade for multiple lesions up to grade III.
AIS, Abbreviated Injury Score.

Urethra injury scale

Grade*	Injury type	Description of injury	AIS-90
I	Contusion	Blood at urethral meatus; urethrography normal	2
II	Stretch injury	Elongation of urethra without extravasation on urethrography	2
III	Partial disruption	Extravasation of urethrography contrast at injury site with visualization in the bladder	2
IV	Complete disruption	Extravasation of urethrography contrast at injury site without visualization in the bladder; <2 cm of urethral separation	3
V	Complete disruption	Complete transection with ≥2 cm urethral separation, or extension into the prostate or vagina	4

*Advance one grade for bilateral injuries up to grade III.
AIS, Abbreviated Injury Score.

Uterus (nonpregnant) injury scale

Grade*	Description of injury	AIS-90
I	Contusion or hematoma	2
II	Superficial laceration (<1 cm)	2
III	Deep laceration (≥1 cm)	3
IV	Laceration involving uterine artery	3
V	Avulsion/devascularization	3

*Advance one grade for multiple injuries up to grade III.
AIS, Abbreviated Injury Score.

Uterus (pregnant) injury scale

Grade*	Description of injury	AIS-90
I	Contusion or hematoma (without placental abruption)	2
II	Superficial laceration (<1 cm) or partial placental abruption <25%	3
III	Deep laceration (≥1 cm) occurring in second trimester or placental abruption >25% but <50%	3
	Deep laceration (≥1 cm) in third trimester	4
IV	Laceration involving uterine artery	4
	Deep laceration (≥1 cm) with >50% placental abruption	4
V	Uterine rupture	
	Second trimester	4
	Third trimester	5
	Complete placental abruption	4–5

*Advance one grade for multiple injuries up to grade III.
AIS, Abbreviated Injury Score.

Fallopian tube injury scale

Grade*	Description of injury	AIS-90
I	Hematoma or contusion	2
II	Laceration <50% circumference	2
III	Laceration ≥50% circumference	2
IV	Transection	2
V	Vascular injury; devascularized segment	2

*Advance one grade for bilateral injuries up to grade III.
AIS, Abbreviated Injury Score.

Ovary injury scale

Grade*	Description of injury	AIS-90
I	Contusion or hematoma	1
II	Superficial laceration (depth <0.5 cm)	2
III	Deep laceration (depth ≥0.5 cm)	3
IV	Partial disruption of blood supply	3
V	Avulsion or complete parenchymal destruction	3

*Advance one grade for bilateral injuries up to grade III.
AIS, Abbreviated Injury Score.

Vagina injury scale

Grade*	Description of injury	AIS-90
I	Contusion or hematoma	1
II	Laceration, superficial (mucosa only)	1
III	Laceration, deep into fat or muscle	2
IV	Laceration, complex, into cervix or peritoneum	3
V	Injury into adjacent organs (anus, rectum, urethra, bladder)	3

*Advance one grade for multiple injuries up to grade III.
AIS, Abbreviated Injury Score.

Vulva injury scale

Grade*	Description of injury	AIS-90
I	Contusion or hematoma	1
II	Laceration, superficial (skin only)	1
III	Laceration, deep (into fat, or muscle)	2
IV	Avulsion: skin, fat, or muscle	3
V	Injury into adjacent organs (anus, rectum, urethra, bladder)	3

*Advance one grade for multiple injuries up to grade III.
AIS, Abbreviated Injury Score.

Testis injury scale

Grade*	Description of injury	AIS-90
I	Contusion or hematoma	1
II	Subclinical laceration of tunica albuginea	1
III	Laceration of tunica albuginea with <50% parenchymal loss	2
IV	Major laceration of tunica albuginea with ≥50% parenchymal loss	2
V	Total testicular destruction or avulsion	2

*Advance one grade for bilateral lesions up to grade V.
AIS, Abbreviated Injury Score.

Scrotum injury scale

Grade	Description of injury	AIS-90
I	Contusion	1
II	Laceration of scrotal diameter <25%	1
III	Laceration of scrotal diameter ≥25%	2
IV	Avulsion <50%	2
V	Avulsion ≥50%	2

AIS, Abbreviated Injury Score.

Penis injury scale

Grade*	Description of injury	AIS-90
I	Cutaneous laceration or contusion	1
II	Buck's fascia (cavernosum) laceration without tissue loss	1
III	Cutaneous avulsion	3
	Laceration through glans or meatus	3
	Cavernosal or urethral defect <2 cm	3
IV	Partial penectomy	3
	Cavernosal or urethral defect ≥2 cm	3
V	Total penectomy	3

*Advance one grade for multiple injuries up to grade III.
AIS, Abbreviated Injury Score.

Peripheral vascular organ injury scale

Grade*	Description of injury	AIS-90
I	Digital artery or vein	1–3
	Palmar artery or vein	1–3
	Deep palmar artery or vein	1–3
	Dorsalis pedis artery	1–3
	Plantar artery or vein	1–3
	Non-named arterial or venous branches	1–3
II	Basilic or cephalic vein	1–3
	Saphenous vein	1–3
	Radial artery	1–3
	Ulnar artery	1–3
III	Axillary vein	2–3
	Superficial or deep femoral vein	2–3
	Popliteal vein	2–3
	Brachial artery	2–3
	Anterior tibial artery	1–3
	Posterior tibial artery	1–3
	Peroneal artery	1–3
	Tibioperoneal trunk	2–3
IV	Superficial or deep femoral artery	3–4
	Popliteal artery	2–3
V	Axillary artery	2–3
	Common femoral artery	3–4

*Increase one grade for multiple grade III or IV injuries involving >50% vessel circumference.
Decrease one grade for <25% vessel circumference disruption for grade IV or V.
AIS, Abbreviated Injury Score.

References

Moore EE, Cogbill TH, Jurkovich GJ, et al. Organ injury scaling III: Chest wall, abdominal vascular, ureter bladder, and urethra. *J Trauma* 1992;33:337.

Moore EE, Cogbill TH, Jurkovich GJ, et al. Organ injury scaling V: Spleen and liver (1994 revision). *J Trauma* 1995;38:323.

Moore EE, Cogbill TH, Malangoni MA, et al. Organ injury scaling. *Surg Clin North Am* 1995;75:293–303.

Moore EE, Cogbill TH, Malangoni MA, et al. Organ injury scaling II: Pancreas, duodenum, small bowel, colon, and rectum. *J Trauma* 1990;30:1427.

Moore EE, Dunn EL, Moore JB, et al. Penetrating abdominal trauma index. *J Trauma* 1981;21:439.

Moore EE, Jurkovich GJ, Knudson MM, et al. Organ injury scaling VI: Extrahepatic biliary, esophagus, stomach, vulva, vagina, uterus (nonpregnant), uterus (pregnant), fallopian tube, and ovary. *J Trauma* 1995;39:1069–1070.

Moore EE, Malangoni MA, Cogbill TH, et al. Organ injury scaling IV: Thoracic vascular, lung, cardiac and diaphragm. *J Trauma* 1994;36:226.

Moore EE, Malangoni MA, Cogbill TH, et al. Organ injury scaling VII: Cervical vascular, peripheral vascular, adrenal, penis testis, and scrotum. *J Trauma* 1996;41:523–524.

Moore EE, Shackford SR, Pachter HL, et al. Organ injury scaling: Spleen, liver and kidney. *J Trauma* 1989;29:1664.

TETANUS PROPHYLAXIS
ANDREW B. PEITZMAN

*T*etanus (lockjaw) is a preventable disease that can be lethal to its victims. It is caused by *Clostridium tetani*, a spore-forming anaerobic bacillus. Under ideal wound conditions, the spore is converted to the vegetative form, which produces an exotoxin, tetanospasmin, which acts on the nervous system. A second toxin, tetanolysin, is also produced, but its role is less clear. The average incubation period for tetanus is 10 days (range, 4 to 21 days). It can appear in 1 to 2 days in severe trauma cases. Attention to tetanus prophylaxis is important in all trauma patients, especially those with multiple injuries or open-extremity trauma.

I. PREVENTION
The prevention of tetanus has two components: proper wound care and immunization.

II. WOUND CHARACTERISTICS AND SUSCEPTIBILITY TO TETANUS.
Traumatic wounds can be classified as tetanus prone or nontetanus prone based on various characteristics of the wound (Table B-1). A wound with one or more of these characteristics is a tetanus-prone wound.

III. WOUND CARE
   A. Aseptic surgical techniques should be used when caring for any wound. All devitalized tissue and foreign bodies must be removed.

   B. Wounds should be left open if any one of the following is present:
     1. Doubt about the adequacy of debridement
     2. A puncture injury
     3. A tetanus-prone wound

TABLE B-1   **Wound Characteristics and Susceptibility to Tetanus**

Wound characteristics	Tetanus-prone wounds	Nontetanus-prone wounds
Age of wound	>6 h	≤6 h
Configuration	Stellate, avulsion, abrasion	Linear
Depth	>1 cm	≤1 cm
Mechanism of injury	Missile, crush, burn, frostbite	Sharp surface (knife, glass)
Signs of infection	Present	Absent
Devitalized tissue	Present	Absent
Contaminants (dirt, feces, grass, saliva)	Present	Absent
Denervated or ischemic tissue	Present	Absent

IV. AGENTS FOR TETANUS IMMUNIZATION

Active immunization against tetanus with tetanus toxoid greatly decreases the risk of the disease. Eighty-eight percent of cases occur in patients who have never been vaccinated. Populations in this country who are less likely to be immunized include older patients, with 75% of the deaths in this country in elderly patients. The prevalence of tetanus immunization in foreign-born persons may be as low as 51%.

- A. **Active immunization** is performed with tetanus toxoid, which can be given as a single or combined agent.
    1. **Types of tetanus toxoid agents**
        a. **Diphtheria and tetanus toxoids and pertussis vaccine adsorbed (DTP or DPT).** This agent is used for patients younger than 7 years of age.
        b. **Diphtheria and tetanus toxoids adsorbed (DT) (pediatric type).** This agent is used for patients younger than 7 years of age and for patients in whom the pertussis vaccine is contraindicated.
        c. **Tetanus and diphtheria toxoids adsorbed (Td) (adult type).** This agent is used in patients 7 years of age or older. This preparation is preferable to tetanus toxoid alone because many adults are susceptible to diphtheria, and the simultaneous administration of diphtheria toxoid will enhance protection against this disease.
        d. **Tetanus toxoid adsorbed (Tt).** This agent is for use only in adults. Tetanus toxoid is a sterile preparation of inactivated toxin. It is available as a fluid or in an adsorbed form. The adsorbed form is preferable because it induces higher antitoxin titers and a longer duration of protection.
        e. **dTaP (diptheria, tetanus with acellular pertussis).** This is a newer preparation recommended for non-allergic adults at 10-year intervals to stem the rise in pertussis ("whooping cough"). It can be used similar to dT.
    2. **Administration.** Agents containing tetanus toxoid adsorbed are administered intramuscularly (IM) in doses of 0.5 mL.
- B. **Passive immunization**
    1. **Agents**
        a. **Tetanus immune globulin (TIG) (human) (Hyper-Tet).** This agent is preferable. The risk of hypersensitivity reactions is minimal because it is a human preparation. The dose for tetanus prophylaxis is 250 to 500 U IM.
        b. **Tetanus antitoxin equine.** This agent has a significant risk of hypersensitivity reactions and should not be used unless TIG (human) is unavailable and the possibility of tetanus outweighs the potential reactions of horse serum. Tests for sensitivity to equine serum should be performed before the administration of equine serum.
    2. **A separate syringe and separate injection site** must be used when Tt and TIG are both administered.

V. IMMUNIZATION GUIDELINES

- A. **Active immunization**
    1. **Infants and children.** For children younger than 7 years of age, immunization requires four injections of DTP or DT. A booster injection (fifth dose) is administered at 4 to 6 years of age (not necessary if fourth dose is given on or after the fourth birthday). A routine booster of Td is indicated at 10-year intervals.
    2. **Adults.** Immunization requires at least three injections of tetanus toxoid. An injection of Td should be repeated every 10 years (although this is somewhat controversial), provided that no significant reactions to Td have occurred.
    3. **Pregnant women.** Active immunization of the pregnant mother during the first 6 months of pregnancy will prevent neonatal tetanus. Two injections of Td are given 2 months apart. After delivery and 6 months after the second dose, the mother is given a third dose of Td to complete her active immunization. An injection of Td should be repeated every 10 years, provided that no significant reactions to Td have occurred.

| TABLE B-2 | Prophylaxis against Tetanus in Wound Management | | | |

	Tetanus-prone wounds		Nontetanus-prone wounds	
History of adsorbed tetanus toxoid (doses)	Td[a,b]	TIG	Td[a,b]	TIG
Unknown or <3	Yes	Yes	Yes	No
≥3[c]	No[d]	No	No[e]	No

[a] For persons 7 years old or older, Td is preferred to tetanus toxoid alone.
[b] For persons younger than 7 years old, DPT (diphtheria-pertussis-tetanus) (or DT [diphtheria-tetanus] if pertussis vaccine is contraindicated) is preferred to tetanus toxoid alone.
[c] If only three doses of fluid toxoid were received previously, a fourth dose, preferably an adsorbed toxoid, should be given.
[d] Yes, if it has been more than 5 years since last dose (more frequent boosters are not needed and can accentuate side effects).
[e] Yes, if it has been more than 10 years since last dose.
Td, tetanus-diphtheria toxoid (adult type); TIG, tetanus immune globulin.

If a child is born to a nonimmunized mother who had no obstetric care, the infant should receive 250 U of TIG. The mother should also receive active and passive immunization.

B. Prophylaxis against tetanus in wound management. In patients with wounds, the guidelines illustrated in Table B-2 should be used to determine whether tetanus toxoid with or without TIG administration is necessary. Major and minor wounds may be involved with tetanus.

The effectiveness of prophylactic antibiotics is unknown. Penicillin delays the onset of tetanus. For patients who need TIG as part of the treatment for tetanus prophylaxis, and TIG is not readily available, penicillin allows a period of 2 days in which to obtain the TIG and begin passive immunization.

VI. CONTRAINDICATIONS
A. Tetanus and diphtheria toxoids
1. **A history of neurologic or severe hypersensitivity** reaction to a previous dose is the only contraindication in a patient with a wound. Local side effects alone do not necessitate discontinuing the use of these toxoids.
2. **Immunization should be postponed** until appropriate skin testing can be performed if a systemic reaction is suspected to represent allergic hypersensitivity.
3. **Passive immunization should be considered** for a tetanus-prone wound if a contraindication to the use of tetanus toxoid exists.
B. Tetanus immune globulin.
If a history of previous systemic reaction to horse serum representing allergic hypersensitivity exists and it is necessary to administer tetanus antitoxin equine, immunization should be withheld until appropriate skin testing is performed.
C. Pertussis vaccine in DTP.
DT, instead of DTP, should be administered if there was a previous adverse reaction after DTP or a single-antigen pertussis vaccination. Adverse reactions include:
1. **Immediate anaphylactic reaction**
2. **Temperature ≥105°F within 48 hours**
3. **Collapse or shocklike state within 48 hours**
4. **Encephalopathy within 7 days**, including severe alterations in consciousness with generalized or focal neurologic signs persisting for >12 hours
5. **Persistent, inconsolable crying lasting ≥3 hours**
6. **High-pitched cry within 48 hours**
7. **Convulsion with or without fever within 3 days**

VII. PATIENT INSTRUCTIONS
   A. Written instructions should be given to the patient regarding
     1. Treatment received, including immunizations administered
     2. Follow-up appointments for:
       a. Wound care
       b. Completion of active immunization if necessary
   B. Each patient should be given a wallet-sized card documenting immunization dosage and date received. The patient should be instructed to carry this card at all times.

AXIOMS

- Wounds should be classified as tetanus prone or nontetanus prone based on characteristics of the wound. If uncertain, administer active immunization.
- Recognize high-risk groups who may not have had the primary immunization series as children: individuals born outside the United States or populations in this country who are secluded for religious or other reasons.
- Elderly patients may have a diminished response to tetanus toxoid.

Bibliography
Agents for immunization. In: *Drug Evaluations Subscription.* Chicago, Ill: American Medical Association; 1991.

American College of Surgeons Committee on Trauma. Advanced Trauma Life Support Course. Tetanus immunization. In: *Advanced Trauma Life Support Course for Physicians.* Chicago, Ill: American College of Surgeons; 2004;7:337–340.

Furste W, Aguirre A. Tetanus. In: Howard RJ, Simmons RL, eds. *Surgical Infectious Disease.* 3rd ed. Norwalk, Conn: Appleton & Lange; 1995.

Rhee P, Nunley MK, Demetriades D, et al. Tetanus and trauma: A review and recommendations. *J Trauma* 2005;58:1082–1088.

Ross SE. *Prophylaxis against Tetanus in Wound Management.* Chicago, Ill: American College of Surgeons Committee on Trauma; 1995.

Webb KP. Tetanus prophylaxis. In Lopez-Viego MA, ed. *The Parkland Trauma Handbook.* Philadelphia, Pa: Mosby—Year Book; 1994.

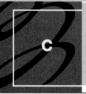

UPMC
University of Pittsburgh
Medical Center

PHYSICIAN ORDER SET

AUTHORIZATION IS GIVEN TO THE PHARMACY TO DISPENSE AND TO THE
NURSE TO ADMINISTER THE GENERIC OR CHEMICAL EQUIVALENT WHEN
THE DRUG IS FILLED BY THE PHARMACY OF THE UPMC HEALTH SYSTEM
HOSPITAL-UNLESS THE PRODUCT NAME IS CIRCLED.

IMPRINT PATIENT IDENTIFICATION HERE

Trauma Surgery: Admission: Non-ICU—Physician Order Set

Nursing Unit: ☐ Regular _____ ☐ Telemetry _____ Attending Physician: _____

Diagnosis: _____ Condition: _____

Allergies: _____

Check All Orders That Apply with a ☒ *& All Handwritten Orders Should Be* **BLOCK PRINTED** *for Clarity*

Communication Orders

☐ 23-Hour observation status ☐ Restraints: Refer to Rastraints Orders Form

☐ Thoraco-lumbar spine (TLS) precautions

☐ C-spine precautions (NO pillow)

☐ Reverse Trendelenberg 30 degrees

☐ Head of bed elevated 30 degrees

☒ Notify house officer of patient arrival to nursing unit

☒ Call physician if any of the following occur:

- Temperature >38.5° or <36° ■ SaO$_2$ <92% ■ Respiratory rate >30 or <10 breaths/min
- Heart rate >120 or <50 beats per minute ■ Urine output <250 mL/8 hours ■ Accucheck glucose <70 or >350 mg%
- Systolic blood pressure <90 or >150 mmHg ■ New onset of lethargy, difficulty waking agitation delirium
- Diastolic blood pressure >100 or <60 mmHg ■ Other: _____

Vital Signs

☐ Cardiac telemetry (only in monitored bed) ☐ Pulse Oximetry: ⇨ ☐ with vitals signs ☐ Continuous

☐ Vital sign checks: ☐ q 4 hours ☐ q 2 hours

☐ Neurological checks: ☐ q 8 hours ☐ q 6 hours ☐ q 4 hours ☐ q 2 hours

☐ Neurovascular checks: ☐ q 8 hours ☐ q 6 hours ☐ q 4 hours ☐ q 2 hours

Activity

☐ Bed rest ☐ Logroll q 2 hours ☐ Out of bed ad lib ☐ Out of bed to chair with assistance (select one): ☐ bid ☐ tid

☐ Overhead Trapeze

☐ Ambulate as tolerated (select all that are appropriate): **May order only if patient does NOT have C-spine precautions.**

☐ No weightbearing limitations

☐ RUE ⇨ ☐ WBAT ☐ NWB ☐ Touch down WB

☐ LUE ⇨ ☐ WBAT ☐ NWB ☐ Touch down WB

☐ RLE ⇨ ☐ WBAT ☐ NWB ☐ Touch down WB ☐ Pivot-transfer only

☐ LLE ⇨ ☐ WBAT ☐ NWB ☐ Touch down WB ☐ Pivot-transfer only

_____ _____
(**BLOCK** Print Name) (Signature)

Date/Time: _____ Pager # _____

Additional Handwritten Orders Should Be Placed at the **End** of This Order Set.

☐ Order Set Faxed to Pharmacy By:

(name/time) Unit: _____

0031-01-U Form ID: PUH-1164 Last Revision Date: 02/17/2007 Page 1 of 5

UPMC
University of Pittsburgh
Medical Center

PHYSICIAN ORDER SET

AUTHORIZATION IS GIVEN TO THE PHARMACY TO DISPENSE AND TO THE

NURSE TO ADMINISTER THE GENERIC OR CHEMICAL EQUIVALENT WHEN

THE DRUG IS FILLED BY THE PHARMACY OF THE UPMC HEALTH SYSTEM

HOSPITAL–UNLESS THE PRODUCT NAME IS CIRCLED.

IMPRINT PATIENT IDENTIFICATION HERE

Trauma Surgery: Admission: Non-ICU—Physician Order Set

Allergies: ___

Patient Care

- [ ] Intake & output q shift
- [ ] Foley to gravity drainage
- [ ] Nasogastric tube to: (Select one) [ ] Low intermittent suction (60–80 mmHg) [ ] Low continuous suction (60–80 mmHg)
- [ ] Remove the nasogastric tube antireflux valve from the blue sump port
- [ ] Chest tube (1) to: (Select one) [ ] 20-cm suction [ ] ___ cm suction [ ] Water seal
- [ ] Chest tube (2) to: (Select one) [ ] 20-cm suction [ ] ___ cm suction [ ] Water seal
- [ ] Thigh-high pneumatic compression devices (SCDs) **on at all times** while patient is in bed
- [ ] Cervical collar on all times [ ] Change cervical collar to Miami J cervical collar
- [ ] Carter pillow (elevate): [ ] RUE [ ] LUE
- [ ] Sling to: [ ] RUE [ ] LUE
- [ ] Abduction pillow between legs
- [ ] Bucks traction to: ___ lb traction
- [ ] Skeletal traction to: ___ lb traction
- [ ] Other: ___

Respiratory Care

- [ ] Respiratory consult [ ] Other: ___
- [ ] Cough and deep breathe Q 2 hours
- [ ] Aerosol face mask ___ % O_2
- [ ] Nasal cannula ___ % O_2
- [ ] Wear oxygen to maintain SaO_2> ___ %
- [ ] Incentive spirometry 10 times/hour while awake

Nutritional Services

- [ ] NPO [ ] NPO except meds [ ] Clear liquids
- [ ] Regular [ ] ___ calorie ADA [ ] Advance diet as tolerated to: ___

Continuous Infusions

- [ ] Cap IV when taking fluids well [ ] Add KCq ___ mEl/Liter to each bag of solution below
- [ ] Dextrose 5%/0.45 sodium chloride (D_5 1/2 NS) at ___ mL/hour [ ] Lactated Ringer's (LR) at ___ mL/hour
- [ ] Dextrose 5%/0.9% sodium chloride (D_5 NS) at ___ mL/hour [ ] 0.9% sodium chloride at ___ mL/hour
- [ ] Dextrose 5% in Lactated Ringer's (D_5 RL) at ___ mL/hour [ ] 0.45% sodium chloride (1/2 NS) at ___ mL/hour

___ (**BLOCK** Print Name) ___ (Signature)

Date/Time: ___ Pager # ___

Additional Handwritten Orders Should Be Placed at the End of This Order Set.
Order Set Faxed to Pharmacy By:
[ ] (name/time) Unit: ___

0031-01-U Form ID: PUH-1164 Last Revision Date: 02/17/2007 Page 2 of 5

UPMC
University of Pittsburgh
Medical Center

PHYSICIAN ORDER SET

AUTHORIZATION IS GIVEN TO THE PHARMACY TO DISPENSE AND TO THE

NURSE TO ADMINISTER THE GENERIC OR CHEMICAL EQUIVALENT WHEN

THE DRUG IS FILLED BY THE PHARMACY OF THE UPMC HEALTH SYSTEM

HOSPITAL-UNLESS THE PRODUCT NAME IS CIRCLED.

IMPRINT PATIENT IDENTIFICATION HERE

Trauma Surgery: Admission: Non-ICU—Physician Order Set

Allergies: _____

Medications   Do **NOT** exceed a total of 4,000 mg of acetaminophen in a 24-hour period.

- ☐ Docusate 100 mg po bid   ☐ Senokot S two tabs po q Hs prn constipation
- ☐ Enoxaparin (**Lovenox**) 30 mg subcutaneous bid (*DVT Prophylaxis*) Do **NOT** substitute.
- ☐ Famotidine (**Pepcid**) 20-mg IV bid until patient is taking po, then discontinue and start Famotidine 20 mg po bid
- ☐ For patients <65 years of age: Prochlorperazine (**Compazine**) 10-mg IV q 6 hours prn for nausea
- ☐ For patients >65 years of age: Ondansetron (**Zofran**) 4-mg IV Q 6 hours PRN nausea
- ☐ Antibiotic for treatment: Dose: _____ Route: _____ Freq: _____
- ☐ See separate PCA order sheet
- ☐ Ibuprofen 600 mg po q 6 hours around the clock for pain   ☐ Acetaminophen 650 mg po/PR q 4 hours prn for fever/mild pain (1–3)
- ☐ Acetaminophen 325 mg/Oxycodone hydrochloride 5 mg (**Percocet**) 1 tablet po q 4 hours prn for moderate pain (4–6)
- ☐ Acetaminophen 325 mg/Oxycodone hydrochloride 5 mg (**Percocet**) 2 tables q 4 hours prn for severe pain (7–10)
- ☐ Acetaminophen 325 mg/Hydrocodone bitattrate 5 mg (**Vicodin**) 1 tablet po q 4 hours prn for moderate pain (4–6)
- ☐ Acetaminophen 325 mg/Hydrocodone bitattrate 5 mg (**Vicodin**) 2 tables po q 4 hours prn for severe pain (7–10)
- ☐ Acetaminophen 325 mg/Oxycodone 5 mg (**Roxiect**) 5 mL po q 4 hours prn for moderate pain (4–6)
- ☐ Acetaminophen 325 mg/Oxycodone 5 mg (**Roxiect**) 10 mL po q 4 hours prn for severe pain (7–10)
- ☐ Morphine 1-mg IV q one hour prn mild to moderate pain (4–6)
- ☐ Morphine 2-mg IV q one hour prn severe pain (7–10)

Labs

Now _____

☐ Lytes	☐ Lytes	☐ PT	☐ Calcium
☐ BUN/Creatinine	☐ BUN/Creatinine	☐ PTT	☐ Hct
☐ Glucose	☐ Glucose	☐ Sodium	☐ _____
☐ CBC. Diff	☐ CBC, Diff	☐ Potassium	☐ _____
☐ Platelet count	☐ Platelet count	☐ Magnesium	☐ _____
☐ CPK/MB q _____ hours x _____		☐ Phosphorus	

- ☐ CPK q _____ hours x _____
- ☐ Troponin I q _____ hours x _____
- ☐ Accucheck glucose q _____ hours x _____
- ☐ Hct q _____ hours x _____
- ☐ Urinalysis

(**BLOCK** Print Name) _____   (Signature) _____

Date/Time _____   Pager# _____

Additional Handwritten Orders Should Be Placed at the End of This Order Set.

☐ **Order Set Faxed to Pharmacy By:**
   (name/time) _____   Unit: _____

0031-01-U   Form ID: PUH-1164   Last Revision Date: 02/17/2007   Page 3 of 5

UPMC
University of Pittsburgh Medical Center   **PHYSICIAN ORDER SET**

AUTHORIZATION IS GIVEN TO THE PHARMACY TO DISPENSE AND TO THE
NURSE TO ADMINISTER THE GENERIC OR CHEMICAL EQUIVALENT WHEN
THE DRUG IS FILLED BY THE PHARMACY OF THE UPMC HEALTH SYSTEM
HOSPITAL-UNLESS THE PRODUCT NAME IS CIRCLED.

IMPRINT PATIENT IDENTIFICATION HERE

Trauma Surgery: Admission: Non-ICU—Physician Order Set

Allergies:

Diagnostic Tests

☐ 12-lead EKG

Radiology

☐ CXR   ☐ In the department   ☐ Portable   ☐ In am (_____/_____/_____) re: _____

☐ CT chest   Clinical indication: _____

☐ Ct head   ☐ In am (_____/_____/_____)   Clinical indication: _____

☐ CT abdomen/pelvis   Clinical indication: _____

☐ MRI:_____   Clinical indication: _____

☐ Other:_____   Clinical indication: _____

Consults

☐ Orthopaedic consult, clinical indication: _____

☐ Spine trauma consult, clinical indication: _____

☐ Neurosurgery consult, clinical indication: _____

☐ Facial service consult, clinical indication: _____

☐ Hand surgery consult, clinical indication: _____

☐ Ophthalmology consult, clinical indication: _____

☐ PMR consult, clinical indication: Status: Postrauma

☐ Psychiatry consult, clinical indication: _____

☐ PT consult, reason: _____

☐ OT consult, reason: _____

☐ Social work consult, reason: _____

☐ Substance abuse treatment referral

_____
(**BLOCK** Print Name)

_____
(Signature)

Date/Time: _____   Pager # _____

Additional Handwritten Orders Should Be Placed at the End of This Order Set.
Order Set Faxed to Pharmacy By:
☐
(name/time)   Unit:

0031-01-U   Form ID: PUH-1164   Last Revision Date: 02/17/2007   Page 4 of 5

UPMC
University of Pittsburgh
Medical Center

PHYSICIAN ORDER SET

AUTHORIZATION IS GIVEN TO THE PHARMACY TO DISPENSE AND TO THE

NURSE TO ADMINISTER THE GENERIC OR CHEMICAL EQUIVALENT WHEN

THE DRUG FILLED BY THE PHARMACY OF THE UPMC HEALTH SYSTEM

HOSPITAL-UNLESS THE PRODUCT NAME IS CIRCLED.

IMPRINT PATIENT IDENTIFICATION HERE

Trauma Surgery: Admission: Non-ICU—Physician Order Set

Allergies:

Additional Orders Should Be BLOCK PRINTED for Clarity	
The following abbreviations are disallowed: u (unit), MS and MSO4 (morphine), MgSO4 (magnesium sulfate), QD (daily), QOD (every other day), IU (international units)	
Other Orders	**Medication Orders**

Safe Prescribing Practices: Verify all orders by reading the order back to the prescriber. Do not use zeros following a decimal point. Use a zero before a decimal point. Order IV medications by dose per time (e.g., mg/h). Order levothyroxine in micrograms (μg), not mg doses

(**BLOCK** Print Name)

(Signature)

Date/Time: Pager #

☐ **Order Set Faxed to Pharmacy By:**
(name/time)   **Unit:**

0031-01-U   Form ID: PUH-1164   Last Revision Date: 02/17/2007   Page 5 of 5

UPMC
University of Pittsburgh
Medical Center

Admission Orders: Trauma ICU

AUTHORIZATION IS GIVEN TO THE PHARMACY TO DISPENSE AND TO THE
NURSE TO ADMINISTER THE GENERIC OR CHEMICAL EQUIVALENT WHEN
THE DRUG IS FILLED BY THE PHARMACY OF UPMC-UNLESS THE PRODUCT
NAME IS CIRCLED.

IMPRINT PATIENT IDENTIFICATION HERE

		Medications	Dose	Route	Frequency/Indication
Admit Unit		☐ Famotidine	20 mg	IV	Q 12 hours
Service		☐ Enoxaparin	30 mg	Subq	Q 12 hours Do <u>NOT</u> Substitute
Diagnosis		☐ Dalteparin	5,000 u	Subq	Q 24 hours
Allergies		☐ Heparin	5,000 u	Subq	Q 12 hours
Condition	☐ Critical ☐ Serious ☐ Fair ☐ Good	☐ Propofol	mg/kg/m	IV	
Vital Signs	Vital signs, I and O, monitoring and turning per ICU standards	☐ Lorazepam	mg	IV	
Activity	☐ Bed rest ☐ Mobilize to chain	☐ Haloperidol	mg	IV	
Precautions	☐ None ☐ C-spine ☐ TLS	☐ Morphine	mg	IV	
	☐ Logroll only	☐ Fentanyl	mg	IV	
Position	☒ Elevate HOB 30° per ICU standards	☐ Phenytoin	mg	IV	
Nutrition	☐ NPO ☐ Ice chips ☐ Sips ☐ TPN	☐ Labeltalol	mg	IV	
Enteral	Product _____ mL/h	☐ Hydralazine	mg	IV	
Devices	☐ Pneumatic compression devices	☐ Metoprolol	mg		
NG tube	☐ Intermittent suction ☐ Continuous ☐ Gravity	☐ Ondansetron	mg	IV	
Chest tubes	☐ Suction ____ cm H₂O ☐ Water seal	☐ Cefazolin	g	IV	
Drains		☐ Acetaminophen	mg		
Traction		☐ Regular insulin sliding scale ☐ 12 units ☐ 20 units ☐ 28 units			
Other					
Dressings		☐ Insulin infusion per unit protocol			
IV Fluids	Maintenance Infusion Rate: _____ mL/h	☐ PCA per order form			
Type	☐ D5W ☐ D5W with KCL ____ mEq/L	☐ Chlorhexedine (0.12%) mouth rinse per unit protocol			
	☐ LR ☐ LR with KCL ____ mEq/L	☐ Titrate propofol to Ramsay sedation scale ☐ 2 ☐ 3 ☐ 4			
	☐ 0.9% NaCl ☐ 0.9% NaCl with KCL ___ mEq/L	☐ BP Rx Threshold ☐ SBP > ☐ MAP > _____ mmHg			
	☐ 0.45% NaCl ☐ 0.45% NaCl with KCL ___ mEq/L	☐ Hold Metoproll or HR <60 bpm or SBP <100 mmHg			
Pharmacy additive	☐ MVI 10 mL/L in IV above	**Electrolytes**			
Other		KCL ☐ Per protocol Target ☐ 3.5 mEq/L ☐ 4.2 mEq/L			
Blood	☐ Type and screen ☐ Hold ____ Units PRBC	Magnesium Sulf ☐ 4-g IV over 4 hours prn Mg⁺² < 2 mEq/L			
Transfuse	____ Units PRBC ____ Units FFP ____ Units Plts	Phosphate ☐ Phos. <1.0 mg/dL 30 mmol over 6 hours—IV			
		☐ Phos. 1.0–2.0 mg/dL 15 mmol over 4 hours—IV			

Phosphate given as KPO₄ unless K >4.0 mEq/L NaPO₄ when K >4.0 mEq/L.

Physician Name (Print) _____

Pager # _____

Physician (Signature) _____

Date: _____ Time: _____

☐ **Order Set Faxed to Pharmacy By:**
(name/time) _____

0031-01-U   Form ID: PUH-1402   Last Revision Date: 08/15/2006   Page 1 of 2

UPMC
University of Pittsburgh
Medical Center

Admission Orders: Trauma ICU

AUTHORIZATION IS GIVEN TO THE PHARMACY TO DISPENSE AND TO THE
NURSE TO ADMINISTER THE GENERIC OR CHEMICAL EQUIVALENT WHEN
THE DRUG IS FILLED BY THE PHARMACY OF THE UPMC-HOSPITAL-UNLESS
THE PRODUCT NAME IS CIRCLED.

IMPRINT PATIENT IDENTIFICATION HERE

Ventilator	☐ AC ☐ IMV ☐ PSV	cm H$_2$O
Settings	RR / Tidal volume / FiO$_2$ / PEEP	
	Bpm / mL / / cm H$_2$O	
Other		
BiPap	Mode IPAP EPAP	
Weaning	☒ Wean ventilator per protocol ☐ Extubate	
Oxygen Rx	☐ AFM % ☐ Nasal cannula L/min	
Toilet	☐ Per respiratory care protocol/pathway	
Directed	☐ Incentive spirometry ☐ PEP ☐ Flutter valve	
	☐ IPPB ☐ CPAP ☐ NT suction	
	Administer directed pulmonary toilet every hours	
Bronchodilator	Administer bronchodilators every hours	
Method	☐ MDI ☐ Nebulizer ☐ IPPB	
Drug	☐	

Diagnostics

Diagnostics	☐ Portable CXR	☐ STAT	☐ In AM
	☐ 12-lead EKG	☐ STAT	☐ In AM
CT scan			
MRI			
X-rays			

Consults

☐ Orthopaedics	☐ Neurosurgery	☐ Plastic Surgery
☐ Maxillofacial Surgery	☐ ENT	☐ Ophthalmology
☐ Rehabilitation Medicine	☐ Physical Therapy	☐ Occupational Therapy
☐ Social Service		

Labs		
STAT	☐ ABG ☐ HCT ☐ Glu ☐ K$^+$ ☐ Na$^+$	
	☐ Ca^{+2} ☐ Lytes ☐ Lactate ☐ BUN/Creatinine	
	☐ Ca/Mg/Phos ☐ LFTs ☐ Bili ☐ Urinalysis	
	☐ Troponin I ☐ CPK/MB	
	☐ CBC ☐ Diff ☐ Platelets ☐ PT/PTT	
Cultures	☐ Blood x 2 ☐ Urine ☐ Blind BAL ☐ Sputum	
Morning Labs	☐ Lytes/BUN/Creatinine ☐ Ca/Mg/Phos	
	☐ Glucose ☐ ABG ☐ CBC	
	☐ CBC ☐ WBC diff ☐ Platelets ☐ PT/PTT	

Monitoring	Frequency	Duration
Glucose every:	hours	x hours
Hematacrit every:	hours	x hours
ABG every:	hours	x hours
Troponin I every:	hours	x hours
every:	hours	x hours

ICU Physician or Primary Service Notifications

☒	Temperature >38.5° or <36°C
☒	Systolic blood pressure <90 mmHg or >160 mmHg
☒	Mean arterial pressure <60 mmHg or >110 mmHg
☒	Urine output <25 mL/h or >300 mL/h
☒	Respiratory rate <10 or >30 breaths/min
☒	Pulse <50 or >120 bpm
☒	Pulse oximetry saturation <90%
☒	Pain score >5 or pain interfering with therapy
☒	Intracranial pressure sustained >30 mmHg

CCM Fellow/Attending Notification

☒	Oliguria unresponsive to fluid challenge within 1 hour
☒	Hypotension unresponsive to fluid challenge within 15 minutes
☒	Hypotension necessitating >20% escalation in vasopressor dosage
☒	CI <2.0 L/min/M^2 unresponsive to fluid challenge within 15 minutes
☒	Worsening oxygenation requiring >10% escalation in FiO$_2$
☒	New or worsening bleeding
☒	New seizures, anisocoria, focal weakness, or unresponsiveness

Physician Name (Print)

Pager #

Physician (Signature)

Date: _____ Time: _____

☐ **Order Set Faxed to Pharmacy By:**
   (name/time)

0031-01-U   Form ID: PUH-1402   Last Revision Date: 08/15/2006   Page 2 of 2

UPMC
University of Pittsburgh
Medical Center

TRAUMA ADMISSION
HISTORY AND PHYSICAL

999900

Date : 2007   ED Arrival Time: _____

History (Mechanism of Injury): ☐ N/A

1. Blunt: ☐ MVC: Driver/Passenger   Restrained/Unrestrained

☐ MCC: Driver/Passenger   Helmet/Unhelmeted   ☐ ATV ☐ Assault ☐ Fall _____(ht) ☐ Ped struck ☐ Other: _____

IMPRINT PATIENT IDENTIFICATION HERE   Page 1 of 4

2. Penetrating: ☒ Firearm ☐ Stab wound ☐ Other: _____

Description of Injury (location, duration, quality, severity, timing, context, signs and symptoms, modifying factors):   ☐ Scene run
27 y/o male gunshot wound to the chest, rt arm, hip with a pneumothorax.

Prehospital care: _____   Location of care: _____

Past Medical History: ☐ Coronary artery disease ☐ COPD ☐ Stroke ☐ DM ☐ Obesity ☐ Hypertension ☐ Asthma ☐ MI ☐ Afib

☐ Cancer: _____   ☐ Other: _____

Home medications: _____

Past Surgical History: _____

Medications: ☐ ASA ☐ Plavix ☐ Coumadin   **Allergies:** ☐ NKDA

☒ Unable to obtain because of the emergent nature of the patient ☐ Unable to obtain because: _____   ☐ No reported medical history

Past Family History: ☐ Coronary artery disease ☐ COPD ☐ Stroke ☐ DM ☐ Obesity ☐ Hypertension ☐ Asthma ☐ MI ☐ Afib

☐ Cancer: _____   ☐ Other: _____   **Relation to patient:** _____

☒ Unable to obtain because of the emergent nature of patient ☐ Unable to obtain because: _____   ☐ No significant family history

Past Social History:
☐ Tobacco _____ppd   ☐ EtOH _____per day/week   ☐ Drugs   Occupation:_____

☒ Unable to obtain because of the emergent nature of patient   ☐ Unable to obtain because: _____

REIVIEW OF SYSTEMS

Constitutional	Neg/Pos	Findings:	Musculoskeletal	Neg/Pos	Findings:
Eyes	Neg/Pos	Findings:	Neurological	Neg/Pos	Findings:
Ears, Nose Mouth/Throat	Neg/Pos	Findings:	Psychiatric	Neg/Pos	Findings:
Cardiovascular	Neg/Pos	Findings:	Endocrine	Neg/Pos	Findings:
Respiratory	Neg/Pos	Findings:	Hematologic/ Lymphatic	Neg/Pos	Findings:
Gastrointestinal	Neg/Pos	Findings:	Skin	Neg/Pos	Findings:
Genitourinary	Neg/Pos	Findings:	Allergic/ Immunologic	Neg/Pos	Findings:

☐ All other systems have been reviewed and are negative   ☒ Unable to obtain because: _____

Initial Trauma Room VS: P: 114   BP: RESP: O$_2$ Saturation: T: Height: Weight:

Primary Survey

Airway: Patent (Yes)/ No   intubation   Breathing: intubation

Circulation: Pulse/Strength   0   1+   2+   Site:

Interventions on the primary survey:

9655-01-U   Form ID: PUH-2233-3670   Last Revision Date: 5/19/2006

Name: _____   Page 1 of 4

NAME:_____ D.O.B:_____ MEDICAL RECORD#: _____ DATE: _____

Glasgow Coma Scale (GCS):

Eye Opening: None 1   **Verbal Response:** None 1   **Motor Response:** None 1   **GCS Total:** 3

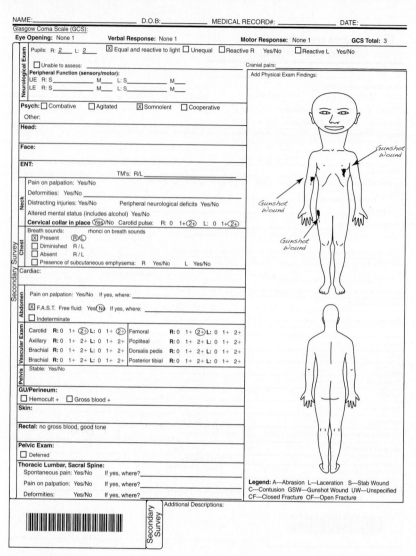

Secondary Survey

Neurological Exam

Pupils: R: _2_ L: _2_   ☒ Equal and reactive to light ☐ Unequal ☐ Reactive R Yes/No   ☐ Reactive L Yes/No

☐ Unable to assess: _____   Cranial pairs:_____

Peripheral Function (sensory/motor):

UE R: S_____ M___ L: S_____ M___

LE R: S_____ M___ L: S_____ M___

Cranial pairs:

Add Physical Exam Findings:

Psych: ☐ Combative ☐ Agitated ☒ Somnolent ☐ Cooperative

Other:

Head:

Face:

ENT:

TM's: R/L_____

Neck

Pain on palpation: Yes/No

Deformity: Yes/No _____

Distracting injuries: Yes/No   Peripheral neurological deficits Yes/No

Altered mental status (includes alcohol) Yes/No

Cervical collar in place ⟨Yes⟩/No Carotid pulse: R: 0 1+⟨2+⟩ L: 0 1+⟨2+⟩

Chest

Breath sounds: rhonci on breath sounds

☒ Present ⟨R⟩⟨L⟩

☐ Diminished R / L

☐ Absent R / L

☐ Presence of subcutaneous emphysema: R Yes/No   L Yes/No

Cardiac:

Abdomen

Pain on palpation: Yes/No If yes, where: _____

☒ F.A.S.T. Free fluid: Yes/⟨No⟩ If yes, where: _____

☐ Indeterminate

Vascular Exam

Carotid	**R:** 0 1+ ⟨2+⟩ **L:** 0 1+ ⟨2+⟩	Femoral	**R:** 0 1+ ⟨2+⟩ **L:** 0 1+ 2+
Axillary	**R:** 0 1+ 2+ **L:** 0 1+ 2+	Popliteal	**R:** 0 1+ 2+ **L:** 0 1+ 2+
Brachial	**R:** 0 1+ 2+ **L:** 0 1+ 2+	Dorsalis pedis	**R:** 0 1+ 2+ **L:** 0 1+ 2+
Brachial	**R:** 0 1+ 2+ **L:** 0 1+ 2+	Posterior tibial	**R:** 0 1+ 2+ **L:** 0 1+ 2+

Pelvis

Stable: Yes/No

GU/Perineum:

☐ Hemocult + ☐ Gross blood +

Skin:

Rectal: no gross blood, good tone

Pelvic Exam:

☐ Deferred

Thoracic Lumbar, Sacral Spine:

Spontaneous pain: Yes/No   If yes, where?_____

Pain on palpation: Yes/No   If yes, where?_____

Deformities: Yes/No   If yes, where?_____

Additional Descriptions:

Secondary Survey

Legend: A—Abrasion L—Laceration S—Stab Wound C—Contusion GSW—Gunshot Wound UW—Unspecified CF—Closed Fracture OF—Open Fracture

Name:

NAME: _____   D.O.B.: _____   MEDICAL RECORD #: _____   DATE: _____

Preliminary Imaging Performed/Reviewed:	Date:	For acute trauma (circle):	Findings:
☒ CXR	2007/01/27	☒ Pending Neg/Pos	_____
☐ Pelvis	_____	☐ Pending Neg/Pos	_____
☐ Neck (simple films)	_____	☐ Pending Neg/Pos	_____
☐ Extremity films	_____	☐ Pending Neg/Pos	_____
☐ CT head	_____	☐ Pending Neg/Pos	_____
☐ CT neck	_____	☐ Pending Neg/Pos	_____
☐ CT chest	_____	☐ Pending Neg/Pos	_____
☐ CT abdomen/pelvis	_____	☐ Pending Neg/Pos	_____
☐ Other: _____	_____	☐ Pending Neg/Pos	_____
☐ Other: _____	_____	☐ Pending Neg/Pos	_____

Name:

9655-01-U

NAME: _____ D.O.B.: _____ MEDICAL RECORD . _____ DATE: _____

A. Injuries and Problems Identified: | **Error**
Date of Diagnosis:
1. 879.8 GUNSHOT WOUNDS, MULTIPLE ☐
2. ☐
3. ☐
4. ☐
5. ☐
6. ☐

B. Injuries and Problems to Rule Out:

C. Plan:
1.

2.

3.

D. Attending Note and Attestation: ☐ Patient to follow up in clinic. Discharge to home.

I saw the patient. I personally examined the patient. I agree with the notes written by the resident.
☐ With the exception of:

☐ With the addition of:

Assessment and Plan

Procedures: ☐ Chest tube 32020 ☐ Intubation 31500 ☐ DPL 49080 ☐ Cricothyroidotomy 31605 ☐ CPR 92950 ☐ Cystogram 51605
☐ Urethrogram 74450 ☐ Thoracotomy 32160 ☐ Arterial line 36620 ☐ Percutan. cent. line 36556 ☐ Cutdown cent. line 36558
☐ Other: _____ ☐ Other: _____ ☐ Other: _____

| Critical Care: | 30–74 min. (99291) | 75–104 min. (99291, 99292×2) | 105–134 min. (99291, 99292×2) | 135–164 min. (99291, 99292×2) | 165–194 min. (99291, 99292×2) | ____ (min.) |

Initial IP: _____ Subsequent Care: _____ 23 H. Admit to Obs: _____ ☐ 99217 Discharge from Obs
☒ 99499 (resus) Admit, discharge same calendar day. ____ ☐ 99238 discharge (<30 min.) ____ (min.) ☐ 99239 discharge (<30 min.) ____ (min.)
☐ No charge **Modifiers:** ☐ –24 E/M unrelated to recent surgery ☐ 25 separate E/M encounter with minor procedure ☐ 57 Decision for surgery within 24 hours

Visit

Signature attests that all four pages have been reviewed and completed.

Housestaff Physician/Other Signature: _____
Title: _____ Pager: _____ Date/Time: _____
Attending Physician Signature: _____
Title: _____ Pager: _____ Date/Time: _____

Name: _____

UPMC University of Pittsburgh Medical Center

200 Lothrop Street
Pittsburgh, PA 15213-2582

TRAUMA CARE FLOW RECORD

Date: _____ Treatment room: _____

Mechanism of injury:
☐ MVC ☐ Stab ☐ Fall
☐ ATV ☐ Assault ☐ Other
☐ GSW ☐ Motorcycle

Arrived by: **Transferred from:**
☐ Self ☐ Home
☐ Air ☐ Scene
☐ Ambulance ☐ Hospital

Details of injury/prehospital report: _____

V.S. at scene: _____
Loss of consciousness: ☐ Yes ☐ No ☐ Unknown

Prehospital interventions:
☐ CPR ☐ In progress
☐ Intubation ☐ Chest tube
☐ O₂ ☐ Ng ☐ Og
☐ Foley
☐ Cervical collar
☐ CID | Total Intake | Output
☐ Backboard | Crystalloid: _____
☐ Splint | Colloid: _____
☐ Medication PTA

Trauma team activated: Level I Time: _____
☐ Yes ☐ No Level II Time: _____

IMPRINT PATIENT IDENTIFICATION HERE

PERSONNEL RESPONSE

	NAME	ARRIVAL TIME
Triage Nurse		
Nurse Recorder		
Primary Trauma Nurse		
Secondary Trauma Nurse		
ED Attending		
Trauma Attending		
Chief Resident		
Team Leader		
CCM/Anesthesia		
Social Service		
Relief Nurse		

Consults	Name	Time called	Returned Call	Time Arrived
Orthopedics				
Neurosurgery				
Eye				
Hand				
Face				

Medical History: _____

Medications: _____

Allergies: _____

Pregnant: Yes No LMP _____
Tetanus: _____

PATIENT ARRIVAL TIME: _____

3272-01-U   FORM 1064-2400-0207A

NAME _____ MEDICAL RECORD _____ DATE _____

NURSING OBSERVATIONS
PATIENT RESPONSE TO TREATMENTS

TIME	B/P CUFF	B/P (ART) LINE	PULSE	RESP SPONT/ASSIST	EKG	SAO₂	O₂	GCS TOTAL	PAIN SCALE	INITIALS

Disposition _____ Time _____
I&O _____ Intake _____ Output _____
Total _____
C-spine precaution ☐

T/L/S precaution ☐

Airway patient ☐ O₂ _____
Intubated ☐
IVs Patient ☐ Patient _____
Fluid _____

VALUABLES
(List above)
☐ With Patient
☐ To Family
☐ Security
☐ Other

CLOTHING
☐ Cut Off
☐ With Patient
☐ To Family
☐ Security
☐ Other

Physician MD Signature: _____
Accompanied by ☐ Rn ☐ PCT ☐ Escort
GCS _____

Last Set V.S. _____
Monitor Rhythm _____
Lacerations Sutured
☐ Done ☐ N/A
Splints in Place
☐ Done ☐ N/A Not Done _____

Transferring Rn _____

LIST BELONGINGS: _____

FINAL DISPOSITION _____ TIME _____

Left Page — MEDICAL RECORD

NAME _____ DATE _____

SECONDARY SURVEY

TIME: _____

Head/Neck _____ TM R ___ L ___

NECK

FACE

GI/GU Abdomen

Rectal _____ Hemocult + −

Pelvis

Musculoskeletal/Skin

LEGEND:

Movement/Pulses
S—Strong
W—Weak
A—Absent

Sensation
P—Present
A—Absent

Pulses
Same as movement

Other
T—Intubated
P—Medication-induced paralysis
UTA—Unable to assess

SCALE FOR PUPIL SIZE

B—Brisk   S—Sluggish   N—Nonreactive

1 2 3 4 5 6 7 8mm

PRIMARY SURVEY

TIME: _____

Respiratory: _____ O₂ _____ LPM

Breath sounds   R   L
Clear   □   □
Diminished   □   □
Absent   □   □

Cardiovascular:

Airway
□ Patent
□ Compromised
□ Obstructed

Neurovascular   MOVEMENT   SENSATION   PULSES
RUE
LUE
RLE
LLE

PROCEDURES

TIME: _____

Endotrach   Size _____ □ BBS _____ □ CO₂ detector change
Nasotrach   Located _____ cm at the _____
Thoracotomy
Cricothyrotomy   Tube size _____
Chest tube   □ R size _____   □ L size _____
FAST

IV ACCESS

□ Central   Size _____ R L Site _____
   Size _____ R L Site _____
□ Peripheral   Size _____ R L Site _____
□ Peripheral   Size _____ R L Site _____
□ Peripheral   Size _____ R L Site _____

GI/GU

NG   OG   \
Foley   Urine Heme + −   HCG + −
DPL   Fluid return _____

LAB RESULTS

Blood Gas   Other
Time Drawn   Time Drawn
O₂ LPM   Hgb/Hct
PH   Glucose
PCO₂   Na
PO₂   K
HCO₃   ETOH
BE   Drug Screen

Labs drawn by: _____   Site: _____   □ Betadine Prep

GLASGOW COMA SCALE

EYE OPENING		
SPONTANEOUS	4
TO VOICE	3
TO PAIN	2
NONE	1
VERBAL RESPONSE		
ORIENTED	5
CONFUSED	4
INAPPROPRIATE WORDS	3
INCOMPREHENSIBLE WDS.	2
NONE	1
MOTOR RESPONSE		
OBEYS COMMANDS	6
LOCALIZES PAIN	5
WITHDRAW TO PAIN	4
FLEXION TO PAIN	3
EXTENSION TO PAIN	2
NONE	1

GCS TOTAL: _____
□ T   □ P

Neurological:

Oriented to:
□ Person   □ Place
□ Time   □ Event

Behavior:

REVISED TRAUMA SCORE

GLASGOW COMA SCALE		
13–15	4
9–12	3
6–8	2
4–5	1
3	0
RESPIRATORY RATE	
10–29	4
>29	3
6–9	2
1–5	1
0	0
SYSTOLIC BLOOD PRESSURE mm Hg	
>89	4
76–89	3
50–75	2
1–49	1
NO PULSE	0

TOTAL RTS:

PUPILS: R   L
SIZE
BRISK
SLUGGISH
UNRESPONSIVE   □   □

Right Page — MEDICAL RECORD

NAME _____ DATE _____

TIME Every 15 min. x 4 then every hour															
EYE OPENING															
SPONTANEOUS	4	4	4	4	4	4	4	4	4	4	4	4	4	4	4
TO VOICE	3	3	3	3	3	3	3	3	3	3	3	3	3	3	3
TO PAIN	2	2	2	2	2	2	2	2	2	2	2	2	2	2	2
NONE	1	1	1	1	1	1	1	1	1	1	1	1	1	1	1
VERBAL RESPONSE															
ORIENTED	5	5	5	5	5	5	5	5	5	5	5	5	5	5	5
CONFUSED	4	4	4	4	4	4	4	4	4	4	4	4	4	4	4
INAPPROPRIATE WORDS	3	3	3	3	3	3	3	3	3	3	3	3	3	3	3
INCOMPREHENSIBLE WORDS	2	2	2	2	2	2	2	2	2	2	2	2	2	2	2
NONE	1	1	1	1	1	1	1	1	1	1	1	1	1	1	1
MOTOR RESPONSE															
OBEYS COMMANDS	6	6	6	6	6	6	6	6	6	6	6	6	6	6	6
LOCATES PAIN	5	5	5	5	5	5	5	5	5	5	5	5	5	5	5
WITHDRAW (PAIN)	4	4	4	4	4	4	4	4	4	4	4	4	4	4	4
FLEXION (PAIN)	3	3	3	3	3	3	3	3	3	3	3	3	3	3	3
EXTENSION (PAIN)	2	2	2	2	2	2	2	2	2	2	2	2	2	2	2
NONE	1	1	1	1	1	1	1	1	1	1	1	1	1	1	1

Right pupil
Left pupil
RUE
LUE
RLE
LLE
T
P

INTAKE

CRYSTALLOID
NS 1 2 3 4 5
LR 1 2 3 4 5
TOTAL

PACKED CELLS   1 2 3 4 5 6 7 8 9 10
               1 2 3 4 5 6 7 8 9 10
TOTAL

OUTPUT

Chest _____ R
NG/OG
EBL
URINE
TOTAL

GCS   PAIN
TOTAL SCALE   TEMP

NURSING OBSERVATIONS
PATIENT RESPONSE TO TREATMENTS

INITIALS

Study

Time _____   Study
□ CXR Supine
□ C-Spine AP
□ Pelvis
□ Cystogram
□ Urethrogram
□ CT   □ Head
       □ Neck
       □ Abd.
       □ Pelvis
□ Other

C-Spine Cleared By:

Cleared   Radiographically   □ Yes   □ No
          Clinically   □ Yes   □ No

Warming Intervention
□ Blankets
□ Level 1 Infuser
□ IV Fluids
□ Lights
□ Bair Hugger

VITAL SIGNS EVERY HOUR

TIME	B/P CUFF	B/P A-LINE	PULSE	EKG	SAO₂	SAO₂	CSR	OSR			

Initials _____ Signature _____   Initials _____ Signature _____

Physician MD Signature: _____

3272-02-U FORM 1064-2400-02078

UPMC
University of Pittsburgh
Medical Center

PHYSICIAN ORDER SET

AUTHORIZATION IS GIVEN TO THE PHARMACY TO DISPENSE AND TO THE
NURSE TO ADMINISTER THE GENERIC OR CHEMICAL EQUIVALENT WHEN
THE DRUG IS FILLED BY THE PHARMACY OF THE UPMC HEALTH SYSTEM
HOSPITAL–UNLESS THE PRODUCT NAME IS CIRCLED.

IMPRINT PATIENT IDENTIFICATION HERE

TRAUMA PATIENT: DISCHARGE ORDERS AND INSTRUCTIONS

Attending physician: _____

Allergies: _____

[X] Discharge to: _____

Injuries:

1	_____	5	_____
2	_____	6	_____
3	_____	7	_____
4	_____	8	_____

Check All Orders That Apply with an [X] . *All Handwritten Orders Should Be* BLOCK PRINTED *for Clarity*

[X] Call **(412) 647-2002** if you experience any of the following or if you have any questions that are not listed below:

- Persistent headache
- Nausea/vomiting
- Dizziness
- Ringing in the ears
- Numbness/tingling

- Abdominal pain
- Warmth at wound site
- Night sweats
- Chest pain
- Fever/chillls

- Shortness of breath
- Visual changes
- Pain not relived with prescribed medicine
- Increased redness or wound drainage
- Significant new problems not specified above

**IF YOU BELIEVE YOU HAVE A LIFE-THREATENING EMERGENCY,
PLEASE CALL 911 OR YOUR LOCAL EMERGENCY MEDICAL SERVICE (EMS)**

CLINIC	ATTENDING PHYSICIAN	WHEN	PLACE	PHONE #
Trauma	TraumaClinic		Falk Clinic 6B	(412) 648-3164 or (412) 648-3167
Orthopaedics				
Neurosurgery				
Other Services				
Other Services				
Services	**Name**		**Phone #**	
Home Care				
Equipment Company				

(BLOCK Print Name) _____

Date/Time: _____

(Signature) _____

Pager #: _____

0031-01-U

Order Set Faxed to Pharmacy By:
[ ] (name/time) _____ Unit: _____

Form ID: PUH-1495   Last Revision Date: 10/01/2006

Page 1 of 3

UPMC
University of Pittsburgh
Medical Center

PHYSICIAN ORDER SET

AUTHORIZATION IS GIVEN TO THE PHARMACY TO DISPENSE AND TO THE
NURSE TO ADMINISTER THE GENERIC OR CHEMICAL EQUIVALENT WHEN
THE DRUG IS FILLED BY THE PHARMACY OF THE UPMC HEALTH SYSTEM
HOSPITAL-UNLESS THE PRODUCT NAME IS CIRCLED.

IMPRINT PATIENT IDENTIFICATION HERE

TRAUMA PATIENT: DISCHARGE ORDERS AND INSTRUCTIONS

Do you have a primary care physician? ☐ No ☐ Yes Name: _____

If yes, notify your primary care physician of your admission to the hospital

Ask if a follow-up appointment in the office of your primary care physician is needed.

Diet: _____

Activity

Walking: ☐ No restrictions ☐ Weightbearing restrictions (check all that are applicable)

☐ Pivot transfer ☐ Touchdown ☐ Nonweightbearing

☐ LLE ☐ RLE ☐ LUE ☐ RUE

Sitting:	☐ No Restrictions	☐ Hip flexion precautions no greater than 30/60/90°	Other: _____
Lifting:	☐ No Restrictions	☐ No lifting greater than (5–10) lb	
Stairs:	☐ No Restrictions	☐ Limit use	
Driving:	☐ No Restrictions	☐ No driving until seen for follow-up	☐ No driving while taking pain medications
Work:	☐ No Restrictions	☐ No work until seen for follow-up	☐ Light duty
School:	☐ No Restrictions	☐ No school until seen for follow-up	☐ May attend, but no physical activity
Bathing:	☐ No Restrictions	☐ May shower ☐ No tub baths	☐ Sponge bathe ONLY
Sexual Activity:	☐ No Restrictions	☐ Restrictions: _____	

Special Care In Instructions (when applicable)

☐ Wound Care/Dressing Changes: _____

☐ Incentive Spirometry (send home with patient) _____

☐ Pin Care _____

☐ Ostomy Care: _____

☐ Drain Care (i.e., flushing drains, recording outputs, bring output #s to clinic): _____

☐ Braces/Slings/Splings: _____

☐ Laboratory Studies: Date and Place to be drawn: _____

PA Trauma Outcome Functional Status

Feeding _____ Expression _____ Locomotion _____ Social interaction _____ Transportation/mobility _____

(**BLOCK** Print Name) _____ (Signature) _____

Date/Time: _____ Pager #: _____

☐ **Order Set Faxed to Pharmacy By:**
(name/time) Unit: _____

0031-01-U Form ID: PUH-1304 Last Revision Date: 10/01/2006 Page 2 of 3

UPMC
University of Pittsburgh
Medical Center

PHYSICIAN ORDER SET

AUTHORIZATION IS GIVEN TO THE PHARMACY TO DISPENSE AND TO THE
NURSE TO ADMINISTER THE GENERIC OR CHEMICAL EQUIVALENT WHEN
THE DRUG IS FILLED BY THE PHARMACY OF THE UPMC HEALTH SYSTEM
HOSPITAL-UNLESS THE PRODUCT NAME IS CIRCLED.

IMPRINT PATIENT IDENTIFICATION HERE

TRAUMA PATIENT: DISCHARGE ORDERS AND INSTRUCTIONS

Medications   *Do **NOT** drive or consume alcoholic beverages while taking pain medications.*
*This **DOES NOT** include Tylenol™ or other antiinflammatory medications.*

Drug _____ Dose _____ Route _____ Frequency _____ Amount Dispenensed _____

Drug _____ Dose _____ Route _____ Frequency _____ Amount Dispenensed _____

Drug _____ Dose _____ Route _____ Frequency _____ Amount Dispenensed _____

Drug _____ Dose _____ Route _____ Frequency _____ Amount Dispenensed _____

Drug _____ Dose _____ Route _____ Frequency _____ Amount Dispenensed _____

Drug _____ Dose _____ Route _____ Frequency _____ Amount Dispenensed _____

Medication Reconciliation

☐ I have reviewed the current list of medications, the new medications ordered, and compared them to the home medication list.

(**BLOCK** Print Name) _____   (Signature) _____

Date/Time: _____   Pager #: _____

Discharge instructions given by: _____ / _____

Registered Nurse (Print Name)   /   Registered Nurse (Signature)   Date

I have received Healthy Lifestyle information material. The information covers the benefits of healthy eating, regular exercise,
and health care tips related to diabetes, stroke, and key points of heart failure management including signs and symptoms
to report to physician, daily weight instruction, daily activity review, and dietary choices. Additional information addresses
smoking cessation, warning signs of cancer, and steps to control and prevent the spread of infection.
Patient verifies understanding of Discharge Instructions and is leaving with all valuables/belongings.

Patient/Significant Other Signature _____   Date/Time _____

Give photocopy of Orders/Instructions to patient.

0031-01-U   Form ID: PUH-1495   Last Revision Date: 10/01/2006

☐ **Order Set Faxed to Pharmacy By:**
   (name/time) _____   Unit: _____

Page 3 of 3

Note: Page numbers followed by f indicate figures; page numbers followed by t indicate tables.